A Practical Guide to

Third Trimester of Pregnancy and Puerperium

A Practical Guide to

Third Trimester of Pregnancy and Puerperium

Editor

Alok Sharma MBBS MD(OBG) MICOG DHA

Registrar, Department of Obstetrics and Gynecology
Kamla Nehru State Hospital for Mother and Child
Indira Gandhi Medical College
Shimla, Himachal Pradesh, India

Foreword

Alka Kriplani

JAYPEE *The Health Sciences Publisher*

New Delhi | London | Philadelphia | Panama

Jaypee Brothers Medical Publishers (P) Ltd

Headquarters
Jaypee Brothers Medical Publishers (P) Ltd
4838/24, Ansari Road, Daryaganj
New Delhi 110 002, India
Phone: +91-11-43574357
Fax: +91-11-43574314
Email: jaypee@jaypeebrothers.com

Overseas Offices

J.P. Medical Ltd
83 Victoria Street, London
SW1H 0HW (UK)
Phone: +44-2031708910
Fax: +02-03-0086180
Email: info@jpmedpub.com

Jaypee-Highlights Medical Publishers Inc
City of Knowledge, Bld. 237, Clayton
Panama City, Panama
Phone: +1 507-301-0496
Fax: +1 507-301-0499
Email: cservice@jphmedical.com

Jaypee Medical Inc.
325 Chestnul Street
Suite 412, Philadelphia, PA 19106, USA
Phone: +1 267-519-9789
Email: support@jpmedus.com

Jaypee Brothers Medical Publishers (P) Ltd
17/1-B Babar Road, Block-B, Shaymali
Mohammadpur, Dhaka-1207
Bangladesh
Mobile: +08801912003485
Email: jaypeedhaka@gmail.com

Jaypee Brothers Medical Publishers (P) Ltd
Bhotahity, Kathmandu
Nepal
Phone: +977-9741283608
Email: kathmandu@jaypeebrothers.com

Website: www.jaypeebrothers.com
Website: www.jaypeedigital.com

Inquiries for bulk sales may be solicited at: jaypee@jaypeebrothers.com

A Practical Guide to Third Trimester of Pregnancy and Puerperium

First Edition: **2016**

ISBN: 978-93-85891-29-8

Printed at Sanat Printers

Dedicated to

"Dear God, whose eternal blessing and divine presence helps us to fulfil all our goals"

My parents, Smt Dhanwanti Devi Sharma and Shri Hans Raj Sharma, who have laid the foundation stone of literacy in me and gave me the courage to face the challenges of the world by inculcating good attributes in me.

My wife, Dr Pratibha Sharma, for her tolerance and understanding of the time away from her during my own career and in editing this textbook. Her constant encouragement, moral support, and love was one of the source of inspiration to me for completing this work.

My brother, Dr Amit Sharma, for guiding me at every step in shaping this book.

Lastly, my lovely daughter, Hiranya Sharma, for her immense patience.

Contributors

EDITOR

Alok Sharma MBBS MD(OBG) MICOG DHA
Registrar, Department of Obstetrics and Gynecology
Kamla Nehru State Hospital for Mother and Child
Indira Gandhi Medical College
Shimla, Himachal Pradesh, India

CONTRIBUTING AUTHORS

Aashima Arora MD DMD
Assistant Professor
Department of Obstetrics and Gynecology
Postgraduate Institute of Medical Education and Research
Chandigarh, India

Parul Arora MD DNB
Research Officer
Department of Obstetrics and Gynecology
Postgraduate Institute of Medical Education and Research
Chandigarh, India

Charmila Ayyavoo MD DGO DFP FICOG
Consultant
Southern Railway Hospital
Director
Aditi Hospital and Parvathy Ayyavoo Fertility Centre
Trichy, Tamil Nadu, India

Rashmi Bagga MD DNB
Professor
Department of Obstetrics and Gynecology
Postgraduate Institute of Medical Education and Research
Chandigarh, India

Naveen Bajaj DM
Consultant Neonatologist
Deep Hospital
Ludhiana, Punjab, India

Geetha D Balsarkar MD DGO DNB FCPS
Professor
Department of Obstetrics and Gynecology
Nowrosjee Wadia Maternity Hospital
Seth Gordhandas Sunderdas Medical College
Mumbai, Maharashtra, India

Pooja K Bandekar MD DNB FCPS DGODFP MRCOG
Professor (Additional) and Head
Department of Obstetrics and Gynecology
Nowrosjee Wadia Maternity Hospital
Seth Gordhandas Sunderdas Medical College
Mumbai, Maharashtra, India

Kawita S Bapat MS FICOG
Director
Department of Obstetrics and Gynecology
One Centre For Gynecological Excellence, Bapat Hospital
Indore, Madhya Pradesh, India

Keshav Benipal MBBS MD
Senior Resident
Department of Obstetrics and Gynecology, Kamla Nehru Hospital
Indira Gandhi Medical College
Shimla, Himachal Pradesh, India

Vandana R Bhuria MD
Assistant Professor
Department of Obstetrics and Gynecology
Pt BDS Post Graduate Institute of Medical Sciences
Rohtak, Haryana, India

Jyoti Bindal MS FACS FICS FICOG LLB PGDHM
Professor and Head
Department of Obstetrics and Gynecology, Gajra Raja Medical College
Gwalior, Madhya Pradesh, India

Parag Biniwale MD FICOG FICMCH
Consultant, Biniwale Clinic
Pune, Maharashtra, India

Veerendrakumar CM MD DNB
Professor and Unit Head
Department of Obstetrics and Gynecology, Vijayanagara Institute of Medical Sciences
Bellary, Karnataka, India

Meenakshi B Chauhan MBBS MS MICOG FICOG
Professor
Department of Obstetrics and Gynecology
Pt BDS Post Graduate Institute of Medical Sciences
Rohtak, Haryana, India

Monica Chauhan MD
Medical Officer, Postpartum Program
Kamla Nehru State Hospital for Mother and Child
Indira Gandhi Medical College
Shimla, Himachal Pradesh, India

Niranjan N Chavan MD FICOG FCPS DGO DFP
Professor and Head
Department of Obstetrics and Gynecology
Lokmanya Tilak Medical College
Mumbai, Maharashtra, India

Nidhika Chhabra MBBS MS
Consultant Obstetrician and Gynecologist, Chhabra Hospital
Ludhiana, Punjab, India

Girindra Chingtham MD Dip Reproductive Medicine Dip Gynecological Endoscopy
Consultant
Department of Obstetrics and Gynecology
Maipakpi Maternity and Child Hospital
Imphal, Manipur, India

Saswati S Choudhury MD FICOG FICMCH
Associate Professor
Department of Obstetrics and Gynecology
Gauhati Medical College
Guwahati, Assam, India

Sanjay D Cruz MD DNB DM
Associate Professor
Department of Medicine
Government Medical College and Hospital
Chandigarh, India

Joshi Suyajna D MD
Professor (Rtd.) and Head
Department of Obstetrics and Gynecology
Vijayanagara Institute of Medical Sciences
Bellary, Karnataka, India

Krishna Dahiya MBBS MD
Professor
Department of Obstetrics and Gynecology
Pt BDS Post Graduate Institute of Medical Sciences
Rohtak, Haryana, India

Monika Dalal MBBS MD
Assistant Professor
Department of Obstetrics and Gynecology
Pt BDS Post Graduate Institute of Medical Sciences
Rohtak, Haryana, India

Jyothika A Desai MD DGO PGDMLE
Senior Consultant
Department of Obstetrics and Gynecology
Dr PR Desai Hospital and CSI Hospital
Bangalore, Karnataka, India

Ajay S Dhawle MD DNB
Specialist Registrar
Department of Obstetrics and Gynecology
St John's Hospital
Livingston, Scotland, UK

Sangeet Kaur Dhillon MD
Assistant Professor
Department of Forensic Medicine
Indira Gandhi Medical College
Shimla, Himachal Pradesh, India

Tanupriya Dogra MBBS DGO
Senior Resident
Department of Obstetrics and Gynecology
Kamla Nehru Hospital
Shimla, Himachal Pradesh, India

Yogita Dogra MBBS MD
Consultant
Department of Obstetrics and Gynecology
Deen Dayal Upadhyay Zonal Hospital
Shimla, Himachal Pradesh, India

Geeta J Doppa MBBS MD
Professor and Head
Department of Obstetrics and Gynecology
KVG Medical College
Sullia, Karnataka, India

Ramaraju H Ediger MBBS MS MICOG FICMCH
Associate Professor
Department of Obstetrics and Gynecology
Vijayanagara Institute of Medical Sciences
Bellary, Karnataka, India

Narotam K Ghezta MDS
Lecturer
HP Government Dental College
Shimla, Himachal Pradesh, India

Ravikanth O Gowder MBBS DGO MS
Assistant Professor
Department of Obstetrics and Gynecology
KVG Medical College
Sullia, Karnataka, India

Kiran Guleria MD DNB MNAMS ICMCH
Director and Professor
Department of Obstetrics and Gynecology
University College of Medical Sciences and GTB Hospital
Delhi, India

Kumud B Gupta MD
Professor and Head
Department of Obstetrics and Gynecology
MM Medical College and Hospital
Kumarhatti, Himachal Pradesh, India

Meeta Gupta MS FICOG
Assistant Professor
Department of Obstetrics and Gynecology
Acharya Shri Chander College of Medical Sciences
Jammu, Jammu and Kashmir, India

Mudita Gupta MBBS MD
Skin Specialist
Department of Dermatology
Deen Dayal Upadhyay Zonal Hospital
Shimla, Himachal Pradesh, India

Neha Gupta MS DNB FMAS
Consultant
Department of Fetal Medicine
Jaypee Hospital
Noida, Uttar Pradesh, India

Sadhana Gupta MS MNAMS FICOG FICMU FICMCH
Senior Consultant
Department of Obstetrics and Gynecology
Jeevan Jyoti Hospital and Medical Research Centre
Gorakhpur, Uttar Pradesh, India

Shubhrita Gupta DNB
Senior Registrar
Lokmanya Tilak Municipal General Hospital and Lokmanya Tilak Municipal Medical College
Mumbai, Maharashtra, India

Yashdeep Gupta MD DM
Assistant Professor
Department of Medicine
Government Medical College and Hospital
Chandigarh, India

Thejavathy GV MD
Professor
Department of Obstetrics and Gynecology
Bhagwan Mahaveer Jain Hospital
Bangalore, Karnataka, India

Saima Iqbal MBBS FCPS
Assistant Professor
Department of Gynecology
Services Institute of Medical Science
Lahore, Pakistan

Kanupriya Jain MD
Assistant Professor
Department of Obstetrics and Gynecology
Dayanand Medical College and Hospital
Ludhiana, Punjab, India

Neerja Jamwal MBBS MD
Consultant, Department of Obstetrics and Gynecology
Kullu Valley Hospital
Kullu, Himachal Pradesh, India

Shashwat K Jani MBBS MS Dip Advanced Laparoscopy
Assistant Professor
Department of Obstetrics and Gynecology
Smt NHL Municipal Medical College
Sheth VS General Hospital
Ahmedabad, Gujarat, India

Nishi Jaswal MBBS MD
Registrar
Department of Immunohematology and Blood Transfusion
Indira Gandhi Medical College
Shimla, Himachal Pradesh, India

Kanupriya Jindal MBBS
Junior Resident
Department of Obstetrics and Gynecology
Kamla Nehru Hospital
Shimla Himachal Pradesh, India

Umesh N Jindal MBBS MD
Director
Department of Reproductive Medicine
Jindal IVF and Sant Memorial Nursing Home
Chandigarh, India

Divya Kadam MS
Consultant
Department of Obstetrics and Gynecology, Ashirwad Nursing Home
Mumbai, Maharashtra, India

Madhvi Kaistha MBBS MD
Assistant Professor
Department of Community Medicine
Gian Sagar Medical College and Hospital
Banur, Punjab, India

Parneet Kaur DGO MD
Associate Professor
Department of Obstetrics and Gynecology
Government Medical College
Patiala, Punjab, India

Rajneet Kaur MD
Associate Professor
Department of Physiology
Dr Rajendra Prasad Goverment Medical College
Kangra, Himachal Pradesh, India

Ram K Kaushal MD
Professor and Head
Department of Pediatrics
Maharishi Markandeshwar Medical College
Kumarhatti, Himachal Pradesh, India

Suvarna S Khadilkar MD DGO FICOG Dip Endocrinology
Consultant Endocrinologist and Gynecologist
Bombay Hospital and Medical Research Center
Mumbai, Maharahtra, India

Shailesh Kore MD DNB FCPS DGO DFP DICOG
Additional Professor and Unit Head
Department of Obstetrics and Gynecology
Lokmanya Tilak Municipal Medical College
Mumbai, Maharashtra, India

Parul J Kotdawala MD FICOG FICMCH
Honorary Endoscopy Surgeon
Department of Obstetrics and Gynecology
VS Hospital and NHL Municipal Medical College
Ahmedabad, Gujarat, India

Alka Kriplani MD FRCOG FAMS FICOG FIMSA FICMCH FCLS
Professor and Head
Department of Obstetrics and Gynecology
All India Institute of Medical Sciences
New Delhi, India

Aswath Kumar MBBS MD FICOG
Dip Advanced Laproscopy
Additional Professor
Department of Obstetrics and Gynecology
Jubilee Mission Medical College
Thrissur, Kerala, India

Pratap Kumar MD DGO
Professor
Department of Obstetrics and Gynecology
Kasturba Medical College
Manipal, Karnataka, India

Shakuntala Kumar MBBS DGO FICOG
Dip Endoscopy
Medical Director and Senior Consultant
Department of Obstetrics and Gynecology
Nulife Hospital, Fortis Hospital
New Delhi, India

Alka Kuthe MBBS DGO
Kuthe Hospital and Maternity Home
Amravati, Maharashtra, India

Jiya Lal MBBS MD DCH
Consultant Pediatrician
Department of Health and Family Welfare
Health Care Centre-Karsog
Mandi, Himachal Pradesh, India

Stephen W Lindow FRCOG
Senior Lecturer and Honorary Consultant
Department of Obstetrics and Gynecology
Hull and East Yorkshire NHS Hospitals
Hull, Yorkshire, United Kingdom

Arti Luthra MS FICOG FICMCH
Director
Luthra Maternity and Infertility Centre
Dehradun, Uttarakhand, India

Manish Machave MD
Consultant, Machave Hospital
Pune, Maharashtra, India

Anjali Mahajan MD
Assistant Professor
Department of Community Medicine
Indira Gandhi Medical College
Shimla, Himachal Pradesh, India

Kapil Malhotra MBBS MD
OBG Specialist
Department of Health and Family Welfare
Netaji Subhash Chandra Bose Government Zonal Hospital
Mandi, Himachal Pradesh, India

Roopa Malik MS
Associate Professor
Department of Obstetrics and Gynecology
Pt BDS Sharma Post Graduate Institute of Medical Sciences
Rohtak, Haryana, India

Kavita Mandrelle DGO MD FICOG
Professor and Head
Department of Obstetrics and Gynecology
Christian Medical College and Hospital
Ludhiana, Punjab, India

Madhuri Mehendale DNB DGO FCPS
Assistant Professor
Lokmanya Tilak Municipal General Hospital and Lokmanya Tilak Municipal Medical College
Mumbai, Maharashtra, India

Reeti Mehra MD FIMSA
Associate Professor
Department of Obstetrics and Gynecology
Government Medical College and Hospital
Chandigarh, India

Sujata Misra MD FICOG
Associate Professor and Unit Head
Department of Obstetrics and Gynecology
Shri Ramachandra Bhanj Medical College
Cuttack, Odisha, India

Jay Mehta MBBS DNB
Resident
Department of Obstetrics and Gynecology
Shri IVF Clinic
Mumbai, Maharashtra, India

Kewal A Mistry MD
Consultant Radiologist
Synergy Institute of Medical Sciences
Dehradun, Uttarakhand, India

Charu Mittal MD DNB
Consultant Gynecologist
Department of Obstetrics and Gynecology
Sahara Multi-Specialty Hospital
Gwalior, Madhya Pradesh, India

Manishi Mittal FRM MD
Consultant
Mittal Maternity and Superspeciality Hospital
Yamunanagar, Haryana, India

Anu Namgyal MBBS MS
Medical Officer Specialist
Regional Hospital
Kullu, Himachal Pradesh, India

Saumya Nanda MD
Assistant Professor
Department of Obstetrics and Gynecology
Institute of Medical Sciences and SUM Hospital
Bhubaneshwar, Odisha, India

Smiti Nanda MBBS MD
Senior Professor and Head
Department of Obstetrics and Gynecology
Pt BDS Post Graduate Institute of Medical Sciences
Rohtak, Haryana, India

Muralidhar V Pai MBBS DGO MD
Professor and Head
Department of Obstetrics and Gynecology
Kasturba Medical College
Manipal, Karnataka, India

Anita Pal MD
Professor
Department of Obstetrics and Gynecology
Kamla Nehru State Hospital For Mother and Child
Shimla, Himachal Pradesh, India

Kiran Pandey MBBS MD FICOG FICMCH FIMSA MAMS
Professor and Head
Department of Obstetrics and Gynecology
Ganesh Shankar Vidyarthi Memorial Medical College
Kanpur, Uttar Pradesh, India

Uma Pandey MD FRCOG
Associate Professor
Department of Obstetrics and Gynecology
Institute of Medical Sciences, Banaras Hindu University
Varanasi, Uttar Pradesh, India

Daizy Pathak MD
Consultant, Reproductive Medicine
Luthra Maternity & Infertility Centre
Dehradun, Uttarakhand, India

Rashmi Patil MS FMAS
Consultant, St Martha's Hospital
Bangalore, Karnataka, India

Sharda Patra MD DNB
Professor
Department of Obstetrics and Gynecology
Lady Hardinge Medical College and Smt SK Hospital
New Delhi, India

Indira Prasad MD
Assisatant Professor
Department of Obstetrics and Gynecology
Lady Harding Medical College
New Delhi, India

Sandeep Puri MBBS MD
Principal and Professor
Department of Medicine
Dayanand Medical College and Hospital
Ludhiana, Punjab, India

Suman Puri MBBS MD FICOG
Professor and Head
Department of Obstetrics and Gynecology
Dayanand Medical College and Hospital
Ludhiana, Punjab, India

Priyangi Purohit MBBS MS
Assistant Professor
Department of Obstetrics and Gynecology
BJ Medical College and Civil Hospital
Ahmedabad, Gujarat, India

Susheela Rani MD PGDMLE FICOG
Medical Director and Consultant
Manjushree Speciality Hospital
Bangalore, Karnataka, India

Rohini Rao MD
Senior Medical Officer
Department of Obstetrics and Gynecology
Kamla Nehru State Hospital for Mother and Child
Shimla, Himachal Pradesh, India

Manisha Rewatkar MBBS MS
Registrar
Department of Obstetrics and Gynecology
Mahatma Gandhi Institute of Medical Sciences
Sewagram, Maharashtra, India

Aradhna Sharma MD
Senior Resident
Department of Pharmacology
Dr. Rajendra Prasad Goverment Medical College
Kangra, Himachal Pradesh, India

K Aparna Sharma MD DNB
Assistant Professor
Department of Obstetrics and Gynecology
All India Institute of Medical Sciences
New Delhi, India

Bali R Sharma MD
Associate Professor
Department of Obstetrics and Gynecology
Indira Gandhi Medical College
Shimla, Himachal Pradesh, India

Chanderdeep Sharma MD
Assistant Professor
Department of Obstetrics and Gynecology
Dr Rajendra Prasad Government Medical College
Kangra, Himachal Pradesh, India

Esha Sharma MBBS MS DNB
Consultant, Ramkrishna IVF Centre
Siliguri, West Bengal, India

Jai B Sharma MD FRCOG FAMS
Professor
Department of Obstetrics and Gynecology
All India Institute of Medical Sciences
New Delhi, India

Nalneesh Sharma MBBS MD
Consultant, Department of Obstetrics and Gynecology
Deen Dayal Upadhyay Zonal Hospital
Shimla, Himachal Pradesh, India

Padam Sharma DPT BOT
Consultant Therapist
Delhi Diabetes Research Centre
New Delhi, India

Pratibha Sharma BDS
Medical Officer-Dental
Deen Dayal Upadhyay Zonal Hospital
Shimla, Himachal Pradesh, India

Shashank Shekhar MBBS MD
Assistant Professor
Department of Obstetrics and Gynecology
All India Institute of Medical Sciences
Jodhpur, Rajasthan, India

Poonam V Shivkumar MBBS MD
Professor and Head
Department of Obstetrics and Gynecology
Mahatma Gandhi Institute of Medical Sciences
Sewagram, Maharashtra, India

Hema J Shobhane MBBS MD FICOG FICMCH
Associate Professor, Department of Obstetrics and Gynecology
Maharani Laxmi Bai Medical College
Jhansi, Uttar Pradesh, India

Laxmi Shrikhande MD FICOG FICMCH FICMU
Director
Shrikhande IVF and Surrogacy Center
Nagpur, Maharashtra, India

Arshdeep Singh MBBS MD DM
Senior Resident
Department of Gastroenterology
Dayanand Medical College and Hospital
Ludhiana, Punjab, India

Savita R Singhal DGO MD FICOG FICMCH
Professor
Department of Obstetrics and Gynecology
Pt BDS Sharma Post Graduate Institute of Medical Sciences
Rohtak, Haryana, India

Atish Singla MBBS
MD Student
Department of Obstetrics and Gynecology
Government Medical College
Patiala, Punjab, India

Rubina Sohail MBBS MCPS FCPS DCPS-HPE
Professor
Department of Gynecology Unit II
Services Institute of Medical Sciences
Lahore, Pakistan

Akanksha Sood MS DNB MRCOG FACOG
Senior Clinical Fellow
Department of Obstetrics and Gynecology
Saint Mary's Hospital
Manchester, United Kingdom

Anuradha Sood MD
Assistant Professor
Department of Microbiology
Dr Rajendra Prasad Government Medical College
Kangra, Himachal Pradesh, India

Ashwani K Sood MD FIAP
Professor, Department of Pediatrics
Indira Gandhi Medical College
Shimla, Himachal Pradesh, India

Geetika G Syal MBBS MD
Consultant, Department of Obstetrics and Gynecology
Simla Sanitarium Hospital
Shimla, Himachal Pradesh, India

Kartik Syal MBBS MD
Assistant Professor
Department of Anesthesia, Critical Care and Pain
Indira Gandhi Medical College
Shimla, Himachal Pradesh, India

Sangeeta T Tajpuriya MBBS MD
Consultant, Rajashree Nursing Home
Nagpur, Maharashtra, India

Navneet Takkar MBBS MS
Associate Professor
Department of Obstetrics and Gynecology
Government Medical College
Chandigarh, India

Pratik Tambe MD FICOG
ART Consultant and Gynecology Endoscopic Surgeon
Nirmiti Fertility and IVF
Mumbai, Maharashtra, India

Amit Tandon MD
Assistant Professor, Department of Obstetrics and Gynecology
Sarojini Naidu Medical College
Agra, Uttar Pradesh, India

Parikshit D Tank MD DNB FCPS DGO DFP MNAMS MICOG MRCOG
Consultant, Department of Obstetrics and Gynecology
Ashwini Maternity and Surgical Hospital, Center for Endoscopy and Assisted Reproduction
Mumbai, Maharashtra, India

Surekha Tayade MD DNB MNAMS FICOG FAIMER Fellow PSG FRI
Professor
Department of Obstetrics and Gynecology
Mahatma Gandhi Institute of Medical Sciences
Sewagram, Maharashtra, India

Nisha Thakur MDS
Lecturer
HP Government Dental College
Shimla, Himachal Pradesh, India

Rajesh K Verma MD
Assistant Professor
Department of Anesthesiology
Indira Gandhi Medical College
Shimla, Himachal Pradesh, India

Gurleen Wander MBBS
Registrar
Department of Obstetrics and Gynecology
Whittington Hospital NHS Trust
London, United Kingdom

Reena J Wani MD MRCOG FICOG DNBE FCPS DGO DFP
Additional Professor
Department of Obstetrics and Gynecology
Topiwala National Medical College and BYL Nair Charitable Hospital
Mumbai, Maharashtra, India

Divya Yadav MS(OBG) FICMCH
Lecturer
SN Medical College
Agra, Uttar Pradesh, India

Manisha Yadav
Senior Resident
Department of Obstetrics and Gynecology
All India Institute of Medical Sciences
New Delhi, India

Foreword

The third trimester of pregnancy is the penultimate time in the experience of pregnancy and childbirth after the initial months of pregnancy; the mother is now looking forward toward a pleasurable conclusion to an incredible journey. After having carried the baby in her womb for all this while, she now already has an emotional connect and registers herself as a mother to the unborn child. This, however, is also a very crucial time for both the mother and the baby when even a small oversight can lead to disastrous consequences.

A book exclusively dedicated to the third trimester is a commendable venture and I would like to congratulate Dr Alok Sharma for having assessed the need and possessing the foresight to make this happen. During the third trimester, the woman undergoes a substantial changes in her physiology which make her vulnerable to develop a number of conditions either de novo or by unmasking of preexisting ailments. These profound changes can only be understood and managed by venturing into not just obstetrics but also medicine and the medicine behind obstetrics.

Starting with the normal physiology and anatomy, then progressing to the normal antenatal, intranatal, and postnatal period, this book follows a very logical and lucid manner of presenting the contents to the reader. From then on, there is an extensive coverage of all the complications that a woman can come across in the third trimester. Each of the topics has been discussed so that there is a basic understanding of "why and how" before providing the "what next?"

The section on neonatal care emphasizes the obstetrician's need to understand the basics of neonatology.

I would like to reiterate that Dr Alok Sharma is the right person with the vision and dynamism backed by a sound knowledge to take this venture to its deserved conclusion. I wish him all the best in this endeavor.

Alka Kriplani MD FRCOG FAMS FICOG FIMSA FICMCH FCLS
Professor and Head, Department of Obstetrics and Gynecology
Director in-charge, WHO-CCR, HRRC, and Family Planning
All India Institute of Medical Sciences, New Delhi, India
President, Federation of Obstetric and Gynaecological Societies of India
Padma Shri Awardee—2015

Preface

I welcome with enthusiasm the opportunity to edit this very first edition of venerable textbook on "*A Practical Guide to Third Trimester of Pregnancy and Puerperium*". I have tried to provide a textbook to help the undergraduates, postgraduates, and practitioners to clarify their doubts and to organize some of the intricacies regarding the subject.

I have assembled a group of contributors, nationally and internationally, with an exceptional range of backgrounds and similar interests. All the contributors has emphasized the latest clinical management approaches with better understanding. They have contributed with the same goal to create a source of information that would help in the care of women in their last phase of pregnancy, during labor, and even after delivery. This textbook not only contains normal physiology but also deals with medical, surgical, and gynecological complications during the third trimester of pregnancy, labor and puerperium.

No two births are the same and no two mothers have the same changes during pregnancy, labor, and puerperium; therefore, it becomes more important to have a textbook which deals with planning and anticipating any possible complication during this phase.

It has been tried to my level best to cover all the relevant aspects pertaining to this phase where an obstetrician may need guidance in decision making, with a multidisciplinary approach to treat the patients in various disorders.

I hope that the aggregate of my efforts would result in a textbook that will be a worthy resource for those who want to care for pregnant women.

Alok Sharma

Acknowledgments

Thanksgiving is a pleasant job, but it is nonetheless difficult where one sincerely tries to put feelings in words. These humble words of expression and gratitude cannot really convey the deep feelings of my heart.

Any attempt to create and produce a textbook, one has to be fortunate enough to have the assistance and support of infinite talented professionals both within and outside the field. To begin with, I am indebted to all the authors for their generous contribution to this book, who despite their busy schedule have provided recent, up-to-date, and evidence-based chapters on various aspects of third trimester of pregnancy and puerperium. Contributors have been selected from different parts of India and abroad, and from various specialties and organizations.

I am especially thankful to Dr Mala Arora for her inspiration and continuous support in conception of this book. It, again, has been a pleasure to work with the dedicated professionals from Jaypee Brothers Medical Publishers (P) Ltd. The publisher has been gracious enough in offering support without any interference, whatsoever, and the team has also ensured that the quality of work is superb. Production of the manuscript would not have been possible without a dedicated team to bring these efforts together.

This acknowledgment would be incomplete without my humble and sincere thanks to my respected and dear father Shri Hans Raj Sharma, who has extended his talents in skillfully coordinating and overseeing the composition. His dedicated attention to detail and organization of the work was vital to the completion of this project and has also brought me in touch with another skill for which I respect and adore him even more.

I am deeply indebted to the unconditional support of Dr Neeraj Choudhary (Senior Acquisition Editor-Corporate), who has brought his considerable intelligence, energetic work ethics, and creativity to this edition. His dedication to creating the best textbook possible equalled my efforts to provide the gracious style to this textbook. This textbook would have not seen the light of the day without untiring efforts of Ms Shweta Tiwari (Editorial Coordinator), Ms Neha Bhatia (Development Editor), and the Editors, Mr Gladden Savieo and Dr Swati Mishra, who skillfully kept my project on track through an array of potential hurdles while doing their jobs sincerely and diligently. I would also acknowledge the work of Mr Birendra Kumar who designed and executed the layout of the book in a very artistic manner.

I would also like to thank Dr Madhu Choudhary from Jaypee Brothers (Senior Content Strategist) whose constant encouragement and valuable suggestions helped me in conceptualizing, initiating, and executing this project. The book has materialized in to a much elaborate and comprehensive title than was planned and anticipated, only with her help. A special note of thanks for Ms Vibha Saraswati, who delivered her baby under my care and also agreed to help us with the various yoga postures, when she came to know about the book. Her help was instrumental in making this chapter easy to understand and will also highlight the importance of yoga during and after pregnancy.

Contents

Section 5: Neonate

Section 6: Obstetrical Complications

Section 7: Medical and Surgical Complications

PLATE 1

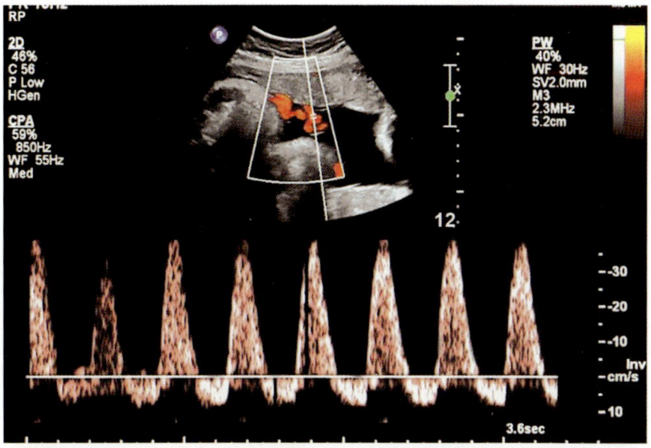

FIG. 6: Reversal of diastolic flow in umbilical artery *(Chapter 6)*.

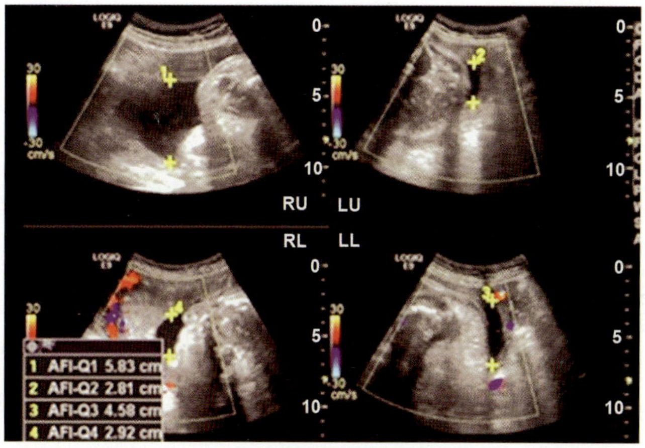

FIG. 8: Amniotic fluid index technique *(Chapter 7)*.

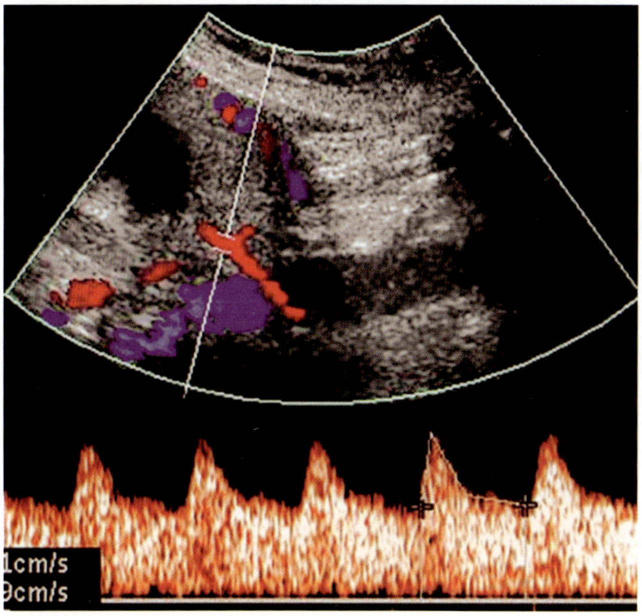

FIG. 7: Normal uterine artery Doppler waveforms *(Chapter 6)*.

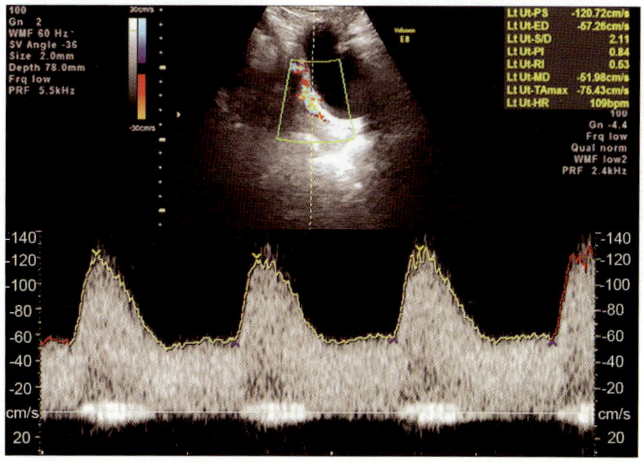

FIG. 9: Uterine artery Doppler *(Chapter 7)*.

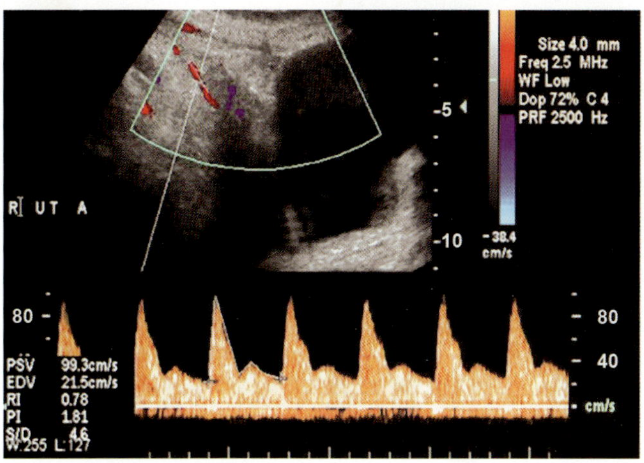

FIG. 8: Early diastolic notch in uterine artery *(Chapter 6)*.

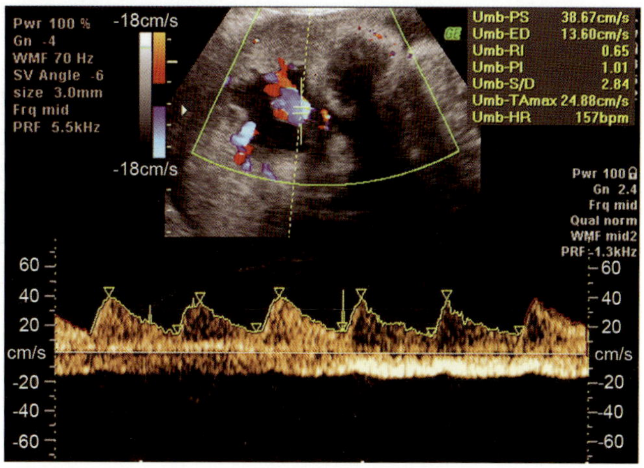

FIG. 10: Umbilical artery Doppler *(Chapter 7)*.

PLATE 2

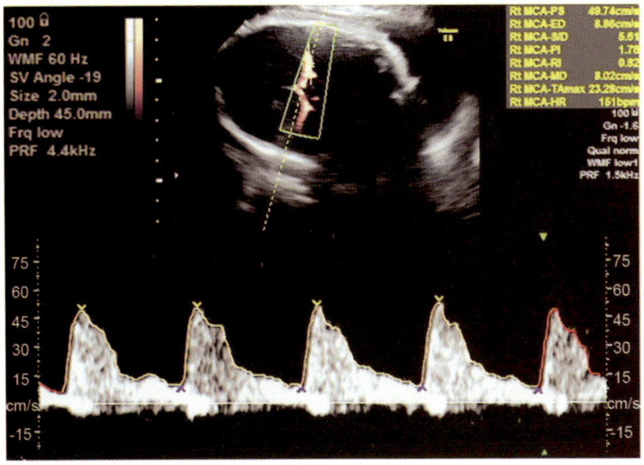

FIG. 11: Middle cerebral artery (MCA) Doppler *(Chapter 7)*.

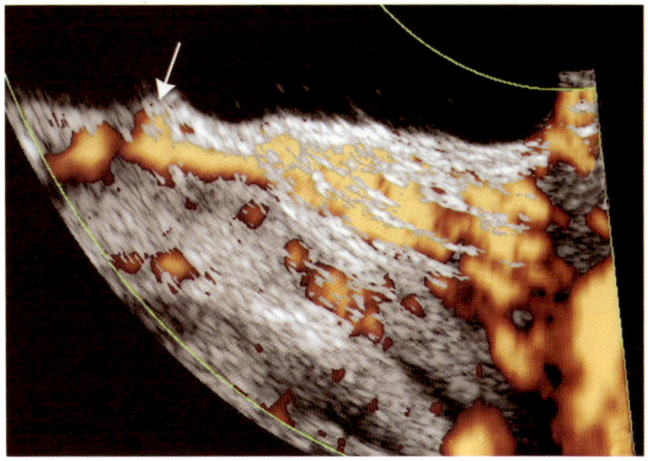

FIG. 17: Arrow indicates thinning or disruption of the hyperechoic serosa-bladder interface *(Chapter 7)*.

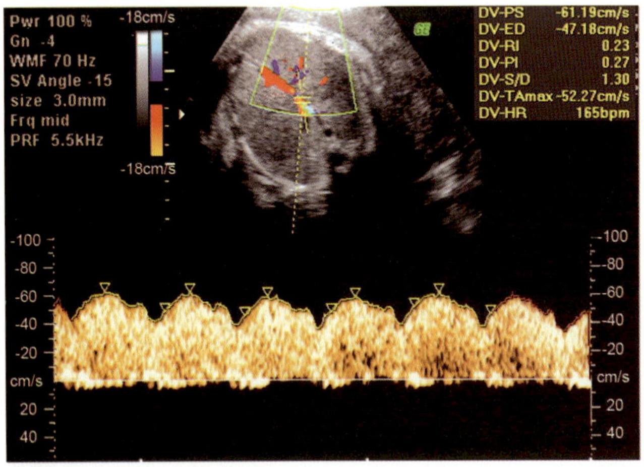

FIG. 12: Ductus venosus Doppler *(Chapter 7)*.

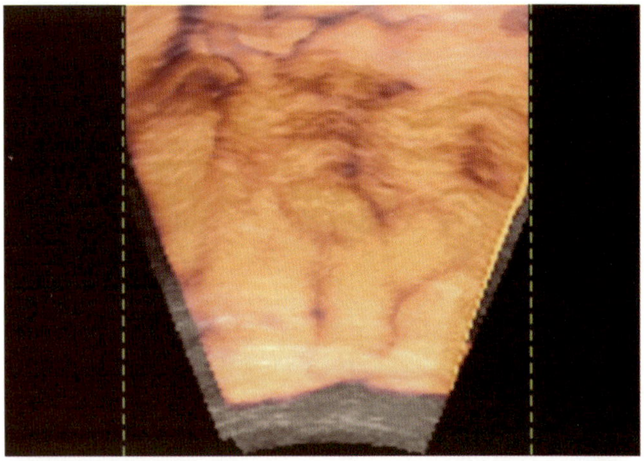

FIG. 18: Numerous coherent vessels involving the whole uterine serosa-bladder junction (basal view) *(Chapter 7)*.

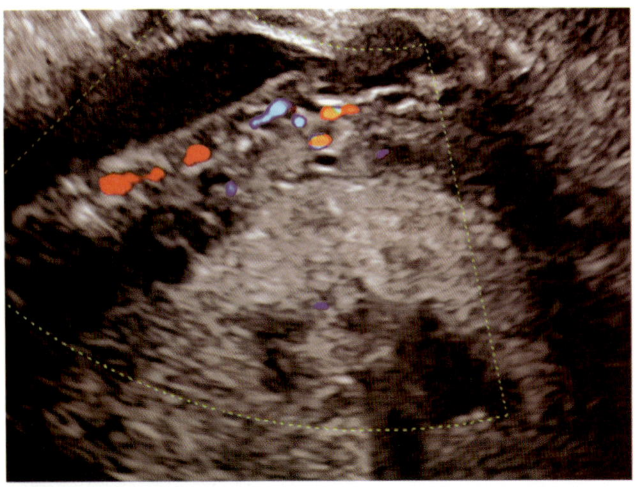

FIG. 16: Hypervascularity of serosa-bladder interface *(Chapter 7)*.

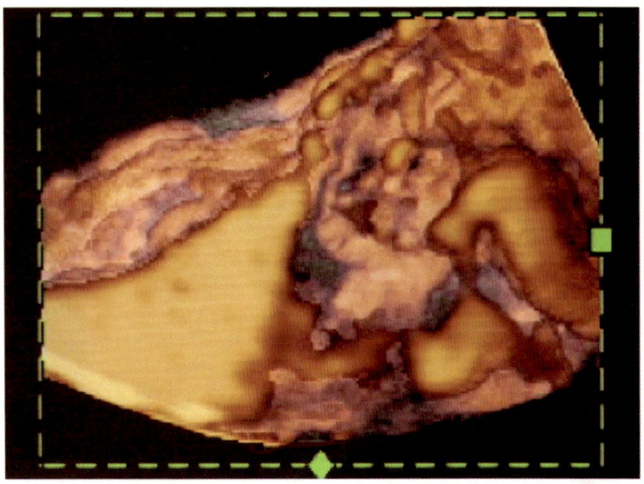

FIG. 19: Hypervascularity (lateral view) *(Chapter 7)*.

PLATE 3

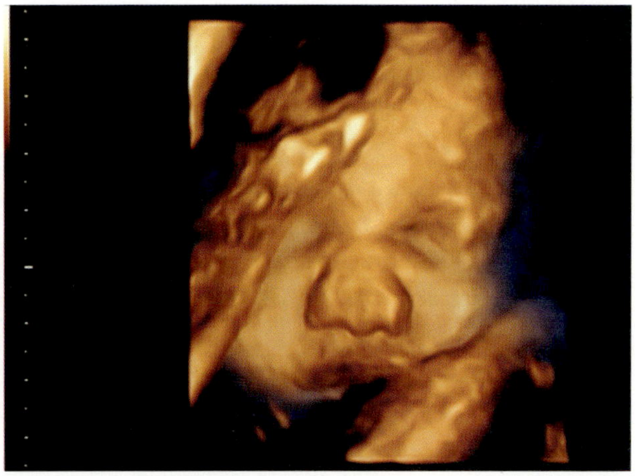

FIG. 21: Three-dimensional ultrasound of face *(Chapter 7)*.

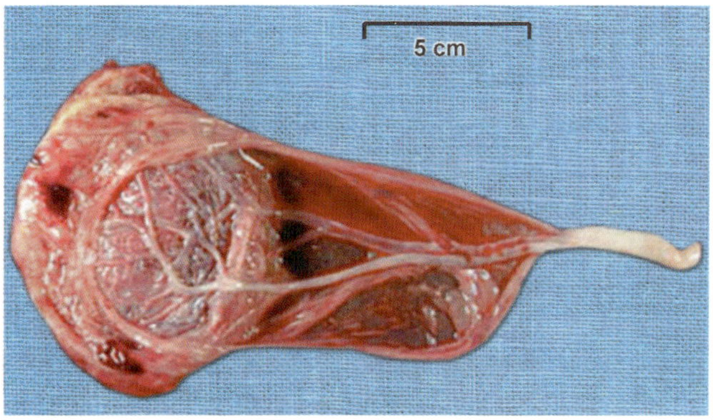

FIG. 3: "Velamentous" insertion of umbilical cord *(Chapter 9)*.

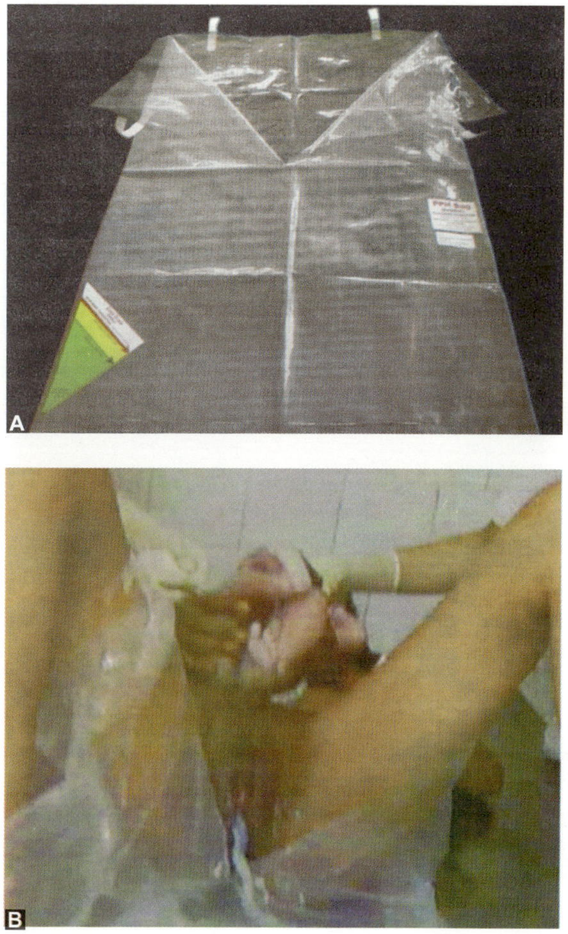

FIGS 1A AND B: **A,** Debdas Bag; **B,** Application of Debdas Bag *(Chapter 23)*.

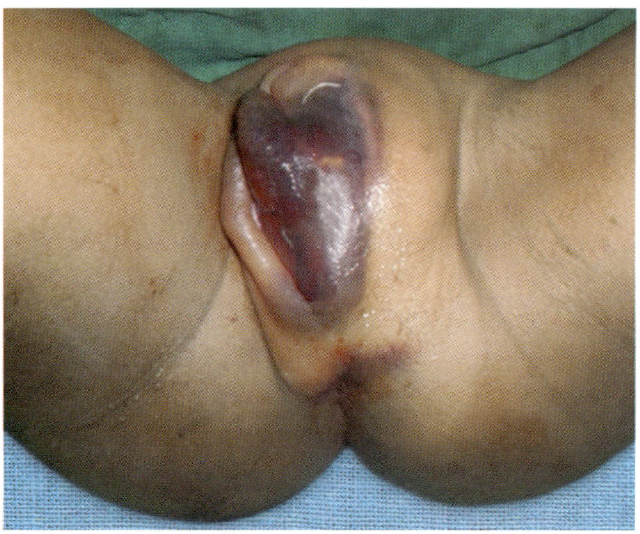

FIG. 1: Vulval hematoma *(Chapter 24)*.

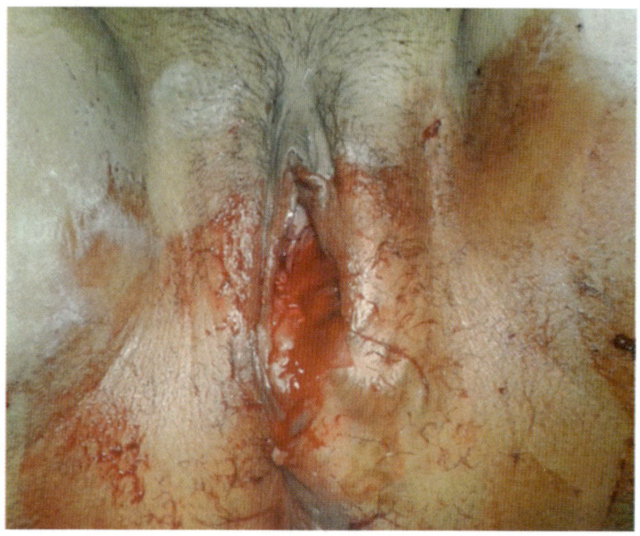

FIG. 2: Paravaginal hematoma *(Chapter 24)*.

PLATE 4

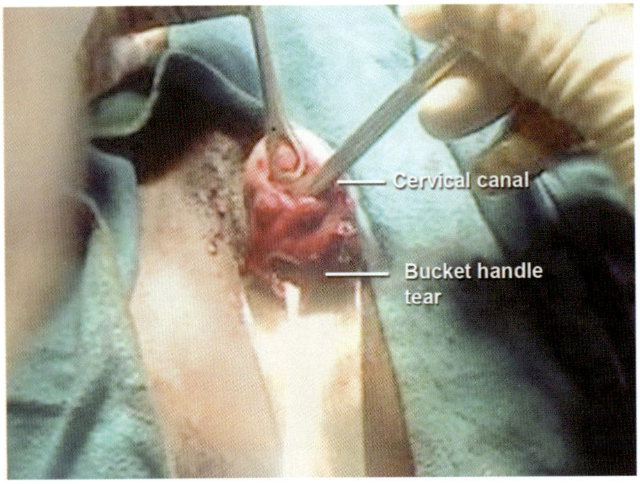

FIG. 3: Bucket handle tear *(Chapter 24)*.

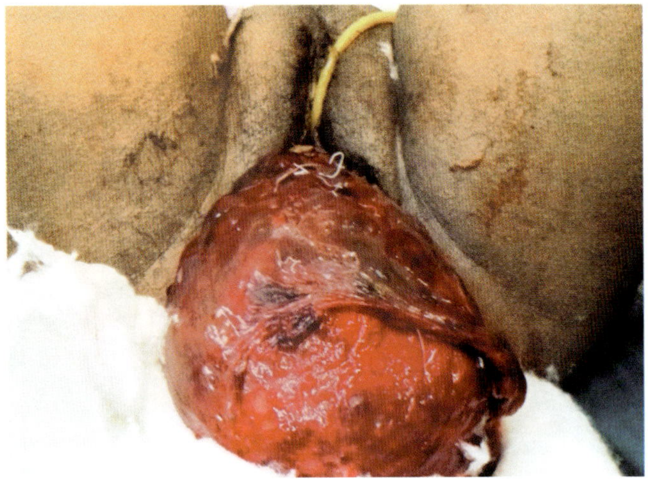

FIG. 3: Acute uterine inversion (complete) *(Chapter 26)*.

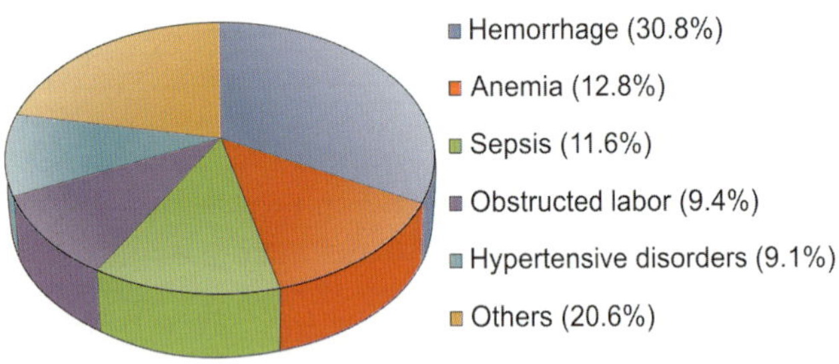

FIG. 1: Leading causes of maternal deaths in Asia *(Chapter 26)*.[1]

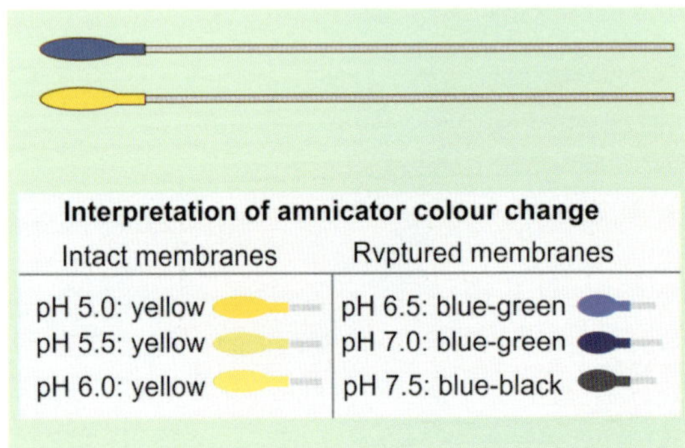

FIG. 2: Color change in amnicator test on premature rupture of membrane *(Chapter 36)*.

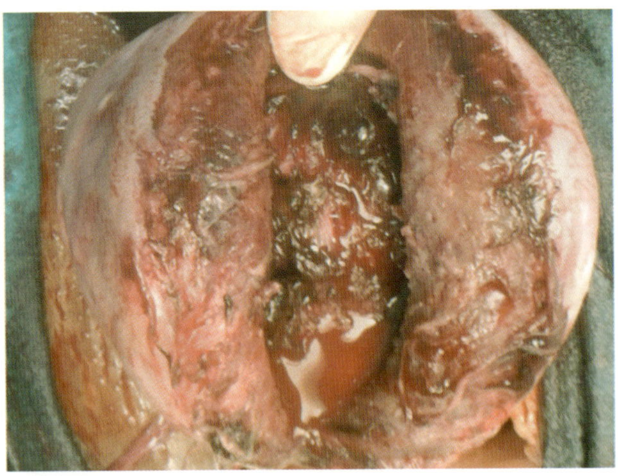

FIG. 2: Uterine rupture in a woman with classical cesarean diagnosed intraoperatively (type of uterine incision was unknown beforehand; a relatively common occurrence in developing countries) *(Chapter 26)*.

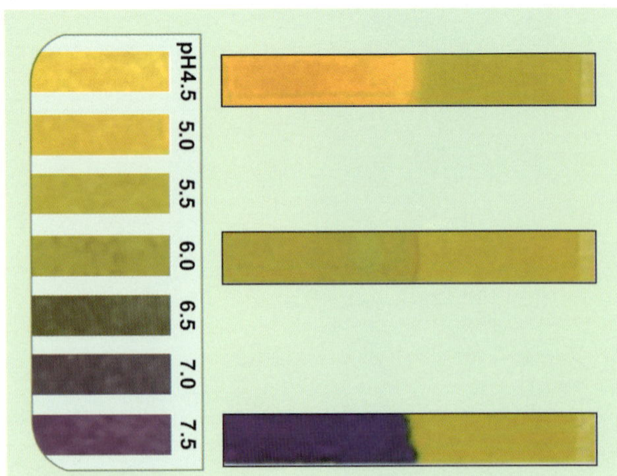

FIG. 3: Nitrazine paper test. Blue color indicates presence of amniotic fluid *(Chapter 36)*.

PLATE 5

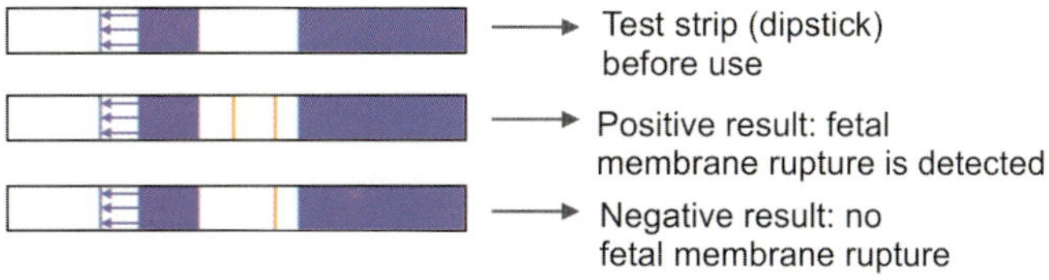

FIG. 5: Interpretation of results on AmniSure dipstick *(Chapter 36)*.

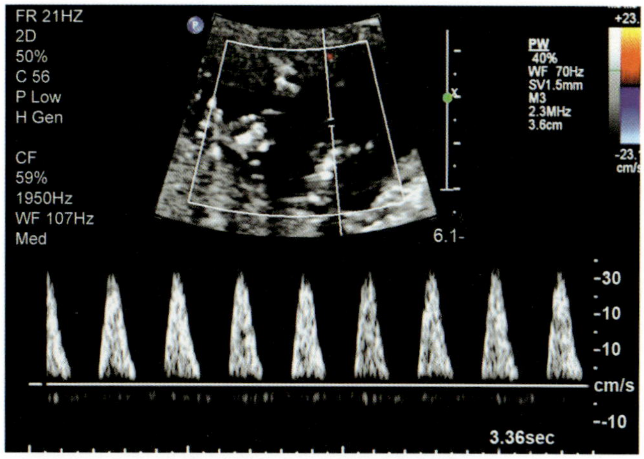

FIG. 3: Absent end-diastolic flow (umbilical artery Doppler) *(Chapter 43)*.

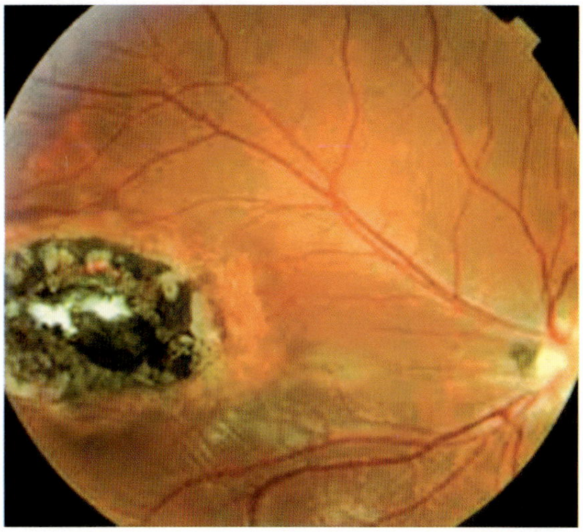

FIG. 6: Endoscopic view of the site of membrane rupture *(Chapter 36)*.

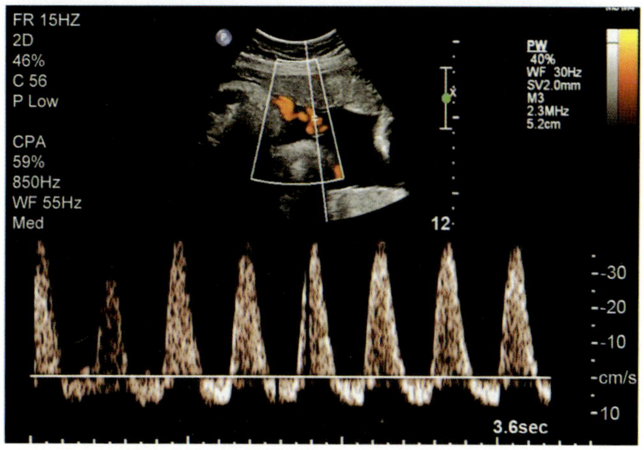

FIG. 4: Reversal of end-diastolic flow (umbilical artery Doppler) *(Chapter 43)*.

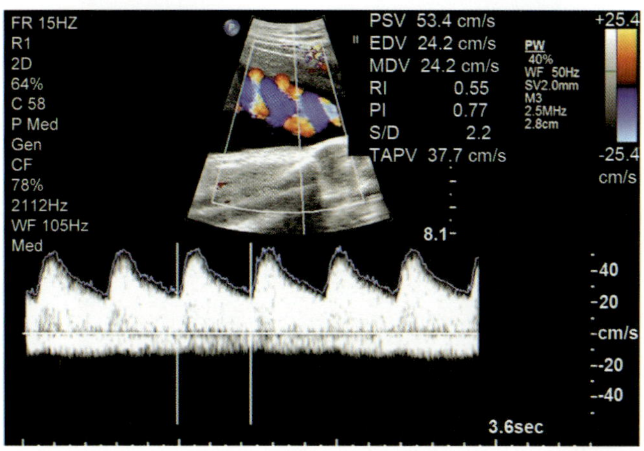

FIG. 2: Normal umbilical artery Doppler *(Chapter 43)*.

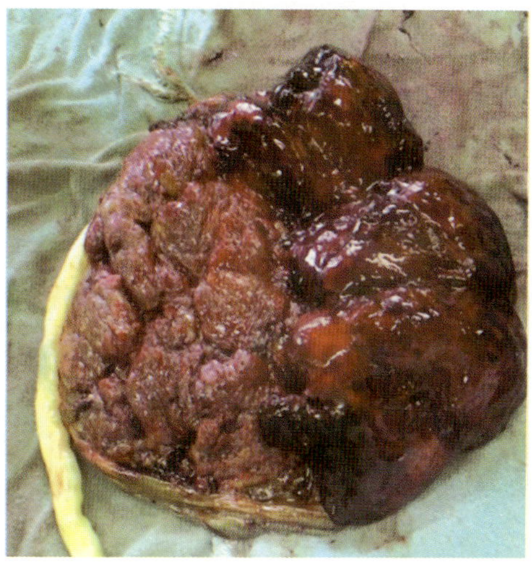

FIG. 3: Placental abruption *(Chapter 45)*.

PLATE 6

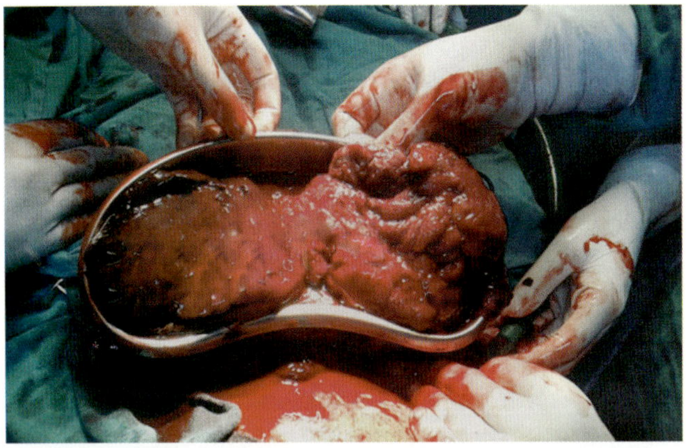

FIG. 4: Placental abruption after cesarean section *(Chapter 45)*.

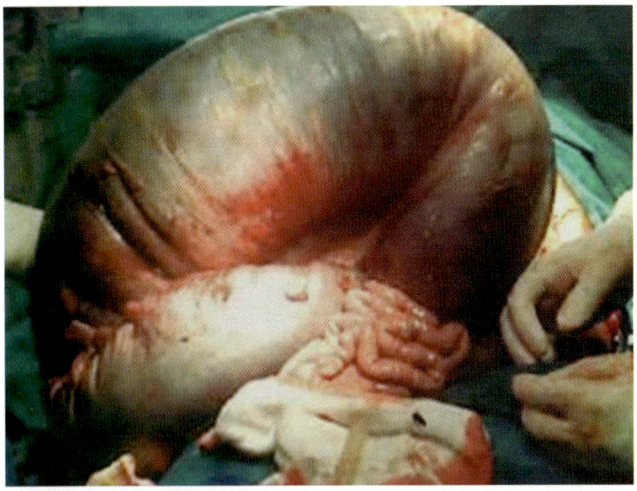

FIG. 2: Massively dilated colon in volvulus *(Chapter 49)*.

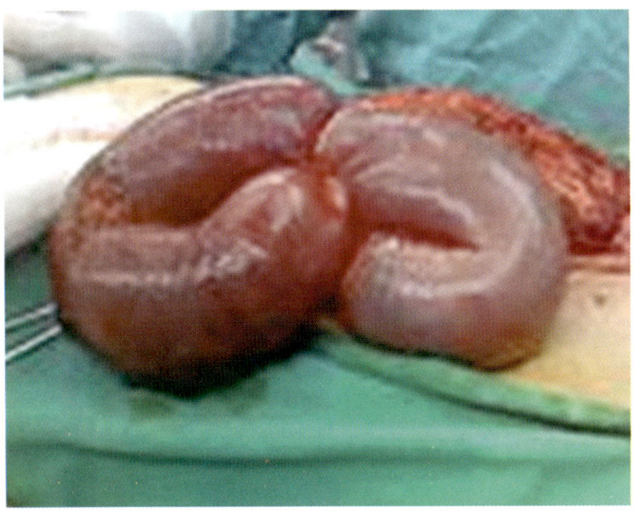

FIG. 3: Picture of colonic pseudo-obstruction *(Chapter 49)*.

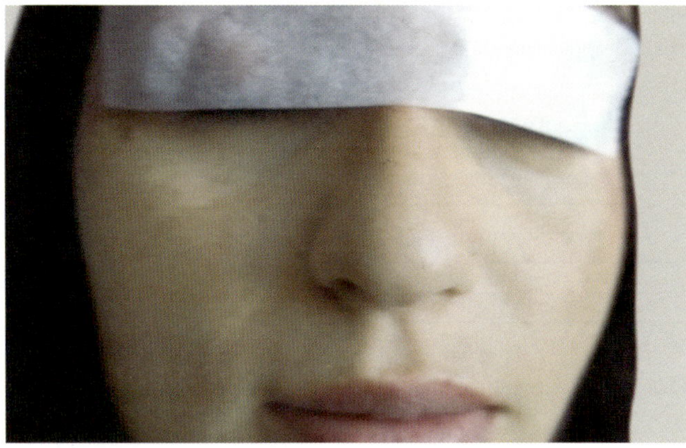

FIG. 1: Chloasma *(Chapter 61)*.

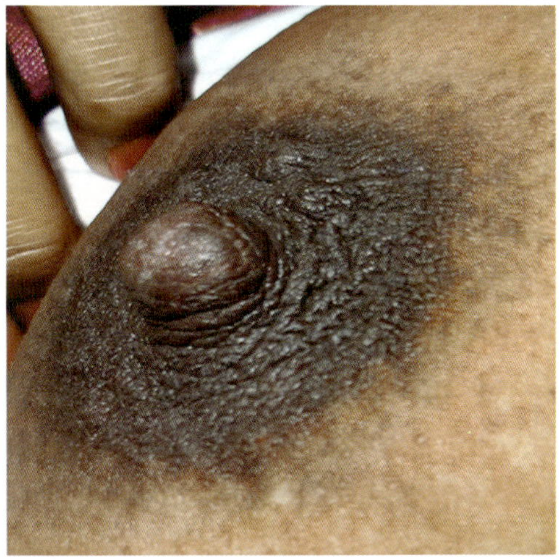

FIG. 2: Secondary areola *(Chapter 61)*.

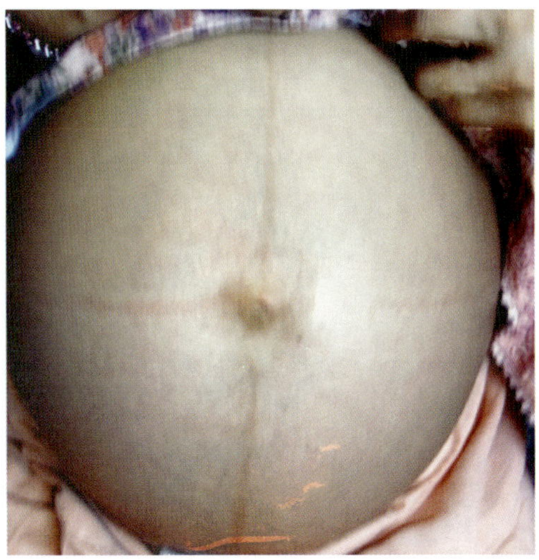

FIG. 3: Linea nigra *(Chapter 61)*.

PLATE 7

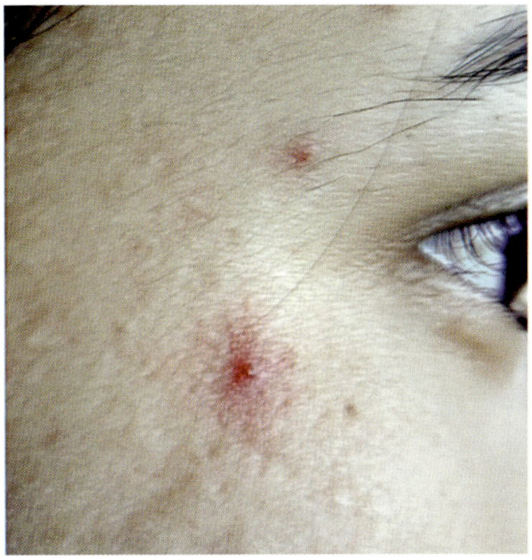

FIG. 4: Spider nevi *(Chapter 61)*.

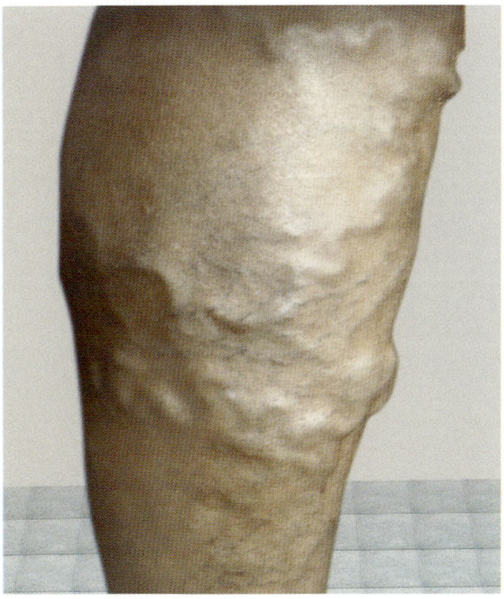

FIG. 5: Varicose veins *(Chapter 61)*.

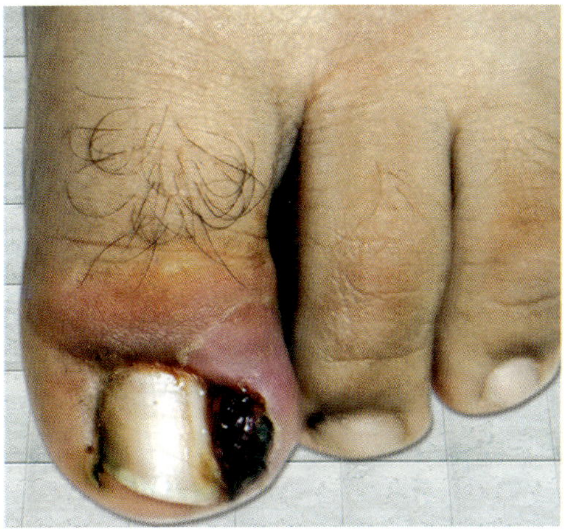

FIG. 6: Granuloma gravidarum *(Chapter 61)*.

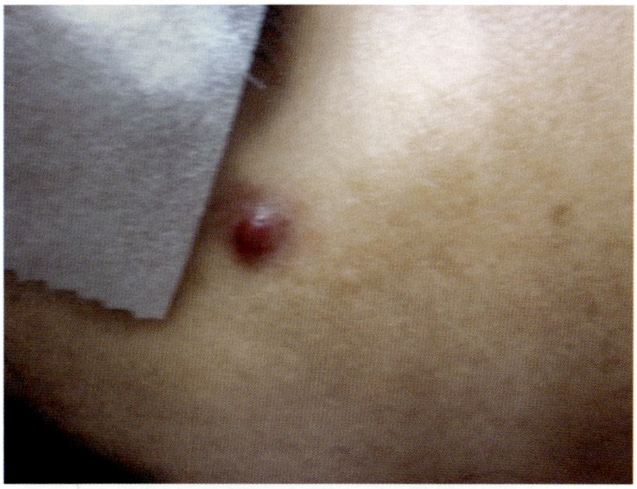

FIG. 7: Hemangioma *(Chapter 61)*.

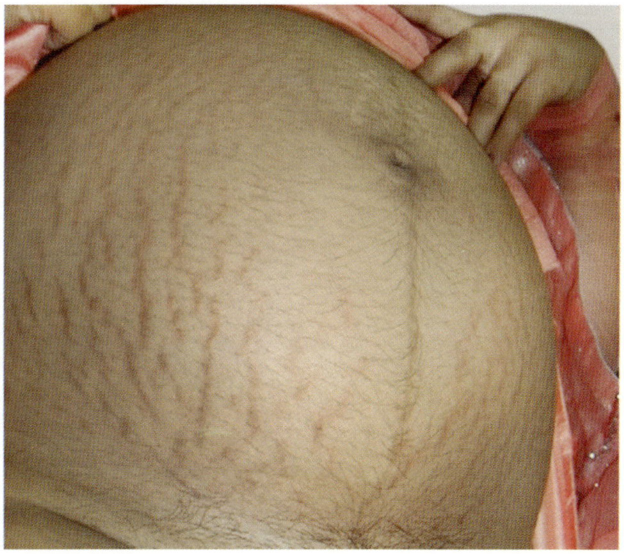

FIG. 8: Striae gravidarum *(Chapter 61)*.

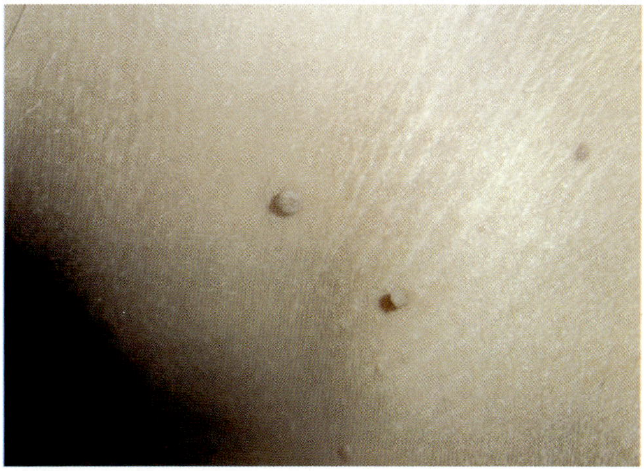

FIG. 9: Molluscum fibrosum gravidarum *(Chapter 61)*.

PLATE 8

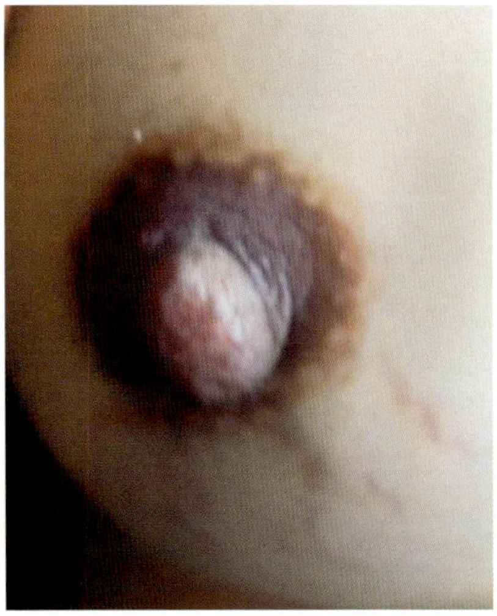

FIG. 10: Montgomery tubercles *(Chapter 61)*.

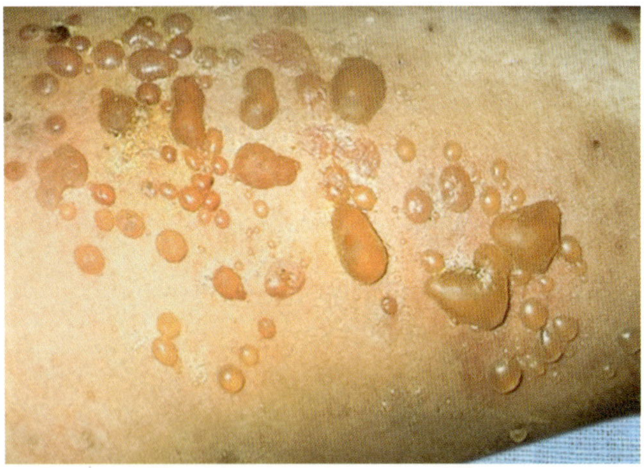

FIG. 11: Vesicles with urticated base in pemphigoid gestationis *(Chapter 61)*.

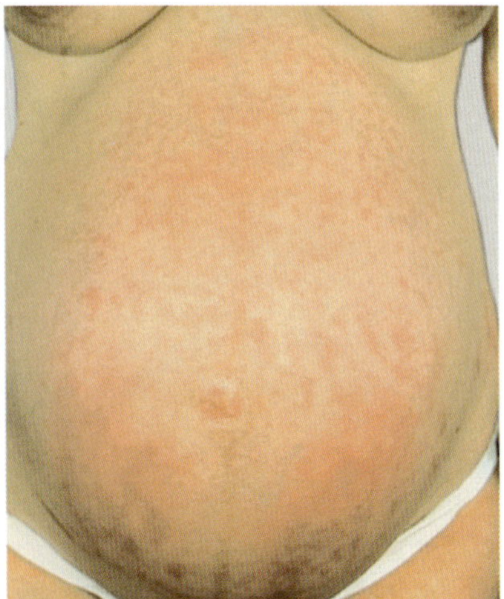

FIG. 12: Periumbilical sparing in pruritic urticarial papules and plaques of pregnancy *(Chapter 61)*.

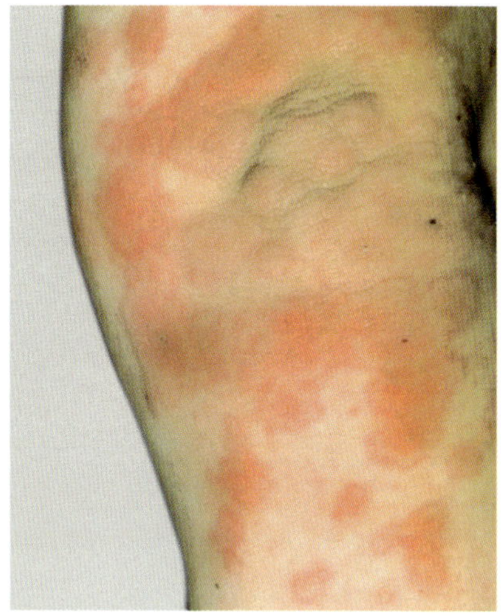

FIG. 13: Urticated papules and plaques in pruritic urticarial papules and plaques of pregnancy *(Chapter 61)*.

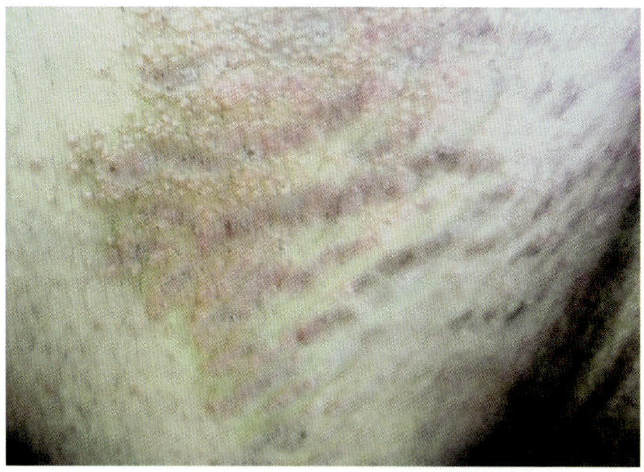

FIG. 14: Atopic eczema of pregnancy (E type) *(Chapter 61)*.

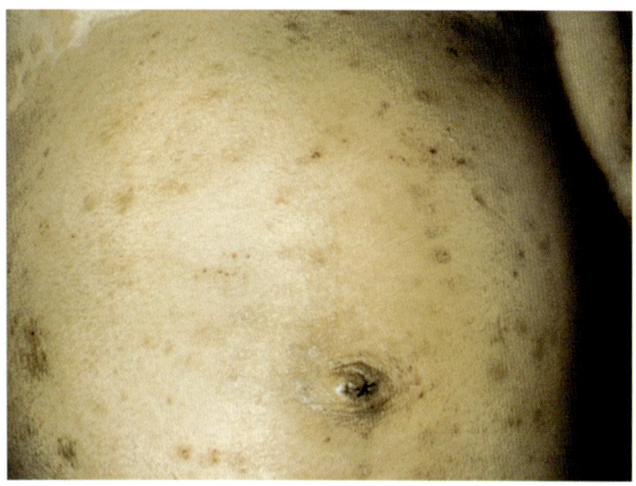

FIG. 15: Atopic eczema of pregnancy (P type) *(Chapter 61)*.

PLATE 9

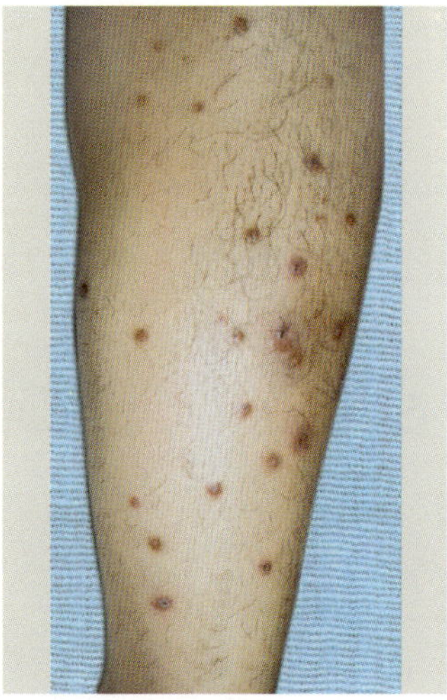

FIG. 16: Prurigo of pregnancy *(Chapter 61)*.

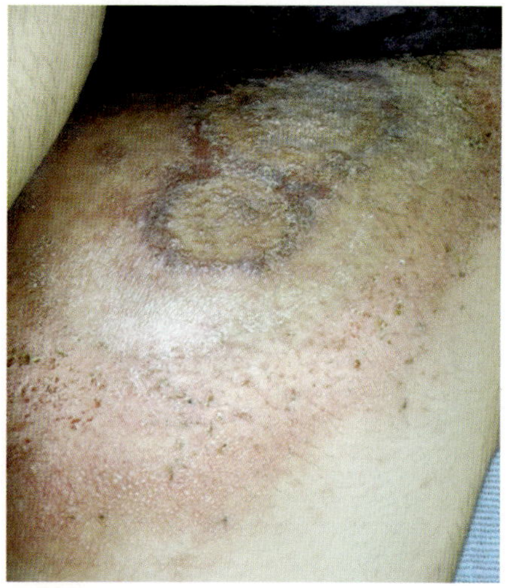

FIG. 18: Subcorneal pustulosis in impetigo herpetiformis *(Chapter 61)*.

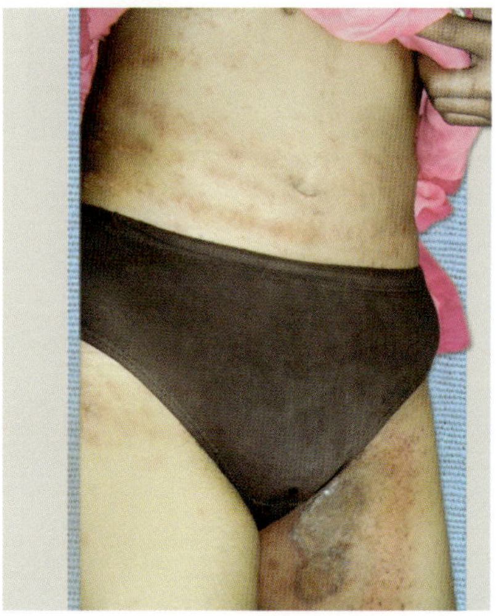

FIG. 17: Centrifugally spreading plaques in intertriginous areas in impetigo herpetiformis *(Chapter 61)*.

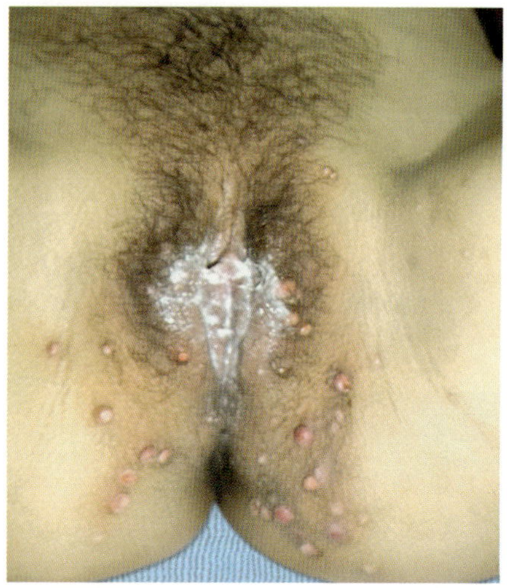

FIG. 19: Curdy discharge in candidiasis and pearly white umbilicated papules of molluscum *(Chapter 61)*.

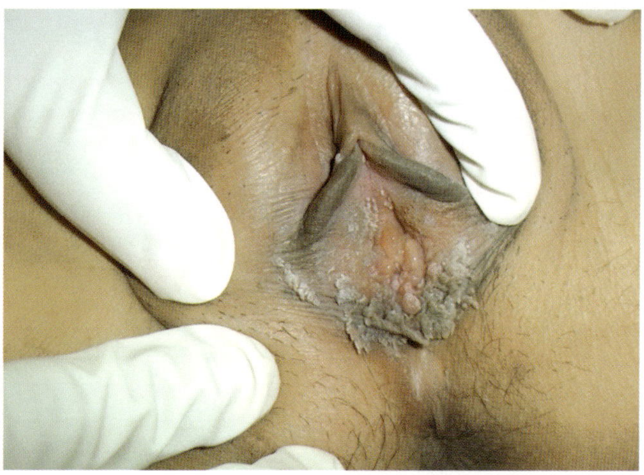

FIG. 20: Exuberant genital warts in pregnancy *(Chapter 61)*.

PLATE 10

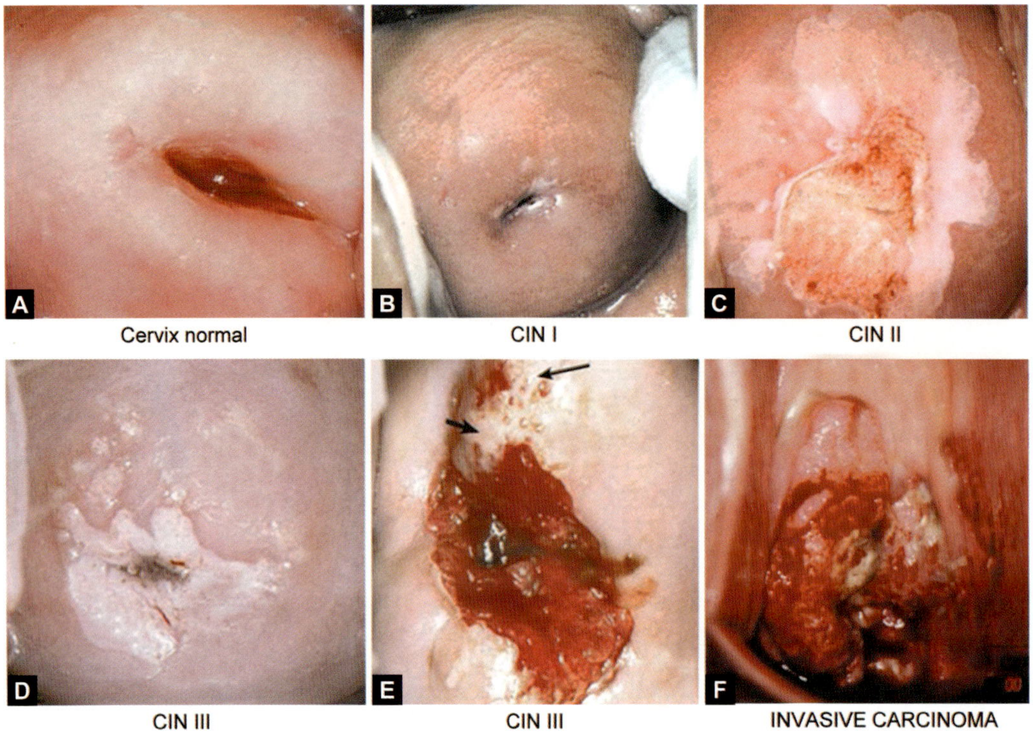

FIGS 1A TO F: Cervical cancer *(Chapter 67)*.

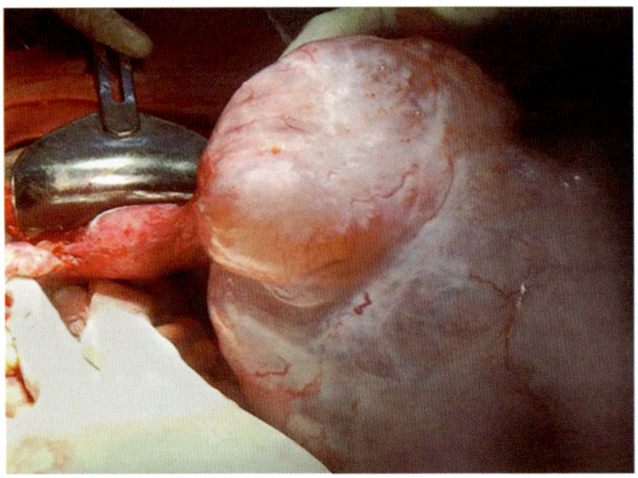

FIG. 2: Ovarian tumor *(Chapter 67)*.

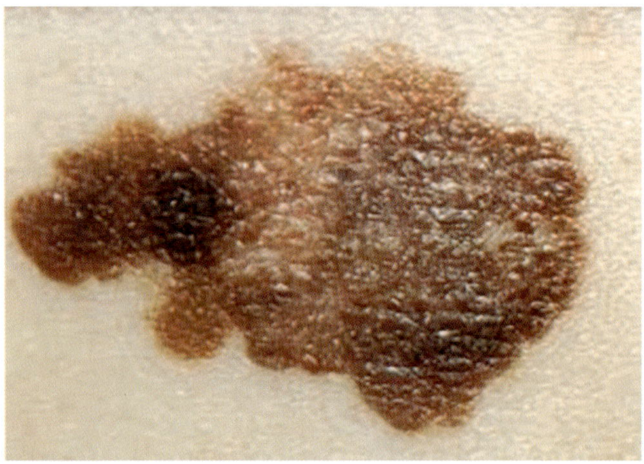

FIG. 3: Malignant melanoma *(Chapter 67)*.

PLATE 11

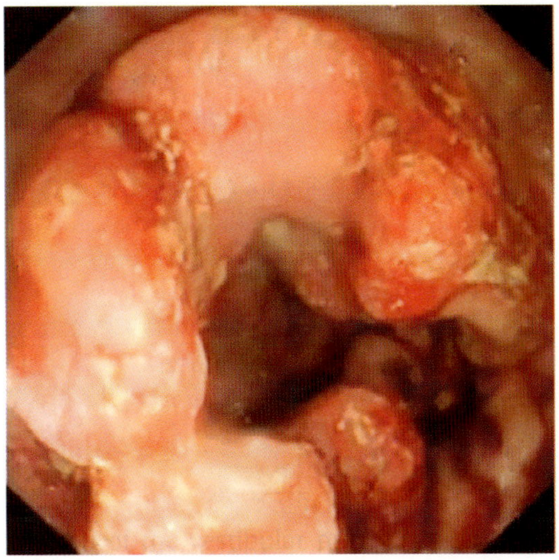

FIG. 4: Colorectal cancer *(Chapter 67)*.

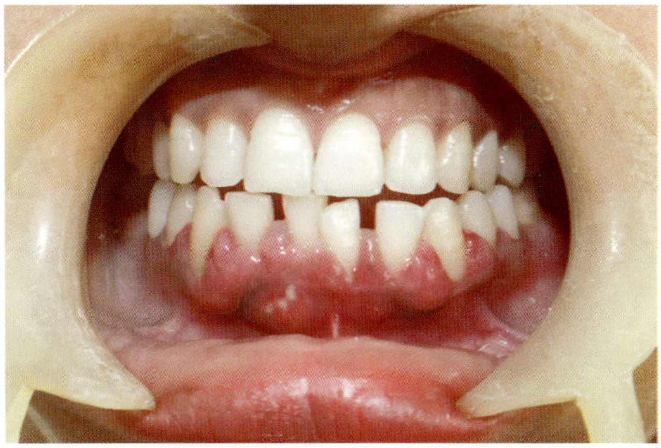

FIG. 1: Pregnancy gingivitis—gingivitis is aggravated due to increase in hormone ***(Chapter 68)***.

Courtesy: Dr Amit Kumar, MDS-Periodontics.

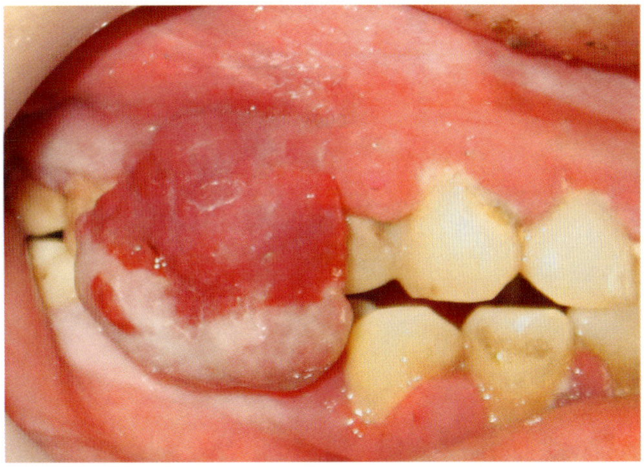

FIG. 2: Pregnancy tumor—it is caused by increased angiogenesis, which is caused by sex hormones, coupled with local factor like plaque ***(Chapter 68)***.

Courtesy: Thakur M, et al. Pregnancy tumor. Kerala Dental Journal. 2012; 35(3):308-10.

Section 1

Anatomy and Physiology

CHAPTER 1

Obstetrics Risk Management

Savita R Singhal, Roopa Malik

INTRODUCTION

Patient safety is our prime concern, particularly when it is an obstetric patient where two lives are involved. There is need of 100% perfection on the part of the healthcare providers, as slight negligence can be a nightmare for patient, family, society, and physician. Since the inception of patient safety concept in 1991, there has been surge in publications on obstetric risk management.

Risk management is the identification, assessment, and prioritization of risk followed by application of resources to minimize and control the occurrence and impact of unfortunate events or to maximize the realization of opportunities.[1] Healthcare staff does not have any intention to harm the patients, in spite of their efforts for patient safety, risks occur in health sector due to medical negligence. There is risk to physician also is in the form of financial loss due to litigation, damage to morale and reputation and about 38% of doctors who are sued suffer from depression.[2] A study at Institute of Medicine, United States (US), reported 44,000–98,000 deaths each year in hospitals as a result of medical errors.[3] The medical negligence is on increase in recent years and cost has almost doubled in United Kingdom (UK), overall expenditure in 1998 was 84 million dollars.[4] Risks in the field of obstetrics are much more as clinical situation can change rapidly, especially during intra- and postpartum periods. As per National Health Survey Litigation Authority, 2012, 49% of total values of claims were for the obstetric speciality.[5] Many obstetricians are abandoning their practice because of higher liability risks, especially in western countries.

TYPES OF RISKS

The risks can be classified broadly into two types:

1. Nonclinical risks
2. Clinical risks.

Nonclinical Risks

Nonclinical risks have least to do with the clinical acumen of the physician and are mainly at the administration level, due to system/equipment failure. Few examples are:

- Shortage of supplies
- Faulty equipment and machinery
- Falling of patient from a trolley
- Hazard due to electricity supply failure
- Baby delivering in toilet commode
- Delay in shifting of patient to operation theater
- Delay in cesarean due to large number of pending emergency cases.

Clinical Risks

The clinical risks are most of the times due to errors at the level of treating physician and team. The errors can be categorized as:

- Intentional errors: These errors are due to:
  - Violation of rules or guidelines
  - As an act of omission
  - Due to lack of knowledge
- Unintentional errors: These errors are mostly due to:
  - Overburden of work, fatigue

- Misinterpretation of clinical findings
- Incorrect history by patient
- Incorrect or partial information at time of patient handoff.

Clinical risks are like if proper consent is not taken, unnecessary cesarean section, incorrect decision regarding obstetric hysterectomy, etc.

OBSTETRIC RISK EVENTS

The common risks events to mother and newborn are:

- Neonatal risks:
  - Birth asphyxia
  - Birth trauma
  - Admission to neonatal intensive care unit (NICU)
  - Fresh still birth
  - Early neonatal death
- Maternal risks: it can occur during antenatal, intra- or postpartum periods
  - Antenatal period:
    - Failure to diagnose thalassemia, heart disease, congenital malformation or malpresentation
    - Maternal morbidity (shifted to intensive care unit, renal failure)
    - Eclampsia in hospitalized patient
    - Scar rupture or uterine rupture
  - Intrapartum period:
    - Prolonged or difficult delivery
    - Inappropriate use of vacuum or forceps
    - Shoulder dystocia
  - Postpartum period:
    - Venous thromboembolism
    - Retained foreign body, swabs, etc.
    - Postpartum hemorrhage
    - Maternal death.

CAUSES OF OBSTETRIC RISK EVENTS

The risks are due to many factors listed below.

Communication Lapses

Communication failures are one of the leading causes of medical errors and as per the Joint Commission on Accreditation of Healthcare Organizations, 72% of obstetric adverse events are due to poor communication.[6] Physician ability to communicate with the patient and among team members is the key for patient safety. Lapses in communication may be due to excessive hierarchy as seen in teaching hospitals, improper intimidation, language barrier, physical environment, and lack of structured communication. Communication lapses can occur at various levels.

Patient-physician Communication

Patient outcome depends a lot on successful communication with the patient. With good communication, especially if it is in her language, patient develops rapport and trust in physician and can come out with certain facts which may help in arriving at correct diagnosis and counseling the patient regarding treatment plan and prognosis. There are various communication models; to discuss all is beyond the scope of this chapter. Few are listed below:

- Partnership model: It is a type of open communication in which physician and patient spend equal time with each other in talking and thus increases patient involvement in healthcare through counseling, in treatment plan, and long-term follow-up.[7] This model helps in reducing the likelihood of litigation
- Acknowledge, Introduce, Duration, Explanation and Thank You model: This model is developed by Studer Group[8] and it comprises: to acknowledge the patient, give your introduction, give reasonable time, explain properly to the patient, and show appreciation for her cooperation
- Rapport, Empathy, Support, Partnership, Explanation, Cultured background, and Trust model: It has seven components: rapport, empathy, support, partnership, explanation, cultured background, and trust.[9]

Physician-physician Communication

Communication of information about patient from one member of healthcare team to another is critical part of patient safety. Structured form of communication, such as Situation, Background, Assessment and Recommendation technique,[10] should be considered. The process includes the interactive communication, limited interruptions, a process for verification, an opportunity to review a relevant data, and discussion between the giver and receiver of the patient's information.

Incomplete Documentation and Record Keeping

Records are the documents or other things that preserve the information and record keeping is an important tool to improve the quality of patient care. Some physicians feel that record keeping is onerous task that prevent them from providing care to patient rather they should remember that it is a key element and is part of professional duty. Electronic health record (EHR) is better than paper health records as EHR has the advantage of improving legibility of prescription, reducing the risk of medication errors, and online accessing of information.[11]

Important points regarding documentations are as follows:

- Entries should be legible
- Entries should be signed with physician's full name and job title

- Records should be complete, e.g., partogram, labor charts, delivery, operation notes
- If any amendment or alteration is required than that should be done without defacing the original entry which should be readable and the amendments are to be signed by physician with name and title
- Always write the accurate time and dates of findings
- Use standard abbreviations
- Always mention the indication of surgery in operative notes
- Notes should be written by physician who is delivering the care
- Records should be completed as early as possible after the care.

Improper Consent

Informed consent is the process of communication between patient and physician that results in the patient's authorization or agreement to undergo a specific medical intervention and the patient must be fully informed in her language before decision to undergo major treatment and it must be documented in written.[12] It has two components:

1. Comprehension
2. Free consent.

Comprehension: It includes patient's awareness, understanding of situation and possibilities, meaning she has been given all options of treatment and prognosis in her own language.

Free consent: It is voluntary choice to authorize someone else to act in certain ways.

In India, sometimes it is seen that the physician gets the consent signed from husband or mother-in-law or any other relative of the patient, but for legal purposes, the consent has to be signed by patient herself before any procedure or treatment. Proxy consent is allowed only in certain situations where patient is not in a position to give the consent due to emergency situation (very sick), not mentally sound or underage.

Fear, Language, and Culture

Atmosphere of trust should be created in the team to avoid the fear among junior members of team. A line must be drawn between acceptable and unacceptable behaviors. One physician should be held responsible for management and he should be easily accessible. In case of nonavailability, a backup person should be identified. Every member of the team should be encouraged to participate and contribute, to transfer of information without reluctance at time of patient handoff. Using standardized medical terminology avoids errors in communication that may occur when colloquialisms are used. The culture of misbehavior with patient and use of abbreviations, other than those that are well known and widely accepted, should be discouraged. Some of the patients may file a complaint against the treating physician regarding misbehavior or delay in examining and providing treatment, which can be tackled by quality care maintaining the standards.

Medication Risk

The incidence of adverse drugs-related injuries varies from 15 to 18.5%.[13,14] The medication risk can be in the form of wrong prescription, dosage and route of administration, omission of the drug or administration of expired drug. Most of the errors occur at the level of ordering the drug and are due to fatigue, stress, lack of knowledge, carelessness, illegible handwriting or inappropriate abbreviations used in prescription. Medication risk can be avoided to some extent by:

- Regular updating of the knowledge regarding dosage and route of administration, contraindications, and interaction with other drugs
- Reconfirmation of name and date of expiry of the drug at the time of administration by nursing staff
- Prescription should be legible, clearly mentioning the dosage, route of administration, and frequency of administration. Clear verbal instruction should be given to the patient regarding how and when to take the medicine and also about interaction with other drugs
- There should be separate boxes for the commonly used, uncommonly used or lifesaving medications to avoid wrong administration.

Fatigue

Inadequate sleep and long working hours result in fatigue which can decrease alertness, affect cognitive function, short-term memory, and impair performance. An adult needs minimal of 5 hours sleep at night. As obstetrics is a busy branch with continuous emergency input, the question is for how many hour the residents can work at a stretch. The Accreditation Council for Graduate Medical Education has suggested 16 hours daily work for first year residents and intermediate level and senior residents may be scheduled for 24 hours of duty.[15] To avoid the errors due to fatigue, there should be back up care in the department. Secondly, the tasks can be postponed if feasible and can be done at a later time. Work efficiency can be increased by altering sleep pattern like going to sleep immediately after night shift, sleep for 2 hours before night shift or if not possible, then a small nap of 45 minutes can help.

Failure to Disclose

Adverse events are unpleasant situation for patient, her family, and the physician, however, timely disclosure of adverse events helps in combating the obstetrics risk. It should be done preferably by the senior member and in the presence of minimum of two team members. Disclosure should be timely in the sense that even if all facts are not available, counsel the attendants that further information will be provided soon. Disclosure should be done at a quiet and confidential setting.[16] It is important that at the time of disclosure, there should be expression of sympathy, apology, and showing concerns regarding the situation of the women. Some developed countries have reported drastic decrease in the legal fees and liability statement when disclosure programs were followed. University of Michigan Health System and Illinois Medical Center at Chicago noticed 50% reduction in legal fees and actions[17,18] once they started following the disclosure programs.

Incomplete Patient Handoff

Patient handoff is a necessary component of risk management and is described as the transfer of patient information and knowledge, along with authority and responsibility from one clinician or team of clinicians to another clinician or team of clinicians during transition of care across the continuum. It should include opportunity to ask questions, clarify and confirm the information being transmitted. Every member of the healthcare team should be encouraged to participate and contribute to the transfer of information without hesitation.[19] Patient handoff should take priority over all the duties except emergencies.[20] Patient handoffs should be complete, clear, and timely and it can be verbal, written or both. Written is always better for documentation purpose. Use of "CUS" words to alert the receiver to level of concern regarding the safety of patient is very important.

- C: I am concerned
- U: I am uncomfortable
- S: I am scared.

Machinery and Equipment Failures

In many instances inadequate instructions or poorly designed equipment/machinery like infusion pumps, monitors, cardiotocography machine, etc. can be underlying cause of patient injury. In such cases, it is often assumed that healthcare provider has made an error but on complete root cause analysis (RCA), technical failures may be revealed as a cause of adverse event.

Administrative Failures

Inadequate administrative policies guiding the delivery of care can be a significant contributing factor in many medical errors. There may be insufficient supplies of drugs, catheters, intravenous sets, etc. leading to delay in treatment and risk to mother. In India, under various schemes run by Government, e.g., Janani Suraksha Yojana (JSY), Janani-Shishu Suraksha Karyakram (JSSK), there is provision of free treatment and free transport to all obstetrics patients, sometimes there may be delay in procurement of the supplies. There is need of strong transport system both for the patients and healthcare personnel to avoid delay in treatment. Organization is also responsible to provide the training about the assigned work to the healthcare providers, especially where new or temporary employees are often used, so as to orient them to the working place and policies of the institute. There may be lack of organizational transfer of knowledge.

PRINCIPLES OF RISK MANAGEMENT

The principles are:

- Patient safety and quality care
- Learn from mistakes
- Develop strategies and guidelines
- Support for staff members.

The aim of risk management is to reduce the harm to the patient by providing safe and quality care which indirectly safeguards the physician from litigation and enquiries. The policy should be not to blame someone but to learn from the mistakes and to make some rules/guidelines so that risk can be avoided, minimized or eliminated in future. Medical staff should be provided with financial and legal support by the administration.

COMPONENTS OF RISK MANAGEMENT

Components of risk management are:

- Risk reporting
- Evaluation of risk events
- Audit of risk events
- Learning from adverse events
- Formulating guidelines
- Funding the risk
- Risk management tools.

Risk Reporting

The risk event can be reported either from a maternity service or from an external source like a national audit. It involves identification of risk after it has happened and list of such events should be maintained and regularly updated by the medical staff. These risk incidents should be well displayed on the maternity dashboards and such events should be reported to risk management team of the hospital without any delay.

Evaluation of Risk Events

The risk events can be evaluated prospectively or retrospectively.

Prospective Risk Evaluation

One of the tools for prospective evaluation of risk events is Failure Mode and Effect Analysis (FMEA). In this, any process is outlined in detail and evaluation is done about the ways in which any step might go wrong (failure modes) and consequences of these failure modes. Contributory factors and controls for each failure modes are also identified. Then, action plan is made keeping in mind priorities of each failure mode.

Retrospective Risk Evaluation

Once a risk event has already happened, a systemic approach for investigation and identification of contributory factors and ways to prevent its recurrence is known as RCA. It is well accepted method. There should be regular staff clinical meetings on maternal mortality or near miss or other adverse events to evaluate the risks.

Audit of Risk Events

Audit of risk events can be done at the regional level from where the risk has been reported or at higher level, e.g., national level. Audit should include the entire important adverse event reporting, the effectiveness and implementation of formulated guidelines and re-audit to make sure the action has had the desired effects, e.g., in UK, there are national audits related to obstetric field most important being Confidential Enquiry into Maternal and Child Health. The reports of these audits are used as a reference for source of learning and service review.

Learning from Adverse Events

This involves sharing of lessons learnt from risk analysis and treatment with other staff members at local level or at a broader level like national level so as to prevent its recurrence. It is also beneficial to the patient and their attendants so as to understand why risk event happened.

Formulating Guidelines

It means to prepare guidelines or policies to decrease the chances of risk happening again and also to limit the damage as a result of risk event which has already occurred. Guidelines may involve providing the orientation and training programs to medical staff, improving infrastructure or manpower. It also includes making protocols for the treatment according to availability of resources and acceptability by the concerned population.

Funding the Risk

There should be some financial support policies by the administration to the affected healthcare providers and sufferer. Administration may also provide medicolegal help to the staff members. Various schemes have been launched in UK to combat these financial claims like Clinical Negligence Scheme Trust, Existing Liabilities Scheme, Liabilities to Third Party Scheme, etc.

Risk Management Tools

Various tools have been devised for management of risks, like:

- Checklist: As humans have limited ability to remember, well designed checklists are very effective in reducing the risk. These are only effective if they are used every time you perform any specific procedure, even if you are fully trained and experienced. The World Health Organization has provided pilot edition of the Safe Childbirth Checklist to support the delivery of essential maternal and perinatal care practices
- Risk management and standard operating procedures: It includes use of various risk management tools, like checklist, communication strategies (closed loop, read back, repeat back), briefings, debriefings, and standard operating procedures for correct use of each procedure
- Nontechnical skills (NOTECHS): NOTECHS is a behavior rating system that allows valid and reliable observation and assessment of various NOTECHS of operating team; surgeon, anesthetist, and nursing staff.[21] The skills which are assessed are as follows:
    - Vigilance and situation awareness:
        - Developing and maintaining a dynamic awareness of the situation in theater based on assembling data from the environment (patient, team, time, displays, equipment), understanding what they mean, and thinking ahead about what may happen next
        - Gathering information
        - Understanding information
        - Projecting and anticipating future state
    - Decision making during surgical crisis:
        - Skills for diagnosing the situation and reaching a judgment in order to choose an appropriate course of action
        - Considering options
        - Selecting and communicating option
        - Implementing and reviewing decisions
    - Communication and interaction:
        - Skills for working in a team context to ensure that the team has an acceptable shared picture of the situation and can complete tasks effectively
        - Exchanging information
        - Establishing a shared understanding
        - Coordinating team activities
    - Leadership and management skills:
        - Leading the team and providing direction, demonstrating high standards of clinical practice

  and care, and being considerate about the needs of individual team members
  - Setting and maintaining standards
  - Supporting others
  - Coping with pressure
- Patient safety programs: Patient safety programs help in combating the medical liabilities and such programs may be developed at level of the institute as per requirement. In UK, National Patient Safety Agency[22] was established in 2001 and US, Australia, and other countries have also set standards, training, and research on issue of patient safety. In one study at New York Presbyterian Hospital, implementation of patient safety programs reduced the compensation from 27 million dollars in 2003–06 to 2.5 million dollars in 2007–09 and sentinel events decreased from 5/1,000 in year 2000 to none in 2008–09.[23]

OBSTETRIC RISK PREVENTION AT DIFFERENT LEVELS

Various steps can be taken at different levels to prevent the risk events in obstetrics.

- Administrative level:
  - Proper and sufficient supply of good quality drugs, equipments, machinery
  - Adequate infrastructure
  - Adequate number of experienced staff
  - Training of staff: Staff should be sent on regular trainings, workshops, and conferences for updating their knowledge of subject
  - Making teams for regular supervision
  - Strong transport system
- Departmental level:
  - Coordination between staff members
  - Assignment of duties, especially for teaching hospitals where multiple levels of working staff is there, so as to fix the responsibility
  - Protocol and guidelines should be issued for management of common clinical conditions
  - Protocols to be displayed in labor wards and emergency
  - Time-to-time staff clinical meetings for discussion of adverse events and mortality
  - Back up for the medical staff in case of emergency due to fatigue, overwork or personnel problems
- Treating team level:
  - Coordination between team members
  - Take written informed consent from the patient
  - Give all treatment options to the patient, let the patient decide about the management
  - Follow the protocols designed in the department
  - If referral needed, early referral is advisable to decrease the morbidity and mortality
  - Complete and proper record keeping should be done by members of treating team with legible signatures
  - Handoff of the patients at the time of change of duties with complete records of the patient
  - Timely disclosure of adverse events
- Individual level:
  - Updating knowledge regularly, by reorientation programs, from internet and journals
  - While communicating with the patient, be polite, explain in detail about the procedure, effects, and side effects of treatment
  - Do not hesitate to take consultation of senior personnel if in doubt
  - Do not be negligent in examining the patient at admission and during care
  - Read literature or watch video before doing any procedure, if not confident
  - Avoid doing duties when fatigued; ask for change of the duties.

EMERGENCY SITUATIONS IN OBSTETRICS

Various obstetric emergency situations, such as postpartum hemorrhage, fetal distress, cord prolapse, shoulder dystocia, eclampsia, and many more, are seen in day-to-day practice. Emergency management in obstetrics is very crucial as most of the mortality and morbidity occurs during the emergencies. For handling the emergencies, there is need for adequate number of trained staff, drug supplies, and equipments. To deal with emergency situations and to decrease the risk events, there is need of:

- Protocols: the protocols should be put in labor room, patient-receiving room or casualty
- Emergency drills and simulation: this is the need of the hour, especially for the hospitals with less working load or frequent change of the supporting staff
- Crash cart: it is important to see that there is adequate number of drugs and it has to be replenished and rechecked periodically for expiry date of the drugs by nursing staff
- Trigger points: department can make some protocols of trigger points and paste it, so that even lower staff can inform when trigger threshold limits are crossed
- Adequate supplies: depending on the workload of the hospital
- Rapid response team: recently, the concept of rapid response team is promoted by various societies like the American Congress of Obstetricians and Gynecologists, Joint Commission, and Association of Women's Health.[24] The rapid response team has four components:
  1. Activators
  2. Responders
  3. Quality improvement
  4. Administrator.

  Activators are individuals who activate the rapid response team and these may be clinical staff, floor staff, or nursing staff or even the clinicians. Responders are the clinicians who attend the patient and provide the treatment. The quality improvement team reviews the activators and responders, and makes recommendations which are implemented by administrators.

Example

A 28-year-old $G_2P_1L_1$ woman with 39 weeks pregnancy reported to emergency with chief complaints of labor pains for past 2 hours. She was examined by the junior resident and was kept for vaginal delivery. Later on, she had decelerations and emergency cesarean section was done in view of fetal distress. A baby of birth weight 4.2 kg was delivered with an Appearance, Pulse, Grimace, Activity, and Respiration/American Pediatric Gross Assessment Record (APGAR) score of 3/10 at birth. Retrospectively, she gave history of gestational diabetes which was managed on diet. The baby was admitted to NICU because of severe birth asphyxia. After a stay of 7 days in NICU, baby expired. Patient filed a legal suit against the hospital for mismanagement.

What do we Learn from this Example?

- The decision for mode of delivery should have been taken by the senior obstetrician as the resident might not have enough knowledge to decide the mode of delivery
- Incomplete history taking: there should have been proper communication with the patient giving adequate time so that she would have given history of gestational diabetes at the time of admission only
- Informed written consent should be obtained regarding the risk of big size baby, gestational diabetes, chances of having fetal distress and its consequences, which could help at time of litigation.

CONCLUSION

Patient safety and quality care is the key factor for risk management. There should be policy of learning from mistakes and not to blame. Adequate supplies, manpower, and infrastructure should be ensured. Staff should be sent on regular trainings, workshops, and conferences for updating their knowledge of subject. Proper communication with patient and among team members is very important. Informed written consent should be taken from the patient. Departmental protocols should be formulated and followed strictly. Patient handoff should take priority over all the duties except emergencies. Risk events should be reported to seniors. Existing policies should be reviewed and new guidelines should be formulated. Medical staff should be provided with financial and legal support by the administration in case of adverse events.

REFERENCES

1. Hubbard WD. How do we know what works? In: The Failure of Risk Management: Why It's Broken and How to Fix It. Hoboken, NJ, John Wiley and Sons; 2009. pp. 37-46.
2. Scholefield H. Risk management in obstetrics. Curr Obstet Gynaecol. 2005;15:237-43.
3. Brennan TA, Leape LL, Laird NM, Hebert L, Localio AR, Lawthers AG, et al. Incidence of adverse events and negligence in hospitalized patients: Results of the Harvard Medical Practice Study 1. N Eng J Med. 1991;324(6):370-6.
4. Fenn P, Diacon S, Gray A, Hodges R, Rickman N. Current cost of medical negligence in NHS hospitals: analysis of claims database. BMJ. 2000;320(7249):1567-71.
5. NHS Litigation Authority. (2012). Ten Years of Maternity Claims: An Analysis of NHS Litigation Authority Data. [online] Available from www.nhsla.com/Safety/Documents/Ten%20Years%20of%20Maternity%20Claims%20-%20An%20Analysis%20of%20the%20NHS%20LA%20Data%20-%20October%202012.pdf. [Accessed May, 2015].
6. The Joint Commission on Accreditation of Healthcare Organizations. (2004). Sentinel Event Alert, Issue 30: Preventing infant death and injury during delivery. [online] Available from www.jointcommission.org/sentinel_event_alert_issue_30_preventing_infant_death_and_injury_during_delivery/default.aspx. [Accessed May, 2015].
7. Roter DL. Patient question asking in physician-patient interaction. Health Psychol. 1984;3(5):395-409.
8. Studer Group. Acknowledge, Introduce, Duration, Explanation, and Thank You (AIDET®): Five Fundamentals of Patient Communication. AIDET Implementation Guide. Gulf Breeze, FL, United States of America: Studer Group; 2005.
9. Mutha S, Allen C, Welch M. Toward Culturally Competent Care: A Toolbox for Teaching Communication Strategies. San Francisco, CA, United States of America: Center for the Health Professions, University of California; 2002.
10. Haig KM, Sutton S, Whittington J. SBAR: a shared mental model for improving communication between clinicians. Jt Comm J Qual Patient Saf. 2006;32(3):167-75.
11. Committee opinion no. 472: Patient safety and the electronic health record. Obstet Gynecol. 2010;116(5):1245-7.
12. ACOG Committee on Ethics. ACOG Committee Opinion No. 439: Informed consent. Obstet Gynecol. 2009;114(2 Pt 1):401-8.
13. Hug BL, Witkowski DJ, Sox CM, Keohane CA, Seger DL, Yoon C, et al. Adverse drug event rates in six community hospitals and potential impact of computerized physician order entry for prevention. J Gen Int Med. 2010;25(1):31-8.
14. Landrigan CD, Parry GJ, Bones CB, Hackbarth AD, Goldman DA, Sharek PJ. Temporal trends in rates of patient harm resulting from medical care. N Eng J Med. 2010;363(22):2124-34.
15. Nasca TJ, Day SH, Amis ES, ACGME Duty Hour Task Force. The new recommendations on duty hours from the ACGME Task Force. N Eng J Med. 2010;363(2):e3.
16. Weiss PM, Miranda F. Transparency, apology and disclosure of adverse outcomes. Obstet Gynecol Clin North Am. 2008;35(1):53-62.
17. Boothman RC, Blackwell AC, Campbell DA, Commiskey E, Anderson S. A better approach to medical malpractice claims? The University of Michigan experience. J Health Lit Sci Law. 2009;2(2):125-59.

18. McDonald TB, Helmchen LA, Smith KM, Centomani N, Guvderson A, Mayer D, et al. Responding to patient safety incidents: the "seven pillars". Qual Saf Health Care. 2010;19(6):e11.
19. ACOG Committee Opinion No. 517: Communication strategies for patient handoff. Obstet Gynecol. 2012;119(2 Pt 1):408-11.
20. William RG, Silverman R, Schwind C, Fortune JB, Sutyak J, Horvath KD, et al. Surgeon information transfer and communication: factors affecting quality and efficiency of inpatient care. Ann Surg. 2007;245(2):159-69.
21. Mishra A, Catchpole K, McCulloch P. The Oxford NOTECHS System: reliability and validity of a tool for measuring teamwork behaviour in the operating theatre. Qual Saf Health Care. 2009;18(2):104-8.
22. NHS National Patient Safety Agency (NPSA). (2001). Transfer of Patient Safety function to the NHS Commissioning Board Special Health Authority. [online] Available from www.npsa.nhs.uk. [Accessed May, 2015].
23. Grunebaum A, Chervenak F, Shupski D. Effect of a comprehensive obstetric patient safety program on compensation payments and sentinel events. Am J Obstet Gynecol. 2011;204(2):97-105.
24. American College of Obstetrician and Gynecologists Committee on Patient Safety and Quality Improvement. Committee opinion no. 590: preparing for clinical emergencies in obstetrics and gynecology. Obstet Gynecol. 2014;123(3):722-5.

CHAPTER 2

Introduction and Physiological Changes

Parneet Kaur, Atish Singla

INTRODUCTION

Pregnancy is a normal healthy condition and simultaneously the most common altered physiologic state to which human beings are subjected to. Maternal physiologic adjustments in pregnancy occur to support the requirements of fetal homeostasis without jeopardizing maternal wellbeing. Maternal systems remodel to deliver substantial energy to the fetus and remove inappropriate waste products. The normal values for many hematological, biochemical, and physiological indices during pregnancy differ markedly from those in the nonpregnant range.

PHYSIOLOGICAL CHANGES IN PREGNANCY

Maternal physiological changes in pregnancy occur as a result of hormonal alterations, mechanical effects of the gravid uterus, increased metabolic and oxygen requirements, metabolic demands of the fetoplacental unit, and hemodynamic alterations associated with the placental circulation. Maternal physiological adaptation to pregnancy may pose challenges to the obstetrician who has to decide whether changes observed during the course of routine prenatal supervision are physiologic or first manifestations of ensuing medical or obstetrical problem. All the body systems are affected to varying extent. Such changes become more significant as pregnancy progresses.

CARDIOVASCULAR SYSTEM

Soon after conception, the maternal cardiovascular system undergoes major adaptations that progress throughout gestation. In conjunction with the increased circulatory burden of pregnancy, these changes may unmask previously unrecognized heart disease and result in significant morbidity and mortality. Most of these changes are almost fully reversed in the weeks and months after delivery.

Heart Rate and Rhythm

Mean heart rate increases by 10–20 beats/min over the course of pregnancy. Most women remain in normal sinus rhythm during pregnancy.[1,2]

Heart

The heart is displaced to the left and upwards and rotated somewhat on its long axis. As a result, the apex is moved somewhat laterally from its usual position, causing a larger cardiac silhouette on chest radiograph.

- All the four cardiac chambers enlarge in size from the first trimester to the end of third trimester
- All heart valves also show enlargement
- All heart sounds are louder and first heart sound is split
- A systolic ejection murmur is normal and is due to turbulence secondary to increased blood flow through normal heart valves
- A diastolic murmur is heard occasionally
- Small pericardial effusions are frequently found which usually resolve after delivery.[1,3,4]

Electrocardiograph and Echocardiograph[3]

Electrocardiographic changes occur in the form of:

- Sinus tachycardia, atrial, and ventricular ectopics
- Rotation of the electrical axis of the heart to the left

- ST segment depression and T wave inversion in inferior and lateral leads.

However, these changes are of no clinical significance. Echocardiographic changes occur in the form of:

- Left ventricular hypertrophy by 12 weeks
- 50% increase in left ventricular mass at term
- 12–14% increase in aortic, pulmonary, and mitral valve sizes.

Cardiac Output

Cardiac output increases by about 30–50% with the first increase noted as early as 5th week of gestation and peaking by mid-to-late pregnancy, after which there is only a slight increase until labor, delivery, and the postpartum period. Cardiac output is increased as a result of increased heart rate and stroke volume (Fig. 1). These parameters are reversed by 6 months postpartum. It may even take a year for the residual effects of cardiovascular remodeling to subside.[1,5-7]

Cardiovascular changes during pregnancy are summarized in table 1. The hemodynamics during labor and puerperium are summarized in tables 2 and 3.

Blood Pressure

Systolic blood pressure does not show a significant drop in pregnancy. It may drop slightly by 6–8%. However, there is marked drop in diastolic pressure. It is reduced in the first two trimesters by up to 20–25% and returns to nonpregnant level by term. This is due to the placenta acting as an arteriovenous shunt, together with peripheral vasodilating factors like estrogen, progesterone, and increased endothelial synthesis of prostaglandin E_2 and prostacyclins.[3]

Supine Hypotension

During late pregnancy when the women in the supine position, the large pregnant uterus rather consistently compresses venous return from the lower body. It may also compress the aorta. The results are that cardiac filling may be reduced with diminished cardiac output. Specifically, Bamber and Dresner[8] found cardiac output at term to increase 1.2 L/min (almost 20%) when a women moved from her back-to-left lateral position. Moreover, in the supine gravid patient, uterine blood flow estimated by Doppler velocimetry decreases by a third.[9] This may directly affect fetal heart rate patterns. A paravertebral collateral circulation can develop that allows blood to bypass the obstructed inferior vena cava. The supine hypotensive syndrome of pregnancy occurs when there is inferior vena caval obstruction further exacerbated by an underdeveloped paravertebral collateral system and insufficient increase in the systemic vascular resistance or heart rate.[1,7]

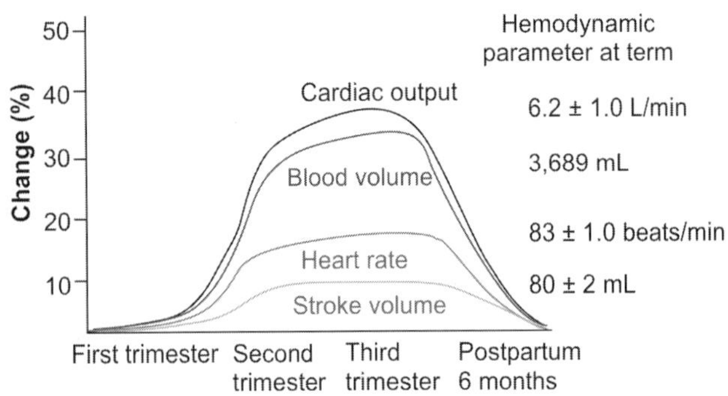

FIG. 1: Changes in cardiac output, stroke volume, and heart rate.[6]

TABLE 1: Cardiovascular changes during pregnancy[5]

Parameter	Percentage of change
Cardiac output	40–50% increase
Stroke volume	30% increase
Heart rate	15–25% increase
Intravascular volume	45% increase
Systemic vascular resistance	20% decrease
Systolic blood pressure	Minimal
Diastolic blood pressure	20% Decrease at midpregnancy Prepregnancy values at term
Central venous pressure	Unchanged
Oxygen consumption	30–40% increase

TABLE 2: Hemodynamics during labor[5]

Parameter	Stage of labor	Percentage of change
Cardiac output	• Latent phase • Active phase • Expulsive phase • Immediate postpartum	• 10% increase • 25% increase • 40% increase • 75–80% increase
Heart rate	• All stages	• Increase
Central venous pressure	• All stages	• Increase

TABLE 3: Hemodynamics during puerperium[5]

Parameter	Postpartum	Percentage of change
Cardiac output	• Within 1 h • 24–48 h • 2 weeks • 12–24 weeks	• 30% above prelabor values • Just below prelabor values • 10% above prepregnant values • Baseline prepregnancy values
Heart rate	• Immediate • 2 weeks	• Decrease • Prepregnant values
Stroke volume	• 48 h • 24 weeks	• Remains above prelabor values • 10% above prepregnant values

This tendency towards stagnation of blood in the lower extremities during the latter part of pregnancy contribute to the dependent edema frequently experienced, development of varicose veins in the legs and vulva, as well as hemorrhoids. They also predispose to deep vein thrombosis.[10]

Preload and Afterload

The increased blood volume delivered to the heart increases the preload. Preload is influenced by maternal position; the supine position results in compression of inferior vena cava and decreased cardiac output. The ability of the normal heart to adapt to chronic volume overload probably prevents pressures from rising in women without heart disease.

Afterload is the force against which the ventricular muscle contracts; typically it is reduced during pregnancy. It can be measured by either measuring the arterial systolic pressure or calculating the systemic vascular resistance.

During pregnancy, there is a fall in systemic vascular resistance. The drop in vascular resistance is mainly due to increased flow in uteroplacental circulation. In addition, the hormonal milieu of pregnancy leads to the secretion of various vasodilators, such as nitric oxide and prostaglandins, which cause drop in vascular resistance.[1,6]

Pregnancy has numerous effects on cardiac evaluation, including changes in the electrocardiogram, chest radiograph, and echocardiogram. Although these minor changes occur in healthy pregnant women at term, symptoms and signs, such as chest pain, syncope, severe arrhythmias, systolic murmur more than grade 3, or diastolic murmur, suggest severe disease and warrant further investigation.

Peripartum Cardiomyopathy

Peripartum cardiomyopathy is defined as the presence of heart failure without any obvious cause in a pregnant woman occurring anytime from 1 month predelivery to 5 months postpartum. If any pregnant or postpartum woman has unexpected and persistent dyspnea or is noted to be having tachypnea or tachycardia and pulmonary embolism has been excluded, she may be having peripartum cardiomyopathy and should be investigated further by a cardiologist.[11]

HEMATOLOGICAL CHANGES

Blood Volume

Blood volume increases significantly during pregnancy. The increase starts at around 6 weeks' gestation and reaches a maximal volume of 4700 to 5200 mL by 32 weeks' gestation. A rapid increase is typically noted until midpregnancy, with a slower increase thereafter. Plasma volume increases by 15% during the first trimester, accelerates in the second trimester, peaks at around 32 weeks reaching up to 50% above nonpregnant levels, and stays elevated until term. It returns to nonpregnant level by 6 days postdelivery.[3,12]

Red Blood Cells

The red cell mass falls during the first 8 weeks of pregnancy, increases back to nonpregnant levels by 16 weeks and then rising to 30% above nonpregnant levels by term. The plasma volume increase is proportionately greater than the increase in red cell mass, and the resulting hemodilution explains the so-called physiological anemia of pregnancy.[3]

The increased blood volume delivered to the ventricle during pregnancy increases the preload and can be estimated by examining ventricular diastolic volume and pressure. The pregnancy-induced hypervolemia has important functions:

- To meet the metabolic demands of the enlarged uterus with its greatly hypertrophied vascular system
- To provide an abundance of nutrients and elements to support the growing placenta and fetus
- To protect the mother and in turn the fetus, against the deleterious effects of impaired venous return in the supine and erect positions
- To safeguard the mother against the adverse effects of blood loss associated with parturition.

Reduced plasma volume expansion has been associated with low-birth weight and intrauterine growth retardation.[1,10]

Hemoglobin Concentration and Hematocrit

Both hemoglobin and hematocrit decreases slightly during pregnancy due to increase in plasma volume which causes hemodilution.[13,14]

Leukocytes

The leucocyte count ranges during pregnancy are higher than nonpregnant values and the upper values approach 15,000/μL. The distribution of cells is also altered. Lymphocytes decrease during pregnancy through the first and second trimester and increases during the third trimester. Specifically, during the third trimester, the percentage of granulocytes and CD8 T lymphocytes are significantly increased along with concomitant reduction in percentage of CD4 T lymphocytes and monocytes. There is an absolute monocytosis during pregnancy, especially in the first trimester, but decreases as gestation advances. Because of the stress of delivery, during labor and early puerperium, white blood cell count may vary from 9,000 to 25,000/μL. By 4 weeks postdelivery, typical white blood cell ranges are similar to those in healthy nonpregnant women.[10,15]

Platelets

Platelets decrease during pregnancy, particularly in the third trimester. This is termed as gestational thrombocytopenia.

This is partly due to hemodilution and partly due to increased platelet activation and accelerated clearance. The platelet count averages about 213,000/μL compared to 250,000/μL in nonpregnant women. It has been recommended that the lower limit of platelet count in late pregnancy should be considered 150,000/μL.[10,15]

Coagulation and Fibrinolysis

Pregnancy is considered a "hypercoagulable state". It is characterized by:

- Increase in all clotting factors except XI and XIII
- Factors II, V, and XII remain unchanged
- Levels of protein S decrease progressively with advancement of gestation
- Resistance to activated protein C occurs in pregnancy
- Bleeding time and clotting time remain unchanged
- Fibrinogen increases to 300–600 mg/dL and averages 450 mg/dL
- Tissue plasminogen activator activity gradually decreases over the course of normal pregnancy
- In pregnancy, activated partial thromboplastin time is usually shortened by up to 4 s in the third trimester
- There are no marked changes in prothrombin time or thrombin time
- Levels of antithrombin remain relatively constant throughout gestation and the early puerperium.

Coagulation factors remain elevated for up to 8–12 weeks postpartum. These physiological changes may be important for minimizing intrapartum blood loss, but they entail an increased risk of thromboembolism during pregnancy and postpartum period.[10,15-17]

Inflammatory Markers

Many tests, which are done to diagnose inflammation cannot be used reliably in pregnancy, as pregnancy is characterized by increased C-reactive proteins, erythrocyte sedimentation rate, and complement factors C-3 and C-4.[10]

Immunological Functions

Pregnancy is thought to be associated with suppression of a variety of humoral and cell-mediated immunological functions to accommodate the foreign semiallogenic fetal graft. Thus there is suppression of T-helper cell and T-cytotoxic cells, which decreases the secretion of interleukin-2, interferon-γ, and tumor necrosis factor-β.[10]

RESPIRATORY SYSTEM

Capillary engorgement of the nasal and pharyngeal mucosa and larynx begins early in the first trimester. This explains why many pregnant women complain of difficulty in nasal breathing, experience more episodes of epistaxis and experience voice changes. The diaphragm rises about 4 cm during pregnancy. The subcostal angle widens appreciably as the transverse diameter of the thoracic cage increases approximately by 2 cm. The thoracic circumference increases by 6 cm, but not sufficiently to prevent a reduction in the residual lung volume created by the elevated lung diaphragm.[16]

Physiology

- Respiratory rate remains unchanged
- The minute ventilation increases by about 40% from 7.5 to 10.5 L/min. The increase in minute ventilation occurs because of enhanced respiratory drive primarily due to stimulatory effects of progesterone, low expiratory reserve volume, and compensatory alkalosis
- Oxygen consumption increases by about 18% from 250 to 300 mL/min
- Tidal volume increases gradually from the first trimester by up to 45% at term
- Functional residual capacity is decreased by 20–30% at term due to reduction of 25% in ERV and 15% in residual volume
- The peak expiratory flow rates increase progressively as gestation advances
- Lung compliance is unaffected by pregnancy, but airway conductance is increased and total pulmonary resistance reduced, as a result of progesterone
- The maximum breathing capacity and forced or timed vital capacity are not altered appreciably.[3,10]

The changes in respiratory system are summarized in table 4.

Blood Gases

Partial pressure of arterial carbon dioxide ($PaCO_2$) decreases to 3.7–4.2 kPa by the end of the first trimester and remains at this level until term. Arterial partial pressure of oxygen (PaO_2) in upright pregnant women is in the region of 14 kPa, higher than that in nonpregnant women. This is

TABLE 4: Changes in pulmonary function during pregnancy

Parameter	Change
Respiratory rate	↔
Minute ventilation	↑
Oxygen consumption	↑
Tidal volume	↑
Functional residual capacity	↓
Expiratory reserve volume	↓
Residual volume	↓
Peak expiratory flow rate	↑
Vital capacity	↔

TABLE 5: Normal arterial blood gas values in pregnancy[3]

Parameter	Values
pH	7.40–7.45
Partial pressure of arterial carbon dioxide ($PaCO_2$)	3.7–4.2 kPa
Arterial partial pressure of oxygen (PaO_2)	13–14 kPa
Bicarbonate (HCO_3)	18–21 mmol/L

due to lower $PaCO_2$ levels, a reduced arteriovenous oxygen difference and a reduction in physiological shunt. To compensate for the respiratory alkalosis, there is reduction in bicarbonate (HCO_3) levels. Thus, reduced $PaCO_2$ from maternal hyperventilation aids carbon dioxide transfer from the fetus to the mother while also facilitating oxygen release to the fetus.[3] Normal arterial blood gas values in pregnancy are shown in table 5.

Oxygen Consumption

As a result of increased fetal and maternal tissue mass and cardiac and respiratory work, peak maternal oxygen consumption can increase by 20–30% at term. Whereas most of the increase in cardiac output occurs early, the increase in oxygen consumption occurs progressively throughout pregnancy.[1]

URINARY SYSTEM

There are significant changes in the urinary tract and renal function. The kidneys enlarge in size by about 1 cm. There is marked dilatation of renal calyces, pelvis, and ureters. As a result of dilatation, the capacity of the renal pelvis and ureter increases from 15 to 75 mL. Unequal ureteral dilatation may result from the cushioning provided to the left ureter by sigmoid colon and perhaps from the greater compression of right ureter as the consequence of dextrorotation of the uterus. Due to the decreased tone of ureters and bladder, stasis of urine is common, predisposing the gravid female to urinary tract infection and bacteriuria.[16]

The glomerular filtration rate (GFR) increases as much as 25% by second week after conception and 50% by the beginning of second trimester and is maintained at this augmented level at least till 36th gestational week. Renal plasma flow increases in during pregnancy, peaking in the third trimester at 60–80% above prepregnancy levels. Primarily because of increased GFR, approximately 60% of women report urinary frequency during pregnancy.[1,3,10]

Iosif et al.[18] reported during pregnancy absolute and functional urethral lengths were found to increase by 6.7 mm and 4.8 mm, respectively. Also, the maximum urethral pressure and the urethral closure pressure also increased throughout pregnancy. Thus, the physiologic changes, which took place within the urethra during pregnancy, were to advantage from standpoint of maintaining continence. Still, women experience some degree of urinary incontinence in third trimester and postpartum period.[19]

Renal Function Tests

- There is decrease in serum creatinine levels during normal pregnancy and a level above 0.9 mg/dL suggests underlying renal disease
- Creatinine clearance is a useful test to estimate the renal function. In nonpregnant patients, the average value is around 110–115 mL/min. During pregnancy, the 24-hour creatinine clearance increases by 25% by 4 weeks after the last menstrual period and by 45% at 9 weeks. During the third trimester, a consistent and significant decrease occurs towards nonpregnant values preceding delivery
- There is also fall in serum urea and uric acid values
- Glycosuria during pregnancy may not be abnormal. The appreciable increase in glomerular filtration, together with impaired tubular reabsorptive capacity for filtered glucose, accounts in most cases for glycosuria
- Proteinuria is not evident during pregnancy except occasionally in slight amounts during or soon after vigorous labor.[3,10,20]

Renal changes of normal pregnancy are summarized in table 6.

TABLE 6: Renal changes of normal pregnancy[21]

Variable	Change in pregnancy
Kidney size	The kidney length increases by 1.0–1.5 cm and kidney volume increases by up to 30%
Hydronephrosis	Physiological dilation of the urinary collecting system with hydronephrosis in up to 80% of women (right >left)
Renal blood flow	Increased by 80% above baseline
Glomerular filtration rate	150–200 mL/min (rises 40–50% above baseline)
Serum creatinine	Falls to 0.4–0.5 mg/dL (n = 0.8)*
Uric acid	Falls to 2–3 mg/dL (n = 4–5)
Blood urea nitrogen	Falls to 8–10 mg/dL (n = 13)*
Sodium	Mild hyponatremia (fall of 4–5 mol/L)
Osmolality	Falls to a new osmotic set point of about 270 mOsm/kg

*Considered normal in a nonpregnant individual, reflects renal impairment in a pregnant women.

GASTROINTESTINAL TRACT

- The gums swell and bleed easily. Incidence of caries is increased
- The lower esophageal sphincter (LES) pressure reduces under the effect of circulating progesterone and therefore the barrier pressure (LES-gastric pressure) is reduced significantly during pregnancy, thus, causing gastro-esophageal reflux, esophagitis, and pyrosis (heartburn)
- Gastric emptying time appears to be unchanged during each trimester and compared with nonpregnant women. During labour, however, and especially after administration of analgesic agents, gastric emptying time may be prolonged. As a result, a major danger of general anesthesia for delivery is regurgitation and aspiration of either food-laden or highly acidic gastric contents
- The stomach and intestines are displaced by the enlarging uterus resulting in alteration of physical findings in certain diseases. The appendix, for instance, may reach the right flank. The implication of this displacement in the correct diagnosis of appendicitis is apparent
- Constipation occurs as a result of delayed small bowel transit and increased water resorption. Thus hemorrhoids are fairly common during pregnancy. Another contributory factor for hemorrhoids is elevated pressure in veins below the level of gravid uterus.[3,16]

Liver

Hepatic blood flow increases substantively as does the portal vein diameter. Total alkaline phosphatase activity almost doubles. The raised alkaline phosphatase are heat stable and are placental in origin.[20] Serum aspartate transaminase, alanine transaminase, γ-glutamyl transferase, and bilirubin levels are slightly lower compared with nonpregnant values.[22] Leucine aminopeptidase is a proteolytic liver enzyme whose serum levels may be increased with liver disease. Its activity is markedly elevated in pregnant women. Pregnancy-induced aminopeptidase has oxytocinase and vasopressinase activity which occasionally causes transient diabetes insipidus.[10]

Gallbladder

During normal pregnancy, the contractility of the gallbladder is reduced, leading to an increased residual volume. Impaired emptying leads to stasis, which is associated with increased bile cholesterol saturation of pregnancy, contribute to increased prevalence of cholesterol gallstones in multiparous women.[3,10]

WEIGHT

The average weight gain during pregnancy is 25–35 pounds, with most of the gain occurring during the last two trimesters. A break-up of weight gained is given in table 7.[23]

TABLE 7: A break-up of weight gain

Fetus	8 lbs
Amniotic fluid, placenta and fetal membranes	4 lbs
Uterus	3 lbs
Breast	2 lbs
Blood and extracellular fluid	5 lbs
Fat accumulation	3–13 lbs

Without prenatal control of diet, the mother's weight gain can be as great as 75 lbs instead of the usual 25–35 lbs. Woman who gain 10% or more of their weight before pregnancy mass are at higher risk for complications, such as gestational diabetes mellitus and pregnancy-induced hypertension.[24] There is now accumulating evidence supporting a link between maternal obesity, or excessive gestational weight gain, and offspring obesity as a neonate, child, adolescent and adulthood, as well as metabolic outcomes including increased risk of insulin resistance, hypertension and dyslipidemia, and other outcomes such as behavioral problems and risk of asthma.[25]

Exercise and Pregnancy

It was observed that during pregnancy all categories of activity decreased except walking which increased by third trimester.[26] But according to the recommendations given by the American College of Obstetricians and Gynecologists for exercise during pregnancy and postpartum period, regular exercise is promoted for its overall health benefits. They recommended the accumulation of 30 minutes or more of moderate intensity physical activity on most, and preferably all, days of the week after medical evaluation and clearance. Similarly, the recommendations note that rapid resumption of activities postpartum have no adverse effects but gradual return to former activities is advised.[27]

ENDOCRINE SYSTEM

Pituitary

There is significant enlargement of pituitary gland during pregnancy. There is increase in number of prolactin-secreting cells, with the proportion of lactotrophs increasing from 1% to 40%. This results in elevated prolactin levels up to 10–20 times those of normal, nonpregnant values.[3]

Maternal serum values of growth hormone increase slowly from approximately 3.5 ng/mL at 10 weeks to plateau after 28 weeks at approximately 14 ng/mL. Growth hormone in amniotic fluid peaks at 14–15 weeks and slowly declines thereafter to reach baseline values after 36 weeks. The main source of growth hormone is pituitary gland in the first trimester of pregnancy but from the beginning of second trimester placenta becomes the principle source. The function of growth hormone during pregnancy is incompletely understood but it appears to have some effect on fetal growth and development of eclampsia.[10]

Thyroid

- The thyroid gland enlarges in size
- There is increased synthesis of thyroid-binding globulin by the liver in pregnancy as a result of high estrogen levels and increased iodine excretion
- This increase leads to a compensatory rise in serum concentrations of total T_4 and T_3
- The levels of free T_4 and T_3 are unaffected, thus euthyroid state is maintained
- Thyroid-stimulating hormone (TSH) levels fall slightly in first trimester then recover later in pregnancy (changes in TSH due to α-human chorionic gonadotropin subunit)
- In general, TSH is useful in screening for thyroid disease. However, it can be misleading when used alone in individuals being monitored for known thyroid disease
- There is iodine deficiency as a result of loss through increased GFR and decreased tubular absorption
- Active transport of iodine to fetoplacental unit and fetal thyroid activity also deplete the maternal iodide pool[3]
- The normal range of TSH during pregnancy is 0.1–2.5 mIU/L during first trimester and 0.2–3.0 mIU/L during second and third trimesters.[28]

Adrenals

- There is an increase in the levels of corticosteroid-binding globulin
- Total and free cortisol rises
- There is increased secretion of aldosterone and by third trimester, 1 mg/day is secreted
- Levels of plasma deoxycorticosterone show a rise
- Maternal plasma levels of both androstenedione and testosterone are slightly elevated
- Levels of adrenocorticotropic hormone also rise after showing a reduction in early pregnancy
- Maternal levels of dehydroepiandrosterone sulfate are decreased.[10]

Pancreas

Beta-cells undergo hyperplasia resulting in increased insulin secretion. Pregnancy is associated with an insulin-resistant condition, similar to that of type II diabetes. Insulin resistance increases with advancing pregnancy due to insulin antagonism by human placental lactogen, cortisol, prolactin, estrogen, and progesterone.[3]

Parathyroids

Parathyroid hormone plasma concentrations decrease during first trimester and then increase gradually throughout the remainder of pregnancy. The action of this hormone on bone resorption, intestinal absorption and kidney reabsorption is to increase extracellular fluid calcium concentration as fetal skeletal mineralization requires approximately 30 g of calcium, primarily during the third trimester.

GENERAL METABOLISM

The general metabolism is increased in pregnancy in response to needs of growing fetus. The metabolic needs of the fetus peak in the third trimester during the phase of greatest growth. Maternal metabolism during early gestation is thus largely anabolic, in essence hoarding nutrients in preparation for the upcoming demands. Late in gestation, maternal metabolism becomes largely catabolic, shunting nutrients to the rapidly growing fetus. The basal metabolic rate increases by about 60% during second half of pregnancy. The energetic cost of pregnancy is highly variable but on an average it is 80,000 kcal. Efforts to achieve good maternal nutritional status preconception as well as throughout gestation best assure a good milieu for fetal growth and development. Energy in excess of fetal needs has a high potential to be stored as maternal fat because of the overall anabolic milieu of pregnancy.[29]

Water Metabolism

- Increased water retention is a normal physiological alteration of pregnancy. It is mediated, at least in part, by a fall in plasma osmolality of approximately 10 mOsm/kg
- At term, the water content of the fetus, placenta and amniotic fluid approximates 3.5 L, another 3.0 L accumulates from increase in maternal blood volume and in the size of uterus and breasts. Thus minimum amount of extra water accumulated during pregnancy by average woman is 6.5 L
- Thus demonstrable pitting edema of the ankles and legs is seen in most pregnant women, especially at the end of the day.[10]

Carbohydrate Metabolism

- Handling of glucose changes dramatically during pregnancy
- Maternal insulin resistance develops, usually early in pregnancy, thereby limiting maternal glucose consumption and allowing shunting of most of the glucose to the fetus
- Insulin sensitivity may decrease as much as 80% during late pregnancy

- Maternal fasting blood sugar decreases by 10% in late pregnancy
- Because of the increased GFR and decreased renal threshold for glucose, there is renal glycosuria, i.e., woman excrete more than 5.5 mmol of glucose in 24 hours
- Therefore, routine use of urinalysis for monitoring glycemic control is unreliable.[3,6]

Protein Metabolism

- Nitrogen balance is altered significantly during pregnancy
- At term, the fetus and the placenta contain about 500 g of protein and the maternal gain is also about 500 g chiefly distributed in the uterus, breast, and the maternal blood
- Shifts in protein metabolism are complex and change gradually throughout gestation so that nitrogen conservation for fetal growth achieves full potential during last quarter of pregnancy
- There is no evidence that woman deposit nitrogen in early gestation. In fact, there is increased nitrogen retention in late pregnancy due to decrease in urea excretion
- A decrease in urea synthesis seems to account for the reduction in urea nitrogen in late pregnancy
- Urea synthesis declines by 45% in the third trimester of pregnancy
- The total plasma protein level falls from 7 to 6 g/L, mainly because plasma albumin level drops from 4 to 3 g/L.[6,21,29]

Fat Metabolism

- An average of 3–4 kg of fat is stored during pregnancy mostly in the abdominal wall, breasts, hip, and thighs
- Because of the insulin resistance in the adipose tissue, lipolysis increases, providing fatty acids as an alternate fuel for maternal consumption and glycerol as a gluconeogenic substrate
- At 10 weeks of pregnancy, serum triacylglycerol levels are 20% higher than nonpregnant women and they reach a value of approximately 3 times that of nonpregnant women by term
- Total cholesterol rises by 25–50% and low-density lipoprotein by 50%
- Pregnancy thus generates a relatively atherogenic lipid profile
- Levels of circulating triglycer ides correlate well with fetal weight, and hyperlipidemia in third trimester is the best predictor of large for gestational age fetus.[6,21,29]

Iron Metabolism

- The iron stores of normal young women are only ~300 mg
- Normal pregnancy is associated with a "demand" of 1,000 mg of additional iron:
  - 500 mg is required to increase maternal red blood cell volume
  - 300 mg are actively transported to fetus and placenta
  - 200 mg are lost through various channels of excretion, primarily the gastrointestinal tract.

Because most iron is used during the latter half of pregnancy, the iron need become large after midpregnancy and averages about 6–7 mg/day.[10,21]

Calcium Metabolism

- The daily maternal requirement of calcium is 1–1.5 g
- During the entire pregnancy, 32 g of calcium is transferred to the fetus
- The requirement goes up during the last 3 months and lactation period and this demand is met by marked increase in efficiency of calcium absorption and by the rates of bone resorption
- The fetus requires approximately 300 mg/day calcium during the third trimester.[10,21]

EYE

- There is increased thickness of cornea due to fluid retention (contact lens intolerance)
- Intraocular pressure decreases which is attributed to increased vitreous outflow.[10]

CENTRAL NERVOUS SYSTEM

There may be pregnancy-related decline in memory which is limited to third trimester. It is transient and resolves after delivery.[30]

Woman also have disturbed sleep pattern, fewer hours of night sleep, and reduced sleep efficiency during pregnancy, beginning from as early as 12 weeks of pregnancy and extending through 2 months postpartum.[31]

Understanding maternal physiology is crucial in understanding the changes and clinical scenarios associated with pregnancy. This knowledge will help us distinguish the physiological and pathological processes during pregnancy. It is important to interpret the investigations in the context of the changed values. Pregnancy-specific ranges should be used in making clinical decisions. Because there is a fall in plasma albumin, thus the drugs which are highly bound to albumin may be increased in free-drug concentration. It is important to consider these effects while prescribing certain drugs.

ANATOMICAL CHANGES IN PREGNANCY

Skin

During pregnancy, skin undergoes a number of changes, mainly thought to be due to hormonal changes.

- Pigmentation: hyperpigmentation occurs in up to 90% of women during pregnancy. This begins in the first trimester and is prominently noticed in areas of normal pigmentation as nipples, areola, perineum, and vulva
- Linea nigra: this appears as an area of pigmentation extending from symphysis pubis to xiphisternum. Although the pigmentation fades after delivery, it rarely returns to prepregnancy levels
- Melasma: it develops in up to 70% of woman, mainly in the second half of pregnancy. It appears as patches of light-brown facial pigmentation usually over forehead, cheeks, upper lip, nose, and chin
- Spider naevi: these present as a central red spot and reddish extensions which radiate outwards like a spider's web and occur on the face, the trunk, and arms. Most appear in early pregnancy and regress following delivery, although in 25% of woman they may persist. Recurrences are known to occur at the same site in subsequent pregnancies
- Striae gravidarum: they appear perpendicular to skin tension lines as pink linear wrinkles. They fade and become white and atrophic, although never disappear completely
- Striae albicans: in multiparous women, silvery lines that represent the cicatrices of previous striae called striae albicans can also be seen. They represent the scar tissue in deeper layers of the skin and are due to stretching and breakdown of the elastic tissue and increase in aldosterone production
- Palmar erythema: it is reddening of the palms at thenar and hypothenar eminencies. This is thought to be due to high levels of estrogen in pregnancy and is seen up to 70% of woman by the third trimester and fade within 1 week of delivery.[3,10]

MUSCULOSKELETAL SYSTEM

Abdominal muscles are stretched to the point of their elastic limit by the end of pregnancy. Occasionally the muscles of the abdominal wall do not withstand the tension to which they are subjected; as a result rectus muscles separate in the midline creating diastasis recti of varying extent.

Pregnant women develop progressive lordosis. Compensating for the anterior position of the enlarging uterus, lordosis shifts the center of gravity back over the lower extremities. The sacroiliac, sacrococcygeal and pubic joints have increased mobility during pregnancy. It may contribute to maternal postural alterations and in turn create lower back discomfort.[10]

BREASTS

Breast changes are more markedly seen in primigravidas compared to multigravidas. In the early weeks of pregnancy, there usually occurs breast tenderness, tingling sensation and paresthesias. After the second month, the breast progressively increases in size. There is marked hypertrophy and proliferation of the ducts under the estrogen and the alveoli under the effect of both estrogen and progesterone. There is also hypertrophy of the connective tissue stroma. Myoepithelial cells become prominent. The weight of each breast at term is 400–800 g.

- Nipple and areola: nipples become considerably larger, more deeply pigmented and more erectile. The areolae become broader and more deeply pigmented with (5–15) small elevations called Montgomery's tubercles which are hypertrophic sebaceous glands. An outer zone of the less marked and irregular pigmented area appears in second trimester and is called secondary areola and is more prominent in primigravida
- Breast secretion: after 12 weeks of gestation, thick yellowish fluid called colostrum can often be expressed from the nipples by gentle massage.

Rarely, the breast may enlarge and become so pathologically extensive, referred to as gigantism, that it may require surgical intervention.[10,21]

REPRODUCTIVE SYSTEM

Uterus

The uterus demonstrates remarkable changes during pregnancy:

- It increases in weight from 70 to 1100 g by term
- In nonpregnant woman, the cavity has a capacity of 10 mL, which is increased by 500–1,000 times by the end of pregnancy
- The uterine blood flow increases from 50 mL/min in nonpregnant state to 750 mL/min near term
- The adult uterus comprises three layers:
    - Inner layer thin circular muscle fibers
    - Outer layer thin long muscle fibers
    - Central layer thick inter locking muscle fibers
- The ratio of muscle to connective tissue increases from the lower part of the uterus to the fundus
- In early pregnancy, uterine growth result from both hyperplasia and hypertrophy, while later hypertrophy accounts for most of increase
- As the pregnancy advanced, the uterus is divided into upper and lower uterine segments. The lower uterine segment corresponds to the isthmus of nonpregnant uterus
- Uterine enlargement is most marked in the fundus
- For the first few weeks, the uterus maintains its original pear shape, but as pregnancy advances, corpus and fundus assume a more globular shape, becoming almost spherical by 12 weeks

- By the end of 12 weeks, the uterus becomes too large to maintain entirely within the pelvis. As the uterus enlarges, it contacts the anterior abdominal wall, displaces the intestines laterally and superiorly and continues to rise, ultimately reaching almost to the liver
- With the ascent of uterus, it usually undergoes rotation to the right. This dextrorotation is caused by the rectosigmoid on the left side of the pelvis.

Cervix

- The cervix becomes softer and swollen in pregnancy because of increased vascularity and edema of the entire cervix, together with hypertrophy and hyperplasia of cervical glands
- The major component of cervix is connective tissue along with small amount of smooth muscle
- The mucus glands becomes distended and secrete mucus which forms a mucus plug that is expelled in labor as the show
- Prostaglandins and collagenase, especially in last weeks of pregnancy, act on collagen fiber make cervix more softer.

Vagina

- The vaginal mucosa becomes thicker during pregnancy
- The vaginal discharge during pregnancy increased due to increase desquamation of the superficial vaginal mucosal cells
- The pH is acidic varying from 3.5 to 6.

Ovaries

- Ovulation ceases during pregnancy and the maturation of new follicles is suspended
- A decidual reaction on and beneath the surface of the ovaries, similar to that found in the endometrial stroma, is common in pregnancy
- The caliber of ovarian veins increase enormously from 0.9 to 2.6 cm at term.[10,16,20]

Obstetricians must be aware at all times about pregnancy-induced changes in all bodily systems, to safeguard against mistaken diagnosis of pathology when none exists.

CONCLUSION

Obstetricians must be aware at all times about pregnancy induced changes in all bodily systems, to safeguard against mistaken diagnosis of pathology when none exists. Understanding maternal physiology is crucial in understanding the changes and clinical scenarios associated with pregnancy. This knowledge will help us distinguish the physiologic and pathologic processes during pregnancy. It is important to interpret the investigations in the context of the changed values. Pregnancy specific ranges should be used in making clinical decisions. Because there is a fall in plasma albumin, thus the drugs which are highly bound to albumin may be increased in free drug concentration. It is important to consider these effects while prescribing certain drugs.

REFERENCES

1. Silversides CK, Colman JM (Eds). Heart Disease in Pregnancy, 2nd edition. Massachusetts, USA: Blackwell Publishing; 2007.
2. Sadaniantz A, Kocheril AG, Emaus SP, Garber CE, Parisi AF. Cardiovascular changes in pregnancy evaluated by two-dimensional and Doppler echocardiography. J Am Soc Echocardiogr. 1992;5(3):253-8.
3. Chandraharan E, Arulkumaran S (Eds). Obstetric and Intrapartum Emergencies: A Practical Guide to Management. London, United Kingdom: Cambridge University Press; 2012.
4. Abduljabbar HS, Marzouki KM, Zawawi TH, Khan AS. Pericardial effusion in normal pregnant women. Acta Obstet Gynecol Scand. 1991;70(4-5):291-4.
5. Kannan M, Vijayanand G. Mitral stenosis and pregnancy: Current concepts in anaesthetic practice. Indian J Anaesth. 2010;54(5):439-44.
6. Liu LX, Arany Z. Maternal cardiac metabolism in pregnancy. Cardiovasc Res. 2014;101(4):545-53.
7. Miller RD (Ed). Miller's Anesthesia, 7th edition. Elsevier Health Sciences; 2007.
8. Bamber JH, Dresner M. Aortocaval compression in pregnancy: the effect of changing the degree and direction of lateral tilt on maternal cardiac output. Anesth Analg. 2003;97(1):256-8.
9. Jeffreys RM, Stepanchak W, Lopez B, Hardis J, Clapp JF. Uterine blood flow during supine rest and exercise after 28 weeks of gestation. BJOG. 2006;113(11):1239-47.
10. Cunningham FG, Leveno KJ, Bloom SL, Spong CY, Dashe JS, Hoffman BL, Casey BM, Sheffield JS editors. Williams Obstetrics. 24th ed. United States of America: The McGraw-Hill Education; 2014.
11. Burt CC, Durbridge J. Management of cardiac disease in pregnancy. Cont Edu Anaesth Crit Care Pain. 2009;9(2):44-7.
12. Ouzounian JG, Elkayam U. Physiologic changes during normal pregnancy and delivery. Cardiol Clin. 2012;30(3):317-29.
13. Ichipi-Ifukor PC, Jacobs J, Ichipi-Ifukor RN, Ewrhe OL. Changes in haematological indices in normal pregnancy. Physiol J. 2013;2013(283814):4-8.
14. Taylor DJ, Lind T. Haematological changes during normal pregnancy: iron induced macrocytosis. Br J Obstet Gynaecol. 1976;83(10):760-7.
15. Chandra S, Tripathi AK, Mishra S, Amzarul M, Vaish AK. Physiological changes in hematological parameters during pregnancy. Indian J hematol Blood Transfus. 2012;28(3):144-6.
16. Daftary SN, Chakravarti S, editors. Manual of Obstetrics: Updated Edition of the Classic Holland & Brews Manual of Obstetrics, 3rd edition. New Delhi, India: Reed Elsevier India Private Limited; 2011.
17. Bremme KA. Haemostatic changes in pregnancy. Best Pract Res Clin Haematol. 2003;16(2):153-68.
18. Iosif S, Ingemarsson I, Ulmsten U. Urodynamic studies in normal pregnancy and in puerperium. Am J Obstet Gynecol. 1980;137(6):696-700.
19. Wesnes SL, Hunskaar S, Bo K, Rortveit G. The effect of urinary incontinence status during pregnancy and delivery mode on incontinence postpartum. A cohort study. BJOG. 2009;116(5):700-7.

20. Padubidri V, Anand E (Eds). Textbook of Obstetrics, 1st edition. New Delhi, India: BI Publications (P) Ltd; 2006.
21. Prakash J. The kidney in pregnancy: A journey of three decades. Indian J Nephrol. 2012;22(3):159-67.
22. Ruiz-Extremera A, Lopez-Garrido MA, Barranco E, Quintero MD, Ocete-Hita E, Muñoz de Rueda P, et al. Activity of hepatic enzymes from week sixteen of pregnancy. Am J Obstet Gynecol. 2005;193(6):2010-6.
23. Guyton AC, Hall JE (Eds). Textbook of Medical Physiology, 12th edition. Haryana, India: Elsevier; 2011.
24. Mottola MF. Exercise prescription for overweight and obese woman: pregnancy and postpartum. Obstet Gynecol Clin North Am. 2009;36(2):301-16.
25. O'Reilly JR, Reynolds RM. The risk of maternal obesity to the long-term health of the offspring. Clin Endocrinol (Oxf). 2013;78(1):9-16.
26. Mottola MF, Campbell MK. Activity patterns during pregnancy. Can J Appl Physiol. 2003;28(4):642-53.
27. Artal R, O'Toole M. Guidelines of the American College of Obstetricians and Gynecologists for exercise during pregnancy and the postpartum period. Br J Sports Med. 2003;37(1):6-12.
28. Bajaj S, Rajput R, Jacb JJ (Eds). Endocrine Disorders during Pregnancy, 1st edition. New Delhi, India: Jaypee Brothers Medical Publishers (P) Ltd; 2013.
29. King JC. Physiology of pregnancy and nutrient metabolism. Am J Clin Nutr. 2000;71(5):1218S-25S.
30. Keenan PA, Yaldoo DT, Stress ME, Fuerst DR, Ginsburg KA. Explicit memory in pregnant women. Am J Obstet Gynecol. 1998;179(3 Pt 1):731-7.
31. Lee KA, Zaffke ME, McEnany G. Parity and sleep patterns during and after pregnancy. Obstet Gynecol. 2000;95(1):14-8.

CHAPTER 3

Fetal Skull and Maternal Pelvis

Yogita Dogra

INTRODUCTION

An understanding of the anatomy of fetal head and maternal pelvis is essential for obstetrical practice. There may be marked variations in anatomical structures in individual women. The maternal passages comprise the bony canal with soft structures which line it and close in its outlet. Since the head presents in such a preponderating proportion of cases, it must be studied in detail and in relation to parturient canal through which it has to pass. As the head is the largest part of fetus, it is more important to know whether greatest diameter of head passes through different planes of the pelvis.

FETAL SKULL

It is formed of vault, face, and base. The vault is composed of soft bones separated by sutures and fontanels. Figures 1 and 2 identify certain regions and landmarks in the fetal skull, which have particular importance for obstetric care because they may form the so-called presenting part of the fetus. The fetal skull is divided into:

- Vertex: a quadrangular area bounded anteriorly by bregma and coronal sutures, behind by the lambda and lambdoid sutures, and laterally by lines passing through parietal eminences
- Brow: an area bounded on one side by anterior fontanel and coronal sutures and on the other side by the root of the nose and supraorbital ridges of either side
- Face: an area bounded on one side by root of the nose and supraorbital ridges and on the other by the junction of the floor of the mouth with neck
- Sinciput is the area lying in front of the anterior fontanel and corresponds to the area of brow
- Occiput is the area between the base of the skull and the posterior fontanel.

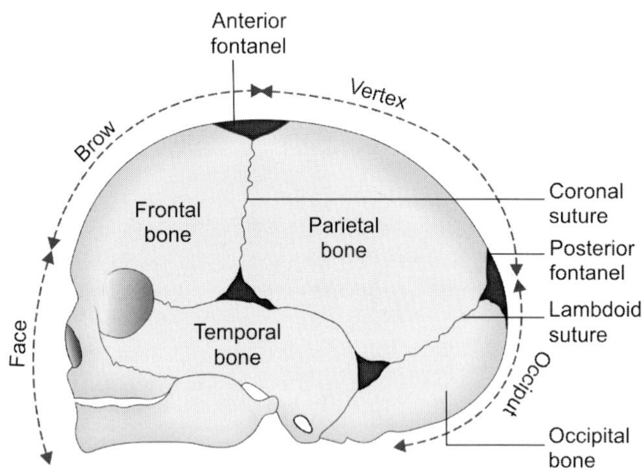

FIG. 1: Bones of the fetal skull—side view facing left.

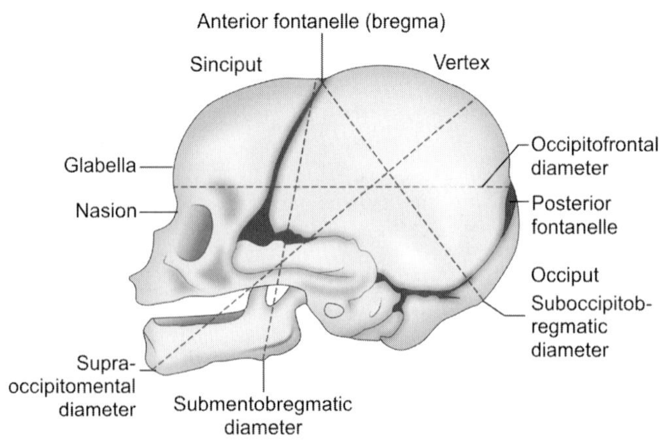

FIG. 2: Lateral view of the fetal skull showing prominent landmarks and anteroposterior diameters.

Sutures of Obstetrical Significance (Fig. 3)

Sutures of obstetrical significance include:
- Sagittal suture lies between two parietal bones
- Coronal sutures run between parietal and frontal bones on either side
- Frontal suture lies between two frontal bones
- Lambdoid sutures separate occipital bone and two parietal bones.

Clinical Importance

- Permits gliding movement of one bone over the other during molding of the head while head passes through the pelvis during labor
- Position of fontanel and sagittal suture can identify attitude and position of vertex
- In deep transverse arrest, the sagittal suture lies transversely at the level of the ischial spines
- Digital palpation of sagittal suture gives an idea of degree of internal rotation of head and degree of molding of head
- In hydrocephalus, suture separation results in finding of islands of bone in a sea of membranes.

Fontanels

A fontanel is a membrane-filled space created by the joining of two or more sutures. Out of six, only two are of obstetric significance (Fig. 3).

Anterior Fontanel (Bregma)

Diamond-shaped area of unossified membrane formed by junction of four sutures. The anteroposterior (AP) and transverse diameters measure 3 cm × 2 cm each.
- Anteriorly: frontal suture
- Posteriorly: sagittal suture
- Laterally, on both side: coronal suture.
  Anterior fontanel ossifies by 18 months after birth.

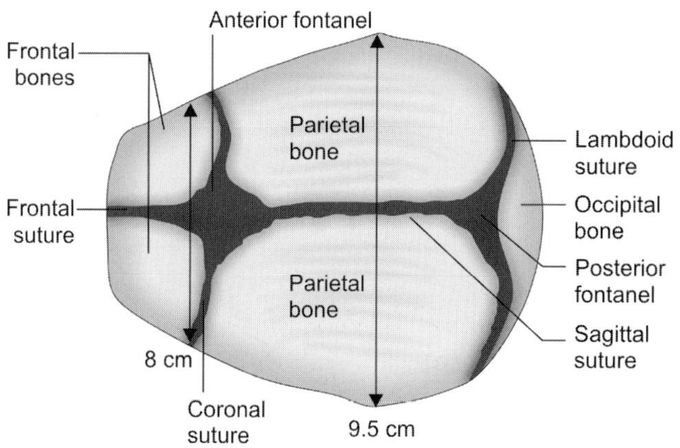

FIG. 3: Regions and landmarks in the fetal skull facing to the left. Notice the average diameters.

Clinical importance

- Degree of flexion can be assessed. On vaginal examination, if it is felt easily, it indicates head is deflexed as in occipitoposterior position
- It helps in molding of head
- Internal rotation of head can be assessed
- Intracranial pressure (ICP) can be roughly assessed after birth. Depression in dehydration and bulging in raised ICP
- Collection of blood and blood transfusion can be performed via superior longitudinal sinus
- Cerebrospinal fluid can be collected from its lateral angles.

Posterior Fontanel (Lambda)

It is Y-shaped triangular depressed area at the junction of three sutures. It measures about 1.2 cm × 1.2 cm.
- Anteriorly: sagittal suture
- Posteriorly: two lambdoid sutures at both sides.
  It ossifies at term.

Clinical importance

- From its relation to the maternal pelvis, position of vertex is determined
- Internal rotation can be assessed
- Degree of flexion can be assessed from its position. On vaginal examination, if it is felt easily and anterior fontanel is not felt, this indicates good flexion of the fetal head.

Diameters of Skull

The engaging diameter of fetal skull depends on the degree of flexion of the presenting part. The AP diameters which may be engaged are discussed below (Fig. 2).

Vertex Presentation

- Suboccipitobregmatic: it extends from the nape of the neck to the center of anterior fontanel, measures 9.5 cm:
  - Attitude: complete flexion
  - Clinical importance: the smallest diameter
- Suboccipitofrontal: it extends from the nape of the neck to root of nose, measures 10 cm:
  - Attitude: incomplete flexion
- Occipitofrontal: it extends from the occipital eminence to the root of the nose (glabella), measures 11.5 cm:
  - Attitude: marked deflexion
  - Clinical importance: this engaging diameter may give rise to prolonged labor.

Brow Presentation

- Mentovertical: it extends from the midpoint of the chin to the highest point on the sagittal suture, measures 14 cm:
  - Attitude: partial extension
  - Clinical importance: baby has to be delivered by cesarean section.

Face Presentation

- Submentovertical: it extends from the junction of the floor of the mouth and neck to the highest point on the sagittal suture, measures 11.5 cm:
  - Attitude: incomplete extension
  - Clinical importance: baby has to be delivered by cesarean section
- Submentobregmatic: it extends from the junction of the floor of mouth and neck to the center of bregma, measures 9.5 cm:
  - Attitude: complete extension
  - Clinical importance: baby has to be delivered by cesarean section

The transverse diameters are (Fig. 3):

- Biparietal diameter: it extends between two parietal eminences, measures 9.5 cm
- Clinical importance: irrespective of position of head, this diameter always engages
- Bitemporal diameter: distance between the anteroinferior ends of the coronal suture, measures 8 cm
- Bimastoid: between tips of mastoid processes, measures 7.5 cm
- Significance: incompressible diameter, it cannot be reduced even by destructive operations
- Supersubparietal: from point placed below one parietal eminence to a point placed above other parietal eminence of opposite side, measures 8.5 cm.

Circumferences of Skull

Circumferences of skull differ according to the attitude of the head (Table 1).

Molding

It is due to compression which the head undergoes during its passage through the resistant birth canal. There is diminution of those diameters most compressed and compensatory elongation of those least compressed. The types of molding and its site in various presentations are shown in figure 4. It is assessed during vaginal examination at two sites—parietal-parietal and parietal-occipital sites. During normal delivery, an alteration of 0.5–1 cm in skull diameter commonly occurs without brain damage. It disappears within few hours after birth. It is a protective mechanism and prevents fetal brain from compression as long as it is not excessive or too rapid.

The degree and direction of molding are determined by a number of factors:

- Size, shape, elasticity, and attitude of the fetal head
- Size and shape of the maternal pelvis
- Presentation and position of the head
- Strength of uterine contractions and duration of labor
- Rate of cervical dilatation and position of the cervix.

TABLE 1: Circumferences of skull

Attitude of the head	Plane of engagement	Circumference
Complete flexion	• Biparietal: suboccipitobregmatic • Shape: almost round	27.5 cm
Deflexed	• Biparietal: occipitofrontal • Shape: oval	34 cm
Incomplete extension	• Biparietal: mentovertical • Shape: bigger oval	37.5 cm
Complete extension	• Biparietal: submentobregmatic • Shape: almost round	27.5 cm

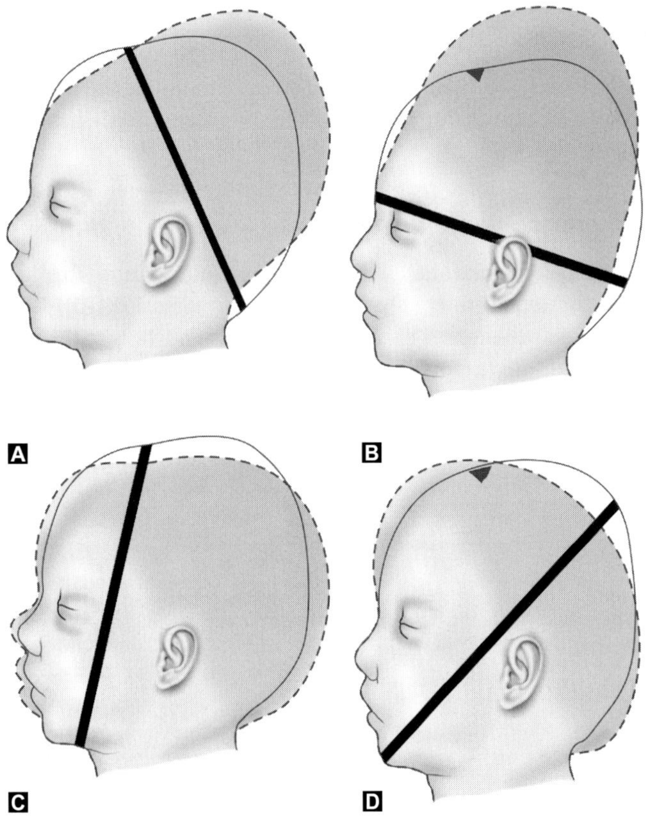

FIGS 4: Types of molding in cephalic presentation shown by dotted line. **A,** head well flexed; **B,** head deflexed (sugar loaf head); **C,** face presentation; and **D,** brow presentation.

Grades of Molding

- Grade 0: the suture lines are separate
- Grade 1: the suture lines meet
- Grade 2: if the sutures overlap but can be reduced with gentle digital pressure
- Grade 3: when the sutures overlap and are irreducible with digital pressure, it is usually pathological.

Molding occurs relatively easily in the soft head of the premature fetus, whereas the hard inelastic fetal head characteristic of prolonged pregnancy resists alteration in shape.

Clinical importance

- Slight molding is inevitable and beneficial. It enables the head to pass more easily through the birth canal
- Shape of the molding can be used to denote the position of the head occupied in the pelvis
- Extreme molding as in obstructed labor may produce intracranial disturbance in the form of tearing of tentorium cerebelli or subdural hemorrhage.

Caput Succedaneum (Fig. 5)

It is localized area of edema on fetal scalp in vertex presentation due to pressure effect of dilating cervical ring and vaginal introitus. It is usually formed after rupture of membranes and during the first stage of labor.

Characteristics

- It is physiological, present at birth, and disappears within 24–36 h
- It is soft, diffuse, and pits on pressure
- No underlying skull bone fracture
- Not limited by sutures (compared from cephalo-hematoma).

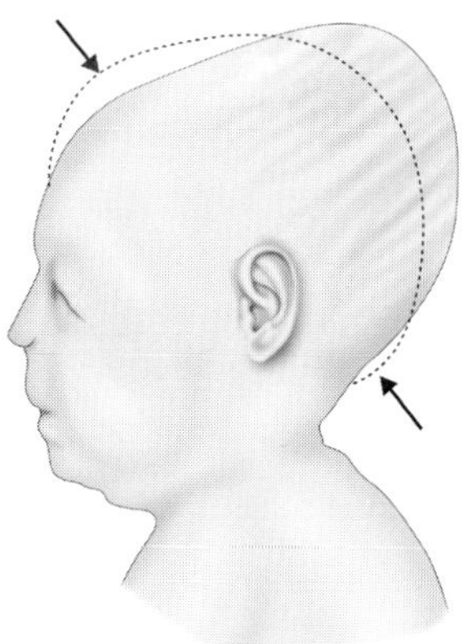

FIG. 5: Formation of caput succedaneum.

Obstetric Importance

- It signifies static position of the head for a long period of time
- Location of caput gives an idea about the position of head occupied in the pelvis and the degree of flexion achieved. In left position, the caput is placed on the right parietal bone and in right position, on left parietal bone
- With increasing flexion, the caput is placed more posteriorly
- In prolonged labor, a large caput suggests disproportion
- Secondary caput succedaneum is formed upon the part of scalp which presents at the vulva and is on the occipital bone near the posterior fontanel.

MATERNAL PELVIS

The bony pelvis is made up of two innominate bones (fusion of ilium, ischium, and pubis)—sacrum and coccyx. The innominate bones are joined to each other at symphysis pubis and to the sacrum by two sacroiliac joints (Fig. 6).

The pelvis is anatomically divided into a false pelvis and a true pelvis.

- False pelvis: it is also known as greater pelvis or pelvis major. Formed by iliac portions of innominate bones and limited above by iliac crests
  - Boundaries (Fig. 7):
    - Posteriorly: lumbar vertebrae
    - Laterally: iliac fossa
    - Anteriorly: anterior abdominal wall
  - Significance: support enlarged uterus during pregnancy.
- True pelvis: it is also known as lesser pelvis or pelvis minor
  - Anteriorly: shallow, formed by symphysis pubis (4 cm)
  - Posteriorly: deep, formed by sacrum and coccyx (11.5 cm).

  It is composed of inlet (brim), cavity, and outlet.

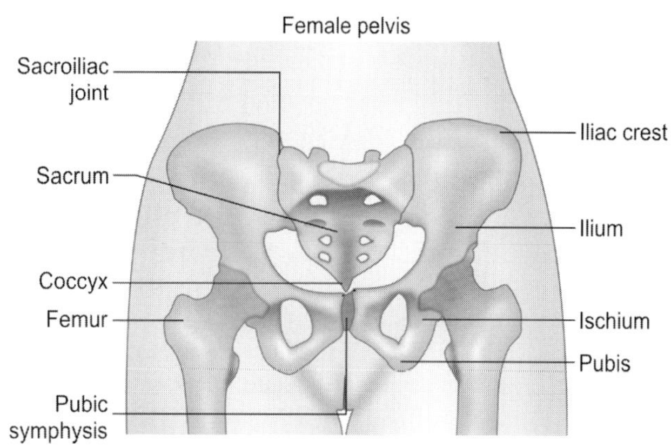

FIG. 6: Bones and joints forming the bony pelvis.

Pelvic Inlet

Pelvic inlet divides the pelvic cavity into false and true pelvis.

Boundaries: from posterior to anterior on each side (Fig. 8):
- Sacral promontory
- Ala of the sacrum
- Sacroiliac joints
- Iliopectineal lines
- Iliopubic eminencies
- Upper border of the superior pubic rami
- Pubic tubercles
- Pubic crests and upper border of symphysis pubis.

Plane: it is an imaginary flat surface, also called superior strait (Figs 9 and 10).

Inclination: in erect posture, pelvis is tilted forwards. The plane of inlet makes an angle of 55° with horizontal and is called angle of inclination (Fig. 9). Radiographically, it is measured as angle between plane of inlet and body of L5 (135°).
- High inclination: when angle of inclination is increased due to sacralization of L5
  - Significance:
    - Delay in engagement because uterine axis fails to coincide with that of inlet
    - Favors occipitoposterior position
    - Difficulty in descent of head because long birth canal and flat sacrum interferes with internal rotation
- Low inclination: the angle of inclination is lessened due to lumbarization of S1
  - Facilitates early engagement.

Sacral angle: it is the angle between true conjugate and first two pieces of sacrum. Normally, it is greater than 90°. If less, sugg ests funneling of pelvis.

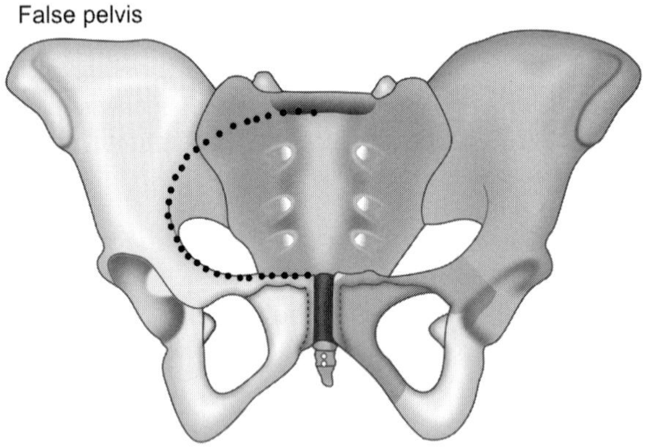

FIG. 7: Pelvic brim dividing the true and false pelvis.

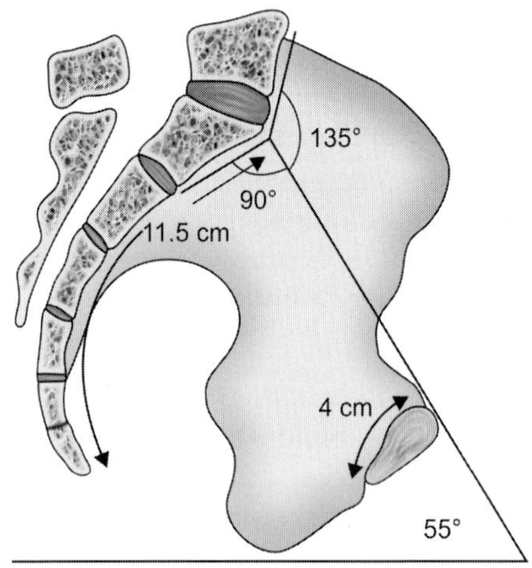

FIG. 9: The plane of inlet, inclination of pelvis and sacral angle.

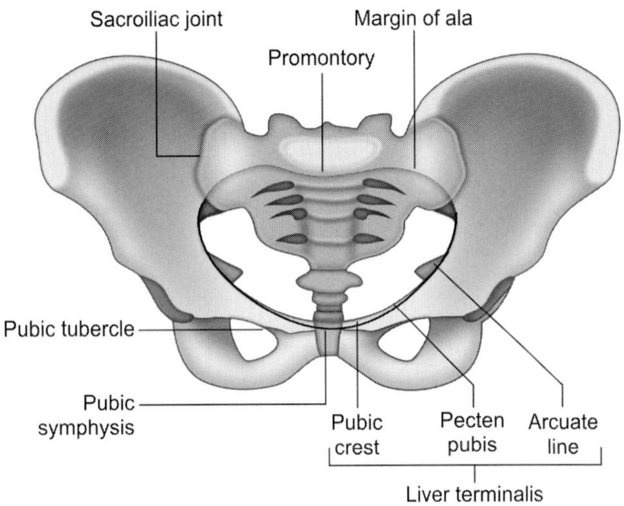

FIG. 8: Pelvic inlet with its boundaries.

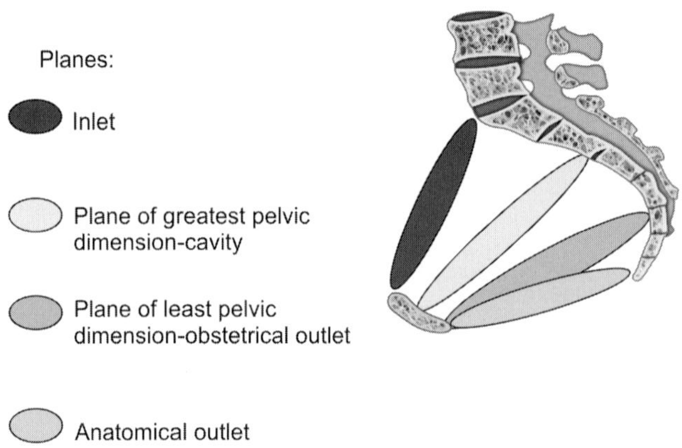

FIG. 10: Planes of pelvis.

Axis: it is a midperpendicular line drawn to plane of inlet.

Direction: downwards and backwards; it passes from the umbilicus to the tip of the coccyx.

Importance: uterine axis should coincide so that force of uterine contractions spread in right direction.

Diameters of Pelvic Inlet

Anteroposterior diameters (Figs 11 and 12)

- True conjugate (anatomical conjugate, conjugate vera): Distance between midpoint of sacral promontory to the inner margin of upper border of pubic symphysis is 11 cm. Its direct measurement can only be made by X-ray pelvimetry

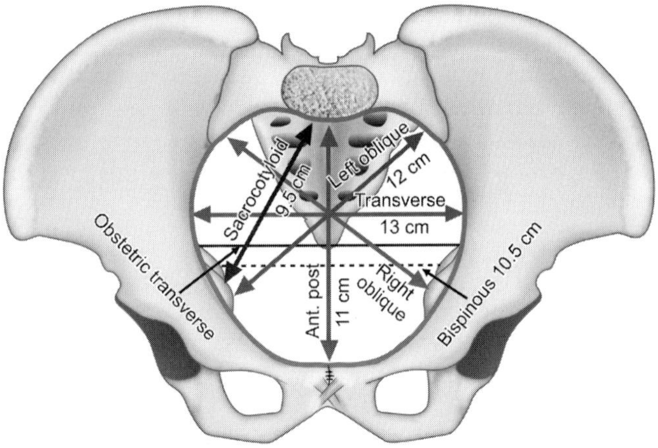

Ant. post, anteroposterior.

FIG. 11: Diameters of the pelvic inlet.

- Obstetric conjugate: distance between midpoint of sacral promontory to prominent bony projection in midline on inner surface of symphysis pubis is 10 cm. It cannot be measured clinically but is calculated by deducing 1.5 cm from diagonal conjugate
- Diagonal conjugate: distance between midpoint of sacral promontory to lower border of symphysis pubis using the tip of the second finger and the point where the index finger meets the pubis is 12 cm (Fig. 13).

Transverse diameter

Distance between the two farthest points on pelvic brim over iliopectineal lines is 13 cm. It lies 4 cm anterior to the promontory and 7 cm behind the symphysis. It is the largest diameter in the pelvis. The head enters the brim through the "available or obstetric transverse" diameter which bisects the AP diameter in the center.

Oblique diameter

Distance between one sacroiliac joint to opposite iliopubic eminence is 12 cm. These are right and left, named according to the sacroiliac joint from which they start.

Sacrocotyloid

Distance between midpoint of sacral promontory to iliopubic eminence is 9.5 cm. It is occupied by the biparietal diameter in a flat pelvis.

Posterior sagittal diameter

It extends from the point of intersection of obstetric conjugate and the transverse diameter to the middle of the sacral promontory (4 cm).

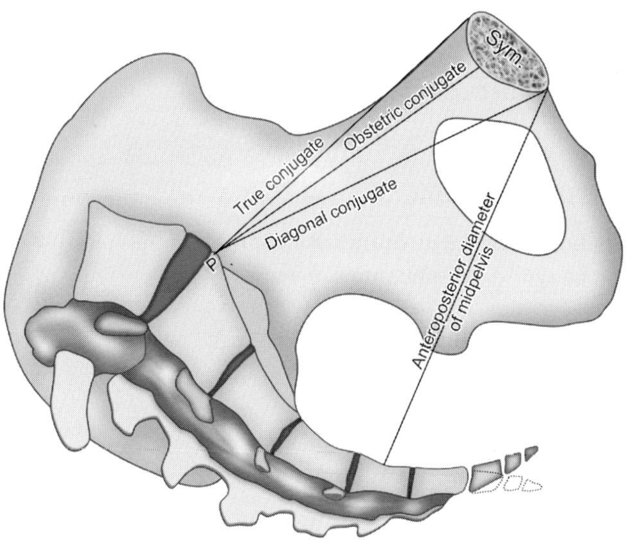

FIG. 12: Anteroposterior diameters of pelvic inlet and midpelvis.

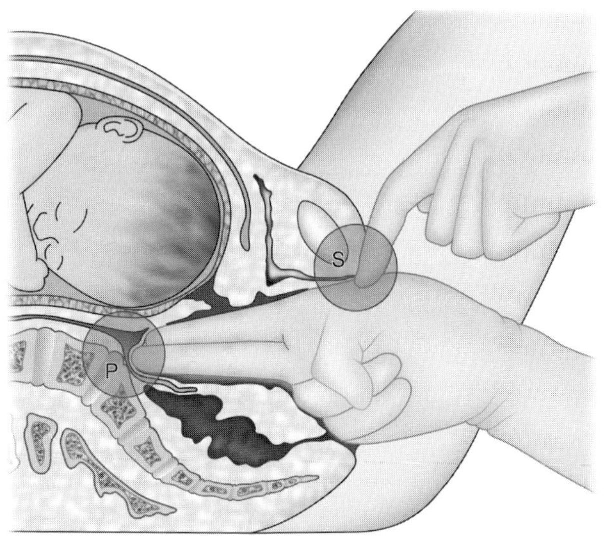

FIG. 13: Vaginal examination to determine the diagonal conjugate.

Pelvic Cavity

Pelvic cavity is the most roomy zone with almost round shape. It forms a curved canal with a shallow anterior wall measuring 4 cm, deep lateral wall 7.5 cm, and a deep posterior wall measuring 11.5 cm (Fig. 9). It is bounded above by inlet and below by plane of least pelvic dimension.

Plane of Greatest Pelvic Dimension (Fig. 10)

Plane of greatest pelvic dimension extends from midpoint of posterior surface of symphysis pubis to junction of second and third sacral vertebrae.

- Axis: downward direction
- Diameters:
  - Anteroposterior diameter: it measures from the midpoint on posterior surface of symphysis pubis to junction of S2 and S3 (12 cm)
  - Transverse diameter: no precise measurement, as points lie over soft tissues covering sacrosciatic notches and obturator foramen (12 cm).

Pelvic Outlet

Obstetric Outlet

It is anteroposteriorly oval (Fig. 14).

Boundaries

- Above: plane of least pelvic dimension
- Below: anatomical outlet
- Anteriorly: deficient at pubic arch
- Lateral walls: ischial bones
- Posterior wall: coccyx.

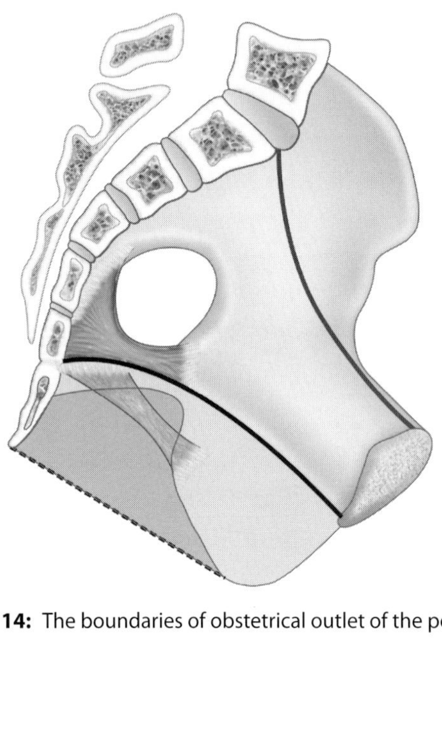

FIG. 14: The boundaries of obstetrical outlet of the pelvis.

Plane

Known as plane of least pelvic dimensions (Fig. 10), it extends from lower border of symphysis pubis to tip of ischial spines and posteriorly to meet the tip of S5. It is the narrowest plane in the pelvis.

At the level of ischial spines:

- The plane of obstetric outlet (plane of the least pelvic dimensions) is at this level
- The levator ani muscles are situated at this level and its ischiococcygeus part is attached to the ischial spines
- The obstetric axis of the pelvis changes its direction
- The head is considered engaged when the vault is felt vaginally at or below this level
- Internal rotation of the head occurs when the occiput is at this level
- Pudendal nerve block is carried out at this level
- The external os of the cervix is located normally
- The vaginal vault is located nearly
- The ring pessary should be applied above this level for treatment of prolapse.

Diameters

- Anteroposterior: it extends from inferior border of symphysis pubis to tip of sacrum (11 cm)
- Transverse diameter (bispinous): distance between tip of two ischial spines (10.5 cm)
- Posterior sagittal: distance between tip of sacrum and midpoint of bispinous diameter (5 cm).

Axis

Direction is almost vertical.

Anatomical Outlet (Bony Outlet)

Anatomical outlet (bony outlet) is diamond shaped.

Boundaries (Fig. 15)

- Anteriorly: lower border of symphysis pubis
- Laterally: ischiopubic rami, ischial tuberosity, sacrotuberous ligament
- Posteriorly: tip of coccyx.

Axis

Downwards and forwards.

Diameters (Fig. 15)

- Anteroposterior: extends from lower border of symphysis pubis to tip of coccyx (13 cm)

- Transverse diameter (intertuberous diameter): measures between inner borders of ischial tuberosities (11 cm)
- Posterior sagittal: AP distance between sacrococcygeal joint and midpoint of transverse diameter of outlet.

Subpubic angle

- Formed by approximation of two descending pubic rami
- 85° in normal female pelvis
- If angle is less, transverse diameter of outlet will also be less.

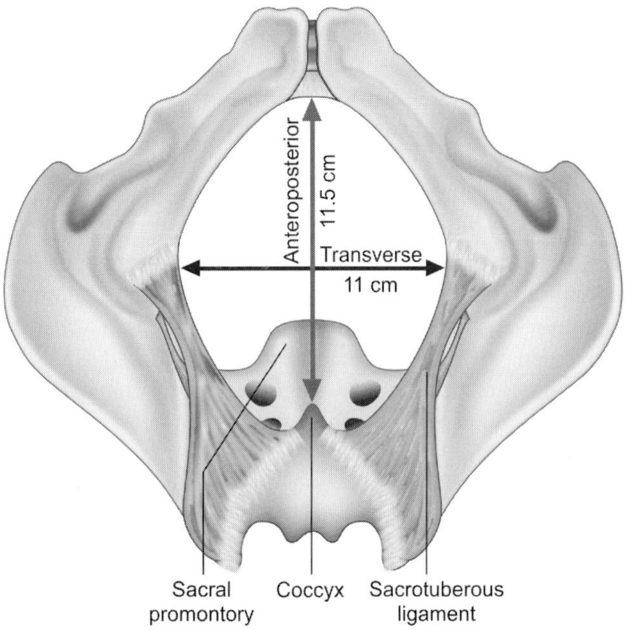

FIG. 15: The boundary of anatomical outlet with its diameters.

Pubic arch

It measures 6 cm in between pubic rami at level of 2 cm below the apex of subpubic arch. Clinically, it is assessed by placing three fingers side by side.

Midpelvis

Segment of the pelvis bounded above by the plane of greatest pelvic dimensions and below by a plane known as midpelvic plane.

Plane (Fig. 16)

Extends from lower margin of symphysis pubis through ischial spines to meet either junction of S4 and S5 or tip of sacrum.

Diameters

- Transverse or bispinous diameter (10.5 cm)
- Anteroposterior (Fig. 13): extends from lower border of symphysis pubis to the point on sacrum at which midpelvic plane meets (11.5 cm)
- Posterior sagittal: extends from midpoint of bispinous diameter to point on sacrum at which midpelvic plane meets (4.5 cm).

Pelvic Axis (Fig. 17)

Anatomical

Also called curve of Carus, it is formed by joining the axes of inlet, cavity, and outlet. It is C-shaped with the concavity directed forwards.

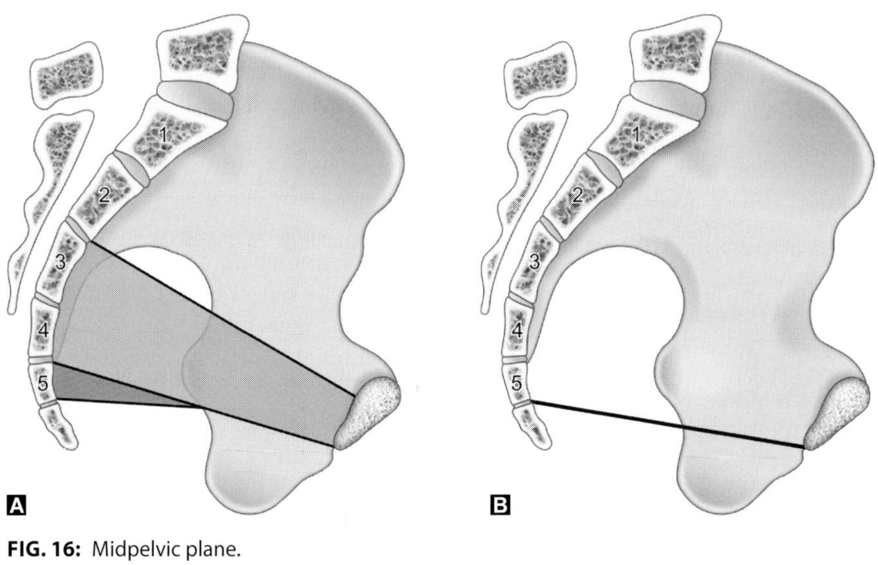

FIG. 16: Midpelvic plane.

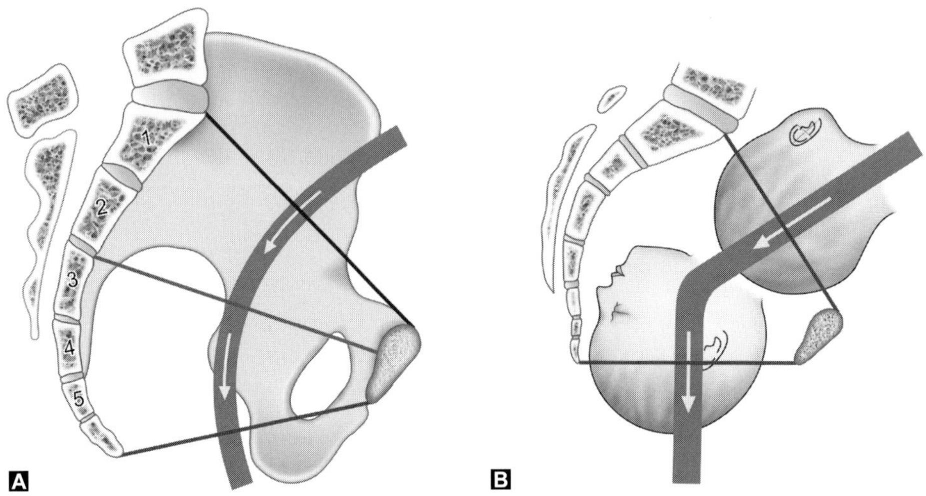

FIGS 17: Pelvic axix. **A,** Curve of Carus; **B,** the actual axis.

Obstetrical

It is through this axis that the fetus negotiates the pelvis.

Direction: downwards and backwards up to level of ischial spines and then abruptly forwards.

Waste Space of Morris

Normally, the subpubic angle is well rounded and if a round disk of diameter 9.5 cm (approximating fetal head) is placed under the subpubic arch, the distance between pubic symphysis and the edge of the disk should not be more than 1 cm. This measurement is the waste space of Morris.

Significance: when it is more than 1 cm, the available AP diameter of the outlet is reduced.

Pelvic Joints

- Symphysis pubis: secondary fibrocartilaginous joint; it has no capsule and no synovial cavity
- Sacroiliac articulation: synovial joint; it has got a capsule and a synovial cavity
- Sacrococcygeal joint: synovial hinge joint.

Physiological Changes in Pelvis in Pregnancy and Labor

During pregnancy, there is remarkable relaxation of pelvic joints. The relaxation of symphysis pubis commences in the first half of pregnancy and increases during the last 3 months.[1] There is increase in width of symphysis pubis, more in multiparas. The upward gliding movement of sacroiliac joint also contributes to the mobility of pelvis at term. AP diameter of the outlet may increase by 1.5–2 cm in lithotomy position. Increase in AP diameter of the inlet during labor is facilitated by rotatory movements of the sacroiliac joints. These changes have been attributed to the success of modified squatting position to hasten second stage of labor.[2] The squatting position may increase the interspinous diameter and pelvic outlet diameters.[3,4]

Muscular Support

The pelvic diaphragm provides considerable support to the pelvic viscera. It is comprised of levator ani (consists of pubococcygeus, puborectalis, and iliococcygeus muscles) and the coccygeus muscle. Vaginal delivery itself is a significant risk factor for damage to the levator ani muscle or to its innervation.[5,6] The pubococcygeus, preferably termed pubovisceral muscle is more commonly damaged.[7,8] Sufficient evidence exists to support that these injuries may predispose to greater risk of pelvic organ prolapse or urinary incontinence.[9-11]

CONCLUSION

During labor, fetus assumes positions and attitudes that are determined in part by the configuration of mother's pelvis. The outcome of labor depends more on the actual pelvic diameters than the shape and type of pelvis. The size, presentation and position of fetus are also important factors in the conduct of labor. Several pelvic diameters can be assessed clinically including diagonal conjugate, prominence of ischial spines, convergence of pelvic side walls, angle of subpubic arch, and sacral curvature. Thus, clinical estimation of adequacy of pelvis can alert the clinician to the possible risk of pelvic dystocia.

REFERENCES

1. Borell U, Fernstrom I. The movements at the sacro-iliac joints and their importance to changes in pelvic dimensions during parturition. Acta Obstet Gynecol Scand. 1957;36(1):42-57.
2. Gardosi J, Hutson N, B-Lynch C. Randomised controlled trial of squatting in the second stage of labour. Lancet. 1989;2(8654):74-7.
3. Russell JG. Moulding of the pelvic outlet. J Obstet Gynaecol Br Commonw. 1969;76(9):817-20.
4. Russell JG. The rationale of primitive delivery positions. Br J Obstet Gynaecol. 1982;89(9):712-5.
5. DeLancey JO, Kearney R, Chou Q, Speights S, Binno S. The appearance of levator ani muscle abnormalities in magnetic resonance images after vaginal delivery. Obstet Gynecol. 2003;101(1):46-53.
6. Weidner AC, Jamison MG, Branham V, South MM, Borawski KM, Romero AA. Neuropathic injury to the levator ani occurs in 1 in 4 primiparous women. Am J Obstet Gynecol. 2006;195(6):1851-6.
7. Lien KC, Mooney B, DeLancey JO, Ashton-Miller JA. Levator ani muscle stretch induced by simulated vaginal birth. Obstet Gynecol. 2004;103(1):31-40.
8. Margulies RU, Huebner M, DeLancey JO. Origin and insertion points involved in levator ani muscle defects. Am J Obstet Gynecol. 2007;196(3):251.el-5.
9. DeLancey JO, Miller JM, Kearney R, Howard D, Reddy P, Umek W, et al. Vaginal birth and de novo stress incontinence: relative contributions of urethral dysfunction and mobility. Obstet Gynecol. 2007;110(2 Pt 1):354-62.
10. DeLancey JO, Morgan DM, Fenner DE, Kearney R, Guire K, Miller JM, et al. Comparison of levator ani muscle defects and function in women with and without pelvic organ prolapsed. Obstet Gynecol. 2007;109(2 Pt 1):295-302.
11. Rortveit G, Daltveit AK, Hannestad YS, Hunskaar S. Vaginal delivery parameters and urinary incontinence: the Norwegian EPINCONT study. Am J Obstet Gynecol. 2003;189(5):1268-74.

CHAPTER 4

Fetus In Utero

Kiran Pandey

INTRODUCTION

In humans, the unborn young from the end of the 8th week after conception to the moment of birth is defined as fetus. Fetal lie, presentation, position, and attitude can be ascertained beyond 28 weeks of pregnancy. However, they are of significance in patients near term or in labor. Assessment of fetus *in utero* helps to decide the mode of termination of pregnancy and foretells the difficulties that may arise during labor. For better understanding of fetus *in utero*, we will discuss it under various subheads in following chapter.

FETAL LIE

Fetal lie is (Figs 1A to C) relationship of the longitudinal axis of the fetus to that of the mother:[1]

- If the two are parallel, then the fetus is said to be in a longitudinal lie (present in over 99% of labor at term)
- If the two are at 90° angles to each other, the fetus is said to be in a transverse lie
- If the fetal and the maternal axes may cross at a 45° angle, forming an oblique lie, which is unstable and always becomes longitudinal or transverse during the course of labor.

Predisposing factors for transverse or oblique lie include multipara, placenta previa, hydramnios, and uterine anomalies.

FETAL PRESENTATION

The portion of the fetal body that is either foremost within the birth canal or in closest proximity to it:[1]

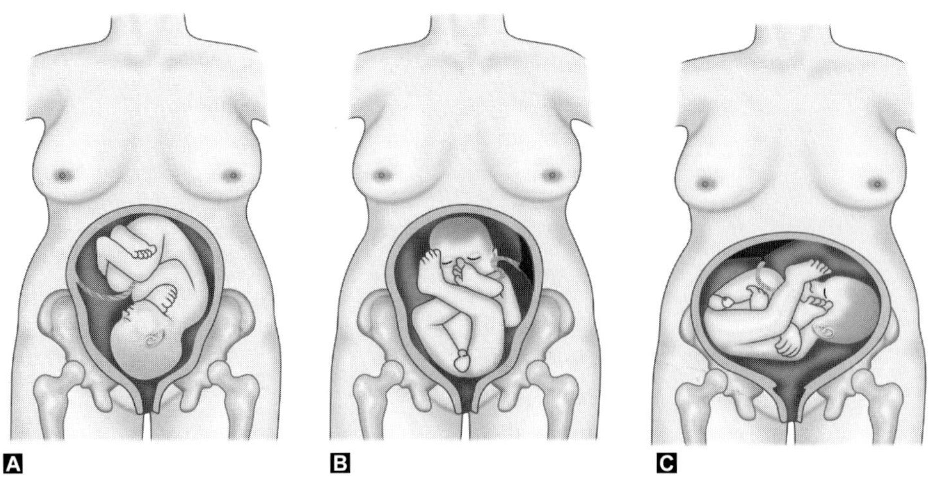

FIGS 1: Lie of the fetus *in utero*: **A,** Longitudinal lie vertex presentation; **B,** longitudinal lie breech presentation, and **C,** transverse lie shoulder presentation.

- In longitudinal lies, the presenting part is either cephalic (96.5%) or podalic (3%) presentations, respectively[2]
- In transverse lie, the shoulder (0.5%) is the presenting part.[2]

Types of Cephalic Presentation

Cephalic presentation is considered normal and occurs in about 96.5% of deliveries. It is due to many factors such as gravitation (head being heavier than breech) and adaptation (smaller circumference of head 27.5 cm as compared to breech 32.5 cm).[2] There are different types of cephalic presentations (Figs 2A to H), which depend on the fetal attitude such as occiput, sinciput, brow, or face depending on the degree of extension.

Types of Breech Presentation

Breech presentation is considered abnormal and occurs about 3% at term. In breech presentation, lie is longitudinal and podalic pole presents at pelvic brim. It is the most common malpresentation. Causes of breech presentation are enumerated in table 1.

Factors responsible for breech presentation are as follows:

- A complete breech presentation (Figs 3A to C) occurs when fetus is in flexed attitude, i.e., both the hips and knees are flexed. It is common in multipara. Presenting part is buttocks, external genitalia, and both feet
- An incomplete breech (Figs 3A to C) can be frank breech (i.e., when the hips are flexed so the legs are straight), footling, or knee. It is common in primipara.

Shoulder Presentation

The shoulder, arm, or trunk may present first if the fetus is in a transverse lie. This type of presentation occurs in 0.5% cases. Transverse lie is more common with premature delivery or multiple pregnancies, twins, polyhydramnios, placenta previa, and contracted pelvis.

Compound Presentation

Compound presentation means prolapse of fetal extremity alongside the presenting part, e.g.,:

- Prolapse of the hand in cephalic presentation (most common)[3]
- Prolapse of lower extremity in cephalic presentation (relatively rare).

Cord Presentation

Cord is present below the presenting part and can be felt per-vaginally lying in the intact bag of membranes. It has to be differentiated from:

- Occult prolapse where cord is present by the side of presenting part and cannot be felt per-vaginally
- Cord prolapse where cord prolapses into the vagina or outside vulva following rupture of membranes.

PRESENTING PART

It is the part which lies over the internal os.

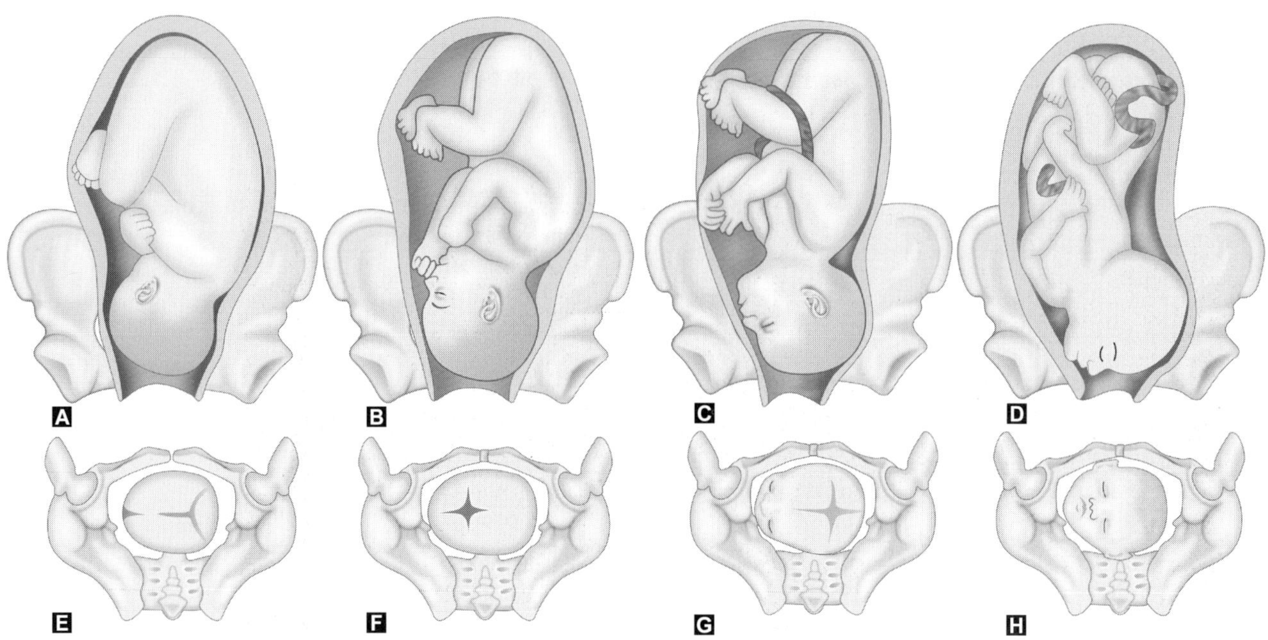

FIGS 2: Types of cephalic presentations: **A,** Vertex presentation; **B,** military presentation; **C,** brow presentation; **D,** face presentation; **E,** complete flexion; **F,** moderate flexion; **G,** poor flexion (extension), and **H,** full extension.

- Cephalic: vertex, brow, or face
- Breech: fetal legs flexed (complete breech), fetal legs extended (frank breech), or foot (footling presentation).

FETAL ATTITUDE

The fetal attitude describes the relationship of the fetus' body parts to one another. The normal fetal attitude is commonly referred to as the fetal position. The head is tucked down to the chest, with arms and legs drawn in towards the center of the chest. Abnormal fetal attitudes may include a head that is extended back or other body parts extended or positioned behind the back. Abnormal fetal attitudes can increase the diameter of the presenting part as it passes through the pelvis, increasing the difficulty of birth. The universal attitude is of flexion.

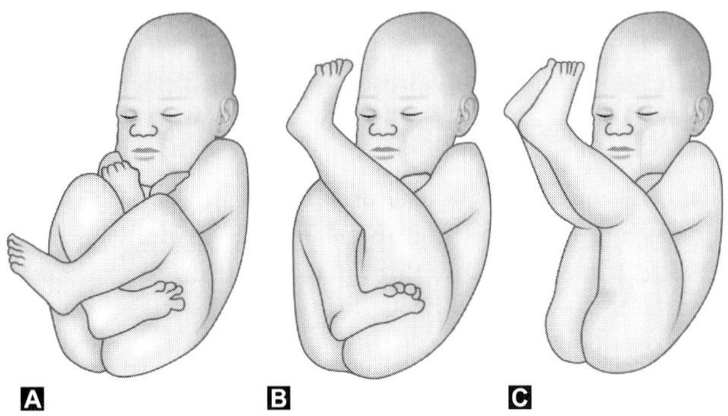

FIGS 3: Types of breech presentation: **A**, Complete breech; **B**, incomplete breech, and **C**, frank breech.

TABLE 1: Factors responsible for breech presentation

Maternal	Fetoplacental
Contracted pelvis	Prematurity
Congenital malformation of uterus	Hydrocephalous
Polyhydramnios	Placenta previa
Oligohydramnios	Twins
Multipara with lax abdominal wall	Anencephaly

DENOMINATOR

It is an arbitrary fixed bony point at the presenting part which comes in relation with the various quadrants of the maternal pelvis. Table 2 shows denominator in relation to various presentations.

POSITIONS

It is the relation of the denominator to the different quadrants of the maternal pelvis. The pelvis is divided in the equal segments of 45°, i.e., it is divided into eight parts (Fig. 4).

In vertex, there are eight positions which are as follows:[2] (1) direct occipitoanterior (2%), (2) direct occipitoposterior (1%), (3) left occipitoanterior (13%), (4) right occipitoanterior (10%), (5) left occipitotransverse (40%), (6) right occipitotransverse (24%), (7) left occipitoposterior (3%) and (8) right occipitoposterior (7%).

In face presentation, there are six positions (Figs 5A to C) which are as follows: mentoanterior: (1) right, (2) left, and (3) direct; and mentoposterior: (4) right, (5) left, and (6) direct.

In breech presentation, sacrum of the fetus is used as the identifying landmark, instead of the occiput. Various positions are as follows:

- Direct sacrum anterior (DSA) means the fetal sacrum is closest to the mother's symphysis
- Left sacrum anterior means the fetal sacrum is closest to the mother's symphysis and rotated slightly to the mother's left (clockwise from DSA). It is the most common
- Right sacrum anterior means the fetal sacrum is closest to the mother's symphysis and rotated slightly to the mother's right (counterclockwise from DSA)
- Right sacrum transverse
- Left sacrum transverse
- Direct sacrum posterior
- Right sacrum posterior
- Left sacrum posterior.

In transverse presentation, position may be:

- Dorsoanterior (most common)
- Dorsoposterior
- Dorsosuperior
- Dorsoinferior.

TABLE 2: Fetal lie, presentation, attitude, and denominator

Lie	Presentation	Attitude	Denominator
Longitudinal	• Vertex • Occipitoanterior • Occipitoposterior	• Flexion • Deflexion	• Occiput • Occiput
Longitudinal	• Brow	• Partial extension	• Frontal eminence
Longitudinal	• Face	• Extension	• Mentum
Longitudinal	• Breech		• Sacrum
Transverse	• Shoulder		• Acromion/scapula

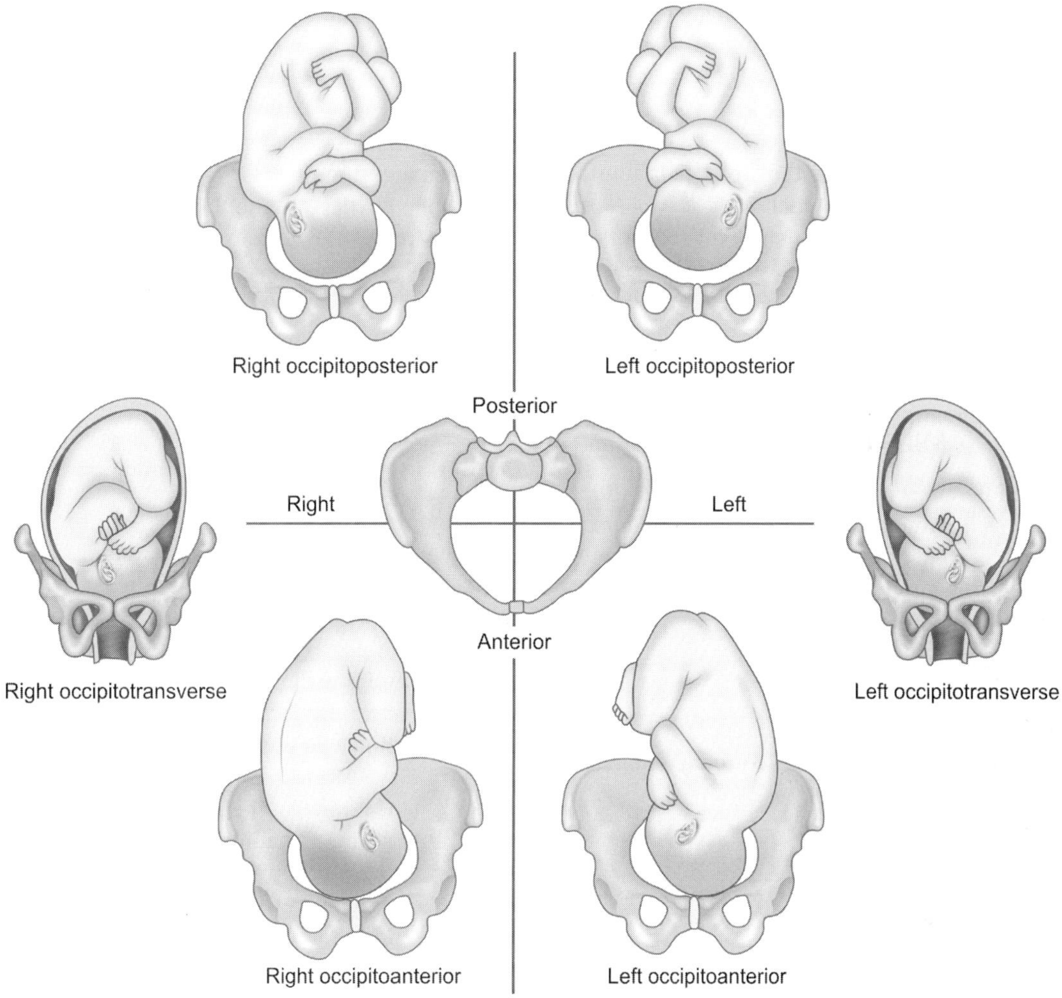

FIG. 4: Various positions of vertex. Lie: longitudinal or vertex; presentation: vertex; reference point: occiput; attitude: complete flexion.

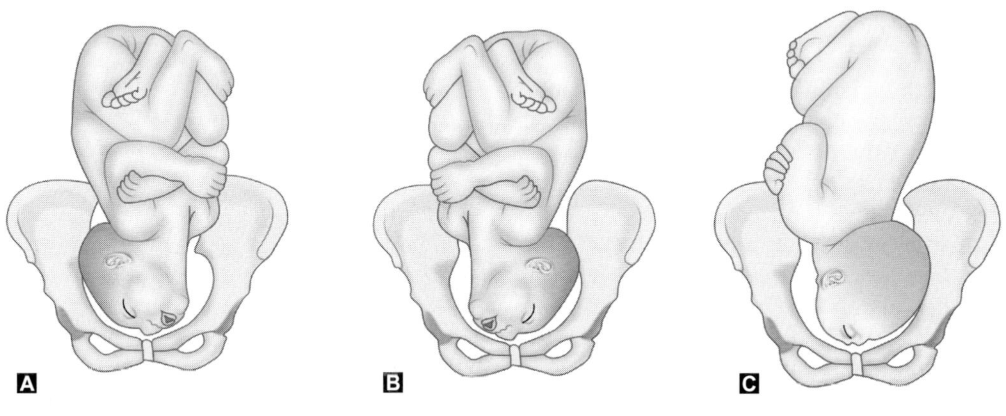

FIGS 5: Various positions of face: **A,** Left mentoanterior; **B,** right mentoanterior; **C,** right mentoposterior.

According to the position of the head, the fetal position is termed right or left.

CEPHALIC PROMINENCE

It is the most prominent part of the head palpable per abdomen. In vertex presentation, when head is well flexed, cephalic prominence is sinciput which is on the opposite side of back; when head is extended, occiput is the cephalic prominence. When head is neither flexed nor extended, no cephalic prominence is felt. This is known as military position.[4]

OBSTETRIC EXAMINATION

To ascertain fetal lie, presentation, attitude, and position, a systematic approach is required. These include abdominal examination and internal examination. In some cases where doubt exists, ultrasonography may be required.

Abdominal Examination

Prerequisites

- Patient's consent should be taken. Proper counseling regarding the procedure to be done
- Bladder should be empty
- Adequate exposure of abdomen should be done
- Patient should be in dorsal position with thigh slightly flexed and abducted
- Examiner should stand on right side of patient
- A female attendant is preferable in case of male examiner
- If the patient is apprehensive, constant reassurance to relieve the anxiety of patients is required.

Inspection

- The uterus is normally visible per abdomen at 12–14 weeks of gestation
- Note the shape of abdomen. The abdomen may be flabby in obese patients or pendulous in multipara. It should be assessed whether the abdomen is longitudinally or transversely distended. Rarely, eversion of uterus may be seen in divarication of recti
- Full bladder may be visible in late pregnancy
- Umbilicus may be normal, inverted, or everted
- Contour of the abdomen: contour of abdomen can be ovoid, cylindrical, or spherical. In cases of occipitoposterior position, abdomen looks flat below the umbilicus
- See for fullness of flanks. it indicates term pregnancy. Fullness of flanks can also be seen in patients with abnormal presentation as in transverse or oblique lie
- Size of the uterus: assess for undue enlargement of uterus which may be seen in multiple pregnancy, polyhydramnios, etc. It also helps to assess bulk of fetus
- Fetal movement: they can be seen after 24 weeks
- Skin changes: look for striae gravidarum, striae albicans, linea nigra, and scars
- Inspection of scars should include:
    - Site of scar, e.g., transverse (Pfannenstiel), longitudinal (paramedian or central), or any other scar of previous surgery
    - Integrity of abdominal scar, i.e., whether healed by primary or secondary intention
    - Any herniation if present.

Palpation

- Fundal height: fundal height (Fig. 6) is palpated with ulnar border of left hand without applying pressure from xiphisternum towards the umbilicus
- Put a mark on uppermost level:
    - Centralize the uterus if deviated
    - Determine the uppermost level of fundus
        - Symphysis pubis: 12 weeks
        - Between symphysis pubis and umbilicus: 16 weeks
        - Umbilicus: 24 weeks
        - At the junction of lower one-third and upper two-third of distance umbilicus and ensiform cartilage: 28 weeks
        - Midpoint between the umbilicus and ensiform cartilage: 30 weeks
        - At the junction of lower two-third and upper one-third of distance umbilicus and ensiform cartilage: 32 weeks

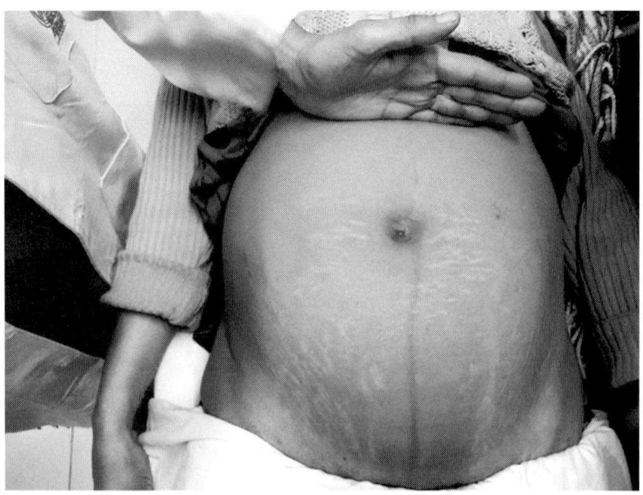

FIG. 6: Fundal height.

  - Midpoint between 32 weeks and 36 weeks: 34 weeks if head is free or 40 weeks if head is engaged (uterus becomes more spherical)
  - Xiphisternum: 36 weeks
- Variations in fundal height measurements are enlisted in table 3
- Assess whether uterus is contracted or relaxed. Uterus may be hard, tender, and tense in concealed hemorrhage
- In cases of post-term pregnancy, height of uterus may be less than period of gestation and hardness of skull bones may be felt and uterus may be full of fetus.

OBSTETRICAL GRIPS/LEOPOLD'S MANEUVERS

- Palpation should be done gently and systematically using flat of the fingers
- It should be done when uterus is relaxed and not during Braxton-hicks contractions or uterine contractions during labor.

First Maneuver: Fundal Palpation

- Palpation should be done facing the patient's head
- Using both hands, palpate the fundal area to determine the pole of the fetus in this part (Fig. 7)
- Breech: broad, hard irregular mass
- Head: smooth, hard globular mass. Head is ballottable in complete breech. It is nonballottable in frank breech due to splinting action of legs
- In case of transverse fundal area is empty, i.e., none of the fetal poles can be identified.

Second Maneuver: Lateral Palpation (Fig. 8)

- Palpation should be done facing patient's face
- Palpation is done along the anterolateral aspects of uterus placing flat of the hands on either side of umbilicus. Both the sides are palpated. Palpate the patient's right side with your left hand and the patient's left side with your right hand. One hand to be fixed while palpation is being done with other hand.
- Feel for the number of fetuses

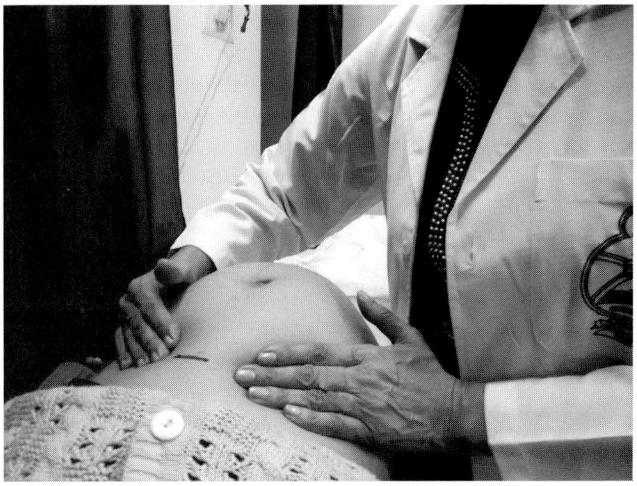

FIG. 7: First maneuver: fundal palpation.

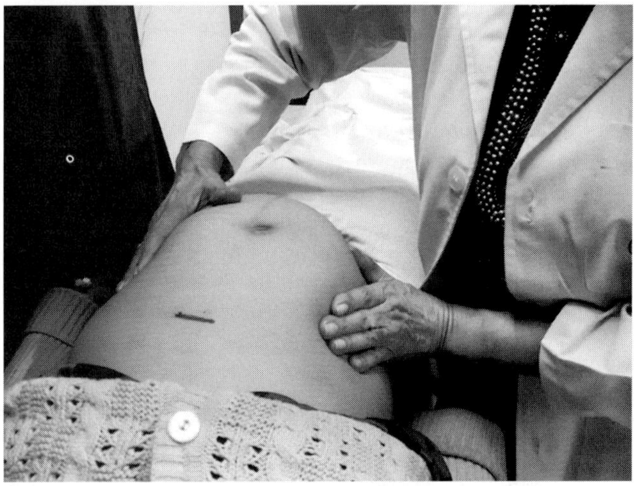

FIG. 8: Second maneuver: lateral palpation.

TABLE 3: Variations in fundal height measurements

More than estimated gestational age	Less than estimated gestational age
• Multiple pregnancy • Error in estimated date of conception • Fetus is healthy but physically large • Gestational diabetes causing a larger baby • Polyhydramnios • Large for gestational age • Hydatidiform mole/hydrops fetalis • Pelvic tumors: ovarian, fibroid • Concealed accidental hemorrhage • Full bladder • If the presenting part is very high	• Fetus descent into the pelvis, seen normally 2–4 weeks before delivery • Error in estimated date of pregnancy based on first day of last menstrual period • Fetus is healthy but physically small • Oligohydramnios • Transverse or oblique lie • Small for gestational age • Intrauterine death • Uterus not centralized

- Feel for the spine and back of the fetus to determine the fetal lie. Smooth, curved, and resistant feel is suggestive of back. Back can be made more prominent by gently pressing the fundus down towards the maternal pelvis
- The limbs site is relatively empty and small knob-like irregular parts may be felt. In occipitoposterior position limbs may be felt on both sides of midline. Limbs may be difficult to palpate in obese or apprehensive patients or if limbs are towards maternal spine
- In cases of transverse lie one can appreciate smooth, hard, and globular mass (head) on one side (lumbar area) and broad, soft, and irregular mass (breech) on other side
- In cases of oblique lie one can appreciate head/breech in the hypochondrium or iliac area on one side and vice-a-versa on the other side
- Anterior shoulder may be felt as a marked prominence above the head. It is near midline in anterior fetal position or away from in posterior position.

Third Maneuver/Second Pelvic Grip/Pawlik's Grip: Presentation Palpation (Fig. 9)

- It is done facing the patient
- Outstretched thumb and four fingers of the right hand are placed over the lower pole of uterus keeping the ulnar border just above symphysis pubis
- Differentiation between head and breech is made similarly as stated earlier
- Pole may be empty in transverse lie
- Maneuver may be difficult to conduct if presenting part is deeply engaged.

Fourth Maneuver/First Pelvic Grip: Presentation Palpation (Fig. 10)

- It should be done facing the patient's feet
- It should be done using four fingers of both the hands and placing them in the lower portion of maternal abdomen on either side of mid-line parallel to inguinal ligament
- Pressure is exerted in the direction of pelvic inlet, i.e., downwards and backwards in manner to approximate the finger tips
- The characteristics to note are presentation, attitude, and engagement
- Differentiate between head and breech as already stated
- Head maturity and size is assessed. This also helps in assessing fetal gestational age to some extent. It may also help to diagnose intrauterine growth restriction
- Attitude of head is seen by the position of sinciput (prominent and pointed) and occiput (smooth and curved)
- In a well flexed attitude sinciput lies above the level of occiput
- The location of cephalic prominence helps to determine attitude, i.e., if back and cephalic prominences are on same side attitude is of extension and if these are on opposite sides attitude is of flexion
- Engagement is determined convergence and divergence of finger tips. When head is engaged only sinciput can be felt abdominally. When head is deeply engaged no poles can be felt abdominally
- In primipara head is usually engaged by 38 completed weeks. However, engagement may also occur during early labor. Head may not be engaged due tocertain conditions (Box 1).

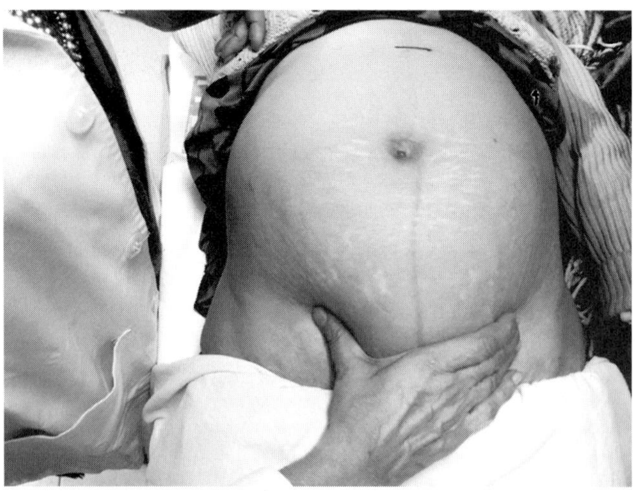

FIG. 9: Third maneuver/second pelvic grip/Pawlik's grip: presentation palpation.

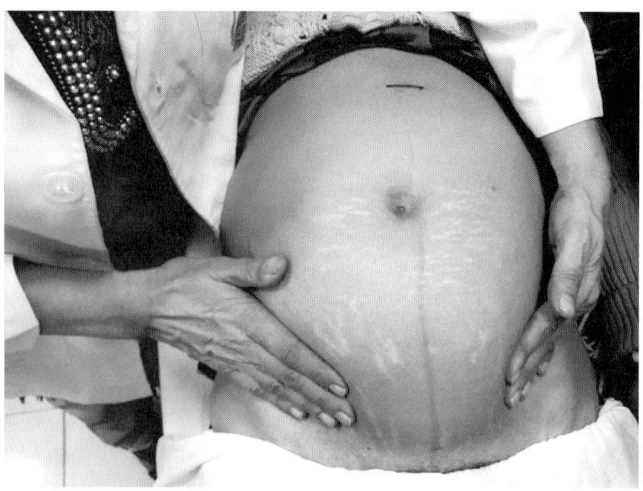

FIG. 10: Fourth maneuver/first pelvic grip: presentation palpation.

Box 1: Causes of nonengagement of head

- Wrong dates
- Deflexed head (occipitoposterior position)
- Contracted pelvis/cephalopelvic disproportion
- Multiple pregnancy
- High inclination of pelvis
- Polyhydramnios
- Placenta previa

Detection of Cephalopelvic Disproportion

Pinard's Test

The patient after evacuating bladder and rectum is placed in a semi-sitting position so that the fetal axis is perpendicular to pelvic brim. With left hand head is pushed downwards and backwards into the pelvis while the fingers of the right hand are put on the symphysis to detect disproportion.[5]

Inference

- No disproportion: head can easily be pushed into maternal pelvis
- Minor disproportion: anterior surface of head is in line with posterior surface of symphysis pubis
- Moderate disproportion: head is in line with anterior surface of symphysis pubis and does not enter maternal pelvis
- Marked disproportion: head overrides symphysis pubis. Vaginal delivery cannot occur.

Muller-Munro-Kerr Method

Patient after evacuating bladder and rectum is placed in dorsal position. The examiner pushes head of fetus into the maternal pelvis with left hand while two fingers of left hand are placed at the level of ischial spine and its thumb over symphysis pubis to detect disproportion.[5]

Inference

- No disproportion: head can easily be pushed up to ischial spine with no overlapping of parietal bones
- Moderate disproportion: head can be pushed but not up to ischial spine. However, parietal bones may be slightly overlapped
- Marked disproportion: head cannot be pushed and overhangs symphysis pubis.

Muller-Hillis Maneuver

Examiner grasps fetal brow and subocciput abdominally and presses fetal head downwards into the maternal pelvis. Head will easily enter pelvis in absence of cephalopelvic disproportion.[5]

FIFTH FORMULA (TABLE 4)

Descent of the head is measured by abdominal palpation and expressed in terms of fifths above the pelvic brim. It is more reliable when large caput formation occurs.[6]

Liquor Assessment

Feel and estimate the amount of liquor. This step requires experience. However, if there is an excessive amount of liquor as in polyhydramnios (Box 2), the uterus will be tense and it will be quite difficult for you to feel for fetal parts. Uterus may be full of fetus in cases of oligohydramnios (Box 3).

Assessment of Scar Tenderness (Figure 11)

Patient with previous lower segment cesarean section (LSCS), not in labor:

- Patient placed in dorsal position
- Patient should be relaxed while patient attention being diverted by indulging patient in conversation
- Scar is present behind the symphysis pubis so to elicit scar tenderness fingers of right hand are insinuated behind pubic symphysis
- The lower pole of uterus is palpated
- Wincing of patient indicates scar tenderness.

Patient with previous LSCS, in labor:

- Scar is palpated in the lower pole of uterus just above the pubic symphysis
- Palpation is done in between the contractions
- Rest of procedure is similar as above.

TABLE 4: Formula of fives

5/5	4/5	3/5	2/5	1/5	0/5
Completely Above	S: High O: Easily felt	S: Easily felt O: Felt	S: Felt O: Just felt	S: Felt O: Not felt	S: Not felt O: Not felt
Head floating	On the brim	Not engaged	Just engaged	Engaged	Deeply engaged
Station ≤5	Station –4	Station –3, –2	Station –1	Station 0	Station ≥+1

Box 2: Causes of polyhydraminos[7]

- Idiopathic (50%)
- Fetal causes:
  - Fetal anomalies, including:
    - Anencephaly
    - Hydrocephaly
    - Tracheoesophageal fistula
    - Esophageal atresia
    - Gastroschisis
    - Duodenal atresia
    - Spina bifida
    - Cleft lip and palate
    - Cystic adenomatoid lung malformation
    - Diaphragmatic hernia
    - Skeletal dysplasias
    - Beckwith-Wiedemann syndrome
    - Multiple congenital anomalies and aneuploidy
    - Twin pregnancy
- Maternal causes:
  - Diabetes mellitus (preexisting and gestational)
  - Rhesus isoimmunization and hydrops fetalis
  - Infection with toxoplasmosis, rubella, cytomegalovirus, herpes simplex, and others

Box 3: Causes of oligohydraminos[8]

- Fetal causes:
  - Urinary tract abnormalities such as bilateral renal agenesis (Potter's syndrome), fetal polycystic kidneys, or congenital urinary tract obstruction
  - Chromosomal anomalies
  - Intrauterine growth restriction
  - Postmaturity
  - Maternal drug intake, e.g., angiotensin-converting enzyme inhibitors, prostaglandin inhibitors
- Maternal causes:
  - Uteroplacental insufficiency
  - Hypertensive disorders
  - Idiopathic

Measurements

Symphysis-fundal Height

Mother should be supine with legs straight, bladder should be empty. Two points are marked: first corresponding to the upper border of symphysis pubis and other upper border of fundus. Distance in between these two is measured (Fig. 12).

- After 24 weeks up to 36 weeks, symphysis-fundal height (SFH) corresponds to number of weeks of gestation ±2 (in a singleton pregnancy with longitudinal lie and a nonobese patient with empty bladder)

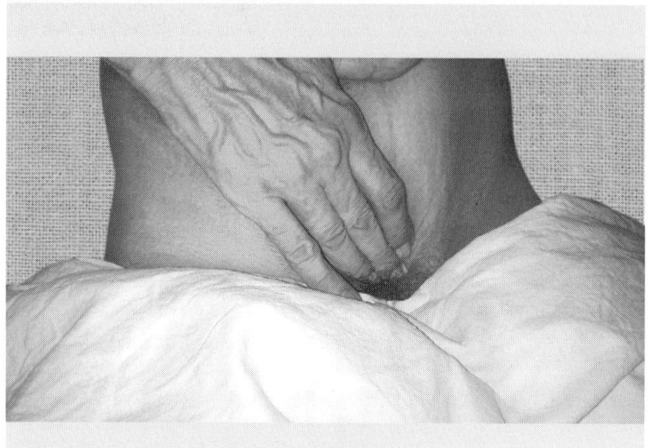

FIG. 11: Assessment of scar tenderness.

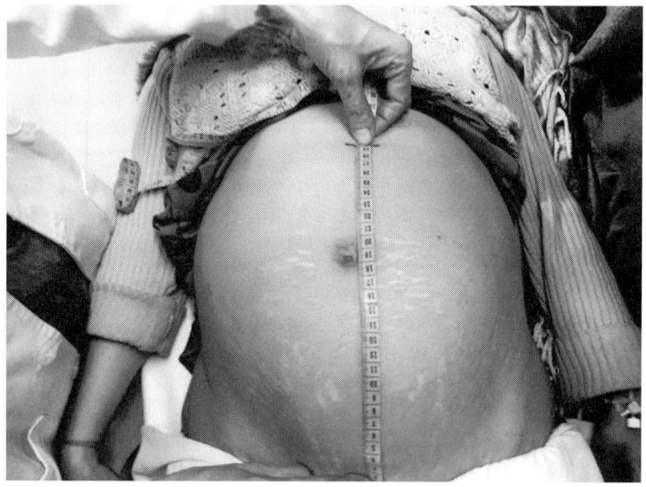

FIG. 12: Measurement of symphysis-fundal height.

- This relationship between growth of uterus and SFH can be expressed on a graph known as gravidogram
- More objective, less interobserver variation.

Abdominal Girth

It is measured in inches at the level of umbilicus. At 30 weeks, it is 30 inches. It increases by 1 inch/week till term (Fig. 13).

Effective fetal weight:

Johnson's formula[4]

- If vertex at or above ischial spine:
  [SFH (cm) - 12] × 155 = Fetal weight (g)
- If vertex below ischial spine:
  [SFH (cm) - 11] × 155 = Fetal weight (g)

Disadvantage: applicable only for vertex presentation.

Cesarean section Dawn's formula

This method uses Dawn's pelvimeter to assess vertical length (L) of gravid uterus measured from superior border of symphysis pubis to upper most level of fundus in cm, transverse diameter (T), i.e., distance between the farthest points at the level of uterine fundus and double abdominal wall thickness (DAWT) (lower abdomen is pinched by left hand and thickness measured in cm by pelvimeter). If DAWT is more than 3 cm excess cm above 3 is subtracted from T and 0.5 of excess is subtracted from L.[9]

Auscultation

Auscultation of fetal heart sounds (Fig. 14) is essential for the diagnosis of live pregnancy. Fetal heart sounds are best heard through left scapular region in vertex and breech presentation. If there is difficulty in localizing fetal heart sounds, then patient is asked to stretch the legs. The localization of fetal heart sounds helps to determine lie, presentation, and position of fetus (Table 5). The rate and rhythm helps to determine whether fetus is in distress.

Assessment in Multiple Pregnancies (Twins)

Inspection

Abdomen is unduly enlarged (barrel shaped).

- Palpation: Fundal height is more than gestational age
    - Abdominal girth is more than normal, average at term
    - Palpation of too many fetal parts
    - Association with polyhydramnios may be seen
    - Finding of two fetal heads or three fetal poles.

Auscultation

Two distinct fetal heart sounds at two separate points with a silent area in between by two observers.

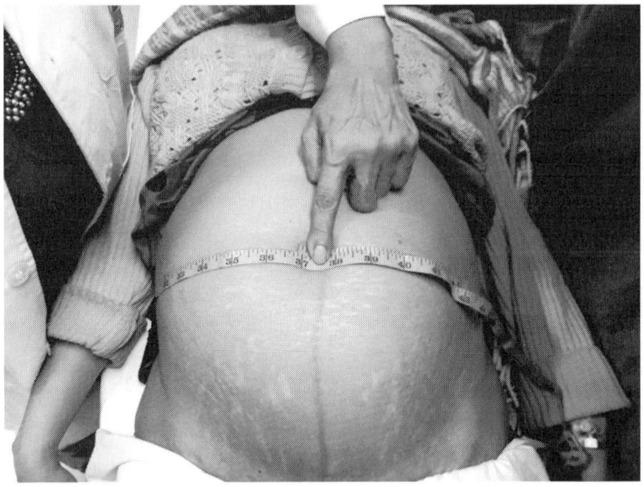

FIG. 13: Measurement of abdominal girth.

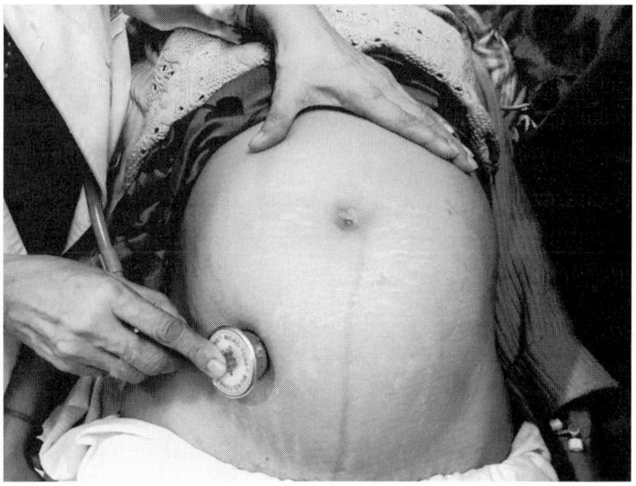

FIG. 14: Auscultation of fetal heart sounds.

TABLE 5: Localization of fetal heart

Fetal position	Localization
• Occipitoanterior position	• Midpoint of spino-umbilical line of same side
• Occipitolateral position	• More laterally same side
• Occipitoposterior position	• Towards maternal flanks on same side with difficulty
• Complete breech	• Around umbilicus in midline
• Frank breech	• Lower level in midline
• Mentoanterior	• Anteriorly towards side of limbs
• Mentoposterior	• Maternal flanks towards side of limbs with difficulty
• Transverse-dorsoanterior	• Centrally below the level of umbilicus
• Transverse-dorsoposterior	• Centrally at higher level of umbilicus

Note: With progress of labor, position of fetal heart becomes more anterior and shifts downwards.

CONCLUSION

Fetus lies in an attitude of flexion. Any deviation in this attitude is an important indicator of deviation from the normal course of progress. The fetal lie is mostly longitudinal (99.5%) with cephalic presentation in 96.5% and breech presentation in 3% cases. Left occipito-anterior is the most common fetal position. Abdominal examination including the Leopold's maneuver and auscultation of fetal heart sounds are the cornerstones of good obstetric clinical assessment. Clinical pelvimetry can be done especially in cases of primigravida with post-term pregnancies. Pregnant patients must be encouraged for periodic antenatal visits to assess the fetal well-being *in utero*.

REFERENCES

1. Cunningham GF, Leveno KJ, Bloom SL, Hauth JC, Rouse DJ, Spong CY. Williams Obstetrics, 23rd edition. Philadelphia: McGraw Hill Health Professions Division; 2010.
2. Dutta DC. Dutta's Textbook of Obstetrics, 7th edition. Kolkata: Hiralal Konwar Medical Publisher; 2011.
3. Goplerud J, Eastman NJ. Compound presentation; a survey of 65 cases. Obstet Gynecol. 1953;1(1):59-66.
4. Balakrishnan S. Textbook of obstetrics, 2nd edition. Hyderabad: Paras Medical Publisher; 2013.
5. Arulkumaran S, Sivanesaratnam V, Chatterjee A, Kumar P. Essentials of Obstetrics, 2nd edition. New Delhi: Jaypee Brothers Medical Publishers; 2011.
6. Baskett TF, Calder AA, Arulkumaran S. Munro Kerr's Operative Obstetrics, 11th edition. Philadelphia: Elsevier Publishers; 2007.
7. Gabbe SG. Fetal and maternal causes of polyhydramnios. In: Gabbe SG, Niebyl JR, Simpson JL (Eds). Obstetrics: Normal and Problem Pregnancies, 6th edition. Philadelphia: Elsevier Saunders; 2012.
8. Johnson JM, Chauhan SP, Ennen CS, Niederhauser A, Magann EF. A comparison of 3 criteria of oligohydramnios in identifying peripartum complications: a secondary analysis. Am J Obstet Gynecol. 2007;197(2):207.e1-7.
9. Dawn CS. Textbook of Obstetrics and Neonatology, 13th edition. Kolkata: Dawn Medical Publisher; 1997.

Section 2

Antepartum

CHAPTER 5

Age and Parity

Shakuntla Kumar, Pratik Tambe, Amit Tandon

INTRODUCTION

The impact of maternal age on pregnancy and the neonate cannot be underestimated. With improvements in healthcare in particular and development of society in general, larger numbers of women are postponing child-bearing until later in their lives. With the availability of assisted reproduction, egg and embryo freezing, we see far greater numbers of elderly primigravidae in current clinical practice.

At the other end of the reproductive spectrum, more teenagers are now falling pregnant, placing their health at risk. The number of teenage pregnancies continues to be significantly high since the past two decades, in spite of concerted multipronged strategies to tackle this problem.

We examine these two critical scenarios and review the peculiar circumstances which accompany these two clinically diverse situations. The incidence of maternal and fetal complications in the antenatal period, the currently available evidences and guidelines, the strategies for screening and coping with these high-risk pregnancies are discussed.

TEENAGE PREGNANCY

Pregnancies occurring before 20 years are known as teenage pregnancies. Worldwide, according to World Health Organization (WHO) statistics, about 16 million women aged 15–19 years deliver every year, which amounts to 11% of total births.

This remains a public health problem because about 70,000 adolescent mothers are dying every year due to teenage pregnancy. The prevalence varies widely in different countries. In India, it was 83 per 1,000 population during the years 2005-10. The National Family Health Survey (NFHS) III 2005-06 has estimated the overall teenage pregnancy incidence in India to be 16%.[1]

Teenage pregnancies in developed countries are out of marriage and are usually due to adolescent sexual habits. However, in developing nations like India, they are due to the traditional custom of early marriage prevalent in several parts of the country which is well accepted by family members and society. Despite the law against marriage of girls before 18 years, according to NHFS III, 47.4% of women in India were child brides with a very high proportion of them living in rural areas.[2]

The WHO has estimated that the risk of death following pregnancy is twice as great for women between 15 and 19 years as compared to the women between the ages of 20 and 24 years. The maternal mortality rate is up to five times higher for 10–14-year-old girls than for women of above 20 years of age.[2]

Teenage pregnancy is also considered as high risk as this is the important period for bone development. Occurrence of pregnancy poses an additional burden on the growing girl and she is strapped of the nutrients by the fetus. As a result, vitamin and mineral deficiency is common. These girls are also more prone to poor antenatal care and illegal abortions.

Current Scenario

- Half of the world's population is under the age of 25 years. Around 1.8 billion are aged 10–25 years, history's largest generation of adolescents, and about 85% live in the developing world

- Most of these girls become sexually active before they turn 20 years of age
- 49% of girls in lesser developed countries get married before they turn 18 years
- 10–40% of young unmarried girls have had an unwanted pregnancy according to community studies
- Some 14 million children all over the world are born every year to young women aged 15–19 years.[3]

Causes

Causes of teenage pregnancies vary in industrialized countries as compared to developing countries. Adolescent sexual behavior, which may also be influenced by alcohol and drugs; and peer pressure to engage in sexual activity early, may be the reason in developed countries.

In developing countries, the causes are:

- Poverty
- Early marriage
- Poor education
- Lack of knowledge regarding reproductive sexual health
- Unaware about available contraceptive options
- Incorrect use of contraception
- Rape/sexual abuse/domestic violence
- Low self-esteem
- Lack of educational ambitions and goals.[3]

According to the third NFHS, adolescents (10–19 years) constitute about 21.5% of the population and more than 47% of girls were already married by 18 years. Trends show that from 1992 to 2006, the percentage of women married by 18 years of age has only reduced from 54 to 47%.[4]

This underlines the need for greater impetus to female education and social awakening regarding the status of the girl child and women in our society.

Impact

The combination of poor nutrition and early childbearing expose young women to serious health-risks during pregnancy and childbirth, including damage to the reproductive tract, pregnancy-related complications, such as anemia, pregnancy-induced hypertension (PIH), preterm labor, cephalopelvic disproportion, maternal mortality, peri- and neonatal mortalities, and low birth weight (LBW).[1,3]

Gortzak-Uzan et al. assessed the perinatal outcome of teenage pregnancy in a large cohort 11,496 patients from 1990 to 1997: 600 (5.2%) were 16–17 years old, 2,097 (18.2%) were 18–19 years old, and the remaining 8,799 (76.6%) were 20–24 years old. Lack of prenatal care was common in the youngest mothers. Rates of preterm delivery (PTD) were 14.2, 9.8, and 8.8% in the three age-groups, respectively ($p < 0.05$). Rates of malformations, small for gestational age (SGA), LBW, and very low birth weight (VLBW) were also significantly higher in the youngest mothers.

A multivariate analysis on LBW was performed to assess the unique contribution of young maternal age, adjusted for potential confounders. Adjusted odds ratios (ORs) for LBW were 1.25 [95% confidence interval (CI) = 1.00–1.56] for maternal age less than 18 years, 2.57 (95% CI = 2.14–3.07) for PIH, 1.55 (95% CI = 1.30–1.84) for lack of prenatal care, and 4.09 (95% CI = 3.2–5.2) for malformations.

They concluded that teenage pregnancy is associated with adverse outcomes, such as LBW, PTD, SGA, and malformations. The risk for LBW was affected mainly by demographic factors (maternal ethnicity, lack of prenatal care) and medical factors (PIH, malformations).[5]

- During adolescence, the body is in a growing stage. If pregnancy occurs during these years, nutrition must suffice the growth of the mother and the baby. The outcomes are influenced by this biological immaturity.[1] Pregnancy comes as an extra burden on the body and leads to negative balance mainly on the spine and pelvis
- Lack of antenatal care: pregnant teenage girls do not receive appropriate prenatal care, more so in rural areas. According to data, only 24 and 31% (NFHS-I and II, respectively) women aged less than 20 years received antenatal care during the first trimester compared to 27 and 37% women in the 20–24 years age group[6]
- Medical and obstetric complications are greater for girls aging 14 years and younger due to underdeveloped pelvis leading to increased obstructed labor and increased incidence of cesarean birth.

According to NFHS III:

- 13% of women (<20 years) reported massive vaginal bleeding and 14% had very high fever
- Younger women (<20 years) reported more symptoms of postpartum complications compared to those aged 20–24 years
- Among children whose weight was reported, 26% were underweight (<2.5 kg) among young mothers (<20 years).

The infant mortality rate, neonatal, postnatal, and child mortality rates were higher in mothers less than 20 years as compared to those aged 20–29 years. An overwhelming majority of studies (9 out of 10) found that PTD, stillbirth, fetal distress, birth asphyxia, anemia, LBW, PIH, and spontaneous abortion were most frequently encountered complications during teenage pregnancy.[7]

Other negative social and medical consequences of teenage pregnancy include lower access to higher education, high divorce rates, premature death of women, population growth, weak and unhealthy children, and single motherhood.[6]

Way Forward

Teenage pregnancy is a complex social issue. There is no single or simple approach that will reduce pregnancy among all groups of teenagers. Because the causes of teen pregnancy are complicated, the strategies should be multipronged.[8]

The following 10 best practices have been identified for practitioners dealing with teen pregnancy prevention:[9]

1. Youth development
2. Involvement of family and other caring adults
3. Male involvement
4. Cultural relevance
5. Community-wide campaigns
6. Service learning programs
7. Programs to improve employment opportunities
8. Sexuality education and acquired immunodeficiency syndrome education programs
9. Outreach in teen pregnancy prevention programs
10. Access to reproductive health services.[10-15]

Recent research by the Alan Guttmacher Institute compared the rates of teenage pregnancy in five developed nations, and their approaches to the issue. It concluded that comprehensive and balanced information about sexuality is one of the hallmarks of countries with lower levels of adolescent pregnancy. Easy access to contraceptives and other reproductive health services were seen to contribute to lower pregnancy rates.

ADVANCED MATERNAL AGE

A woman who is pregnant for the first time after 35 years or more, is considered an elderly primigravida. With various socioeconomic issues taking precedence over childbearing, delaying childbirth is increasingly becoming common and traditionally, such pregnancies are considered as high risk.[16] Effective birth control, advances in assisted reproductive technology (ART), delayed marriage, increasing rates of divorce followed by remarriage, and women's pursuit of higher education and career advancement all contribute to this trend.

The past three decades have seen significant increases in maternal age at childbirth in many high-income countries. The proportion of first births to women aged 35 years and over in the United States (US) increased nearly eight times from 1970 to 2006. In 2006, about 1 out of 12 first births were to women aged 35 years and over compared with 1 out of 100 in 1970. In 2009, the birth rate in the US continued to rise in women aged 40–44 years. In Europe, the percentage of live births to mothers aged 35 years and over in United Kingdom (UK) rose from 8.7 in 1990 to 19.3 in 2004.[17-19]

Advanced maternal age (AMA) is associated with a range of adverse pregnancy outcomes including LBW, preterm birth, stillbirths, unexplained fetal death, and increased rates of cesarean section. The majority of studies documents an increased risk of adverse pregnancy outcome in advanced age women, some studies have yielded inconsistent conclusions about both the specific outcomes adversely affected by maternal age and the strength of the association. There is limited consensus among studies as to the precise maternal age when the increase in the risk of adverse pregnancy outcome becomes clinically important. Some studies have reported that the association only becomes significant at age greater than 40 years, while others suggest that age more than or equal to 35 years is the cut-off for increased risk.

Contemporary older mothers tend to be well educated, of higher socioeconomic status, and of lower parity than older mothers from the recent past. In addition, ART may have also contributed to rise in the number of pregnancies in women in their forties. Social advantages may ameliorate some of the adverse effects of AMA on perinatal outcome. Currently, older women who become pregnant are more often primiparous and of better socioeconomic status while in the past they were more often multiparous and of low socioeconomic status.[20]

Kenny et al. performed a population-based cohort study using data on all singleton births in 2004-08 from the North Western Perinatal Survey based at the University of Manchester, UK.[21] The study cohort consisted of 215,344 births: 122,307 mothers (54.19%) were aged 20–29 years, 62,371 mothers (27.63%) were aged 30–34 years, 33,966 mothers (15.05%) were aged 35–39 years, and 7,066 mothers (3.13%) were aged more than or equal to 40 years.

Women aged more than 40 years at delivery were at increased risk of stillbirth [risk ratio (RR) = 1.83; 95% CI = 1.37–2.43], preterm (RR = 1.25; 95% CI = 1.14–1.36) and very preterm birth (RR = 1.29; 95% CI = 1.08–1.55), macrosomia (RR = 1.31; 95% CI = 1.12–1.54), extremely large for gestational age (RR = 1.40; 95% CI = 1.25–1.58) and cesarean delivery (RR = 1.83; 95% CI = 1.77–1.90).[21]

Complications Related to Late Pregnancy

As women age, they have a greater opportunity to acquire conditions that can influence their health and the health of the fetus. Therefore, women aged 35 years or older are expected to have twice the rates of antepartum hospitalization than their younger counterparts.[20,22] The two most common medical problems complicating pregnancy are: hypertension (pre-existing and pregnancy-related) and diabetes (pregestational and gestational).[20]

Hypertension

Hypertension is the most frequent medical problem encountered in pregnancy with older women. The incidence of preeclampsia in the general obstetric population is 3–4%, which increases to 5–10% in women over age 40 years and is as high as 35% in women over age 50 years.[23] With careful monitoring and appropriately timed intervention, maternal and fetal morbidity and mortality can be reduced, but this is associated with an increase in preterm birth, SGA infants, and cesarean delivery.[22,24]

Diabetes Mellitus

The prevalence of diabetes increases with maternal age; the rates of both pre-existing diabetes mellitus and gestational diabetes increase three- to sixfold in older women when compared to women in their early age-group.[20,22] Pre-existing diabetes is associated with an increased risk of congenital anomalies, perinatal mortality, and perinatal morbidity, while the most common complication from gestational diabetes is macrosomia.[25]

Abnormal Placentation

Placental abruption and placental previa do occur more commonly in older women, with a large portion of this risk associated with increasing parity. Gilbert et al.[20] found 10-fold increased risk of placenta previa in nulliparous women 40 years of age or older when compared to women aged 20–29 years, although the absolute risk of this was small (0.25 vs. 0.03%).

Perinatal Morbidity

In the past several years, it has been observed that AMA is responsible for a substantial increase in the rate of LBW and PTD. It was found that nulliparous women aged 35–40 years with singleton gestations had a near twofold increased risk of PTD, and a 1.7-fold increased risk of delivering a SGA baby compared to women aged 20–24 years. Smoking has been associated with an increased perinatal morbidity in all age groups, but the risk is particularly high in smoker's aged 30–39 years.[26]

Perinatal Mortality

Retrospectively, a significant proportion of perinatal deaths seen in older women were related to an increase in lethal congenital and chromosomal anomalies. But now in the developed world, the increased perinatal mortality experienced by older women, is largely due to nonanomalous fetal deaths and perinatal losses associated with multiple gestations. Many studies have shown that there is an increased risk of unexplained fetal death among older gravida, even after controlling for risk factors such as hypertension, diabetes, antepartum bleeding, and multiple gestation.[27,28]

Dysfunctional Labor and Cesarean Delivery

Women aged 35 years or older are more likely to be delivered by cesarean section. The cesarean delivery rate increases with the advancing age.[20,27] The reasons for this are multifactorial, while there appears to be a linear relationship between dysfunction labor and maternal age; other factors found responsible are increased risk of medical complications, inductions of labor, and malpositions seen in older gravida.

Maternal Mortality

While advancing maternal age is associated with an increased risk of maternal mortality, in industrialized countries, this is still a rare event.[28] The most common causes of death were related to hypertension, hemorrhage, and thromboembolism.[23,29] In nonindustrialized nations where maternal mortality is many fold higher, the lack of adequate care contributes substantially to these maternal losses, and plays a much larger role than maternal characteristics.[30]

Stillbirth

The risk of stillbirth is lowest amongst women between the ages of 15 and 35 years. It increases considerably beyond that interval in women at the extremes of reproductive age spectrum.[31]

According to Fretts et al., AMA is an independent risk factor for fetal death. After controlling for other risk factors, such as placenta previa, abruption, previous abortion, and prior fetal deaths, women at or above 35 years of age were twice as high at risk for fetal death as their younger counterparts. Women older than 40 years have further increased risk.[32,33]

Huang et al., by using McGill Obstetrical Neonatal Database, found that 60% of unexplained stillbirths occurred after 36 years. In a separate study, they showed that increased risk of unexplained stillbirths late in pregnancy was significantly higher in women aged 35 years or older. Older women were at a statistically significant increased risk for "unexplained" fetal death (OR = 2.2; 95% CI = 1.3–3.8); women aged 35 years or older had approximately 1 in 440 births end in unexplained fetal death, compared to 1 in 1,000 births for women younger than 35 years.[27]

Women who were 35 years or older had a statistically significant increase in the frequency of multiple gestation, hypertension, diabetes mellitus, placenta previa, placental abruption, previous abortion, and previous fetal death.[34] Hence, increased antepartum surveillance is indicated in these women of advanced age.[35]

Advanced maternal age was found to be an independent risk factor for fetal death at 28–31 weeks. Women of advanced age are at higher risk of stillbirth throughout gestation and the risk peaked between 37 and 41 weeks. It was found that AMA was associated with increased rates of PTD, LBW, and VLBW.[36,37] Nulliparous women aged 40 years or over have a higher risk of operative delivery (cesarean, forceps, and vacuum deliveries: 61%) than do younger nulliparous women (35%).[20] This increase occurs in spite of LBW and gestational age and may be explained by the increase in other complications of pregnancy, low threshold of physician, and patient anxiety and preference.

Maternal overweight, obesity, and smoking are the most important potentially modifiable risk factors for stillbirth. Culturally appropriate preconception care and quality antenatal care that is accessible to all women has the potential to reduce stillbirth rates in high-income countries.

The stillbirth risk associated with maternal age can be somewhat addressed through increased awareness and careful consideration to the most appropriate time to have children. Based on the available data, timely induction of labor at or near term for older mothers is likely to be associated with a reduction in stillbirth risk without increasing the likelihood of birth by cesarean section. Public education and awareness on special risks in pregnancy at older age is useful in women who tend to postpone motherhood.[38]

Fetal Growth Restriction

Advanced maternal age is an independent risk factor for intrauterine growth restriction (IUGR). Hence, women aged 35 years or older should be screened for IUGR.[32,39,40]

Advanced maternal age has been found to be an important sociodemographic determinant for IUGR. In this study, parity was also found to be a risk factor for IUGR with primiparous women at higher risk of delivering IUGR babies.[40]

The uterine vasculature in older women fails to sufficiently adapt to increased hemodynamic demands of pregnancy.[32] Histopathological examination of the placenta has highlighted the role of maternal age in placental ageing.

Grandmultiparity

Grandmultiparity is defined as parity more than or equal to 5 (including previous delivery). In developed countries, currently grandmultiparity is becoming rare (3–4% of all births).[41]

In India, the incidence of grandmultiparity was found to be 2.7% in a study. Most of these women were in age group 26–30 years. Marriage in young age, concept of large family size, desire for a male child, and lack of other source of recreation contribute to grandmultiparity at a lower age in our country.[42]

Grandmultiparity is associated with low socioeconomic status and low education status, poor prenatal care, smoking and alcohol consumption. Grandmultiparas had increased rate of insulin-dependent gestational diabetes.[43] Most of these women have anemia, hypoproteinemia, and calcium deficiency due to rapid succession of pregnancy and lactation.

However, according to Yasmeen et al., grandmultiparity is not an independent risk factor for poor pregnancy outcome. They concluded that it carries no significant risk of obstetric and neonatal complications, especially in settings where modern obstetrical care is readily available.[44] With improvement in socioeconomic state and better standard of antenatal care, grandmultiparity does not lead to additional obstetric or perinatal risk.[45]

CONCLUSION

Pregnancy at extremes of reproductive age remains a challenge to healthcare professionals including obstetricians, midwives, internists, and to health and family welfare planning officials. With high-quality evidence and good delivery of antenatal care, coupled with social awareness, dissemination of information on reproductive rights and contraception, there may be improvement in maternal and neonatal outcomes in the years to come.

REFERENCES

1. Kamini S, Avvaru KV. Teenage pregnancy: maternal and fetal outcomes. Int Org Sci Res J Dent Med Sci. 2014;13(4):41-4.
2. Ghose S, John LB. Obstetrics and psychosocial outcome of teenage pregnancy. J Evol Med Den Sci. 2013;2(45):8745-8.
3. The United Nations Children's Fund (UNICEF). (2009). Child Protection: Teenage Pregnancies. Plan Your Future: Plan Your Families. Young People and Family Planning. [online] Available from www.unicef.org/malaysia/Factsheet-Child-Protection-Preventing-Teenage-Pregnancies-Family-Planning.pdf. [Accessed June, 2015].
4. Ministry of Health and Family Welfare, Government of India; World Health Organization. Reproductive and Sexual Health of Young People in India: Secondary Analysis of data from National Family Health Surveys of India - 1,2,3(1992-2006) for the age group 15-24 years. 2009.
5. Gortzak-Uzan L, Hallak M, Press F, Katz M, Shoham-Vardi I. Teenage pregnancy: risk factors for adverse perinatal outcome. J Matern Fetal Med. 2001;10(6):393-7.
6. Raj AD, Rabi B, Amudha P, Teijlingen VE, Glyn C. (2010). Factors associated with teenage pregnancy in South Asia: a systematic review. [online] Available from hsj.gr/medicine/factors-associated-with-teenage-pregnancy-in-south-asia-a-systematic-review.php?aid=3616. [Accessed June, 2015].
7. Domenico DM, Jones KH. (2007). Adolescent pregnancy in America, causes and responses. [online] Available from specialpopulations.org/Vol%2030-1%20Chapters/JVSNEVol30-1_Fall07_Domenico.pdf. [Accessed June, 2015].
8. Kirby D. Emerging answers: research findings on programs to reduce teen pregnancy (summary). Am J Health Edu. 2001;32(6):348-55.
9. Johns MJ, Moncla F, Gong EJ. Teenage pregnancy prevention programs. J Extens. 2000;38(4):4FEA1.
10. Card JJ, Niego S, Mallari A, Farrell WS. The program archive on sexuality, health & adolescence: Promising "prevention programs in a box". Fam Plann Perspect. 1996;28(5):210-20.
11. Franklin C, Corcoran J. Preventing adolescent pregnancy: a review of programs and practices. Soc Work. 2000;45(1):40-52.
12. Hutchins J. Promising approaches to preventing teen pregnancy. In: Kreinin T, Kuhn S, Rodgers AB, Hutchins J (Eds). Get Organized: A Guide to Preventing Teen Pregnancy. Washington DC, USA: The National Campaign to Prevent Teen Pregnancy; 1999. pp. 5-28.

13. Miller BC. Families Matter: A Research Synthesis of Family Influences on Adolescent Pregnancy. Washington DC, USA: The National Campaign to Prevent Teen Pregnancy; 1998.
14. Moore KA, Sugland BW, Blumenthal C, Glei D, Snyder N. Adolescent Pregnancy Prevention Programs: Interventions and Evaluations. Washington DC, USA: Child Trends Incorporation; 1995.
15. Sonenstein FL, Stewart K, Lindberg LD, Pernas M, Williams S. Involving Males in Preventing Teen Pregnancy. A guide for Program Planners. Washington DC, USA: The Urban Institute; 1997.
16. Hook EB, Cross PK, Jackson L, et al. Maternal age-specific rates of 47, +21 and other cytogenetic abnormalities diagnosed in the first trimester of pregnancy in chorionic villous biopsy specimens: comparison with rates expected from observations at amniocentesis. Am J Hum Genet. 1988;42:797.
17. Huang L, Sauve R, Birkett N, Fergusson D, van Walraven C. Maternal age and risk of stillbirth: a systematic review. CMAJ. 2008;178(2):165-72.
18. Mathews TJ, Hamilton BE. Mean age of mother, 1970-2000. Natl Vital Stat Rep. 2002;51(1):1-13.
19. Martin JA, Hamilton BE, Sutton PD, Ventura SJ, Menacker F, Kirmeyer S, et al. (2009). Births: Final Data for 2006. National Vital Statistics Reports, volume 57, number 7. [online] Available from www.cdc.gov/nchs/data/nvsr/nvsr57/nvsr57_07.pdf. [Accessed June, 2015].
20. Gilbert WM, Nesbitt TS, Danielsen B. Childbearing beyond age 40: pregnancy outcome in 24,032 cases. Obstet Gynecol. 1999;93(1):9-14.
21. Kenny LC, Lavender T, McNamee R, O'Neill SM, Mills T, Khashan AS. Advanced maternal age and adverse pregnancy outcome: evidence from a large contemporary cohort. PLoS One. 2013;8(2):e56583.
22. Seoud MA, Nassar AH, Usta IM, Melhem Z, Kazma A, Khalil AM. Impact of advanced maternal age on pregnancy outcome. Am J Perinatol. 2002;19(1):1-8.
23. Callaghan WM, Berg CJ. Pregnancy-related mortality among women aged 35 years and older, United States, 1991-1997. Obstet Gynecol. 2003;102(5 Pt 1):1015-21.
24. Zeitlin JA, Ancel PY, Saurel-Cubizolles MJ, Papiemik E. Are risk factors the same for small for gestational age versus other preterm births? Am J Obstet Gynecol. 2001;185(1):208-15.
25. Casey BM, Lucas MJ, McIntire DD, Leveno KJ. Pregnancy outcomes in women with gestational diabetes compared with the general obstetric population. Obstet Gynecol. 1997;90(6):869-73.
26. Salihu HM, Shumpert MN, Aliyu MH, Kirby RS, Alexander GR. Smoking-associated fetal morbidity among older gravidas: a population study. Acta Obstet Gynecol Scand. 2005;84(4):329-34.
27. Hung DY, Usher RH, Kramer MS, Yang H, Morin L, Fretts RC. Determinants of unexplained antepartum fetal deaths. Obstet Gynecol. 2000;95(2):215-21.
28. Frøen JF, Arnestad M, Frey K, Vege A, Saugstad OD, Stray-Pedersen B. Risk factors for sudden intrauterine unexplained death: epidemiological characteristics of singleton cases in Oslo, Norway, 1986-1995. Am J Obstet Gynecol. 2001;184(4):694-702.
29. Callaway LK, Lust K, McIntyre HD. Pregnancy outcomes in women of very advanced maternal age. Aust N Z J Obstet Gynaecol. 2005;45(1):12-6.
30. Ghosh MK. Maternal mortality. A global perspective. J Reprod Med. 2001;46(5):427-33.
31. Balayla J, Azoulay L, Assayag J, Benjamin A, Abenhaim HA. Effect of maternal age on the risk of stillbirth: a population-based short study on 37 million births in the United States. Am J Perinatol. 2011;28(8):643-50.
32. Odibo AO, Nelson D, Stamilio DM, Sehdev HM, Macones GA. Advanced maternal age is an independent risk factor for intrauterine growth restriction. Am J Perinatol. 2006;23(5):325-8.
33. Lavery JP. Placenta previa. Clin Obstet Gynecol. 1990;33(3):414-21.
34. Ananth CV, Wilcox AJ, Savits DA, Bowes WA, Luther ER. Effect of maternal age and parity on the risk of uteroplacental bleeding disorders in pregnancy. Obstet Gynecol. 1996;88(4 Pt 1):511-6.
35. Signore C, Freeman RK, Spong CY. Antenatal testing-a reevaluation: executive summary of a Eunice Kennedy Shriver National Institute of Child Health and Human Development workshop. Obstet Gynecol. 2009;113(3):687-701.
36. Fretts RC, Usher RH. Fetal death in women in the older reproductive age group. Contemp Rev Obstet Gynaecol. 1997;9:173-9.
37. Fretts RC, Schmittdiel J, McLean FH, Usher RH, Goldman MB. Increased maternal age and the risk of fetal death. N Engl J Med. 1995;333(15):953-7.
38. Flenady V, Middleton P, Smith GC, Duke W, Erwich JJ, Khong TY, et al. Stillbirths: the way forward in high-income countries. 2011;377(9778):1703-17.
39. Carolan M, Frankowska D. Advanced maternal age and adverse perinatal outcome: a review of the evidence. Midwifery. 2011;27(6):793-801.
40. Jahan MK, Shafiquzzaman M, Nahar K, Rahman M, Sultana N, Rahman MM, et al. Outcome of pregnancy in women 35 years of age and above. Mymensingh Med J. 2009;18(1):7-12.
41. Bai J, Wong FW, Bauman A, Mohsin M. Parity and pregnancy outcomes. Am J Obstet Gynecol. 2002;186(2):274-8.
42. Sultan S, Ojha J. Grand multiparity still an obstetric challenge--a clinical study of grand multipara in a tertiary care center. J Evol Med Den Sci. 2013;2(39):7423-30.
43. Roman H, Robillard PY, Verspyck E, Hulsey TC, Marpeau L, Barau G. Obstetric and neonatal outcomes in grand multiparity. Obstet Gynecol. 2004;103(6):1294-9.
44. Yasmeen L, Rasheed T, Syed S. Is grandmultiparity still a risk factor for obstetric complications? Ann Pak Inst Med Sci. 2010;6(1):58-61.
45. Fayed HM, Abid SF, Stevens B. Risk factors in extreme grand multiparity. Int J Gynaecol Obstet. 1993;41(1):17-22.

CHAPTER 6

Antepartum Surveillance of Fetal Well-being

Meenakshi B Chauhan

INTRODUCTION

The assessment of fetal well-being during pregnancy is one of the most important objectives of prenatal care. Antepartum fetal surveillance helps in timely detection of morbid changes in the fetal status followed by adequate interventions to prevent fetal death or disability (American College of Obstetricians and Gynecologists).[1] Antepartum surveillance is especially important in high risk pregnancies (Table 1). The methods used to detect and evaluate fetal hypoxia are as follows:

- Clinical methods:
  - Maternal weight gain
  - Fetal growth:
    - Fundal height
    - Abdominal girth
  - Daily fetal movement count (DFMC)
- Nonstress test (NST)
- Contraction stress test (CST)
- Biophysical profile (BPP)
- Modified BPP(MBPP)
- Doppler studies of umbilical, uterine, and cerebral arteries and veins.

However, there are limitations to the generalized use of these tests. In the first place, there is no ideal single test that can detect all fetal problems. Secondly, these tests are not absolutely specific and their interpretation can lead to iatrogenic preterm delivery and increased neonatal morbidity. Finally, many times they give false-negative results and have no beneficial effects.

Indeed, the only testing modality for which there is level of evidence I for effect in the use of umbilical artery (UA) Doppler as a means of surveillance of growth-restricted fetuses.[2]

TABLE 1: Indications of antepartum surveillance

Previous obstetric history	
Maternal	• Hypertensive disorder of pregnancy • Placental abruption
Fetal	• Intra-uterine growth restriction • Stillbirth
Current pregnancy	
Maternal	• Post-term pregnancy • Hypertensive disorder of pregnancy • Diabetes mellitus • Preterm premature rupture of membrane • Chronic abruption • Isoimmunization • Abnormal maternal serum screening (human chorionic gonadotropin or α-fetoprotein >2.0 multiples of the median) in absence of confirmed fetal anomaly • Vaginal bleeding • Morbid obesity • Advanced maternal age • Assisted reproductive technology • Antiphospholipid antibody syndrome
Fetal	• Decreased fetal movement • Intrauterine growth restriction • Oligohydramnios/polyhydramnios • Multiple pregnancy • Rh isoimmunization • Fetal infections

INITIATION

Prenatal assessment of the fetal condition has two objectives: (1) to exclude fetal abnormality (done predominantly in the first half of pregnancy) and (2) to monitor the condition of the presumed normal fetus, with a view of determining the optimal time for delivery.[3] The timing of initiation should be individualized and reflect the risk factor(s) associated with that pregnancy. The obstetric history, severity of complication in the present pregnancy, and available neonatal care facilities have to be taken into account. On an average, surveillance is generally recommended at 32 weeks if there is a single risk factor causing minimal-to-moderate risk for antepartum fetal death. When there are severe or more than one risk factor, monitoring may be started at 26–28 weeks.

FREQUENCY

Frequency of testing should also be individualized. The maternal age, gestational age, previous obstetric history, and presence or absence of underlying current medical and/or obstetrical complications should be taken into account. The testing is usually performed once or twice weekly. However, it may be done daily or even more frequently to maximize gestation age and at the same time avoiding significant morbidity in preterm fetus.[4]

METHODS

Clinical Assessment

- Weight gain: maternal weight gain during pregnancy can be very variable and is not a significant indicator of fetal well-being
- Symphysio-fundal height can be a good marker for monitoring fetal growth
- Abdominal girth is not always reliable.

Fetal Kick Count

To keep an account of maternal perception of fetal movement (FM), this is the simplest and most inexpensive method of evaluating fetal well-being. The periods of fetal activity lasts for about 40 minutes and period of rest about 20 minutes. As many as 30 gross movements may occur in 1 hour. Peak activity is between 9.00 PM and 1.00 AM a time which coincides with a period of low maternal plasma glucose level. The different methods used are as follows:

- Cardiff count to 10 (Pearson, Weaver):[5] patients are instructed to begin counting FMs until they reach 10 movements. If the 10 movements are noticed in 10 hours or less, the fetus is in good health. Modified protocols include those of Liston (count to 6 h)[6] and Moore (count to 2 h)[7]
- Daily FM count: the woman is instructed to count for 1-hour duration in the morning, afternoon, and evening after meals. Daily fetal movement count is calculated by multiplying the sum by 4 and it should be more than 10.

Women who report decreased FMs (<6 distinct movements within 2 h) should have an evaluation of maternal and fetal status. The firstline fetal tests include the NST and BPP. When the NST is normal and there are no risk factors, women should continue with DFMC. If the NST is normal and risk factors are identified, e.g., gestational hypertension or suspicion of small for gestational age fetus or oligohydramnios, further testing within 24 hours (ultrasound or BPP) is recommended. In situations where the NST is atypical or abnormal, further testing (BPP or CST) should be performed as soon as possible.

Nonstress Test

It is most commonly used for antepartum evaluation of fetal status. It is the graphic recording of fetal heart rate (FHR) acceleration in response to FM. This response is a reflex that involves the cerebral cortex and is affected by physiologic or pathologic influences on the fetal brain. This reflex is most commonly suppressed by fetal sleep or hypoxia. Thus, absence of accelerations during a NST must be considered a consequence of fetal hypoxia until proved otherwise. It is noninvasive, easily performed and interpreted and is readily accepted by the patient. In most cases, a normal NST is predictive of good perinatal outcome for 1 week (providing the maternal-fetal condition remains stable), except in women with insulin dependent diabetes or with a postdates pregnancy, in which case NSTs are recommended at least twice weekly.[8-10]

Cardiotocography machine works on the principle of Doppler and FHR is represented on a graph paper.

Procedure[11]

- Patient is made to lie in semirecumbent position
- The equipment is applied to maternal abdomen and the uterine activity and FHR is traced for 20 minutes
- An event marker is given to the patient to mark the perceived FMs on the graph every time she feels FM.

Interpretation

- Reactive NST (Fig. 1): two or more FHR accelerations of at least 15 beats per minute and lasting at least 15 seconds from baseline within a 20-minute period usually occurring with episodes of fetal activity. No late deceleration
- Nonreactive NST (Fig. 2): if no spontaneous FM occurs during the initial 20 minutes of observation, the test is continued for another 20 minutes, and during this period FM is provoked by external manipulation. If there is no acceleration, test is considered nonreactive
- Equivocal: if the quality of monitor tracing is inadequate for interpretation.

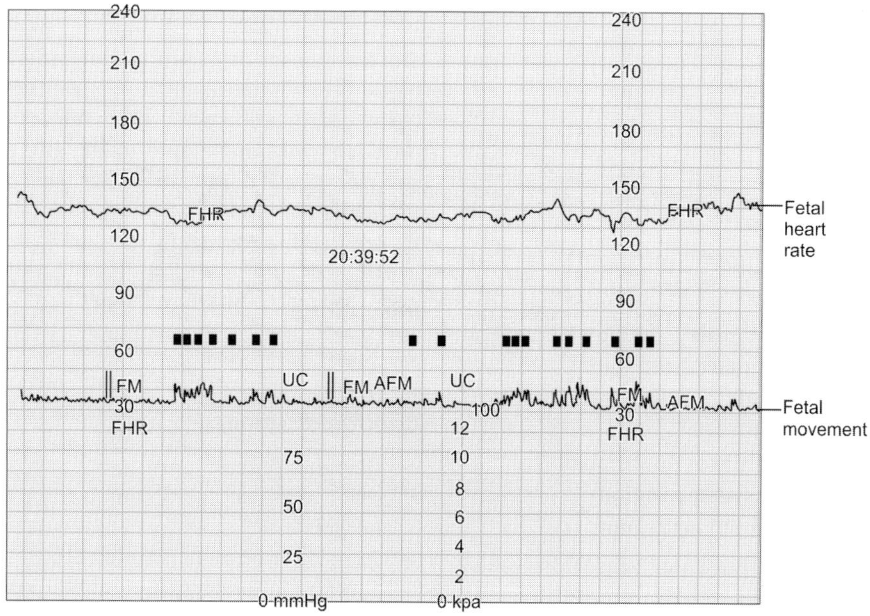

FHR, fetal heart rate; FM, fetal movement; UC, uterine contraction; AFM, auto fetal movement.

FIG. 1: Reactive nonstress test: acceleration of fetal heart of 15 beats per minute or more, lasting 15 seconds or more.

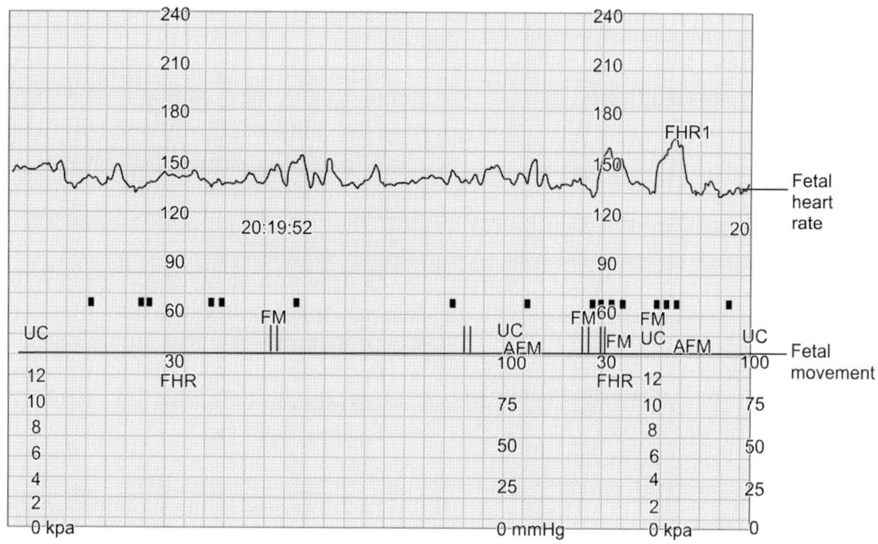

FHR, fetal heart rate; FM, fetal movement; UC, uterine contraction; AFM, auto fetal movement.

FIG. 2: Nonreactive nonstress test: there is decreased variability, no acceleration in association with fetal movements.

Variables of Nonstress Test

- Baseline FHR
- Variability of FHR
- Presence or absence of accelerations
- Presence or absence of decelerations.

Baseline FHR: mean FHR between peaks and depression (normal 110–160 beats per minute).

- Tachycardia: mean FHR more than 160 beats per minute. In the presence of good variability, tachycardia is not a sign of fetal distress

Causes:
- Maternal fever
- Fetal hypoxia
- Fetal anemia
- Amnionitis
- Fetal tachyarrhythmias
- Fetal heart failure
- Drugs:
  - Beta-sympathomimetics
  - Parasympatholytics
- Rebound transient tachycardia following a deceleration accompanied by decreased variability

- Bradycardia: mean FHR less than 110 beats per minute

Causes:
- Congenital heart block (little or no variability)
- Occiput posterior or transverse position
- Fetal hypoxia with or without academia
- Maternal hypothermia.

Fetal Heart Rate Variability

- Fetal heart rate variability is beat-to-beat oscillations of baseline FHR excluding accelerations and decelerations. Normal variation is 5–25 beats per minute
- Less than 5 beats per minute for 40 minutes are abnormal.

If the NST is nonreactive along with adequate variability, it is a false-positive result. While a nonreactive test with decreased or absent variability denotes fetal hypoxia.

Accelerations

Presence of accelerations is a reliable sign of fetal health, while its absence denotes fetal sleep or compromise.

Decelerations

A decrease in FHR below baseline by 15 beats per minute or more is found in 50% of NST. If it is nonrepetitive, brief or less than 30 seconds, it is normal. If it is repetitive, more than or equal to 3 in 20 minutes or lasting for more than or equal to 1 minute, it denotes fetal compromise.

Vibroacoustic Stimulation Test

Vibroacoustic stimulation (VAS) test has also been added to the protocol to perform the NST. It uses stimulation with an artificial larynx which produces a stimulus of approximately 80–82 Hz over the fetal head during 1–3 seconds. A healthy fetus will respond with sudden movement (startle response) followed by acceleration of the FHR. This method was designed to decrease the time spent in the performance of NST.

Contraction Stress Test

This test is based on experimental evidence that uteroplacental blood flow decreases markedly during uterine contractions (UCs) creating a hypoxic state. A fetus with chronic or acute problem will not be able to tolerate a decrease in oxygen supply and will demonstrate this by decelerations of the FHR following contractions. The results of CST are categorized as shown in table 2 and figures 3 and 4.

Indications

- Nonreactive NST

Contraindications

- Placenta previa
- Prior classical cesarean section or extensive uterine surgery
- Preterm rupture of membranes
- Preterm labor or patients at high risk of preterm labor
- Multiple gestation
- Cervical incompetence.

Procedure

Cardiotocography machine is applied to the maternal abdomen and uterine activity and FHR is observed for 15–20 minutes.

Intravenous oxytocin is started at 0.5 mL/min. The rate is doubled every 15–20 minutes until three contractions lasting 40–60 seconds occur within a period of 10 minutes. Patients showing spontaneous uterine activity of sufficient duration and frequency do not require oxytocin. Nipple stimulation may also be used in place of oxytocin (nipple stimulation test).

Contraction stress test is used infrequently for primary fetal surveillance because of:
- Long duration of test, and intravenous access[12]
- Requirement of continuous supervision by trained personnel
- Existence of risks.

TABLE 2: Interpretation of contraction stress test

Negative (normal)	No late or significant variable deceleration
Positive (abnormal)	Late deceleration following 50% on more of contraction
Equivocal (suspicious)	Intermittent late or significant variable decelerations
Equivocal (hyperstimulatory)	Deceleration occurs in presence of contractions more frequent than every 2 min or last longer than 90 s
Unsatisfactory	Contractions fewer than three in 10 min or uninterpretable tracing

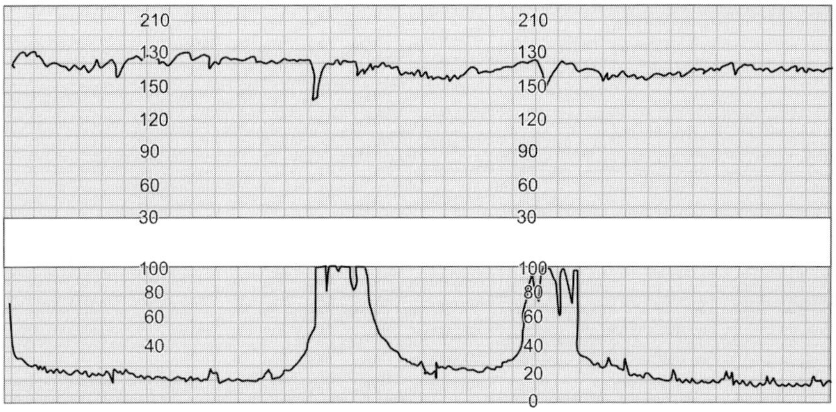

FIG. 3: Negative contraction stress test: adequate variability; no deceleration with uterine contractions.

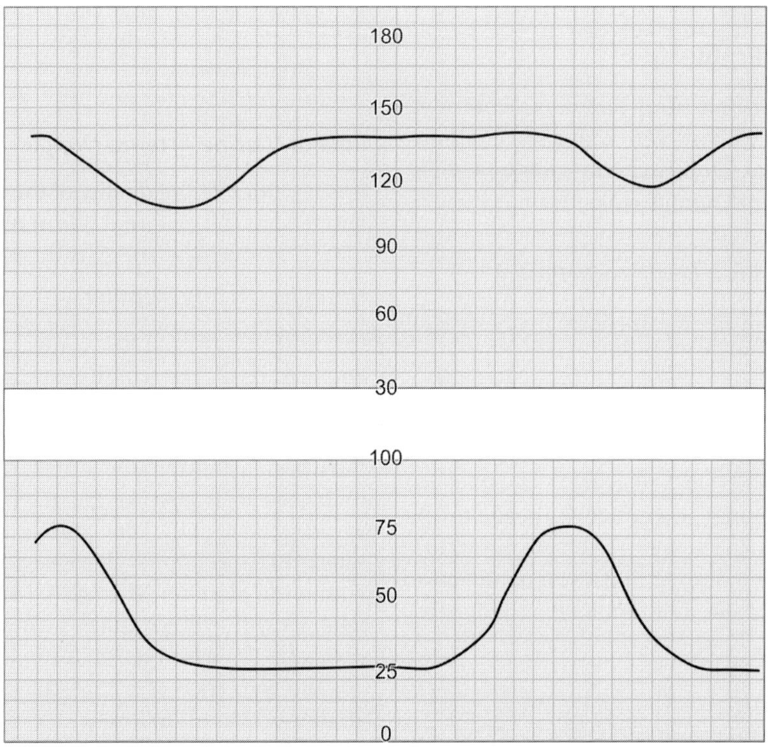

FIG. 4: Positive contraction stress test absent variability; deceleration present with uterine contraction.

The advantage of the CST is that it most closely approximates intrapartum surveillance of the fetus at risk.[13]

Biophysical Profile

It combines NST along with four sonographic variables (Table 3).[14] Each of the five variables is assigned a numerical value of 2 (if present or normal) and 0 (if absent or abnormal). The BPP variables are dependent on activity of certain areas of fetal central nervous system that respond to hypoxia. BPP can predict adverse outcome more precisely than NST and it can be used where NST is nonreactive. Biophysical profile should not be performed within 48–96 hours of administration of corticosteroids as they decrease the BPP transiently.

TABLE 3: Biophysical Profile (Manning's Score)

Biophysical variable	Score 2	Score 0
Nonstress test	Two or more accelerations of 15 or more beats per minute for 15 or more seconds in 20-40 min	Nil or one acceleration in 20-40 min
Fetal breathing movements	One or more episodes of rhythmic breathing episode lasting for 30 s or more within 30 min	Less than 30 s of breathing in 30 min
Fetal movement	Three or more discrete body or limb movements within 30 min	Less than three discrete movements in 30 min
Fetal tone	One or more episode of limb extension or opening or closing of a hand within 30 min	No movements or no extension or flexion in 30 min
Amniotic fluid volume	Single vertical pocket of >2 cm	Largest single vertical pocket <2 cm

Limitations

- Expensive
- Time consuming
- Subjective
- Not validated for fetuses less than 32 weeks.

Modified Biophysical Profile

This combines the observation of an index of acute fetal hypoxia—the NST with or without VAS, with a second index indicative of chronic fetal problems—the amniotic fluid indexes. It takes only about 10 minutes to perform.

Guidelines for Using Modified Biophysical Profile

- If both NST and the fluid volume are normal, weekly fetal surveillance may be done with MBPP
- If both tests are abdominal and pregnancy is beyond 36 weeks, termination of pregnancy is indicated
- If amniotic fluid is decreased but the NST is reactive, a search for indicators of placental insufficiency or undiagnosed ruptured membranes need to be undertaken
- If amniotic fluid volume is normal, and NST is nonreactive, further testing with Doppler, CST or full BPP is indicated.

Doppler Studies

With Doppler studies, fetal and maternal vessels are interrogated with ultrasound waves. The frequency shift caused by moving red cells is submitted to spectrographic analysis and represented graphically as a waveform which show change in velocity of blood. Velocity is greater in systole than in diastole. When peripheral vascular resistance is low, a good amount of blood flow occurs during diastole but when resistance is high, most of the blood flow will occur during systole and diastolic flow will be minimal. Thus, a simple visual analysis of the waveforms provides a qualitative measurement of the resistance to flow in the vessels that are being examined.

Role of Umbilical and Middle Cerebral Artery Doppler

- As complementary to other methods of fetal surveillance
- As a follow-up test when the results shown by other tests are equivocal
- Will precisely determine the need to deliver
- To identify women at risk of placental insufficiency
- Middle cerebral artery (MCA) is used to evaluate severity of fetal anemia.

Role of Uterine Arteries Doppler

It is an index of the quality of the uteroplacental circulation and reflects the maternal side of placental circulation.

Umbilical Artery Doppler

In normal pregnancy, fetal umbilical circulation is characterized by continuous forward flow, i.e., low resistance, to the placenta, which improves with gestational age as primary, secondary and tertiary branching continues, thus decreasing resistance to flow all the way to term.[15,16] Increased resistance is characterized by abnormal systolic to diastolic (S/D) ratio, pulsatility index (PI), or resistive index (RI) and implies decreased functioning vascular units within the placenta. The limited availability of substrates for fetal growth will produce a compensatory hemodynamic response, known as centralization of flow (Figs 5 and 6).

The sequence of events thus observed by the Doppler studies of UA is as follows:

- Increased UA resistance without centralization of flow
- Increased UA resistance with centralization of flow
- Absent UA diastolic flow
- Reversed UA diastolic flow
- Alteration in venous circulation.

Interpretation of changes in UA Doppler is given in table 4.

Uterine Artery Doppler

One of the most important physiological adaptations of the pregnancy is invasion of spiral arteries by cytotrophoblast.

TABLE 4: Interpretation of Doppler study of umbilical artery

Increased umbilical artery (UA) resistance without centralization of flow	• Systolic to diastolic (S/D) ratio of UA above normal limits • S/D ratio in middle cerebral artery (MCA) will remain normal	• Close fetal surveillance
Increased UA resistance with centralization of blood flow	• Brain sparing effect • MCA S/D ratio < UA S/D ratio • MCA becomes a low-resistance vessel	• Closer surveillance • Not an indication of immediate delivery
Absent UA diastolic flow	• UA blood flow occur only during systolic • Mild metabolic acidosis	• Intra-uterine life should be maintained only if expectancy is better than delivery
Reversed UA diastolic flow	• Blood flow is revered during diastole	• To be delivered immediately

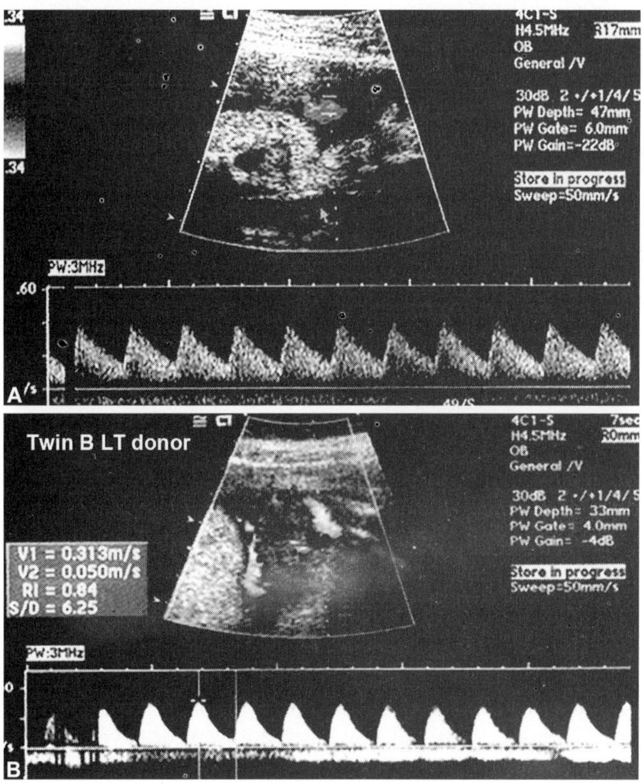

FIGS 5: A, Normal umbilical artery waveform and **B,** abnormal umbilical artery waveforms showing absent diastolic flow.

This increases their diameter from 15–20 μm to approximately 300–500 μm. Thus, transformation of a high-resistance vascular system to one of low resistance and high capacitance

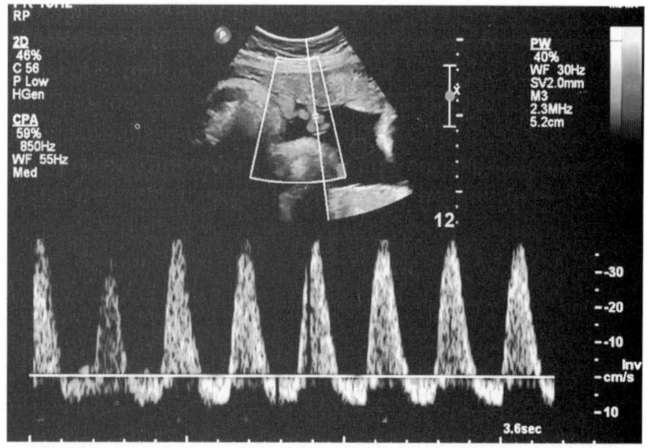

FIG. 6: Reversal of diastolic flow in umbilical artery *(For color version, see Plate 1).*

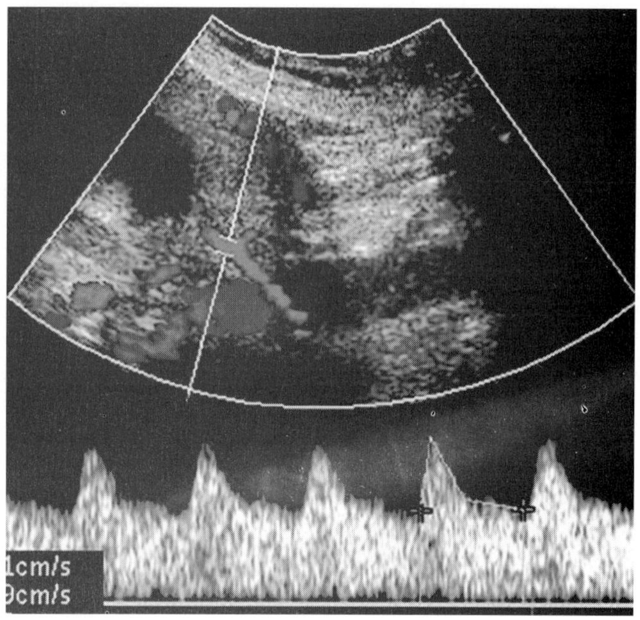

FIG. 7: Normal uterine artery Doppler waveforms *(For color version, see Plate 1).*

occurs. This results in 10-fold increase in blood flow (Fig. 7). Abnormalities in this fundamental component of normal placentation are associated with pregnancy complications like pre-eclampsia, fetal growth restriction (FGR), preterm labor and intra-uterine fetal death.

Several indices are available to assess the changes in resistance to flow in the uterine arteries. They are similar to those used in the evaluation of UA flow (S/D ratio, PI, and RI) plus early diastolic notching (Fig. 8). The notch is an index of increased impedance to flow and corresponds to a brief sharp decrease in velocity before the beginning of diastole

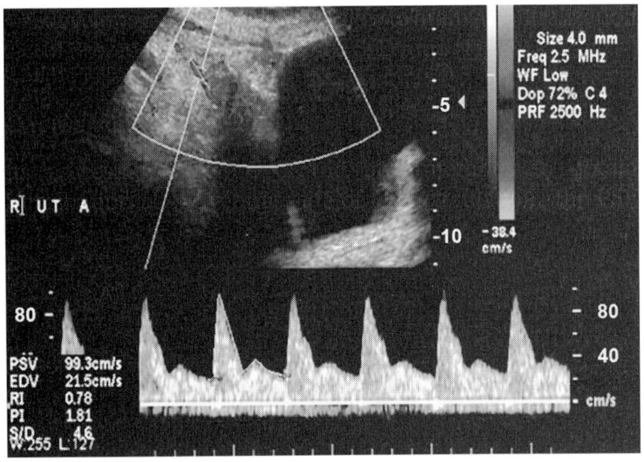

FIG. 8: Early diastolic notch in uterine artery *(For color version, see Plate 1).*

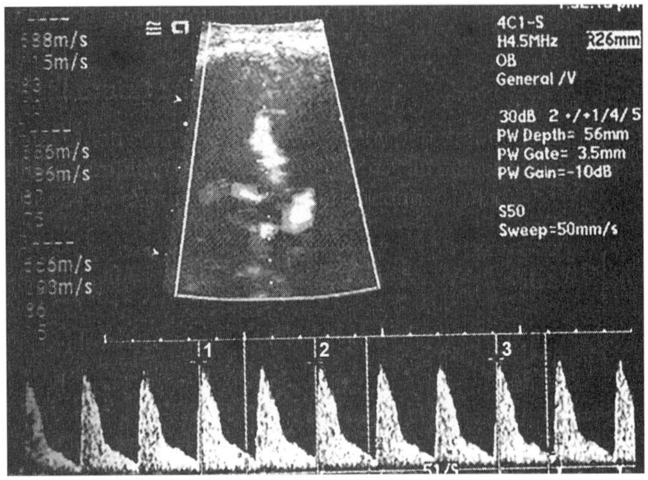

FIG. 9: Normal middle cerebral artery Doppler waveform showing high resistance to flow.

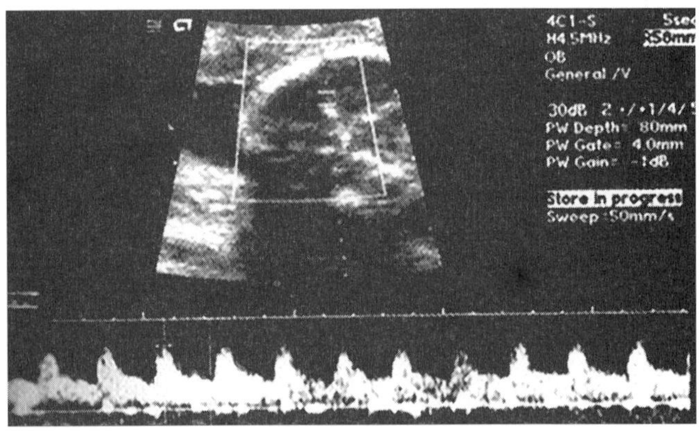

FIG. 10: Abundant flow in middle cerebral artery showing centralization of flow.

with a nadir smaller than the peak diastolic velocity. The pathological threshold values for different indices of uterine artery resistance are:
- Systolic to diastolic ratio more than 3.0 after 30 weeks
- Resistive index more than 0.56
- Presence of protodiastolic notch in the placental ipsilateral side at 20 weeks or in the contralateral side after 26 weeks
- Pulsatility index more than 1.56.

Abnormal placentation occurs long before the clinical appearance of obstetrical complications. Thus, uterine artery Doppler can be used as screening test particularly for pre-eclampsia, FGR, and abnormal pregnancy outcome. Abnormal uterine artery Doppler after 24 weeks of gestation is associated with development of pre-eclampsia and intrauterine growth restriction (IUGR). The positive-predictive value of this test is low but it has got a high negative-predictive value.

Middle Cerebral Artery

Many authors conclude that MCA peak systolic velocity (PSV) is highly correlated with severe fetal anemia (sensitivity as high as 100%).[17-19]

This is very useful for Rh-isoimmunized fetuses, but can be useful in compromised fetuses also.
- Middle cerebral artery waveform show minimal diastolic flow (high-resistant vessel) as shown in figure 9
- With impaired blood flow, compensatory response develops resulting increased flow to brain—centralization of flow resulting in decreased S/D ratio (Fig. 10).

Ductus Venosus Doppler

Its assessment is one of the best methods to obtain information about venous side of fetal circulation. The PSV in ductus venosus is in the range of 40–80 cm/sec (Fig. 11A). When the foramen ovale closes during atrial contraction, the ductus venosus waveform reflects the pressure on the right atrial (RA) and the atrial contraction in the waveform is a reflection of the right ventricular preload.

If fetal compromise occurs due to placental insufficiency, in its final stage the academia affect the fetal cardiac function causing an increase in right ventricular preload. This results in interrupted forward flow due to absent or reversed flow during atrial contraction revealing poor fetal health and morbid neonatal outcome (Fig. 11B).

Fetal Blood Sampling

Fetal blood sampling can be done by percutaneous umbilical blood sampling (cordocentesis). This can be performed easily after 24 weeks under ultrasound guidance (Box 1).

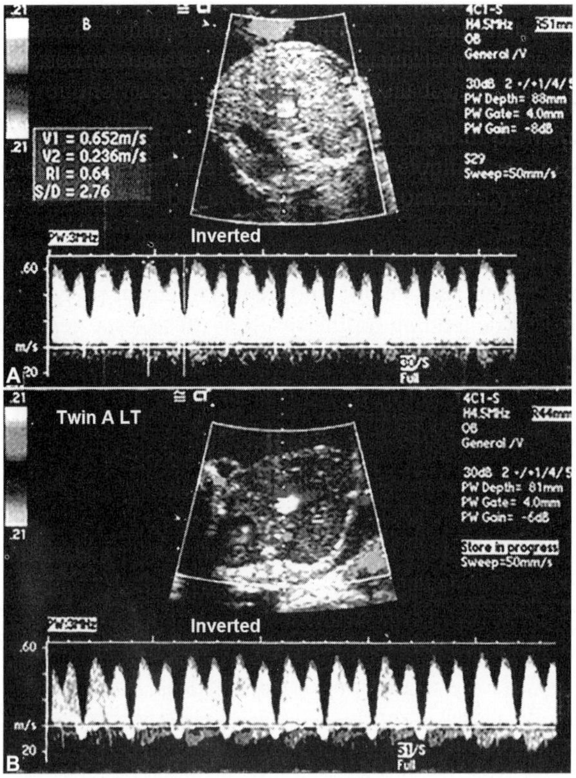

FIGS 11: Ductus venosus waveforms: **A,** Normal and **B,** abnormal showing interrupted and reversed forward flow during atrial systole.

Box 1: Indications for cordocentesis

- Rapid karyotyping in fetuses with structural abnormalities discovered during ultrasound
- Fetal hemolytic disease
- Suspected fetal viral injection
- Nonimmune hydrops
- Suspected fetal thrombocytopenia
- Twin-to-twin transfusion
- Suspected fetal hemoglobinopathy

Main risks are bleeding from puncture site and vagal reflex causing severe bradycardia.

The use of cordocentesis has declined with the use of other noninvasive methods for fetal diagnosis.

Placental Grading

The Grannum classification of placental grading[20] according to senescent charges seen on ultrasound examination has been used for some to reduce perinatal mortality. However, it is not routinely used as there is no consensus on its use.

Fetal lung maturation tests: they can be used in premature fetuses to predict the chances of developing respiratory distress syndrome but are not often used practically.

RECOMMENDATIONS[21]

Recommendation I: Fetal Movement Counting

- Daily monitoring of FMs starting at 26–32 weeks should be done in all pregnancies with risk factors for adverse perinatal outcome (level of evidence I-A)
- Healthy pregnant women without risk factors should be made aware of the significance of FMs in the third trimester and asked to perform a FM count if they perceive decreased movements (level of evidence I-B)
- Women who do not perceive six movements in an interval of 2 hours require further antenatal testing and should contact their caregivers or hospital as soon as possible (level of evidence III-B)
- Women who report decreased FMs (<6 distinct movements within 2 hours) should have a complete evaluation of maternal and fetal status, including NST and/or BPP. Prior to considering an intervention for fetal well-being, an anatomical scan to rule out a fetal malformation should be done, if one has not already been done. Management should be based upon the following:
    - NST is normal and there are no risk factors: the woman should continue with DFMC (level of evidence III-B)
    - NST is normal and risk factors or clinical suspicion of IUGR/oligohydramnios is identified: an ultrasound for either full BPP or amniotic fluid volume assessment within 24 hours. The woman should continue with DFMC (level of evidence III-B)
    - NST is atypical/abnormal: further testing (BPP and/or CST and assessment of amniotic fluid volume) should be performed as soon as possible (level of evidence III-B).

Recommendation II: Nonstress Test

- Antepartum NST may be considered when risk factors for adverse perinatal outcome are present (level of evidence III-B)
- In the presence of a normal NST, usual FM patterns, and absence of suspected oligohydramnios, it is not necessary to conduct a BPP or CST (level of evidence III-B)
- A normal NST should be classified and documented by an appropriately trained and designated individual as soon as possible (ideally within 24 hours). For atypical or abnormal NSTs, the nurse should inform the attending physician (or primarycare provider) at the time that the classification is apparent. An abnormal NST should be viewed by the attending physician (or primarycare provider) and documented immediately (level of evidence III-B).

Recommendation III: Contraction Stress Test

- The CST should be considered in the presence of an atypical NST as a proxy for the adequacy of intrapartum

uteroplacental function and together with the clinical circumstances, will aid in decision making about timing and mode of delivery (level of evidence III-B)
- The CST should not be performed when vaginal delivery is contraindicated (level of evidence III-B)
- The CST should be performed in a setting where emergency cesarean section is available (level of evidence III-B).

Recommendation IV: Biophysical Profile

- In pregnancies at increased risk for adverse perinatal outcome and where facilities and expertise exist, BPP is recommended for evaluation of fetal well-being (level of evidence I-A)
- When an abnormal BPP is obtained, the responsible physician or delegate should be informed immediately. Further management will be determined by the overall clinical situation (level of evidence III-B).

Recommendation V: Uterine Artery Doppler

- Where facilities and expertise exist, UA Doppler may be performed at the time of 17–22 weeks' gestation detailed anatomical ultrasound scan in women with the following factors for adverse perinatal outcome (level of evidence II-A)
- Women with a positive UA Doppler screen should have the following:
  - A double marker screen (for α-fetoprotein and β-human chorionic gonadotropin) if at or before 18 weeks' gestation (level of evidence III-C)
  - A second UA Doppler at 24–26 weeks. If the UA Doppler is positive at the second scan, the woman should be referred to a maternal-fetal medicine specialist for management (level of evidence III-C).

Recommendation VI: Umbilical Artery Doppler

- Umbilical artery Doppler should not be used as a screening tool in healthy pregnancies, as it has not been shown to be of value in this group (level of evidence I-A)
- Umbilical artery Doppler should be available for assessment of the fetal placental circulation in pregnant women with suspected placental insufficiency. Fetal UA Doppler assessment should be considered at time of referral for suspected growth restriction, or during follow-up for suspected placental pathology (level of evidence I-A)
- Depending on other clinical factors, reduced, absent, or reversed UA end-diastolic flow is an indication for enhanced fetal surveillance or delivery. If delivery is delayed to improve fetal lung maturity with maternal administration of glucocorticoids, intensive fetal surveillance until delivery is suggested for those fetuses with reversed end-diastolic flow (level of evidence II-1B).

CONCLUSION

Antepartum fetal surveillance is important especially in high risk pregnancies. A battery of testing modalities can be used which include fetal movement assessment, nonstress test, contraction stress test, fetal biophysical profile, and umbilical artery Doppler velocimetry. Initiation of testing at 32–34 weeks of gestation is appropriate for most pregnancies. A reassuring test should be repeated periodically depending on the high risk factors. The management of pregnancy is planned depending on the result of these tests, gestational age, amount of liquor, and maternal conditions.

REFERENCES

1. ACOG practice bulletin. Antepartum fetal surveillance. Number 9, October 1999, (replaces Technical Bulletin Number 188, January 1994). Clinical management guidelines for obstetrician-gynecologists. Int J Gynaecol Obstet. 2000;68(2):175-85.
2. Williams KP, Farquharson DF, Bebbington M, Dansereau J, Galerneau F, Wilson RD, et al. Screening for fetal well-being in a high-risk pregnant population comparing the nonstress test with umbilical artery Doppler velocimetry: a randomized controlled clinical trial. Am J Obstet Gynecol. 2003;188(5):1366-71.
3. James DK, Steer PJ, Weiner CP, Gonik B. High Risk Pregnancy: Management Options, 3rd ed. Philadelphia, PA, USA: Elsevier Saunders; 2006.
4. Miller DA, Rabello YA, Paul RH. The modified biophysical profile: antepartum testing in the 1990s. Am J Obstet Gynecol. 1996;174(3):812-7.
5. Pearson JF, Weaver JB. Fetal activity and fetal wellbeing: an evaluation. Br Med J. 1976;1(6021):1305-7.
6. Baskett TF, Liston RM. Fetal movement monitoring: clinical application. Clin Perinatol. 1989;16(3):613-25.
7. Moore TR, Piacquadio K. A prospective evaluation of fetal movement screening to reduce the incidence of antepartum fetal death. Am J Obstet Gynecol. 1989;160(5 Pt 1):1075-80.
8. Hannah ME, Hannah WJ, Hellmann J, Hewson S, Milner R, Willan A. Induction of labor as compared with serial antenatal monitoring in post-term pregnancy. A randomized controlled trial. The Canadian Multicenter Post-term Pregnancy Trial Group. N Engl J Med. 1992;326(24):1587-92.
9. Barrett JM, Salyer SL, Boehm FH. The nonstress test: an evaluation of 1,000 patients. Am J Obstet Gynecol. 1981;141(2):153-7.
10. Miller JM, Horger EO. Antepartum heart rate testing in diabetic pregnancy. J Reprod Med. 1985;30(7):515-8.
11. Cito G, Luisi S, Mezzesimi A, Cavicchioli C, Calonaci G, Petraglia F. Maternal position during non-stress test and fetal heart rate patterns. Acta Obstet Gynecol Scand. 2005;84(4):335-8.
12. Miller DA. Antepartum testing. Clin Obstet Gynecol. 1998;41(3):647-53.
13. Lagrew DC. The contraction stress test. Clin Obstet Gynecol. 1995;38(1):11-25.
14. Manning FA. Dynamic ultrasound-based fetal assessment: the fetal biophysical profile score. Clin Obstet Gynecol. 1995;38(1):26-44.
15. Adamson SL. Arterial pressure, vascular input impedance, and resistance as determinants of pulsatile blood flow in the umbilical artery. Eur J Obstet Gynecol Reprod Biol. 1999;84(2):119-25.
16. Kingdom JC, Burrell SJ, Kaufmann P. Pathology and clinical implications of abnormal umbilical artery Doppler waveforms. Ultrasound Obstet Gynecol. 1997;9(4):271-86.

17. Mari G, Deter RL, Carpenter RL, Rahman F, Zimmerman R, Moise KJ, et al. Noninvasive diagnosis by Doppler ultrasonography of fetal anemia due to maternal red-cell alloimmunization. Collaborative Group for Doppler Assessment of the Blood Velocity in Anemic Fetuses. N Engl J Med. 2000;342(1):9-14.
18. Kutschera J, Tomaselli J, Urlesberger B, Maurer U, Hausler M, Gradnitzer E, et al. Absent or reversed end-diastolic blood flow in the umbilical artery and abnormal Doppler cerebroplacental ratio--cognitive, neurological and somatic development at 3 to 6 years. Early Hum Dev. 2002;69(1-2):47-56.
19. Detti L, Mari G, Akiyama M, Cosmi E, Moise KJ, Stefor T, et al. Longitudinal assessment of the middle cerebral artery peak systolic velocity in healthy fetuses and in fetuses at risk for anemia. Am J Obstet Gynecol. 2002;187(4):937-9.
20. Grannum PA, Berkowitz RL, Hobbins JC. The ultrasonic changes in the maturing placenta and their relation to fetal pulmonic maturity. Am J Obstet Gynecol. 1979;133(8):915-22.
21. Society of Obstetricians and Gynaecologists of Canada. Antenatal Fetal Surveillance. J Obstet Gynaecol Can. 2007;29(9 Suppl 4):s9-24.

CHAPTER 7

Imaging in Third Trimester

Neha Gupta

INTRODUCTION

Since the first application of ultrasound in 1958 by Ian Donald and coworkers, it has now become part and parcel of modern day obstetrics. With the advances in technology and computer processing, it is crucial for the assessment of fetal anatomy, growth, and well being.

There are three types of sonographic evaluation for the second and 3rd trimester:

1. Standard second or third trimester examinations
2. Limited examination: it is performed when a specific question requires investigation, e.g., amniotic fluid assessment, placental localization
3. Specialized examinations: a detailed anatomic evaluation. Other specialized examinations might include fetal Doppler ultrasound, biophysical profile, fetal echocardiogram, or additional biometric measurements.

Sonography should be performed for valid clinical indication and with lowest possible exposure settings: the ALARA (as low as reasonably achievable) principle (American Institute of Ultrasound in Medicine 2008).[1] All women undergoing sonographic examination should be explained about its limitations.

The main indications of second and third trimester ultrasound examinations[2] are as mentioned in box 1. This chapter will restrict to main use of imaging in the third trimester.

Box 1: Indications for second and third trimester ultrasonography

- Estimation of gestational age
- Evaluation of fetal growth
- Evaluation of vaginal bleeding
- Evaluation of cervical insufficiency
- Evaluation of abdominal and pelvic pain
- Determination of fetal presentation
- Evaluation of suspected multiple gestation
- Adjunct to amniocentesis or other procedure
- Significant discrepancy between uterine size and clinical dates
- Evaluation of pelvic mass
- Examination of suspected hydatidiform mole
- Adjunct to cervical cerclage placement
- Evaluation of suspected ectopic pregnancy
- Evaluation of suspected fetal death
- Evaluation of suspected uterine abnormality
- Evaluation for fetal well-being
- Evaluation of suspected amniotic fluid abnormalities
- Evaluation of suspected placental abruption
- Adjunct to external cephalic version
- Evaluation for premature rupture of membranes or premature labor
- Evaluation for abnormal biomechanical markers
- Follow-up evaluation of a fetal anomaly
- Follow-up evaluation of placental location for suspected placenta previa
- Evaluation for those with a history of previous congenital anomaly
- Evaluation of fetal condition in late registrants for prenatal care
- To assess findings that may increase the risk of aneuploidy
- To screen for fetal anomalies

CLINICAL APPLICATIONS

Estimation of Gestational Age

The accurate dating of pregnancy is necessary for determination of viability in cases of premature labor, intrauterine growth restriction (IUGR), or induction as in cases of postdates.

First trimester crown-rump length (CRL) is the most accurate means for dating the pregnancy followed by head circumference (HC) when CRL is greater than 84 mm. But what to do when the patient first presents in the third trimester? The precision of prediction of gestational age (GA) by different parameters is mentioned in table 1.

A combination of biometric parameters, like biparietal diameter (BPD), HC, abdominal circumference (AC), and femoral length (FL), should be used than just a single parameter. A follow-up interval scan to assign accurate due date is done at 2–3 weeks.[3]

- Fetal pulmonary system has a relatively late maturation and the risk of respiratory distress syndrome (RDS) is practically zero once a fetus has completed 39 menstrual weeks. Criteria to determine pulmonary maturity include:[4]
    - Fetal heart beat documented for 20 weeks by stethoscope or 30 weeks by Doppler
    - Passage of 36 weeks since a positive serum or urinary pregnancy test
    - Crown-rump length at 6–11 weeks support GA more than or equal to 39 weeks
    - Sonographic measurement at 12–20 weeks support GA more than or equal to 39 weeks
- Additional GA markers, alone are insufficiently accurate to determine GA but serve as a confirmatory marker that the dates assigned on the basis of biometric parameters is fairly accurate:
    - Distal femoral epiphysis not seen before 28 weeks but is seen in 94% fetuses at 34 weeks[5]
    - Proximal tibial epiphysis, not seen before 34 weeks, but is seen in 100% of fetuses beyond 39 weeks[5]
    - Transverse cerebellar diameter and foot length (spared in IUGR)
    - Colonic haustrations, presence indicates at least 30 weeks of GA

TABLE 1: Precision of predictors of gestational age in the second and third trimesters

Predictor	Gestational age interval (in weeks)			
	14–20	20–26	26–32	32–42
Biparietal diameter (BPD)	1.4 (108)	2.1 (81)	3.8 (100)	4.1 (171)
Corrected BPD	1.2 (100)	1.9 (78)	3.3 (85)	3.8 (85)
Femoral length	1.4 (100)	2.5 (79)	3.1 (104)	3.5 (174)
Head circumference	1.2 (100)	1.9 (78)	3.4 (85)	3.8 (85)
Abdominal circumference	2.1 (98)	3.7 (83)	3.0 (101)	4.5 (166)

Note: Numbers are 2 standard deviations (SDs; in weeks) for predicted gestational age based on number of patients (indicated in parentheses).

- Placental grading has no role
- Others being small intestinal peristalsis, colonic echogenicity.

Fetal Well-being

Estimation of Fetal Weight

Formulas and nomograms are based on the combinations of BPD, HC, AC, and FL.

Biparietal diameter: BPD (Fig. 1) is measured at level of cavum septum pellucidi and ventricular atrium, from outer to outer/outer to inner edge of the skull, depending on which charts you are using.

Head circumference: it can be taken in two ways:

1. Ellipse method (Fig. 2): it is an automated method, depends on which machine you are using (whether the machine has it or not)
2. Derived from measurements of occipitofrontal diameter (OFD) and BPD (Fig. 2).

It is the most reliable parameters for estimating menstrual age because of its shape independence, its ease of measurement (and therefore accuracy), and its predictive value for GA. It can predict menstrual age to within 1 week [2 standard deviations (SDs)] before 20 weeks' gestation to 3.8 weeks (2 SDs) in the late third trimester.

Transventricular plane is used; should have cavum septum pellucidi, posterior horn of ventricle. Biparietal diameter and OFD are measured from outer to outer portions of the vault of the skull. It actually depends on what software/chart you are using:

Abdominal circumference: AC is the most variable measurement, and taken at the skin line on a transverse view

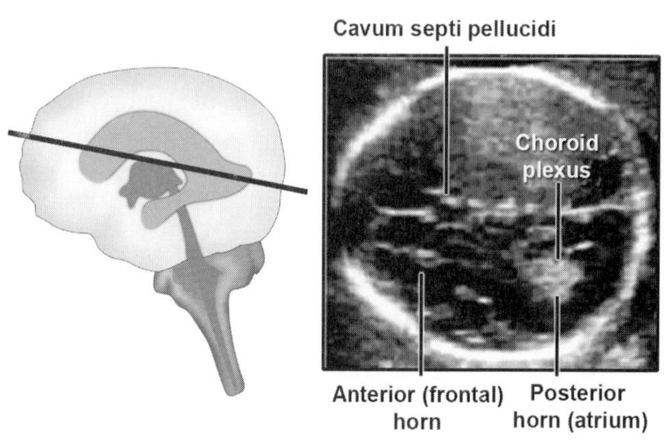

FIG. 1: The transventricular plane obtained by a transverse scan at the level of the cavum septum pellucidum will demonstrate the lateral borders of the anterior (or frontal) horns, the medial and lateral borders of the posterior horns (or atria) of the lateral ventricles, the choroid plexuses and the Sylvian fissures.

at the level of junction of the umbilical vein, portal sinus, and fetal stomach, when visible (Fig. 3).

Two methods:
1. Ellipse method (Fig. 3)
2. Anteroposterior abdominal diameter and transverse abdominal diameter.

Femoral length: long-axis of the shaft excluding distal femoral epiphysis (Fig. 4).[6,7]

Commonly used formulas are Hadlock and Shephard. Hadlock is better than Shephard as based on three fetal parameters (HC, AC, FL), thereby reducing the error by 15–25%.

Abnormalities of the Growth

Intrauterine growth restriction with estimated fetal weight less than 5th percentile and low gestational age (LGA) more than 95th percentile for the GA: these are beyond the scope of this chapter.

Interval Growth Velocity

Minimum interval between scans to be kept is 3 weeks to reduce the false positive diagnosis of abnormal growth to check whether maintaining its growth velocity or plateauing or falling off the curve (Fig. 5).[8,9]

The author use growth curves introduced by Yudkin et al. at her center.[9] This shows an early-onset IUGR, but the growth velocity has been maintained.

Amniotic Fluid Estimation

Evaluation of amniotic fluid is an integral part of evaluation of IUGR or post-term pregnancy. The factors involved in regulating amniotic fluid volume (AFV) are still not completely understood. There are six proposed pathways (Brace, 1997)[10] for fluid movement into and out of the amniotic cavity as enumerated in table 2.

Two main methods are used to measure amniotic fluid:
1. Deepest vertical pocket (Fig. 6): the concept of measuring single deepest amniotic fluid pocket free of umbilical cord and fetal parts [maximum vertical pocket (MVP)] was introduced by Chamberlain in 1984.[11] It is the best method for evaluation of amniotic fluid in multifetal pregnancies:
   i. Oligohydramnios: MVP less than 2 cm (MVP <3 cm in each sac in multifetal pregnancies)
   ii. Polyhydramnios: MVP more than 8 cm
2. Amniotic fluid index (AFI) (Box 2, Figs 7 and 8): sum of the deepest amniotic fluid pockets measured in the four

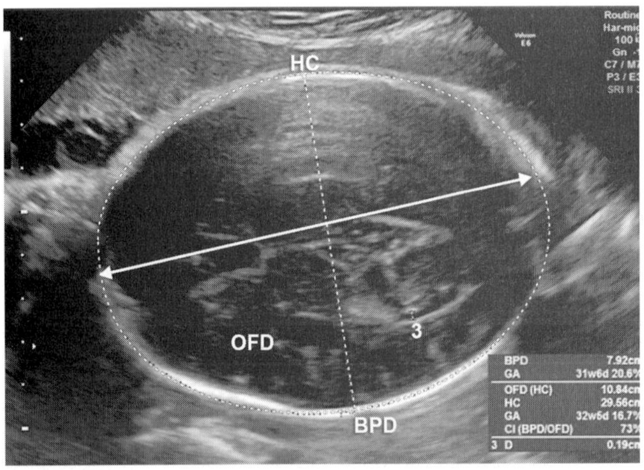

FIG. 2: Head circumference measurement showing ellipse as well as biparietal diameter and occipitofrontal diameter method.

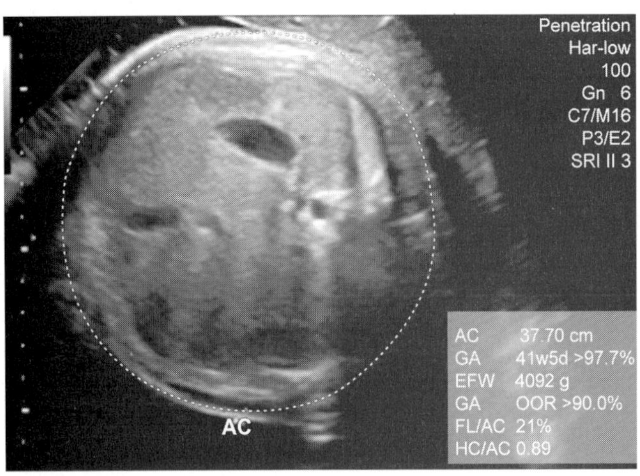

FIG. 3: Abdominal circumference measurement by the use of ellipse method.

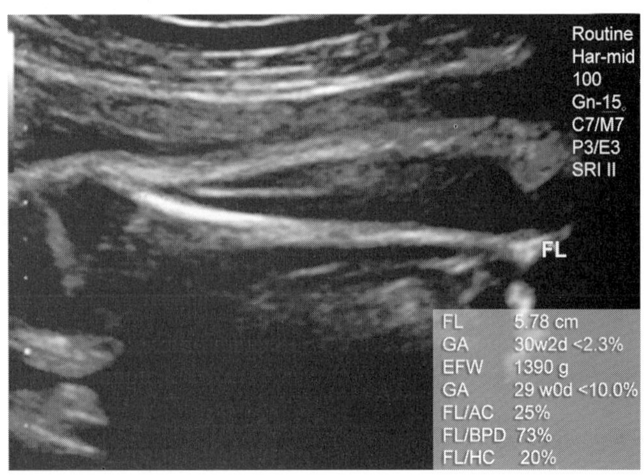

FIG. 4: Femoral length measurement.[7]

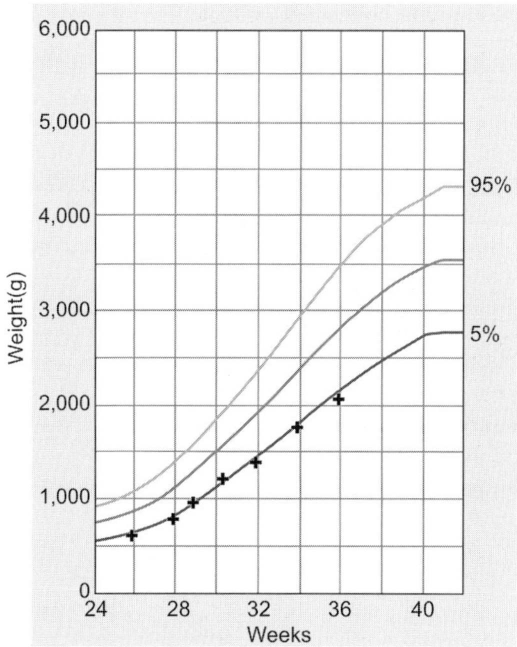

FIG. 5: Estimated fetal weight.[9]

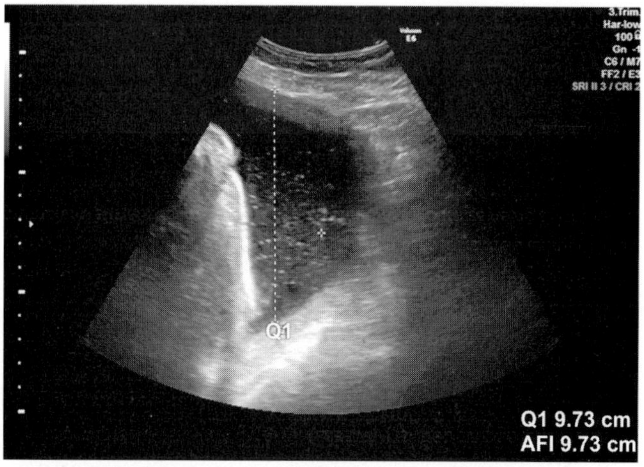

FIG. 6: Deepest vertical pocket: single deepest amniotic fluid pocket free of umbilical cord and fetal parts (maximum vertical pocket).

TABLE 2: Pathways for amniotic fluid movement in and out of amniotic cavity

Pathway	mL/day to the fetus	mL/day to amniotic fluid
Fetal swallowing	500–1,000	–
Oral secretions	–	25
Secretions from the respiratory tract	170	170
Fetal urination	–	800–1,200
Intramembranous flow across the placenta, umbilical cord, and fetals	200–500	–
Transmembraneous flow from the amniotic cavity into the uterine circulation	–	10

Box 2: Amniotic fluid index technique[13]

- Position patient supine
- A linear, curvilinear, or sector transducer can be used
- Divide the uterus into four quadrants using the maternal sagittal midline vertically, and arbitrary transverse line approximately halfway between the symphysis pubis and the upper edge of the uterine fundus (Fig. 7)
- The transducer must be kept parallel to the maternal sagittal plane and perpendicular to the maternal coronal plane throughout
- The deepest unobstructed and clear pocket of amniotic fluid is visualized, and the image frozen. The ultrasound calipers are manipulated to measure the pocket in a strictly vertical direction
- The process is repeated in each of four quadrants and the pocket measurements summed = AFI
- If the AFI is <8 cm, perform the four quadrant evaluation three times and average the values:
  - Oligohydramnios: AFI <8 cm
  - Polyhydramnios: AFI >24 cm

quadrants of the gravid uterus was introduced by Phelan in 1987.[12,13] The range of AFI across gestation is depicted in table 3.[14]

Pitfalls in the measurement of amniotic fluid

- Excessive transducer pressure can cause 21% decrease in AFI
- Avoid pockets with umbilical cord: color Doppler assists in this regard
- Obesity as fat scatters ultrasound beam, thereby erroneously decreasing AFI
- Free-floating particles due to vernix make amniotic fluid less conspicuous.

Biophysical Profile

The main aim of fetal surveillance is to identify fetuses at risk of intrauterine death and to identify these potential threats early enough to allow interventions to prevent adverse outcomes.

The nonstress test (NST) is the most frequently used method. A reactive NST is indicative that fetus is not asphyxiated at that time with high false positive rates of 50–75.[15]

The biophysical profile (BPP) (Table 4) gives a more complete evaluation of the state of fetal health.[16]

The gradual hypoxia concept:[17] biophysical activities that appear first in the fetal life are the last to disappear in asphyxiated or in intraamniotic infection.

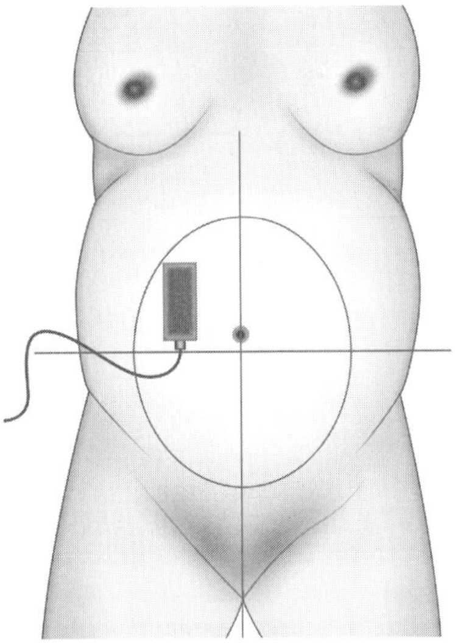

FIG. 7: The uterus divided into four quadrants between the symphysis pubis and the upper edge of the uterine fundus.

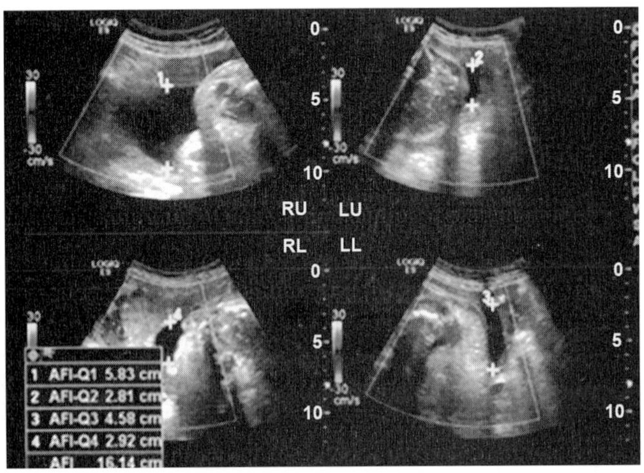

FIG. 8: Amniotic fluid index technique *(For color version, see Plate 1)*.

TABLE 3: Amniotic fluid index values in normal pregnancy[14]

Weeks	2.5th percentile	5th percentile	Median	95th percentile	97th percentile
16	7.3	7.9	12.1	18.5	20.1
17	7.7	8.3	12.7	19.4	21.1
18	8.0	8.7	13.3	20.2	22.0
19	8.3	9.0	13.7	20.7	22.5
20	8.6	9.3	14.1	21.2	23.0
21	8.8	9.5	14.3	21.4	23.3
22	8.9	9.7	14.5	21.6	23.5
23	9.0	9.8	14.6	21.8	23.7
24	9.0	9.8	14.7	21.9	23.8
25	8.9	9.7	14.7	22.1	24.0
26	8.9	9.7	14.7	22.3	24.2
27	8.5	9.5	14.6	22.6	24.5
28	8.6	9.4	14.6	22.8	24.9
29	8.4	9.2	14.5	23.1	25.4
30	8.2	9.0	14.5	23.4	25.8
31	7.9	8.8	14.4	23.8	26.3
32	7.7	8.6	14.4	24.2	26.9
33	7.4	8.3	14.3	24.5	27.4
34	7.2	8.1	14.2	24.8	27.8
35	7.0	7.9	14.0	24.9	27.9
36	6.8	7.7	13.8	24.9	27.9
37	6.6	7.5	13.5	24.4	27.5
38	6.5	7.3	13.2	23.9	26.9
39	6.4	7.2	12.7	22.6	25.5
40	6.3	7.1	12.3	21.4	24.0
41	6.3	7.0	11.6	19.4	21.6
42	6.3	6.9	11.0	17.5	19.2

TABLE 4: Biophysical profile

Biophysical variable	Normal (score = 2)	Abnormal (score = 0)
Fetal breathing movements	One or more episodes of ≥20 s within 30 min	Absent or no episode of ≥20 s within 30 min
Gross body movements	Two or more discrete body/limb movements within 30 min (episodes of active continuous movement considered as a single movement)	Less than two episodes of body/limb movements within 30 min
Fetal tone	One or more episodes of active extension with return to flexion of fetal limb(s) or trunk (opening and closing of hand considered normal tone)	Slow extension with return to partial flexion, movement of limb in full extension, absent fetal movement, partially open fetal hand
Reactive fetal heart rate (FHR)	Two or more episodes of acceleration of ≥15 beats/min and of >15 s associated with fetal movement within 20 min	One or more episodes of acceleration of FHR or acceleration of <15 beats/min within 20 min
Qualitative amniotic fluid volume	One or more pockets of fluid measuring ≥2 cm in vertical axis	Either no pockets or largest pocket <2 cm in vertical axis

The first to get compromised in fetal hypoxia are fetal heart reactivity and fetal breathing movements followed by fetal movements and then fetal tone.

Modified biophysical profile:[18] this denotes a testing scheme using the NST with evaluation of amniotic fluid. Thus, this modification assesses both the most sensitive acute marker (fetal heart tracing) and chronic marker (AFV) of fetal well-being.

Hemodynamic Modifications

Both arterial and venous Doppler have been used to identify fetuses with IUGR and also to obtain additional information for planning delivery of fetuses at risk.

Fetal arterial Doppler

- Uterine artery Doppler: there is progressive decrease in impedance with advancing gestation. The uterine artery can be imaged as it crosses hypogastric artery and vein just before it enters uterine-cervical junction. Doppler to be taken as it crosses hypogastric artery and before it divides into uterine and cervical branches (Fig. 9):
  - An increasing uterine pulsatility index (PI) is suggestive of increasing impedance in uterine circulation as in IUGR and pre-eclampsia cases and signifies failed or inadequate invasion of maternal spiral arterioles in the second wave of invasion around 16 weeks
  - A mean uterine artery PI more than 95th percentile is suggestive of placental insufficiency and warrants close monitoring of fetal Dopplers.
- Umbilical artery Doppler: it reflects the status of the placental circulation. It is normally a low-diastolic impedance circulation with increase in the end-diastolic flow with advancing gestation[19]

  The most common measure of GA-specific umbilical artery resistance is:
  - Systolic/diastolic ratio
  - Pulsatility index: (S – D)/M
  - Resistance index (RI): (S – D)/S.

  Doppler artery waveforms are taken from a freely floating loop of cord. Waveforms obtained from placental end shows lower values of ratio than at fetal end (Fig. 10). In cases of placental insufficiency in IUGR, initially there is increase in umbilical artery PI-absent end-diastolic flow (AEDF) and ultimately reversed end-diastolic flow. Reversed end-diastolic flow denotes advanced stage of fetal compromise and is associated with more than 70% obliteration of placental arterial circulation.[20]
- Middle cerebral circulation: the cerebral circulation is a high impedance circulation with continuous forward flow throughout the cardiac cycle
  - In the presence of fetal hypoxemia, central redistribution of blood flow occur, resulting in an increased blood flow to the brain, heart, and adrenals, and a reduction in flow to the peripheral and placental circulations. The blood flow redistribution is known as the brain-sparing effect[21]
  - Circle of Willis can be imaged at the transverse plane of fetal head at the base of the skull. In this plane, proximal and distal middle cerebral arteries are seen in the long axis with their course almost parallel to the insonating ultrasound beam
  - Middle cerebral artery (MCA) waveforms obtained from the proximal portion of the vessel after its origin from the circle of the Willis (Fig. 11)
  - Thus, it is helpful in the assessment of IUGR:[22]
    - In the preterm small for gestational age (SGA) fetus, MCA Doppler has limited accuracy to predict acidemia and adverse outcome and should not be used to time delivery

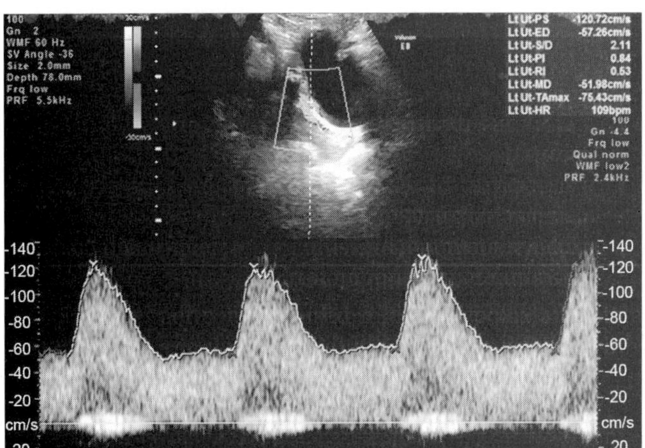

FIG. 9: Uterine artery Doppler *(For color version, see Plate 1).*

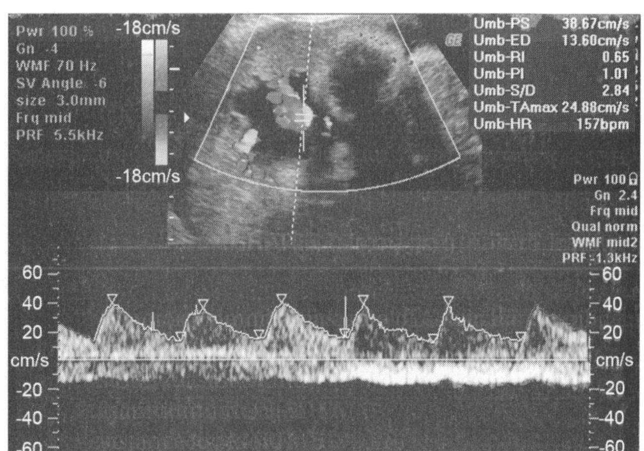

FIG. 10: Umbilical artery Doppler *(For color version, see Plate 1).*

- In the term SGA fetus with normal umbilical artery Doppler, an abnormal MCA Doppler (PI <5th centile) has moderate predictive value for acidosis at birth and should be used to time delivery
- Reduced MCA PI or MCA PI/umbilical artery PI (cerebroplacental ratio <1) is, therefore, an early sign of fetal hypoxia in SGA fetuses

- In Rh-isoimmunized pregnancy and anemia due to Parvovirus B19 infection, the MCA-peak systolic velocity (MCA-PSV) more than 1.5 multiple of median is suggestive of fetal anemia.

Fetal venous Doppler: Doppler waveforms obtained from the central venous circulation in the fetus reflects the physiologic status of the right ventricle:

- Ductus venosus: it can be easily obtained from a transverse view of the fetal abdomen at the same anatomic plane of the AC (Fig. 12). The presence of turbulence on color flow Doppler helps in identifying the ductus venosus. It has a biphasic form. The presence of positive "a" is suggestive of forward flow and is reassuring sign
- Umbilical vein: with severe right ventricular dysfunction, atrial contraction generates reverse flow in the venous system, and hence, pulsatile flow in the umbilical vein and negative "a" wave in the ductus venosus

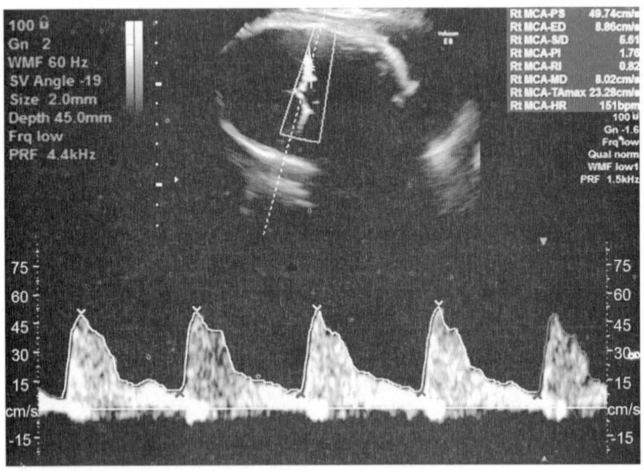

FIG. 11: Middle cerebral artery (MCA) Doppler *(For color version, see Plate 2).*

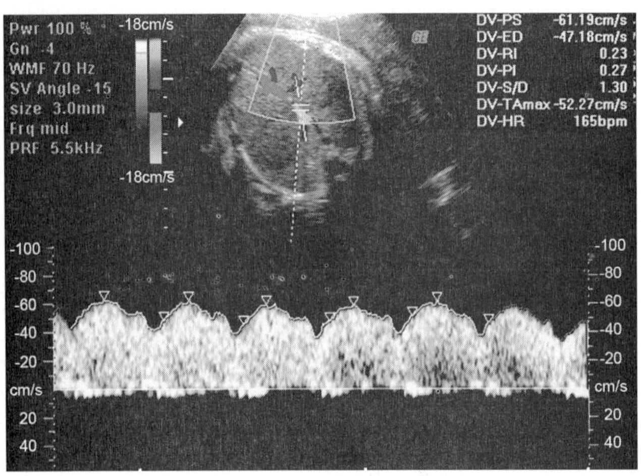

FIG. 12: Ductus venosus Doppler *(For color version, see Plate 2).*

Fetal Doppler and IUGR: in IUGR, there is sequential deterioration of arterial Dopplers followed by venous Dopplers, then abnormal cardiotocographic tracings and then, BPP. However, these sequential patterns are seen in 20% preterm fetuses.[23] Once centralization occurs, no specific trend can be seen in the observational period.

OTHER APPLICATIONS

Placenta

Placenta previa exists when the placenta is inserted wholly or in parts into the lower segment of the uterus. It is classified by ultrasound imaging according to what is relevant clinically:

- If the placenta lies over the internal cervical os, it is considered a major previa
- If the leading edge of the placenta is in the lower uterine segment (LUS) but not covering the cervical os, minor or partial previa exists.

Localization

Transvaginal scans (TVS) improve the accuracy of placental localization and are safe, so the suspected diagnosis of placenta previa at 20 weeks of gestation by abdominal scan should be confirmed by TVS:

- TVS is better at localization of low lying placenta [sensitivity = 87.5%, specificity = 98.8%, positive-predictive value = 93.3%, negative-predictive value = 97.6%, false-negative rate = 2.33%][24]
- All women require follow-up imaging if the placenta covers or overlaps the cervical os at 20 weeks of gestation[25]
- Women with a previous cesarean section (CS) require a higher index of suspicion as there are two problems to be excluded: placenta previa and placenta accreta. If the placenta lies anteriorly and reaches the cervical os at 20 weeks, a follow-up scan can help identify if it is implanted into the CS scar.[25]

Follow-up of Low Lying Placenta

- Women who bleed should be managed individually according to their needs
- In cases of asymptomatic women with suspected minor previa, follow-up imaging can be left until 36 weeks of gestation
- In cases with asymptomatic suspected major placenta previa or a question of placenta accreta, imaging should

be performed at around 32 weeks of gestation to clarify the diagnosis and allow planning for third-trimester management, further imaging, and delivery.[25]

Morbidly Adherent Placenta

A morbidly adherent placenta (MAP) includes placenta accreta, increta, and percreta as it penetrates through the decidua basalis into and then through the myometrium and up till the serosa.

There has been increase in the incidence of MAP over the years. The main risk factors being age greater than 35 years, previous curettage, multiparity, and previous lower segment cesarean section (LSCS).

The incidence of MAP increases with increase in number of LSCS:[25]

- Without previa 0.04%
- With placenta previa 9.3%
- Previa with previous CS 24%
- Four CSs 67%.

Role of Ultrasound in Diagnosis of Morbidly Adherent Placenta[26]

Features on gray scale:

- Loss of the retroplacental sonolucent zone (Fig. 13)
- Irregular retroplacental sonolucent zone
- Thinning or disruption of the hyperechoic serosa-bladder interface (Fig. 14)
- Presence of focal exophytic masses invading the urinary bladder
- Abnormal placental lacunae (Fig. 15).

Features on color Doppler:

- Diffuse or focal lacunar flow
- Vascular lakes with turbulent flow (PSV >15 cm/s)
- Hypervascularity of serosa-bladder interface (Fig. 16)

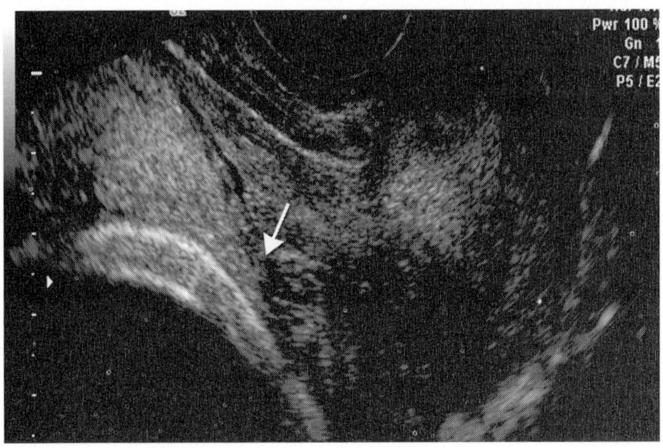

FIG. 13: Arrow indicates loss of retroplacental zone.

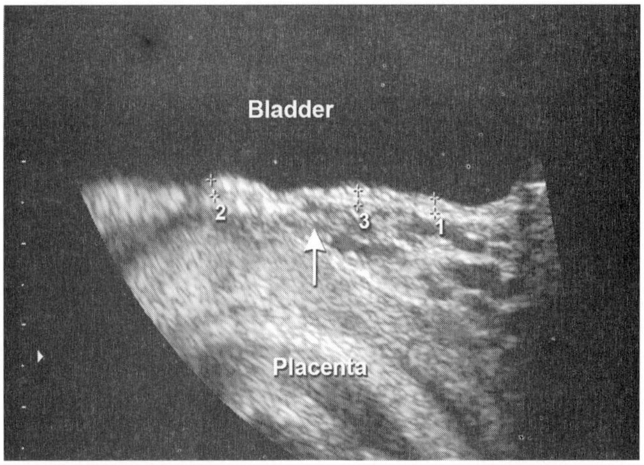

FIG. 14: Arrow indicates thinning or disruption of the hyperechoic serosa-bladder interface.

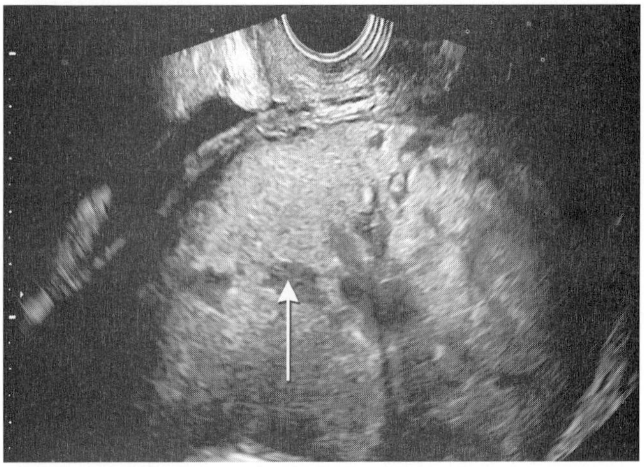

FIG. 15: Arrow indicates abnormal placental lacunae.

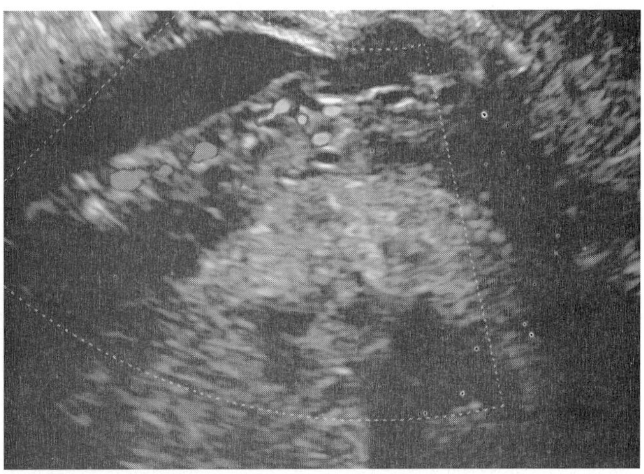

FIG. 16: Hypervascularity of serosa-bladder interface *(For color version, see Plate 2).*

- Markedly dilated vessels over peripheral subplacental zone
- Thinning or disruption of the hyperechoic serosa-bladder interface (Fig. 17).

Features on three-dimensional (3D) power Doppler:[25]

- Numerous coherent vessels involving the whole uterine serosa-bladder junction (basal view: fig. 18)
- Hypervascularity (lateral view: fig. 19)
- Inseparable cotyledonal, intervillous circulations, chaotic branching, detour vessels (lateral view: fig. 19).

Diagnosis of MAP is important as it helps in proper planning. The different risks and treatment options should have been discussed and a plan agreed, which should be reflected clearly in the consent form. This should include the anticipated skin and uterine incisions and whether conservative management of the placenta or proceeding straight to hysterectomy is preferred in the situation where accreta is confirmed at surgery. Additional possible interventions in the case of massive hemorrhage should also be discussed, including cell salvage and interventional radiology when available.

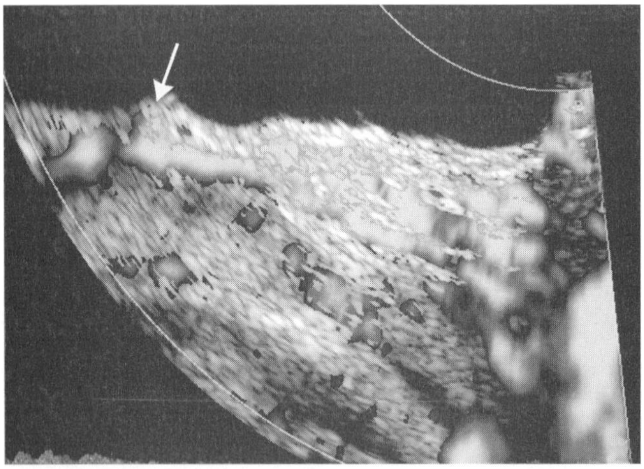

FIG. 17: Arrow indicates thinning or disruption of the hyperechoic serosa-bladder interface *(For color version, see Plate 2)*.

Cervix

Cervix can be measured by transabdominal, transperineal, and transvaginal techniques. There is no doubt as laid down by various studies that TVS is the most accurate way to measure cervical length.

- Clean transvaginal probe, placed in an aseptic probe cover (condom) filled with ultrasonographic gel, is inserted into the anterior fornix of the vagina
- Obtain a sagittal long axis view of the endocervical canal, along its entire length
- Withdraw the probe until the image is blurred and apply just enough pressure to restore the image, avoiding excess pressure, which can elongate the cervix
- Enlarge the image so that the cervix occupies two-thirds of the picture, with both the external and the internal os clearly visible
- Measure the cervical length from the internal to the external os along the endocervical canal (take at least three measurements and record the shortest, best measurement in millimeters; Fig. 20)
- Apply transfundal pressure for 15 seconds and record the cervical length again
- Describe the presence of funneling (opening) of the internal os
- Cervix and measure its length and width.

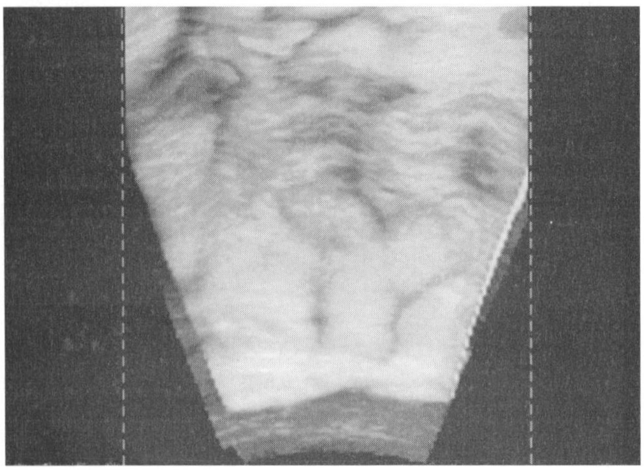

FIG. 18: Numerous coherent vessels involving the whole uterine serosa-bladder junction (basal view) *(For color version, see Plate 2)*.

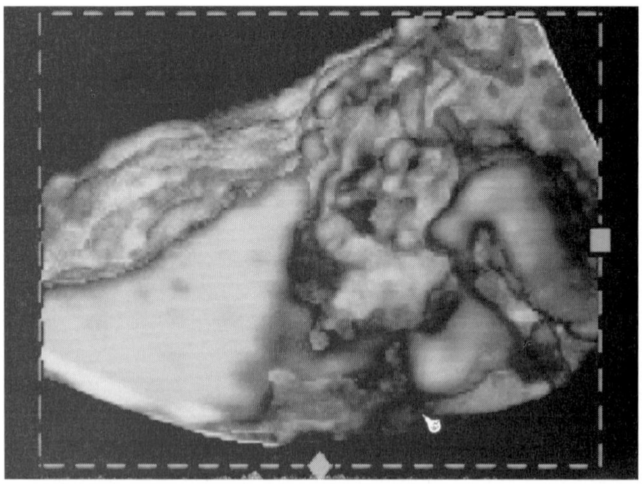

FIG. 19: Hypervascularity (lateral view) *(For color version, see Plate 2)*.

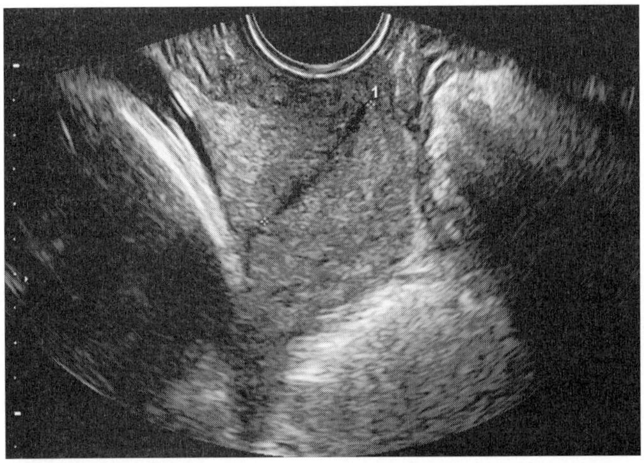

FIG. 20: Transvaginal-cervical measurement from internal to external os.

Normal Findings

Transvaginal sonography has been shown to be superior to manual examination for evaluating the cervix. Various cervical parameters have been evaluated, but cervical length is the most reproducible and reliable measurement.

If the cervical canal is curved, the cervical length can be measured on a straight line between the internal and external os or as the sum of two straight lines that follow the curve.

Normal cervical length is 25–50 mm at 14–30 weeks' GA in singleton pregnancies. A cervical length more than 25–30 mm is a reassuring.

After 30 weeks, the cervix progressively shortens in preparation for term labor, so that a length of 15–24 mm can be physiological in asymptomatic women.

In normal pregnancies, the cervical canal and the internal os are closed, and the length of the cervix is the only measurement to be made.

The length may change dynamically during a 5–10-minute examination, and in some cases, funneling of the upper cervical canal may appear and resolve. It occurs in women having contractions, and similarly, the cervix may shorten in response to transfundal pressure in an otherwise normal cervix.

In multiple pregnancies, cervical length measured at 14–19 weeks is similar to that in singleton pregnancies, but in multiple pregnancies, the cervix is progressively much shorter, starting from 20 weeks' GA.

Indications as given by fetal medicine foundation, United Kingdom

- Prediction of the likelihood of delivery within the subsequent 7 days in women presenting with threatened preterm labor
- In pregnancies complicated by polyhydramnios, cervical assessment helps to indicate whether amniodrainage is required or not
- In females planned for CS, cervical assessment can help to decide whether to carry out at 37–38 weeks or delay up to 38–39 weeks
- In female undergoing induction of labor, cervical assessment helps to predict induction-delivery interval and likelihood of vaginal delivery
- In prolonged pregnancies, measurement of cervical length at 41 weeks can predict the likelihood of spontaneous onset of labor and vaginal delivery in the subsequent 10 days.

Cesarean Scar

There is controversy regarding the measurement of cesarean scar thickness for deciding whether to give a trial of vaginal birth after cesarean (VBAC) or not. A recent meta-analysis involving 12 studies and 1,834 women showed that no cut-off value could be established LUS thickness more than 3.5 mm good sensitivity but poor specificity.[26] Various models have been created to predict the likelihood of a successful VBAC. Predicting successful VBAC section using a model based on cesarean scar features examined by transvaginal sonography was given by Naji O, et al. in 2013. This type of models (Table 5) can act as a guide for predicting the likelihood of success of VBAC but clinical sense always has to be taken into account.

Three-dimensional and Four-dimensional Ultrasound Imaging

Three-dimensional and four-dimensional (4D) ultrasound-imaging has seen a rapid development due to advancement of the machine and the softwares. The advantage being entire data can be saved in few volumes and is much easier to work offline and reconstruct after the patient has left. It is much useful in evaluating malformations in much detail that are picked on two-dimensional (2D) imaging.

Three-dimensional reconstruction of the face (Fig. 21) is one of the first applications that is quite popular. With the advancing gestation due to enlarging fetus, crowding of fetal parts, and decreasing liquor, 3D evaluation of all the organs is not possible. However, in the third trimester, seeing the real form of face in 3D or 4D (3D in real time), helps in parent-fetal bonding as actually facial expressions of the fetus, hand-to-mouth movements can be seen.

We are routinely doing 3D evaluation of face in the well-being as seeing the baby live like a human is a very nice feeling for the parents.

TABLE 5: Predicting successful vaginal birth after cesarean section using a model based on cesarean scar features examined by transvaginal sonography

Parameter	Failed vaginal birth after cesarean (VBAC) (n = 47)	Successful VBAC (n = 74)
Age (years)	33 (20, 28, 35, 43)	32 (21.0, 29.0, 34.0, 39.0)
Body mass index (kg/m^2)	25 (19, 23, 29, 40)	27 (18.0, 24.0, 30.0, 41.0)
Previous VBAC	3 (6.4)	25 (33.8)
Residual myometrial thickness (mm):		
First trimester	5.5 (3.0, 4.8, 6.4, 9.1)	5.9 (2.8, 3.5, 5.9, 7.6)
Second trimester	2.8 (0.5, 2.6, 3.1, 4.2)	4.2 (2.6, 3.0, 4.6, 6.3)
Third trimester	2.5 (0.5, 2.4, 2.6, 3.8)	3.6 (3.2, 2.6, 3.9, 5.9)
Delta RMT: first trimester – second trimester (mm)	2.8 (0.1, 2.1, 3.4, 6.2)	0.8 (0.1, 0.4, 1.2, 4.7)
Gestational age at delivery (weeks)	39 (31, 38, 40, 42)	40 (38, 40, 41, 42)
Birth weight (g)	3170 (1495, 2926, 3600, 4756)	3488 (2420, 3125, 3700, 4540)
Spontaneous onset of labor	30 (63.8)	57 (77.0)
Use of syntocinon	12 (25.5)	2 (2.7)
Use of prostaglandin	9 (19.1)	8 (10.8)

VBAC, vaginal birth after cesarean.

Note: Data is given as median (minimum, first quartile, third quartile, maximum) or n (%).

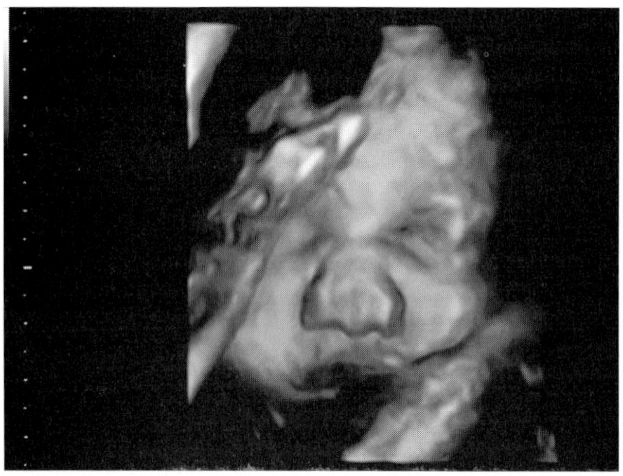

FIG. 21: Three-dimensional ultrasound of face ***(For color version, see Plate 3)***.

Role of Computed Tomography and Magnetic Resonance Imaging

Computed tomography (CT) is relatively contraindicated during pregnancy as dose of radiation exposure is about 10 mGy (1 rad) and of abdominopelvic is 30 mGy (3 rad). The permissible limit is 50 mGy (5 rad) by National Council on Radiation and Protection and Measurements. Therefore, when the benefits outweigh the risks, then only diagnostic imaging with CT should be considered. Generally, limited to the evaluation of acute maternal abdomen when magnetic resonance imaging is not available.

Magnetic resonance imaging provides better contrast resolution, no ionizing radiation and imaging in more than one plane. It is used for evaluation of cases with placenta accreta, for evaluation of fetal anomalies, especially central nervous system and kidney when the sonography provides diagnostic dilemma. However, the fetal movements interfere with the acquisition of good quality images.

CONCLUSION

The imaging in the third trimester is for the assessment of fetal growth and its growth velocity which is further added on by the use of Dopplers. This helps in management decisions whether to continue with expectant management or to timely deliver, especially in high risk settings before a stillbirth occurs.

REFERENCES

1. Fowlkes JB; Bioeffects Committee of the American Institute of Ultrasound in Medicine. American Institute of Ultrasound in Medicine consensus report on potential bioeffects of diagnostic ultrasound: executive summary. J Ultrasound Med. 2008;27(4):503-15.
2. American College of Obstetricians and Gynecologists. ACOG Practice Bulletin No. 101: Ultrasonography in pregnancy. Obstet Gynecol. 2009;113(2 Pt 1):451-61.
3. Butt K, Lim K; Society of Obstetricians and Gynaecologists of Canada. Determination of gestational age by ultrasound. J Obstet Gynaecol Can. 2014;36(2):171-81.
4. ACOG educational bulletin. Assessment of fetal lung maturity. Number 230, November 1996. Committee on Educational Bulletins of the American College of Obstetricians and Gynecologists. Int J Gynaecol Obstet. 1997;56(2):191-8.

5. Chinn DH, Bolding DB, Callen PW, Gross BH, Filly RA. Ultrasonographic identification of fetal lower extremity epiphyseal ossification centers. Radiology. 1983;147(3):815-8.
6. American Institute of Ultrasound in Medicine. AIUM Practice Guideline for the performance of an antepartum obstetric ultrasound examination. J Ultrasound Med. 2003;22(10):1116-25.
7. Bensen CB, Doubilet PM. Sonographic prediction of gestational age: accuracy of second- and third-trimester fetal measurements. AJR Am J Roentgenol. 1991;157(6):1275-7.
8. Reece EA, Goldstein I, Hobbins JC (Eds). Fundamentals of Obstetric and Gynecologic Ultrasound. Stamford, CT, USA: Appleton & Lange; 1994.
9. Yudkin PL, Aboualfa M, Eyre JA, Redman CW, Wilkinson AR. New birthweight and head circumference centiles for gestational ages 24 to 42 weeks. Early Hum Dev. 1987;15(1):45-52.
10. Brace RA. Physiology of amniotic fluid volume regulation. Clin Obstet Gynecol. 1997;40(2):280-9.
11. Chamberlain PF, Manning FA, Morrison I, Harman CR, Lange IR. Ultrasound evaluation of amniotic fluid volume. I. The relationship of marginal and decreased amniotic fluid outcomes to perinatal outcome. Am J Obstet Gynecol. 1984;150(3):245-9.
12. Phelan JP, Smith CV, Broussard P, Small M. Amniotic fluid volume assessment with the four-quadrant technique at 36-42 weeks' gestation. J Reprod Med. 1987;32(7):540-2.
13. Moore TR. Clinical assessment of amniotic fluid. Clin Obstet Gynecol. 1997;40:300-7.
14. Moore TR, Cayle JE. The amniotic fluid index in normal human pregnancy. Am J Obstet Gynecol. 1990;162(5):1168-73.
15. Evertson LR, Gauthier RJ, Schifrin BS, Paul RH. Antepartum fetal heart testing. I. Evolution of the nonstress test. Am J Obstet Gynecol. 1979;133(1):29-33.
16. Manning FA, Platt LD, Sipos L. Antepartum fetal evaluation: development of a fetal biophysical profile. Am J Obstet Gynecol. 1980;136(6):787-95.
17. Vintzileos AM, Fleming AD, Scorza WE, Wolf EJ, Balducci J, Campbell WA, et al. Relationship between fetal biophysical activities and umbilical cord blood gas values. Am J Obstet Gynecol. 1991;165(3):707-13.
18. Nagoette MP, Towers CV, Asrat T, Freeman RK. Perinatal outcome with the modified biophysical profile. Am J Obstet Gynecol. 1994;170(6):1672-6.
19. Fleischer A, Sculmann H, Farmakides G, Bracero L, Blattner P, Randolph G. Umbilical artery waveforms and intrauterine growth retardation. Am J Obstet Gynecol. 1985;151(4):502-5.
20. Creasy RK, Resnick R. Intrauterine growth retardation. In: Creasy RK, Resnick R, Iams JD, Lockwood CJ, Moore TR (Eds). Creasy and Resnick's Maternal-Fetal Medicine: Principles and Practice, 6th edition. Philadelphia, PA, USA: WB Saunders; 2009.
21. Mari G, Deter RL. Middle cerebral artery flow velocity waveforms in normal and small-for-gestational-age fetuses. Am J Obstet Gynecol. 1992;166(4):1262-70.
22. Royal College of Obstetricians and Gynaecologists. (2014). The investigation and management of the small-for-gestational-age fetus. Green-top guidelines no. 31. [online] Available from: www.rcog.org.uk/globalassets/documents/guidelines/gtg_31.pdf. [Accessed November, 2015].
23. Baschat AA, Gembruch U, Reiss I, Gortner L, Weiner CP, Harman CR. Relationship between arterial and venous Doppler and perinatal outcome in fetal growth restriction. Ultrasound Obstet Gynecol. 2000;16(5):407-13.
24. Leerentveld RA, Gilberts EC, Arnold MJ, Wladimiroff JW. Accuracy and safety of transvaginal sonographic placental localization. Obstet Gynecol. 1990;76(5 Pt 1):759-62.
25. Royal College of Obstetricians and Gynaecologists. (2011). Placenta praevia, placenta praevia accrete and vasa paevia: diagnosis and management. Green-top guideline no. 27. [online] Available from: www.rcog.org.uk/globalassets/documents/guidelines/gtg_27.pdf. [Accessed November, 2015].
26. Jastrow N, Chaillet N, Roberge S, Morency AM, Lacasse Y, Bujold E. Sonographic lower uterine segment thickness and risk of uterine scar defect: a systematic review. J Obstet Gynaecol Can. 2010;32(4):321-7.

CHAPTER 8

Pregnancy after Assisted Reproductive Techniques Including Third Party Conception

Umesh N Jindal

INTRODUCTION

Beginning of third trimester of pregnancy is like the end of a seemingly unending dark tunnel through which an infertile couple passes to fulfill their long cherished dream of getting a baby. These couples have often undergone many surgeries, injections, and procedures, spanning over many years. In addition to the physical and psychological burden, huge financial expenses are involved.

Even in young couples who have conceived spontaneously, planning for delivery starts with the beginning of third trimester. There are apprehensions regarding mode and place of delivery, the care of newborn and the expenses involved. There is the fear of the unknown, which grips the expectant mother, her family ,and even attending physician.

Are pregnancies conceived through assisted reproductive techniques (ARTs) any different than the spontaneously conceived pregnancies? What special care do these women require for a successful outcome? Do all ART babies require neonatal intensive care unit (NICU) facilities? What are the legal formalities for pregnancies conceived through third party reproduction? These are very pertinent questions for which there are not many answers in literature.

In United Kingdom, according to updated National Institute for Health and Care Excellence (NICE) guidelines, the ART pregnancies are not treated any differently than spontaneously conceived pregnancies. In fact, the mode of conception is kept confidential.[1] At the same time, medical literature is replete with adverse maternal and perinatal outcomes in ART pregnancies. There are increased chances of multiple pregnancy, pregnancy induced hypertension (PIH), gestational diabetes mellitus (GDM), antepartum hemorrhage (APH), intra-uterine growth retardation (IUGR), and preterm birth. The delivery is more likely to be operative and requirement of NICU care is more frequent.[2]

IMPORTANT FACTORS HAVING SIGNIFICANT BEARING ON OUTCOME AND MANAGEMENT

Assisted reproductive technique pregnancy with preceding history of infertility is a very heterogeneous group. A vast number of confounding variables which may affect outcome exist. The factors may be related to the etiology of infertility or other incidental or associated medical conditions. The treatments and procedures required are also likely to have some impact on outcome. All other antenatal problems which may occur in any spontaneously conceived pregnancy can affect ART pregnancies also. Table 1 categorizes various

TABLE 1: Various factors likely to have an influence on pregnancy outcome

Type of ART pregnancy	Factors contributing to adverse outcome

• Spontaneous conception after infertility, medical or surgical interventions, or bad obstetric history	• Pre-existing patient profile
	• Etiology of infertility
	• Surgical intervention
	• Medical conditions pre-existing
	• Previous obstetric history
	• Higher average age
	• Higher average BMI
	• Average higher S/E status
	• Etiology of infertility:
	  ○ Polycystic ovarian syndrome
	  ○ Endometriosis
	  ○ Adenomyosis
	  ○ Fibroids
	  ○ Tuberculosis
	  ○ Uterine malformations
	  ○ Unexplained infertility

Continued

Continued

Type of ART pregnancy	Factors contributing to adverse outcome
• First and second trimester events	• Threatened abortion • Embryo reduction • Cervical cerclage • Amniocentesis/CVS
• Multiple pregnancy	• Twins • Triplets or higher order
• Medicines for ART and complications	• Ovulation induction agents • Ovarian hyperstimulation syndrome • Luteal support
• Conception after intra-uterine insemination	• No known additional problems than above
• ART conceptions: ○ IVF or ICSI ○ Fresh day 2–3 embryo transfer ○ Fresh blastocyst transfer ○ Frozen day 2–3 (slow) ○ Frozen day 2–3 (vitrified) ○ Frozen blastocyst ○ IVM ○ Oocyte frozen and ICSI ○ Assisted hatching ○ Different media ○ PGD/PGS	• Impact of various procedures, media, duration of ex vivo life, invasiveness of procedures, etc. on pregnancy outcome not well understood and studied. • Difficult to isolate from problems in patient profile. Short follow-up
• Third party reproduction ○ IUI-D ○ Ovum donation ○ Embryo donation ○ Surrogacy	• Require appropriate consents at the time of procedure to take care of any legal objections later on. Only surrogacy will require additional procedures for handing over the baby

ART, assisted reproductive technique; BMI, body mass index; CVS, chorionic villus sampling; ICSI, intracytoplasmic sperm injection; IVM, *in vitro* maturation; PGD, preimplantation genetic diagnosis; PGS, preimplantation genetic screening; IUI-D, intra-uterine insemination with donor sperm.

factors and ART procedures which may have bearing on the outcome.

Important factors having significant bearing on outcome and management are discussed below.

Spontaneous Pregnancy after Infertility

Infertility is a heterogeneous condition resulting from variety of underlying pathologies. These conditions are likely to have impact on the pregnancy outcome as well. Infertile couples may be at increased risk for obstetric complications even if they conceive spontaneously with or without medical or surgical interventions. It is important to separate out the baseline risk in infertile women who have not undergone any ART procedure.[3] In a recent meta-analysis comprising of 19,983 births in infertile and 1,249,775 births in fertile women, the incidence of preterm labor was 8.2 and 5.4% in the two groups, respectively [Odds ratio (OR) 1.38, 95% confidence interval (CI): 1.25–1.54]. In the same group, OR for small for gestational age (SGA) was 1.24 (95% CI: 1.12–1.36) and low birth weight (LBW) was 1.30 (95% CI: 1.16–1.45).[4]

In another study, subfertile women conceiving without ART had increased odds of PIH 1.29, (CI 1.02–1.61), APH (OR 1.41; CI 1.05–1.89), perinatal death (OR 2.19; CI 1.10–4.36), LBW (OR 1.44; CI 1.11–1.85), preterm birth (OR 1.32; CI 1.05–1.67), very preterm birth (OR 2.37; CI 1.35–4.13), and cesarean delivery (OR 1.56; CI 1.37–1.77).[5] There was no increased risk of premature rupture of membranes (PROM), SGA, or postpartum hemorrhage (PPH). However, increased risk of placental abnormalities including abruption [relative risk (RR) 1.6; 95% CI 1.1–2.5] and placenta previa (RR 3.0; 95% CI 2.0–4.7) have also been reported.[6]

An excellent study recently concluded that was based on 281,157 pregnancies included in the national register of Japan in which pregnancy outcome was compared among women who achieved pregnancies through ovulation induction, intra-uterine insemination (IUI) and *in vitro* fertilization (IVF) or intracytoplasmic sperm injection and spontaneously conceived women who were matched for age, parity, height, weight, smoking, and alcohol. They were also controlled for pre-existing maternal adverse factors such as respiratory, cardiovascular, diabetes, hypertension, thyroid, renal, and gynecological diseases. Maternal age and body mass index (BMI) tended to be higher in the ART group. There was increased incidence of placenta previa and preterm delivery and this was independent of the type of ART procedure (OR 2.20; CI 1.68–2.87). A marked increase in the incidence of placenta accreta (OR 2.67; 95% CI 1.42–5.03) was also observed. The authors concluded that the adverse outcome was related to the pre-existing maternal complications and are independent of the ART procedure employed.[7]

The mechanism for these adverse perinatal outcome is increased average age and BMI, hypertension, thyroid disease and in Indian population, diabetes. Presence of fibroids, adenomyosis, and uterine malformations which are relatively more common in infertile group also worsens the prognosis. These women are more likely to have undergone corrective surgical procedures for these conditions. Moreover, repeated diagnostic procedures, like cervical dilatation, hysteroscopy, etc., may result in cervical incompetence. Previous bad obstetric history may indicate presence of antiphospholipid syndrome or inherited thrombophilia which may be responsible for severe IUGR and PIH. Even endometriosis has been known to affect implantation, placentation, and adverse perinatal outcome.[8]

Polycystic ovarian syndrome (PCOS) is very common disease and is responsible for nearly 30% of all infertility. Pregnancy outcome in PCOS has been studied widely. A recent meta-analysis based on 27 studies and in 4,982 women reported higher risk of developing GDM (OR 3.43; 95% CI 2.49–4.74), PIH (OR 3.43; 95% CI 2.49–4.74), preterm birth (OR 1.93; CI 1.45–2.57), cesarean section (OR 1.74; 95% CI 1.38–2.11), higher admission to NICU (OR 2.32; CI 1.40–3.85) as compared to controls.[9]

Management of any ART pregnancy begins with assessment of all those possible prepregnancy factors which may affect outcome and complications. In addition to these, the etiology of infertility and its impact on pregnancy outcome has to be taken into consideration. All these factors should be clearly defined and noted down on the antenatal record.

First and Second Trimester Events

Threatened Abortion

First and second trimester events, like threatened abortions, have a direct impact on third trimester complications. The incidence of vaginal bleeding is fairly common in ART pregnancies (25–30%). In a retrospective case-control study of women reaching third trimester, the incidence of history of intra-uterine hematoma (IUH) during first trimester was 13.5%. In women with IUH, the OR of gestational hypertension was 2.60, pre-eclampsia 2.8, PPH 3.1, placenta previa 8.7, oligohydramnios 5.8, and preterm delivery 2.1 and all these ratios were significantly higher than the control group, i.e., ART pregnancies reaching third trimester and without history of IUH.[10] Increased risk for preterm PROM and LBW (OR 1.78), IUGR (OR 1.54), perinatal mortality (OR 2.15), and LBW (OR 1.83) was observed in women with history of IUH.[11]

In women with history of vaginal bleeding, especially with IUH, third trimester has to be carefully monitored. Third trimester is likely to be associated with a significantly higher complication and obstetrician should be at look out for these.

Embryo Reduction

During embryo transfer, two or three embryos are transferred in order to achieve a higher pregnancy rate. This leads to an increased incidence of twins' (20–30%) and triplets' pregnancy (5–7%). Spontaneous reduction of multiple pregnancy right from early to late gestations is a common phenomenon. Iatrogenic embryo reduction is also frequently practiced. The incidence of spontaneous pregnancy reduction is nearly (18.8%) at less than 12 weeks, 15.8% in twins, 24.5% in triplets, and 38.4% in quadruplets. Nearly 80% reductions occur within 9 weeks.[12,13]

The spontaneous reduction group has a better prognosis as compared to ongoing twin or triplet pregnancies but have higher incidence of LBW, preterm delivery as compared to original singleton or twins. The adverse outcome is related to the period of gestation of reduction. The later the demise the worse is the effect on outcome.

Multifetal pregnancy reduction (MFPR) done can also improve outcome in multiple pregnancy similar to the spontaneous pregnancy reduction.[14,15] Still these women may have higher complication rate as compared to singleton or nonreduced twins. Interestingly, the reduced gestational sacs, placentas and fetuses are retained as fetus papyraceous or compressus. Their expulsion should be ensured at the time of delivery. Very rarely, these are completely absorbed.

Amniocentesis and Chorionic Villus Biopsy

The women undergoing ART are older in age and may require invasive prenatal testing more frequently. There is no evidence in literature for increased complications or effect on maternal or perinatal outcome which may be attributed to invasive diagnostic procedures other than that due to IVF or inherent problem in patient.[16] There is a 1% risk of abortion but that occurs within 1 month.

Cervical Cerclage

Incidence of cervical incompetence has been reported to be higher in women with PCOS especially in black (17.5%) and South-Asian women (7.8%).[17] The incidence is also higher in women with infertility and ART because of higher rate of interventions and associated bad obstetric history. A woman reaching third trimester with cervical suture is very high risk candidate for preterm delivery. These babies are more likely to need NICU admission especially in cases with multiple fetuses. Many of these women will require long-term hospital admission to prevent onset of preterm labor.

Multiple Pregnancy

Multiple embryos are transferred in order to achieve a higher chance of success. Nearly 21.8% of all ART pregnancies reaching third trimester have more than one fetus. In those countries where the restriction on number of embryo transferred is not imposed, the incidence is much higher.[18-20]

Assisted reproductive technique singleton pregnancies are at higher risk for all obstetric complications as compared to naturally conceived pregnancies. Furthermore, twin pregnancies whether conceived naturally or through ART have much higher risk of adverse maternal and perinatal outcome. Multiple pregnancies resulting from ART have slightly higher risk of all complications and adverse perinatal outcome as compared to naturally conceived twins especially prematurity and LBW. Women with IVF pregnancies and carrying twins or triplets need special care. The cervix should be regularly monitored sonographically for any evidence of cervical shortening. Hospitalization and tocolysis may be required. Betamethasone administration should be done at 28–30 weeks for enhancing lung maturity. One should not wait for the onset of labor pains or PROM for administration of steroids. These women need delivery in a tertiary care center which is attached to a good NICU. Timely referral to such a center is life saving for the babies. There is significant financial burden in the neonatal care of preterm and very preterm twins and this may run into lakhs. The requirement of additional funds should be explained in the very beginning to these couples.

Assisted Reproductive Techniques Procedures

Conception after Intra-uterine Insemination

There are many studies which have compared obstetric outcome after IUI with spontaneously conceived pregnancies or ART pregnancies. Studies have compared outcome of pregnancies conceived with donor sperm (IUI-D) and those in whom sperm has been obtained from husband. No increased adverse maternal or perinatal risks were attributable to the procedure over and above of those expected due to the high risk patient profile or presence of multiple pregnancy.[21,22]

Conception after In Vitro Fertilization-intracytoplasmic Sperm Injection

The impact of various procedures, media, day of transfer, frozen transfer, etc. has been studied extensively. It is very difficult to isolate the impact of procedures from the prepregnancy risk factors, multiple pregnancy, etc. However, it is reassuring that the various IVF procedures do not have a direct impact on maternal complications or perinatal outcome. The management of third trimester of any type of ART pregnancy, fresh or frozen embryo transfer, day 3, or blastocyst is no different than any other high risk pregnancy.

Third Party Reproduction

Intra-uterine insemination with donor sperm

In general, the outcome is good. Women are young and have less chance of associated morbidity. No special treatment or precautions are required. There are no legal formalities. According to the Indian Guidelines, children resulting from IUI-D with appropriate consent of husband have full legal rights similar to naturally conceived children.[23] There is no legal requirement for disclosure of source of semen. On the other hand, confidentiality should be maintained.

Ovum donation and embryo donation

Women with oocyte donation are older and many of them even beyond 50 years. Many women requesting ovum donation have smaller uterus, have sex chromosome abnormalities like Turner's syndrome. In adequately screened women which excludes prepregnancy high risk factors, the outcome of pregnancy is similar to other ART pregnancies. There is no legal restriction or formalities which need to be done at the time of delivery. The ovum donation is treated at par with sperm donation.

Two categories of women with ovum donation need special mention.

Ovum donation in older women especially above 50 years of age is associated with very high risk of maternal complications. There is very high risk of pre-eclampsia, gestational hypertension, preterm delivery, placenta previa, and PPH. Pre-IVF selection for fitness for pregnancy is very important in this group. Relatively higher maternal morbidity and mortality rate is reported in these women mainly due to age factor.

In women with Turner's syndrome a higher risk of hypertensive disorders (20.5%) is reported. Potentially life-threatening complications, like aortic dissection, regurgitation of the tricuspid, and mitral valve, are known to occur. Neonatal outcomes are reassuring; however, with a preterm birth rate which is similar to other pregnancies. Prepregnancy evaluation for coarctation of aorta or other significant cardiac lesion should be done in all cases of Turner's syndrome.

All ovum donation pregnancies in Turner's syndrome who did not have prepregnancy evaluation of cardiovascular risks by echocardiography or thoracic magnetic imaging, etc. should be considered very high risk for cardiovascular complications and maternal mortality due to aortic dissection. They should have appropriate consultation and investigations during pregnancy if not done earlier. They should have overnight blood pressure monitoring associated and very close follow-up during pregnancy in a unit associated with cardiac intensive care.[24-26]

Surrogacy

The last and the most controversial of ART pregnancies is surrogacy. In general, the pregnancy outcome is good, less complications, and lower risk of cesarean delivery. Most surrogate contracts are successfully executed and there is little difficulty in handing over the babies.[27] According to the Indian Council of Medical Research guidelines and ART draft bill 2015, the birth notification has to be sent in the name of the commissioning couple. The surrogate should be admitted in her own name. Delivery register should maintain delivery in her name with details of the commissioning couple for which she has agreed to be the gestational carrier. The baby should be handed over to commissioning couple in hospital after taking proper consent. Recently, surrogacy has been banned for foreigners in India.

CONCLUSION

The ART pregnancies are very precious and high risk pregnancies. There are lot of prepregnancy risk factors which are associated in these women namely higher age, higher weight, blood pressure, diabetes, etc. Presence of multiple pregnancy is common and one of the major reasons for adverse perinatal outcome in these women. Third party reproduction does not add additional medical or legal requirements except in cases of surrogacy. Women above 40 years constitute a very high risk group and have much higher maternal complication rate.

REFERENCES

1 National Institute for Health and Care Excellence. Clinical Guidance 62 (2010), Antenatal care – Routine care for the healthy pregnant woman. [online] Available from: http://www.nice.org.uk/nicemedia/live/11947/40115/40115.pdf.

2 Pandey S, Shetty A, Hamilton M, Bhattacharya S, Maheshwari A. Obstetric and perinatal outcomes in singleton pregnancies resulting from IVF/ICSI: a systematic review and meta-analysis. Hum Reprod Update. 2012;18(5):485-503.

3 Saunders DM, Mathews M, Lancaster PA.The Australian Register: current research and future role. A preliminary report. Ann N Y Acad Sci. 1988;541:7-21.

4 Messerlian C, Maclagan L, Basso O. Infertility and the risk of adverse pregnancy outcomes: a systematic review and meta-analysis. Hum Reprod. 2013;28(1):125-37.

5 Jaques AM, Amor DJ, Baker HW, Healy DL, Ukoumunne OC, Breheny S, et al. Adverse obstetric and perinatal outcomes in sub-fertile women conceiving without assisted reproductive technologies. Fertil Steril. 2010;94(7):2674-9.

6 Welmerink DB, Voigt LF, Daling JR, Mueller BA. Infertility treatment use in relation to selected adverse birth outcomes. Fertil Steril. 2010;94(7):2580-6.

7 Hayashi M, Nakai A, Satoh S, Matsuda Y. Adverse obstetric and perinatal outcomes of singleton pregnancies may be related to maternal factors associated with infertility rather than the type of assisted reproductive technology procedure used. Fertil Steril. 2012;98(4):922-8.

8 Lin H, Leng JH, Liu JT, Lang JH. Obstetric outcomes in Chinese women with endometriosis: a retrospective cohort study. Chin Med J (Engl). 2015;128(4):455-8.

9 Qin JZ, Pang LH, Li MJ, Fan XJ, Huang RD, Chen HY. Obstetric complications in women with PCOS. Reprod Biol Endocrinol. 2013;11:56.

10 Xiang L, Wei Z, Wu J, Zhou P, Xiang H, Cao Y. Clinical significance of first-trimester intrauterine haematomas detected in pregnancies achieved by IVF-embryo transfer. Reprod Biomed Online. 2014;29(4):445-51.

11 Saraswat L, Bhattacharya S, Maheshwari A, Bhattacharya S. Maternal and perinatal outcome in women with threatened miscarriage in the first trimester: a systematic review. BJOG. 2010;117(3):245-57.

12 Hvidtjørn D, Grove J, Schendel D, Vaeth M, Ernst E, Nielsen L, et al. 'Vanishing embryo syndrome' in IVF/ICSI. Hum Reprod. 2005;20(9):2550-1.

13 Oloyede OA, Iketubosin F, Bamgbopa K. Spontaneous fetal reduction and early pregnancy complications in multiple pregnancies following in vitro fertilization. Int J Gynaecol Obstet. 2012;119(1):57-60.

14 Haas J, Mohr Sasson A, Barzilay E, Mazaki Tovi S, Orvieto R, Weisz B, et al. Perinatal outcome after fetal reduction from twin to singleton: to reduce or not to reduce? Fertil Steril. 2015;103(2):428-32.

15 Shiva M, Mohammadi Yeganeh L, Mirzaagha E, Chehrazi M, Bagheri Lankarani N. Comparison of the outcomes between reduced and non-reduced triplet pregnancies achieved by Assisted Reproductive Technology. Aust N Z J Obstet Gynaecol. 2014;54(5):424-7.

16 Würfel W, Haas-Andela H, Krüsmann G, Rothenaicher M, Hirsch P, Kwapisz HK, et al. Prenatal diagnosis by amniocentesis in 82 pregnancies after in vitro fertilization. Eur J Obstet Gynecol Reprod Biol. 1992;44(1):47-52.

17 Feigenbaum SL, Crites Y, Hararah MK, Yamamoto MP, Yang J, Lo JC. Prevalence of cervical insufficiency in polycystic ovarian syndrome. Hum Reprod. 2012;27(9):2837-42.

18 Qin J, Wang H, Sheng X, Liang D, Tan H, Xia J. Pregnancy-related complications and adverse pregnancy outcomes in multiple pregnancies resulting from assisted reproductive technology: a meta-analysis of cohort studies. Fertil Steril. 2015;103:1492-508.

19 Sullivan EA, Zegers-Hochschild F, Mansour R, Ishihara O, de Mouzon J, Nygren KG, et al. International Committee for Monitoring Assisted Reproductive Technologies (ICMART) world report: assisted reproductive technology 2004. Hum Reprod. 2013;28(5):1375-90.

20 Ferraretti AP, Goossens V, Kupka M, Bhattacharya S, de Mouzon J, Castilla JA, et al. Assisted reproductive technology in Europe, 2009: results generated from European registers by ESHRE. Hum Reprod. 2013;28(9):2318-31.

21 Nuojua-Huttunen S, Gissler M, Martikainen H, Tuomivaara L. Obstetric and perinatal outcome of pregnancies after intrauterine insemination. Hum Reprod. 1999;14(8):2110-5.

22 De Sutter P, Veldeman L, Kok P, Szymczak N, Van der Elst J, Dhont M. Comparison of outcome of pregnancy after intra-uterine insemination (IUI) and IVF. Hum Reprod. 2005;20(6):1642-6.

23 Indian Council of Medical Research. National Guidelines for Accreditation, Supervision & Regulation of ART Clinics. [online] Available from: icmr.nic.in/art/art_clinics.htm. [Accessed December, 2015].

24 Hagman A, Loft A, Wennerholm UB, Pinborg A, Bergh C, Aittomäki K, et al. Obstetric and neonatal outcome after oocyte donation in 106 women with Turner syndrome: a Nordic cohort study. Hum Reprod. 2013;28(6):1598-609.

25 Bondy C. Pregnancy and cardiovascular risk for women with Turner syndrome. Womens Health (Lond Engl). 2014;10(4):469-76.

26 Chevalier N, Letur H, Lelannou D, Ohl J, Cornet D, Chalas-Boissonnas C, et al. Materno-fetal cardiovascular complications in Turner syndrome after oocyte donation: insufficient prepregnancy screening and pregnancy follow-up are associated with poor outcome. J Clin Endocrinol Metab. 2011;96(2):E260-7.

27 Söderström-Anttila V, Wennerholm UB, Loft A, Pinborg A, Aittomäki K, Romundstad LB, et al. Surrogacy: outcomes for surrogate mothers, children and the resulting families-a systematic review. Hum Reprod Update. 2015 Oct 9. [Epub ahead of print].

CHAPTER 9

Intra-uterine Fetal Death

Alka Kuthe

INTRODUCTION

Intra-uterine fetal death (IUFD) refers to babies with no signs of life *in utero*. Fetal death, as defined by the World Health Organization (WHO) in 1950 and revised by the working group formed by the American Academy of Pediatrics and the American College of Obstetricians and Gynecologists (ACOG) in 1988, is a death prior to the complete expulsion or extraction from its mother of a product of human conception, irrespective of duration of pregnancy, which is not an induced termination of pregnancy.[1] Death is indicated by the absence of all signs of life such as beating of the heart or pulsation of the umbilical cord or the definite movement of voluntary muscles. When a fetus does not survive but dies during birth or during the last half of pregnancy, it is known as Intra-uterine death. It embraces all fetal deaths weighing 500 g or more occurring both during pregnancy (antepartum) and during labor (intrapartum).[2] We come across number of definitions in different parts of the world. For statistical use, WHO recommends that IUFD occurring after 20 weeks or fetal weight more than 500 g when gestational age is not known, should be classified as fetal death.[1] It is a separate entity and needs to be distinguished from early pregnancy loss or spontaneous abortion. It is further divided into early (20–27 weeks) and late (28 weeks or more) fetal deaths.

TERMINOLOGY[3]

The WHO defines stillbirth as a "fetal death late in pregnancy" and allows each country to define the gestational age at which a fetal death is considered as a stillbirth for reporting purposes. As a result, some countries define stillbirth as early as 16 weeks of gestation, whereas others use a threshold as late as 28 weeks.

According to the International Classification of Diseases, revision 10, an early fetal death is death of a fetus weighing at least 500 g (or if birth weight is unavailable then after 22 weeks gestation or with a crown-heel length of 25 cm or more), while late fetal death is defined as death of a fetus weighing at least 1,000 g (or a gestational age of 28 weeks or a crown-heel length of 35 cm or more). Late fetal deaths are recommended by the WHO as the measure for international comparison.

The Perinatal Mortality Surveillance Report (Confidential Enquiry into Maternal and Child Health, 2011) defines stillbirth as a baby delivered without signs of life after 23^{+6} completed weeks of pregnancy. This definition was accepted by the Royal College of Obstetricians and Gynecologists (RCOG) in their 2010 Green-top Guideline.[4]

The National Perinatal Epidemiology Centre's perinatal death notification form defines stillbirth as "a baby delivered without signs of life from 24 weeks gestation and/or more than 500 g".

The Stillbirths Registration Act (1994) applies "in relation to a child born weighing 500 g or more or having a gestational age of 24 weeks or more who shows no signs of life".

American College of Obstetricians and Gynecologist defines stillbirth as fetal death occurring during pregnancy at 20 weeks of gestation or later. IUFD refers to babies with no signs of life *in utero*. There is general agreement between the above bodies on this definition. In this guideline, stillbirth is taken to refer to a baby delivered without signs of life from 24 weeks gestation and IUFD is taken to refer to death *in utero* after 24 weeks gestation.

INCIDENCE

The incidence of IUFD varies in different parts of the world according to the gestational age used for reporting the death. The death rate also gets affected by the standard of the healthcare services and variety of socioeconomic factors in different regions of the world. In the developed world, 1 in 200 infants is stillborn.[3] Many a times, they are under-reported in developing countries. The average fetal mortality reported by the National Centre for Health Statistics, United States, for the year 2003 was 6.9 per 1,000 births.[1] In 2009, the stillbirth rate in England, Wales, and Northern Ireland was 5.2 per 1,000 total births, a rate that shows only a slight downward trend since 2000 (Centre for Maternal and Child Enquiries, 2011).[5] In Ireland, around 350 stillbirths are registered every year.[3] The incidence has gradually declined mainly due to periconceptional, antenatal, and intranatal cares coupled with advanced prenatal diagnostic techniques which allow selective termination in congenital anomalies.

CAUSES

The cause of Intra-uterine death is unexplained in 15–35% of all cases. In cases where a cause is clearly determined, it can be referred to fetal, maternal, or placental pathology as shown in table 1.[6] With advances in obstetrics, clinical genetics, maternal-fetal and neonatal medicine, and perinatal pathology, a number of stillbirths that previously would have been categorized as "unexplained" can now be labeled as the result of specific cause. The subsequent pregnancy following the Intra-uterine death can be efficiently and comparatively easily managed if the cause of the death is known.

- Maternal causes:
  - Advanced maternal age
  - Postmaturity
  - Hypertensive disorders
  - Antepartum hemorrhage
  - Infection
  - Uterine rupture
  - Maternal trauma or death
  - Severe anemia
  - Rh disease
  - Diabetes
  - Systemic lupus erythematosus (SLE)
  - Antiphospholipid antibody syndrome
  - Hemoglobinopathies
  - Inherited thrombophilias
- Fetal causes:
  - Infections: viruses, bacteria, protozoa
  - Intra-uterine growth restriction
  - Multiple gestations
  - Hydrops fetalis
  - Congenital malformations
  - Genetic abnormality
- Placental causes:
  - Placental insufficiency
  - Abruption
  - Premature rupture of membranes
  - Cord accident
  - Vasa previa
  - Fetomaternal hemorrhage.

TABLE 1: Categories and causes of fetal death[7-10]

Fetal: 25–40%	Chromosomal anomalies, nonchromosomal birth defects, nonimmune hydrops, infections—viruses, bacteria, protozoa
Placental: 25–35%	Prematurely ruptured membranes, abruption, fetomaternal hemorrhage, cord accident, placental insufficiency, intrapartum asphyxia, previa, twin-twin transfusion, chorioamnionitis
Maternal: 5–10%	Age >35 years, obesity, hypertensive disorders, diabetes, thyroid disorder, antiphospholipid antibodies, thrombophilias, renal disease, preterm labor, abnormal labor, infections and sepsis, uterine rupture, postterm pregnancy, smoking, illicit drugs, and alcohol
Unexplained: 15–35%	---

Many fetal deaths due to placental abnormalities could also be categorized as having underlying maternal or fetal causes.[6] Placental abruption is associated with approximately half of the cases of hypertension and thus can be considered as maternal cause. Similarly, placental insufficiency found in aneuploidy could be considered as fetal cause.

The above causes can operate individually or can coexist. Let us see how they can lead to such undesirable event.

Maternal Causes

They are responsible for 5–10% fetal deaths. Because of this fact, they are underestimated. Placental abruption or isoimmunization is often considered due to placental and fetal factors. Hypertensive disorders and diabetes are the two most common maternal disorders responsible for 5–8% stillbirths.[6,11,12]

Hypertensive Disorders (Preeclampsia, Eclampsia, Chronic Hypertension, Chronic Nephritis)

One of the most common causes leading to fetal demise is preeclampsia. Because of the hypertensive spasm of the vessels supplying the maternal placental site, there occurs significant reduction in placental blood flow. This leads to placental insufficiency. The oxygen supply to the baby is markedly reduced. It is the small, growth restricted baby, the result of the inadequacy of its own placenta, who is most likely to die *in utero* before labor.

Chronic hypertension causes similar chain of events but the prognosis on the whole is somewhat better, provided preeclampsia does not supervene. Associated overweight and obesity are the increased risks for stillbirth.

Chronic nephritis, although an uncommon complication of pregnancy, has a very bad prognosis for the growing fetus who frequently dies *in utero* before, even the stage of viability is reached due to placental infarction and progressive hypoxia.

Antepartum Hemorrhage

Acute placental insufficiency may be the consequence of both abruption placenta and placenta previa of any degree leading to Intra-uterine death. Placental abruption is the most common single diagnosable cause of fetal death. Fretts and Usher (1997) found abruption to be the cause of death in 14% of stillborns.[6,12]

Severe Anemia

It is frequently met in tropics and can be because of different etiological factors. If left untreated, may cause Intra-uterine death due to maternal hypoxemia.

Diabetes

Apart from impaired glucose metabolism and its consequences on the different body systems, the disease also affects vasculature. Though the exact cause of fetal death is not clear, hypoglycemia, hypoxia, and acidosis are often associated with preeclampsia, polyhydramnios, congenital malformation, and maternal ketosis leading to fetal death.[2]

Fever

Hyperpyrexia, i.e., a body temperature over 103°F, due to any cause can directly kill the fetus *in utero*. Malaria may cause fetal death due to placental insufficiency due to placental parasitization or due to direct effect of high fever.[1]

Maternal Infections

Hepatitis, toxoplasmosis, influenza, mumps, herpes simplex, poliomyelitis, and rarely syphilis may cause fetal death.

Antiphospholipid Antibody Syndrome

Presence of lupus anticoagulant and anticardiolipin antibodies are blamed to give rise to increased fetal loss. Decidual vasculopathy with fibrinoid necrosis, placental vascular atherosis, and intervillous thrombosis are the pathological changes held responsible to cause placental infarction, fetal growth restriction (FGR), recurrent abortion, and fetal death. Very few of the otherwise unexplained stillbirths can be attributed solely to the autoantibodies and other thrombophilias, although women with these are more prone for adverse pregnancy outcome.[6,9]

Hereditary Thrombophilias

They have been associated with abruption placenta, Intra-uterine growth restriction; and Intra-uterine death.

Postmaturity

Postmaturity, as a cause for Intra-uterine death is disappointing to accept; as in such cases, there is no particular disease in either mother or baby and the tragic result might have been definitely prevented by timely successful induction of labor combining clinical judgment and ultrasonography/Doppler technique.

Extremes of Reproductive Age

They are definitely associated with higher fetal death rate even when adjusted for known associations such as maternal medical disorders and congenital anomalies.[6,13-15]

Rh-incompatibility

Rh-isoimmunization leading to excessive hemolysis of fetal red blood cells produces fetal anemia, hypoxia, and heart failure. Nonimmune hydrops is also important.

Iatrogenic

- External version: though rarely tried these days, it may result in true knot of the cord or entanglement of the cord round the neck or limbs of the fetus causing death of the fetus
- Excessive dosage of the drug: the use of quinine beyond therapeutic level may lead to fetal death.[2]

Placental Causes

Fetomaternal Hemorrhage

Although usually it occurs spontaneously, it is common with severe maternal trauma.

Placental and Membrane Infection

It is usually associated with fetal infection. Malaria and tuberculosis are the exceptions. Chorioamnionitis is characterized by mononuclear and polymorphonuclear leukocytic infiltration of the chorion. Preterm stillbirths are mole commonly associated with such infections that include aerobic, anaerobic bacteria, as well as ureaplasma and mycoplasma.

Placental Infarcts

These are the areas of fibrinoid trophoblastic degeneration progressing towards calcification and ischemic infarction from spiral artery occlusion. Marginal and subchorionic infarcts are common but of no importance.

Twin-to-twin Transfusion Syndrome

It is the most common factor responsible for fetal death in monochorionic multifetal pregnancy.

Placental Insufficiency

It is more often diagnosed in order to explain the so-called idiopathic cases of Intra-uterine death but in about a fifth of cases of Intra-uterine death, no definite cause can be found.

Fetal Causes

Fetal Chromosomal Abnormalities and Malformations

The reported incidence of major congenital malformations in stillborns is highly variable. It depends on whether autopsy was performed and if so the training, experience, and interest of pathologist.[6,16] Faye-Peterson and associates (1999) found that a third of fetal loss was caused by structural anomalies.[6,17] Neural tube defects, hydrops, isolated hydrocephalus, and complex congenital heart disease were the most common. Major structural anomalies, hydrops, and aneuploidy are particularly amenable to antenatal diagnosis. The severe degree of malformations proves lethal to the life of the fetus. Fetal malformations may cause death before, during, or after labor depending upon their nature and extent. They constitute nearly 25–40% of all stillbirths.

Fetal Infections

Stillbirths caused by infections are also common, especially when ascending bacterial infection of amniotic fluid and placenta takes place. In indigent and inner-city women, congenital syphilis can be a common cause of fetal death.[6] Infection with rubella, varicella, listeriosis, borreliosis, toxoplasmosis, cytomegalovirus, and parvovirus-B19 are potentially lethal infections.

Idiopathic Causes

In about 15–35% of cases, the cause remains obscure in spite of thorough clinical workup. In about 0–8% of subsequent pregnancies, the mishap recurs pointing towards diabetes, Rh-incompatibility, syphilis, antiphospholipid syndrome, chronic nephritis, and hereditary thrombophilias as a predisposing factor.[2] There are certain risk factors that were recently reviewed by Reddy (2007) and Silver (2007) which increase the chance for IUFD.[6,9,10] They may be responsible for unexplained (sudden unexplained Intra-uterine death). They are as follows:

- Nulliparity
- Multiparity (>5 pregnancies)
- Smoking cigarettes, tobacco use, drinking alcohol, or use of illegal (street) drugs, such as cocaine, during pregnancy
- Black race women have more than twice the rate of stillbirth than that of Caucasian females[10]
- Obesity
- Being 35 years old or older, or being a teenager
- Use of drugs for the treatment of fertility/analgesics during pregnancy
- Fourfold increase in multifetal pregnancies (ACOG, 2009)[18]
- Previous stillbirth
- Intra-uterine FGR
- Health disorders such as diabetes, high blood pressure, cholestasis (liver disease), and history suggestive of clotting disorder
- Preconceptional weight greater than 70 kg
- Less than 3 prenatal office visits/late prenatal care
- Thrombophilia and aneuploidy as the underlying pathology
- Injury during pregnancy such as from a fall, car accident, or physical abuse
- Low socioeconomic status.

Bukowski and associates (2009) linked excessive rates of stillbirth infants with fetal macrosomies, defined as growth potential more than 90th percentile.[6,19] A systematic review by Fretts in 2005 identified 15 risk factors for stillbirth. The most common that cannot be corrected during prenatal care were preconceptional obesity, socioeconomic status, and advanced maternal age.[20] Advanced maternal age and obesity, and their association with higher incidence of medical disorders, like diabetes and hypertension and congenital anomalies, increase the risk of stillbirth. However, the correlation of fetal death with prepregnancy birth weight and maternal age persists even after adjustment of these confounding variables. The stillbirths found in these mothers, particularly in prepregnancy overweight women are mostly unexplained and the risk is more at later gestations (term stillbirths) probably due to greater placental dysfunction. The excess risk is independent of weight gain during pregnancy and obesity-related diseases.[1] In a study quoted by Stephansoon et al., they could not explain the increased risk associated with low socioeconomic class on the basis of age, race, weight, body mass index, and cigarette smoking.[21]

The relative frequency of the causes of stillbirth is different depending on the gestational age when the fetal death occurs. Between 24 weeks and 28 weeks, the most common causes of fetal death are infection, abruption placenta, congenital fetal abnormalities, and unexplained fetal death. Between 28 weeks and 36 weeks, the most common reasons are unexplained, FGR, and abruptio placenta. After 37 weeks, the most common etiologies are unexplained, FGR and abruption placenta but the frequency of unexplained stillbirths increases markedly when compared with the 28–36 weeks' group (Fretts, 2005).[20]

SIGNS AND SYMPTOMS

Certain signs and symptoms may give clue in clinching diagnosis of IUFD, such as:

- The mother may give history that the baby has stopped moving for a length of time
- The uterus does not increase in size over period of time but on the contrary the fundal height decreases which is less for the period of amenorrhea (if dates have been crosschecked with ultrasound)
- Uterine tone is diminished and the uterus feels flaccid. Braxton Hicks contractions are not easily felt
- The heartbeat cannot be heard either by stethoscope or with a special heart monitor
- On ultrasound examination, the baby is not found moving and the fetal heart pulsations are not seen
- Retrogression of the positive breast changes that occur during pregnancy is evident following death of the fetus
- Egg shell crackling of the fetal head is noticed although it is a late sign.

DIAGNOSIS

History and physical examination are of moderate value in the diagnosis of Intra-uterine death. In most patients, the only symptom is diminished fetal movement. An inability to obtain fetal heart suggests Intra-uterine death. However, auscultation of the fetal heart by Pinard stethoscope or Doppler is inaccurate and this together with cardiotocography should not be used to investigate suspected IUFD. Intra-uterine death is confirmed by visualization of the fetal heart and the absence of cardiac activity by real-time ultrasound.

Macerated stillbirth nearly always indicates fetal death in early pregnancy and not in labor, and in most cases is caused by hypoxia. On the other hand, fresh stillbirth, i.e., nonmacerated, usually indicates death due to hypoxia or trauma or both. This distinction is very much important while eliciting past obstetric history or in attempting to pinpoint a particular cause for stillbirth.

Maceration is a destructive aseptic process which first reveals itself by blistering and peeling of the fetal skin. This appears between 12 and 24 hours after fetal death. The process involves the whole body, giving rise to the characteristic radiological signs. The ligaments are softened because of which the vertebral column is liable to sag or collapse, especially when the patient is in erect posture. The ribs may concertina together and the skull bones, already loosened in their mutual attachments, overlap each other at the sutures because of the shrinkage of the brain within (Spalding's sign). It usually takes a week or more for Spalding's sign to appear after Intra-uterine death. Though it is the most definite out of all radiological signs, it loses its importance if the membranes are already ruptured or if the labor is in progress. Two X-rays taken within several hours with identical positioning may show total absence of fetal movements if the pictures are superimposed. This is highly suggestive of fetal death. X-ray also shows gas bubbles in the heart, aorta, vena cava, liver, umbilical cord, and abdominal cavity. These signs are very reliable in the diagnosis of Intra-uterine death and appear within first few days and provide the first conclusive evidence.

Table 2 shows relation between time since fetal death, grade, and features of maceration.

INVESTIGATIONS

Before investigating, parents should be counseled that:

- In almost half of stillbirths, no specific cause is found
- When a cause is found, it can definitely help in preventing IUFD in future pregnancy
- Correlation between abnormal blood test and postmortem examination should be made as an abnormal test, result is not necessarily related to the IUFD
- Sometimes further investigation is necessary.

Sonography

- When the pregnant patient complains of diminished or no fetal movements, then in addition to obtaining careful history and clinical examination, the patient should be immediately subjected to sonography (biophysical profile) and color Doppler (umbilical artery Doppler velocimetry) if necessary to confirm the cause and diagnosis. Thus real-time ultrasonography and Doppler study are essential investigations for an accurate diagnosis of IUFD. The sonography report reveals:

TABLE 2: Time of fetal death and grade of maceration[22]

Grade	Features	Time since fetal death
0	"Parboiled" reddened skin	<8 hours
I	Skin slippage and peeling	>8 hours
II	Extensive skin peeling, red serous effusions in chest and abdomen	2–7 days
III	Liver yellow-brown, turbid effusions	≥8 days

- Lack of fetal movements (including cardiac) during a requisite period of careful observation, which is a strong presumptive evidence of fetal death
- Oligohydramnios and collapsed cranial bones gradually become evident. Sonography allows direct visualization of the fetal heart, and views can be supplemented with color Doppler of the heart and umbilical cord. Use of ultrasound also facilitates visualization of other secondary features, such as fetal hydrops, polyhydramnios, anhydramnios, and skin edema (RCOG, 2010).[4]

X-ray of Abdomen

Straight X-ray of abdomen is rarely done nowadays. The following features may be found in varying degrees either singly or in combination.

- Spalding's sign: the irregular overlapping of the cranial bones on one another is due to liquefaction of the brain matter and softening of the ligamentous structures supporting the vault. It usually appears 7 days after death. Similar features may be found in extrauterine pregnancy with the fetus alive
- Hyperflexion of the spine: it is more common. In some cases hyperextension of the neck is seen
- Crowding of the ribs shadows with loss of normal parallelism
- Appearance of gas shadow (Robert's sign): gas in the heart chambers and great vessels may appear as early as 12 h but difficult to interpret. When they are detected provide conclusive evidence (Figs 1 and 2).[23]

In addition to the above, laboratory tests should be recommended:

- To assess maternal well-being
- To diagnose the condition
- To determine the cause of death
- The chance of recurrence
- To estimate the blood fibrinogen level and partial thromboplastin time and possible means of avoiding further pregnancy complications.[4,24,25]

Even identification of a sporadic cause can bring emotional closure and facilitate parental recovery.

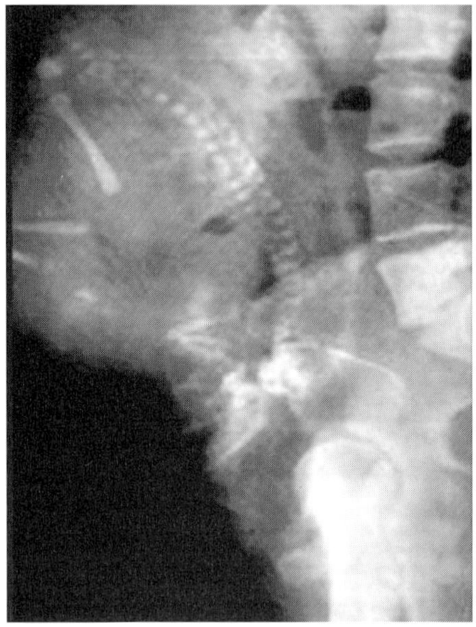

FIG. 1 Intra-uterine fetal death: gas presents in cardiac chambers, abdominal aorta and superior mesenteric artery. This early sign is diagnostic of Intra-uterine death. Spalding's sign is not yet visible.

Courtesy: Dr E Sweet.

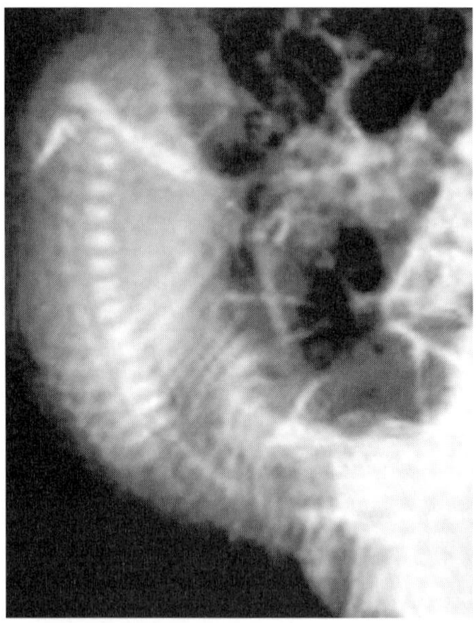

FIG. 2 Intra-uterine fetal death during labor at 41 and half weeks gestation: the first stage was prolonged and fetus died in slightly less than 24 hours before this picture was taken. Note the gas shadows in the thoracic and abdominal aorta and both common iliac vessels.

Courtesy: Dr E Sweet.

Other Maternal Tests

Hematological Examination

Hematological examination consists of ABO and Rh grouping, complete blood count, venereal disease research laboratory test, human immunodeficiency virus, total immunoglobulin, serum glucose measurement. Glycosylated hemoglobin, renal functions test (urea, creatinine, and uric acid estimation), thyroid profile, TORCH (toxoplasmosis, rubella, cytomegalovirus and herpes simplex), antiphospholipid antibodies, and lupus anticoagulant testing if required. Anti-(D)-antibody test (if mother is Rh-negative); maternal blood should be tested for detection of fetal erythrocytes (Kleihauer-Betke test). Elevated uric acid levels early in the third trimester in preeclamptic women have been associated with perinatal death and it is therefore recommended to evaluate the contribution of preeclampsia to the death.[24] Abnormal renal function is an indicator of possible SLE, which is associated with a significant increase in fetal morbidity and mortality.

Routine Urine Examination

Risks associated with Intra-uterine dead fetus can be life-threatening like. they are described below.

Infection

The dead tissue favors the growth of gas-forming organisms like *C. Welchii* with fatal consequences. This is unlikely as long as membranes are intact but once the membranes rupture the risk increases.

Blood coagulation disorders

In around 10–20% cases, as the dead fetus is retained *in utero* for more than 4 weeks, the patient may land up into coagulation disorders [disseminated intravascular coagulation (DIC), a syndrome set-off by a number of medical conditions including malignancy, infection, and liver disease, and leads to consumption of clotting factors in the blood]. Thus, there is a possibility of defibrination from "silent" DIC. Though it was first noticed in the case of fetal death due to Rh iso-immunization of the mother, however, its possibility in other etiologies as mentioned before cannot be forgotten. It occurs due to gradual absorption of thromboplastin, liberated from the dead tissues of placenta and decidua into the maternal circulation. Fortunately, before the disorder develops, the onset of labor, whether spontaneous or induced, is anticipated. In multiple gestations, one stillbirth can be dangerous to the other unborn baby or babies.

Psychological trauma

The mental loss to the patient/couple/family cannot be measured but a proper counseling showing empathetic attitude can give relief.

During labor

There are possibilities of uterine inertia, retained placenta, and postpartum hemorrhage. Medicine used for treatment can have side effects in the form of heavy bleeding, pain, fever, rigors, vomiting, diarrhea, etc.

BREAKING THE NEWS

When a diagnosis is confirmed, if a woman is alone, it is desired to call her relatives before conveying the facts. They are told in a timely and empathetic manner in a consulting room and not in a passage. Everything needs to be explained in a compassionate manner and transparency should be maintained. Simple words should be used while explaining instead of complicated medical terminologies. Patient and relatives need to be given the opportunity and space to talk about their loss. It has been shown that parents value acceptance and recognition of their emotions. After informing the details about the fetomaternal condition, it is mandatory to take signature of the patient and the accompanying relatives with date and time.

PREVENTION

The role of obstetrician in the prevention of fetal death starts with identification of patients with risk factors and subjecting them to screening in first and second trimester, their careful and systematic follow-up clinically and with serial ultrasound examination. As in many of the cases, causes are unknown and total prevention is difficult. Therefore, any effect of effectively reducing the incidence of macerated stillbirth will depend upon the early diagnosis and prompt management of pregnancy-induced hypertension, preeclampsia, eclampsia, careful management of diabetes, judicious and timely use of labor induction methods in cases of Rh-isoimmunization and in established postmaturity. Treatment for high blood pressure, diabetes should be preferably started in consultation with physician. It is the small baby who by its unsatisfactory growth calls for our attention towards inadequacy of its own placenta because of which he is most likely to die *in utero* before labor. Similarly, infarction of the placenta makes the fetus progressively hypoxic causing irreversible damage leading to Intra-uterine death. It is, therefore, very much important to foresee this catastrophic event and deliver the baby before its unfavorable Intra-uterine environment kills it. For this, 24 hours urinary estriol levels for three consecutive days are of great help to detect the disaster in advance.[23] Errors are likely to occur in collection and the whole specimen may not be forwarded to laboratory. Therefore, it is better to do creatinine excretion rate as well which remains fairly constant and any discrepancy quickly indicates that 24-hours collection is not complete. There is unfortunately great variation in what we regard as normal estriol excretion. For this, in modern medicine, it is better to make use of sonography at least once a week and sometimes twice a week in high-risk cases. Symptoms of bacterial infection, such as from a dental abscess, in pregnant women should be timely recognized and immediately treated. Umbilical cord constriction may be recognized and discovered by ultrasound.

Importance of Antenatal Classes

Antenatal classes can be routinely planned to educate the pregnant women. Along with diet and other useful tips, fact to be conveyed is that the blood supply to the fetus is through the placenta and umbilical cord. This can be impaired by placental aging, hypertension or diabetes in pregnancy, placental separation, kinking of the cord, etc. If the blood supply of the baby is impaired for significant period, irreparable damage including neurological and even death can result. Therefore, in order to prevent this catastrophic event, there is a need of proper periconceptional care, regular antenatal care, and high-risk pregnancy screening.

MANAGEMENT

Intra-uterine death is an extremely traumatic moment for the patient and her family. Therefore, the diagnosis should be confirmed before breaking the news. The diagnosis having been established beyond doubt from the clinical evidences of absent fetal heart sounds, absent fetal movements, cessation of uterine growth, and recession of the signs of continuation of pregnancy supported by sonographical techniques as mentioned above, one is faced with the selection of the following alternatives of management. But before that, once the Intra-uterine death has been confirmed, the patient and her relatives should be informed of her condition. Often, allowing them to see the lack of cardiac activity helps them to accept the diagnosis. But still they are likely to be upset. For that, as said before, proper counseling regarding, probable cause of death, the need for investigations, management protocol, autopsy after the birth of the infant, and further management is done.

The management can be of two types:[2]

1. Expectant (noninterference)
2. Expeditious (interference).

Expectant

In about 80% of cases, spontaneous expulsion occurs within 2 weeks after death of the fetus. But the patient should be assured of safety of noninterference. A course of antibiotics may be advised to prevent the infection. The patient may remain at home with this advice and get admitted in the hospital once she gets labor pains. Fibrinogen levels should be done every week. A falling blood fibrinogen level approaching 150 mg/dL demands immediate admission for controlled heparin infusion.[2]

Expeditious

In the following indications, interference is indicated:

- Psychological upset and social pressure: it is the most common psychological trauma along with the fear associated with the dead fetus inside the uterus and the social pressure may make the obstetrician to urgently intervene
- Infection: at times, manifestations of infection may call for interference
- Falling blood fibrinogen level: in those patients who do not go in spontaneous labor, there is a risk, although quit less of hypofibrinogenemia and consumptive coagulopathy, usually after 3–4 weeks of retention of dead fetus. The patient needs urgent admission for correcting the levels well above the critical values before interference
- Prolongation of pregnancy beyond 2 weeks: there is a tendency of pregnancy to get prolonged beyond 2 weeks. In order to prevent complications associated with retention of dead fetus, the patient needs admission for interference.

SCHEME OF MANAGEMENT OF INTRA-UTERINE FETAL DEATH (FLOWCHART 1)[2]

The dead fetus preferably should be delivered by medical induction. The methods used for the termination depends upon two important findings on per vaginum examination, such as, whether (i) the cervix is unripe or (ii) the cervix is ripe.

Again, the response to induction or the induction delivery interval varies depending upon the parity, the gestational age, the mode of previous delivery, and again if the previous delivery is by cesarean section, whether it is a recurrent type of indication. In general, the body gets easily rid of the dead fetus. Therefore the vaginal route is preferred, unless there is some absolute contraindication for that. As said earlier on, the methods of induction are of two types:

- If the cervix is not ripe:
  - Vaginal prostaglandin E_2 (PGE_2) gel/suppositories
  - Synthetic PGE_1 analog: tablet misoprostol (vaginally or orally).
- If cervix is ripe:
  - Amniotomy
  - Oxytocin intravenous (IV)
  - Methyl-prostaglandin F2α IV.

Before induction, patient must be counseled regarding different methods of induction of labor available and more important the expected induction-delivery interval. Labor can be induced by oxytocin infusion in titrating doses or with the use of prostaglandins (PGs) for preinduction cervical ripening followed by IV oxytocin drip. Patients with a history of a prior cesarean delivery should be treated carefully because of the risk of uterine rupture, just as in any birth following cesarean delivery.

Prostaglandins

When the cervix is unfavorable or in pregnancies remote from term, PGs are generally more effective than oxytocin alone. In a study comparing intravaginal misoprostol to oxytocin alone in women with late fetal deaths, the average

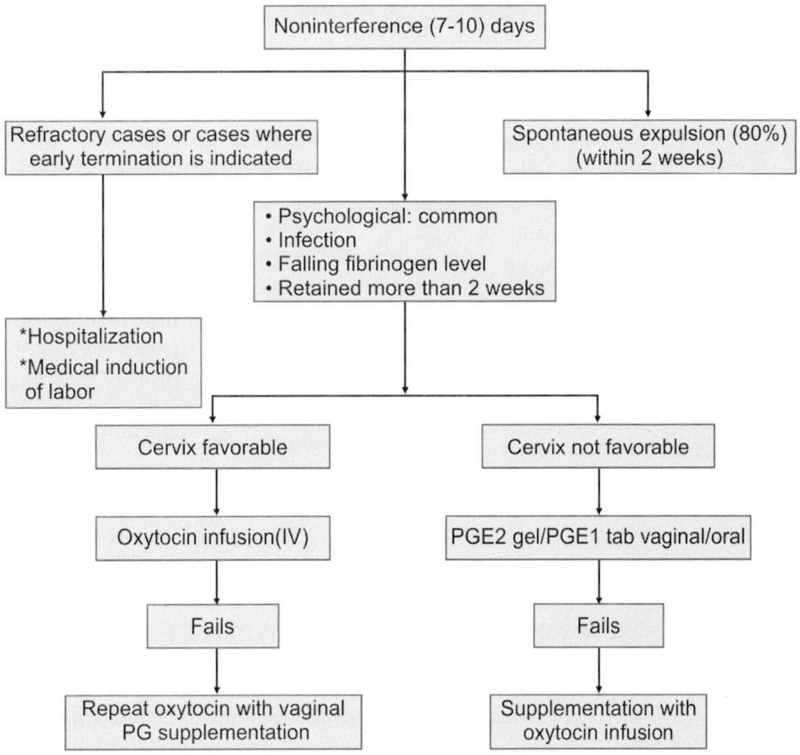

IV, intravenous; PG, prostaglandin.

FLOWCHART 1 Scheme of management of Intra-uterine death.[2]

induction-delivery interval was 14.8 hours and 31 hours in the misoprostol and oxytocin group respectively when the Bishop's score was less than 6. The difference was insignificant when the Bishop's score was more than 6 or membranes were ruptured. PGE_2, F2α, misoprostol (synthetic analog of PGE_1) have all been used for induction of labor. Vaginal administration of PGE_2 gel/suppositories is very effective for induction where the cervix is unfavorable/unripe. This may have to be repeated after 6–8 hours depending upon the response. Misoprostol can be used in preference to PGE_2 because of equivalent safety and efficacy with lower cost.[4] It can be used orally as well as vaginally, and has good shelf life at room temperature. In Intra-uterine death before 28 weeks, misoprostol (PGE_1) tablet either inserted vaginally or orally (400 µg) to be repeated 4–6 hourly if needed, and/or oxytocin is also found effective. In women with Intra-uterine death after 28 weeks' gestation, lower doses of PGs should be used. The procedure may be supplemented with IV oxytocin drip. In women with no uterine scar, misoprostol (25 µg) 4–6 hourly, may be dispensed for ripening after 28 weeks' gestation. For women with a prior cesarean delivery, mechanical ripening can be carried out with a Foley's catheter, and induction can be continued by carefully monitored oxytocin drip. Pain management in patients undergoing induction of labor for Intra-uterine death is normally easier than in patients with live fetuses. Analgesics can be used for successful pain control. If required, epidural analgesia should be offered. Mifepristone (RU-486), an anti-progesterone has been used for induction of labor in women with fetal death with reasonable efficacy. Its combination with misoprostol increases the efficacy and reduces the induction delivery interval significantly. Wagaarachchi et al. found that the combined use of mifepristone and misoprostol was not only safe but it also reduces induction-delivery interval less than any of the other induction regimens in use.[26] In a series of 96 patients with IUFD after 24 weeks, 200 mg of oral mifepristone was followed by 200 µg of intravaginal misoprostol 24–48 hours later. It was further followed by oral doses as 200 µg every 3 hours for 4 doses. In a pregnancy more than 34 weeks, each dose of misoprostol was reduced to 100 µg. With the first dose of misoprostol, 92.7% women delivered within 36 hours and 98.9% within 72 hours. Mild side effects were noted in 8% of patients.[26] Different regimens with varying doses of both drugs have been tried with successful result and significantly less gastrointestinal side effects.

In low-resource settings, labor can be induced with insertion of a Foley's catheter and extra-amniotic infusion of normal saline (rarely used now-a-days). In hardcore cases, which were diagnosed in the middle trimester of pregnancy (not to be performed on any uterus <6 weeks gestation) and who were least likely to go into labor as a result of oxytocin drip induction, intra-amniotic injection of 20% sodium chloride was used in the past. The method, though fairly simple, is not without danger as may be expected and patients with cardiac or renal disease, as well as preeclampsia, are particularly at risk due to increased maternal serum sodium concentration up to 160 mEq/L, increased volume and osmolarity, and on top of this, an antidiuretic effect following this injection. Cardiac patients may be precipitated into pulmonary edema and the patients with renal disease may become anuric. Fatal cases of severe brain damage have been reported in the past. This is the reason why wider adoption of this method was discouraged.

Oxytocin Infusion

Where the cervix is favorable, oxytocin infusion can be safely and effectively used in titrated doses. Initially, IV drip can be started with 5 units of oxytocin in 500 mL of Ringer's lactate. The rate of drops can be adjusted depending upon the response. Two bottles can be administered consecutively at a time. In case of no response, an increasing dose of oxytocin should be used on the following day. The drip needs to be monitored so as to avoid hypertonus and the resulting rupture of the uterus. The risk of fluid retention due to antidiuretic effect with high dose of oxytocin should be always kept in mind. Hence not more than two bottles should be infused at a time and fluid overload is avoided. If the uterus does not respond, same procedure can be repeated after vaginal administration of PG. If repeated attempts fail to start labor, one should try to exclude the possibility of secondary abdominal pregnancy.

Risks of inducing labor include infection, damage to the uterus, and heavy bleeding. If there is too much blood loss, the patient may need a blood transfusion. If the patient is anemic and particularly has rare blood group (Rh-negative) or if the coagulation profile shows abnormal result, it is safe to keep her blood cross-matched prior to induction to meet demand in case of emergency. Tissue may be left in the uterus after the fetus is delivered. One may face a need to do a dilation and curettage procedure to remove this tissue.

Place of Cesarean Section

As far as possible cesarean section is avoided for delivering Intra-uterine dead baby. It is indicated in case of major degree of placenta previa, transverse lie, previous cesarean section (two or more), and in rare instances where attempts of vaginal birth fail. Thus, its role is limited.

Puerperal Care

The patient should be monitored in the puerperal period with care and empathy. The couple needs support. The possible cause of fetal death needs to be explained in simple words if one is not sure about the exact cause of the tragic event. The usual advice regarding diet and medicines (iron, calcium, antihypertensive if required) is given. Suppression of lactation is of psychological importance for some women following IUFD. If suppression is necessary, dopamine agonists are first-line agents to suppress lactation. Cabergoline is superior to bromocriptine (cabergoline 1 mg/day for 14 days). Dopamine agonists should not be given to women with hypertension or preeclampsia. Estrogens should not be used to suppress lactation.[3,4] The patient is called in the postpartum clinic after 6 weeks to review various investigation reports and counseling for future pregnancy. Women should be routinely assessed for thromboprophylaxis but IUFD is not a risk factor. Heparin thromboprophylaxis should be discussed with a hematologist if the woman has DIC. Established guidelines should be followed for thromboprophylaxis. Given the association of late IUFD with obesity, advanced maternal age, infection, and maternal disease, it is likely that many women with IUFD fall into the moderate- or high-risk categories.[4]

EVALUATION OF THE DEAD FETUS

About one-fourth of fetal deaths remain unexplained in spite of proper evaluation. Therefore, thorough evaluation and thereby accurate diagnosis about the cause of the fetal death is the duty of treating doctor. After knowing it, the couple can mentally prepare for the loss. It will also help in counseling the patient regarding the need for prenatal diagnosis and preconception management in future pregnancy. An attempt to prevent a similar outcome in the pregnancy by proper and timely intervention can be made.[18] At the same time, prompt therapy can be immediately instituted. This must include a detailed history, clinical examination, laboratory evaluation to exclude maternal disease, cytogenetic studies before and after delivery, examination of the newborn, placenta, membranes, and autopsy.

History

Relevant maternal and obstetric factors must be searched in that particular case keeping in mind the risk factors. Detail family history regarding pregnancy losses, congenital malformations, mental retardation, diabetes, consanguinity, etc., should be meticulously elicited.

Clinical Examination

A detail examination of the fetus, placenta, and membranes should be performed after the delivery, and the findings recorded in the chart. The positive prenatal events should be noted down. Photographs should be taken for record whenever possible. A "fetogram" (a radiograph of the fetus), magnetic resonance imaging (MRI), and sonography may also be considered.[6,18] These records would be especially important in providing anatomical information if full autopsy is denied by the parents. A protocol for examination of stillborn as practiced by Parkland Hospital (Table 3) would help in writing down the observations.

Autopsy

An autopsy is an important component of evaluation and may provide an important clue as regards the cause of fetal death. Therefore, the patients should be offered and encouraged to consent for a full autopsy. A gross external examination combined with photography, radiography, MRI, bacterial cultures, and selective use of chromosomal and histopathological studies would help to come to a conclusion.[6,9,10] The time of death may be approximately determined by examination of the infant and assessing degree of maceration. Incerpi et al. showed that an autopsy could reduce the incidence of unexplained birth by 10%.[27] A complete autopsy is much more likely to yield valuable information. Studies showed that autopsy results changed the recurrence risk estimates and parental counseling in 25–50% of cases.[6,10,17] However, if consent for an autopsy is denied, an MRI may be performed if feasible. In many centers, maternal records and autopsy findings are reviewed on monthly basis by a stillbirth committee formed for this special purpose. The cause of death is determined based on the available evidence. Parents are then contacted and offered counseling regarding the cause of death, recurrence risk, if any, and action plan to prevent its recurrence in subsequent pregnancies.

Laboratory Evaluation[6]

About 35% of stillborns are discovered to have major structural anomalies[28] by chromosomal studies and autopsy findings. Approximately 20% have dysmorphic features or skeletal abnormalities and 8% have chromosomal

TABLE 3: Protocol for examination of stillborn[6,7]

Infant description	• Malformations, skin staining, degree of maceration • Color: pale, plethoric
Umbilical cord	• Prolapse, entanglement: neck, arms, legs, hematoma or strictures, number of vessels, length • Wharton jelly: normal, absent
Amniotic fluid	• Color: meconium, blood • Consistency • Volume
Placenta	• Weight, staining: meconium, adherent clots, structural abnormalities: circumvallate or accessory lobes, velamentous insertion (Fig. 3), Edema: hydropic changes
Membranes	• Stained: meconium, cloudy, thickening

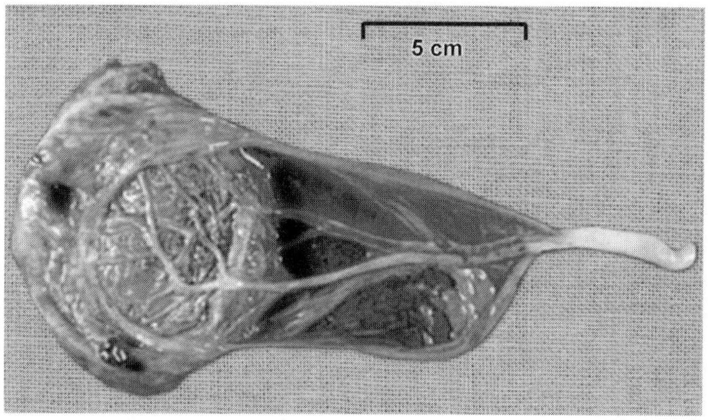

FIG. 3: "Velamentous" insertion of umbilical cord ***(For color version, see Plate 3)***.

abnormalities.[29,30] The ACOG 2009 recommends karyotyping of all stillborns.[18] In the absence of morphological anomalies, up to 5% of stillborn babies will have chromosomal abnormalities.[31] Before taking postmortem fetal tissue or fluid sample, appropriate consent needs to be taken. As per the recommendations of ACOG 2009, either placental block or umbilical cord segment or internal fetal-tissue specimen, such as costochondral junction or patella, can be selected for cytogenetic studies if blood cannot be obtained.[18]

Psychological Aspects

Fetal death is a psychological trauma for the parents and the family. The delivery and other management issues add further stress. The woman needs to be closely monitored as she is at increased risk of postpartum depression.

Pregnancy after Previous Fetal Death

A stillbirth rate of 22.7 per 1,000 in women with prior fetal death has been reported by a population-based Missouri Study.[32] According to Silver (2007), losses associated with placental insufficiency and preterm labor are more likely to repeat in the next pregnancy compared to that associated with multiple gestation and infection.[9] The low-risk woman who has had an unexplained stillbirth has a pregnancy risk increased risk explained about 10-fold. The risk of a stillbirth after 37 weeks is only 1.8 per 1,000 as most losses are found in earlier weeks of gestation.[6] Losses that take place earlier are associated with higher recurrence. Maternal diabetes, chronic hypertension, or some thrombophilias increase the risk of recurrence in addition to hereditary disorders.

Prenatal Evaluation

The calculation of recurrent risk depends upon the knowledge of the cause of death, i.e., infections and cord accidents are less likely to recur while the familial Di George syndrome and aneuploidy have 50% and 1% recurrence rates, respectively.[6] The management plan can also be made beforehand, i.e., aneuploidy and Di George syndrome can be detected in the next pregnancy by chorionic villous sampling or amniocentesis. Maternal medical diseases leading to stillbirth can be easily diagnosed and stringent control in the preconception period or early in pregnancy may improve outcome in the next pregnancy. Tight preconceptional glucose control in diabetic women and stringent blood pressure control or early intervention in pregnancy induce hypertension/chronic hypertension to prevent 10% recurrence of placental abruption are the good examples of preventive strategies.[33] There is some evidence to show that recurrent fetal loss due to antiphospholipid antibodies can be minimized with treatment, especially if placental deficiency, growth restriction or placental infarction were responsible to cause fetal death.[6,9]

MANAGEMENT OF SUBSEQUENT PREGNANCY

According to Reddy (2007), fetal sonographic assessment at midpregnancy or even before that, followed by serial growth monitoring beginning at 28 weeks, can detect FGR which is responsible for almost half of the fetal deaths.[9] Study on fetal biophysical testing by Weeks and colleagues (1995) concluded that antepartum surveillance in the otherwise healthy woman with a previous stillbirth should begin at 32 weeks.[6,34] The ACOG 2009 also support the recommendation as it decreases the iatrogenic preterm delivery rate.[18]

CONCLUSION

Intra-uterine fetal death is a grave, traumatic event for the patient, her family as well as for the treating doctor. Therefore efforts should be made to prevent it. If it occurs, despite the utmost efforts and due care then prompt diagnosis, with determination of cause and timely interference to deliver the baby should be made to prevent the possible complications. Postpartum support along with systematic evaluation of the dead fetus/placenta and advice regarding subsequent pregnancy are the basic important steps in the management, to reduce the recurrence in the subsequent pregnancy.

REFERENCES

1. Mishra R. Post-term pregnancy and intrauterine fetal death. In: Ian Donald's Practical Obstetric Problems, 7th edition. Philadelphia, PA, USA: Lippincott Williams & Wilkins; 2014. pp. 422-6.
2. Dutta DC. Preterm labour, preterm rupture of the membranes, post-maturity, intrauterine death of the fetus. In: Hiralal K (Ed). Textbook of Obstetrics, 6th edition. Kolkata, India: New Central Book Agency (P) Ltd.; 2006. pp. 322-5.
3. Institute of Obstetricians and Gynaecologists, Royal College of Physicians of Ireland, Directorate of Strategy and Clinical Programmes, Health Service Executive. (2013). Clinical Practice Guideline: Investigation and Management of Late Fetal Intrauterine Death and Stillbirth. [online] Available from: www.rcpi.ie/content/docs/000001/668_5_media.pdf. [Accessed June, 2015].
4. Royal College of Obstetricians and Gynaecologists (RCOG). (2010). Late Intrauterine Fetal Death and Stillbirth: in Setting Standards to Improve Women's Health. Green-top Guideline No 55 [online] Available from: www.rcog.org.uk/globalassets/documents/guidelines/gtg_55.pdf. [Accessed June, 2015].
5. Centre for Maternal and Child Enquiries (CMACE). (2011). Perinatal Mortality 2009. [online] Available from: www.hqip.org.uk/assets/NCAPOP-Library/CMACE-Reports/35.-March-2011-Perinatal-Mortality-2009.pdf. [Accessed June, 2015].
6. Cunningham FG, Leveno KJ, Bloom SL, Hauth JC, Rouse DJ, Spong CY (Eds). Diseases and injuries of the fetus and newborn. In: William's Obstetrics, 23rd edition. Philadelphia, PA, USA: McGraw Hill Publication; 2009. pp. 630-3.
7. Cunningham FG, Hollier LM. Fetal death. In: Williams Obstetrics, 20th edition. Norwalk, CT, USA: Appleton & Lange; 1997.
8. Eller AG, Branch DW, Byrne JL. Stillbirth at term. Obstet Gynecol. 2006;108(2):442-7.
9. Reddy UM. Prediction and prevention of recurrent stillbirth. Obstet Gynecol. 2007;110(5):1151-64.
10. Silver RM. Fetal death. Obstet Gynecol. 2007;109(1):153-67.
11. Alessandri LM, Stanley FJ, Garner JB, Newnham J, Walters BN. A case-control study of unexplained antepartum stillbirths. Br J Obstet Gynaecol. 1992;99(9):711-8.
12. Fretts RC, Usher RH. Causes of fetal death in women of advanced maternal age. Obstet Gynecol. 1997;89(1):40-5.
13. Bateman BT, Simpson LL. Higher rate of stillbirth at the extremes of reproductive age: a large nationwide sample of deliveries in the United States. Am J Obstet Gynecol. 2006;194(3):840-5.
14. Reddy UM, Ko CW, Willinger M. Maternal age and the risk of stillbirth throughout pregnancy in the United States. Am J Obstet Gynecol. 2006;195(3):764-6.
15. Wyatt PR, Owolabi T, Meier C, Huang T. Age-specific risk of fetal loss observed in a second trimester serum screening population. Am J Obstet Gynecol. 2005;192(1):240-6.
16. Cartlidge PH, Dawson AT, Stewart JH, Vujanic GM. Value and quality of perinatal and infant postmortem examination: cohort analysis of 400 consecutive deaths. BMJ. 1995;310(6973):155-8.
17. Faye-Petersen OM, Guinn DA, Wenstrom KD. Value of perinatal autopsy. Obstet Gynecol. 1999;94(6):915-20.
18. American College of Obstetricians and Gynecologists (ACOGs) Practice Bulletin No. 102: management of stillbirth. Obstet Gynecol. 2009;113(3):748-61.
19. Bukowski R, Malone FD, Porter TF, et al. Fetal macrosomia increases risk of stillbirth. Am J Obstet Gynecol. 2009. [In Press].
20. Andres SR. Antepartum care of the high-risk pregnancy. In: Arias F, Bhide A, Arulkumaran S, Damania K, Daftary S (Eds). Practical Guide to High Risk Pregnancy and Delivery, 3rd edition. Philadelphia, PA, USA: Elsevier; 2012. pp. 13-4.
21. Stephansoon O, Dickman PW, Johansson AL, Cnattingius S. The influence of socioeconomic status on stillbirth risk in Sweden. Int J Epidemiol. 2001;30(6):1296-301.
22. Langley FA. The perinatal postmortem examination. J Clin Pathol. 1971;24(2):159-69.
23. Donald I (Ed). Abortion and intrauterine death. In: Practical Obstetrics Problems, 4th edition. London, UK: Lloyd-Luke Medical Books Limited; 1974. pp. 78-84.
24. Flenady V, King J, Charles A, Gardener G, Ellwood D, Day K, et al. (2009). The Perinatal Society of Australia and New Zealand (PSANZ). Clinical

Practice Guideline for Perinatal Mortality. [online] Available from: www.psanzpnmsig.org. [Accessed June, 2015].

25. British Colombia Reproductive Care Program. (2000). Perinatal Mortality Guideline 5: Investigation and Assessment of Stillbirths. [online] Available from: www.perinatalservicesbc.ca/NR/rdonlyres/20DAEEFB-E282-42A6-A22C-97D1890BAD46/0/PerinatalMortalityStillbirthInvestAssess5.pdf. [Accessed June, 2015].
26. Wagaarachchi PT, Ashok PW, Narvekar NN, Smith NC, Templeton A. Medical management of late intrauterine death using a combination of mifepristone and misoprostol. BJOG. 2002;109(4):443-7.
27. Incerpi MH, Miler DA, Samadi R, Settlage RH, Goodwin TM. Stillbirth evaluation: what tests are needed? Am J Obstet Gynecol. 1998;178(6):1121-5.
28. Faye-Petersen OM, Guinn DA, Wenstrom KD. Value of perinatal autopsy. Obstet Gynecol. 1999;94(6):915-20.
29. Pauli RM, Reiser CA. Wisconsin Stillbirth Service Program: II. Analysis of diagnoses and diagnostic categories in the first 1,000 referrals. Am J Med Genet. 1994;50(2):135-53.
30. Saller DN, Lesser KB, Harrel U, Rogers BB, Oyer CE. The clinical utility of the perinatal autopsy. JAMA. 1995;273(8):663-5.
31. Korteweg FJ, Bouman K, Erwich JJ, Timmer A, Veeger NJ, Ravise JM, et al: Cytogenetic analysis after evaluation of 750 fetal deaths: Proposal for diagnostic workup. Obstet Gynecol. 2008;111(4):865-74.
32. Sharma PP, Salihu HM, Oyelese Y, Ananth CV, Kirby RS. Is race a determinant of stillbirth recurrence? Obstet Gynecol. 2006;107(2 Pt 1):391-7.
33. Pritchard JA, Cunningham FG, Pritchard SA, Mason RA. On reducing the frequency of severe abruptio placentae. Am J Obstet Gynecol. 1991;165(5 Pt 1):1345-51.
34. Weeks JW, Asrat T, Morgan MA, Nageotte M, Thomas SJ, Freeman RK. Antepartum surveillance for a history of stillbirth: when to begin? Am J Obstet Gynecol. 1995;172(2 Pt 1):486-92.

Section 3

Intrapartum

CHAPTER 10

Drugs and Prostaglandins

Meeta Gupta, Nalneesh Sharma, Kanupriya Jindal

INTRODUCTION

Prostaglandins were first discovered in 1935 and have since then been the subject of intense scientific investigation and experiments. Prostaglandins modulate a wide range of physiological processes in man, but in particular, they play key roles in reproductive processes including ovulation, menstruation, implantation, and labor. They induce myometrial contractility[1] and extracellular matrix changes associated with cervical ripening,[2] thereby regulating the final common pathway characterized by increased uterine activity and cervical dilatation. These properties have been exploited to produce pharmacological agents with prostaglandin against activity for use in the induction of labor, and agents with antagonistic properties for use as tocolytics to treat preterm labor. The stimuli for the synthesis and output of prostaglandins vary and include physiological processes, bacterial products such as lipopolysaccharide, and tissue injury. These stimuli may act through the upregulation of the genetic message for the cyclooxygenase type 2 (COX-2) enzyme. Alternatively, they may exert the same effect through cytokines that regulate the host inflammatory response.

PHARMACOLOGIC AGENTS FOR CERVICAL RIPENING OR LABOR INDUCTION

Pharmacological agents along with mechanical agents has been seen to be more effective for cervical ripening than for labor induction but the cost of combination therapy is additive. Various prostaglandins, their doses, and routes of administration has been extensively studied for cervical ripening and labor induction.

Prostaglandins

They act on cervix and enable ripening by various mechanisms:

- Increase the activity of collagenase in cervix
- Alter the extracellular ground substance of cervix
- Increase the levels of elastase, glycosaminoglycan, dermatan sulfate, and hyaluronic acid in the cervix
- Cervical smooth muscle relaxation facilitates dilation
- Allow for an increase in intracellular calcium levels, causing myometrial contractions.

Risks Associated with Use of Prostaglandins

- Uterine hyperstimulation
- Maternal side effects like nausea, vomiting, diarrhea, and fever.

Prostaglandin E_2 (Dinoprostone)

Prostaglandin E_2 (PGE_2) is most commonly used. It is available in two forms: dinoprostone gel that contains 0.5 mg of dinoprostone and dinoprostone inserts (cervidil) that contains 10 mg of dinoprostone in pessary form.

- Its local applications help in initially cervical softening effacement and dilation by altering the extracellular ground substance of cervix
- Alters the smooth muscle of the cervix and uterus
- Causes gap-function formation which is necessary for the coordinated uterine contractions of labor.

A systemic review that included at least 5,000 pregnancies from more than 70 prospective trials suggested that PGE_2 is superior to placebo or therapy in enhancing cervical effacement and dilation. It is a vaginal gel for local application.[3]

Actions

Uterine stimulation: it stimulates the myometrium of the gravid uterus similar to contractions seen in the uterus at term. Whether this action results from a direct effect of dinoprostone on the myometrium has not been determined.

Other actions: it is also capable of stimulating smooth muscle of gastrointestinal tract (GIT) in humans, so may be responsible for the vomiting and or diarrhea that is occasionally seen with use of dinoprostone. In laboratory animals, as well as in humans, its large doses can lower blood, probably as a result of its effect on smooth muscle of the vascular system. It can also elevate body temperature, however, with the dose of dinoprostone used in cervical ripening these effects have not been seen.

Pharmacokinetics

Absorption: vaginally, it is quickly absorbed. Peak plasma concentrations of the gel formulation are achieved in 30–45 minutes. It is 73% bound to human plasma albumin. The increase in prostaglandin metabolites in plasma was significantly greater with the vaginal gel than with the vaginal tablet suggesting that the gel may have greater bioavailability.

Distribution and metabolism: it is rapidly metabolized to 13,14-dihydro-15-keto PGE_2, which is converted to 13,14-dihydro, 15-keto prostaglandin A2. It is completely metabolized in human lungs and the resulting metabolites are further metabolized in the liver and kidney.

Elimination: the drug and its metabolites are excreted primarily by the kidney with a small amount excreted in the feces.

Preclinical Safety Data

Carcinogenesis, mutagenesis, and impairment of fertility carcinogenic bioassay studies have not been conducted in animals with dinoprostone due to the limited indication for use and short duration of administration. No evidence of mutagenicity was observed in the micronucleus test or Ames assay.

Indications

The vaginal gel is indicated for labor induction in term and near term pregnant women who have favorable induction features and who have a singleton pregnancy with a vertex presentation.

Dosage and Administration

For labor induction at or near term, the initial dose of 1 mg of vaginal gel should be administered by gentle expulsion of the entire contents of the syringe into the posterior fornix. Patient should remain in supine condition for at least 30 minutes. After 6 hours, a second dose may be repeated if necessary:
- 2 mg in case of absence of initial dose
- 1 mg to augment an already present response to the initial dose.

Contraindications

- Known hypersensitivity to prostaglandins or any other constituent of the gel
- In case of:
    - Multiple pregnancy
    - Grand multiparity (6 or more previous term pregnancies)
    - History of difficult labor and/or traumatic delivery
    - Engagement of head has not taken place
    - Ruptured chorioamniotic membranes
    - Previous uterine surgery like cesarean section or hysterotomy
    - Cephalopelvic disproportion (CPD)
    - Fetal distress
    - Cardiotocography suggesting fetal compromise
    - Lower genital tract infections
    - Hyperactive or hypertonic uterine patterns
    - Nonvertex presentations
    - Unexplained vaginal bleeding during present pregnancy.

Adverse Reactions

- Maternal adverse reactions
- Fetal adverse reactions

Maternal adverse reactions

- Hypersensitivity
- Systemic: fever
- GIT: diarrhea, nausea, vomiting
- Musculoskeleton and connective tissues: backache
- Pregnancy and puerperium uterine contractile disorders (increased frequency, tone or duration), uterine rupture
- Postabortal: endometriosis unusual in uterine bleeding.

Fetal adverse reactions

Still birth, fetal distress, altered fetal heart rate (FHR).

Rare increased risk of postpartum disseminated intravascular coagulation has been described in patients whose labor was induced by any pharmacological means (dinoprostone or oxytocin) though appears to be very rare (<1 per 1,000 labors).

Special Precautions

It is recommended that continuous electronic monitoring of uterine activity and FHR should be employed in patients with labor induction. PGE_2 vaginal gel should be used with precaution in patients with previous chorionic villus sampling and compromised hepatic, renal, or in patients with history of asthma, or glaucoma, or raised intraocular pressure.

Intracervical placement of PGE_2 gel may result in advent disruption and subsequent embolization of antigenic tissue causing, in rare circumstances, the development of anaphylactoid syndrome of pregnancy (amniotic fluid embolism).

Technique of Placement of Dinoprostone Gel

Patient selection:
- Afebrile
- Not active vaginal bleeding
- FHR tracing is reassuring
- Informed consent taken
- Bishop score is less than 4.

Bring gel to room temperature before application as per manufacture's instruction. Monitor FHR and uterine activity continuously starting 15–30 minutes before gel introduction and continuing for 30–120 minutes after gel insertion.

Introduce the gel into the cervix as follows:
- If the cervix is uneffaced, use the 20 mm endocervical catheter to introduce the gel into the endocervix just below the level of the internal os
- If cervix is 50% effaced, use the 10 mm endocervical catheter
- After application of the gel, the patient should remain recumbent for 30 minutes before being allowed to ambulate
- May repeat every 6 hours up to 3 doses in 24 hours.

Endpoints of ripening include strong uterine contractions, a Bishop score of more than or equal to 8, or a change in maternal or fetal status.

Maximum recommended dosage is 1.5 mg of dinoprostone (3 doses) in 24 hours. Do not start oxytocin for 6–12 hours after placement of the last dose, to allow spontaneous onset of labor and protect the uterus from overstimulation.[4]

Misoprostol

Misoprostol has been extensively investigated in the past few years for use in cervical ripening and labor induction. Marketed as a gastric cytoprotective agent, the drug is also an effective, safe, and inexpensive agent for cervical ripening and labor induction, although it is not Food and Drug Administration-labeled for that purpose.[5-14]

It is a synthetic analog of PGE_1 and is a cheap and safe drug for cervical ripening. When given orally, it is rapidly absorbed by the GIT and undergoes de-esterification to its free acid, which is responsible for its clinical activity. The peak concentration and half-life of misoprostol acid, the active metabolite, are 12 minutes and 21 minutes, respectively.[14] The total systemic bioavailability of vaginally administered misoprostol is 3 times greater than that of orally administered misoprostol.[15]

Clinical trials indicate the optimal dose and dosing interval is 25 mg intravaginally every 4–6 hours. Higher doses or shorter intervals are associated with higher incidence of side effects, especially hyperstimulation syndrome, defined as contractions lasting longer than 90 seconds, or more than 5 contractions in 10 minutes. Risk also include tachysystole defined as 6 or more uterine contractions in 10 minutes for 2 consecutive 10-minute period[9] and hypersystole, a single contraction of at least 2 minutes' duration. However, maternal outcomes, such as the need for cesarean delivery because of FHR abnormalities, the arrest of labor, or the need for terbutaline administration were not significantly different between the misoprostol group and the dinoprostone and oxytocin control groups.[5] Although the incidence of meconium staining was found in some studies to be higher with misoprostol, overall neonatal outcomes, including the frequency of meconium aspiration syndrome, the incidence of 5-minute Apgar scores below 7, and the rate of neonatal resuscitation or admission to a neonatal intensive care unit, showed no significant differences between groups.[14] They can be managed by changing the maternal position and administering oxygen by face mask, terbutaline (0.25 mg) subcutaneously, or both. The incidence of hyperstimulation varies between 1 and 10%, depending on the dose of misoprostol and the frequency of administration.

Finally, uterine rupture in women within previous cesarean section is also a possible complication, limiting its use to women who do not have a uterine scar. Other uncommon complications resulting from misoprostol use include uterine rupture and fetal demise, but not at rates higher than in control subjects.[16] Maternal effects, such as nausea, vomiting or diarrhea, are uncommon.[17,18] The primary advantages of misoprostol are cost and convenience.

The optimal regimen for intravaginal misoprostol has not been firmly established. Most clinical trials used 25–100 µg prepared from oral tablets and inserted intravaginally. Misoprostol comes in 100 or 200 µg tablets, and the desired dose can be prepared in the pharmacy by dividing the tablet, which is then inserted into the posterior fornix. The most common dose is 50 µg, inserted either once or every 4–6 hours; however, inserting 25 µg every 6 hours is associated with the fewest side effects.[15,16] The maximum cumulative dosage of misoprostol has not been established, but a total dosage of up to 600 µg has been used safely in one clinical trial.[14] When oxytocin augmentation is necessary, a minimal interval of 3 hours is recommended after the last misoprostol dose.[14] Continuous fetal monitoring is currently recommended for at least 3 hours after misoprostol application before the patient is allowed to ambulate.

Oral misoprostol is well tolerated for the management of upper GIT dysfunction. For this reason, oral administration of misoprostol for cervical ripening and labor induction has been tried. Investigators found that a single oral dose of 200 µg or a 50 µg dose given orally every 4 hours was effective, and adverse effects were no different from those in control subjects.[17-19] More studies are in progress to determine the optimal dosing regimen and to further define the safety and effectiveness of oral administration for induction of labor.

Informed consent should always be obtained from patients who are given misoprostol. No fetotoxic, teratogenic, or carcinogenic effects have been observed in animal studies, and no untoward direct effects on neonates have been noted so far in any of the clinical trials.[13,17,18]

Technique for Intravaginal Application of Misoprostol Tablets

After passing urine, patient is placed in lithotomy position. After taking full aseptic precautions, the 25 mg tablet is introduced intravaginally, without using any gel which may prevent tablet from dissolving. The patient should remain in recumbent position for 30 minutes. Monitor fetal heart sound and uterine activity continuously for at least 3 hours after application. If oxytocin augmentation is required, a minimum interval of 3 hours is recommended after last misoprostol dose.

Associated adverse risks include hyperstimulation of uterine muscles and maternal side effects like nausea, vomiting, fever and diarrhea. Use of vaginal prostaglandins increased the likelihood of a vaginal delivery in next 24 hours, but there is an associated increased rate of uterine hyperstimulation and accompanying FHR changes.[19]

It is not recommended in patient with previous uterine scar.

Oxytocin

It is a neurohormone that originates in the hypothalamus and is secreted by the posterior lobe of pituitary gland. This octapeptide is secreted in a pulsatile manner. It binds to uterine receptors to produce uterine contractions, but has no direct effect on the cervix. It has a half-life of 5–12 minutes, a time to steady plasma concentration of 40 minutes, and a steady-state uterine response of 30 minutes or longer. The uterus is increasingly responsive to oxytocin as pregnancy progresses. The number of oxytocin receptors in the uterus increases by 100-fold at 32 weeks and by 300-fold at the onset of labor. This increasing concentration of oxytocin receptors in the myometrium and deciduas is responsible for its variability in response as pregnancy progresses. Traditionally, it has been held that oxytocin levels reach a steady state level within 15–20 minutes of beginning an infusion or increasing the dosage.

It activates the phospholipase C-inositol pathway and increases intracellular calcium levels stimulating contractions in myometrial smooth muscles. In addition, it also directly stimulates the decidual prostaglandin production. An increased level of prostaglandin F2α metabolite was demonstrated in women who underwent successful oxytocin induction of labor, whereas this increase was not present in failed induction. Other areas of the body that show a response to oxytocin include breast, vascular smooth muscle, and kidney. Oxytocin stimulates contraction of the myoepithelium that surrounds the alveoli of the mammary gland, which leads to the milk ejection reflex.

At dosages typically used for the induction of labor, there is not a demonstrable effect on vascular smooth muscle tone. Intravenous (IV) boluses of as little as 0.5 IU transiently decreases peripheral vascular tone, however, which leads to hypotension, likewise, at low dosages, oxytocin exerts negligible effect on renal function.

It can be administered by any route. It is also absorbed by the buccal and nasal mucosa. When administered orally, it is rapidly inactivated by trypsin. The IV route is used almost exclusively to stimulate the pregnant uterus because it allows precise measurement of the amount of drug when side effects occur. The physiological dose of oxytocin to produce regular uterine contraction is 8–12 mU/min. The ideal dosing regimen of oxytocin is not known and there are both low- and high-dose protocols.

The low-dose regimen begins with 1–2 mU/min, increased incrementally by 1–2 mU at 30-minute intervals. The high-dose regimen commences with a dose of 4–6 mU/min, with dose increments of 4–6 mU/min every 15–30 minutes.

The benefits of the low-dose regimen include less risk of tachysystole and the use of a smaller overall dose. However, high-dose oxytocin has been associated with an increase in uterine tachysystole with associated FHR changes. Because mixing methods vary, the rate of infusion should always be documented in mU/min rather than mL/hour.

Fetal monitoring is indicated before beginning the infusion to assess the baseline level of uterine activity and fetal status. Either external or internal monitoring is acceptable as long as uterine activity and FHR are documented adequately. Tracings should be inspected carefully for any evidence of hyperstimulation as manifested by increased baseline tone, tachysystole, or the onset of late decelerations.

Starting doses have ranged from 0.5 mU/min to 2 mU/min with some as much as 6 mU/min. Increments of dose increase have ranged from as low as 1–2 mU/min to as high as 6 mU/min, with adjustments for increased uterine activity. Time interval between increases has ranged from 15 to 40 minutes.

Based on recent pharmacokinetic data, many obstetricians have moved to a regimen whereby the dose of oxytocin is increased by 1–2 mU/min every 40 minutes.

Advantage of this regime derive from not increasing the oxytocin dose before steady state levels of oxytocin have been reached. This leads to lower total dosage of oxytocin required in addition to a lower incidence of hyperstimulation than can result from increasing the oxytocin dose before steady state is reached.

Side Effects

With proper administration and monitoring, oxytocin is a very safe medication. However, still there is always the potential of adverse occurrence. Uterine hyperstimulation is the most common complication met. It may present as tachysystole with more than 5 contractions in 10 minutes, contractions of longer than 90-second duration, or an increase in the baseline uterine tone. The decreased intervillous blood flow associated with hyperstimulation ultimately leads to decreased oxygen transfer to fetus, as indicated by the appearance of the decelerations.

Oxytocin infusion should be discontinued immediately in the presence of hyperstimulation. If there is evidence of fetal distress, standard intrauterine resuscitation measures should be instituted including oxygen administration and positioning the patient in the left lateral decubitus position.

Uterine rupture is an uncommon complication when oxytocin in used properly. Factors that may reduce this risk include avoiding oxytocin use in grand multipara, use of internal uterine pressure monitoring for patients with previous cesarean delivery, and avoiding its use in obstructed labors.

Water intoxication is an uncommon complication, and may be avoided with proper management. The minimum effective dose of oxytocin may be used to avoid the antidiuretic hormone effects of high-dose oxytocin. The risk of water intoxication increases in women who have received large volumes of free water; therefore, 5% dextrose solution without electrolytes generally should not be used during labor induction. Symptoms occur as the plasma sodium concentration falls below 120–125 mEq/L and may include nausea and vomiting, mental status changes, and ultimately seizures and coma; mild instances of water intoxication can be treated by discontinuing the hypotonic fluid and restricting fluid intake. With severe symptomatology, correction of hyponatremia by saline infusion may be necessary. The more recent literature has not identified any correlation between oxytocin induction and neonatal hyperbilirubinemia.

Mifepristone

It is an antiprogestrone agent. Progesterone inhibits contractions of the uterus while mifepristone counteracts this action. Results of seven undergoing trials of women treated with mifepristone have that these women are more likely to have a favorable cervix and delivery within 48–96 hours and less likely to undergo cesarean section. But little information is available about fetal outcome and maternal side effects. Thus there is insufficient information to support the use of mifepristone for cervical ripening.

Relaxin

The hormone relaxin is thought to promote cervical ripening. But there is insufficient data to support its use at present.

PROGRAMMED LABOR

The protocol of programmed labor was first introduced by Daftary et al. in the period of 2000-2007.[20,21] Programmed labor protocol rest on the incorporation of three principles:

1. Active management of labor
2. Synergistic application of analgesics and antispasmodics during active phase to facilitate its progress
3. Monitoring the progress of labor on a pictogram alongside a standard nomogram to detect dysfunctional labor and to adopt timely intervention.

The medication protocol for programmed labor begins only after the patient enters the active phase of labor. The starting point of active phase of labor is identified on the basis of clinical evaluation, when following parameters are satisfied:

- Cervical dilatation is 3 cm or more and cervical effacement is more than 50%
- The uterine contractions come at a frequency of at least 3/10 min and last for 35–45 s
- Head should be engaged
- There should be no clinical suspicion of CPD
- The patient may be in early labor and may have 'show'.

Medications Used in Programmed Labor

Combinations of drugs are used to provide effective pain relief (labor analgesia) coupled with antispasmodic drugs which help cervical softening, yielding, and dilatation.

Metho d

- Start an IV infusion line with 5% ringer lactate solution at the rate about 20 drops/min
- Ensure that the pains are optimal, i.e., 3–4 sustained pains/10 min. If necessary, 2 units of oxytocin can be added to drip to ensure optimal pains
- Dilute an ampoule of 30 mg pentazocine/fortwin with a diluent like normal saline/distilled water. Similarly, dilute an ampoule of diazepam (valium/calmpose) in 10 mL of diluent

- Administer one-fifth of each drug, i.e., 6 mg of fortwin and 2 mg of diazepam slowly in bolus form through the tubing of infusion line
- Administer injection tramadol in the dose of 1 mg/kg body weight intramuscularly along with an antispasmodic injection drotaverine 40 mg
- Progress of labor is to be monitored by charting maternal and fetal parameters and assess progress of labor according to documentation on partogram
- When the patient is in advanced labor, i.e., she complains of bearing down sensation and cervix is almost 7–8 cm dilated, this is the right time to administer injection ketamine
- Injection ketamine is given in dose of 0.25–0.50 mg/kg body weight diluted in 10 mL of normal saline, given slowly over few minutes through the tubing of the infusion line until the desired effect is attained.

Advantages

Optimizing labor protocol or programmed labor protocol leads to shorter labors; analgesia is quite effective and side effects of drugs are minimal and safe for the fetus as well.

- The doubling of the rate of cervical dilatation and, therefore, decrease first in the stage of labor can be attributed to the action of drotaverine. It is a superior cervical dilatation agent than other antispasmodics like epidosin or buscopan
- Tramadol has been found to be an effective analgesia in labor without having a deleterious effect on the mother and the fetus
- The incorporation of partogram into the protocol of programmed labor helped to eliminate the ill effects of prolonged labors, and prompted earlier recognition of dystocia and implementation of measures at the same time.

CONCLUSION

Prostaglandins exert the characteristic prelabor structural changes that occur in the cervix. They are key players in the initiation of labor and also participate in the mediation of the initial uterine contractions and overall control of labor. Beyond the first stage of labor, their role is not clearly understood, especially given that their production is downregulated by oxytocin. Intravaginal prostaglandin is the method of choice for the induction of labor. It is an acceptable and effective vehicle for both cervical ripening and the stimulation of labor, although it must be used with great caution in women with uterine scars and in pregnancies complicated by intrauterine growth restriction. It is especially valuable and effective in women who present for induction with a low Bishop score. Intracervical and extraamniotic administrations of prostaglandin are generally regarded as invasive and are not recommended for routine induction of labor.

REFERENCES

1. Wikland M, Lindblom B, Hammarstöm S, Wiqvist N. The effect of prostaglandin I on the contractility of the term pregnant human myometrium. Prostaglandins. 1983;26(6):905-16.
2. Rajabi MR, Dodge GR, Soloman S, Poole AR. Immunochemical and immunohistochemical evidence of estrogen-mediated collagenolysis as a mechanism of cervical dilatation in the guinea pig at parturition. Endocrinology. 1991;128(1):371-8.
3. Kelly AJ, Kavanagh J, Thomas J. Vaginal prostaglandins (PGE2 and PGF2a) for induction of labour at term. Cochrane Database Syst Rev. 2001;(2):CD003101.
4. Nuutila M, Kajanoja P. Local administration of prostaglandin E2 for cervical ripening and labor induction: the appropriate route and dose. Acta Obstet Gynecol Scand. 1996;75(2):135-8.
5. Sanchez-Ramos L, Kaunitz AM, Wears RL, Delke I, Gaudier FL. Misoprostol for cervical ripening and labor induction: a meta-analysis. Obstet Gynecol. 1997;89(4):633-42.
6. Sanchez-Ramos L, Kaunitz AM, Del Valle GO, Delke I, Schroeder PA, Briones DK. Labor induction with the prostaglandin E1 methyl analogue misoprostol versus oxytocin: a randomized trial. Obstet Gynecol. 1993;81(3):332-6.
7. Varaklis K, Gumina R, Stubblefield PG. Randomized controlled trial of vaginal misoprostol and intracervical prostaglandin E2 gel for induction of labor at term. Obstet Gynecol. 1995;86(4 Pt 1):541-4.
8. Wing DA, Jones MM, Rahall A, Goodwin TM, Paul RH. A comparison of misoprostol and prostaglandin E2 gel for preinduction cervical ripening and labor induction. Am J Obstet Gynecol. 1995;172(6):1804-10.
9. Wing DA, Rahall A, Jones MM, Goodwin TM, Paul RH. Misoprostol: an effective agent for cervical ripening and labor induction. Am J Obstet Gynecol. 1995;172(6):1811-6.
10. Chuck FJ, Huffaker BJ. Labor induction with intravaginal misoprostol versus intracervical prostaglandin E2 gel (Prepidil gel): randomized comparison. Am J Obstet Gynecol. 1995;173(4):1137-42.
11. Wing DA, Paul RH. A comparison of differing dosing regimens of vaginally administered misoprostol for preinduction cervical ripening and labor induction. Am J Obstet Gynecol. 1996;175(1):158-64 [Erratum in Am J Obstet Gynecol. 1997;176(6):1423].
12. Kramer RL, Gilson GJ, Morrison DS, Martin D, Gonzales JL, Qualls CR. A randomized trial of misoprostol and oxytocin for induction of labor: safety and efficacy. Obstet Gynecol. 1997;89(3):387-91.
13. Montvale NJ. Physicians' Desk Reference, 53rd edition. USA: Medical Economics Company; 1999. pp. 2951-3.
14. Zieman M, Fong SK, Benowitz NL, Banskter D, Darney PD. Absorption kinetics of misoprostol with oral or vaginal administration. Obstet Gynecol. 1997;90(1):88-92.
15. Bennett BB. Uterine rupture during induction of labor at term with intravaginal misoprostol. Obstet Gynecol. 1997;89(5 Pt 2):832-3.
16. Ngai SW, To WK, Lao T, Ho PC. Cervical priming with oral misoprostol in pre-labor rupture of membranes at term. Obstet Gynecol. 1996;87(6):923-6.
17. Windrim R, Bennett K, Mundle W, Young DC. Oral administration of misoprostol for labor induction: a randomized controlled trial. Obstet Gynecol. 1997;89(3):392-7.

18. Hofmeyr GJ. Misoprostol administered vaginally for cervical ripening and labour induction in the third trimester [Cochrane Review on CD-ROM]. Oxford, England: Cochrane Library Update Software; 1998. Issue 3.
19. Wing DA, Paul RH. Misoprostol for cervical ripening and labor induction: the clinician's perspective and guide to success. Contemp Obstet Gynecol. 1999;44:46-61.
20. Mir S, Aziz R. Programmed labour and its outcome. JK-Practitioner. 2011;16(1-2):39-42.
21. Daftary SN, Desai SV, Thanawala U, Bhide A, Levi J, Patki A, et al. Programmed labor--indigenous protocol to optimize labor outcome. South Asian Fed Obstet Gynecol. 2009;1(1):61-4.

CHAPTER 11

Induction of Labor

Shailesh Kore, Rashmi Patil, Divya Kadam

INTRODUCTION

The word "induction" has its origin from the word *inducere* which means lead into and induction of labor (IOL) simply means lead into labor. Though nature controls most aspects of labor, but sometimes nature needs to be lead.

Induction of labor is defined as the stimulation of uterine contractions by artificial means prior to its spontaneous onset at a viable gestational age, with the aim of achieving vaginal delivery with or without intact membranes.

In modern obstetrics, IOL is a common procedure and current statistics show that incidence varies between 9.5 and 33.7% of all pregnancies.[1] The overall incidence of labor induction is also on the rise.[1] Since past few decades, the use and misuse of induction has been subject of controversy and debate.

HISTORICAL ASPECTS

Induction of labor has been practiced by obstetricians for centuries. Various methods, such as digital stretching of cervix, stimulation of nipples, massage of uterus, use of tents and rubber tubing, have been reported in the literature.

Other methods, like use of castor oil, enema, and a warm water bath, have been the traditional methods generally used for IOL.

The rupture of forewaters as method for induction was used by Denman in 1756 for cases of contracted pelvis. Hind water rupture with Drew-Smythe catheter was introduced in 1931. Theobald first used pitocin for induction in 1952. Turnbull and Anderson introduced the titration method for oxytocin administration. Prostaglandins (PGs) were first isolated way back in 1935 by Ulf von Euler at Karolinska Institute in Stockholm.

TERMINOLOGIES[2]

- Cervical ripening: It is the use of pharmacologic or other means to soften, efface, and/or dilate the cervix to increase the likelihood of a vaginal delivery after labor induction.
- Augmentation: It is the enhancement of uterine contractions in a pregnant woman who is already in labor.
- Tachysystole: It refers to more than six contractions per 10-minute period averaged over 30 minutes. This is further subdivided into two categories, one with and one without fetal heart rate (FHR) changes.
- Hypertonus: : This refers to excessive uterine contractions lasting more than 120 seconds without FHR changes. This term should be abandoned and has been replaced in this guideline by tachysystole without FHR changes.
- Hyperstimulation: This refers to excessive uterine contractions (tachysystole or hypertonus) with abnormal FHR changes. This term has been used in multiple induction studies. It should be abandoned and has been replaced in this guideline by tachysystole with FHR changes.

PHYSIOLOGICAL BASIS FOR INDUCTION OF LABOR

The onset of spontaneous labor is a result of changes which occur in the uterus and cervix together before the actual commencement of labor and is known as prelabor. During this phase of prelabor, there is an increase in uterine contractility and alteration in shape and compliance of the cervix which is otherwise known as cervical ripening.

Caldeyro-Barcia demonstrated that there is a progressive increase in uterine contractility from about 35 weeks gestation culminating in clinical labor at term. In addition to the uterine changes, the cervix transforms from a rigid sphincter to a soft compliant structure capable of undergoing effacement and dilatation. Both of these processes are mandatory for the onset of spontaneous labor and successful delivery. If induction has to be successful, it must be as physiological as possible. A proposed induction would be easier later in pregnancy closer to the term and onset of spontaneous labor. An unfavorable cervix represents the greatest challenge with regards to labor induction.

Indications

Induction of labor needs to be considered when the advantages of delivering the baby clearly outweighs expectant management; is a safer option for the baby, the mother, or both; and when there are no absolute indications for cesarean section (CS) and no contraindications for vaginal delivery.

Maternal Indications

- Prolonged pregnancy
- Prelabor rupture of membranes
- Medical disorders: Pregnancy-induced hypertension (PIH), diabetes mellitus
- Abruptio placentae.

Fetal Indications

- Intrauterine fetal death
- Presence of fetal growth restriction
- Fetal congenital anomaly needing specialized neonatal care, or when continuation of pregnancy would compromise fetal health.

Other Indications

- Convenience of patient and physician
- Distance from the hospital.

Contraindications

- Cephalopelvic disproportion
- Previous classical cesarean scar
- Significant prior uterine surgery
- Malpresentations
- Abnormal placentation: Placenta previa, vasa previa
- Active genital herpes
- Severe fetal growth restriction/nonreassuring fetal status
- Cervical cancer.

Preinduction of Labor Assessment

- Maternal history
- Confirmation of gestation either by reliable menstrual dates supported by early ultrasound examination
- Abdominal examination to confirm presentation and engagement
- Assessment of pelvis and membrane status
- Cervical assessment by vaginal examination
- Fetal wellbeing assessment
- Ruling out any contraindications
- Urgency of IOL.

The Cervix

The status of cervix is pivotal in determining the success of induction. The cervix has a unique composition which facilitates its various roles during pregnancy and labor-cellular portion and extracellular matrix. The distal portion has greater connective tissue as compared to the part close to the myometrium which is richer in the cellular component.

The stroma of the cervix mainly consists of connective tissue (type 1, 2, 3, and 4 collagen; glycosaminoglycans (GAGs), elastin, and proteoglycans) and little smooth muscle. The exact mechanisms leading to cervical ripening is still not clearly defined, but it is mainly the amount and composition of GAGs and proteoglycans in the matrix which gets altered and hence, direct application of PGs which modify collagen by altering the GAGs are used extensively for labor induction. Other possible interactants in the ripening process are cytokines mainly interleukin-8 (IL-8), platelet-activating factor, monocyte chemotactic protein-1, and nitric oxide.

- Collagen: Collagen is mainly in two forms: type I (70%) and type II (30%) and is arranged in the form of a triple helix. In the nonpregnant cervix, these are arranged in a dense and irregular fashion
- Elastin: These fibers are arranged parallel to and between the collagen fibers and play an important role in taking the pregnancy to term by keeping the os closed
- Decorin: This is a GAG and its relative proportion to collagen is important in the remodeling of the cervix at labor
- Hyaluronic acid: This is the most important proteoglycan which is responsible for the increased water content of the cervix.

Changes During Pregnancy

Following changes become evident during pregnancy:

- Collagen is reorganized and consolidated in early pregnancy with proliferation and hyperplasia of the cellular component
- Near the onset of labor, an overall decrease in the concentration of collagen occurs with dispersion and remodeling into fine fibers, making the cervix softer in consistency
- Increases in decorin levels and physiologic cell death are in part responsible for this process

- Hyaluronic acid levels increase, thereby increasing the water content of the cervix and causes a loosening and dispersal of the fibers
- Chemotactic response at term leads to an influx of neutrophils and an increased levels of cytokines (IL-1β and IL-8) which in turn release collagenases and elastases to allow effacement
- Mechanical forces of uterine contractions extend the elastin and allow dilatation.

Scoring System

Because the process of cervical ripening and the onset of labor is a gradual one occurring over several weeks, it is important to recognize that the further this process has progressed, the easier and more successful it will be to induce labor.

This quantifiable method of cervical favorability was described by Bishop more than 50 years ago (Table 1). To put it in its most simple terms, if the Bishop score[3] is high (>9) reflecting a high degree of cervical ripeness, IOL is usually successful and on the other hand, if it is low (<4), it is much more difficult to induce labor and consequently, higher likelihood of failure.

Other scoring systems include Lange scoring, Fields scoring index, Burnett scoring index, Friedman scoring system, Dhall scoring system, etc. (Tables 2 and 3).

Transvaginal sonography for prediction of cervical favorability by measuring cervical length was studied by many authors[4] but none of these tests have been found to be superior to Bishop score.[5]

TABLE 1: Bishop score

Cervical features	Bishop score			
	0	1–2	3–4	5–6
Dilatation (cm)	0	1	2	3
Effacement (%)	0–30	40–50	60–70	80
Station	−3	−2	−1/0	+1/+2
Consistency	Firm	Medium	Soft	
Position	Posterior	Mid	Anterior	

TABLE 2: Modified Bishop score (Burnett)

Cervical features	Bishop score			
	0	1	2	3
Dilatation (cm)	<1	1–2	2–4	>4
Length of the cervix (cm)	>4	2–4	1–2	<1
Station	−3	−2	−1/0	+1/+2
Consistency	Firm	Average	Soft	
Position	Posterior	Mid/Anterior		

TABLE 3: Lange score (score >5 is favorable)

Station	−3	−2	−1, 0	+1, +2
Points	0	1	2	3
Dilatation of cervix (cm)	0	1–2	3–4	>4
Points	0	2	4	6
Length of cervix (cm)	3	2	1	0
Points	0	1	2	3

Other factors which have higher cervical favorability include multiparity, body mass index less than 30 and fetal weight less than 3.5 kg.[6]

INDUCTION METHODS

Various methods of cervical ripening and IOL used for initiating labour at or around term are as follow:

- Pharmacological method
- Mechanical techniques
- Other methods.

Pharmacological Method

Prostaglandins

Prostaglandins are group of modified long chain hydroxyl fatty acids. The main analogs used for induction are E_1 and E_2. They have potent oxytocic activity on pregnant uterus. PGs not only help in cervical ripening, but also initiate uterine contractions. Since PGs have lack of selectivity on target organs, they act on several organs producing undesirable effects. Also, PGs are rapidly metabolized in the body, so have short duration of action. The inherent chemical instability of PGs leads to unpredictable shelf life of the drug.

In 1960s, Karim et al.[7] were the first to study the use of PGs for labor induction. Thereafter, a variety of administration routes of PGs had been explored including oral, intravenous (IV), sublingual, rectal, intra-amniotic, extra-amniotic, intracervical, endocervical, and vaginal. The vaginal route was found to be the most acceptable, and is now the preferred choice by obstetricians all over the world.

Prostaglandin E_2

Orally, PGE_2 tablet have been used for IOL. Tablet containing 0.5 mg of PGE_2 are given at 30–60 minutes interval. The dose may be increased depending on response and improvement in Bishop score.

Dinoprostone (PGE_2) gel is the most commonly employed PG in obstetrics for IOL. This PG helps not only in cervical ripening process, but also for myometrial contractions. It acts by increasing levels of water and hygroscopic mucopolysaccharides like hyaluronic acid in the cervix.

Generally, two routes of administration have been used: intravaginal and intracervical. Intracervical administration is associated with more chances of tachysystole and fetal distress and hence, not recommended (National Institute for Health and Care Excellence guidelines).

Prostaglandin E_2, dinoprostone is available as a gel containing 0.5 mg of dinoprostone in 2.5 mL of triacetin and colloidal silicon dioxide gel in a prefilled applicator. Peak absorption of the drug occurs within 30–45 minutes of application. If there is no improvement in Bishop score, repeat doses may be given at 6-hour intervals, with a maximum 24-hour dose of 1.5-mg dinoprostone (three doses).

Cervidil, a sustained-release 10 mg dinoprostone vaginal insert, has also received Food and Drug Administration (FDA) approval and is commercially available. The vaginal insert consists of a thin, flat, polymeric hydrogel rectangular chip (29 mm × 9.5 mm × 0.8 mm) with a long tail to facilitate easy removal from the vagina. Each insert contains 10 mg of dinoprostone in a dried polymer matrix that releases dinoprostone at a controlled rate of 0.3 mg/h over 10–12 hours when almost 75% of patients require only a single application. Cervidil is placed in the posterior fornix transversely and is removed after the onset of labor or after 12 hours of application. Patient has to recline for almost 2 hours after application.

Prostaglandin E_1

Misoprostol is the PGE_1 analog which, unlike PGE_2, is stable at room temperature, is effective if taken orally and is also considerably cheaper than the alternative PGs available. The American College of Obstetricians and Gynecologists (ACOG; 2000) has recommended the use of this drug because of proven safety and efficacy. The recommended dose by ACOG 1999 is 25 µg (one-fourth of 100 µg tablet) inserted in the posterior vaginal fornix at 4–6 hour intervals. The tablet need not be moistened with water before application.[8] Oral dose of around 25–100 µg is also as effective[9] but has the disadvantage that it cannot be removed in case of hyperstimulation. The World Health Organization (WHO) recommends 25 mg misoprostol, every 2 hours orally or every 6 hour vaginally.

Contraindications for use of prostaglandins[10-12]

- Known hypersensitivity to PGs
- History of previous uterine surgery
- Grand multiparity
- Signs of fetal compromise on cardiotocography (CTG)
- Any contraindication to vaginal birth
- Multiple pregnancies
- Malpresentations.

Use caution in women with

- Asthma due to potential bronchoconstriction
- Ruptured membranes: use gel with caution
- Oxytocin administration
- Epilepsy
- Cardiovascular disease
- Raised intraocular pressure, glaucoma.

Precautions and monitoring

- Encourage voiding prior to insertion
- Avoid oxytocin drip for at least 6 hour after vaginal PG insertion
- Perform CTG for confirmation of fetal wellbeing
- Perform CTG after insertion (minimum 30 minutes)
- Temperature, blood pressure (BP), pulse, per vaginum loss, uterine activity—hourly for 4 hours
- Advise the woman to inform as contractions commence and confirm fetal wellbeing with continuous CTG
- Reassess the patient after 6 hours.

Possible adverse effects

- Gastrointestinal (e.g., nausea, vomiting, abdominal cramps), back pain, fever
- Increased intraocular pressure in women with a history of glaucoma
- Uterine hypercontractility (> six contractions in 10 minutes, or contractions lasting >2 minutes)
- Placental abruption
- Uterine rupture.

Management of uterine hypercontractility (hyperstimulation)

The following interventions may need to be implemented:

- Maternal position should be changed
- Continuous CTG monitoring
- Administration of emergency tocolysis: 250 µg subcutaneous terbutaline
- Manual removal of the gel/tablet
- Fetal scalp blood sampling, if possible
- Cesarean section, if hypercontractility and fetal compromise persist.

Oxytocin

Oxytocin is a nonapeptide originating in the hypothalamus and secreted by the posterior lobe of the pituitary gland. In 1906, Dale[13] observed that extracts from the posterior lobe of the pituitary gland caused myometrial contractions. Synthetic oxytocin was synthesized much later in 1955 by du Vigneud et al.[14] and is the most frequently used agent for labor induction and augmentation all over the world. Synthetic oxytocin is clear colorless fluid and should be stored at 2–80°C in airtight container. Oxytocin activates the phospholipase C/inositol pathway, thus increasing intracellular calcium, thereby stimulating uterine contractions.

The plasma half-life of oxytocin is only 5 minutes, because of the high activity of placental oxytocinase, and steady-state levels are achieved after 40 minutes of continuous IV infusion.[15] Due to the appearance of oxytocin receptors in the myometrium, the uterus starts to respond to oxytocin at approximately 20 weeks' gestation and increases from then on and is maximum around term. The major disadvantage of oxytocin is that it often does not promote cervical ripening, and it is, hence, usually not effective in patients with unripe cervices. Oxytocin is often used following amniotomy giving best results.

Though administration by intramuscular, intranasal or buccal route is possible, continuous intravascular route is preferred and acceptable, as it allows constant level and close titration.

Dose

- Oxytocin is titrated to the minimum dose possible which can achieve an optimum uterine activity causing maximum of three to four contractions in 10 minutes
- Record the dose of oxytocin delivered (i.e., mIU/min).

Most commonly, *oxytocin* is initiated at a dosage of 1 mIU/min, with increases of 1 or 2 mIU/min every 20–30 minutes until a maximum administration rate of 16–32 mIU/min is reached or adequate uterine activity is present. Many protocols for oxytocin infusion have been reported. A more conservative mode of infusion calls for a starting dose of 0.5 mIU/min with similar dose, increases at intervals of 60 minutes. Another protocol by O'driscoll[16] uses starting doses of 6 mIU/min with equal increases of 6 mIU/min (Table 4).

Computer-controlled oxytocin infusion, developed by Willcount and co-workers delivers pulse dose of oxytocin through feedback loop mechanism accounting for changes in the uterine activity. Overall dose of oxytocin is significantly reduced, but equipment is not readily available for clinicians.

The most common side effect of oxytocin infusion is increased uterine contractility and FHR deceleration. This may require emergency CS and hence, monitoring of FHR and uterine contractions is a must. Placental abruption, uterine rupture, precipitate labor and cervical lacerations are also known complications. Water intoxication, a result of the antidiuretic effect of oxytocin, can occur when large volumes of electrolyte-free fluids are infused. Water intoxication can lead to convulsions, coma, and even death and hence, the infusion of high amount of diluted solution should be kept under check.

TABLE 4: Oxytocin regimen[3]

Regimen	Starting dose (mIU/min)	Increment (mIU/min)	Dose interval (min)
Low dose	0.5–2	1–2	15–30
High dose	6	6, 3, 1	15–40

TABLE 5: Oxytocin protocol

Aims and objective	Every 10 minutes (three contractions), each of 40–80 mmHg strength, lasting for 45 s, with resting tone <20 mmHg, helping in adequate progress of labor
Initial dose	0.5 mIU/min
Increment	Dose double every 30–60 min
Maximum dose	6–20 mIU/min

Suggested oxytocin protocol: oxytocin 5 units should be diluted with 1,000 mL of normal saline, making a solution of 0.5 mU/mL (Table 5).

If uterine hypercontractility with associated signs of fetal compromise:
- Decrease or discontinue oxytocin
- Position woman on her left side
- Increase IV fluids.

Others

Nitric acid donors: Studies have shown that the nitric oxide metabolites are upregulated in the uterine cervix during initiation of labor and leads to cervical ripening without any action on myometrium. Recent studies using nitric oxide donors [isosorbide monotitrate and glyceryl trinitrate (GTN)] have shown enhancement of cervical ripening.[17] The role of these agents in cervical ripening and labor induction is presently investigational.[18]

Antiprogestins (mifepristone): Progesterone is considered as hormone required for maintenance pregnancy. On this basis, studies have been done to see whether mifepristone which is progesterone-receptor antagonist can be used for IOL. More research is required to establish its use/role in induction.[19]

Relaxin: Relaxin is a polypeptide hormone, administered either vaginally or intracervically, and is effective in cervical ripening but is still under trials and is not yet used commercially.[20]

Cytokines: The role of cytokines in cervical ripening, especially IL8, is currently under investigation.[21]

Estrogens: Dehydroepiandrosterone sulfate.

Mechanical Techniques

Mechanical methods, mainly effective in causing cervical dilation, have been used for many years to induce labor. In 1810, James et al. utilized amniotomy to induce labor. Amniotomy and other mechanical methods remained the methods of labor induction most commonly employed until the 20th century.

The mechanical stimulation of the endocervical canal has been shown to trigger the release of PGs. The more common mechanical methods include membrane sweeping, amniotomy, balloon-tipped catheters, hygroscopic dilators (laminaria).

Membrane Sweeping

- Digital separation of the fetal membranes from the lower uterine segment via vaginal examination (this stimulates intrauterine PG synthesis)
- If done from 38 to 40 weeks onwards, it significantly reduced pregnancies beyond 41 weeks.[22]

Contraindications

- Low-lying placenta
- Elective cesarean.

Amniotomy, or Artificial Rupture of the Amniotic Membranes

This method was first used by Denman in 1756 for cases of contracted pelvis; being known as "English method". Artificial rupture of membranes (ARM) is often followed by secondary intervention with IV oxytocin after 4 hours.

Indications

- Cervix is favorable, if Bishop score is more than 7
- Augmentation is needed when labour progress is unsatisfactory due to inadequate contractions; and consider oxytocin in the following situations:
    - Multiparous women: If no contractions after 2 hours
    - Nulliparous women: Immediately following ARM as few women will commence contractions spontaneously unless the cervical score is 7 or more[23]
- To observe the color and amount of liquor as clinically indicated.

Within the next 12 hours, labor should begin and birth should occur within 18 hours so that the risk of ascending infection is reduced.

Procedure

- Perform abdominal examination
- Perform vaginal examination; identify the cervix and membranes via vaginal examination. Where the head is high, chances of cord prolapsed should be in mind
- Appropriate instrument to rupture the membranes (e.g., Amnihook or Alligator forceps)
- Record the FHR immediately following ARM and continue to record every 15–30 minutes until the woman is established in labor
- Record the FHR every 30 minutes
- Continuous CTG, if indicated.

Transcervical Catheters

Although various balloon catheters have been described, Foley's catheters with 24-F/26-F are the most commonly used.

The catheter is placed through the internal os and downward traction is created by taping the catheter to the thigh. If after 12 hours, the catheter has not spontaneously fallen out, obstetric review is indicated. Extra-amniotic saline infusion is a modification using Foley's catheter, and it consists of saline infusion at the rate of 60 mL/h in the extra-amniotic space. Either of the methods in successful cervical dilatation and can be used as an adjunct with other pharmacological techniques.[24]

Contraindication

Low-lying placenta.

Cautions

- Antepartum bleeding
- Rupture of membranes
- Cervicitis.

Hygroscopic Dilators (Laminaria)

Natural and synthetic laminaria have been shown to be effective in cervical ripening. Although their safety and efficacy have been established in the second trimester, it can also be used during the third trimester of pregnancy.[25] Laminaria tents are derived from a plant *Laminaria japonica* which has hygroscopic properties. They are placed intracervically and the largest possible size is introduced along with a few gauzes soaked in water in the vagina. The moisture facilitates the swelling of the laminaria and thus, cervical dilatation.

Other Methods

- Stimulation of nipple (manual or by breast pump)
- Giving hot bath
- Castor oil
- Intra-amniotic injection of ecbolic solutions like hypertonic saline, hypertonic glucose, etc.

RISK ASSOCIATED WITH INDUCTION OF LABOR

- Failed IOL: induction is generally considered failed if latent phase of labor is prolonged beyond 18 hours. In case of failed induction, following measures can be taken:
    - Review the individual clinical circumstances
    - Assess fetal wellbeing using CTG
    - Discuss options for care with the woman

- If appropriate, consider discharging home for 24 hours followed by second attempt at IOL
- Cesarean section

- Uterine hypertonicity:
  - Attempt removal of any remaining dinoprostone gel
  - Stop oxytocin infusion while reassessing labor and fetal state
  - Left lateral position
  - Assess BP and FHR
  - Commence IV hydration if not contraindicated by maternal condition
  - Pelvic examination to assess cervical dilation
  - If persists use tocolytics: Terbutaline 250 µg subcutaneously; salbutamol 100 µg by slow IV injection, sublingual GTN spray 400 µg, if clinically indicated perform emergency CS
- Cord prolapse:
  - Is a potential risk at the time of membrane rupture, especially with ARM and an obstetric emergency
  - Precautions should include:
    - Assessment of engagement of the presenting part
    - Caution during ARM if the baby's head is high.
- Uterine rupture:
  - An uncommon event with IOL
  - Uterine rupture is a life-threatening event for mother and baby
  - If suspected, prepare for an emergency CS, uterine repair or hysterectomy
- Sepsis: Risk of sepsis is more in case of premature rupture of membranes, fetal death, prolonged labor, repeated and mechanical methods.
- Antepartum hemorrhage: This is possible following rupture of membranes causing sudden release of liquor, particularly in cases of hydramnios. Partial detachment of placenta and rupture of vasa previa can occur in mechanical methods of induction, particularly when placenta is low lying.
- Amniotic fluid embolism: Risk can be greatly reduced by starting oxytocin only after rupture of membranes.
- Fetal complications: Like sepsis, fetal pneumonia, iatrogenic prematurity, and neonatal jaundice.

WORLD HEALTH ORGANIZATION 2011: GENERAL PRINCIPLES

- Induction of labor should be performed only when there is a clear medical indication for it and the expected benefits outweigh its potential harms
- In applying the recommendations, consideration must be given to the actual condition, wishes and preferences of each woman, with emphasis being placed on cervical status, the specific method of IOL and associated conditions, such as parity and rupture of membranes
- Induction of labor should be performed with caution since the procedure carries the risk of uterine hyperstimulation, rupture, and fetal distress
- Wherever IOL is carried out, facilities should be available for assessing maternal and fetal wellbeing
- Women receiving oxytocin, misoprostol or other PGs, should never be left unattended
- Failed IOL does not necessarily indicate CS
- Wherever possible, IOL should be carried out in facilities where CS can be performed.

World Health Organization Recommendations 2011[26]

- Induction of labor in women at or beyond term:
  - IOL is recommended for women who are known with certainty to have reached 41 weeks (>40 weeks + 7 days) of gestation (low-quality evidence; weak recommendation)
  - IOL is not recommended for women with an uncomplicated pregnancy at gestational age less than 41 weeks (low-quality evidence; weak recommendation)
- Induction of labor in women with gestational diabetes: If gestational diabetes is the only abnormality, IOL before 41 weeks of gestations is not recommended (very-low-quality evidence; weak recommendation)
- Induction of labor for suspected fetal macrosomia: IOL at term is not recommended for suspected fetal macrosomia (low-quality evidence; weak recommendation)
- Induction of labor in women with prelabor rupture of membranes at term: IOL is recommended for women with prelabor rupture of membranes at term (high-quality evidence; strong recommendation)
- Induction of labor in women with uncomplicated twin pregnancy at or near term: None.

Other Recommendations

- Oral misoprostol (25 µg, 2 hourly) is recommended for IOL (moderate-quality evidence; strong recommendation)
- Vaginal low-dose misoprostol (25 µg, 6 hourly) is recommended for IOL (moderate-quality evidence; weak recommendation)
- Misoprostol is not recommended for women with previous CS (low-quality evidence; strong recommendation).

CONCLUSION

There is definite increase in the incidence of induction of labor due to various reasons now-a-days, majority of them being the medical disorders in pregnancy. Also, availability of better diagnostic facilities leads to early diagnosis helping in timely intervention. Most of the obstetricians are opting for misoprostol and PGE2 gel as their choice for cervical ripening and induction, and oxytocin for augmentation of labor. Nevertheless, there cannot be a fixed approach and the choice of inducing agent needs to be individualized, after detailed evaluation of each patient.

REFERENCES

1. World Health Organization (WHO). (2010). WHO Global Survey on Maternal and Perinatal Health. Induction of Labour Data. [online]. Available from www.who.int/reproductivehealth/topics/maternal_perinatal/globalsurvey/en/. [Accessed September, 2015].
2. Macones GA, Hankins GD, Spong CY, Hauth J, Moore T. The 2008 National Institute of Child Health and Human Development workshop report on electronic fetal monitoring: update on definitions, interpretation, and research guidelines. Obstet Gynecol. 2008;112:661-6.
3. Society of Obstetricians and Gynaecologists of Canada (SOGC). SOGC clinical practice guideline. Induction of labour at term (No 107). J Obstet Gynaecol Can. 2001:1-12.3.
4. Hatfield AS, Sanchez-Ramoz L, Kaunitz AM. Sonographic cervical assessment to predict the success of labor: a systemic review with meta-analysis. Am J Obstet Gynecol. 2007;197(2):186-92.
5. Crane JM. Transvaginal sonography cervical length and successful labour induction. Obstet Gynaecol. 2006;107:60S.
6. Pevzner L, Rumney P, Petersen R, Wing D. Predicting a successful induction of labor: a secondary analysis of misoprostol vaginal insert trial. Abstract no. 218. Presented at 29th Annual Meeting of the Society for Maternal-Fetal Medicine, January 26-31, 2009. San Diego, CA, USA: Washington, DC.
7. Karim SM, Trussell RR, Patel RC, Hillier K. Response of pregnant human uterus to prostaglandin-F_2-alpha-induction of labour. BMJ. 1968;4(5631):621-3.
8. Sanchez-Ramos L, Danner CJ, Delke I, Kaunitz AM. The effect of tablet moistening on labor induction with intravaginal misoprostol: a randomized trial. Obstet Gynecol. 2002;99(6):1080-4.
9. Wing DA, Park MR, Paul RH. A randomized comparison of oral and vaginal misoprostol for labor induction. Obstet Gynecol. 2000;95(6 Pt 1):905-8.
10. MIMS Online. Prostin E2 Vaginal Gel [Pfizer]. 2008 [cited 2011 June 6]. Available from: https://www.mimsonline.com.au. [Accessed September, 2015].
11. MIMS Online. Cervidil Pessary [CSL]. 2006 [cited 2011 June 6]. Available from: https://www.mimsonline.com.au. [Accessed September, 2015].
12. Australian Medicines Handbook. (2011). Dinoprostone. [online]. Available from www.health.qld.gov.au/qcg/documents/g_iol5-1.pdf. [Accessed September, 2015].
13. Dale HH. On some physiological actions of ergot. J Physiol. 1906;34(3):163-206.
14. Du Vigneud, Swan JM, et al. The synthesis of oxytocin. J Am Chem Soc. 1953;75:4879.
15. Seitchik J, Amico J, Robinson AG, Castillo M. Oxytocin augmentation of dysfunctional labor. IV. Oxytocin pharmacokinetics. Am J Obstet Gynecol. 1984;150(3):225-8.
16. O'Driscoll K, Foley M, MacDonald D. Active management of labor as an alternative to cesarean section for dystocia. Obstet Gynecol. 1984;63(4):485-90.
17. Chanrachakul B, Herabutya Y, Punyavachira P. Potential efficacy of nitric acid for cervical ripening in pregnancy at term. Int J Gynaecol Obstet. 2000;71(3):217-9.
18. Thompson AJ, Lunan CB, Cameron AD, Cameron IT, Greer IA, Norman JE. Nitric oxide donors induce ripening of the human uterine cervix: a randomised controlled trial. Br J Obstet Gynaecol. 1997;104(9):1054-7.
19. Frydman R, Lelaidier C, Baton-Saint-Mleux C, Fernandez H, Vial M, Bourget P. Labor induction in women at term with mifepristone (RU 486): a double-blind, randomized, placebo-controlled study. Obstet Gynecol. 1992;80(6):972-5.
20. Brennand JE, Calder AA, Leitch CR, Greer IA, Chou MM, MacKenzie IZ. Recombinant human relaxin as a cervical ripening agent. Br J Obstet Gynaecol. 1997;104(7):775-80.
21. Chwalisz K, Sholz P, Hegele-Hartung CH, et al. Cervical ripening with interleukin 1β and tumor necrosis factor-α (TNF) in pregnant guinea pigs [abstract S27]. Society for Gynecological Investigation, Scientific Program and Abstracts, 40th Annual Meeting, Toronto, Ontario, 1993.
22. Boulvain M, Stan C, Irion O. Membrane sweeping for induction of labour. Cochrane Database Syst Rev. 2005;(1):CD000451.
23. Subramanian D, Penna L. Induction of labour. In: Arulkumaran S, Warren R (Eds). Best Practice Labour and Delivery. Cambridge, UK: Cambridge University Press; 2009. pp. 195-206.
24. Sherman DJ, Frenkel E, Tovbin J, Arieli S, Caspi E, Bukovsky I. Ripening of the unfavorable cervix with extraamniotic catheter balloon: Clinical experience and review. Obstet Gynecol Surv. 1996;51(10):621-7.
25. Hale RW, Pion RJ. Laminaria: an underutilized clinical adjunct. Clin Obstet Gynecol. 1972;15(3):829-50.
26. World Health Organization. (2011). WHO recommendations for induction of labor. [online] Available from: at:http://www.who.int/reproductivehealth/publications/maternal_perinatal_health/ 9789241501156/en/.

CHAPTER 12

Anesthesia and Analgesia

Kartik Syal

INTRODUCTION

Anesthesia and analgesia form an important aspect of culmination of long process of pregnancy and childbirth in the form of providing either analgesia during normal delivery or anesthesia for operative delivery. Along with this, anesthesia and/or analgesia in third trimester can also be needed for emergency operative procedures other than delivery.

PHYSIOLOGICAL CHANGES IN PREGNANCY AFFECTING ANESTHESIA

Cardiovascular System

The increase in cardiac output by up to 30–50% at 34 weeks, along with increase in stroke volume by nearly 30% by the time cervical dilatation is 8 cm,[1] have two major implications on anesthesia.

First and foremost is that compensated heart diseases can present itself during pregnancy and can get aggravated during labor. Anesthetic drugs have profound effects on heart, from myocardial suppression to changes in heart rate and in afterload and preload; all these can cause heart-related morbidity and even mortality. Second effect, even in healthy pregnant heart is that due to increase in cardiac output, the induction by intravenous (IV) agents is faster and by inhalational agents is slower.

Also, fall in hematocrit (15%) due to increase in plasma volume by almost 50%[2] keeps mother relatively safe in view of blood loss during delivery, which may be around 500 mL in uncomplicated cases. Even a blood loss of around 1,000 mL during cesarean section is well tolerated by most pregnant patients, until and unless any comorbidity is present.

Aortocaval Occlusion (Supine Hypotension Syndrome)

Pregnant patients having nausea, hypotension, and dizziness in supine position were researched and it was hypothesized in 1935 that it was due to inferior vena cava compression.[3] Later on, studies confirmed the compression of inferior vena cava and even aorta by enlarging uterus (after 20 weeks), causing decreased preload and hypotension. Angiography even revealed that there is excessive flow in collateral circulation through epidural and azygous veins. This compensation along with vasoconstriction of blood vessels prevent symptoms in around 90% of pregnant patients even till term.[4] However, during anesthesia, especially regional anesthesia, there is vasodilation and relaxation of abdominal muscles causing increased uterine pressure on great vessels leading to profound decrease in preload and hypotension, many-a-times needing intervention in the form of vasoconstrictors and fluid bolus. Mechanical means of patient positioned with left side tilt (15° at least to >30° for maximal effect) or manually pushing uterus to left side should be used with variable benefit.[5] In some cases, this compression can even cause placental blood flow insufficiency due to congestion in placental veins due to increased upward flow pressure and also due to aortic compression causing retarded flow. In one study, it was shown that there is up to 20% increase in intervillous blood flow on changing the position from supine to left tilt.[6]

Respiratory System

With the abdominal cavity expanding with growing fetus, the expiratory reserve volume is reduced by 25% and residual volume by 15%, reducing total functional residual capacity (FRC) by 20%. This decrease is maximum in third trimester and can cause symptoms in supine position. This, along with increased oxygen (O_2) demand makes pregnant patients prone to early desaturation on apnea. Also, capillary engorgement due to progesterone and increased retention of body fluid causes airway mucosal edema. These factors put an obstetric patient in great danger during intubation, with enlarged breasts (difficult laryngoscopy) and airway edema (including of false and true vocal cords) making intubation difficult, and changed respiratory physiology lowers threshold to hypoxia.

There is steady increase in minute ventilation to keep up with oxygen demand of growing fetus. This along with decreased FRC causes faster induction and depth of inhalational anesthesia. Hyperventilation is common in labor pains, causing respiratory alkalosis leading even to apnea and decrease in oxygen saturation in between the contractions. Opioids in any route can potentiate apnea and can further decrease the saturation levels though in clinically used concentrations and doses, it is insignificant.

Gastrointestinal System

Physiological lower esophageal sphincter is not effective in pregnancy as expanding uterus pushes it to thoracic cavity, distorting its shape and progesterone relaxes its smooth muscles. Though it was earlier believed that progesterone also delays gastric emptying, but large scale studies have refuted this finding.[7] These changes along with increased abdominal pressure necessitates aspiration prophylaxis and rapid sequence induction in most pregnant patients to prevent regurgitation and aspiration, described as Mendelson syndrome.

Other Physiological Changes in Pregnancy

Exaggerated lumbar lordosis, prominent abdomen, engorged epidural vessels, edema, and epidural fat deposition make regional anesthesia (spinal and epidural) difficult and dictates dose reduction of local anesthetic agents. With these anatomical changes, there is also increased sensitivity to local anesthetic agents due to progesterone. Thus, lower doses are used and complications like significant hypotension and bradycardia, bloody needle taps and failure to reach spinal or epidural space are more common.

LABOR ANALGESIA

In a joint statement given in 1992, the American Anesthesiologists and Obstetrics and Gynecologists Society stated, "Labor pains are one of the most distressing pains a human being may have to bear; there is no other circumstance where it is considered acceptable for a person to experience such severe pain, amenable to safe intervention, while under a physician's care. Hence option of labor analgesia should be given to all pregnant females".[8]

This advisory given long time back changed the outlook towards labor analgesia from being given to those who demanded to being offered to all.

Physiology of Labor Pains

In the first stage of labor, myometrial ischemia due to uterine contractions causes release of pain transmitters like bradykinin, histamine, and serotonin. Also, there is stretching of mechanoreceptors in lower uterine segment and cervix. From these, the visceral pain impulses travel in A-δ and C nerve fibers through paracervical ganglion and hypogastric plexus to cause pain in T_{10}-L_1 spinal cord segments. The pain is poorly localized, over entire abdomen and may be transmitted to legs and gluteus. The pain in second stage is exaggerated extension of pain in first stage and has principally somatic localized component. Distension of pelvic structures and perineum due to birthing fetus causes relative ischemia and even micro- and macroinjuries causing pain. Somatic pain is carried by branches of pudendal nerve in S_2-S_4 dermatomes.

The severity of this pain has been described as "distressing", "horrible" or "excruciating" by most females during and after labor.[9] Even when reported on objective pain scores like McGill pain questionnaires, labor pain is one of the most intense pain.[10]

Severe pain leads to sympathetic stimulation, which can cause increase in catecholamines and cortisol levels, decreasing uterine contractions along with decrease in placental perfusion. This along with increased oxygen consumption and increased cardiac output can cause increase in lactic acids causing maternal metabolic acidosis. These factors may combine to cause significant fetal acidemia and fetal hypoxia, especially in patients with comorbid heart or pulmonary conditions.

Interventions to Reduce Labor Pain

Bromage PR summarizing labor analgesia, stated, "Superficially obstetric anesthesia appears to be a simple field with a limited range of interest, but it is a deceptively demanding subspecialty. Not only are two patients involved in each anesthetic administration but also the dynamic events of normal labor require that the muscles concerned with delivery retain their power and coordination to the full".[11]

Figure 1 shows diagrammatic representation of various interventions to reduce labor pains.

History of Labor Analgesia

In 1847, James Young Simpson administered the first obstetric general anesthetic using ether. His action was widely criticized concerning maternal and fetal safety. The concept of labor analgesia was popularized by John Snow who delivered Queen Victoria's eighth child under chloroform analgesia in 1853.[12] The history of labor analgesia progressed through the use of nitrous oxide (N_2O) by Klikovitch in Russia, use of morphine, hyoscine and later, pethidine and finally the use of regional technique by Aburel in 1931.[13]

The preferred technique of labor analgesia should be safe to mother and fetus, effective and controllable, predictable in its effects and should have a high technical success rate; also it should not weaken uterine contractions or maternal bearing down. Modern neuraxial labor analgesia reflects a shift in obstetrical analgesia, thinking away from a simple focus on pain relief towards a focus on the overall quality of analgesia.[14]

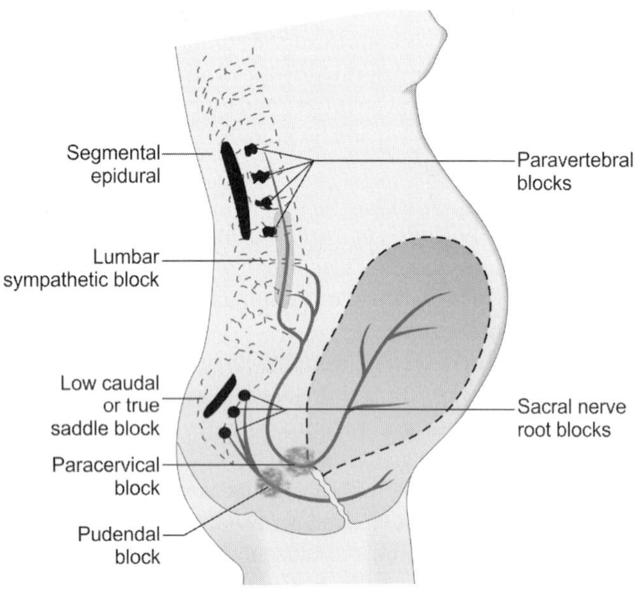

FIG. 1: Interventions to reduce labor pains.

Table 1 enumerates different nonpharmacological and pharmacological ways to provide labor analgesia.

Nonpharmacological Means

Transcutaneous electrical nerve stimulation, continuous support in labor, psychological preparation, touch and massage, water bath, intradermal sterile water injections, acupuncture and hypnosis, all may be beneficial for the management of pain during labor.[15] However, there have been no proven scientific data analysis of the quality of pain relief offered by these techniques and conclusive data is lacking. The only consistent benefit appears to be a reduction in requirement of pharmacological means of analgesia. Psychological preparations of the patient with professionals, in many studies, have shown to have a positive influence in pregnant patients to bear pain. Transcutaneous electrical nerve stimulation involves excitation of sensory nerves, decreasing impulses from pain pathways due to cross-conductions and has also been shown to increase endogenous opioids production, thus providing some benefit during active phase of labor.

Pharmacological Means

Systemic opioids have been used for long remain the most widely used medications for labor analgesia. Pethidine has enjoyed a widespread popularity in this regard, now recently being challenged by availability of better agents like fentanyl (1–2 μg/kg slow IV) and its derivatives which are suitable to be administered by patient-controlled IV pumps as well. Butorphanol 1 mg IV or intramuscular (IM) is also a popular agent for providing pain relief. Other agents include ketamine (up to 1 mg/kg slow IV), tramadol (1–2 mg/kg IM or slow IV), etc., which can be used in ways to combine the advantages of each other. The technique remains popular as no specialized equipment is required and it is easy to administer; forming the basis of "programmed labor".

TABLE 1: Different ways to provide labor analgesia

Nonpharmacological	Pharmacological		
	Inhalational	Systemic	Regional
• Birthing preparation • Hypnosis • Transcutaneous electrical nerve stimulation • Acupuncture • Electroanalgesia • Hydrotherapy • Aromatherapy	• Entonox • Sevoflurane • Desflurane • Trilene • Methoxyflurane	• Opioids • Sedatives • Ketamine • Tramadol	• Epidural • Subarachnoid block (spinal) • Combined spinal epidural • Lumbar sympathetic block • Paracervical block • Pudendal block

Programmed Labor

Programmed labor is an optimized labor protocol to ensure smooth progress of labor resulting in the vaginal delivery of a healthy baby through judicious use of labor inducers, appropriate obstetric-analgesic regimen, and partographic monitoring. It is suitable for low-risk primigravidae and can be carried out by the obstetrician in the active phase of labor by combining different drugs in doses lower than conventional individual doses. This minimizes the occurrence of adverse effects associated with any of them and supplementation can be continued till after delivery. A simple regime described as follows:[16]

- Injection diazepam 2 mg IV (total: 10 mg)
- Injection tramadol 50 mg IM (total: 100 mg)
- Injection pentazocine 6 mg IV (total: 30 mg)
- Injection drotaverine 40 mg IV every 2 hours (maximum: 3 doses)
- Injection ketamine 0.25–0.50 mg/kg IV (maximum: 1 mg/kg or 100 mg in 30 minutes) slow.

Programmed labor has been shown to produce good analgesia and amnesia, shorten the period of labor, decrease operative delivery and blood loss as well as improve uterine flow.

Inhalational Analgesia

Inhalational analgesia through face mask was the earliest form of obstetric analgesia, using subanesthetic concentrations of inhalational anesthetic agents, including N_2O. The advantages include that the mother remains awake with protective laryngeal reflexes, technique is self-administered (which makes it safe, as face mask falls when patient goes to deepen plane) and progress of labor is unaltered. Several inhalational agents, both gaseous and volatile, have been used successfully in labor. The earliest to be used were ether, chloroform, and cyclopropane, followed by trichloroethylene and methoxyflurane. Enflurane, isoflurane, sevoflurane, and desflurane are more recent additions; with entonox (50% N_2O + 50% O_2) still the most widely used, but sevoflurane is believed to be the best agent. The disadvantage of using volatile agents is that sophisticated equipment is needed to administer these agents in a controlled way. Also, there is atmospheric pollution and chances of deepening of anesthetic depth and aspiration if face mask is held by someone other than patient herself.

Regional Analgesia

Central neuraxial analgesia is the most versatile method of labor analgesia and is currently the gold standard technique for pain control in obstetrics.[17] The use of neuraxial techniques has increased dramatically in the last 20 years. Local anesthetics alone were used for many years, but are now generally administered in lower concentrations in combination with opioids to provide effective, synergistic analgesia whilst reducing some of the unwanted side effects of local anesthetics, such as motor block. Regional analgesia is effective in preventing the increase in catecholamines associated with labor pain. Therefore, the sympathetic overactivity, which may lead to decrease in uterine blood flow and dysrhythmic contractions, is successfully blunted by regional analgesia by providing effective pain relief. Also, this pain relief allows parturient to be awake and be able to participate in labor and delivery.

Regional anesthesia may be administered by the anesthetist using epidural, subarachnoid (spinal) block, combined spinal epidural or lumbar sympathetic block. Paracervical block, pudendal block, and local perineal infiltration are forms of labor analgesia practiced by obstetricians themselves.

Epidural labor analgesia

The most important indication for labor analgesia remains maternal request for pain relief. Others would include maternal and fetal indications which by themselves warrant an anesthetic management of labor analgesia, specifically epidural analgesia. Despite the supposed availability of many options, epidural analgesia remains the only effective technique to relieve severe pain as well as offer therapeutic benefits for high-risk parturients. Obstetric patients with previous cesarean section, anticipated difficult airway, multiple pregnancy, and obesity stand to benefit with an indwelling epidural catheter, in face of an emergency cesarean section. Preeclamptic parturients derive additional benefit by virtue of improved placental blood flow and blood pressure control. The same stands for parturients with cardiac and pulmonary disease where drastic hemodynamic changes during labor are avoided, thereby preserving both maternal and fetal well-being. Specific fetal indications include prematurity and small-for-date babies where the resultant improved maternal oxygen saturation and relaxed pelvic floor muscles allow a controlled and less traumatic delivery. There is also a reduced risk of intracerebral bleeding and improvement in acid base status of the baby.

This technique necessitates vigilant monitoring, including fetal monitoring, necessary resuscitation equipment, and trained staff. Contrary to former practice of inserting the epidural catheter once labor was established, presently maternal request predominantly governs the timing of epidural insertion,[18] with the obstetrician's approval. In cases where therapeutic benefits are expected, especially in cardiac patients and in preeclampsia patients, the epidural catheter should be inserted as soon as possible, even along with induction.

Most commonly, a mid-lumbar (L_{2-4}) midline placement is preferred (Fig. 2). T_{10}-L_1 dermatomes are blocked to relieve pain of uterine contractions and cervical dilatation while S_2-S_4 segments need to be blocked to relieve pain of vaginal and perineal distension. Caudal approach to epidural space through sacral hiatus is restricted to use in patients nearing delivery with contraindication to spinal anesthesia. Contraindications include patient refusal, local anesthetic allergy, coagulopathies [drug or disease-induced, e.g., hemolysis, elevated liver enzymes, and low platelet count (HELLP) syndrome], infection at the site of insertion, and obstetric hemorrhage and moderate-to-severe hypovolemia.

The preparation of patient should ideally begin in the antenatal period, with detailed counseling sessions with both the anesthetist as well as the obstetrician, to allay anxiety and discuss the benefits as well as risks along with preanesthetic check-up. A full informed consent explaining procedure, complications (urinary retention, shivering, etc.) and inadequacies (incomplete pain relief, ambulation problems, etc.) is mandatory before administering any form of labor analgesia, more so in regional techniques.

Various regimes include intermittent bolus epidural analgesia (patient or anesthetist controlled epidural analgesia) with or without basal local anesthetic infusion, continuous infusion epidural analgesia (at rate of 8–15 mL/h), opioid alone or addition of opioid to local anesthetics; which decreases latency, prolongs duration, improves quality of analgesia, and allows lower doses of both drugs to be used.

Drugs commonly used are bupivacaine in concentrations varying from 0.06 to 0.125% and ropivacaine 0.06–0.15% with or without opioids, which are fentanyl 50–100 µg in 10 mL saline (or 1–2 µg/mL) and sufentanil 10–25 µg in 10 mL saline. Use of lignocaine is generally confined to initial test dose or second stage of labor, avoiding concentrations more than 1%. The use of lower concentrations or opioids alone as in combined spinal epidural is what has come to be known as "walking epidural". The proposed advantages of ambulation in labor include the parturient's enjoyment of mobility, autonomy and self-control in labor, increased uterine activity and increased intensity of contractions, decreased frequency of contractions, decreased pain, decreased duration of the first stage of labor, decreased incidence of fetal heart rate (FHR) abnormalities, and decreased incidence of operative and/or assisted deliveries.[19]

The blood pressure is measured every 3–5 minutes after administration of doses of local anesthetic for 15–20 minutes or until hemodynamically stable and subsequently every 15–30 minutes. Other monitoring may include pulse oximetry, FHR monitoring, hourly change in position, sensory level of analgesia, Visual Analog Scale scores and intensity of motor block, and other adverse effects like urinary retention.

Labor analgesia using subarachnoid (spinal) space

Subarachnoid space (Fig. 2) is utilized more often now as an addition to epidural injection (combined spinal epidural analgesia) due to its rapid reliable effect. Opioid like 25 µg fentanyl with low dose (2.5 mg) bupivacaine in a concentration of 0.1% can be used for practically immediate relief of pain, and gives time for epidural to act. Isolated spinal analgesia in above doses can also be used, especially in patients coming for labor analgesia with almost full dilatation. But if we increase the concentration or dose of local anesthetic agents given in intrathecal (spinal) space, we will have loss of motor power and increased rate of instrumental deliveries. Also, increase in opioids cause increased incidence of their side effects, especially pruritis. Continuous spinal anesthesia is not used these days due to high incidence of infection and neurological complications.

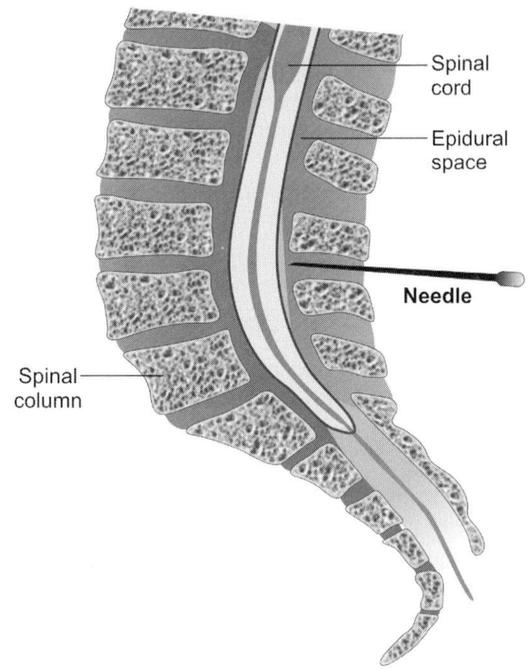

FIG. 2: Epidural and subarachnoid space.

Other regional techniques

Lumbar sympathetic block

Bilateral paravertebral lumbar sympathetic block at level of L_2, though effective, is seldom used due to its limited duration and technical difficulty.

Paracervical block

This block is given by injecting local anesthetic agents into vaginal fornices lateral to the cervix. As it is simple to perform and can provide good analgesia in 40–80% of patients, it is still used by many obstetricians. Though the most deterrent complication is high incidence of fetal bradycardia after this block due to uterine vasoconstriction and high fetal local anesthetic concentration. Hematoma, sacral neuropathy, and abscess being the other complications.

Pudendal nerve block

Especially used for instrumental deliveries by obstetricians, it has been superseded by more reliable and safer spinal or epidural blocks. Bilateral nerve is blocked behind ischial spines adjacent to lateral vaginal walls by 10–15 mL of 1% lignocaine. Failure or partial block in 40–50% of cases and hematoma formation are complications associated with this block.

Care during Regional Analgesia

- Hypotension may occur and lead to decrease in uteroplacental flow if persistent. Maintenance of normovolemia and infusion of around 250 mL Ringer's lactate takes care of this problem
- Abolishing of Ferguson reflex[20] leading to delay in delivery has not been established in humans.[21] But the second stage (American College of Obstetricians and Gynecologists) as long as 3 hours for nulliparous and 2 hours for parous patients are taken as normal. There are reports variable for assessing increase in instrumental deliveries with labor analgesia, generally higher incidence with increasing concentration of local anesthetic agents.[22] At high concentration of local anesthetic agents, dense block may occur leading to higher rates of instrumentation. A recent Cochrane review indicate, that overall there is delay (study of 13 trials combined) as well as increased incidence of instrumental deliveries (23 trials assessed) with use of regional labor analgesia techniques.[23] Though no increase in rates of cesarean section was found, which is more affected by maternal and fetal factors and obstetrical management[24]
- As it is commonly called as "walking epidural", patient is allowed and motivated to ambulate, but weakness and paresthesia contradicts unsupported ambulation
- Incidence of shivering increases with use of regional techniques in labor, from 10–20 to 20–50%. The reasons are multifactorial from anxiety to low-temperature fluids to exposed maternal surface. But, the main reason is shifting of core temperature to periphery by regional anesthesia, mainly in epidural along with loss of sympathetically-mediated vasoconstriction
- Maternal hyperthermia in contrast to shivering can also be seen in some patients, averaging around 1°C over 7–10 hours. Hypothesis of this phenomenon being resetting of thermoregulation center and imbalance between heat loss and production
- Opioids, when used alone in regional anesthesia can cause their own side effects like pruritis, nausea, vomiting, and respiratory depression in neonate. These effects occur rarely when opioids are used as adjuncts to local anesthetic agents. Still some recommend omission of opioids from epidural top ups when full dilatation is achieved
- Backache: though concern have been raised of possibility of regional techniques causing backaches or aggravating the same, large prospective studies have refuted these claims[25]
- Urinary retention: it has been seen that during labor, there is inadequate urinary evacuation due to pain and neurohormonal changes, causing increased chances of postnatal urinary complaints. This can be aggravated by decreased or total loss of bladder sensation by regional anesthesia techniques, a problem which can be solved by frequent encouragement to evacuate or intermittent catheterization
- Other complications of regional techniques include total or partial failure, unintentional dural puncture, extensive neuroblockade, and intravascular injection of drug
- The effect on breastfeeding has not been well established with conflicting studies available.[26] There has been hypothesis suggesting problems in breastfeeding with regional labor analgesia techniques due to drugs used, fetal neurohormonal changes as well as increased need of oxytocin infusions.

ANESTHESIA IN THIRD TRIMESTER

Anesthesia for Cesarean Section

Anesthesia technique for cesarean section is complicated by various variables like urgency, indication, fasting status, comorbid conditions, and maternal wish.

General Anesthesia

The use of this technique for routine cesarean section is declining with time due to following reasons:

- Airway problems: difficulty in intubation and ventilation is the most dreaded complication in general anesthesia. Enlarged breasts, buccal fat depositions, mucosal edema, and capillary engorgement make ventilation, laryngoscopy, and intubation difficult in obstetrics cases. This along with the fact that these patients are prone to sudden desaturation due to higher demand and decreased reserve make mother and fetus highly prone for hypoxia. Capillary engorgement also may lead to oral bleeding with laryngoscopy making further attempts to intubation more difficult.

  Thus, difficult intubation tray along with supraglottic airway devices like laryngeal mask airway (laryngeal airway devices) should always be kept by the anesthesiologist. Also, preoxygenation of 100% oxygen for 3–5 minutes or eight vital capacity breaths is necessary.
- Aspiration: ever since Mendelson[27] described aspiration, many studies have confirmed high incidence of aspiration in pregnant patients, going even up to 15%.

Acidic gastric contents (pH <2.5) and failure of lower esophageal sphincter to effectively work can lead to pulmonary complications. This is aggravated by failure or delay in securing airway causing higher volume aspiration (>25 mL significant).

These two airway-related complications lead to more than half of anesthesia-related deaths in cesarean section. In one survey spreading over 5 years, it was found that general anesthesia was associated with 16 times more case fatality rate than regional anesthesia, though this difference since then has decreased due to better airway management and aids to intubation.[28] These facts have led to use of regional anesthesia technique for routine cesarean section in most institutes.

- Multiple drugs: giving general anesthesia involves addition of multiple drugs into maternal and fetal circulations. In standard doses, the drugs rarely have significant effects, but chances of neonatal respiratory and central depression remain. Also, unknown teratogenic and neurohormonal influence of drugs further complicates this choice of anesthesia
- Awareness: patients counseled and consenting for regional anesthesia knows that they will be awake and aware of their surgery to some extent at least till extraction of baby. But, patients going for general anesthesia also can have awareness because of tendency of keeping anesthetic drugs on the lower side in view of fetal safety. This should be explained to the patient and should be included in the consent to avoid legal matters in the future.

To decrease the incidence of awareness, N_2O (40–66%) combined with volatile anesthetic agents [<1 minimum alveolar concentration (MAC)] or ketamine (in doses up to 1 mg/kg) can be used.

Advantages of general anesthesia

- Immediate onset of anesthesia; induction takes only around 15 seconds
- Anesthetist with multitude of drugs is in full control of hemodynamics of the patient
- Motionless patient is an aid to the surgeon.

Indications for general anesthesia

- Dire maternal and fetal emergency, like profound fetal bradycardia, cord prolapse with fetal compromise, uncontrolled eclampsia, etc.
- Coagulopathy and other contraindications to regional anesthesia
- Maternal wish
- Acute severe maternal hypovolemia
- Inadequate regional anesthesia.

General considerations in conduct of general anesthesia

- Fasting period: more the period, better it is. Most advocate a fasting period of at least 8 hours for elective surgery. A dextrose maintenance drip can be started to prevent catabolism if this fasting period exceeds
- Premedication: light premedication with benzodiazepines, like oral midazolam or lorazepam should be given to prevent anxiety and sympathetic activation
- Aspiration prophylaxis: H_2-receptor antagonist (ranitidine 150 mg oral or 50 mg IV) and metoclopramide 10 mg (oral or IV) is given as standard procedure a night before and 30 minutes before surgery. Nonparticulate antacids, like 30 mL of 0.3 M sodium citrate can be used to increase the pH of gastric contents and decrease the ill effects of aspiration
- Rapid sequence induction: after adequate preoxygenation, rapid sequence induction with cricoid pressure is used to prevent regurgitation
- Sedatives and analgesics are kept in balance of providing anesthesia to mother and avoiding neonatal depression. Once baby is extracted full doses of short-acting agents can be given keeping in mind early start of breastfeeding is prudent
- In cases of full stomach, patients extubation too can cause aspiration. So, it should be done only after recovery of reflexes and in lateral, head down position
- Conduct of general anesthesia can have fluctuations in hemodynamics due to sympathetic stimulations during laryngoscopy, intubation and extubation. This can have detrimental effects on patients with cardiac diseases and in patients with hypertensive disorders
- Halothane, especially and other inhalational agents can cause uterine relaxation if given at concentrations higher than MAC. This can be beneficial in difficult to extract cases but may lead to uterine atony and postpartum hemorrhage.

Spinal Anesthesia for Cesarean Section

It involves injection of local anesthetic agents (bupivacaine or ropivacaine generally) with or without adjuncts (opioids like fentanyl mostly) into subarachnoid space with the help of spinal needle in complete sterile condition under full hemodynamic monitoring. Spinal anesthesia is the most used technique for cesarean section due to following reasons:

- Quick onset (around 5–10 minutes with commonly used 0.5% heavy bupivacaine)
- Simple to perform with easily identifiable target, which is cerebrospinal fluid (CSF)
- Reliable with good quality regional anesthesia
- With small manipulation in dose and head tilt using heavy local anesthetic agents, anesthetist can vary the spread of block
- No direct effect of drug on fetus
- Good intraoperative conditions.

Complications associated with spinal anesthesia

- Hypotension: hypotension is generally associated with spinal anesthesia and necessitates fluid bolus and dose of vasoconstrictors. Preloading with 10–15 mL/kg of Ringer's lactate or normal saline, left lateral position and elevated legs can help in decreasing the incidence and severity of hypotension. Ephedrine is one of the most favored vasopressor due to its lesser vasoconstriction in uterine vessels. Phenylephrine in doses of 50–100 μg IV is recommended now due to its better and prolonged maintenance of blood pressure. Prolonged significant hypotension can cause fetal acidosis and morbidity
- High spinal: hormonal and mechanical factors in pregnancy decrease the need of local anesthetic agents for regional anesthesia. Higher doses can cause hypotension, bradycardia and even loss of consciousness, needing ventilatory and hemodynamic support
- Postdural-puncture headache: this is related to breach in dura caused by spinal or less frequently but more drastically by larger epidural needle, leading to continuous leakage of CSF. The pain typically occurs in fronto-occipital region, within 24–48 hours of regional anesthesia, increases with sitting or standing, and is usually of thumping type. Its incidence has decreased from over 50% to less than 10% with the use of smaller diameter atraumatic (splitting Whitacre type rather than cutting Quincke type) spinal needles of sizes 25 gauge and above.[29] But in cases of inadvertent dural puncture with 16 gauge or 18 gauge epidural needle, the incidence goes up to even 70%, warranting prophylactic steps, like proper hydration, analgesics, caffeine, bed rest, and even epidural fluids and blood patch to be considered. Treatment of established postdural-puncture headache (PDPH) involves all these interventions. Caffeine in doses of 300–500 mg/day (one glass of strong coffee contains around 50–100 mg caffeine) is effective due to vasoconstriction of cerebral vessels. Sumatriptan is also used due to similar reason. Desmopressin and adrenocorticotropic hormone have also been tried but not recommended. The most effective treatment is injecting 20 mL of self blood in the epidural space which clots and seals the dural opening and prevents leakage and symptoms are relieved. Chances of infection, invasive procedure, need of two doctors simultaneously (one for venipuncture and other for epidural injection), and relapse of pain due to clot dislodgment are points against this treatment approach. Hence, it is left for severe resistant cases. Epidural fluid and dextran have also been used with short-term success
- Persistent neurological symptoms: present day drugs are not associated with any persistent neurological symptoms except if injected directly into neural tissue ignoring excruciating pain on injection. These were related to use of chloroprocaine and continuous lignocaine anesthesia
- Limited anesthesia time is also one of the factors leading to more frequent use of epidural technique. Continuous spinal anesthesia is not recommended due to neurological complications; hence, anesthesia and analgesia time is limited by duration of effect of single shot local anesthetic agent.

Epidural Anesthesia for Cesarean Section

Epidural anesthesia involves injection of local anesthetic agents into epidural space. The space is further from nerves, thus the dose of drug injected is higher and time taken to effect is also longer. This restricts its usefulness in emergency cases, like fetal distress. The greatest advantage of this technique is that it can be extended from providing labor analgesia to operative anesthesia to postoperative analgesia. Around 15–18 mL of 2% lignocaine or bupivacaine (concentration >0.25%) is needed for operative procedures (T4 level needed).

Complications associated with epidural anesthesia

- As there is no clear endpoint other than loss of resistance through ligamentum flavum, which itself is edematous and lax in pregnancy, a good "feel" of reaching epidural space is not appreciated. This can cause failure and dural puncture leading to PDPH
- Intraspinal injection of epidural dose will cause high spinal and will require intensive care unit care
- Migration of epidural catheter to intrathecal or intravascular position is a known fact and so drug should be injected always after negative aspiration
- Hypotension can occur but less in severity and incidence compared from spinal anesthesia due to slow onset of effect. However, precautions, like preloading and monitoring, are essential
- Postdural-puncture headache due to inadvertent dural puncture has been discussed
- Patchiness of effect is common with plain epidural technique due to reasons like intraspace adhesions, septas, etc.

General Considerations of Regional Anesthesia

- Regional anesthesia can be converted to general anesthesia due to reasons, like partial effect, prolongation of surgery, etc., hence full preparation as for general anesthesia are to be undertaken
- Both techniques can be combined to take advantage of fast onset of spinal anesthesia and prolonged action of epidural technique. Thus, low doses are needed in spinal anesthesia which prevents most of its complications. Addition of spinal dose accelerates anesthesia time

and provides profound block which is sometimes not available with epidural anesthesia

- Coagulopathy contraindicates regional anesthesia. Platelet counts 50,000/μL for spinal and 75,000/μL for epidural are taken as minimum acceptable limit
- Technically, more difficult in pregnant patients due to exaggerated lumbar lordosis and lumbar and epidural fat depositions
- More chances of bloody tap due to engorged vessels in pregnancy. Significant hematoma formation is rare but if it evolves urgent diagnosis and evacuation is mandatory to prevent any neurological catastrophe
- As in all operative procedures, consent form an important legal document in cases of cesarean section. In cases of severe labor pains, consent should also be taken from closest relative present considering the patient may be biased towards some approach due to the severest form of pain
- There are four operative steps where in spite of T4 level of anesthesia, patient may feel distressed:
  1. Stretching of rectus sheath compared from dissecting it
  2. Uterine fundal pressure during extraction of baby, due to pressure on ribs and thorax
  3. Exteriorization of uterus to view uterine incision, due to stretching of peritoneum
  4. Paracolic gutters sweeping.

  This justifies use of analgesics and sedatives like opioids after extraction of baby. Ketamine in doses till 1 mg/kg can be used safely to blunt these responses even with fetus *in utero*.
- Nausea and vomiting are frequently encountered and should be managed with good level of anesthesia, maintenance of blood pressure, and prophylactic metoclopramide and ranitidine. Ondansetron (60–100 μg/kg IV) and low-dose propofol (20 mg IV) can be used.

Anesthesia for Retained Placenta

Regional anesthesia till T7 segment is the technique of choice. Extension of epidural catheter being used for analgesia can also be done. Spinal anesthesia using 10 mg of hyperbaric (heavy) bupivacaine with or without fentanyl (10–25 μg) can be used safely and reliably. To provide tocolysis, 50–100 μg IV boluses of glyceryl trinitrate can be given every minute monitoring blood pressure. General anesthesia using inhalational volatile agents, especially halothane, can also be used.

Anesthesia for Nonobstetric Cases

Only emergency surgeries should be undertaken in the third trimester of pregnancy. Considerations already covered for cesarean section hold true for nonobstetric cases too. Effects of drugs on fetus are insignificant but continuous FHR should be monitored. Regional anesthetic technique is preferred over general anesthesia, if surgical indication allows. Hypoxia, acidosis, and hypotension should be avoided.

EFFECTS OF MATERNAL ANESTHESIA AND ANALGESIA ON FETUS

Anesthesia and analgesic agents when used in standard doses and route are safe and mostly have insignificant clinical effects on fetus. If excessive doses for deep anesthesia are given, it can lead to respiratory and central depression in fetus. Fetal morbidity and mortality due to anesthesia is catastrophic due to complications of anesthesia, like profound hypotension, leading to inadequate blood flow to fetus, hypoxia due to inability to ventilate and intubate, toxic doses of local anesthetic agents erroneously given via IV route.

Inhalational Agents including Nitrous Oxide

Agents, like halothane, isoflurane, etc., can be used under their MAC without any significant effect on fetus. Use of N_2O in labor is in consequential for the fetus as excretion through lungs is very rapid. N_2O interferes with deoxyribonucleic acid synthesis by inactivating its cofactor vitamin B_{12}, but its use for a short duration during labor and delivery is clinically insignificant. Its use can have indirect effect due to hypoxia in fetus if nitrous oxygen mixture is given for labor analgesia along with opioids.

Opioids

Opioids enter fetal circulation according to their lipid solubility. Commonly used opioids in labor and delivery are fentanyl and its derivatives alfentanil, sufentanil, and remifentanil. Lipid solubility of these agents and high concentration of albumin in fetus can cause its accumulation and respiratory depression of fetus. The significance of this is when these agents are used at high dose, using IV route, e.g., doses exceeding 400 μg for fentanyl. Use of other opioids, like butorphanol, nalbuphine, pentazocine, etc., can be undertaken safely during delivery in standard doses, taking care to prevent respiratory depression and indirect effects of hypoxia to the fetus.

Local Anesthetic Agents

Local anesthetic agents in use for regional techniques of analgesia and anesthesia are lignocaine, bupivacaine, and ropivacaine. Though bupivacaine and ropivacaine are more lipophilic and hence, more prone for fetal accumulation, in clinical practice lignocaine is the one which can cause its toxic effects in fetus in concentrations more than 10 μg/mL. Higher protein binding, higher placental tissue uptake, and less frequent bolus doses prevent bupivacaine and ropivacaine toxicity. As these agents are weak bases they get trapped in weakly acidic pH of fetus, which becomes significant in fetal distress when fetal pH is further decreased.

Adjuncts in Regional Anesthesia

Other than opioids, clonidine, neostigmine, and adrenaline can be used as adjuncts to local anesthetic agents for labor analgesia as well as for regional anesthesia. Clonidine is a α_2-agonist which prolongs the action of local anesthetic agents and also improves quality of analgesia by acting in dorsal horn of spinal cord. Though found to be safe and effective for use in labor analgesia, cumulative doses exceeding 150 μg may lead to maternal hypotension, bradycardia, and fetal bradycardia.[30]

Neostigmine acts on the spinal cholinergic receptors but is not frequently used due to side effects, like nausea, vomiting, and sedation at clinically useful doses.

Adrenaline can also be added to local anesthetic agents, especially lignocaine due to variety of effects, like reduced vascular absorption, reduced risk of local anesthetic toxicity, greater intensity and quality of block, and prolongation of lignocaine block. In spite of these beneficial effects, adrenaline is rarely used in obstetrics as it is seen that doses exceeding 50 μg in epidural space can cause uteroplacental insufficiency, reduced uterine activity, and prolongation of labor. IV injection of as small as 15 μg of adrenaline can cause maternal and fetal cardiovascular stimulation leading to erroneous diagnosis as well as uteroplacental vasoconstriction. Small less than 40 μg adrenaline in diluted concentration (1:200,000 and above) can be used in epidural technique after ensuring lack of direct intravascular administration.

CONCLUSION

Pain is considered an important determinant of patients' wellbeing; it being characterised as 5th vital sign. In all conditions, healthcare providers work towards reducing pain and thereby suffering of a patient coming to them. Except in the situation of labor where the intent of providing analgesia to a parturient is probably still lacking in developing nations, specially the situation prevalent in India. The same is aggravated by customs of not interfering with the natural process of child birth. It is duty of obstetricians and anesthetists to combine as a team to give options of pain relief as many safe and efficient means are available as discussed in the chapter.

REFERENCES

1. Robson SC, Dunlop W, Boys RJ, Hunter S. Cardiac output during labour. Br Med J (Clin Res Ed). 1987;295(6607):1169-72.
2. Taylor DJ, Lind T. Red cell mass during and after normal pregnancy. Br J Obstet Gynaecol. 1979;86(5):364-70.
3. Ahltorp G. [On problems in the supine position in pregnant women]. Acta Obstet Gynecol Scand. 1935;15:295-341.
4. Kinsella SM, Lohmann G. Supine hypotension syndrome. Obstet Gynecol. 1994;83(5 Pt 1):774-88.
5. Kinsella SM, Whitwam JG, Spencer JA. Aortic compression by the uterus: identification with the Finapres digital arterial pressure instrument. Br J Obstet Gynaecol. 1990;97(8):700-5.
6. Kauppila A, Koskinen M, Puolakka J, Tuimala R, Kuikka J. Decreased intervillous and unchanged myometrial blood flow in supine recumbency. Obstet Gynecol. 1980;55(2):203-5.
7. O'Sullivan G. The stomach--fact and fantasy: eating and drinking during labour. Int Anesthesiol Clin. 1994;32(2):31-44.
8. American College of Obstetricians and Gynecologists (ACOG). Committee on Obstetrics: Maternal and Fetal Medicine. Pain Relief during Labor. ACOG opinion number 118. Washington, DC, USA: ACOG; 1992.
9. Brown ST, Campbell D, Kurtz A. Characteristics of labor pain at two stages of cervical dilation. Pain. 1989;38(3):289-95.
10. Melzack R, Taenzer P, Feldman P, Finch RA. Labour is still painful after prepared childbirth training. Can Med Assoc J. 1981;125(4):357-63.
11. Bromage PR. Epidural analgesia. Philadelphia, PA, USA: Saunders; 1978. p. 513.
12. Snow J. On administration of chloroform in during parturition. Assoc Med J. 1853;1(23):500-2.
13. Curelaru I, Sandu L. Eugen Bogdan Aburel (1899-1975). The pioneer of regional analgesia for pain relief in childbirth. Anaesthesia. 1982;37(6):663-9.
14. Wong CA. Advances in labor analgesia. Int J Womens Health. 2009;1:139-54.
15. Simkin PP, O'hara M. Nonpharmacologic relief of pain during labor: systematic reviews of five methods. Am J Obstet Gynecol. 2002;186(5 Suppl Nature):S131-59.
16. Daftary SN, Desai SV, Thanawala U, Bhide A, Levi J, Patki A, et al. Programmed Labor--indigenous protocol to optimize labor outcome. South Asian Feder Obstet Gynecol. 2009;1(1):61-4.
17. Hawkins JL. Epidural analgesia for labor and delivery. N Engl J Med. 2010;362(16):1503-10.
18. Ohel G, Gonen R, Vaida S, Barak S, Gaitini L. Early versus late initiation of epidural analgesia in labor: does it increase the risk of cesarean section? A randomized trial. Am J Obstet Gynecol. 2006;194(3):600-5.
19. Chamberlain G, Stewart M. Walking through labour. Br Med J (Clin Res Ed). 1987;295(6602):802.
20. Ferguson JK. A study of the motility of the intact uterus at term. Surg Gynecol Obstet. 1941;73:359-66.
21. Saunders NJ, Spiby H, Gilbert L, Fraser RB, Hall JM, Mutton PM, et al. Oxytocin infusion during second stage of labour in primiparous women using epidural analgesia: a randomised double blind pacebo controlled trial. BMJ. 1989;299(6713):1423-6.
22. Ismail S. Labor analgesia: an update on the effect of epidural analgesia on labor outcome: Review article. J Obstet Anaes Crit Care. 2013;3(2):70-3.

23. Anim-Somuah M, Smyth RM, Jones L. Epidural versus non-epidural or no analgesia in labour. Cochrane Database Syst Rev. 2011;(12):CD000331.
24. Segal S, Su M, Gilbert P. The effect of a rapid change in availability of epidural analgesia on the cesarean delivery rate: a meta-analysis. Am J Obstet Gynecol. 2000;183(4):974-8.
25. Breen TW, Ransil BJ, Groves PA, Oriol NE. Factors associated with back pain after childbirth. Anesthesiology. 1994;81(1):29-34.
26. Szabo AL. Review article: Intrapartum neuraxial analgesia and breastfeeding outcomes: limitations of current knowledge. Anesth Analg. 2013;116(2):399-405.
27. Mendelson CL. The aspiration of stomach contents into the lungs during obstetric anesthesia. Am J Obstet Gynecol. 1946;52:191-205.
28. Chestnut DH. Anesthesia and maternal mortality. Anesthesiology. 1997;86(2):273-6.
29. Turnbull DK, Shepherd DB. Post-dural puncture headache: pathogenesis, prevention and treatment. Br J Anaesth. 2003;91(5):718-29.
30. Syal K, Syal GG, Chauhan G, Gupta KB. Clonidine as an adjunct in epidural labour analgesia using bupivacaine: maternal and neonatal outcome. J Paed Obs Gynae. 2010;1(10):385-8.

CHAPTER 13

Normal Labor and Vaginal Delivery

Jyothika A Desai, Thejavathy GV

INTRODUCTION

Labor actually means hard work and it is quite appropriate to term it that way because of the tiring (hardship) process the woman goes through, and the force with which the uterine muscle contracts to deliver the fetus. Labor and delivery are normal physiologic processes. Only about 50% of high-risk, pregnancy related complications are identified before screening and admission for labor. Careful evaluation of both the mother and fetus upon presentation to the labor and delivery suite is important. Attention to the principles of normal labor and maternal-fetal physiology are necessary to avoid unnecessary interventions in the labor and delivery process. Normal labor can be defined as a physiological process during which the fetus and placenta along with the membranes are delivered by effective uterine contractions through a completely effaced and dilated cervix. Normal labor is a retrospective clinical diagnosis made by proper history and physical examination of the parturient woman.[1]

Evaluation of the patient presenting with symptoms of labor includes:
- History
- Physical examination
- Selected laboratory tests
- Fetal assessment.

A clinical impression and management plan are formulated from the information obtained.

HISTORY OF THE PRESENT LABOR

The onset, frequency, duration, and intensity of uterine contractions should be determined. Contractions that effect progressive cervical effacement and dilation are usually regular and intense (the patient may no longer be able to walk or talk during these contractions). They usually are accompanied by a "bloody show," the passage of blood-tinged mucus from the effacing cervix. Braxton Hicks contractions are experienced by many women during the last week of pregnancy. These are usually irregular, mild, not well organized, and do not result in cervical change. Factors that differentiate true labor from false or prodromal labor are given in Table 1.

Rupture of Membranes

The status of the fetal membranes must be determined if it is not reported as part of initial presentation. The patient may present with leaking fluid alone or in conjunction with uterine contractions. The time of occurrence is important, because prolonged rupture increases the risk of chorioamnionitis. The patient may report a large gush of fluid with continued leakage, leaving little doubt as to its source. Such a history is reliable in more than 90% of patients. The patient may report

TABLE 1: Differences between true and false labor pains

True Labor	False Labor
• Contractions occur at regular intervals • Location of pain is in the back and abdomen • Interval slowly reduces or shortens • Intensity keeps increasing • Associated with cervical effacement and dilatation • Progress of labor not affected by enema or sedation	• Contractions occur at irregular intervals • It is mostly in lower abdomen • Interval remains irregular • It remains the same • No associated changes in the cervix • Pain usually subsides after enema and/or sedation

merely increased moisture on her underclothes, which leads to uncertainty about whether this moisture represents urine, vaginal secretions, cervical mucus, or amniotic fluid. Confirmation of rupture of membranes (ROM) may include physical examination, laboratory testing, and ultrasonography.

Vaginal Bleeding

The extent, if any, of vaginal bleeding should be ascertained. Spotting or blood-tinged mucus is common in normal labor. Heavy vaginal bleeding merits complete investigation because it may be abnormal and reflect a significant disorder.

Fetal Movement

The initial assessment of the patient reporting symptoms of labor should include questions about the level of her fetus's movement. Most patients are aware of their fetus's baseline level of activity. If the patient reports a significant or progressive decrease in fetal movement from her normal baseline, fetal well-being must be ascertained.

Such evaluations can involve fetal monitoring with a nonstress test, a contraction stress test, or biophysical profile. Fetal movement-counting protocols are often used routinely in the third trimester as a screen for fetal well-being.

HISTORY OF PRESENT PREGNANCY

The history of the present pregnancy should be obtained by interviewing the patient in labor and by reviewing the prenatal record. The prenatal record may be from one's own institution or from an outside source. The patient, of course, may have had no prenatal care or have no record of it. If a prenatal record is available, important items should be verified with the patient.

Gestational Age

Gestational age is best determined from data in the prenatal record. The later the patient presents for initial prenatal care, the more difficult it becomes to accurately determine the estimated gestational age (EGA). Patients presenting for initial prenatal care at more than 24 weeks of gestation are considered to have inherently unreliable dates. Important landmarks for determining gestational age include. The first day of the last menstrual period (LMP)—the estimated date of confinement (EDC) is calculated as 40 weeks or 280 days from this date. The date of last ovulation (as determined by an ovulation prediction kit or basal body temperature chart), or the date of conception (if known precisely), with the EDC calculated as 38 weeks from this date, early ultrasound measurement of crown-rump length at 6–12 weeks of gestation (accurate to within 3 days), the average of multiple biometric measurements on fetal ultrasound between 12 weeks and 20 weeks of gestation (accurate to within 10 days), fetal heart tones, first heard with a Doppler instrument at 10–12 weeks of gestation or with a fetoscope at 18–20 weeks of gestation, quickening (maternally perceived fetal movement), which occurs at approximately 18–20 weeks of gestation in primigravidas, uterine size before 16 weeks of EGA, as determined by an experienced clinician. Accurate dating requires evaluation during the first half of pregnancy.

The patient presenting in labor with an uncertain LMP and no prenatal care may be difficult to date with accuracy. Uncertain gestational age presents a significant problem because of different management strategies for term, preterm, and post-term pregnancies. In these situations, the only alternative is to use ultrasonography in the labor and delivery suite, realizing that it may, at best, be accurate to within only ±3 weeks of gestation in the last trimester.

History of Past Pregnancies

Each past pregnancy and its duration and outcome should be reviewed. Particular attention should be paid to preterm deliveries, operative deliveries, prolonged or difficult labors, shoulder dystocias (15% risk of recurrence), malpresentation, eclampsia or pre-eclampsia (5–40% risk of recurrence), placental abruption or placenta previa (risk increases with age, parity, and prior cesarean delivery), and blood loss requiring transfusion. Other medical facilities may need to be contacted for records to verify or clarify certain points.

Medical History

All active medical problems should be evaluated and the extent of the disease determined. The stress of labor can aggravate many medical problems and jeopardize both maternal and fetal well-being.

Psychosocial and Emotional History

Labor is a stressful physical and psychological event, and understanding the patient's psychosocial and emotional status and history will help in planning for her care and maintaining her sense of control. How the patient wishes, to be addressed should be determined. Her preparation and plans for labor and birth should be discussed. The patient's labor support person(s) and their preparation should be identified. Questions about substance and alcohol use or abuse, intimate partner violence, and diagnosis and treatment of psychiatric disorders should be included. This part of the history must be obtained from the patient without any family or support persons present.

PHYSICAL EXAMINATION

Although active labor is not the optimal setting for a comprehensive physical examination, a focused examination with emphasis on the abdomen and pelvis can be performed between painful contractions. Any signs of intercurrent medical illness or abnormalities of major organ systems should be elicited and carefully noted. Special note should be taken of those parts of the physical examination that may generate abnormal findings because of that individual patient's history.

The following have to be checked when a woman comes to the hospital at term complaining of pains:

- Checking on her prenatal records
- Detailed history of the pain, frequency and duration
- Any history of watery discharge or bleeding per vaginum
- Appreciation of fetal movements.

Physical examination of the patient will include:

- Maternal vital signs like pulse, temperature, pallor, and blood pressure
- Systemic examination of cardiovascular, respiratory and central nervous system.

OBSTETRIC EXAMINATION

- Presence of uterine contractions.
- Abdominal examination with Leopold maneuver, fundal grip, feeling the podalic pole, lateral grips, with back on one side and limbs on the other side, first pelvic grip appreciating the cephalic pole and the second pelvic grip making sure whether the head is engaged or not.
- Auscultation of the fetal heart sounds, its rate and regularity.
- Pelvic examination is done to assess the cervical length, dilatation, consistency, position and station of the fetal head. Pelvis is also assessed clinically for its adequacy at the inlet, mid pelvis and outlet to rule out cephalopelvic disproportion.

Only after the examination has been completed, we will know whether the patient is in true labor or not.

Sometimes accurate diagnosis of labor at term may be difficult especially in the latent phase of labor. A repeat examination by the same person 2 hours later will confirm the diagnosis. Educating the patient in the antenatal period about labor and childbirth will definitely help in cooperation of the patient, and the obstetrician will be able to do her job better in a relaxed environment. It is also important to have an attendant who is close to the patient throughout labor to reassure her and reduce the stress and strain of labor.

For all practical purposes, labor has been divided into four stages.

First Stage of Labor

It begins with the onset of regular uterine contractions and ends with full dilatation of the cervix. On an average, it is about 10–12 hours in a primigravida and 5–6 hours in a multipara.

Progress of labor was analyzed and a curve developed by Friedman (1954) after studying labor in 100 consecutive primigravidae in spontaneous labor at term. In his landmark study of 500 primigravidae, he subdivided the first stage into an early latent phase and a rapid active phase according to the curve of cervical dilatation.

The duration of latent phase is variable and is associated with little cervical dilatation (up to 3 cm) and effacement from 3 cm to about less than 0.5 cm. This is followed by the active phase where the cervix dilates from 3 to 10 cm, i.e., full cervical dilatation.

The active phase of cervical dilatation is divided into an acceleration phase, phase of maximum slope and a deceleration phase (Fig. 1).

Second Stage of Labor

The second stage of labor begins with full dilatation of the cervix and is completed with delivery of the newborn. The duration is about 1–2 hours in a primigravida and about 1 hour in a multigravida. In multipara, more than 1 hour without regional anesthesia and 2 hours with regional anesthesia is prolonged second stage.

Third Stage of Labor

The time taken from the delivery of the fetus to the delivery of the placenta and membranes is termed the third stage of labor. Most times the placenta is delivered or expelled within 10 minutes of the delivery of the baby. Sometimes it may take a little longer, up to 30 minutes in both nulliparous and multiparous women. Earlier one would wait for spontaneous separation and expulsion of the placenta, which is called expectant management of the third stage, but now active management is preferred over expectant as blood loss is reduced with diminished risk of postpartum hemorrhage. The third stage of labor is considered prolonged if it is more than 30 minutes. Anything more than 2 hours without

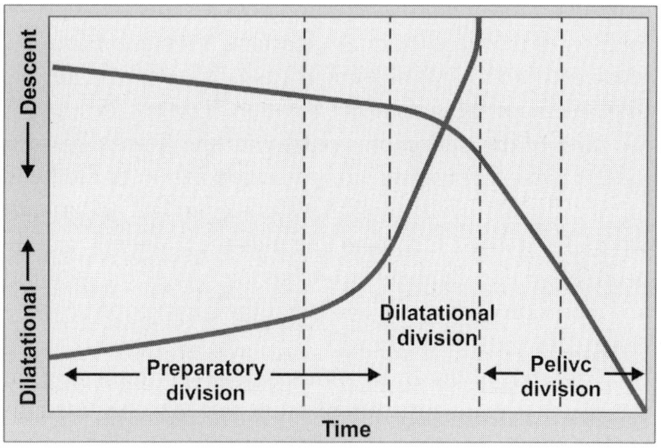

FIG. 1: Graphical representation of normal labor.

regional anesthesia or 3 hours with regional anesthesia in a nullipara is called prolonged second stage.

Fourth Stage of Labor

It is the period of 1 hour after the delivery of the placenta. It is a very critical period where the patient is kept under close observation for any excessive bleeding per vaginum.

Proper management of normal labor is important in developed and developing countries, especially in developing countries, where prolonged and neglected labor is associated with high maternal morbidity and mortality.

MECHANISMS OF LABOR IN THE VERTEX PRESENTATION

The process of labor and delivery is marked by characteristic changes in fetal position or cardinal movements in relation to the maternal pelvis. These spontaneous adjustments are made to effect efficient passage through the pelvis as the fetus descends (Fig. 2). Engagement is the descent of the largest transverse diameter, the biparietal diameter, to a level below the pelvic inlet. An occiput below the ischial spines is engaged. Descent of the head is a discontinuous process occurring throughout labor. Because the transverse diameter of the pelvic inlet is wider than the anteroposterior (AP) diameter, and because the greatest diameter of the unflexed fetal head is the AP diameter, in most instances, the fetus enters the pelvis in an occiput transverse alignment. Flexion decreases the AP diameter of the fetal head. It occurs as the head encounters the levator muscle sling, thereby decreasing the diameter by approximately 1.5–2.5 cm (occipitomental, 12.0 cm, to occipitofrontal, 10.5 cm). Later, further flexion occurs, reducing the diameter to 9.5 cm (suboccipitobregmatic). Internal rotation occurs in the midpelvis. The architecture of the midpelvic passageway changes so that the AP diameter of the maternal pelvis at this level is greater than the transverse diameter. The fetus accommodates to this change by rotation of the head from a transverse orientation (occiput transverse) to an AP alignment (usually occiput anterior), thus accomplishing internal rotation. Further descent to the level of the perineum occurs with the head aligned in the AP plane. Crowning: after internal rotation of the head, further descent occurs until the suboccipút lies underneath the pubic arch. At this stage, the maximum diameter of the head (biparietal diameter) stretches the vulval outlet without any recession of the head even after the contraction is over—called "crowning of the head".

Extension of the head allows delivery of the head from the usual occiput anterior position through the introitus. Little actual descent occurs with extrusion of the head because the head is delivered by a reversal of the flexion that occurred as it entered the pelvis. The face appears over the perineal body, while the symphysis pubis acts as the fulcrum on which the occiput impinges. Restitution: it is the visible passive movement of the head due to untwisting of the neck sustained during internal rotation. Movement of restitution occurs rotating the head through $1/8^{th}$ of a circle in the direction opposite to that of internal rotation. The occiput thus points to the maternal thigh of the corresponding side to which it originally lay. External rotation occurs after delivery of the head, when the fetal head rotates back, or restitutes, toward the original transverse orientation (external rotation or restitution, when the biacromial diameter (fetal shoulders) is aligned in an AP orientation with the greatest diameter of the pelvic outlet. The remainder of the delivery proceeds with presentation of the anterior shoulder beneath the symphysis pubis and the posterior shoulder across the posterior fourchette. Birth of shoulders and trunk: after the shoulders are positioned in AP diameter of the outlet, further descent takes place until the anterior shoulder escapes below the symphysis pubis first. By a movement of lateral flexion of the spine, the posterior shoulder sweeps over the perineum. Rest of the trunk is then expelled out by lateral flexion.

The steps in mechanism of normal labor are:

- Engagement
- Descent
- Flexion
- Internal rotation and crowning
- Extension
- Restitution
- External Rotation

It can be remember by mnemonic: engaged Decent Females In England Returns Egypt.

MANAGEMENT OF FIRST STAGE OF LABOR

- Once true labor is confirmed, the patient is admitted to the labor ward
- Basic tests like hemoglobin, blood group to be rechecked
- Admission NST in places where it is possible
- Preparation of the perineum
- Informed consents for labor and various instrumental procedures.

Management of the patient in labor is based on these principles:

- Maternal position
- Monitoring of the mother
- Monitoring the fetus
- Hydration
- Maintenance of partogram
- Pain relief
- Amniotomy
- Smooth muscle relaxants?
- Augmentation of labor.

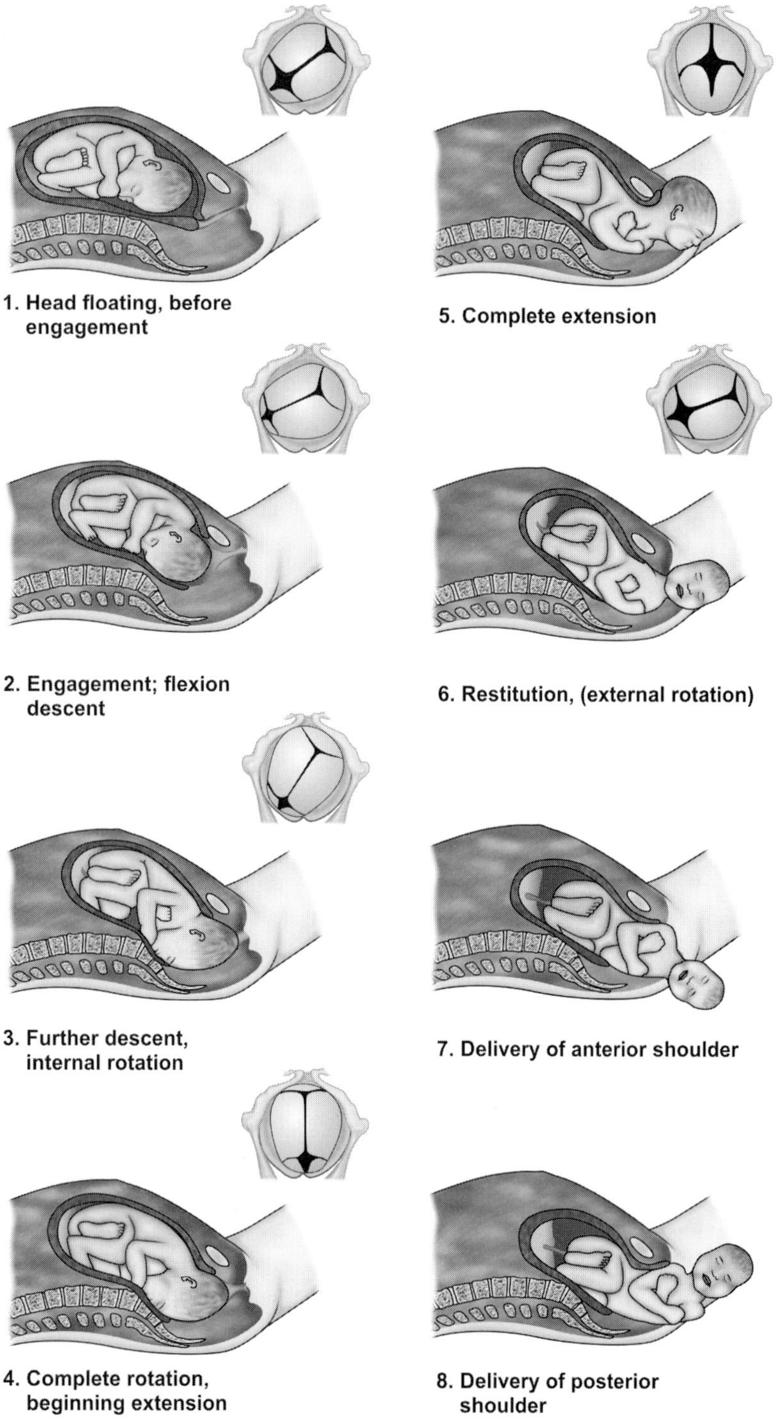

FIG. 2: Mechanism of labor

Maternal Position

Maternal position in labor has consequences for both maternal comfort and fetal well-being. The dorsal supine position with the gravid uterus resting on the aorta and inferior vena cava can cause decreased cardiac output and relative placental hypoperfusion. Patients in the latent phase of labor frequently are most comfortable if they are allowed to be out of bed and walking. No significant risk of fetal compromise exists, as long as an initial monitoring strip is reassuring and the membranes are intact or the presenting part is well-applied to the cervix. Studies comparing patients who were ambulatory during the active phase of labor versus those who were confined to bed have found some acceleration of the first stage of labor and decreased numbers of operative deliveries in the ambulatory group, with equal fetal outcomes. In the late active phase, it was difficult to keep the ambulatory group walking. Patients who have freedom of movement in labor will find positions that are most comfortable to them and thereby minimize their pain. The patient's labor support person, doula, or registered nurse is critical in helping the patient become comfortably positioned during labor. If it becomes necessary, bed rest on the patient's side rather than on her back is recommended and allows intermittent or continuous fetal monitoring to be performed. One study showed that continuous fetal monitoring may be carried out in the ambulatory patient by telemetry with no difference in fetal outcome, but significantly less subjective pain than in control subjects.

Monitoring of the Mother

- Maternal vital signs: pulse, temperature and blood pressure should be checked every 4 hours
- Frequency, intensity and duration of uterine contractions should be recorded
- The descent of the fetal head, in fifths palpable above the pelvic brim is noted
- Vaginal examination about cervical length, dilatation, position, consistency and station of the fetal head in relation to the ischial spines to be followed every 3–4 hours
- Bladder care: making the patient frequently empty her bladder and noting the urine output.

Monitoring of the Fetus

- Fetal heart is monitored every 30 minutes in the first stage. It is checked immediately after a uterine contraction according to ACOG guidelines 2007
- Regularity, rate and any deceleration should be checked
- Fetal heart can be monitored either by the fetoscope, stethoscope, Doppler or by electronic fetal monitoring.

Hydration

- Patient is not given any solid food in active labor
- Only clear oral fluids are recommended
- Intravascular fluids (Ringer's lactate/dextrose normal saline) can be given at the rate of 60–120 mL/hour.

Partogram

- All the parameters, maternal and fetal, should be plotted on the partogram and labor progress monitored by the partogram.[1] Maintaining a partogram helps in early identification of abnormal labor by plotting the alert line and the action line (Fig. 3)
- In order to identify women who are heading for prolonged labor, a line of acceptable progress is drawn on the partogram called the alert line. If the rate of dilatation of cervix falls to the right of this line, the progress is not normal (slow). In a primigravida, cervical dilatation is about 1–1.2 cm/hour, and in a multigravida, it is about 1.5–2.0 cm/hour. Not all progress at the same pace, hence a certain grace period is given before any action is taken and is based on the line drawn parallel about 1–4 hours to the right of the alert line, called the action line
- Descent of the fetal head in active labor is about 1 cm/hour in primigravidae and 2 cm/hour in multigravidae. Descent is maximum in the deceleration phase, which is after 6 cm of cervical dilatation
- Abnormal labor can be diagnosed early and appropriate steps taken to avoid complications in mother and baby.

Pain Relief

- It can be given in the form of systemic opioid analgesics: pethidine (meperidine), or regional analgesia by epidural route (fentanyl, remifentanil).

Amniotomy

- Artificial ROM is not done as a routine.
- It can be done to augment labor and to reduce the duration of labor.
- The cervix should be at least 4–5 cm dilated, well-effaced and head should be well-applied to the cervix for amniotomy to be done.

Use of Smooth Muscle Relaxants

- Smooth muscle relaxants are not universally used for cervical dilatation.
- However, where there is no contraindication, they can be used to reduce the duration of labor (drotaverine, hyoscine hydrochloride and valethamate bromide).

Augmentation of Labor

- Augmentation of labor can be done either by amniotomy or by oxytocin drip.
- About 5 units in 500 mL of Ringer's lactate/Dextrose normal saline with an infusion rate not exceeding 30–40 mL/hour.
- Drip rate adjusted to get physiological uterine contractions (once in every 3 minutes lasting for 40–60 seconds).

As labor pains increase, there is further descent and flexion of the fetal head with the chin touching the fetal

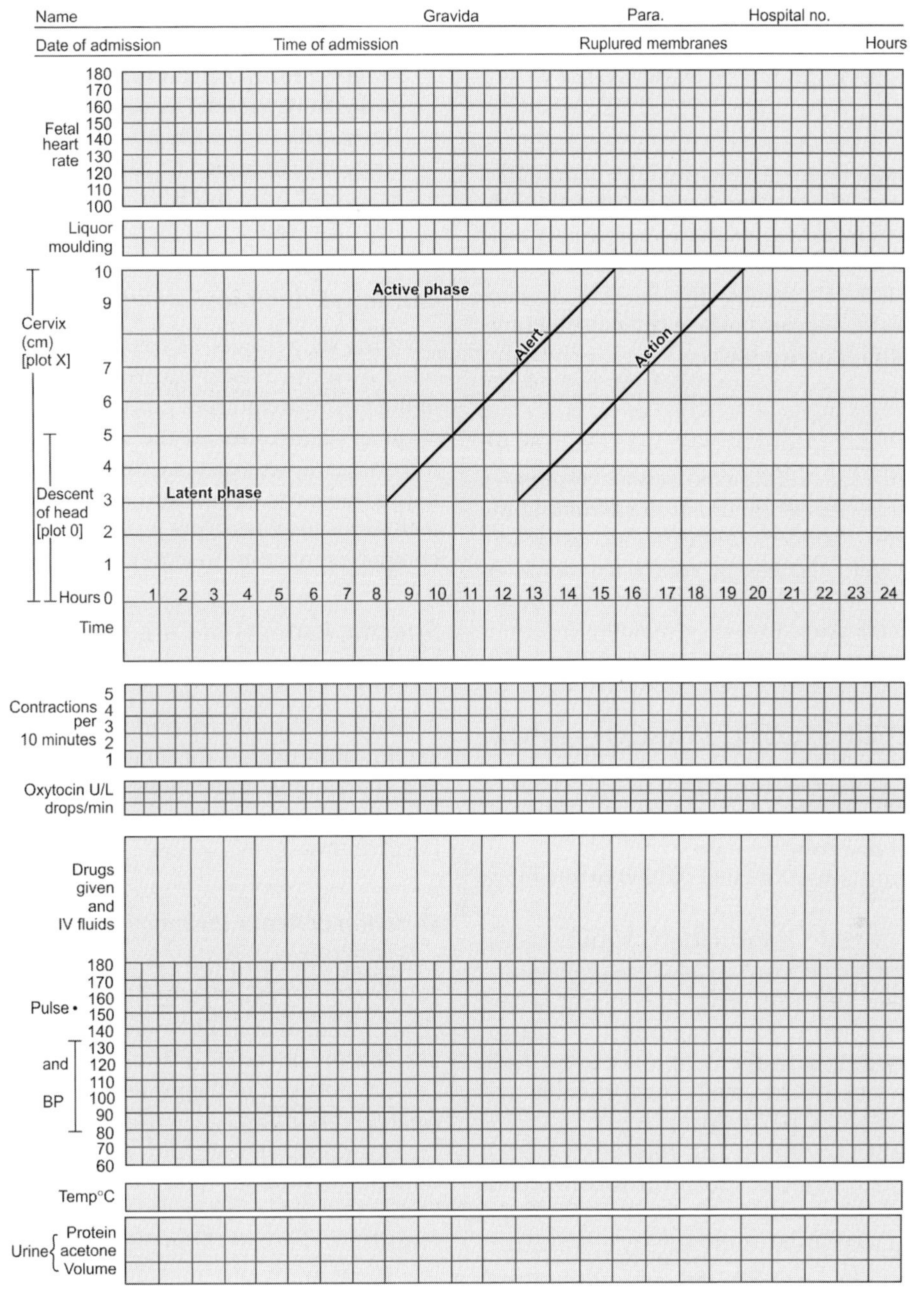

FIG. 3: Partogram.

thorax. Once the fetal head touches the pelvic floor, there is internal rotation, which is one-fourth or three-fourths of a circle, depending on whether it is occipito-anterior or occipito-posterior position.

- The fetal head usually enters the pelvic inlet either transversely or obliquely, the sagittal suture remaining parallel to the axis but not midway between the pubic symphysis and sacral promontory
- If the sagittal suture is closer to the sacral promontory, it is called anterior asynclitism and anterior parietal bone is felt per vaginum. If it is closer to the pubic symphysis, it is called posterior asynclitism and posterior parietal bone is easily palpated
- A moderate degree of asynclitism is usually present in normal labor, if it is severe as in some cases, the chances

of cephalopelvic disproportion are increased even in a pelvis of normal size.

Caput Succedaneum

- In vertex presentation, sometimes, when the membranes are absent, there is swelling of the portion of the fetal scalp in contact with the unyielding, resistant cervical os, usually a few millimeters in thickness, but occasionally big, as in prolonged labor. It usually resolves in a few days. It is not bound by the sutural margins unlike a cephalhematoma, which takes a few months to resolve.

Molding

- It is the change in the shape of the fetal head by compressive forces from outside. This is important in shortening the engaging diameter, (suboccipitobregmatic), especially in women with mild degrees of contracted pelvis or asynclitism and is brought about by overlapping of the sutures of the fetal skull. Excessive molding indicates gross disproportion and should be avoided.

MANAGEMENT OF SECOND STAGE OF LABOR

The second stage of labor is regarded as the climax of the birthing process. It extends from full dilatation of the cervix to the birth of the baby.

During the second stage of labor, skilled attendants should:[2,3]

- Continuously provide information, support, and encouragement to the woman and her companion
- Encourage active pushing once the urge to bear down is present, with encouragement to adopt any position preferred by the woman, except lying supine which risks aortocaval compression and reduced uteroplacental perfusion
- Premature pushing without full dilatation of the cervix is seen with occipito-posterior positions of the head
- Listen to the fetal heart frequently (every 15 minutes in low risk/every 5 minutes or after each contraction in high-risk) in between contractions to detect bradycardia
- Check the maternal pulse and blood pressure
- Observe progressive descent and rotation of the presenting part. This includes observing progressive distension of the perineum and visibility of the presenting part, and a vaginal examination where progress appears to be slow
- Conduct the delivery with perineal support to avoid tears and use of episiotomy only where a tear is very likely. A policy of restricted episiotomy should be followed
- Be ready to augment contractions with an intravenous oxytocin infusion during the second stage where contractions have become infrequent and where the fetal heart rate remains normal
- Be ready to undertake instrumental vaginal delivery (vacuum or forceps) where indicated
- See that the bladder is kept empty during the second stage.

Guiding Principles

As with all aspects of maternity care, in accordance with a rights-based approach, the individual needs of the woman and her companion during the second stage of labor should be taken into consideration, tailoring highest quality care to the individual's needs. A particularly important aspect is information and communication that prepare the woman and her labor companion of what to expect during labor and delivery.

Specific Aspects of Care in the Second Stage

Initiation of Active Pushing

A woman should be encouraged to push when the cervix is fully dilated, the fetal head is on the pelvic floor, and she feels an urge to bear down. Even when she feels the urge, pushing should only be encouraged during contractions.

Duration of Active Pushing in the Second Stage of Labor

Primiparous women should not actively push for more than 2 hours and multiparous women for more than 1 hour, due to an increased risk of birth asphyxia and maternal sepsis associated with prolonged labor. Lack of descent of the presenting part may also indicate obstructed labor.

Intervention should be considered promptly, options evaluated and acted upon, before these indicated time periods if the maternal and/or fetal condition deviates from the normal.

Maternal and Fetal Monitoring during the Second Stage

Maternal parameters should be monitored during the second stage of labor especially for specific indications such as a history of high blood pressure, etc.

Equipment in good working order and devices that simplify detection of the fetal heart, should be available at the recommended frequency. The frequency of fetal heart auscultation should be every 5-10 minutes or more often when bradycardia is suspected. One can get good information about the condition of the fetus, by auscultating immediately after a contraction.

Pinard stethoscope (fetoscope) may be adequate in very quiet labor rooms, but it is often difficult to use reliably owing to extraneous noise or maternal obesity and especially in the second stage because of the woman's naturally vigorous movements. Wide availability of handheld Doppler devices with battery backup should be used in above cases.

Position of the Woman during the Second Stage of Labor

The following positions may be adopted:
- Dorsal with 15° left lateral tilt (widely used)
- Lateral
- All fours.

Use of Oxytocin during the Second Stage of Labor

Intravenous oxytocin should be administered in the presence of inadequate uterine contractions.

Pain Relief during the Second Stage of Labor

Pain relief options must be discussed with the woman prior to the onset of labor. The need for pain relief is highly variable between individuals and should be individually assessed (inhalation analgesics/narcotics/epidural analgesia). While psychosocial interventions such as having a birth companion and provision of supportive care may reduce the need for analgesia, the second stage, thankfully is usually short and self-limiting.

Local anesthesia should be used for perineal infiltration prior to cutting an episiotomy, and the practice of cutting an incision without anesthesia is to be deprecated. For instrumental delivery, a pudendal block may be indicated, especially for forceps delivery.

Episiotomy

An episiotomy is an incision made into the perineum for the purpose of enlarging the soft tissue outlet at crowning (Figs 4 and 5).

Reviews have demonstrated that a policy of restricted episiotomy (episiotomy only when necessary) has better maternal outcomes than a policy of routine episiotomy.

Delivery of the Head

Slow delivery of the head is conducted in between uterine contractions.

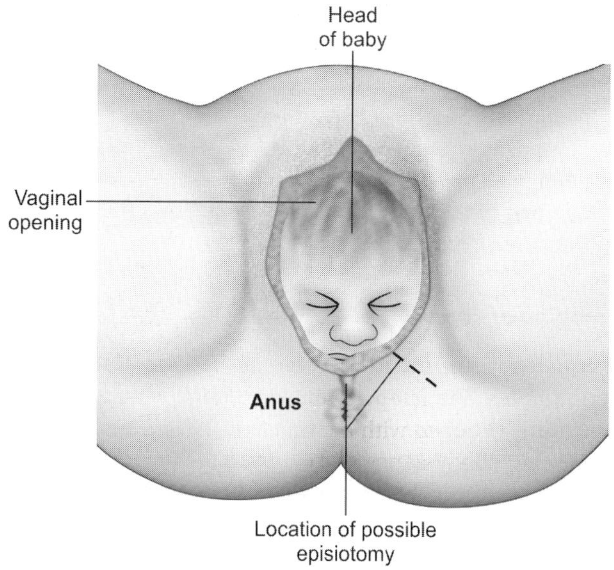

FIG. 4: Timing of episiotomy (i.e., crowning of head).

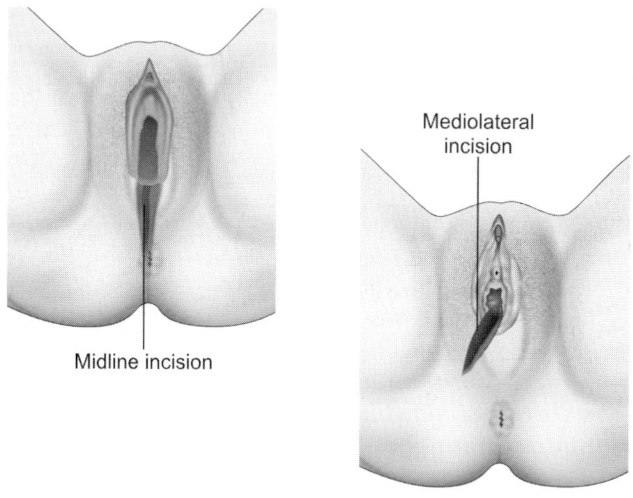

FIG. 5: Types of episiotomy.

Ritgen Maneuver

By the time the head distends the vulva and perineum enough to open the vaginal introitus to a diameter of 5 cm or more, one hand: a towel-draped, gloved hand may exert forward pressure on the chin of the fetus through the perineum just in front of the coccyx; the other hand: exerts pressure superiorly against the occiput. Oronasopharyngeal suction is done following delivery of the head.

Delivery of Shoulder and Body

- Following delivery of the head, restitution and external rotation occur and the occiput turns towards one of the maternal thighs.

- The neck is checked for a nuchal cord and if present released.
- The head is gently grasped by both hands and depressed posteriorly till anterior shoulder is released.
- The posterior shoulder is then released by drawing the head in an upward direction.

The rest of the body almost always follows the shoulder without any difficulty.

Clamping of Cord

After delivery, the infant is placed at the level of the vagina for 3 minutes. The fetoplacental circulation is not occluded. The cord is clamped with a distance of 4–5 cm between two clamps and at a distance of 3 cm from the baby's abdomen. Delaying the clamping till pulsations stops will allow the baby to receive an additional 80 mL of blood. Active management of the third stage of labor advocates delayed clamping of the cord.

MANAGEMENT OF THIRD STAGE OF LABOR

After the birth of the baby, the size and tone of the uterus is noted. If it is firm with no unusual bleeding, wait for the placenta to separate. Undue traction on the cord before separation of the placenta is not exerted as it can cause unnecessary complications.

The signs of placental separation are:

- The uterus contracts and rises
- The cord suddenly lengthens
- A gush of blood is seen.

This can take about 1–5 minutes to 30 minutes from the delivery of the newborn up and is considered normal.

There are two ways of managing the third stage.

- Expectant management where we wait for spontaneous separation and expulsion of the placenta.
- Active management of labor includes:
  - Administration of a uterotonic, preferably oxytocin 10 units, given in 500 mL Ringer's lactate at 10 mL/min for first few minutes and then 1–2 mL/min
  - Controlled cord traction and asking the patient to slightly bear down facilitating expulsion of placenta
  - Uterine massage to make the uterus contract and retract and reduce the volume of blood loss
- Confirm if the fetal membranes have come out in toto. Check the placenta on the maternal surface to make sure no fragments are left behind
- Inspect the perineum, vagina and paraurethral area for any tears.
- Episiotomy if given is sutured in layers.

FOURTH STAGE OF LABOR[4,5]

This is about an hour after delivery of the placenta. This is a very important period to keep a check on the delivered patient.

Maternal vital signs like pulse and blood pressure should be recorded immediately after the delivery and every 15 minutes up to 1 hour.

A watch on the tone of the uterus and amount of vaginal bleeding should be kept.

This is the time when mother-baby bonding should be encouraged and the first breast-feed initiated.

After monitoring the mother's vitals, checking for any excessive bleeding, rechecking on an empty bladder and initiation of breast-feeding, the mother and baby can be shifted to the ward and a relieved and relaxed obstetrician take leave.

CONCLUSION

The process of vaginal delivery involves a practice of watchful expectancy. Most women deliver healthy babies without much assistance, but the crux of obstetrics lies in detecting and managing successfully those women whose labor is abnormal. In recent years, the importance of a Doula in providing comfort to the laboring woman has been duly recognized. More women opt for vaginal delivery today as the fear of pain has been effectively banished by epidural analgesia. The strict use of the modified partogram helps in early identification and prompt management of abnormal labours. Restricted use of episiotomy is advocated wherever feasible but a timely, needed episiotomy should not be denied either. Active management of the third stage of labor avoids excessive loss of blood which the average Indian woman can ill afford. In short, the obstetrician should spare no efforts to make birthing an enjoyable experience for the laboring woman.

REFERENCES

1. World Health Organization. Making Pregnancy Safer: the Critical Role of the Skilled Attendant. A Joint Statement by WHO, ICM and FIGO. Geneva: WHO; 2004.
2. Roberts J, Hanson L. Best practices in second stage labor care: maternal bearing down and positioning. J Midwifery Womens Health. 2007;52(3):238-45.
3. Gupta J, Hofmeyr G. Position for women during second stage of labour. Cochrane Database Syst Rev. 2004(1):CD002006.
4. Hodnett ED, Gates S, Hofmeyr GJ, Sakala C, Weston J. Continuous support for women during childbirth. Cochrane Database Syst Rev. 2011(2):CD003766.
5. National Institute for Health and Clinical Excellence. Intrapartum Care. Care of healthy women and their babies during childbirth. NICE clinical guideline, September 2007.

CHAPTER 14

Fluid Management in Labor

Vandana R Bhuria

INTRODUCTION

The process of labor may be considered as a physical endurance event. As adequate hydration is useful for peak athletic performance, it is logical, therefore, adequate hydration contributes to an effective labor. Optimal hydration during labor has not yet been defined. For the high-risk mothers, fluid and electrolyte balance in labor forms the mainstay of the intrapartum or the perioperative care. Thus, it becomes important to understand the physiological changes that occur during normal and abnormal pregnancy. These physiological changes, indirectly, influence the fluid management in labor and also the immediate postpartum period.[1]

Through this chapter, we will discuss various aspects of fluid management in normal labor and other medical and obstetric disorders of the mother.

PHYSIOLOGICAL CHANGES IN PREGNANCY IN HEMATOLOGICAL SYSTEM

Plasma volume increases to the extent of 40–50% in pregnancy and red blood cell (RBC) volume is increased to the extent of 20–30%. This disproportionate increase in plasma and RBC volume produces a state of hemodilution in pregnancy. This relative hemodilution is beneficial to the mother as it protects the mother against the adverse effects of blood loss during delivery. Again, diminished blood viscosity due to relative hemodilution will ensure optimum gaseous exchange between maternal and fetal circulations.

FLUIDS IN LABOR

Oral Intake versus Parenteral Fluids

Once labor has been established, the gastric emptying time is remarkably prolonged. So, traditionally, solid food is withheld during labor and delivery. Oral intake is restricted in many labor and delivery units in response to work by Mendelson in the 1940s. Mendelson emphasized the risk of aspiration and further lung damage if unanticipated general anesthesia is required in laboring patients. Since the 1940s, with better general anesthetic techniques and greater use of regional anesthesia, there has been a considerable change in obstetrical anesthesia. With improved anesthesia techniques, however, aspiration complications have become too rare to study; and some providers feel restricting clear liquids for laboring women is unjustified.[2]

The National Institute for Health and Clinical Excellence Intrapartum Guidelines

Women may drink during established labor and be informed that isotonic drinks may be more beneficial than water.

According to American Academy of Pediatrics and the American College of Obstetricians and Gynecologists (2002), sips of clear liquids, occasional ice chips, and lip moisturizers are permitted.

Cochrane Pregnancy and Childbirth Group's Trial Register (February 2013) was advised by some authors.[3] They included nine randomized control trials. The authors concluded that although the administration of intravenous (IV) fluids compared with oral intake alone demonstrated a reduction in the duration of labor, this finding emerged from only two trials. Other trials suggested that if a policy of no oral intake is applied, then the duration of labor in nulliparous women may be shortened by the administration of IV fluids at a rate of 250 mL/h rather than 125 mL/h.

Although routine administration of IV fluids to laboring women is a widely adopted policy, but it has not been adequately elucidated. No definite consensus has been set on the type or volume of fluids that are required, or indeed whether intravenous fluids are at all necessary. Women should be allowed to take oral fluids during labor so that they can adequately hydrate themselves.

Furthermore, excessive volume of intravenous fluids may pose risks to both the mother and the newborn. Dextrose-containing fluids reduce the sodium levels (hyponatremia) of both the laboring mothers and their newborns.

Water intoxication is associated with iatrogenic fluid overload, prolonged administration of oxytocin in hypotonic solutions, and after excessive oral intake of fluids by the mother.[4] Authors[4] have reported a case of neonatal seizures due to maternal water intoxication in labor as patient had taken 3–4 L of water over an 8-hour period during labor. Water concentration equilibrates across the placenta; hence, in situation of maternal hyponatremia and water intoxication, the fetus is also hyponatremic. Fetal antidiuretic hormone (ADH) levels rise just before the onset of labor and are markedly elevated during labor. Cerebral squeeze resulting from the labor and birth process stimulates the hypersecretion of ADH in the fetus. High levels of ADH and limited renal capacity leads to the newborn being unable to handle water overload resulting in hyponatremia. Thus, fluid intake during labor needs careful monitoring to avoid water intoxication and further maternal and fetal hyponatremia.

FLUID MANAGEMENT IN PREECLAMPSIA

Fluid management for the patient with pregnancy-induced hypertension presents a challenge for the obstetrician, especially for the patient with preeclampsia. The etiology and pathophysiology of pregnancy-induced hypertension are incompletely understood.[5] The patient with preeclampsia is often in positive fluid balance and excess fluid is mainly in the interstitial space due to salt retention, low-oncotic pressure, and increased capillary permeability. In marked contrast, the plasma volume is usually reduced and there is hemoconcentration. The colloid osmotic pressure of plasma is reduced in these patients due to hypoproteinemia. As a result, there is a considerable controversy regarding fluid therapy in patient with preeclampsia.

In general, pregnancy-induced hypertension is characterized by failure to achieve the normal pregnancy associated plasma volume expansion which is combined with manifestations of excess interstitial fluid. The paradox of intravascular volume depletion combined with increased extracellular volume leads to divergent opinions regarding optimal fluid management. Volume replacement has been advocated by some[6,7] because of intravascular hypovolemia, whereas others[8,9] have recommended volume restriction and even diuretics because of the extracellular fluid excess. A combined obstetric and anesthetic approach is required for optimal fluid management in case of pregnancy-induced hypertension and preeclampsia. Management plans differ and should be tailored according to the specific clinical situation.

Uncomplicated Preeclampsia

Preeclampsia is an unpredictable condition, so high-dependency care is advised for all patients of preeclampsia, regardless of severity.

Crystalloid or Colloid

In preeclampsia, the serum oncotic protein level are low, thus, reducing the colloid oncotic pressure of plasma (COP_P).

Colloid infusion (synthetic product or human albumin solution) initially increases the colloid osmotic pressure in contrast to the crystalloids which dilute the oncotic protein, thereby reducing the COP_P. It is thought that the rise in COP_P after colloid infusion will draw fluid back into circulation and some have argued that colloid infusion may contribute to fluid overload, particularly in the postpartum period.[10] In contrast, crystalloid will move more quickly across the endothelium into the interstitial space.[11] The initial improvement in hemodynamics with colloids might later reverse, and therefore lead to increased edema.[12] So, the crystalloid solutions are the mainstay of fluid therapy in the preeclamptic patients.

Hartmann's Solution (Ringer's Lactate) or Normal Saline?

Reid and colleagues[13] conducted a study and found plasma-volume expansion is greater and more sustained with normal saline (NS) than with Hartmann's solution. However, diuresis occurs more quickly and to a greater degree with Hartmann's solution. They suggested that Hartmann's solution might be more suitable for women with preeclampsia but specific research would be necessary to confirm this.

To conclude, in uncomplicated preeclampsia, crystalloid infusion limited to between 75 and 125 mL/h throughout the intrapartum and early postpartum period (12–24 hours) is appropriate.[14,15] The precise nature of a conservative fluid regimen varies from unit to unit. Some employ a simple formula, such as a maximum of 2.5 L in 24 hours or 1 mL/kg/h[16] whereas other prefers to calculate the rate as previous hour's urine output (UO) plus 40 mL or 1 mL/kg/h.

Once patient is able to tolerate oral intake, it is sensible to allow free oral fluids with a steady decline in IV fluid in line with this.

Preeclampsia Complicated with Oliguria

Renal pathology in preeclampsia comprises of three components:

1. Prerenal component: reduced renal blood flow secondary to reduced circulating volume
2. Intrinsic renal component: afferent arteriolar vasoconstriction and glomerular damage, secondary to deposition of fibrinogen degradation product in the capillary bed. Acute tubular necrosis may develop in patient with placental abruption and severe hypovolaemia.
3. Postrenal component: there may be a small effect from ureteric compression in late labor.

The alteration in renal function affects both water homeostasis (oliguria/anuria) and ability to excrete metabolites (decreased creatinine clearance). These two often occur simultaneously, but some degree of dissociation may exist. Patient can have oliguria without any alteration in intrinsic renal function (creatinine clearance) or there can be marked increase in serum creatinine levels with a good fluid output being maintained.

Also, remember that oliguria does not necessarily indicate severe volume depletion, particularly around time of delivery. It may, simply be the physiological response to stress (mediated through arginine vasopressin release from posterior pituitary) or be the indicator of severe glomerular damage.

Management of Oliguria

First step in the management is to find out the cause in patients of oliguria. Blockade of urinary catheter should be ruled out in patients of sudden onset anuria. Often, it is simply physiological anuria but it can be a sign of worsening preeclampsia. Complete blood screen should be repeated to test for hemolysis, elevated liver enzymes, and low platelet count (HELLP) syndrome. More rarely, it might reflect occult hemorrhage or sepsis which should be properly diagnosed and treated.

Moderate Oliguria in Absence of Hemolysis, Elevated Liver Enzymes, and Low Platelet Count Syndrome

Because magnesium is cleared almost exclusively by renal clearance, infusion of magnesium should be reduced by half, if oliguria develops to avoid toxic accumulation in blood[12] (Flowchart 1). Close monitoring of patient including vitals and input-output charting 1 hourly should be done with a watchful expectancy for pulmonary edema.

Severe Oliguria Associated with HELLP Syndrome

Severe oliguria (UO <10 mL/h for 2 h) with HELLP syndrome becomes an indicator for invasive monitoring. Central venous pressure (CVP) is a guide to circulating blood volume.

If CVP indicates grossly underfilled vascular component, Hartmann's solution should be infused (250 mL over 30 min). This will promote diuresis in 25% of patients. If there is no response to fluid infusion, then furosemide infusion (5 mg/h) can be used (Flowchart 1). Fluid replacement may be required if UO is more than 200 mL/h.

If the vascular compartment is filled, then most likely possibility is intrinsic renal component (afferent arteriolar spasm or glomerular capillary damage). Dopamine infusion in such cases is advocated at the rate of 3 μg/kg/min as it will treat any arteriolar vasoconstriction. Management of oliguria is formulated in Flowchart 1.

Pulmonary Edema

Pulmonary edema associated with pregnancy-induced hypertension occurs after delivery in 70–80% of cases.[17] Postpartum mobilization of interstitial fluids contribute to the occurrence of pulmonary edema by increasing pulmonary capillary wedge pressure.[8]

The associated increase in hydrostatic pressure, decrease in colloid osmotic pressure, and increase in vascular permeability resulting from endothelial damage,[5] all combine to increase the risk of pulmonary edema. Lehmann and coresearchers[18] in the 1980s suggested that it is highly probable that the chance of pulmonary edema is increased by excessive IV fluid infusion.

It may also be made more likely by pre-existing cardiac disease and certain medications, such as β-mimetic tocolytics.

Management

Once pulmonary edema is diagnosed, it is important to distinguish between acute respiratory distress syndrome-type respiratory problems from cardiogenic forms (silent myocardial infarct, gestational cardiomyopathy, etc.), particularly in elderly or diabetic women.[19]

A complete respiratory and cardiovascular examination should be performed including pulse rate, respiratory rate, blood pressure, oxygen saturation, presence of cardiac murmurs, and added respiratory sounds. Plain chest radiograph is considered to be the most sensitive indicator of detecting early pulmonary edema. Also, include arterial blood gas analysis, electrocardiogram, and cardiac enzymes among the investigations. Echocardiography should be considered if doubt exists about ventricular function (cardiogenic pulmonary edema). Patient should be kept under continuous monitoring with cardiovascular/respiratory observations and continuous pulse oximetry.

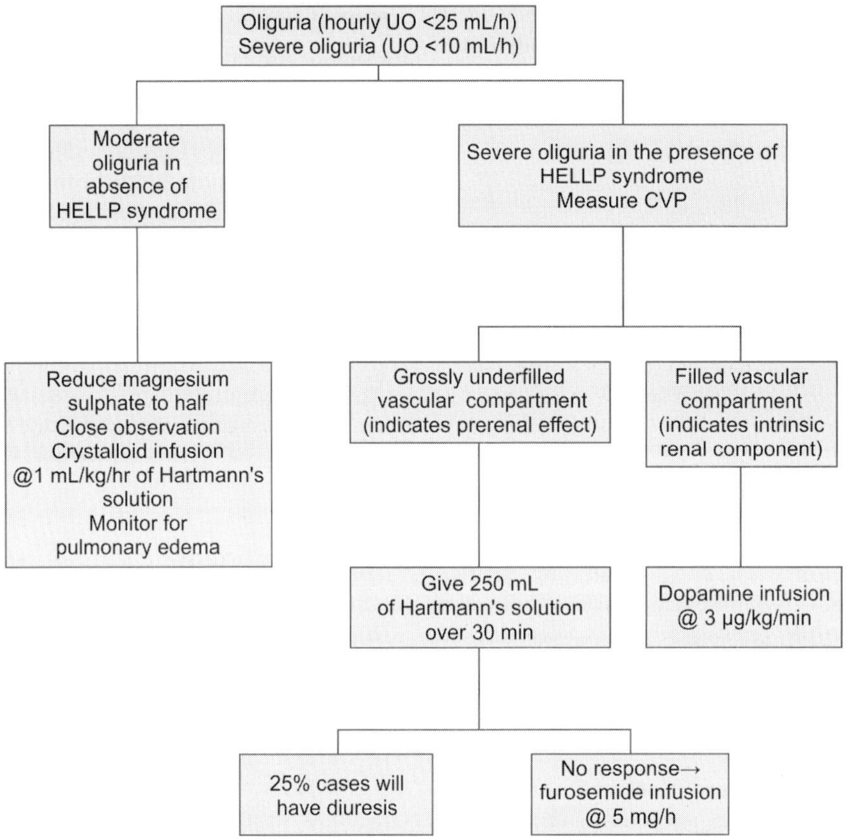

UO, urine output; HELLP, hemolysis, elevated liver enzymes, and low platelet count syndrome; CVP, central venous pressure.

FLOWCHART 1 Management of oliguria.

Management constitutes of supplemental oxygen by face mask, fluid restriction, diuretics and possibly, vasodilators to facilitate afterload reduction. Where there is evidence of fluid overload, intravenous furosemide should be given while monitoring the patient for cardiovascular collapse if the intravascular compartment is depleted. Furosemide acts by reducing the pulmonary artery pressure as well as promoting diuresis. In severe cases, continuous positive airway pressure ventilation may be beneficial.

A multidisciplinary approach involving respiratory physicians, obstetric anesthetists, and intensive care units should be carried out in severe complicated cases of pulmonary edema.

CARDIAC PATIENTS IN LABOR

Intrapartum Hemodynamics in Cardiac Patient

Cardiovascular physiological changes associated with pregnancy are magnified in labor. Each uterine contraction is associated with an expulsion of 300–500 mL blood from uterus into general circulation, adding to preload.[20] This is accompanied by increase in stroke volume and subsequently, cardiac output. Overall, cardiac output in active labor is increased by approximately 2.5 L/min into the range of 7–8 L/min.[21] In association with uterine contractions, blood pressure and CVP are also elevated.

Immediately, postdelivery, there is significant increase in cardiac output, probably as a result of the dramatically reduced vena-caval obstruction by the uterus and the autotransfusion from the contracted uterus.

Once a cardiac patient is in labor, careful monitoring is required with a close attention on the fluid management because patients can be sensitive to both hypo- and hypervolemias. Most women even with mild heart disease should be monitored throughout labor with complete cardiorespiratory assessment (pulse rate, respiratory rate, blood pressure, jugular venous pressure, any added respiratory sounds, cardiac murmurs) and oxygen saturation by using monitors.

In more severe cases, invasive blood pressure and CVP monitoring can also be helpful if substantial blood loss is anticipated and in patients of severe valvular disease or evidence of pulmonary hypertension. Continuous electronic fetal monitoring is recommended.

Intravenous fluid therapy is safer with CVP monitoring. Rate of fluid administration should be 0.5–1 mL/kg/h. Rate should not exceed 75 mL/h. For oxytocin administration, concentrated drip should be used (10 units in 500 mL).

MATERNAL KETOSIS

Maternal ketosis and further ketonuria is a common indication of fluid administration in labor. Dehydration associated with increased muscular activity in labor without adequate oral intake leads to raised levels of ketones in blood and urine (ketosis). Effect of ketosis on mother and baby is not clear. It is, also, not clear whether ketosis during labor is a normal physiological response, or if women with ketosis during labor require intervention (such as IV or oral fluids).[22] The association between marked ketosis and prolonged labor is well known. However, which is the cause or which is the effect is not clearly understood. Adverse effects of ketosis for the mother include increased likelihood of augmentation of labor, forceps-assisted delivery, and postpartum blood loss.[23] Management strategies for ketosis in labor may include encouraging oral fluid intake, IV fluids, and no intervention.

In low-risk women, where there is normal progression of labor, ketosis, as such, does not require any treatment. Oral fluid intake during labor should be encouraged. Adverse effects of additional oral intake during labor include nausea and vomiting in labor and also, excessive fluid intake within a short-time period can cause hyponatremia in both mother and the fetus.

Most common fluids used for IV fluid therapy are crystalloids based fluids of dextrose/glucose, NS, and Ringer's lactate. However, IV fluid therapy is, also, not without adverse effects. The use of large quantity and volume of IV glucose (>25 g) in laboring women can lead to maternal hyperglycemia and iatrogenic hyperinsulinism in fetus, as well as subsequent postnatal hypoglycemia and jaundice.[23] Excessive administration of IV fluids can also lead to dilutional hyponatremia in both mother and neonate. Other reported adverse effects include decreased fetal blood pH and increased fetal lactate, headache, nausea, maternal fluid overload, slowing of labor, and difficulty in establishment of breastfeeding.[23]

Also, IV fluids in labor decreases ambulation of patient and also associated with local pain and discomfort at the cannula site.

REGIONAL ANESTHESIA

The chemical sympathectomy that follows epidural blockade can cause hypotension, especially if mother is hypovolemic. Regional anesthesia leads to peripheral enlargement of vascular compartment and can cause hypotension due to pooling of blood in periphery. To avoid this dangerous hypotension, it is advisable to preload patient with 500–1000 mL of crystalloids.

ANEMIA

Moderate-to-severe anemic patients, who do not have cardiopulmonary-renal decompensation, do not require any special modification in the management of fluid and electrolytes.

HEMORRHAGE AND HEMORRHAGIC SHOCK

Bleeding in obstetric patient requires prompt and adequate treatment to decrease maternal mortality and morbidity. Blood transfusion, secondary to hemorrhage during gestation is relatively common occurring in 1–2% of pregnancies. Although uterine atony is the leading cause of significant bleeding requiring transfusion, retained placenta, trauma, placenta previa, and abruptio placentae are also important etiologies.[24]

The physiological changes in hematological system during pregnancy allow most patient to tolerate the inevitable blood loss associated with delivery. In early stages of hemorrhage, heart rate, myocardial contractility, and vascular tone increases to improve oxygen delivery. There is redistribution of cardiac output, thereby selectively maintaining perfusion to the adrenal gland, brain, and heart at the expense of other organs, including the uterus. Before delivery, such shunting may lead to fetal hypoxia and distress. With continued blood loss and delayed or inadequate resuscitation, further changes occur resulting in an increased permeability and leakage of fluid back into interstitial space. Finally, organ ischemia is the end result.

Initial step in the management is aggressive volume replacement. At the same time, cause of hemorrhage and shock should be sought and appropriate steps should be taken to treat the cause.

Crystalloid solutions are the most commonly used fluids in the initial fluid resuscitation. Ringer's lactate and 0.9% sodium chloride (NS) are two most common crystalloid solutions. They distribute primarily throughout the extravascular space, expanding both the intravascular and interstitial compartments. Roughly for each liter of blood loss, approximately 3 L of crystalloid are required.

Ringer's lactate has the advantage of containing small quantities of additional electrolytes and lactate. American College of Surgeons have recommended it as the initial fluid for resuscitation. NS has the potential for causing hyperchloremic acidosis, thus, making it second choice for fluid resuscitation. Significant blood loss resulting in decreased oxygen carrying capacity requires blood transfusion.

Packed RBCs are the component of choice for the treatment of hypovolemic shock due to hemorrhage. One unit of packed RBCs is expected to increase the hemoglobin by 0.8–1 g/dL. Fresh frozen plasma may be used to prevent coagulopathy.

DIABETES

- Avoid extremes of maternal glycemia
- Avoid dehydration and ketosis.

Blood glucose monitoring in diabetic patient should be done on hourly basis. Blood glucose levels should be maintained between 80 and 100 mg/dL. To control blood glucose, 1 L of 5% dextrose drip is started with 10 units of soluble insulin (neutralizing drip). Insulin infusion rate is 1 U/h for blood glucose of 70–130 mg/dL, 2 U/h for blood glucose of 130–160 mg/dL and 3 U/h for blood glucose of 160–200 mg/dL (Table 1). It is convenient to use motorized syringe pumps for insulin infusion.

If blood sugar levels are below 70 mg/dL, then 5% dextrose drip should be started to prevent hypoglycemia.

Syntocinon, if required, for augmentation of labor in diabetic patients should be given via a separate IV access.

According to the National Institute for Health and Clinical Excellence guidelines 2008, during labor, capillary blood glucose should be maintained between 4 and 7 mmol/L and be monitored on hourly basis.

Women with type 1 diabetes mellitus should be considered for IV dextrose and insulin infusion from the onset of established labor.

Diabetic Ketoacidosis

Diabetic ketoacidosis (DKA) represents acutely decompensated diabetes. Immediate goals include replacement of insulin, fluid, and electrolytes. After a rapid assessment of patient, blood glucose, and ketones, large amount of IV fluids without glucose are rapidly administered to reduce dehydration and to replace electrolytes.

- NS is the fluid of choice and about 1–2 L are infused over 30–60 minutes. After that, assessment for intravascular volume is made and IV fluids are administered at 200–250 mL/h (4–6 L in first 12 hours). 5% dextrose in NS is given when blood glucose is 200 mg/dL
- 6-hourly potassium levels should be done
- We should aim to maintain serum potassium levels at 3.4–4.8 mmol/L. If reduced, 10 mL of 20% potassium chloride in 10% dextrose at the rate of 125 mL/h should be infused
- Intravascular hemodynamic monitoring is preferred to reduce risk of pulmonary edema.

TABLE 1: General guidelines for insulin infusion rates

Blood glucose	Regular insulin
70–130 mg/dL	1 U/h
130–160 mg/dL	2 U/h
160–200 mg/dL	3 U/h

PRETERM LABOR

It is now realized that initial therapy for a preterm labor is hydration and saline loading has emerged as first line of treatment in some centers.[25] In addition to routine oral intake, an infusion of 1,500–2,000 mL/24 h is given. Tocolytic agent ritodrine can cause pulmonary edema when infused with saline and one needs to be cautious. 5% albumin is another good option for a sustained volume expansion.

INDUCTION AND AUGMENTATION

Antidiuretic property of oxytocin leads to retention of water and hyponatremia, especially if the delivery solution is glucose. Studies have shown a reduced cord blood sodium and higher neonatal jaundice when glucose is used. NS is the preferred solution for oxytocin infusion and a policy of using concentrated infusion with an eye on limiting total fluid inputs will be beneficial.

FETAL DISTRESS

In a mistaken belief of providing energy during fetal asphyxia, many institutions have a policy of infusing the concentrated glucose (10% dextrose). Studies have shown that hypoxia is more harmful to fetal brain after maternal feeding or glucose infusion compared to starving, due to anaerobic oxidation of glucose resulting in lactate accumulation and cerebral edema.[26] Acute maternal hyperglycemia (>150 mg/dL) before delivery has a high risk of perinatal asphyxia. Glucose and Ringer's lactate are best avoided and small quantities of saline infusion to expand the blood volume can help by increasing the uteroplacental perfusion. Oxygen and lateral position to restore the cardiac output are other beneficial measures.

WHY FLUID MANAGEMENT?

Pregnancy is "accelerated starvation syndrome". The effect is accentuated in labor by the muscular exertion and forced starvation. The average plasma ketone level in nonpregnant state is 0.13 mmol/L compared to 0.43 mmol/L during pregnancy.[27] Early morning ketonuria was found in 7% of normal pregnant women using Ketostix (indicates presence of acetoacetic acid in urine at concentrations >1.0 mmol/L). About 40% women in labor show positive reaction to Ketostix.[28] This is a milder state of starvation, but a large glucose loading to cover it may lead to iatrogenic hyperinsulinemia and resultant postnatal hypoglycemia in the fetus. Although a small infusion of 5% glucose does not produce significant hyperglycemia in either the mother or the fetus, a cumulatively high dose of glucose infusion (especially in long-protracted labor) causes a significant rise in lactate concentration and significant fall in fetal pH.[29]

Since the ability to excrete water is impaired during labor, an assessment based on UO may be fallacious. The laboring patient has an insensible loss of free water through the skin and lungs (more with panting in final stages of labor). The sweating represents significant hypotonic loss (sweat sodium 0.3%). These issues become more relevant in long labors and especially where the intake is restricted.

RECOMMENDATIONS

To avoid ketosis as a result of prolonged labor, small amounts of glucose may be given slowly. However, a large amount of glucose is avoided with an upper limit of total glucose kept at 6.15% g/h (a 500 mL of 5% dextrose solution has 25 g of glucose). Morton et al. compared 1 L of sodium chloride, Ringer's lactate, dextrose 5% in water, dextrose 10% in water in women with ketonuria and observed that both dextrose and Ringer's lactate raise lactate, and concluded that sodium chloride is best and total dextrose per hour should be less than 25 g.[30] IV fluids are seldom necessary in first 12 hours of labor and total input is kept less than 3,000 g. For expansion of plasma volume, the choice is crystalloid solution like NS. Ringer's lactate is also a good choice in volume replacements of hemorrhages, but in protracted labors, the lactate may be harmful for compromised fetus.

CONCLUSION

To avoid complications, selection of the fluids must be based on the knowledge of the physiological circulatory volume changes during pregnancy and of any medical or obstetric disorder in the mother that would affect fluid balance of internal milieu. Inappropriate fluid administration without adequate knowledge can be detrimental for the mother as well as the neonate.

REFERENCES

1. O'Sullivan G, Scrutton M. NPO during labor. Is there any scientific validation? Anesthesiol Clin North America. 2003;21(1):87-98.
2. Varney H (Ed). Varney's midwifery, 3rd edition. Boston, USA: Blackwell Scientific Incorporation; 1997. p. 146.
3. Dawood F, Dowswell T, Quenby S. Intravenous fluids for reducing the duration of labour in low risk nulliparous women. Cochrane Database Sys Rev. 2013;(6):CD007715.
4. Shivashankar G, Coe A, Satodia P. Neonatal seizure due to maternal water intoxication in labour--a case report. Infant. 2008;4(6):196-97.
5. Roberts JM, Taylor RN, Musci TJ, Rodgers GM, Hubel CA, McLaughlin MK. Preeclampsia: an endothelial cell disorder. Am J Obstet Gynecol. 1989;161(5):1200-4.
6. Cotton DB, Longmire S, Jones MM, Dorman KF, Tessem J, Joyce TH. Cardiovascular alterations in severe pregnancy-induced hypertension: effects of intravenous nitroglycerin coupled with blood volume expansion. Am J Obstet Gynecol. 1986;154(5):1053-9.
7. Wasserstrum N. Issues in fluid management during labor: maternal plasma volume status and volume loading. Clin Obstet Gynecol. 1992;35(3):514-26.
8. Hankins SD, Wendel GD, Cunningham FG, Leveno KJ. Longitudinal evaluation of hemodynamic changes in eclampsia. Am J Obstet Gynecol. 1984;150(5 Pt 1):506-12.
9. Pearson JF. Fluid balance in severe pre-eclampsia. Br J Hosp Med. 1992;48(1):47-51.
10. Moise KJ, Cotton DB. The use of colloid osmotic pressure in pregnancy. Clin Perinatol. 1986;13(4):827-42.
11. Brown MA, Zammit VC, Lowe SA. Capillary permeability and extracellular fluid volumes in pregnancy-induced hypertension. Clin Sci (Lond). 1989;77(6):599-604.
12. Cunningham FG (Ed). Hypertensive disorders of pregnancy. In: Williams Obstetrics, 21st edition. New York, USA: McGraw Hill Medical Publishing; 2003. pp. 567-618.
13. Reid F, Lobo DN, Williams RN, Rowlands BJ, Allison SP. (Ab)normal saline and physiological Hartmann's solution: a randomized double-blind crossover study. Clin Sci (Lond). 2003;104(1):17-24.
14. Jones MM, Longmire S, Cotton DB, Dorman KF, Skjonsby BS, Joyce. Influence of crystalloid versus colloid infusion on peripartum colloid osmotic pressure changes. Obstet Gynecol. 1986;68(5):659-61.
15. Kirshon B, Moise KJ, Cotton DB, Longmire S, Jones M, Tessem J, et al. Role of volume expansion in severe pre-eclampsia. Surg Gynecol Obstet. 1988;167(5):367-71.
16. O'Donnell E, Grady K, Cox C. Eclampsia, pre-eclampsia, HELLP, fatty liver and hepatic rupture. In: Howell C, Grady K, Cox C, Johnson RB (Eds). Managing Obstetric Emergencies and Trauma: The MOET Course Manual, 2nd edition. Cambridge, USA: Cambridge University Press; 2007. pp. 66-72.
17. Sibai BH, Mabie BC, Harvey CJ, Gonzalez AR. Pulmonary edema in severe preeclampsia-eclampsia: analysis of thirty-seven consecutive cases. Am J Obstet Gynecol. 1987;156(5):1174-9.
18. Lehmann DK, Mabie WC, Miller JM, Pernoll ML. The epidemiology and pathology of maternal mortality: Charity Hospital of Louisiana in New Orleans, 1965-1984. Obstet Gynecol. 1987;69(6):833-40.
19. Scissione AC, Ivester T, Largoza M, Manley J, Shlossman P, Colmorgen GH. Acute pulmonary edema in pregnancy. Obstet Gynecol. 2003;101(3):511-5.
20. Adams JQ, Alexander AM. Alterations in cardiovascular physiology during labor. Obstet Gynecol 1958;12(5):542-9.
21. Kjeldsen J. Hemodynamic investigations during labor and delivery. Acta Obstet Gynecol Scand Suppl. 1979;89:1-252.
22. Toohill J, Soong B, Flenady V. Interventions for ketosis during labour. Cochrane Database Syst Rev. 2008;(3):CD004230.
23. Foulkes J, Dumoulin JG. The effects of ketonuria in labour. Br J Clin Pract. 1985;39(2):59-62.
24. Kamani AA, McMorland GH, Wadsworth LD. Utilization of red blood cell transfusion in an obstetric setting. Am J Obstet Gynecol. 1988;159(5):1177-81.
25. American College of Obstetricians and Gynecologists. ACOG Practice Bulletin. Assessment of risk factors for preterm birth. Clinical management guidelines for obstetrician-gynecologists. Number 31, October 2001. (Replaces Technical Bulletin number 206, June 1995; Committee Opinion number 172, May 1996; Committee Opinion number 187, September 1997; Committee Opinion number 198, February 1998; and Committee Opinion number 251, January 2001). Obstet Gynecol. 2001;98(4):709-16.

26. Kenepp NB, Kumar S, Shelley WC, Stanley CA, Gabbe SG, Gutsche BB. Fetal and neonatal hazards of maternal hydration with 5% dextrose before caesarean section. Lancet. 1982;1(8282):1150-2.
27. Paterson P, Sheath J, Taft P, Wood C. Maternal and foetal ketone concentrations in plasma and urine. Lancet. 1967;1(7495):862-5.
28. Dumoulin JG, Foulkes JE. Ketonuria during labor. Br J Obstet Gynaecol. 1984;91(2):97-8.
29. Lawrence GF, Brown VA, Parsons RJ, Cooke ID. Feto-maternal consequences of high-dose glucose infusion during labour. Br J Obstet Gynaecol. 1982;89(1):27-32.
30. Morton KE, Jackson MC, Gillmer MD. A comparison of the effects of four intravenous solutions for the treatment of ketonuria during labour. Br J Obstet Gynaecol. 1985;92(5):473-9.

CHAPTER 15

Partograph

Tanupriya Dogra

INTRODUCTION AND HISTORY

It can be defined as graphical representation of events of labor which encompass the progress of labor along with the condition of mother and fetus.

It was introduced by Wolf in 1946; reinforced by Friedman and he also illustrated the sigmoid characteristics of the curve. Muller added the concept of fetal station.

ADVANTAGES

- It is practical screening tool for helping doctors and staff
- Pictorial display and hence easy and quick to grasp
- Regular observations made on fetus and mother which aids early recognition of problems in either
- It prevents prolonged labor and its sequel
- Hand over is precise
- It gives quantifiable clinical observation in determining need for instrumental or cesarean delivery.[2]

DISADVANTAGES

- It does not identify other risk factors which may be present before labor starts
- Risk of infection following repeated vaginal examinations
- Calls for vaginal examination by same individual to keep range of error to a minimum.

WHO MODEL OF PARTOGRAPH: PRINCIPLES

Better to use partograph with preset alert and action lines:

- Latent phase of labor should not last more than 8 hours
- Active phase starts at 3 cm dilatation of cervix
- During active phase, rate of cervical dilatation should not be less than 1 cm per hour
- Lag time of 4 hours between slowing of labor and need for intervention is unlikely to compromise the fetus or mother and avoids unnecessary intervention
- Vaginal examination 4 hourly is recommended.[4]

COMPONENTS OF PARTOGRAPH

- Record of progress of labor
- Fetal record
- Maternal record (see Fig. 1).

Progress of Labor

- Dilatation of cervix
- Descent of fetal head
- Uterine contraction.

Cervical Dilatation

It follows a sigmoid or S-shaped curve which has latent and active phase. Active phase is further divided into acceleration phase, phase of maximum slope, deceleration phase. Latent phase is that part of labor which is accompanied by orientation, coordination and polarization of uterine contractions and preparation of cervix for active phase.

Acceleration phase is short and variable.

Phase of maximum slope is a major portion of cervical dilatation.

Deceleration phase reflects fetopelvic relationships (Fig. 2).

Plotting cervical dilatation on partograph: it is recorded in the center of graph. Along left side are the figures 0–10 against squares with each square representing 1 cm dilatation. At the bottom of the graph along the X-axis are the numbers 0–24 with

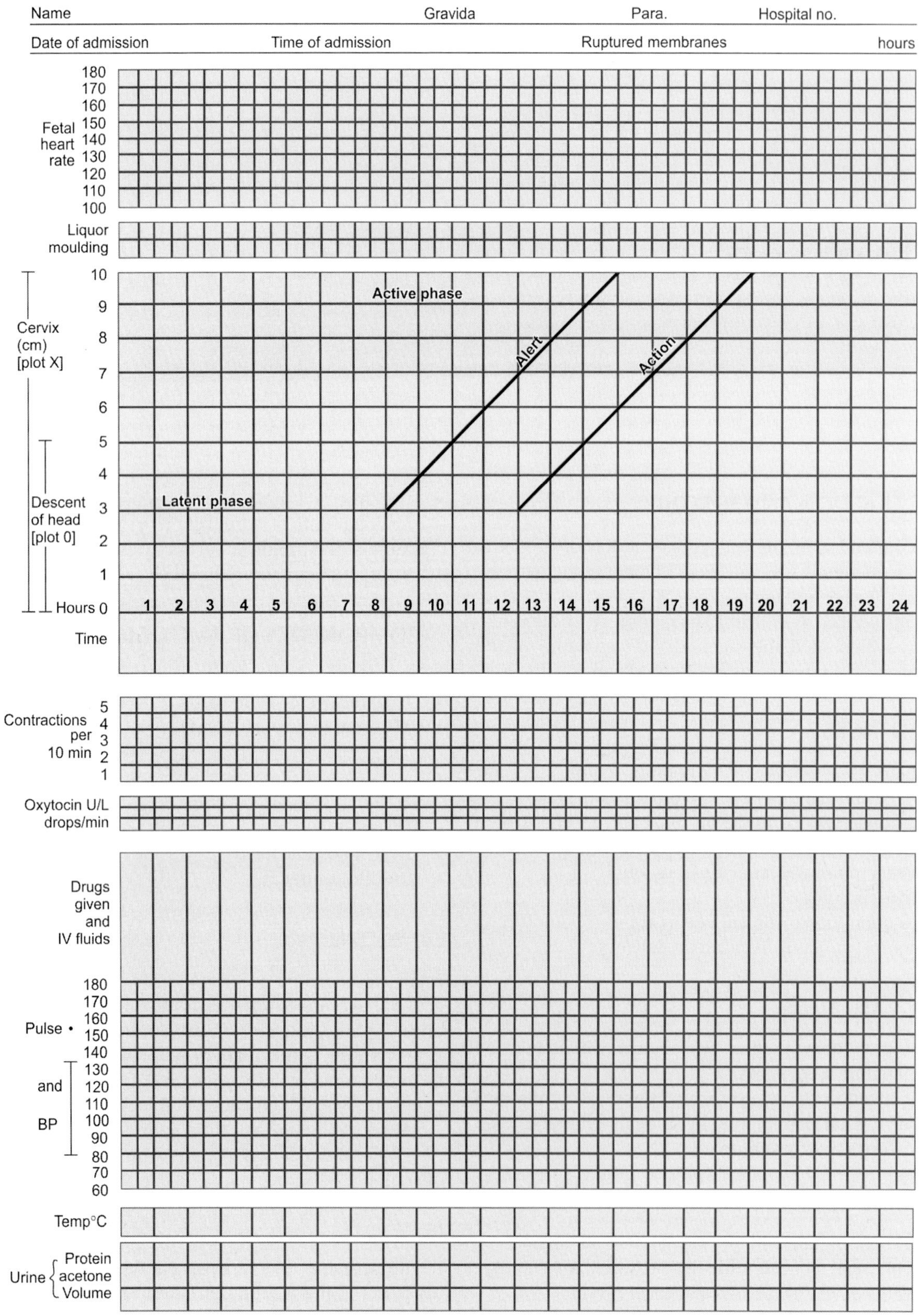

FIG. 1: Partograph. Components of the partograph can be divided into three parts: part I—fetal condition (at top); part II—progress of labor (middle); part III—maternal condition (bottom).

each square representing 1 hour. First vaginal examination is plotted as an X. Thereafter, vaginal examination done 4 hourly unless contraindicated. In partograph, latent phase is demarcated from active phase by a heavy line. In active phase is an alert line, straight line drawn from 3 cm to 10 cm over 7 hours. Four hours to the right of alert line is action line which serves as the critical line, where specific action needs to be taken.[3]

Descent of Fetal Head

The level of head is best measured by abdominal palpation as the number of fifths. Five fifth measured by the width of five fingers is equivalent to a floating head that is above pelvic brim and zero fifth to one that is deeply engaged.

Abdominal assessment may be less accurate; it is more reliable as it ensures that the descent perceived is true descent and not a false impression due to either molding or excessive caput formation.

Descent pattern in normal labor traces a hyperbolic curve.

Uterine Contractions

Half hourly observations were made. Frequency of contractions is assessed by number of contractions in 10 minutes time. If contraction duration less than 20 seconds square is dotted, between 20 seconds and 40 seconds square is cross hatched, more than 40 seconds square is blackened.

Fetal Record

- Fetal heart rate: recorded half hourly and should be heard for at least 1 minute. Normal range 110–160 bpm
- Membranes and liquor: status of membranes and color of liquor are recorded. I for intact, C for clear liquor, M for meconium stained liquor, A for absent liquor

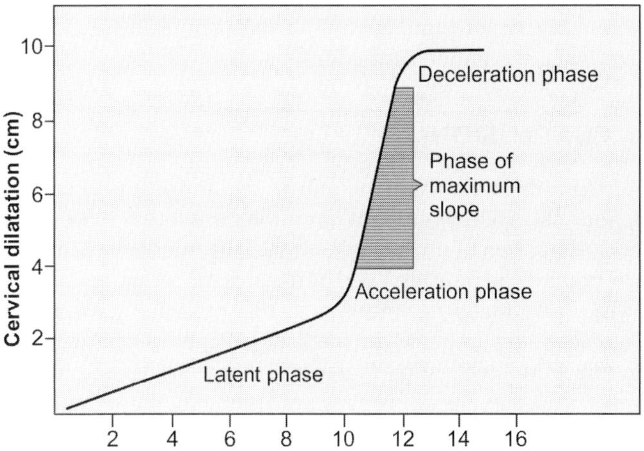

FIG. 2: Cervical dilatation pattern.

- Molding of fetal skull bones: it is an important indicator of pelvic adequacy (Fig. 3).

0 – Skull bones are separate and sutures are easily felt.
1 + – Bones are just touching each other.
2 + – Overlapping of bone not reducible.
3 + – Bones are overlapping irreducibly.

Maternal Record

- Pulse: half hourly
- Blood pressure and temperature 4 hourly or earlier if indicated
- Urine volume 4 hourly and tested for albumin and ketones
- Drugs, oxytocin and intravenous (IV) fluids given.

IMPLEMENTATION

Its implementation implies a functioning referral system with essential obstetrics system in place. The staff should fulfill the minimum training criteria:

- Adequate training in midwifery to observe and conduct normal delivery

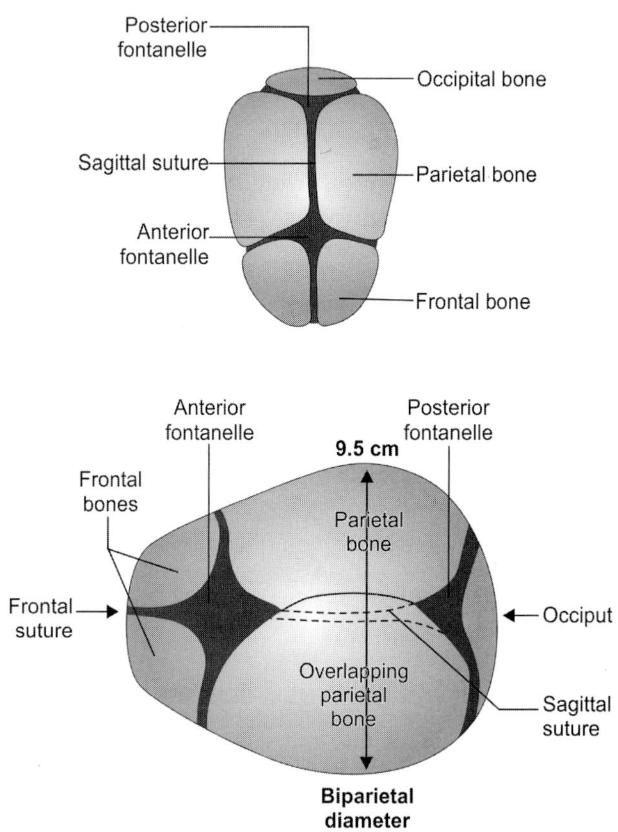

FIG. 3: Molding.

- Be able to perform vaginal examinations and accurately assess cervical dilatation
- Be able to plot cervical dilatation on graph.

ACTIVE MANAGEMENT OF LABOR

Two main components:

1. Organizational component: requires antenatal education of patient and relatives regarding birthing process. Emotional support is given.
2. Medical component:
   - Ensure only term uncomplicated nulliparous included
   - Diagnosis of labor to exclude early admission
   - Cervical examination to ensure adequate progress
   - Timely amniotomy
   - Oxytocin augmentation accordingly.

DISORDERS OF LABOR

- Protraction disorders:
  - Dilatation—if cervical dilatation of less than 1 cm/hr
  - Protracted descent
- Arrest disorders:
  - No dilatation for ≥2 hours
  - No descent for >2 hours.

Table 1 shows three variables with use of partograph. Partograph helps in early detection of these disorders and management accordingly.

MODIFIED PARTOGRAPH

WHO has introduced two modifications (fig 4).

1. Removal of latent phase of labor.
2. Active phase starts at 4 cm of cervical dilatation.

It is used to alleviate below mentioned disadvantage:

- Since prolonged latent phase is relatively infrequent and not usually associated with poor perinatal outcome, usefulness of recording latent phase of labor in partograph is questioned.[1,5]

PAPERLESS PARTOGRAM

Invented by Dr AK Debdas of Jamshedpur, Jharkhand, India.

It is a technique used for monitoring the progress of labor before delivery. It only records the expected time of delivery (ETD), the alert ETD and action ETD for accurate and precise intervention.

TABLE 1: Detection and reduction of prolonged labor

Variable	Before partograph	After partograph
Prolonged labor	6.4%	3.4%
Augmentation of labor	20.7%	9.1%
Emergency cesarean section	9.9%	8.3%

It also makes the application of Freidman formula simple and easy to understand so that even auxiliary nursing midwives (ANMs) can ensure safe delivery.

Applications

It is designed for use by midwives/clinicians in low resource area.

Advantages

- Uses a simple two-step calculation
- Adapted to local needs; require only basic addition and reading of a clock/watch
- Use of potential to simplify and improve the way clinicians prevent prolonged labor
- Not as time consuming for users, only requires 20 seconds to read
- Prompts users to work towards a roughly on-time delivery
- Inexpensive, convenient.

Principles

- Using the golden Freidman formula: dilatation of cervix in active phase of labor at 1 cm/hour. Therefore, removing the unnecessary complexity from WHO partogram while keeping the original concept intact

  Clinician simply adds 6 hours to the time at which woman becomes dilated to 4 cm to find alert ETD. Both ETDs should be written in big letters on the case management sheet, the action ETD circle in red (Fig. 5).
- Mean duration of delivery after alert ETD was 4.3 hours which was similar to WHO partogram.[8]

At the time of alert ETD, clinician is sensitized to the fact that the woman has not yet delivered and if current facility lacks C-section capabilities make arrangements for transportation to higher center.

At the time of action ETD if woman has yet not delivered, she is at risk for prolonged labor than either of medical or surgical intervention needed.[6,7]

CONCLUSION

Partograph is easy and helpful in monitoring progress of labour alongwith condition of mother and fetus. There is an early detection of protracted or arrest disorders. Accordingly the patient can be intervened by oxytocin or cesarean section. WHO introduced newer concept like modified partograph is also being initiated in institutes. Paperless partograph is one step ahead in partographs as very easily used in low resource areas. Its concept remain same as partograph. By using partograph we can save lives of many laboring mothers and fetus thereby reducing maternal mortality rate. So its use should be encouraged in laboring mothers in hospitals.

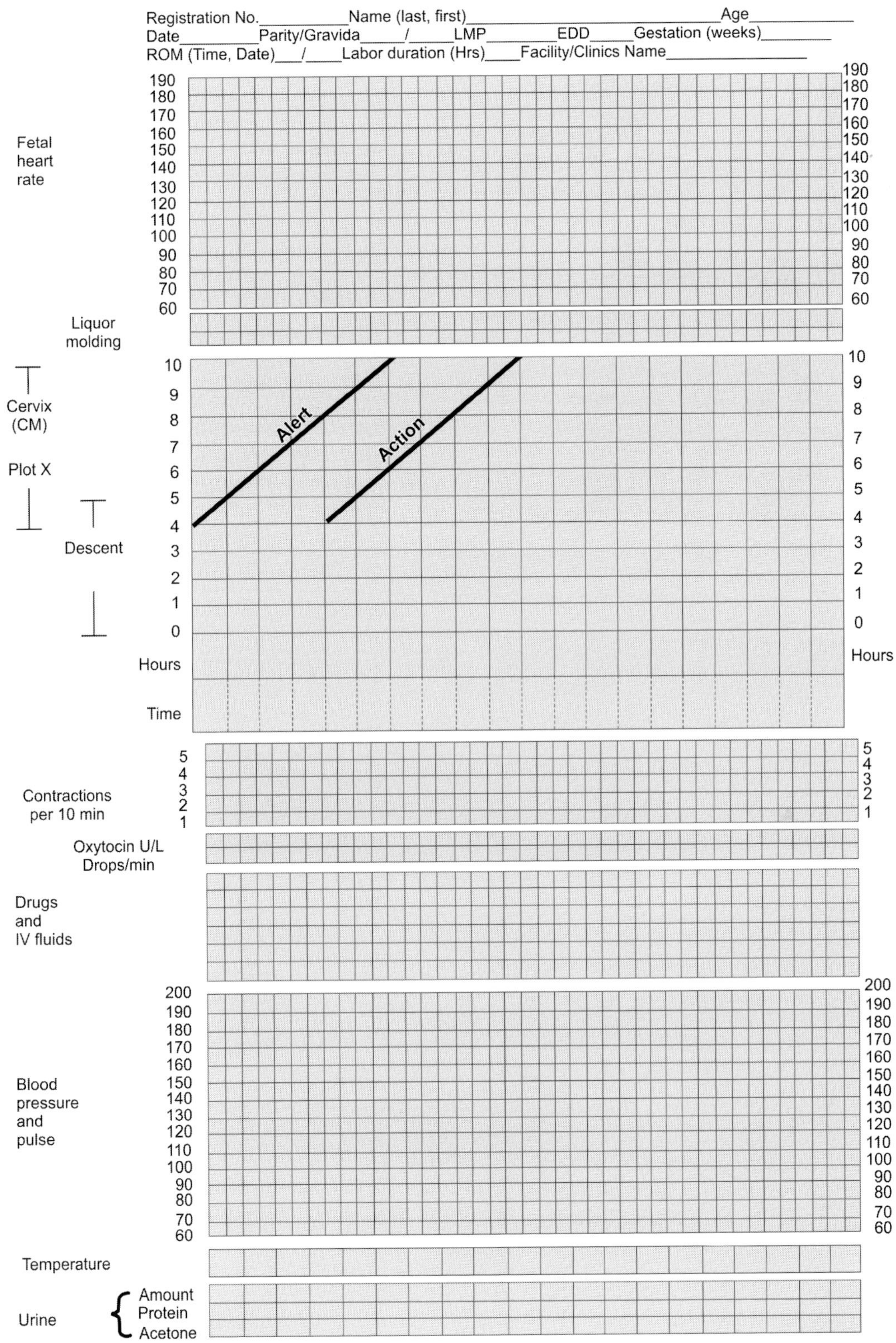

FIG. 4: WHO modified partograph.

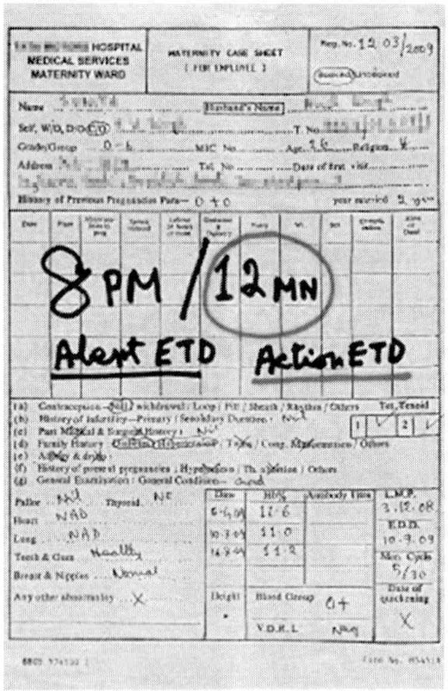

FIG. 5: Paperless partogram.

REFERENCES

1. Reproductive Health 2013, 10:23. Published 18/ 04/2013.
2. Cunningham FG, Leveno KJ, Bloom SL, Hauth JC, Gilstrap LC, Wenstrom KD (Eds). Dystocia. Williams Obstetrics, 22nd edition. New York: McGraw Hill; 2005. pp. 495-524.
3. Freidman EA. Graphic analysis of labor. Am J Obstet Gynecol. 1954;68:1568.
4. World Health Organization. Preventing Prolonged Labor: A Practical Guide. The Partograph. Part 1: Principles and Strategy (WHO/FHE/MSM/93.8); Part II: User's Manual (WHO/FHE/MSM/93.9). Geneva: World Health Organization; 1993.
5. Cohen WR. Controversies in assessment of labour progress in obstetrics and gynecology; 2006 pp. 231-43.
6. J Family Med Prim Care. 2013 Jan- Mar;2(1):47-49. Doi :10.4103/2249-4863.109944.
7. Debdas AK. Paperless partogram. 41st Annual Scientific Session 2008; Sri Lanka College of Obstetricians and Gynecologists. SLJOG. 2008;30:124.
8. Journal of Education and Practice ISSN 2222-1735 (Paper) ISSN 2222-288X Vol.6, No.8, 2015.

CHAPTER 16

Episiotomy

Laxmi Shrikhande, Surekha Tayade,Rohini Rao

INTRODUCTION

The episiotomy is the planned surgical incision of the perineum performed to widen the vaginal opening during the late second stage of labor.[1]

The term episiotomy is derived from the Greek words *episton* meaning "pubic region" and *tomy* meaning "to cut". Episiotomy is synonymously used with perineotomy. It is the most common obstetric operation performed worldwide.

Episiotomy was first described in 1742, suggesting that it was done to prevent the severe perineal tears.[2] It was introduced in the mid-19th century to the United States. In 1920, at a meeting of American Gynecological Society in Chicago, DeLee publicly advocated the adoption of mediolateral episiotomy for deliveries of all nulliparous women.[3]

THE RATIONALES FOR EPISIOTOMY

- Maternal:
    - Shortening of second stage (decreases maternal exhaustion)
    - Decreases the blood loss
    - Preservation of pelvic floor injuries
    - Prevention of uterine prolapsed
    - Prevention of muscle relaxation of perineum and pelvic floor leading to improved sexual function and reduced risk of urinary and fecal incontinence
- Fetal:
    - Prevention of asphyxia
    - Prevention of cranial trauma
    - Prevention of cerebral hemorrhage
    - Prevention of mental retardation
    - Decreases the incidence of shoulder dystocia.

INDICATIONS

Routine episiotomy is not recommended in every case even in primigravida. A constant supervision during labor, especially during the second stage, reduces both indications and incidence of episiotomy.

- Rigid (inelastic) perineum: in elderly primigravidas, the inelastic perineum can cause delay in descent of presenting part or even arrest
- Anticipating perineal tear:
    - Breech delivery
    - Big baby
    - Face to pubis delivery
    - Shoulder dystocia
- Operative delivery: ventouse and forceps delivery
- Previous perineal surgery: perineal reconstructive surgery, pelvic floor repair
- To cut short the second stage:
    - Prolonged second stage
    - Cardiac disease
    - Fetal distress in second stage.

The American College of Obstetricians and Gynecologists (ACOG) in 2006 has advocated the "restricted use of episiotomy" during labor, with physicians encouraged to use clinical judgment to decide when the procedure is necessary. According to the ACOG, "the available data does not support the routine use of episiotomy". However, episiotomy should be performed/considered if:

- Severe maternal lacerations anticipating severe perineal trauma (third or fourth degree tears). Expediting the difficult deliverers in which suspected maternal and/or fetal compromise is suspected
- An episiotomy should be performed in instrumental birth, shoulder dystocia, breech, or suspected fetal compromise

- Episiotomy should not be offered routinely at vaginal birth following third or fourth degree traumas
- Median episiotomy is associated with higher rates of injury to anal sphincter and rectum as compared to mediolateral episiotomy. Mediolateral episiotomy may be preferred to midline episiotomy when clinically indicated.

Recent studies have shown that the indications for episiotomy were based on limited data. Episiotomy does not prevent pelvic floor damage, and thus did not decrease the rate of urinary incontinence and sphincter dysfunctions. There is increased maternal blood loss, increased dyspareunia, suture placement and wound complications. There was general underestimation of the adverse consequences associated with the procedure, including extension to third or fourth degree tears. Thus, few studies have suggested that women who have an episiotomy do not have significantly improved labor, delivery, and recovery compared with those who do not have episiotomy.[4]

The National Institute for Health and Care Excellence and Royal College of Obstetricians and Gynaecologists published similar guidelines in 2007 recommending against routine episiotomy and advocating mediolateral episiotomy whenever indicated.[5]

CONTRAINDICATIONS

The relative contraindications of the episiotomy include:

- Inflammatory bowel disease
- Severe perineal malformations
- Lymphogranuloma venereum
- Coagulation disorders, such as idiopathic thrombocytopenic purpura.

TIMING OF EPISIOTOMY

The timing to perform an appropriate episiotomy should be well judged. Neither it should be too early as it will cause more blood loss, nor it should be too late as it will not prevent invisible lacerations and will fail to protect the pelvic floor. The episiotomy should be given when the perineum is bulging, thinned, and stretched during contraction just prior to crowning of the head.

TYPES OF EPISIOTOMY

The following are the types of episiotomy:

- Mediolateral episiotomy
- Median (midline) episiotomy
- Lateral episiotomy
- J-shaped episiotomy.

Mediolateral Episiotomy

An incision is made at the posterior fourchette and is continued downwards and outwards either to the right or to the left at an angle of at least 45° to the perineal body. The incision angle may approach 90° (perpendicular to the posterior fourchette) if it is given at the peak of the contraction and the perineum is stretched significantly by the fetal head, so that on relaxation of the perineum, the angle will approach 45°. It is mostly 3–4 cm in length. It is in a straight line and about 2.5 cm from the anus.

Median (Midline) Episiotomy

An incision is made vertically along the median raphe of perineum starting from posterior fourchette towards the anus, but not including the fibers of the rectal sphincter capsule. It is commonly made just before delivery of the presenting part, at that time the perineum is thinned and stretched.

A comparison between median and mediolateral episiotomy has been outlined in table 1.

Lateral Episiotomy

An incision is commenced about 1 cm away from the center of fourchette and is directed downwards and laterally. It may injure the Bartholin duct and is totally condemned.

TABLE 1: Comparison between median and mediolateral episiotomy

	Median episiotomy	Mediolateral episiotomy
Muscles	Muscles are cut	Muscles are not cut
Blood loss	Minimal	Slightly more
Repair	Easy	Slightly difficult; chances of hematoma formation, if not repaired properly
Healing	Fast	Takes time
Postoperative comfort	More comfort	Less comfort
Wound disruption	Not common	Relatively more
Dyspareunia	Rare	Comparatively more
Rectal involvement	If extension occurs rectum is involved	Rare
Incision extension	If needed, it cannot be extended	Incision can be extended if needed: as in manipulative deliveries and also in abnormal presentations and positions.

J-shaped Episiotomy

A vertical incision is started from the center of the fourchette and is directed downwards and posteriorly along the midline for about 1.5 cm and then the incision is directed downwards and outwards at 5 or 7 o'clock position. J-shaped episiotomy was started to avoid the injury to anal sphincter. But as the apposition is not perfect and the wound sometimes become puckered, so this kind of episiotomy is neither widely done nor accepted by the physicians.

STEPS FOR MEDIOLATERAL EPISIOTOMY

Preliminaries

The perineum should be cleaned with povidone-iodine lotion and then draped properly. For local anesthesia, the incisional site is infiltrated with 10 mL of 1% lignocaine solution as shown in figure 1A.

Procedure

The index and the middle finger are introduced into the vagina. The fingers are placed between the presenting part and the perineum. The incision can either be given by curved scissors or straight blunt tip pointed sharp scissors. The incision should be given at the height of uterine contraction because at that point the accurate idea of the extent of the incision can be made from the stretched perineum. The incision should be in a straight line starting from center of the fourchette directed downwards and outwards either to the left or right side and about 2.5 cm away from anus (Fig. 1B).

Structures cut are:

- Posterior vaginal wall
- Superficial and deep transverse perineal muscles, bulbospongiosus and part of levator ani
- Fascia covering the muscles
- Transverse perineal branch of pudendal nerve and vessels
- Subcutaneous tissue and perineal skin.

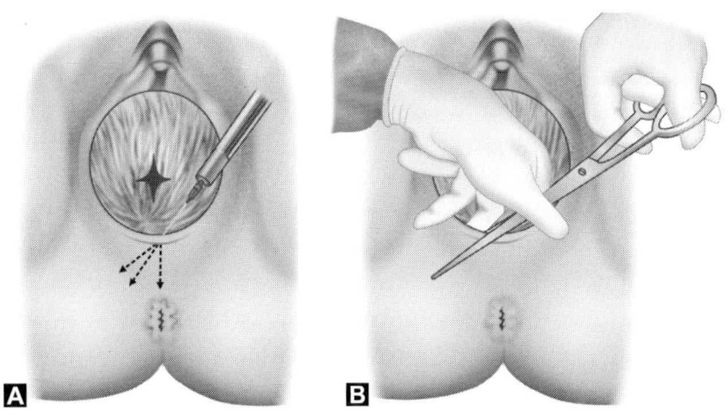

FIG. 1: Steps of mediolateral episiotomy. **A,** Perineal infiltration with local anaesthetic solution in a fan shaped manner; **B,** Cutting the perineum after two fingers are insinuated between perineum and fetal head.

Repair timing

The repair should be done soon after expulsion of placenta. If repair is done before the expulsion it may cause disruption of the wound.

Prerequisites

The patient is given lithotomy position. A good light source should be present. The whole of the perineum along with episiotomy is cleaned and washed with antiseptic lotion. The delivery provider should examine the vagina for blood clots and the episiotomy site. The patient is then draped and repair is to be done under strict aseptic conditions.

Repair

The repair is done in following order:

- The submucosal tissue and mucosa of vagina
- Perineal muscles
- Subcutaneous tissue and skin.

The index and the middle finger are placed in the vagina for retraction, the apex is to be identified and the first suture is taken approximately 1 cm proximal to the apex. The vaginal mucosa and the submucosal tissue are re-approximated in a locked or nonlocked continuous fashion. The incision should be closed in such a way that the anatomy is maintained and the hymenal ring is re-approximated accurately. In deeper episiotomy or laceration the perineum requires additional submucosal sutures to approximate the dead space. The perineal muscles with the fascial sheath of the muscles are repaired in interrupted fashion before closure of the subcutaneous tissue and skin, which is repaired either by subcuticular stitches or interrupted sutures as shown in figure 2.

While repairing the episiotomy, continuous attention must be paid to achieve the hemostasis along with the obliteration of the dead space with minimal injury and tissue destruction.

POSTOPERATIVE CARE AND MANAGEMENT

The episiotomy should be kept dry and clean, the dressing of the wound should be done each time following micturition and defecation. The wound should be cleaned from front to back (vaginal orifices towards anal opening) and is done by cotton swab soaked with antiseptic solution. After cleaning the wound, antiseptic ointment is to be applied. For the relief of the pain at the wound, site magnesium sulfate ($MgSO_4$) compressions, infrared heat application, or use of icepacks to decrease the pain and swelling can be done. Analgesic drugs are also required to reduce the pain.

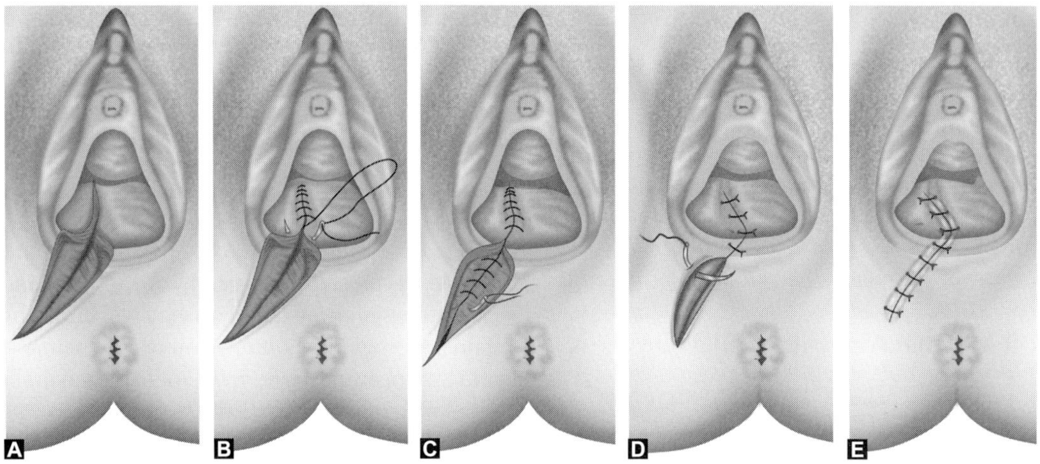

FIG. 2: Steps of repair of episiotomy. **A,** Wound on inspection; **B,** Repair of vaginal mucosa after placing the anchor stitch above the wound apex and vaginal mucosa is stitched in continuous interlocking fashion up to the hymen ring; **C,** Repair of perineal muscles by interrupted sutures; **D,** Apposition of the skin margins; **E,** Repaired wound on inspection.

During the last decade it has been found that the long-lasting and complete pain relief is found with cold sitz bath than the warm sitz bath.[6]

- Patient is advised to be ambulatory after 24 hours
- She is allowed to roll over from side to side and back to side
- She is allowed to sit with her thighs appose and not to feed the baby by sitting cross legged.

Stitch Removal

The wound is sutured by catgut or dexon which is absorbed (are dissolved) and need not to be removed. But if nylon or silk (nonabsorbable material) is used, then stitches should be removed (cut) on 6th day.

Complications of Episiotomy

It includes the following:

- Immediate complications
- Remote complications.

Immediate Complications

Bleeding

The perineum has extensive vasculature and due to the physiological changes of pregnancy and labor, the blood supply is increased and thus, bleeding is the most common complication. As episiotomy incision is given at the time of crowing, so sometimes, the blood vessels are invisible because of compression due to the presenting part. Following delivery, the episiotomy site should be inspected properly for the arterial bleeding and if any arterial bleeding is found, ligation should be done.

Extension to higher-order lacerations

There are many factors which are associated in increased risk of laceration. They include the following:

- Inadequate incision
- Episiotomy not timed properly
- Uncontrolled delivery
- Fetopelvic disproportion
- Shoulder dystocia
- Fetal anomalies
- Malpresentations and malpositions
- Previous injury to reproductive tract.

In primiparous women, the risk of third and fourth degree lacerations is 1% without episiotomy and with mediolateral episiotomy; it is 9% and is raised to 20% in a midline episiotomy.[7] So, by giving the midline episiotomy, the major risk is extension of the laceration into rectum.

There should be a quick and gentle examination of the episiotomy site after the placenta is out as it is very important. Failure to identify the laceration or the extensions can lead to infection, dehiscence, fistula formation, and fecal incontinence.

Infection

The site of episiotomy is frequently contaminated during the process of delivery by the fecal matter and is heavily colonized by the bacteria, thus there is significant risk of infection.

The manifestations of infection occur within 7 days following delivery.

The clinical features are:

- Rise in temperature
- Local tenderness at wound site
- Purulent or malodorous discharge
- Wound is moist, red, and swollen.

Most of the infections are localized and respond to wound care and antibiotics. In rare cases, there could be abscess formation for which drainage is required and sometimes, necrotizing fasciitis may develop.

Dehiscence

Infrequently, the episiotomy repair may undergo dehiscence. The dehiscence can occur with or without the infection or hematoma formation. It may also occur due to the faulty repair. The small dehiscence heals spontaneously by secondary healing. For this, daily dressing of the wound is done till the infection subsides totally. Then the healthy granulation tissue is formed and healing takes place by new margin formation. However, many dehiscence may require suturing under local anesthesia by using cutting needle with nylon thread after saucerizing and debridement of all the necrotic tissue. The postdressing and parenteral antibiotic therapy is necessary.

Remote Complications

- Dyspareunia: narrow vaginal introitus due to faulty repair can cause dyspareunia
- Scar endometriosis: it is a very rare clinical entity.

CONCLUSION

Episiotomy should not be considered a taboo and there is a clear evidence to advocate the restricted use of episiotomy during labour with physicians encouraged to use clinical judgement before embarking on the episiotomy. The policy of restricted use of episiotomy has considerably reduced the maternal morbidity without any increase in adverse neonatal outcome. Thus the policy of restricted use of episiotomy may be adopted as a norm for singleton vaginal term deliveries to improve the maternal outcome. Mediolateral episiotomy should be preferred compared to median when clinically indicated.

REFERENCES

1. Thacker SB, Banta HD. Benefits and risks of episiotomy: an interpretative review of the English language literature, 1860-1980. Obstet Gynecol Surv. 1983;38(6):322-38.
2. Ould SF. A Treatise on Midwifery in Three Parts. Dublin, Ireland: O Nelson & C Connor; 1742.
3. DeLee JB. The prophylactic forceps operation. Am J Obstet Gynecol. 1920;1:34-44.
4. American College of Obstetricians and Gynecologists. ACOG Practice Bulletin. Episiotomy. Clinical Management Guidelines for Obstetrician-Gynecologists. Number 71, April 2006. Obstet Gynecol. 2006;107(4):957-62.
5. National Collaborating Centre for Women's and Children's Health. (2007). Intrapartum care: care of healthy women and their babies during childbirth. [online] Available from: stratog.rcog.org.uk/files/rcog-corp/elearn/128970/134293/Intrapartum_care_NICE.pdf. [Accessed February, 2016].
6. Ramler D, Roberts J. A comparison of cold and warm sitz baths for relief of postpartum perineal pain. J Obstet Gynecol Neonatal Nurs. 1986;15:471-4.
7. Owen J, Hauth JC. Episiotomy infection and dehiscence. In: Gilstrap LC III, Faro S (Eds). Infections in Pregnancy. New York, USA: Alan R Liss; 1990.

CHAPTER 17

Intrapartum Fetal Surveillance

Surekha Tayade

INTRODUCTION

It was way back in 17th century that fetal heart sounds (FHS) were first discovered by Marsac and soon, Killian proposed that fetal heart rate (FHR) could be used to determine fetal well-being. This idea went unnoticed until 1818, when Kergaradee suggested that FHS could be used to determine fetal viability and life (Grant, 1989).[1] In 1833, Evory Kennedy published guidelines for fetal distress and recommended auscultation of the FHR as a tool of intrapartum monitoring. DeLee-Hillis Fetoscope since its invention in 1924, remained at the forefront of intrapartum fetal monitoring for the next half-century.

In the 1960s, electronic fetal monitoring (EFM) system was made commercially available in the United States by Hon and also in other parts of the world by other researchers. In spite of controversies comparing cardiotocography (CTG) with intermittent auscultation, CTG continues to be widely used today as a routine monitor of fetal well-being in labor rooms worldwide. Although, the majority of perinatal, morbidity and mortality may not be prevented by improved fetal monitoring in labor (Nelson, 1996),[2] failures to identify abnormal FHR patterns and lack of appropriate actions are considered to be significant contributing factors (Maternal and Child Health Resource Consortium ,1997–99).

AIM OF INTRAPARTUM FETAL SURVEILLANCE

The principal aim of intrapartum fetal surveillance is to prevent adverse perinatal outcomes arising from fetal metabolic acidosis related to labor. As the fetal brain modulates the FHR through an interplay of sympathetic and parasympathetic forces, FHR monitoring can be used to determine whether or not a fetus is well oxygenated.[3]

In the absence of risk factors, fetal heart surveillance by continuous EFM has not proven benefit. It may, however increase the possibilities of interventions in a normal spontaneous labor lasting less than 12 hours in the active phase. The avoidance of adverse fetal outcomes is the objective of intrapartum fetal monitoring. This objective is common to all hospitals providing maternity services. It is indisputable that monitoring of the fetal heart is an essential part of the care of the fetus during labor. The modalities to be used is a topic of discussion and research in most obstetric setups.

Although EFM has been available since the late 1960s, it has not been proven to improve fetal outcome. However, it has not yet been replaced by a more effective method of fetal surveillance. For monitoring to be effective it must be performed correctly, its results interpreted satisfactorily, and this interpretation must provoke an appropriate response (Grant, 1989).[1]

Intrapartum fetal monitoring was developed in the 1960s to identify events that might result in hypoxic ischemic encephalopathy, cerebral palsy, or fetal death. Continuous EFM, using external or internal transducers, became a part of routine maternity care during the 1970s; by 2002, about 85% of live were monitored by it.

SELECTION OF INTRAPARTUM SURVEILLANCE METHOD (FLOWCHART 1)

Fetal surveillance includes both electronic methods of monitoring fetal well-being (e.g., cardiotocograph) and nonelectronic methods (e.g., fetal blood sampling). Fetal heart rate monitoring can occur via intermittent auscultation or continuous cardiotocograph.[3] Intermittent auscultation of fetal heart employs the use of a Doppler assessment of FHR

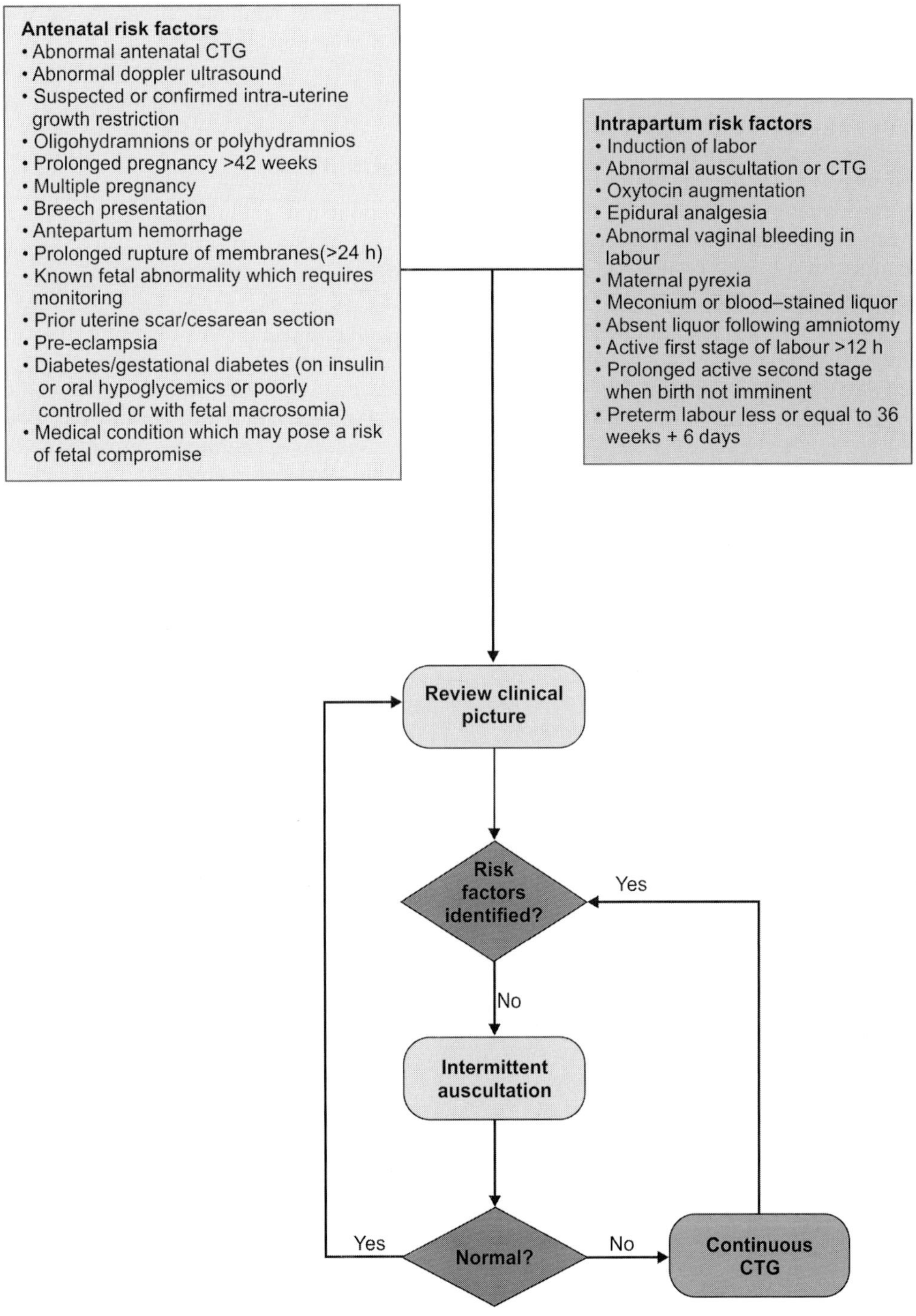

CTG, cardiotocography.

FLOWCHART 1: A chart showing choice of intrapartum fetal monitoring.[1,2]

during labor at defined timed intervals. It is equivalent to continuous EFM in screening for fetal compromise in low-risk patients. Safety in using structured intermittent auscultation is based on a nurse-to-patient ratio of 1:1 and an established technique for intermittent auscultation for each institution.[4]

Cardiotocography is a complex technology applied for surveillance of the fetus during pregnancy, labor, and delivery. The FHR and the frequency of the uterine contractions can be continuously monitored. There are two methods of monitoring the FHR: the external method, in which an ultrasound transducer is placed on the mother's abdomen by an elastic belt, and the internal method, in which electrocardiographic leads are attached directly to the fetus after rupture of the membranes. The uterine activity is monitored by an external tocotransducer or by an intrauterine catheter; the transducers or electrodes are connected to a cardiotocograph where the FHR and the frequency and duration of the contractions are displayed. Both are recorded in a continuous tracing on paper.[5]

The labor admission test is a CTG of 20–30 minutes of duration, carried out when the woman is admitted to the labor ward. It is part of the admission assessment of a woman. The test was introduced as a risk screening in early labor, to detect the compromised fetus on admission and to select the women in need of continuous EFM during labor. The test is commonly used for screening in many countries.[6,7]

There are several considerations when choosing a method of intrapartum fetal monitoring. The most important is the antepartum profile of the patient. Apart from this, certain high-risk factors in the intrapartum period will also determine the use of surveillance method (Table 1). Existence of risk factor precludes the use of continuous EFM.

Continuous EFM may adversely affect the labor process and maternal satisfaction by decreasing maternal mobility, physical contact with her partner, and time with the labor nurse compared with structured intermittent auscultation.

However, the perception that structured intermittent auscultation increases medicolegal risk, the lack of hospital staff trained in structured intermittent auscultation, and the economic benefit of continuous EFM from decreased use of nursing staff may promote the use of continuous EFM. Continuous EFM should be used when there are abnormalities in structured intermittent auscultation or for high-risk patients.[8]

EQUIPMENT

- Doppler ultrasound and/or cardiotocograph (CTG)
- Transducer gel (warmed)
- Progress notes and/or partogram.

PROCEDURE

- Determine the indication for fetal monitoring
- Discuss fetal monitoring with the woman and obtain permission to commence. Provide the "Fetal Monitoring during Pregnancy and Labor" pamphlet if appropriate
- Perform abdominal palpation to determine lie and presentation unless contraindicated (e.g., antepartum hemorrhage, abruption)
- Give the woman an opportunity to empty her bladder
- The woman should be in an upright to lateral position (not supine)
- If performing intermittent auscultation, ensure the volume is turned on and apply probe to abdomen where the anterior shoulder of the fetus is positioned
- If performing a CTG check, the accurate date and time has been set on the CTG machine and the paper speed is set on 1 cm/minute. Ensure the CTG is labeled with the woman's name, unique record number, and date/time

TABLE 1: Antenatal and intrapartum high-risk factors warranting continuous electronic fetal monitoring

Antenatal risk factors	Intrapartum risk factors
• Abnormal antenatal CTG • Abnormal Doppler umbilical artery velocimetry • Suspected or confirmed intrauterine growth restriction • Oligohydramnios or polyhydramnios • Prolonged pregnancy • Multiple pregnancy • Breech presentation • Antepartum hemorrhage • Prolonged rupture of membranes(≥24 hours) • Known fetal abnormality which requires monitoring • Uterine scar (e.g., previous cesarean section) • Hypertensive disorders of pregnancy (pre-eclampsia, essential hypertension) • Gestational diabetes mellitus (poorly controlled, on medication or with fetal macrosomia) • Other current or past obstetric or medical condition which constitutes risk to the fetus • Decreased fetal movements • Morbid obesity (BMI ≥40) • Maternal age ≥42 years • Abnormalities of maternal serum screening associated with an increased risk of poor perinatal outcomes (e.g., low PAPP-A <0.4 MoM)	• Induction of labor with prostaglandins/oxytocin • Abnormal fetal heart rate on auscultation or CTG • Oxytocin augmentation • Epidural analgesia • Abnormal vaginal bleeding in labor • Maternal pyrexia >38°C • Meconium or blood-stained liquor • Absent liquor following amniotomy • Active first stage of labor >12 hours (i.e., regular uterine activity, cervix 4 cm or more dilated) • Active second stage (i.e., pushing)

CTG, cardiotocography; PAPP, pregnancy associated plasma protein-A; BMI, body mass index.

of commencement. Record the maternal heart rate at the commencement of the CTG in order to differentiate between maternal and FHR
- Place the two elastic belts around the abdomen and secure. Position the tocotransducer firmly on the abdomen over the fundus. Apply the transducer gel to the ultrasound transducer and firmly attach over the position of the anterior shoulder of the fetus
- Set the tocotransducer at a uterine resting tone baseline level of 20 mm of mercury
- Record on the trace anything, which may influence the FHR or uterine activity including maternal medications, movement, changes in position, fetal movements, contractions/Braxton Hicks contractions, drinks/food ingested, use of illicit drugs or cigarettes
- Documentation of findings must be recorded in the patient notes and if a CTG is performed all features of the CTG must be documented including:[3,9]
    - Baseline heart rate
    - Variability, accelerations, and decelerations
    - An assessment of the trace as normal, abnormal or pathological
- If the CTG monitoring is continuous, all features must be documented in the patient notes every hour in addition to the review and documentation schedule
- All FHR/CTG abnormalities must be reported to the shift coordinator and the obstetric team and measures initiated, where appropriate, to improve fetal status.

INDICATIONS

Admission Cardiotocography

There is insufficient evidence to recommend routine use of an admission CTG for women identified at the onset of labor as having low risk of developing fetal compromise.

Intermittent Auscultation

Intermittent auscultation is mandatory for all women at the onset of labor as identified as low risk of developing fetal compromise.

When performing intermittent auscultation:
- Use a Doppler ultrasound
- The speaker mode must be turned on
- Each auscultation episode should be performed for at least a full minute commencing during a contraction and continuing for at least 30 seconds after the contraction has finished
- Fetal heart rate auscultation should be undertaken:
    - At least every 15–30 minutes in the active phase of the first stage of labor
    - At least every 5 minutes in the second stage of labor until active pushing
    - Toward the end and for at least 30 seconds after each contraction during active pushing in the second stage of labor.

Continuous Electronic Fetal Monitoring

Continuous EFM is recommended when risk factors for fetal compromise have been detected during pregnancy, are detected at the onset of labor, or develop during labor.[3,9]

When continuous EFM is undertaken
- Cardiotocography should be reviewed at least every 15 minutes
- Cardiotocography trace should be signed every 15 minutes
- Cardiotocography should be signed by the lead clinician each time the woman is reviewed and a plan of care written in the maternal notes
- Cardiotocography trace should be reviewed by a second clinician every hour and signed to ensure critical review of the trace.

Any intrapartum events that may affect FHR (e.g., vaginal examination, fetal blood sampling, or epidural insertion) should be noted on both the CTG, and the maternal notes including date, time, and signature.

Continuous EFM can be interrupted for periods of up to 15 minutes to allow personal care (e.g., toilet, shower). Interruptions should be infrequent and not occur immediately after an intervention that might be expected to alter the FHR (e.g., amniotomy, epidural insertion or top-up).[10] Whilst not recommended in low-risk women if a clinician initiates EFM in the first stage of labor. In a low-risk women, it should only:
- Be undertaken for a minimum of 20 minutes
- The episode of EFM should be discontinued if the CTG is normal.

Indications for Continuous Electronic Fetal Monitoring

These can be antenatal and postnatal risk factors mentioned in table 1.

CARDIOTOCOGRAPHY INTERPRETATION

There are four main features that should be systematically examined to assist with the interpretation of the CTG.

1. Baseline rate
2. Baseline variability
3. Accelerations
4. Decelerations.

Baseline Fetal Heart Rate (Fig. 1)

Baseline FHR is the mean level of the FHR when this is stable, excluding accelerations and decelerations. It is a resting FHR when the fetus is not moving and in the absence of uterine

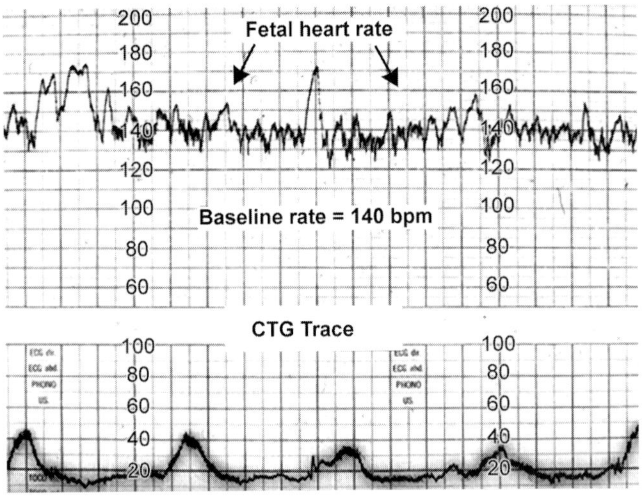

FIG. 1: Baseline fetal heart rate.

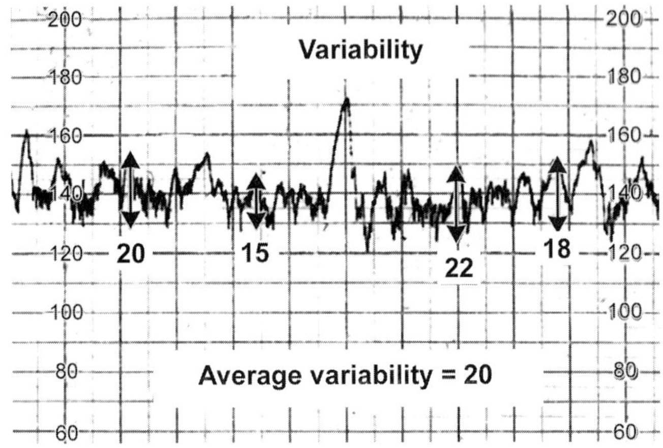

FIG. 2: Baseline variability.

activity. It is determined over a time period of 5–10 minutes, expressed as beats per minute. Preterm fetuses tend to have values towards the upper end of the normal range.

- Normal FHR baseline: 110–160 beats per minute
- Tachycardia: FHR baseline is greater than 160 beats per minute
- Bradycardia: FHR baseline is less than 110 beats per minute.

Fetal tachycardia can be caused by:

- Fetal hypoxia
- Chorioamnionitis—if maternal fever also present
- Hyperthyroidism
- Fetal or maternal anemia, fetal tachyarrhythmia.

Mild bradycardia between 100 and 120 beats per minute is common in the following situations:

- Postdate gestation
- Occiput posterior or transverse presentations

Severe prolonged bradycardia (<80 beats per minute for >3 minutes) indicates severe hypoxia.

Causes of prolonged severe bradycardia are:[1]

- Prolonged cord compression
- Cord prolapse
- Epidural and spinal anesthesia
- Maternal seizures
- Rapid fetal descent.

Baseline Variability (Fig. 2)

Baseline variability is the minor fluctuations in baseline FHR. It is assessed by estimating the difference in beats per minute between the highest peak and lowest trough of fluctuation in one-minute segments of the trace (3–5 cycles/min).

Variability is visually quantitated as the amplitude of peak-to-trough in beats per minute.

- Absent: amplitude range undetectable
- Minimal: amplitude range detectable but 5 beats per minute or fewer
- Moderate (normal): amplitude range 6–25 beats per minute
- Marked: amplitude range greater than 25 beats per minute.

Reduced variability can be caused by:

- Fetus sleeping: this should last no longer than 40 minutes—most common cause
- Fetal acidosis (due to hypoxia): more likely if late decelerations also present
- Fetal tachycardia
- Drugs: opiates, benzodiazepine, methyldopa, magnesium sulfate
- Prematurity: variability is reduced at earlier gestation (<28 weeks)
- Congenital heart abnormalities.

Accelerations (Fig. 3)

Accelerations are transient increases in FHR of 15 beats per minute or more above the baseline and lasting 15 seconds. Accelerations in preterm fetuses may be of lesser amplitude and shorter duration.

Decelerations (Fig. 4)

Decelerations are transient episodes of decrease of FHR below the baseline of more than 15 beats per minute lasting at least 15 seconds, which are:

- Early deceleration: uniform, repetitive decrease of FHR with slow onset early in the contraction and slow return to baseline by the end of a contraction (i.e., start and finish in the contraction). It may indicate head compression and maybe considered as physiological

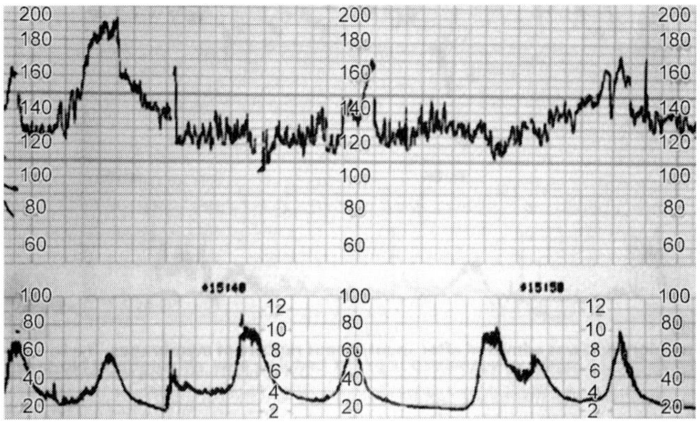

FIG. 3: Accelerations.

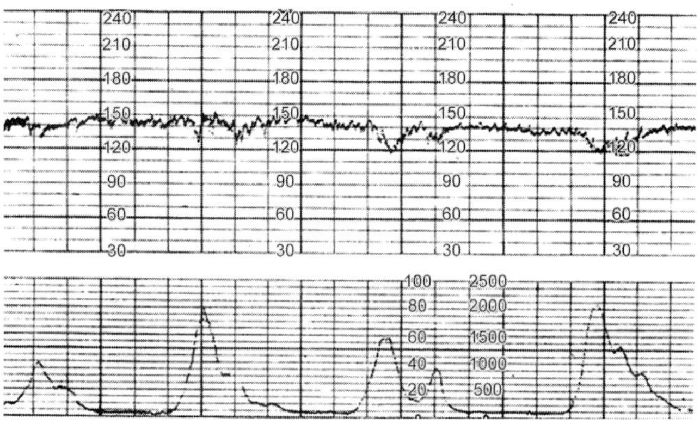

FIG. 4: Decelerations.

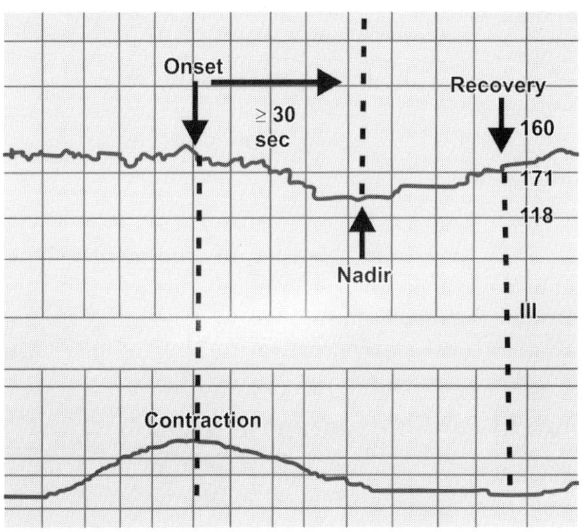

FIG. 5: Late decelerations.

- Late decelerations (Fig. 5): are uniform, repetitive decrease of FHR with, usually, slow onset mid to end of the contraction and nadir more than 20 seconds after the peak of the contraction and ending after the contraction
  - Variable: repetitive or intermittent decrease of FHR with rapid onset and recovery. Time relationships with contraction cycle may be variable but most commonly occur simultaneously with contractions
  - Complicated variable decelerations: the following additional features indicate the likelihood of fetal hypoxia:
    - Rising baseline rate or fetal tachycardia
    - Reducing baseline variability
    - Slow return to baseline FHR after the end of the contraction
    - Large amplitude (by 60 beats per minute or to 60 beats per minute) and/or long duration (60 seconds)
    - Loss of pre- and postdeceleration shouldering (abrupt brief increases in FHR baseline)
    - Presence of postdeceleration smooth overshoots (temporary increases in FHR above baseline)
- Prolonged decelerations: a decrease of FHR below the baseline or more than 15 beats per minute for longer than 90 seconds but less than 5 minutes.

FEATURES OF NORMAL AND ABNORMAL CARDIOTOCOGRAPHY (TABLE 2)

The normal CTG associated with a low probability of fetal compromise has the following features:

- Baseline rate 110–160 beats per minute
- Baseline variability of 5–25 beats per minute
- Accelerations 15 beats per minute for 15 seconds
- No decelerations.

All other CTGs are by this definition are abnormal and require further evaluation taking into account the full clinical picture.

The following features are unlikely to be associated with significant fetal compromise when occurring in isolation, however, the CTG is still considered abnormal and close observation should continue in addition to discussion of the features with the obstetric registrar/lead obstetrician:

- Baseline rate 100–109 beats per minute
- Absence of accelerations
- Early decelerations
- Variable decelerations without complicating features.

The following features may be associated with significant fetal compromise and require further action:

- Fetal tachycardia
- Reduced baseline variability
- Complicated variable decelerations
- Late decelerations
- Prolonged decelerations.

The following features are very likely to be associated with significant fetal compromise and require immediate management, which may include urgent delivery:

TABLE 2: Classification of fetal heart rate trace features

Feature	Baseline (bmp)	Variability (bmp)	Decelerations	Accelerations
Reassuring	110–160	≥5	None	Present
Nonreassuring	100–190 161–180	<5 for 40–90 min	• Typical variable decelerations with over 50% of contractions, for over 90% min • Single prolonged deceleration for up to 3 min	The absence of accelerations with otherwise normal trace is of uncertain significance
Abnormal	<100 >180 Sinusoidal pattern ≥10 min	<5 for 90 min	• Either atypical variable decelerations with over 50% of contractions or late decelerations, both for over 30 min • Single prolonged decelerations for more than 3 min	

- Prolonged bradycardia (<100 beats per minute for >5 minutes)
- Absent baseline variability
- Sinusoidal pattern
- Complicated variable decelerations with reduced baseline variability
- Late decelerations with reduced variability.

High-quality recording of uterine activity is required for meaningful interpretation. Standard terms and definitions should be used to describe FHR pattern. Interpretation of the FHR trace should take into consideration the stage of labor, maternal and fetal condition and identified risk factors. Table 3 shows the mnemonic for interpretation of continuous EFM.

MANAGEMENT OF THE ABNORMAL FETAL HEART RATE PATTERN

Immediate management Includes:
- Identify any reversible cause and initiate appropriate action (e.g., reposition mother to relieve cord compression or maternal hypotension, correct maternal hypotension, cessation of oxytocin and/or tocolysis)
- Initiation or maintenance of EFM
- Consideration of further fetal evaluation (e.g., fetal scalp blood sampling) or birth if a significant abnormality exists.[3,9]

Expedite birth when following is present:
- Significant fetal acidosis is suspected
- There is clear evidence of serious fetal compromise (fetal blood sampling should not be undertaken at this time)
- Cardiotocography abnormalities are of a degree requiring further assessment and fetal blood sampling is contraindicated.[3,9]

Standardization of Fetal Heart Rate Monitoring Protocols

Standard protocols for both intermittent and continuous FHR monitoring are important to:

TABLE 3: DR C BRAVADO mnemonic for interpretation of continuous electronic fetal monitoring[11]

DR	Determine risk	High, medium, or low-risk (i.e., risk in terms of the clinical situation)
C	Contractions	Rate, rhythm, frequency, duration, intensity, and resting tone
BRA	Baseline rate	Bradycardia (<110 bpm), normal (110–160 bpm), or tachycardia (>160 bpm); rising baseline
V	Variability	Reflects central nervous system activity: absent, minimal, moderate, or marked
A	Accelerations	Spontaneous; stimulated; none rises from the baseline of ≥15 bpm, lasting ≥15 seconds. Preterm: ≥10 bpm, lasting ≥10 seconds
D	Decelerations	Absent, early, variable, late, or prolonged
O	Overall assessment and written plan	Stoplight algorithm (Flowchart. 1) assessment includes implementing an appropriate management plan

bpm, beats per minute.

- Improve consistent transfer of information between clinicians
- Reduce the opportunity for error
- Enable a consistent approach to teaching and interpretation.

Standard Cardiotocography Protocols

Paper speed
- 1 cm per minute.

Settings
- Date and time settings should be checked as valid prior to use
- Clinicians should be aware that different manufacturers use different vertical axis scales and this can change the perception of FHR variability
- Alarm parameters should be verified prior to use.

Notating the Cardiotocography

- Cardiotocography should be labeled with the mother's name, unique record number, and date and time of commencement
- Events that may affect the FHR should be noted at the time on the CTG, in the health record with maternal pulse date, time, and signature
- Any clinician who is asked to provide an opinion on a trace should:
  - Note their interpretation of the trace (normal/abnormal) on the CTG
  - Note their interpretation of the trace and proposed actions in the health record
  - Include date, time, and signature.

Storage

- The CTG should be stored securely, either electronically or with the maternal health record
- Fetal heart rate traces related to possible adverse outcomes should be:
  - Photocopied to preserve readability over time
  - Retained for 28 years
  - Stored with consideration of avoiding intense heat, light, or moisture.

FETAL STIMULATION TESTS (TABLE 4)

Various methods of stimulation have been proposed to arouse the fetus from the sleep cycle or rest-activity cycle. If the fetus can be aroused sufficiently, such stimulations may be useful when used in conjunction with tests for fetal well-being. Such interventions should be documented on the CTG.

TABLE 4: Fetal stimulation tests

Test	Recommendation
Digital stimulation	Digital stimulation of the fetal scalp by the healthcare professional during a vaginal examination may be considered as an adjunct to continuous fetal heart rate monitoring[12-14]
Vibroacoustic stimulation	There is insufficient evidence to recommend vibroacoustic stimulation for fetal assessment in labor in the presence of a nonreassuring fetal heart rate trace[15]
Maternal glucose ingestion	There is no evidence that antenatal maternal glucose administration make tests of fetal well-being more effective[16]
Manual fetal manipulation	In view of the lack of demonstrated benefits, the time needed to perform the procedure and the concern for potential trauma to the mother and fetus; this procedure is not currently recommended[17]

How to Interpret and Act

How to act on abnormal cardiotocography interpretations is represented in flowchart 2.

INTRAPARTUM FETAL BLOOD SAMPLING (TABLE 5)

Units using EFM are strongly encouraged to have intrapartum fetal blood sampling facilities. If fetal blood sampling is not available or is inappropriate, decisions regarding delivery should take into account the severity of the FHR abnormality and the clinical circumstances. If fetal blood sampling not possible or inappropriate, then encourage the woman to adopt left lateral position (Table 6). Check blood pressure and give 500 mL crystalloid (intravenous) if appropriate.[1,18]

EXPEDITE DELIVERY

The urgency and mode of delivery should take into account the severity of the FHR and the clinical circumstances. Ideally, delivery should occur within 30 minutes.

TABLE 5: Characteristics of fetal blood sampling

Characteristic	Comment
Contraindications	• Not generally recommended for pregnancies less than 34 weeks • Clear evidence on continuous cardiotocography of serious sustained fetal compromise • Fetal bleeding disorders (e.g., suspected fetal thrombocytopenia) • Face presentation • Maternal infection (e.g., human immunodefeciency virus, hepatitis viruses, herpes simplex, and intrauterine sepsis)
Sample collection	• Woman positioned: ○ Left lateral position ○ Lithotomy with a wedge in place
Interpretation[5]	• Fetal blood sampling should be interpreted taking into account:[1] ○ Any previous measurement ○ The rate of progress in labor ○ Other clinical circumstances • Umbilical cord arterial and venous blood should be collected at the time of birth to confirm acid-base status when: ○ Fetal blood sampling has been performed intrapartum ○ Fetal compromise has been identified by fetal heart rate trace

CTG, cardiotocography; HIV, human immunodeficiency virus; FHR, fetal heart rate.

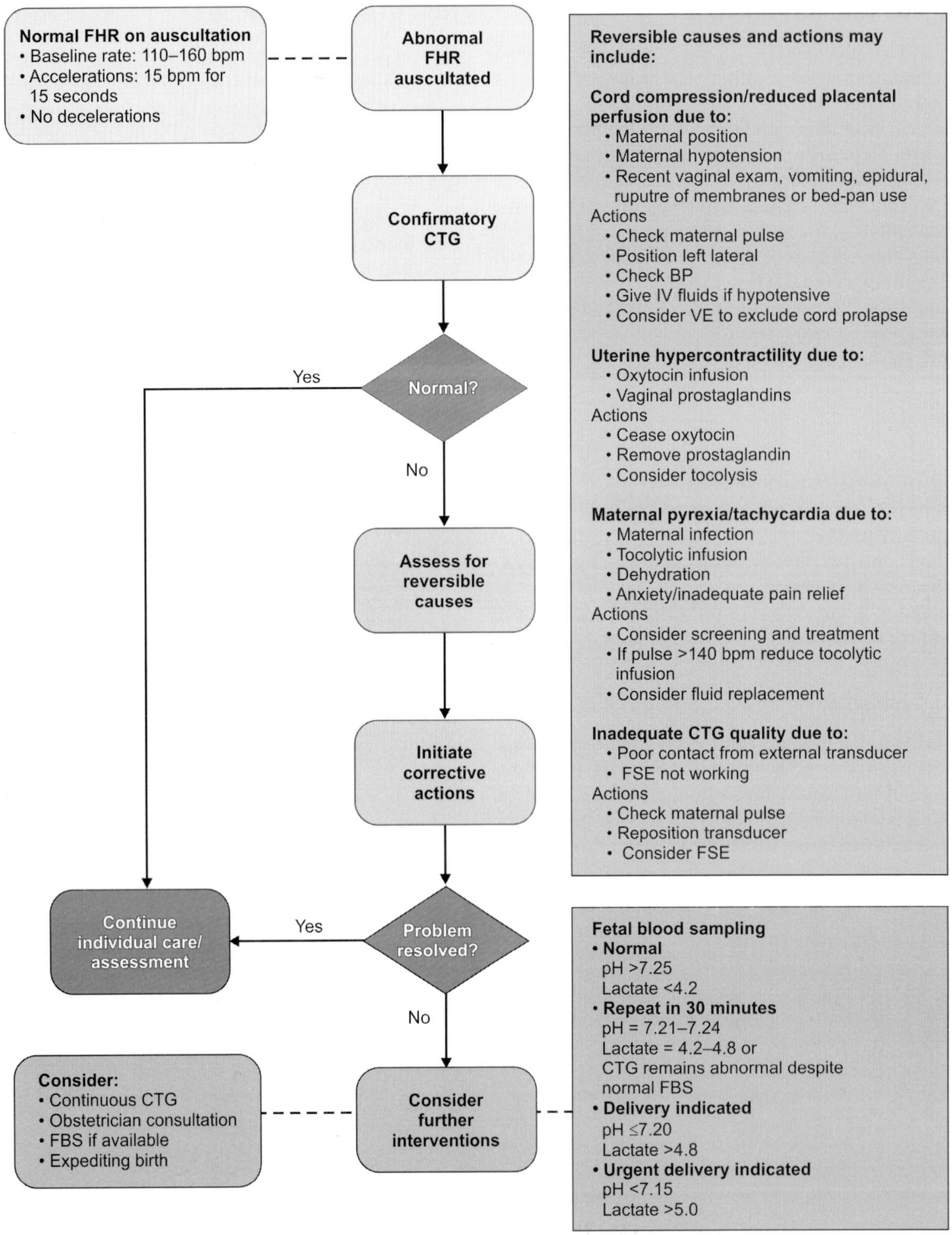

FHR, fetal heart rate; IV, intravenous; FBS, fetal blood sampling; BP, blood pressure; VE, vaginal examination; FSE, fetal scalp electrode; bpm, beat per minute.

FLOWCHART 2: How to act on abnormal cardiotocography interpretations.

TABLE 6: Interpretation of fetal blood sampling

Interpretation	pH 4	Lactate (mmol/L)
Normal	≥7.25	<4.2
Repeat in 30 min	7.21–7.24	4.2–4.8
Birth expedited	≤7.20	>4.8
Urgent birth indicated	<7.15	>5.0

Delivery should be expedited where:
- Significant fetal acidosis is suspected
- There is clear evidence of serious fetal compromise (fetal blood sampling not appropriate)
- Cardiotocography abnormalities require further assessment, but fetal blood sampling is considered clinically inappropriate or not feasible.

CONCLUSION

The primary goal of all obstetricians is to minimize the deleterious effects of labor on the mother, and at the same time, prevent adverse fetal outcomes. EFM, also known as CTG, helps in timely intervention and helps in achieving the standard care. Low-risk women can be managed with intermittent auscultation. In the modern era where litigations are on rise, CTG can also be used as defensive medicine. But, at the same time, we should understand its limitations. Despite the evidences, proving that the rates of cerebral palsy and perinatal death rate have remained the same, EFM has become the standard tool for assessing the oxygenation status of a fetus in labor and will remain the tool for monitoring in years to come.

REFERENCES

1. Grant A. Monitoring the fetus during labour. In: Chalmers I, Enkin M, Keirse MJNC, (Eds). Effective Care in Pregnancy and Childbirth. Oxford: Oxford University Press; 1989. pp 846-82.
2. Nelson KB, Dambrosia JM, Ting TY, Grether JK. Uncertain value of electronic fetal monitoring in predicting cerebral palsy. N Eng J Med. 1996;334:613-8.
3. The Royal Australian and New Zealand College of Obstetricians and Gynaecologists. Intrapartum fetal surveillance. Clinical Guidelines—2nd ed. 2009.
4. Liston R, Sawchuck D, Young D; the Society of Obstetrics and Gynaecologists of Canada, and the British Columbia Perinatal Health Program. Fetal health surveillance: antepartum and intrapartum consensus guideline. No. 197 (replaces No. 90 and No. 112). J Obstet Gynaecol Can. 2007;29(9 Suppl 4):S3-S56.
5. Tucker SM. Fetal monitoring and assessment. St. Louis: Mosby; 2000.
6. Ingemarsson I, Arulkumaran S, Ingemarsson E, Tambyraja RL, Ratnam SS. Admission test: a screening test for fetal distress in labor. Obstet Gynecol. 1986;68:800-6.
7. Phelan JP. Labor admission test. Clin Perinatol. 1994;21:879-85.
8. Kripke CC. Why are we using electronic fetal monitoring? Am Fam Physician. 1999;59(9):2416, 2421-2422.
9. The Women's. (2008). Clinical Practice Guidelines: Cardiotocograph (CTG) interpretation and response. [online] Available from: https://thewomens.r.worldssl.net/images/uploads/downloadable-records/clinical-guidelines/ctg-interpretation-and-response_040614.pdf [Accessed on December, 2015].
10. King Edward Memorial Hospital. (2010). Clinical guidelines: obstetrics and midwifery. Fetal heart rate monitoring: intrapartum. [online] Available from: http://www.kemh.health.wa.gov.au/development/manuals/O&G_guidelines/sectionb/5/b5.6.pdf [Accessed on December, 2015].
11. Hinshaw K, Ullal A. Peripartum and intrapartum assessment of the fetus. Anaesth Intensive Care Med. 2007;8(8):331-6.
12. ACOG practice bulletin No. 106: intrapartum fetal heart rate monitoring: nomenclature, interpretation, and general management principles. Obstet Gynecol. 2009;114(1):192-202.
13. National Institute for Health and Care Excellence. (2007). Intrapartum care: care of healthy women and their babies during childbirth clinical guideline. [online] Available from: https://www.nice.org.uk/guidance/cg55 [Accessed on December, 2015].
14. Liston R, Sawchuck D, Young D; Society of Obstetricians and Gynecologists of Canada SCPG. Fetal health surveillance: antepartum and intrapartum consensus guideline. J Obstet Gynaecol Can. 2007;29(9 Suppl 4):S3-56.
15. East C, Chan F, Colditz P, Begg I. Fetal pulse oximetry for fetal assessment in labour. Cochrane Database Syst Rev. 2007;2:CD004075.
16. Tan K, Sabapathy A. Fetal manipulation for facilitating tests of fetal wellbeing. Cochrane Database Syst Rev. 2001;4:CD003396.
17. Tan K, Sabapathy A. Maternal glucose administration for facilitating tests of fetal wellbeing. Cochrane Database Syst Rev. 2001;4:CD003397.
18. Impey L, Reynolds M, MacQuillan K, Gates S, Murphy J, Sheil O. Admission Cardiotocography: A randomised controlled trial. Lancet. 2003;361:465-70.

CHAPTER 18

Abnormal Uterine Action in Labor

Jyoti Bindal

INTRODUCTION

Labor and delivery is a complex physiologic process causing the expelling of the products of conception. This process is characterized by increased frequency, intensity, and duration of uterine contractions. Effective Uterine contractions are essential prerequisite and key responsible factor for the initiation and progress of labor leading to vaginal delivery. In normal labor, uterine contractions bring about demonstrable effacement and dilatation of the cervix with continuous decent of the presenting part. Uterine contractions are brought about by a number of intercellular alterations in the fetal membranes, decidua, and myometrium.[1,2] which are thought to be initiated by complex interactions between various endogenous factors or agents such as progesterone, estrogen, oxytocin, prostaglandins, relaxin, calcium ions and cyclic adenosine monophosphate.[3,4]

The basic elements or components of uterine contraction are baseline tone, active pressure, frequency, and duration. Uterine activity in spontaneous labor has a wide variation due to various factors: parity, age, race, fetal weight, maternal height and weight, fetal presentation, number of fetus, presence of scar on uterus, any associated medical disorder in pregnancy, etc. Additionally, certain extrinsic factors, such as administration of drugs; epidural anesthesia; retention of urine; rupture of membranes; and change in posture can also affect uterine contractions.[5]

The first stage of labor can be divided into the latent phase and the active phase. Latent phase is usually of several hour duration during which the cervix undergoes softening and effacement with slight dilatation.

Latent phase is characterized by uterine contractions of mild intensity with short duration. The frequency of these contractions is variable.

During active phase, the cervix dilates more rapidly and the presenting part descends. Baseline pressure or basal tone is the pressure at the lowest point of the tracing existing between contractions. Active pressure or amplitude is the difference between the pressure at the peak of a contraction and the basal pressure.

During normal labor, the uterine contractions occur every 3–4 minutes, and each contraction increases the intrauterine pressure 25–75 mmHg above a baseline of 5–20 mmHg.

The uterine blood flow is minimal during the ascending phase of a uterine contraction and stabilizes after the peak intensity is reached. The flow then returns to the pre-contraction level or above. The blood entrapped in the intervillous space acts as a reservoir and is likely to play an important role in the oxygenation of the fetus during the periods of reduced blood flow.

Abnormalities of uterine work and maternal expulsive efforts are a common cause of aberrant labor patterns. Lack of progress can be due to uterine dysfunction. Undue prolongation of labor may contribute to perinatal morbidity and mortality.

TYPES OF ABNORMAL UTERINE ACTION (TABLES 1–4)

Hypotonic Uterine Dysfunction

In this condition, there is no basal hypertonicity and the uterine contractions have a normal gradient pattern. As the rise in pressure during contractions is below average, the dilatation of cervix is prolonged.

Hypertonic Uterine Dysfunction

Here the basal tone of uterine activity is elevated. In some cases, the midsegment of the uterus has more contractions

TABLE 1: Diagnostic questions in cases of suspected dysfunctional labor

Question	Possible pathology	Treatment options
1. Is patient in true labor?	• Prelabor or false labor	• Serial observation, simple enema, sedation
2. Is the progress tardy?	• Inefficient pains, disproportion occipito-posterior position and fetal macrosomia	• Partogram shows tardy progress in active phase. • Consider oxytocin drip, amniotomy, analgesia LSCS for disproportion
3. Are the membranes ruptured?	• Chorioamnionitis, cord prolapsed	• Antibiotics, labor induction, LSCS
4. Is there an undiagnosed?	• Android/anthropoid pelvis	• Trial of labor, oxytocin stimulation, face to pubes delivery forceps/ventouse, LSCS
5. Is the fetus macrosomic generalized/locally?	• Fetal weight >3,800 g • Diabetic mother, postdatism • Hydrocephalus, sacral tumor • Distended fetal bladder	• Trial labor/vaginal assisted delivery/cesarean section
6. Is there an obstructed labor?	• Contracted pelvis, cephalopelvic disproportion, fetal malpresentation/malposition, Müllerian anomaly, pelvic neoplasm, placenta previa	• Avoid traumatic vaginal delivery/operative for cesarean section
7. Are the pains inefficient?	• Hypotonic uterine activity	• Consider use of prostaglandins/oxytocin infusion

LSCS, lower segment cesarean section

TABLE 2: Common clinical finding in women with ineffective labor

- Inadequate cervical dilation or fetal descent
  - Protracted labor—slow progress
  - Arrested labor—no progress
  - Inadequate expulsive effort—ineffective pushing
- Fetopelvic disproportion
  - Excessive fetal size
  - Inadequate pelvic capacity
  - Malpresentation or position of the fetus
- Ruptured membranes without labor

TABLE 3: Abnormal labor patterns, diagnostic criteria and methods of treatment

Labor	Diagnostic criteria		Preferred Treatment	Exceptional Treatment
	Nulliparas	Multiparas		
Prolongation disorder Prolonged latent phase	>20 h	>14 h	Bed rest	Oxytocin or cesarean delivery for urgent problems
Protraction disorders Protracted active-phase dilalation Protracted descent	<1.2 cm/h <1 cm/h	1.5 cm/h <2 cm/h	Expectant and support	Cesarean delivery for CPD
Arrest disorders Prolonged deceleration phase Secondary arrest of dilatation Arrest of descent	 >3 h >2 h >1 h	 >1 h >2 h >1 h	Evaluate for CPD: CPD: cesarean No CPD: oxytocin	Rest, if exhausted Cesarean delivery
Failure of descent	No descent in deceleration phase or second stage			

CPD, cephalopelvic disproportion.
Source: Modified from Cohen, 1983.

TABLE 4: Abnormalities of labor

Abnormality	Criteria for diagnosis
Prolonged latent phase	
Nulliparous	>20 h
Multiparous	>14 h
Protracted active phase	
Nulliparous	<1.2 cm/h
Multiparous	<1.5 cm/h
Secondary arrest of dilation	Cessation of dilatation for more hours
Prolonged deceleration phase	
Nulliparous	>3 h
Multiparous	>1 h
Failure to descent	Not descent
Protracted descent	
Nulliparous	<1 cm/h
Multiparous	<2 cm/h
Arrest of descent	Cessation of descent for 1 h or more
Precipitate labor	
Nulliparous Dilation and descent	>5 cm/h
Multiparous Dilation and descent	>10 cm/h

than the fundus. Impulses may originate in each corner, and there can be complete asynchronism of impulses.

Incoordinate Uterine Contractions

Incoordinate uterine contractions are not synonymous with inefficient uterine contractions. Incoordinate uterine contractions are defined on the basis of irregular frequency of contractions or irregularity of the shape of contractions in tocographic tracings. Minor degrees of incoordination are seen in patients in early labor.

Tetanic Contractions

They denote hypertonic uterine activity with hypersystole or polysystole. A few contractions merging together to form a sustained contraction lasting for a few minutes is called a tetanic contraction. The duration of this tetanic contraction can be anything from 2 minutes to 3 minutes. It is not seen in spontaneous normal labor and is usually brought about by the use of oxytocics during the induction or augmentation of labor.

When the contractions do not merge but the baseline pressure is elevated more than 20 mmHg for more than 3 min, it is called hypertonic uterine activity, denoting increased tone of the uterus.

The tetanic contractions will cutoff the perfusion to the retroplacental pool of blood and hypertonic uterine activity will reduce the perfusion. Such action can cause transient fetal heart rate changes unless remedial action is taken by stopping the oxytocin and/or by giving a uterine relaxant, especially if it is associated with severe fetal bradycardia or fetal tachycardia.[6]

If the contraction frequency is more than one every 2 minutes, it is called polysystole or hypersystole and is usually caused by higher than necessary levels of oxytocin. If dose of oxytocin is further increased, it usually results in hypertonic uterine activity and further excess in the drug infusion results in tetanic contraction. Such uterine hyperstimulation can occur without the dose of oxytocin being increased due to increase in sensitivity of uterus to oxytocin with the advance of labor.[7]

Polysystole is also observed in some patients with abruption placentae. The polysystolic contractions indicate the uterine irritability caused by the seeping of blood into myometrium.

Polarity

The uterus does not have a pacemaker which can be demonstrated anatomically or functionally or with the use of pharmacological agents. The uterine contractions start in the fundus, near a cornu, and propagate down to the body of uterus.

Based on polarity, abnormal uterine action can be classified into two major groups:

Normal polarity: in normal polarity, there is neuromuscular coordination between the dominant upper uterine segment and the passive lower uterine segment. When the upper segment contracts and the lower segment relaxes, it can be drawn up over the fetal pole during the first stage. While during second and third stage, it relaxes so that fetus and placenta are delivered unrestrictedly.

- Hypotonic uterine dysfunction: when the action is too weak:
  - Primary hypotonic inertia, which leads to delayed first stage of labor
  - Secondary inertia, which delayed second or third stage of labor
- Hypertonic uterine dysfunction: when the action is too strong:
  - Precipitate labor: primary or secondary
  - Obstructed labor.

Abnormal polarity: this is true incoordinate uterine action or hypertonic uterine dysfunction.

- Primary hypertonic inertia
- Lower segment dominance
- Contraction ring or localized tonic contraction
- Generalized tonic contraction
- Cervical dystocia: primary type

Normal Polarity

- Hypotonic uterine dysfunction: when the action is too weak, the strength, duration, and frequency of uterine contractions are diminished and the contractions are ineffective.
  - Primary hypotonic uterine inertia: primary hypotonic dysfunction is caused by:
    - Etiology:
      - Elderly primigravida
      - Malpresentation and malposition
      - Emotional factors such as fear, etc.
      - Uterine malformations such as unicornuate or bicornuate uterus
      - Over-distention such as hydramnios or multiple pregnancy
      - Dystocia dystrophica

    Diagnosis can be made out by weak contractions, which are short lived and occur at long intervals. Pain is weak and dilatation of cervix is not effective.
    - Management:
      - Mother and fetus are closely monitored
      - Partogram is maintained
      - Nutrition, hydration, sedatives, and analgesics are given as and when needed
      - Periodical limited vaginal examination is done, necessary antibiotics if needed are given
      - Oxytocics are given in minimal effective dilutions with careful monitoring of uterine action, blood pressure, urinary output, and fetal heart rate
      - Intervention is done if there are any signs of fetal distress or maternal distress
  - Secondary hypotonic uterine inertia:
    - Etiology
      - Usually occurs in multipara, in second or third stage of labor
      - Causes can be uterine fatigue, disproportion, or malpresentation
      - Sedatives like morphine can be a cause

    Diagnosis can be made on the basis of weakening contractions, which may disappear totally leaving labor stranded.
    - Management:
      - Patient may be given sedation in first stage
      - Oxytocin may be started to promote uterine activity
      - Active intervention may be needed if atony returns.
- Hypertonic uterine dysfunction: this may lead to:
  - Precipitate labor:
    - May be spontaneous (primary) or secondary to oxytocin stimulation (iatrogenic)
    - Here the whole process is shortened by dilatation and expulsion occurring simultaneously, due to diminished resistance in the birth canal. In primary precipitate labor, effective uterine contractions occur but are unobserved by the patient, as they are painless. Second stage is precipitated after sudden violent pains
    - Risks of precipitate labor will include lacerations of cervix and perineum, shock, hemorrhage, sepsis, intracranial injury of fetus, or even death of fetus due to sudden delivery without support, leading to fall, etc.
    - When precipitate labor is diagnosed, initially measures may be tried to inhibit uterine contractions, failing which delivery should be controlled with a liberal episiotomy
  - Obstructed labor:
    - In some cases, first stage of labor progresses, in fact, there could be even weak uterine contractions, but as soon as second stage is reached, typical picture of obstructed labor is revealed. Due to obstruction in lower pelvis, upper uterine segment acts more and more strongly both during contractions and relaxations. Slowly relaxation disappears completely, upper segment becomes short and thick, while the lower segment is distended and thinned out. Ultimately, retraction ring, Bandl's ring and rupture may follow unless active intervention is made.

Abnormal Polarity

- Incoordinate uterine action
  - Types:
    - Localized tonic contraction (Schroeder's ring)
    - Generalized tonic contraction (uterine tetany)
    - Cervical dystocia and rigidity
    - Primary, functional, or spasmodic rigidity
    - Secondary rigidity or organic rigidity.

SIGNS OF CEPHALOPELVIC DISPROPORTION

- Abdominal examination
  - Large fetal size
  - Fetal head overriding the pubic symphysis
- Pelvic examination
  - Cervix shrinking after amniotomy
  - Edema of the cervix
  - Head not well applied against the cervix
  - Head not engaged with leading point at -2 station
  - Caput formation
  - Molding (cranial bones overlapping)
  - Deflexion (anterior fontanelle easily palpable)
  - Asynclitism (sagittal suture is not in the middle of the pelvis)

- Other
  - Maternal pushing before complete dilation
  - Early decelerations
  - Negative Hillis-Müller test
  - Reverse Hillis-Müller test.

CLINICAL PELVIMETRY FINDING SUGGESTIVE OF CEPHALOPELVIC DISPROPORTION

- Narrow subpubic arch
- Bi-ischial diameter less than 8 cm
- Prominent ischial spines
- Flat sacrum
- Diagonal conjugate diameter less than 11.5 cm

Causes of Labor Abnormalities

- Power
  - Hypotonic dysfunction
  - Hypertonic dysfunction
  - Poor maternal expulsive efforts
- Passenger
  - Size
  - Presentation
  - Position
  - Attitude
  - Congenital abnormality
- Pelvis
  - Cephalopelvic disproportion
  - Absolute
  - Relative.

Oxytocin Administration for Induction or Augmentation of Labor

- Dilute 10 U of oxytocin in 1000 mL of normal saline
- Use continuous intravenous piggyback administration with Harvard pump or similar device
- If the cervix is already dilated, monitor with pressure catheter and scalp electrode
- Initiate oxytocin infusion at 0.5–1.0 mU/minute
- Increase the dose by IU every 40–60 minutes, until an adequate pattern of contractions is achieved.

Condition for Cervical Ripening, Induction, and Augmentation of Labor

- A clear indication for the procedure
- Vertex presentation
- Bishop cervical score less than 4
- Reactive nonstress test
- No evidence of cephalopelvic disproportion
- No placenta previa.

Common Indication for Cervical Ripening, Induction, and Augmentation of Labor

- Maternal medical problem
  - Hypertension
  - Diabetes
  - Renal disease
  - Sickle cell disease
- Obstetric complications
  - Premature rupture of membranes
  - Post-term pregnancy
- Fetal problems
  - Fetal demise
  - Fetal macrosomia
  - Suspected fetal jeopardy
  - Fetal growth retardation
  - Congenital abnormalities
- Patient safety
  - Cervix dilated 4 cm or more
  - History of rapid labors
- Patient convenience.

Conditions for Operative Vaginal Delivery (forceps or vacuum) in Cases of Presumed Fetal Jeopardy or Prolonged Second Stage of Labor

- Cervix completely dilated and membranes ruptured
- Fetal head engaged: the biparietal diameter has passed through the pelvic inlet
- The leading bony point (not the caput) of the fetal head is at station +2 or lower; be aware that in occiput posterior positions, the leading point of the skull may be at +2 station and the head still unengaged
- Estimated fetal weight less than 4,000 g
- Precise knowledge by ultrasound of the position of the fetal head and the fetal spine
- Adequate clinical pelvimetry
- Easy application and articulation of forceps.

CONCLUSION

Labor abnormalities are easily recognized by using Freidman's curve. However, this is only the first step in the analysis of this problem. It is very important to recognize whether the labor abnormalities are due to conditions affecting the power of expulsive forces, fetal passenger, or the maternal pelvis. Cephalopelvic disproportion is also a form or cause of dystocia. It should be distinctly recognized from lack of progress or failure to progress. Diagnosis of cephalopelvic disproportion involves documentation of adequate uterine work or intrauterine pressure; presence of clinical signs; abnormal clinical pelvimetry; and negative results of Hillis-Müller maneuver. Secondary arrest of cervical dilation is the most common abnormality of the active phase of labor. Primary causes of uterine dysfunction remain epidural analgesia, chorioamnionitis, maternal position during labor, birthing position in second stage of labor, and prematurely ruptured membranes at term. General principles of management of abnormal uterine action are based on the principles that it is well understood that prolonged labor left to the whims of nature may result in higher perinatal mortality. In certain types of dystocia, judicious use of diluted oxytocin infusion is rewarding. In appropriate cases, resorting to cesarean section is far more preferable than difficult vaginal delivery.

REFERENCES

1. Barry E, Schwarz F, Schultz M, MacDonald PC, Johnston JM. Initiation of human parturition III. Fetal membrane content of prostaglandin E2 and F2α precursor. Obstet Gynecol. 1975;46:564-8.
2. Grieves SA, Liggins GC. Phospholipase A activity in human and ovine uterine tissues. Prostaglandins. 1976;12:229-41.
3. Roy AC, Kottegoda SR, Ratnam SS. Another look at initiation of human parturition. Aust NZ J Obstet Gynecol. 1985.25:94-100.
4. Drover JW, Casper RF. Current review : Initiation of parturition in humans. Can Med Assoc J. 1983;128:387-91.
5. Gibb DMF, Arulkumaran S. Uterine contractions and the fetus. In: John Studd, (Ed). Progress in Obstetrics and Gynecology, vol 6. Edinburgh: Churchill Livingstone; 1987. pp 133-5.
6. Ingemarsson I, Arulkumaran S, Ratnam SS. Bolus injection of terbutaline in term labor. 2. Effect on uterine activity. Am J Obstet Gynecol. 1985;153:865-9.
7. Sica Blanco Y, Sala NL. Oxytocin. Proceedings of an International Symposium. London. Pergamon Press; 1961. p 127.

CHAPTER 19

Abnormal Labor

Muralidhar V Pai

INTRODUCTION

Dystocia results from abnormalities in the interplay of uterine function, fetal size, fetal position, and the maternal pelvis. Recognition of risk factors and causes are critical for proper treatment. Appropriate management of dystocia reduces maternal and fetal morbidity and prevents unnecessary cesarean deliveries.

Any deviation from normal labor is abnormal labor. That means one should know as to what constitutes normal labor. Labor is considered to be normal when at term pregnant woman presenting with vertex, goes into spontaneous onset of labor and delivers vaginally, without undue delay and with minimal aids a healthy baby. It goes without saying that there should be no maternal morbidity also.

The irregular painless contractions of earlier trimesters culminate into more frequent, coordinated, and painful contractions of true labor towards term. Cervix responds by effacement and dilation. Before active labor sets in, there is a variable period of latent phase.

DEFINITIONS

- Dystocia: difficult labor and childbirth
- Prolonged latent phase:
  - Nulliparous patient: more than 12–20 hours
  - Multiparous patient: more than 8–14 hours.

  Note that it is often difficult to determine the time of onset of the latent phase because of the increased uterine activity (false labor) that occurs 3–4 days before the onset of spontaneous labor.[1]

  Latent phase is generally complete when cervical dilation reaches 3–4 cm, with variable cervical effacement.
- Protraction disorder:[2]
  - Rate of dilation less than 1.2 cm/h in a primiparous patient
  - Rate of dilation less than 1.5 cm/h in a multiparous patient
  - Adequate contractions must be present
- Secondary arrest of labor:[2,3]
  - No change in cervical dilation over 2 hours of active-phase labor with evidence of adequate contraction
  - No descent of fetal presenting part after 1 hour of complete dilation and effacement of the cervix
- Prolonged second stage of labor:[3,4]
  - More than 2 hours in nulliparous patient without regional anesthesia
  - More than 3 hours in nulliparous patient with regional anesthesia
  - More than 1 hour in multiparous patient without regional anesthesia
  - More than 2 hours in multiparous patient with regional anesthesia
- Precipitous labor:
  - Delivery occurs in 1 hour or less after the onset of active labor.

PATHOPHYSIOLOGY

Dystocia occurs as a result of abnormal functions of and interactions between:

- Power: contractions or maternal effort

- Passenger: Position, size, and presentation of the fetus
- Passage: Maternal pelvic architecture and soft tissues.

ETIOLOGY

Associated risks factors for dystocia include:[5,6]

- Advanced maternal age
- Maternal diabetes/hypertension
- Short maternal stature
- Maternal pelvic contractures or tumors
- Infertility or nulligravity
- Premature rupture of the membranes or oligohydramnios
- Chorioamnionitis
- High station at the end of complete dilation and effacement
- Malposition of the fetus
- Previous perinatal death
- Macrosomic infants
- Regional anesthesia.

Physician and/or patient anxiety due to prior or current pregnancy complications can result in prematurely labeling the labor as "failure to progress".

EPIDEMIOLOGY

Dystocia complicates 8–11% of vertex deliveries in the first and second stages of labor. The leading indication for primary cesarean delivery (CD) in the United States is dystocia or "failure to progress".[7]

Successful management of abnormal labor to effect safe vaginal delivery will result in reduced CD rate.

EVALUATION

History and Physical

- Obtaining accurate history from the patient at antepartum visits is helpful in identifying risk factors
- A physical examination to assess pelvic anatomy helps predict pelvic-outlet abnormalities.

Leopold's maneuvers before labor can determine fetal position.

A physical examination in labor assesses:

- Progress of cervical dilation and effacement over time position
- The presenting part and rate of descent in birth canal.

Tests

Ultrasound evaluation is used frequently to assess:

- Estimated fetal weight
- Amniotic fluid index
- Biophysical profile
- Uterine anomalies or pelvic tumors
- Position of fetus and placenta.

Prolonged Latent Phase

Different studies have quoted different criteria for prolonged latent phase and in primi it is between 12 and 20 hours and in multi between 8 and 14 hours. Prolonged latent phase may be associated with an increased risk for subsequent labor abnormalities, CD, low, Apgar scores, and need for neonatal resuscitation.

Traditionally, labor events are categorized into three stages as follows:

1. First stage: Stage of dilatation when cervix dilates from 0 to 10 cm
2. Second stage: Stage of fetal delivery (after 10 cm dilatation and spontaneous rupture of membranes)
3. Third stage: Stage of placental delivery.

It is prudent to consider a fourth stage of labor, comprising the hour immediately following delivery of the placenta, during which uterus undergoes permanent contraction and retraction and lots of hemodynamic changes occur in mother.

When cervix dilates up to 4 cm, labor is considered to have entered active phase. Thereafter, it dilates at the rate of 1–1.2 cm in primi and 1.5 cm in multi. Progressive descent of the head occurs in the absence of cephalopelvic disproportion (CPD), almost at similar rate. Plotting the progress of labor in partogram is the most objective way to recognize and manage any deviation from the normalcy.

The modified World Health Organization partogram is devoid of recording latent phase of labor, which varies widely between patients. The recording starts at 4 cm of dilatation. Alert line is drawn on the basis of normal dilatation of cervix (1 cm/h after 4 cm) and an action line is drawn 4 hours to the right of alert line. Progress should be assessed at regular intervals as follows:

- General parameters like pulse, blood pressure, respiration 1–2 hours depending on the medical complications present
- Uterine contractions and descent of the head every half hour
- Fetal heart every 15 minutes, soon after the contractions subside
- Vaginal examination every 4 hours to note the cervical dilatation, status of the membranes and station of the head, presence of caput or molding.

ABNORMALITIES OF THE FIRST STAGE

The abnormalities of first stage are categorized as follows:

- Cervical dilatation disorders:
  - Protracted active phase
  - Secondary arrest of dilatation
  - Precipitate labor
- Descent disorders:
  - Protracted descent
  - Arrest of descent
- Obstructed labor.

Dilatation Disorders

In protracted active-phase dilatation, plot crosses initially alert line and later action line if no intervention is taken, whereas in secondary arrest of dilatation, initially cervix dilates normally, but thereafter stops for more than 2 hours in the active phase of labor. Both of these conditions may be due to:

- Undiagnosed CPD
- Uterine inertia
- Epidural anesthesia
- In coordinate uterine contraction:
  - With normal polarity: Bandl's ring (usually due to obstruction)
  - With abnormal polarity: Constriction ring, spastic lower segment, colicky uterus, generalized contraction, asymmetric uterine contraction and cervical dystocia.

Precipitate labor is one where all stages of labor are completed in 2 hours and usually this happens in cases of cervical insufficiency or preterm labor.

Descent Disorders

In protracted descent, head descent is tardy throughout whereas in secondary arrest, there is normal progress of descent of the fetal head initially followed by arrest. Following may be the causes of descent disorders:

- Undiagnosed CPD
- Malpresentation (face or brow)
- Malposition (occipito-posterior)
- Mechanical obstruction.

Obstructed Labor

It is defined as a labor that gets arrested due to a mechanical obstruction despite good uterine contractions.

The cause of obstructed labor may be any one or combination of the following:

Fault in Passage

- CPD
- Soft-tissue obstructions:
  - Cervical dystocia
  - Fibroid uterus
  - Ovarian tumors.

Fault in Passenger

- Neglected shoulder presentation
- Brow/mento-posterior position
- Congenital malformations
- Big baby
- Compound presentation.

Abnormal Labor Should be Anticipated in the Following

- Elderly primi
- Prolonged pregnancy
- Overdistended uterus (either due to polyhydramnios or big baby)
- Contracted pelvis
- PROM
- Induced labor
- Medical disorders of pregnancy, especially gestational diabetes mellitus and pre-eclampsia
- Injudicious use of sedation/oxytocin.

Clinical Features of Abnormal Labor

- Mother may have features of ketoacidosis (especially in obstructed labor)
- Bandl's ring/constriction ring may be present
- Uterus may be tense and tender (except in inertia)
- Fetal parts not well made out (as the uterus is overactive)
- Fetal heart rate disturbances.

Management of Abnormalities of the First Stage

Whenever there is prolonged or tardy cervical dilatation or descent is present (the graph crossing the alert line of partogram), patient is reassessed both abdominally and bimanually as follows:

- Per abdominal (PA): For contractions, descent of head, fetal heart rate
- Per vaginal (PV): To rule out CPD, assess station and position of head, application of cervix to head, membrane status:
  - If CPD is present, patient is taken up for emergency cesarean section
  - If inertia presents, artificial rupture of membranes may be performed followed by oxytocin infusion, provided there are no signs of obstructed labor and fetal distress.

Ideally the graph should not be allowed to cross the action line, if however it crosses, then immediate cesarean section should be performed.

Obstructed labor is prevented by ruling out CPD and soft-tissue obstructions before the patient enters into active phase of labor. However, when diagnosed in labor, ketoacidosis should be corrected, patient may be given pethidine to alleviate anxiety. Since it is not due to the problem of power, there is no role of augmentation of labor using oxytocin. Immediate cesarean section under general anesthesia is appropriate management. There is no role for destructive operations in modern obstetrics.

Most of the problems due to incoordinate uterine action are managed by cesarean section under general anesthesia, so also cervical dystocia.

Problem of precipitate labor is management by close monitoring of the patient in first stage and controlled delivery of the head using outlet forceps to avoid intracranial hemorrhage.

ABNORMALITIES OF THE SECOND STAGE

Abnormalities of Rotation and Descent

Descent and rotation of the fetal head occur concurrently with cervical dilation and many-a-times completed before full dilatation of the cervix. It can take up to 3 hours to descend from 0 to +3 station and an additional 30 minutes for delivery.

The normal duration of second stage is considered by many to be up to 2 hours in primi and 1 hour in multi. However, it would be prudent to diagnose the problem of failure of descent and rotation much before these limits. The abnormalities of rotation and descent in second stage suggest the following:

- Passage:
  - Rare midpelvic contraction
  - Soft-tissue obstruction (pelvic tumor)
  - Lax levator ani muscle tone
- Power:
  - Inadequate uterine contractions
  - Failure of secondary powers (due to maternal exhaustion)
- Passenger:
  - Malpresentation or position (brow, occipito-posterior, mento-posterior)
  - Congenital anomalies (anencephaly, hydrocephaly)
  - Marked degrees of asynclitism.

Effect of Abnormal Labor on Mother

- Exhaustion
- Dehydration/acidosis
- Injuries
- Postpartum hemorrhage
- Sepsis.

Effect on Fetus

- Asphyxia
- Acidosis
- Intracranial hemorrhage
- Infection
- Increased perinatal loss.

Management of Abnormalities of the Second Stage

Reassessment even as late as second stage is important and following are assessed:

- Uterine contractions to rule out inertia
- Pelvis to rule out midcavity/outlet contraction
- Cervix to note the dilatation, application to presenting part, edema
- Head to rule out caput, pathological molding, and malrotation.

Depending on finding the management may be stimulation for uterine contractions using oxytocin, hastening the delivery using outlet forceps or vacuum. If the pelvis below the arrest of head not conducive for autorotation of the head and if large caput and pathological molding is present, then CD is a better option. There is no role for forceps or manual rotation of head in modern obstetrics.

Shoulder Dystocia

When the shoulders are not delivered 1 minute after the delivery of the head, it is considered as shoulder dystocia. It occurs in 0.24–2.00% of vaginal deliveries.

Diagnosis

Clinical manifestations

- Fetal shoulder fails to deliver after delivery of fetal head in spite of routine maneuvers
- Impaction of fetal shoulder behind the pubic symphysis
- Turtle sign: Retraction of fetal head onto perineum after its delivery and before the shoulders can be delivered
- Occurs in 0.6–1.7% deliveries per year.[8]

Risk Factors[9]

- Postdates pregnancy
- Pregestational or gestational diabetes mellitus
- Macrosomic infant
- Maternal obesity
- Prolonged second stage of labor
- Failed attempt at vacuum or forceps delivery
- Prior infant with shoulder dystocia.

Majority of shoulder dystocia cases occur in fetuses weighing less than 4,000 g and without other risk factors.

Treatment

Procedures: prompt action is required to avoid maternal or fetal compromise:[10]

- Stop maternal pushing and call for anesthesia/pediatrics
- Cut generous episiotomy
- Avoid excessive traction on fetal head
- Never use fundal pressure.

Mazzanti technique

- Direct suprapubic pressure against fetal shoulder
- Dislodges shoulder from under symphysis.

McRoberts maneuver

- Hyperflexion of maternal hips against abdomen
- This results in straightening of the lumbar sacral angle and anterior rotation of pubic symphysis
- Dislodges impacted shoulder in 90% of attempts
- Often used in conjunction with Mazzanti technique.

Rubin technique

Apply pressure laterally through abdomen against anterior shoulder: attempt to move shoulder girdle into oblique position.

Woods maneuver

- Apply pressure via vagina directly to anterior surface of posterior shoulder to rotate into oblique position or
- Apply pressure via vagina directly to posterior surface of posterior shoulder to rotate it forward
- Variant of Woods maneuver applies pressure to the posterior surface of the anterior shoulder to move it into oblique position.

Delivery of posterior arm

- Physician passes hand under posterior shoulder
- Fetal forearm flexed by applying pressure to antecubital fossa
- Forearm grasped and swept across the chest and out
- Anterior shoulder delivered using suprapubic pressure and gentle downward traction on the fetal head.

Zavanelli maneuver

- Use Zavanelli maneuver if all above attempts are unsuccessful
- Fetal head rotated to occiput anterior position and flexed
- Constant, firm pressure maintained on vertex to push fetal head cephalad as far as possible
- Proceed with immediate CD.

Complications

- Fracture of fetal humerus or clavicle
- Facial nerve or brachial plexus injury to fetus
- Fetal anoxia or death from prolonged delivery or compressed cord
- Increase in maternal birth canal injuries
- Maternal femoral nerve injury from overzealous flexion of hips
- Increase in maternal blood loss.

ABNORMALITIES OF THE THIRD STAGE

Retained Placenta

When the placenta is not delivered 30 minutes after the delivery of the fetus, it is called retained placenta. Placenta may be retained either because it is not separated, in which situation one may start oxytocin and wait for the contractions to set in and encourage natural mechanism of separating the placenta or it may be due to simple adherent placenta which needs manual removal under general anesthesia. Morbidly adherent placenta (accreta or percreta variety) may need peripartum hysterectomy.

Postpartum Hemorrhage

When the amount of bleeding exceeds 500 mL or sufficient to cause maternal shock, it is considered as postpartum hemorrhage. It may be due to atony or trauma or both. Prompt resuscitation of the patient with fluids and component therapy and management of atony with oxytocics and trauma with suturing the tears and lacerations is needed to control mild cases. In severe cases, one may have to consider drastic steps, like step-wise devascularization or even hysterectomy. If the patient is stable, one may consider uterine artery embolization.

Inversion of the Uterus

It is a rare but dramatic complication. It must be recognized and corrected promptly to avoid serious long-term morbidity. Causes of uterine inversion are: atomicity, fundal implantation of the placenta, and excessive cord traction. There are three degrees of inversion:

1. Dimpling of fundus or depression of posterior wall, but they remain above os
2. Fundus or a portion pass through cervix, but remain inside vagina
3. Endometrium with or without attached placenta visible outside vulva.

Patient is in the risk of neurogenic shock due to tension on nerves because of the pull on infundibulo pelvic ligament, pressure on ovaries ,and peritoneal irritation.

Immediate reinversion may be attempted using tocolytic drugs. The uterus is reinverted with gentle but firm and persistent pressure applied on the fundus to elevate it into the vagina. Whether to remove the placenta before reinversion is controversial. In Johnson technique, reinversion is easier if the placenta is not in place.

In some cases, laparotomy is needed and after opening, the first step is to grasp the round ligaments about 1 inch into the inverted uterus and exert traction, while an assistant elevates the uterus with a hand in the vagina. This procedure is described by Huntington. If this fails, one may resort to Haultain procedure in which a longitudinal incision is made posteriorly through the inverted fundus, allowing ample room to reinvert the fundus.

CONCLUSION

Any deviation from normal labor is abnormal labor. To detect the deviation one should closely monitor the labor using partogram. Once the labor progress crosses the alert line, one should reassess the uterine contractions to diagnose any incoordination, descent of the head to rule out cephalopelvic disproportion or obstructed labor, cervical dilatation and its application to head to rule out cervical dystocia, excessive caput and pathological moulding. It is also important to look for any evidence of fetal distress by CTG and color of the liquor after performing artificial rupture of membranes. Should there be any doubt regarding the progress or evidence of fetal distress it is prudent to perform immediate caesarean delivery in the interest of mother and baby. It is better to avoid shoulder dystocia by planned caesarean delivery in suspected cases, however if one is faced with it then appropriate maneuvers should be performed to deliver the baby. One must follows principles of active management of third stage of labor to avoid postpartum hemorrhage.

REFERENCES

1. Hendricks CH, Brenner WE, Kraus G. The normal cervical dilatation pattern in late pregnancy and labor. Am J Obstet Gynecol. 1970;106(7):1065-82.
2. Friedman EA. Labor: Clinical Evaluation and Management, 2nd edition. New York, USA: Appleton-Century-Crofts; 1978.
3. Kilpatrick SJ, Laros RK. Characteristics of normal labor. Obstet Gynecol. 1989;74(1):85-7.
4. Zhand J, Yancey MK, Klebanoff, MA, Schwarz J, Schweitzer D. Does epidural analgesia prolong labor and increase risk of cesarean delivery? A natural experiment. Am J Obstet Gynecol. 2001;185(1):128-34.
5. Sheiner E, Levy A, Feinstein U, Hershkovitz R, Hallak M, Mazor M. Obstetric risk factors for failure to progress in the first versus the second stage of labor. J Matern Fetal Neonatal Med. 2002;11(6):409-13.
6. Howell CJ. Epidural versus non-epidural analgesia for pain relief in labour. Cochrane Database Syst Rev. 2003;(2):CD000331.
7. Detailed diagnoses and procedures, National Hospital Discharge Survey, 1987. Vital Health Stat. 1989;(100):1-304.
8. American College of Obstetricians and Gynecologists: ACOG practice bulletin no. 40: shoulder dystocia. Obstet Gynecol. 2002;100(5):1045-50.
9. Baskett TF, Allen AC. Perinatal implications of shoulder dystocia. Obstet Gynecol. 1995;86(1):14-7.
10. Naef RW, Morrison JC. Guidelines for the management of shoulder dystocia. J Perinatol. 1994;14(6):435-41.

CHAPTER 20

Operative Vaginal Delivery

Parag Biniwale, Manish Machave, Reeti Mehra

INTRODUCTION

Operative vaginal delivery (OVD) refers to a delivery in which the operator uses forceps or a vacuum device to assist the mother in transitioning the fetus to extrauterine life. The instrument is designed to be applied to the fetal head, and then the operator uses traction to extract the fetus, typically during a contraction while the mother is pushing.

The first instrumental deliveries were performed to extract fetuses from parturients who were at high risk of maternal mortality due to prolonged and/or obstructed labor. In these cases, saving the mother's life took precedence over possible harm to the fetus. The focus of these procedures has changed as a result of modern obstetrical practices that have drastically reduced the risk of intrapartum maternal mortality and major morbidity. Decisions regarding use of instrumental delivery are now also based upon the fetal/neonatal impact of these procedures and can reduce the need of cesarean birth.

INCIDENCE

In the USA, 3.5% of all deliveries are accomplished via an operative vaginal approach. The overall rate of OVD has been diminishing, but the proportion of OVDs conducted by vacuum-assisted births has been increasing and is more than 4 times the rate of forceps-assisted births. In the US, rate of forceps delivery decreased from 17.7% in 1980 to 4.5% in 2006 whereas vacuum delivery increased to 8.4%. This may be explicable by increase in fear of medicolegal cases and by lack of training.[1]

In recent years, the success rate for OVDs has been quite high (99%). This likely reflects appropriate choice of candidates for this intervention.

The reduced use of OVD, increased use of cesarean delivery at many teaching institutions has reduced the resident competency in OVD. The important questions facing our specialty today are whether we want to passively witness OVD become "a lost art" while the cesarean delivery rate continues to climb, or whether we should actively attempt to reverse the current trend, and, if so, how.

INDICATIONS FOR OPERATIVE VAGINAL DELIVERY

The Royal College of Obstetricians and Gynecologists (RCOG) practice bulletin 2011[2] outlined the following indications for OVD (forceps or vacuum), recognizing that no indication is absolute; cesarean delivery is also an option in these clinical settings.

Maternal Indications

- Inadequate expulsive efforts
- Maternal exhaustion (distress)
- Where expulsive efforts (Valsalva) are to be avoided: To shorten and reduce the effects of the second stage of labor on medical conditions (e.g., cardiac disease Class III/IV, hypertensive crises, myasthenia gravis, spinal cord injury patients at risk of autonomic dysreflexia, proliferative retinopathy).

Fetal Indications

- Nonreassuring fetal condition as evidenced by fetal bradycardia or tachycardia in second stage
- After coming head of the breech
- Abruptio placentae or cord prolapse in second stage.

Other Indications

Prolonged second stage of labor (nullipara >2 hour; multipara >1 hour, add 1 hour more, if patient is in epidural analgesia).

OPERATIVE VAGINAL DELIVERY

Operative vaginal delivery refers to any delivery process which is assisted by vaginal operations. Delivery by forceps, ventouse and destructive operations generally included (Table 1).

TABLE 1: Classification of operative vaginal deliveries[3,4]

Type of procedure	Criteria
Outlet	• Scalp is visible at the introitus without separating the labia • Fetal skull has reached the level of the pelvic floor • Sagittal suture is in the direct anteroposterior diameter or in the right or left occiput anterior or posterior position • Fetal head is at or on the perineum • Rotation is ≤45°
Low	• Leading point of the fetal skull (station) is station +2/+5 or more, but has not as yet reached the pelvic floor: • Rotation is ≤45° • Rotation is >45°
Midpelvic	• The head is engaged in the pelvis but the presenting part is above +2 station
High	• (Not included in this classification)

Pre-requisites for Operative Vaginal Delivery (Table 2)

Fetal and Maternal Criteria

- Fetal criteria:
    - Fetal head engaged (head is <1/5 palpable per abdomen)
    - The cervix must be fully dilated
    - The membranes must be ruptured
    - Fetal head position and station is exactly known
    - Pelvis deemed adequate
- Maternal criteria:
    - Bladder must be emptied
    - Adequate maternal analgesia (regional block for midcavity or pudendal block)
    - Informed consent (verbal or written) with prior clear explanation
- Other criteria:
    - Experienced operator
    - Aseptic techniques
    - Back-up plan in case of failure
    - Presence of a neonatologist
    - Willingness to abandon the procedure when difficulties faced.

Forceps

The forceps can be used to assist in extraction of the head in vertex presentation, face in mentoanterior position and the after coming head in breech presentation. Forceps was invented early in the 17th century by Peter I or Peter II of the Chamberlains family. In present day practice, the commonly used forceps used are:

- Long-curved forceps
- Short-curved or outlet forceps, also called Wrigley's forceps
- Kielland's forceps.

TABLE 2: Pre-requisites for operative vaginal delivery (forceps or vacuum application)[4,5]

Maternal criteria	Fetal criteria	Uteroplacental criteria	Other criteria
Adequate analgesia	Vertex presentation	Cervix fully dilated	An experienced operator who is fully acquainted with the use of the instrument
Patient in the lithotomy position	The fetal head must be engaged in the pelvis	Membranes ruptured	Ability to monitor fetal well-being continuously
Bladder empty	The position of the fetal head must be known with certainty. The attitude of the fetal head and the presence of caput succedaneum and/or molding should be noted	No placenta previa	The capability to perform an emergency cesarean delivery, if required
Clinical pelvimetry must be adequate in dimension	The station of the fetal head must be ≥ 0/+5		
Consent obtained	The estimated fetal weight must be documented (ideally 2,500–4,500 g)		

Long- and Short-curved Forceps

The long-curved forceps measures 37 cm in length, distance between the tips is 2.5 cm and widest distance is 9.5 cm. The blades are fenestrated to provide a good grip on the fetal head and avoid slippage during extraction of the fetal head. The parts of the forceps are: blades, shank, handle and lock, and are called right or left in relation to the maternal pelvis in which they lie. The long-curved forceps may have a slot for the axis traction device. The blades have an upper pelvic curve and an inner fetal curve which grasps the fetal head. The lock is commonly the English lock which can be applied, only when the left blade is applied first.

The outlet forceps is also similar in every respect except for a shorter length of the shanks and is meant to be applied when the fetal head is on the perineum.

The Kielland's forceps can be applied in relation to the position of the fetal head, i.e., in a cephalic manner. It can correct asynclitism. It is a diminishing art and is technically difficult to apply and can cause considerable maternal trauma, which is primarily why it has lost its popularity and in modern day, most obstetricians are not familiar with its use.

Obstetrical forceps applied to the fetal head perform the following functions:
- Traction
- Rotation
- Flexion
- Extension.

When one or more of these functions is attempted, there is simultaneous fetal head compression. Head compression is the undesirable factor associated with the use of forceps. Proper technique including accurate application and correct traction, can minimize compressive forces.

Technique

Safe and effective use of forceps depends on good technique. Assemble the forceps before application. Ensure that the parts fit together and lock well. Lubricate the blades of the forceps. Wearing sterile gloves, insert two fingers of the right hand into the vagina on the side of the fetal head. Slide the left blade gently between the head and fingers to rest on the side of the head (Figs 1A and B).

Repeat the same maneuver on the other side, using the left hand and the right blade of the forceps (Fig. 2).

Depress the handles and lock the forceps. Difficulty in locking usually indicates that the application is incorrect. In this case, remove the blades and recheck the position of the head. Reapply only if rotation is confirmed.

After locking, apply steady traction inferiorly and posteriorly till the vertex reaches the pelvic floor, then directly posteriorly till the subocciput hinges under the symphysis pubis and then upwards and forwards to deliver the vertex and the face. Traction is given only with each contraction. After delivery of the head remove the right blade first followed by the left one.[6]

Complications of Forceps Operation

The complications of the forceps' operation are mostly related to the faulty technique and to the indication for which the forceps are applied rather than the instrument. The hazards are grouped into:
- Maternal complications
- Fetal complications.

Maternal Complications

- Immediate:
  - Injury: vaginal laceration or sulcus tear, cervical tear, extension of episiotomy to involve the vaginal vault, complete perineal tear

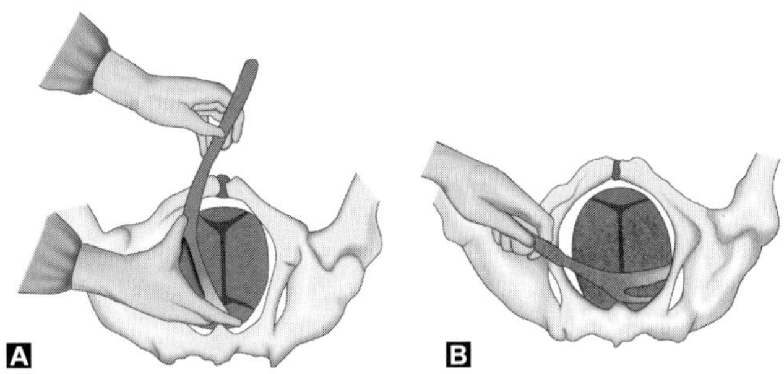

FIGS 1A AND B: Applying the left blade of the forceps.

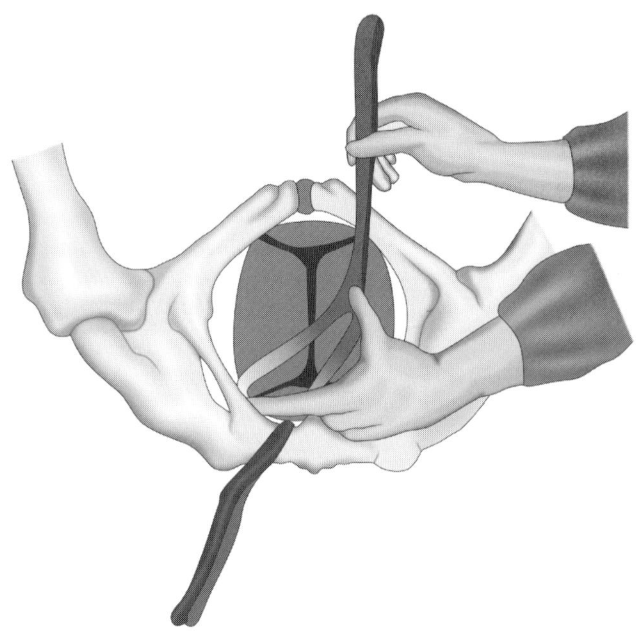

FIG. 2: Applying the right blade of the forceps.

    - Nerve injury: femoral nerve, lumbosacral trunk (L2,3,4 or L4,5) with midforceps delivery
    - Postpartum hemorrhage may be:
        - Traumatic
        - Atonic, requiring blood transfusion
        - Both, may cause shock
    - Anesthetic complications (following local or general anesthesia)
    - Puerperal sepsis and maternal morbidity
- Remote:
    - Painful perineal scars
    - Dyspareunia
    - Low back-ache
    - Genital prolapse
    - Stress urinary incontinence
    - Anal sphincter dysfunction.

Fetal Complications

- Immediate:
    - Asphyxia
    - Facial bruising
    - Intracranial hemorrhage (rupture of the great vein of Galen)
    - Cephalohematoma
    - Facial palsy
    - Skull fractures
    - Cervical spine injury (rotational forceps).
- Remote:
    - Cerebral or spastic palsy due to residual cerebral injury (rare).

Prophylactic Forceps (Elective)

This type of forceps operation was named after De Lee. It refers to forceps delivery only to shorten the second stage of labor when maternal and/or fetal complications are anticipated. The indications are:

- Eclampsia
- Heart disease
- Previous history of cesarean section
- Postmaturity
- Low-birth-weight baby
- To curtail the painful second stage.

It prevents possible fetal cerebral injury due to pressure on the perineum and spares the other from the strain of bearing down efforts. Prophylactic forceps should not be applied until the criteria of low forceps are fulfilled.

Trial Forceps

It is a tentative attempt of forceps delivery in a case of suspected midpelvic contraction with a preamble declaration of abandoning it in favor of cesarean section, if moderate traction fails to overcome the resistance. The procedure should be conducted in an operation theater keeping everything ready for cesarean section. The conduct of the fetal head, the delivery, is completed vaginally, if not cesarean section is done immediately. Many unnecessary cesarean sections or difficult vaginal deliveries can thus be avoided.

Failed Forceps

When a deliberate attempt in vaginal delivery with forceps has failed to expedite the process, it is called failed forceps. It is often due to poor clinical judgment and skill. Failure in the operative delivery may be due to improper application.

Causes: the common causes are:

- In completely dilated cervix
- Unrotated occipitoposterior position
- Cephalopelvic disproportion (CPD)
- Unrecognized malpresentation (brow) or hydrocephalus
- Constriction ring
- Clinically big baby (>4 kg)
- Maternal body mass index (BMI) >30.

Prevention: it is a preventable condition. Only through skill and judgment, proper selection of the case ideal for forceps can be identified. Even if applied in wrong cases, one should resist the temptation to give forcible traction in an attempt to hide the mistake.

Management:

- To assess the effect on the mother and the fetus
- To start a Ringer's solution drip and to arrange for blood transfusion, if required
- To administer parenteral antibiotic
- To exclude rupture of the uterus
- The procedure is abandoned and delivery is done by cesarean section
- Laparotomy should be done in a case with rupture of uterus.

Ventouse

Ventouse is an instrumental device designed to assist delivery by creating a vacuum between it and the fetal scalp. The pulling force is dragging the cranium; while in forceps, the pulling force is directly transmitted to the base of the skull.

Technique

A useful mnemonic, which was initially developed for forceps deliveries, has been adapted for vacuum extraction.[1] This mnemonic is the first 10 letters of the English alphabet. A copy is included at the end of this chapter (in Appendix 1) for use in the operative vaginal birth workshop and may be copied for use on the labor and delivery ward.

APPENDIX 1: Prerequisites for applying ventouse

A	Anesthesia assistance	• Adequate pain relief • Neonatal support
B	Bladder	• Bladder empty
C	Cervix	• Fully dilated, membranes ruptured
D	Determine	• Position, station and pelvic adequacy • Think possible shoulder dystocia
E	Equipment	• Inspect vacuum cup, pump and tubing • Check pressure
F	Fontanel	• Position the cup over the posterior fontanel • Sweep finger around cup to clear maternal tissue
G	Gentle traction	• 0.2 kg/cm^2 initially and between contractions and increase pressure to 0.8 kg/cm^2 • Pull with contractions only, as contraction begins, prompt the woman for good expulsive effort • Traction in axis of birth canal and perpendicular to the cup
H	Halt	• No progress with 3 traction-aided contractions • Vacuum pops off 3 times • No significant progress after 20 minutes of operative vaginal delivery (OVD)
I	Incision	• Consider episiotomy, if laceration imminent
J	Jaw	• Remove vacuum when jaw is reachable or delivery assured

The vacuum should be applied with rigorous adherence to the mnemonic provided. It is important that the indication is clear and well understood by the parents. Consent of the woman must be obtained and properly documented.

- Provide emotional support and encouragement
- Analgesia is not essential but may be desirable, if available
- The bladder should be empty. If the woman is not able to void, consider catheterization
- Final confirmation of full dilatation and fetal position should be made
- The proper function of the vacuum equipment should be determined before the cup is applied
- The cup is applied by compressing it in an anteroposterior diameter and then introducing it into the posterior fourchette, while protecting the maternal tissues and making space with the opposite hand at the flexion point which is 3 cm from the posterior fontanel (Fig. 3).
- If using a 6 cm cup, to be over the flexion point, the leading edge should be 3 cm from the anterior fontanel (Figs 4 and 5).

Contraindications

- Contraindications of ventouse:
    - Any presentation other than vertex (face brow, breech)

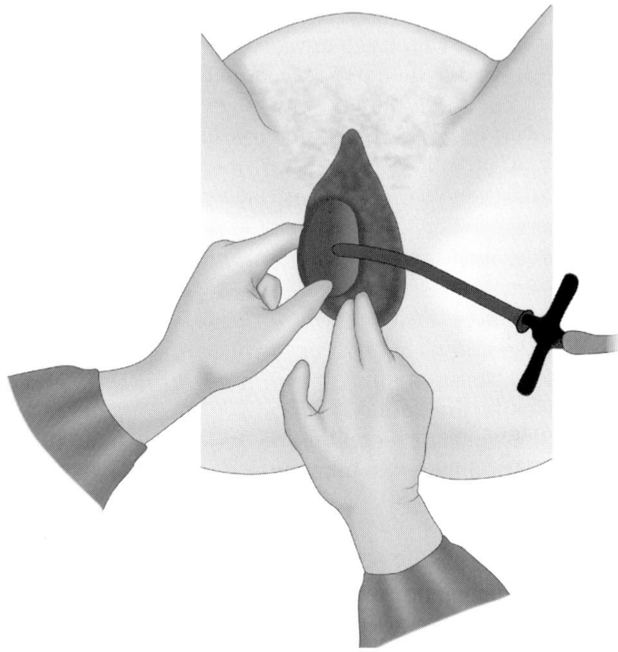

FIG. 3: Applying a vacuum cup.

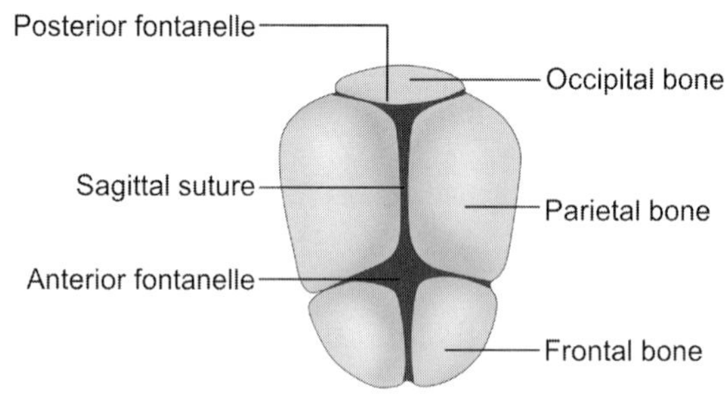

FIG. 4: Identifying the flexion point.

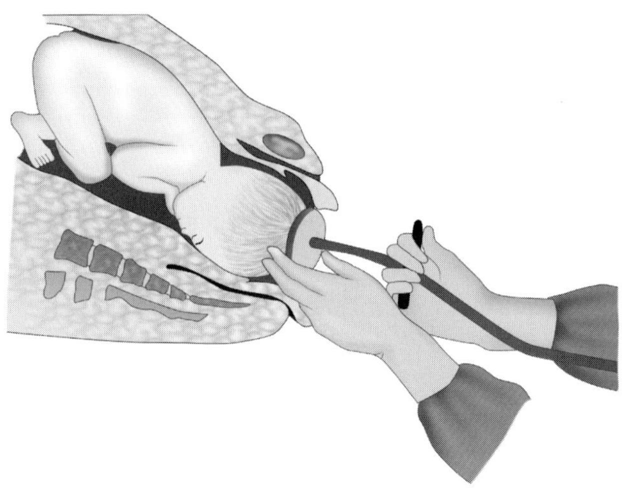

FIG. 5: The application and traction of ventouse.

 - Preterm fetus (<34 weeks). Chance of scalp avulsion or subaponeurotic hemorrhage
 - Suspected fetal coagulation disorder
 - Suspected fetal macrosomia (>4 kg)
- Contraindications for OVD (both for ventouse or forceps):
 - Unengaged fetal head
 - Obvious
 - Fetus having bleeding diathesis (hemophilia).

Vacuum Failure

Before undertaking any attempt at OVD, consider the risk of failure for vaginal delivery and the potential for other complications, such as shoulder dystocia and postpartum hemorrhage. Ensure adequate assistance is present, if such complications should occur. Consider the fetal status before making your attempt to deliver the baby and the time necessary to initiate a cesarean section, if the procedure fails. Under circumstances in which fetal well-being is suspect and/or the potential for success of an OVD is in doubt, proceed directly to cesarean section, if available. If times permits, consider transfer to the next level of care. Whenever operative delivery is considered, a healthcare provider skilled in newborn resuscitation should be present at the birth. This person's sole responsibility must be the care of the newborn.

The vacuum procedure has failed when descent or delivery has not been accomplished. The procedure should be abandoned at this point, and an alternate method of delivery should be selected.

- When to halt—beware:
 - 3 pulls over 3 contractions, no progress abandon procedure
 - 3 pop-offs: after 1, reassess carefully before reapplying
 - After 20 minutes of application with no progress reassess.

The above recommendations should be considered the maximal limits. The incidence of scalp trauma is increased when the cup application is greater than 10 minutes compared to less than 10 minutes. It is imperative that some descent is observed with each pull. If these limits are approached, progress does not occur or there is evidence of scalp trauma, the procedure should be abandoned.

Vacuum versus Forceps Delivery

The relative benefits and risks for vacuum versus forceps delivery has been the subject of much study and debate. The proper comparison is not of vacuum with spontaneous delivery, but of vacuum with other OVD methods or cesarean section.

The potential risk of maternal soft-tissue trauma can be best prevented by avoiding traumatic insertion of the device, by frequent checking for maternal soft-tissue entrapment, by controlling for vacuum slippage or pop-off, by controlling the rate of descent and by controlling delivery over the perineum. Episiotomy is not obligatory with forceps or vacuum, but is more common with forceps. A Cochrane Systematic Review of nine randomized controlled studies involving 1,368 primiparous and multiparous women showed that soft vacuum extractor cups compared with rigid cups were associated with a significant increase in the rate of failure [odds ratios (OR) = 1.6; 95% confidence interval (CI) = 1.2–2.3], but a significant reduction in puerperal scalp trauma (OR = 0.4; 95% CI = 0.3–0.6).[7]

Fetal scalp trauma (hemorrhage and laceration) can best be prevented by avoiding excessive, incorrect or prolonged traction and by avoiding rotational forces. Vacuum traction should be applied intermittently, and coordinated to the maternal expulsive effort. The correct angle of traction through the axis of parturition must be followed. The vacuum should not be used to apply rotational forces.

Assessment of pelvic adequacy is mandatory. Abnormalities of the position or attitude of the vertex can result in relative CPD. The station of the presenting vertex should be assessed both abdominally and pelvically. The presence of a large caput may confuse the assessment of descent, and may indicate the possibility of relative CPD.

One serious potential complication of vacuum extractions is subgaleal or subaponeurotic hemorrhage. The suture lines of the skull do not limit hemorrhage into the subaponeurotic (subgaleal) space, as they do in cephalohematoma. As a result, subgaleal hemorrhages can extend from the brow ridge to the nuchal ridge and from ear to ear, covering the entire calvarium, with a potential volume of several hundred milliliters. This volume loss can produce profound, irreversible and fatal hypovolemic shock to the newborn; it can be fatal. Statistically, subgaleal hemorrhage occurs in approximately 1 in 1,000 normal spontaneous vaginal deliveries and in 46 in 1,000 vacuum extractions. Failure to recognize high pelvic station and/or CPD, and exceeding the recommended limits for the attempted vacuum extraction, are the two common healthcare provider errors associated with subgaleal hemorrhage.

The relative merits of vacuum extraction and forceps have been evaluated in a Cochrane Systematic Review of 10 randomized controlled trials, involving 2,923 primiparous and multiparous women.[8] Vacuum extraction compared with forceps is:

- More likely to fail delivery with:
 - The selected instrument (OR = 1.7; 95% CI = 1.3–2.2)
- More likely to be associated with:
 - Cephalohematoma (OR = 2.4; 95% CI = 1.7–3.4)
 - Retinal hemorrhage (OR = 2.0; 95% CI = 1.3–3.0)
 - Maternal worries about baby (OR = 2.2; 95% CI = 1.2–3.9)
- Less likely to be associated with:
 - Significant maternal perineal and vaginal trauma (OR = 0.4; 95% CI = 0. 3–0.5)

- No more likely to be associated with:
  - Delivery by cesarean section (OR = 0.6; 95% CI = 0.3–1.0)
  - Low 5-minute Apgar scores (OR = 1.7; 95% CI = 1.0–2.8)
  - The need for phototherapy (OR = 1.1; 95% CI = 0.7–1.8).

DOCUMENTATION

The indication, definition and method of operative technique employed must be clearly and completely documented in all operative deliveries.[9,10] The position and station of the fetal head at the commencement of the intervention must be stated. A written note should be prepared for both the woman's and the baby's charts. The need for the intervention must be:

- Convincing
- Compelling
- Documented.

Suggested format for a chart note that may also serve as a template to dictate a delivery summary:

- Date and time of birth
- Name of physician or other primary healthcare provider
- Indication for operative delivery
- Record of informed discussion with the woman of the risks, benefits and options
- Position and station of the fetal head and method of assessment (i.e., vaginally and/or abdominally)
- Amount of molding and caput present
- Assessment of maternal pelvis
- Assessment of fetal heart rate and contractions
- Type of analgesia or anesthesia used, if any
- Use of episiotomy, description and timing, and details of repair
- Ease of application of vacuum or forceps
- Number of attempts and duration of traction for forceps and duration of application for vacuum (start and stop time noted), and force used
- Apgar score
- Results of cord blood analysis, if done
- Neonatal resuscitation activities, if needed
- Description of maternal and neonatal injuries, if any.

CARE AFTER OPERATIVE VAGINAL BIRTH

- Active third stage management
- Prepare for newborn resuscitation
- Umbilical arterial blood gas analysis, where laboratory facilities exist
- Examination for maternal trauma
- Examination for neonatal trauma:
  - Scalp trauma
  - Signs of cerebral irritation (poor sucking, listless)
  - Signs of scalp swelling, cephalohematoma or subaponeurotic bleeds
  - The newborn should be examined carefully at the time of the initial newborn examination. Careful monitoring should be continued in the immediate neonatal period and, at minimum, a second full examination of the newborn should be completed prior to discharge. Any abnormal findings will require further investigation
- Documentation of the indication, definition and method of operative technique
- Review birth with the family.

SUMMARY OF RECOMMENDATIONS BY ROYAL COLLEGE OF OBSTETRICIANS AND GYNAECOLOGISTS 2011

All women should be encouraged to have continuous support during labor as this can reduce the need for OVD. Use of upright or lateral positions and avoiding epidural analgesia can reduce the need for OVD. Delayed pushing in primiparous women with an epidural can reduce the need for rotational and midcavity deliveries. These recommendations have *Level A Evidence*. A recent Cochrane Review concluded that using a partogram[11] does not lead to a reduction in the incidence of operative births and use of oxytocin in second stage also does not reduce OVD.[12] A meta-analysis demonstrated that primiparous women who received epidurals were likely to have fewer rotational or midcavity operative interventions when pushing was delayed for 1–2 hours or until they had a strong urge to push.[13]

Women should be informed in the antenatal period about OVD, especially during their first pregnancy. For deliveries in the delivery room, verbal consent should be obtained before an OVD and the discussion documented in the notes. If circumstances allow, written consent may also be obtained. Written consent should be obtained for trial of OVD in theater.[2]

An OVD should be performed by an operator who has the knowledge, experience and skills necessary to assess and to use the instruments and manage complications that may arise. The operator should choose the instrument most appropriate to the clinical circumstances and their level of skill. Forceps and vacuum extraction are associated with different benefits and risks.

Failed delivery with selected instrument is more likely with vacuum extraction. The options available for rotational delivery include Kielland's forceps, manual rotation followed by direct traction forceps or rotational vacuum extraction. Rotational deliveries should be performed by experienced operators, with the choice depending on the expertise of the individual operator.

Operative vaginal births that have a higher risk of failure should be considered a trial and conducted in a place where immediate recourse to cesarean section can be undertaken. Higher rates of failure are associated with:

- Maternal BMI over 30
- Estimated fetal weight over 4,000 g or clinically big baby
- Occipitoposterior position
- Midcavity delivery or when one-fifths of the head palpable per abdomen.

The use of sequential instruments is associated with an increased risk of trauma to the infant; however, the operator must balance the risks of a cesarean section following failed vacuum extraction with the risks of forceps delivery following failed vacuum extraction. Obstetricians should be aware of increased neonatal morbidity with failed OVD and/or sequential use of instruments and should inform the neonatologist when this occurs to ensure appropriate management of the baby.

There are insufficient data to justify the use of prophylactic antibiotics in OVD. Good standards of hygiene and aseptic techniques are recommended.

Women should be reassessed after an OVD for risk factors for venous thromboembolism and, if appropriate, thromboprophylaxis should be prescribed.

There is a need for evidence-based guidelines, including standardized documentation of operative vaginal procedures. Training strategies for junior practitioners to acquire these skills and for experienced practitioners to maintain and disseminate their skills should be prioritized.

REFERENCES

1. Yeomans ER. Operative vaginal delivery. Obstet Gynecol. 2010;115(3):645-53.
2. Royal College of Obstetricians and Gynaecologists (RCOG). (2011). Operative vaginal delivery (Green-top Guidelines No. 26). [online] Available from www.rcog.org.uk/en/guidelines-research-services/guidelines/gtg26/. [Accessed December, 2015].
3. American College of Obstetricians and Gynecologists. (2000). ACOG Practice Bulletin No. 17: Operative vaginal delivery. [online] Available from www.goforitcourse.com/uploads/1/7/2/5/17251206/pb017.pdf. [Accessed December, 2015].
4. The Royal Australian and New Zealand College of Obstetricians and Gynaecologists (RANZCOG). (2015). College Statement C-Obs 16: Instrumental vaginal delivery. [online] Available from www. ranzcog.edu.au/publications/statements/C-obs16.pdf. [Accessed December, 2015].
5. The Royal Australian and New Zealand College of Obstetricians and Gynaecologists (RANZCOG). (2015). College Statement C-Obs 13: Guidelines for use of rotational forceps. [online] Available from www. ranzcog.edu.au/doc/rotational-forceps.html. [Accessed December, 2015].
6. World Health Organization (WHO). Managing Complications in Pregnancy and Childbirth: A Guide for Midwives and Doctors. Geneva, Switzerland: World Health Organization; 2003.
7. Johanson RB, Menon V. Soft versus rigid vacuum extractor cups for assisted vaginal delivery. Cochrane Database Syst Rev. 2000;(2):CD000446.
8. Johanson RB, Menon BK. Vacuum extraction versus forceps for assisted vaginal delivery. Cochrane Database Syst Rev. 2000;(2):CD000224.
9. Bachman J, Johanson R, Menon V. A vacuum operation needs to be documented in the same manner as any other operative procedure. Forceps delivery correspondence. J Am Acad Fam Pract. 1989;29:4.
10. Touqmatchi D, Boret T, Nicopoullous J. The quality of operative consenting against RCOG advice as standard. J Obstet Gynaecol. 2010;30(2):159-65.
11. Lavender T, Hart A, Smyth RM. Effect of partogram use on outcomes for women in spontaneous labour at term. Cochrane Database Syst Rev. 2008;(4):CD005461.
12. Costley PL, East CE. Oxytocin augmentation of labour in women with epidural analgesia for reducing operative deliveries. Cochrane Database Syst Rev. 2013;7:CD009241.
13. Roberts CL, Torvaldsen S, Cameron CA, Olive E. Delayed versus early pushing in women with epidural analgesia: a systematic review and meta-analysis. BJOG. 2004;111(12):1333-40.

CHAPTER 21

Cesarean Delivery: Recent Advances

Parul J Kotdawala, Girindra Chingtham, Priyangi Purohit

INTRODUCTION

Cesarean section (CS) is the most widely performed major procedure worldwide. Its advent and application has saved the lives of both mothers and infants over the years. Interestingly the rising incidence of cesarean deliveries over the last three decades has caused great concern and consternation among the health providers.

Cesarean section is the delivery of an infant, alive or dead, through an abdominal uterine incision after the period of viability. When it is done prior to the age of viability of the fetus, it is called hysterotomy.

HISTORY

Various tales have been passed on through generations regarding the origin of CS. In *Greek* mythology, it was believed that the God of Medicine, *Aesculapius* was born through his mother's abdomen by his father, *Apollo* (Fig. 1).[1] Similar myths are reported or passed down in folklores originating from China, India, Egypt, Rome and several other places.

The word "cesarean" has been interpreted in various ways. Probably originated from the Latin word "cedere" meaning to "cut open", it is also thought to have derived from Julius Caesar. Some myths abound that the great Julius Caesar was delivered by this procedure. This however, seems unlikely as his mother Aurelia, is reported to have delivered many more children vaginally after Julius Caesar's birth and lived for many years after his birth. It is also presumed to be derived from an ancient Roman custom that pregnant women would not be interred with her baby inside. The baby had to be removed even if it was dead and both bodies were then buried separately. This custom was enacted as a Roman law known as "Lex Regia" by King Pompilus, and was later known as "Lex Caesarea" under the ruling of Julius Caesar.

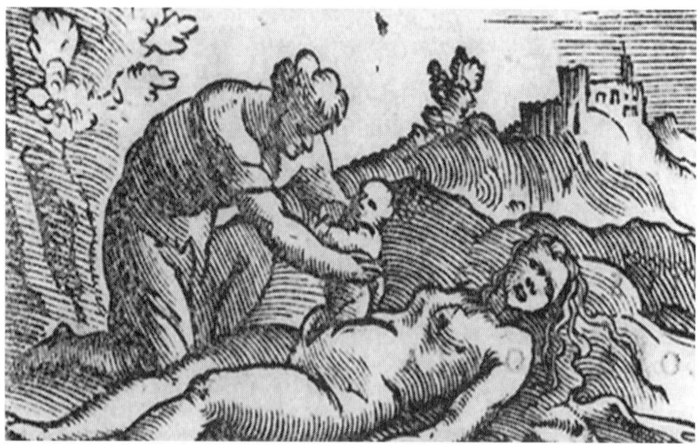

FIG. 1: The extraction of *Asclepius* from the abdomen of his mother *Coronis* by his father *Apollo*. Woodcut from the 1549 edition of Alessandro Beneditti's De Re Medica.[1]

Jacob Nufer, a sow-gelder from Switzerland is supposed to have performed abdominal delivery in the year 1500, on his wife who was unable to deliver her baby after remaining in labor for several days despite assistance from as many as 13 midwives! This is the first reported instance of both the mother and baby surviving an operative abdominal delivery. The authenticity of this is questioned by a few historians as this incident was recorded many years after it happened.

The ancient cesarean techniques were not well documented and as years passed by, each of them became questionable. Mention may be made of a cesarean technique employed by *Banyoro* tribal surgeons in Uganda which *Felkin RW*, a British traveler observed in 1879 (Fig. 2).[2] The

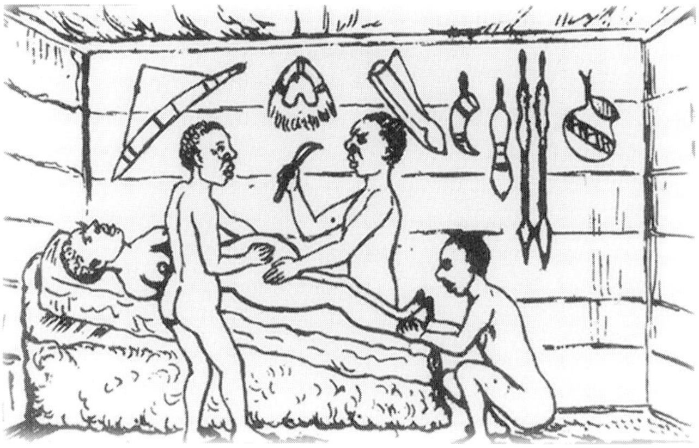

FIG. 2: Banyoro tribe performing childbirth in Uganda, as observed by Felkin RW in 1879.[2]

tribal surgeons first used banana wine to semi-intoxicate the pregnant woman and then washed their hands and cleaned her abdomen with the same banana wine before starting the surgery. A midline vertical incision was given starting from just above the symphysis pubis to just below the umbilicus opening the whole abdomen and uterus at a go. Amniotic fluid was allowed to escape and any bleeding points stopped with the application of red hot irons. Uterine incision was then completed with the help of an assistant by retracting the abdominal wall with his hands and hooking his two fingers into the uterus. Baby was delivered, and after cutting the cord, was handed over to the assistant. The surgeon removed the placenta and dilated the cervix (probably to allow the lochia to drain). He then squeezed the uterus till it contracted but did not suture it. Abdominal wall was closed with iron needles 7, the wound dressing was performed with some root paste and a bandage of cloth wrapped tightly around the wound. After 6 days, the needles were removed. Felkin observed the patient for 11 days and till he left for his country; both the mother and child were alive. Most of the features that we saw in the transformation of modern cesarean technique were visible in this *Banyoro* tribe's method ranging from anesthesia, asepsis, lower midline abdominal incision, hemostasis, manual massage of uterus to closure of the abdominal wall, and wound care.

Earlier in 1876, *Eduardo Porro* of Pavia, Italy performed CS followed by subtotal hysterectomy in order to control uterine hemorrhage and prevent systemic infection at the cost of a woman's future fertility. But, soon the need for removing the uterus to control hemorrhage was avoided with the advent of uterine sutures. In 1882, *Max Sanger*, a German Gynecologist advocated that suturing of the uterus was essential both for reducing hemorrhage as well as infection which had great impact on maternal mortality and morbidity. He used silver wire stitches that produced minimal tissue reaction for suturing uterus. For this contribution, he has been referred to as the *Father of Modern CS*.

Ferdinand Kehrer (1837-1914) of Heidelberg is one of the under-acknowledged contributors to the development of the modern CS. In 1881, he performed a transverse lower segment CS, but it did not become popular. It was not till *Munro Kerr* in 1926 who brought about the transformation of lower segment transverse uterine incision in contrast to classical vertical incision.[3-5]

INCIDENCE

Since 1950 the CS rates are on the rise in spite of effort to keep them at the lowest possible level, and the CS has now become the most common major surgery performed worldwide. World Health Organization (WHO), in its consensus meeting where more than 80 countries were represented, has concluded that a rate of more than 15% is of no benefit to the woman or her child, and has recommended that the CS rates be kept between 5% and 15% to reduce maternal and neonatal morbidity and mortality. Less than 5% CS rate generally denotes poor infrastructure and lack of adequate emergency services in the area. The average number of cesarean deliveries has been put at 16% worldwide. In developing countries, the average is at 6%, while in developed nations, it is at 30%. In India, CS rates have increased from 2.9% in 1992–93 to 7.1% in 1998–99 and further rise to 10.2% in 2005–06.[6] The trend in China also shows an increasing graph from about 8.9% in 1994–94 to around 24.8% in 2001–02.[7] In United States (US) about 1.3 million women undergo CS annually with an average of 32%.[8]

INDICATIONS

The reasons for performing CS were quite different a century ago compared to current practice. The earliest CSs were performed solely for saving the unborn child when the mother was dying or had already died. When performed on a living woman, the maternal mortality was almost guaranteed. Hence there was general reluctance to perform a CS both among the doctors and among the patient community. This led to development of various destructive procedures, like craniotomy for the delivery of a dead child or where there was gross fetopelvic disproportion. In the early 20th century, the development of safer technique along with advent of 3 A's: anesthesia, antiseptics, and antibiotics changed the perception a bout CS. From performing only when vaginal delivery was not possible, gradually the CS started being employed for a variety of indications. The procedure has become so safe now that there are some noises being made that the CS should be the mode of delivery in all pregnancies, citing pelvic floor damage as a sequel of vaginal delivery.

The most common indications for CS can be broadly considered in three headings: (1) passage (maternal-pelvis anatomy), (2) passenger (fetus), and (3) pressure (maternal-uterine activity). We can also consider them as mandatory (absolute) and relative (elective) indications.

Maternal Indications

Absolute

- Contracted pelvis
- Cephalopelvic disproportion (CPD)
- Major degree placenta previa, type III and IV and also type IIB posterior
- Vasa previa
- Abruptio placentae in patients not in labor with alive fetus
- Previous classical CS
- Previous hysterectomy
- Previous history of intracavitatory myomectomy
- Obstruction in the birth canal, like cervical or lower uterine segment fibroid, carcinoma of the cervix, large ovarian cyst incarcerated in the pelvis and in rare cases, impacted rudimentary horn of the uterus in the pelvis.

Relative

- Cervical dystocia
- Previous CS
- Hypertensive disorders of pregnancy
- Medical disorders, like cardiovascular disease, diabetes, etc.
- Human immunodeficiency virus (HIV), hepatitis B, C positive mothers
- Maternal request
- Gross kyphosis and other neuromuscular disorders affecting lower extremities.

Fetal Indications

Absolute

- Umbilical cord prolapse
- Fetal malpresentation with no gross malformations incompatible with life
- Severe oligohydramnios
- Chorioamnionitis
- Demonstrable fetal hypoxia or impending fetal demise.

Relative

- Breech presentation
- Twins
- Fetus conceived through assisted reproductive technology (ART)
- Early Doppler changes in fetal vessels in ultrasound.[9,10]

When we analyze the changes in indications for performing a CS over the years, we notice a distinct pattern emerging. In the latter half of 20th century, the routine list of indications for a CS used to read, in order of frequency; CPD, fetal distress, cervical dystocia, placenta previa, preeclampsia/eclampsia, and then other indications. Obstructed labor and nonreassuring fetal heart rate pattern used to be the most common reasons for performing cesarean in the past. In recent years, maternal request and babies conceived through ART or mothers who conceive at a very late age are adding to the tally of indications for cesarean. In a small survey conducted in our hospital (Smt. SCL Hospital, Smt. Nathiba Hargovandas Lakhmichand Municipal Medical College, Ahmedabad, Gujarat, India), we found the frequency of indications as; almost all data published in last two decades show these four indications (as shown in Table 1) adding up to 75–80%.

TABLE 1: The common indications for cesarean section

Indications	Frequency (%)
Previous cesarean section	28.0
Fetal distress	25.3
Breech	10.7
Cephalopelvic disproportion	10.7
Obstructed labor	05.3
Placenta previa	05.3
Nonprogress of labor	02.7
Pregnancy-induced hypertension	02.7
Others	09.3

As you can see in Table 1, the four most common indications, namely "previous CS", "fetal distress", "breech" and CPD constitute 75% of all indications. Previous CS has grown as number one indication and many published data shows its frequency at 30–40% of all CS! Hence if the overall incidence needs to be curtailed, a focus on these four indications will have the desired impact. The rest of the list (as shown in Table 1) has such small numbers that any focus there may not impact overall incidence. So we need to avoid a primary CS and also bring in a policy of vaginal birth after cesarean (VBAC), close fetal monitoring, promote vaginal breech delivery, and bring in a routine use of partogram to impact these four indications in a bid to reduce the spiraling CS rates.

ANESTHESIA

Earlier, CSs were generally performed under general anesthesia (GA). With higher safety profile of regional analgesia and associated low maternal and neonatal morbidity and mortality, there is a distinct preference for regional blocks (spinal/epidural) for anesthesia during CS.[11] Choice of anesthesia at the time of CS depend on various factors including emergency conditions, maternal preference, and medical diseases associated with pregnancy.

General Anesthesia

Towards the end of the 20th century and onwards, there has been a significant drop in the use of GA during cesarean deliveries. Some of the indications for GA are: failed regional anesthesia, where regional anesthesia is contraindicated, life-threatening fetal conditions and maternal request.[12] The US data shows GA being employed in less than 5% of elective cesarean deliveries as compared to 15–30% emergency situations.[11] There may be airway problems arising out of the anatomical and physiological changes that occur during pregnancy leading to difficult intubation at times.[13] Aspiration is also one of the complications that can occur in obstetric patients under GA. Risk factors include prolonged gastric emptying time in labor, increased intra-abdominal pressure due to the gravid uterus and relaxation of the lower esophageal sphincter due to high progesterone level in pregnancy. To decrease this, prophylaxis against acid aspiration before anesthesia and rapid sequence induction with thiopental and sugammadex (shorter-acting relaxant) is being increasingly used.[14-17]

Regional Anesthesia

Some of the regional techniques commonly used for CS are single-shot spinal anesthesia, epidural anesthesia, and combined spinal-epidural (CSE) anesthesia. Use of continuous spinal anesthesia for cesarean delivery have been reported but with limited success. There are various advantages of regional anesthesia, like avoiding a difficult intubation, use of lesser drugs compared to GA as well as allowing the mother to be awake to witness the delivery of her baby. It is now the preferred choice of anesthesia for cesarean deliveries.[18]

TYPES OF CESAREAN SECTION (FIGURE 3)

Cesarean section has been divided into three categories:
1. Low-transverse CS
2. Low-vertical CS
3. Classical CS.

The most common cesarean technique performed worldwide with universal acceptance is the Munro-Kerr technique of lower-segment CS. But the new technique, Misgav-Ladach (Stark) technique has shown many advantages over conventional Munro-Kerr's and is accepted as the most evidence-based technique in current practice (Table 2).

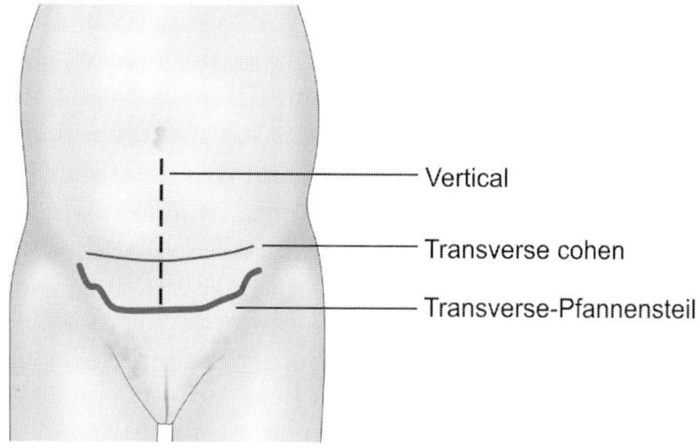

FIG. 3: Type of skin incisions for cesarean section.

MISGAV-LADACH/STARK TECHNIQUE

This technique was developed by Dr. Michael Stark and his team at the Misgav Ladach Hospital in Jerusalem. This technique makes a cesarean delivery faster, with reduced blood loss, less postoperative analgesic requirements and quicker postoperative recovery. The main aim of introducing this technique was to minimize trauma to the tissues by reducing unnecessary dissection.[9,10] The important steps of the procedure are:

- Joel-Cohen skin incision and abdominal opening technique:
  - A straight transverse skin incision about 3–4 cm above the symphysis pubis
  - Subcutaneous tissue is cut only in the middle 1 inch
  - Small cut in rectus sheath by knife
  - Extension of the cut laterally by the push of a semi-opened scissors

TABLE 2: Comparison of three common incisions of cesarean section

	Low-transverse incision	Low-vertical incision	Classical incision
Advantage	• Unlikely to rupture during a subsequent birth • Makes vaginal birth after cesarean (VBAC) possible for subsequent pregnancy • Less blood loss • Easier to repair	• Can be extended upward to make a larger incision if needed	• May be the only choice in these situations: ○ Implantation of a placenta previa on the lower anterior of uterine wall ○ Presence of dense adhesion from previous surgery ○ Transverse lie of a large fetus with the shoulder impacted in the mother's pelvis
Disadvantage	• Limited ability to extend laterally to enlarge the incision	• Slightly more likely to rupture during a subsequent birth • A tear may extend the incision downward into the cervix	• Most likely of the uterine incision to rupture during a subsequent birth • Eliminates VBAC as an option for birth of a subsequent infant

- Opening the peritoneum by stretching it with fingers
- Pulling apart the peritoneum, rectus muscles and the subcutaneous tissues as one
- Small transverse incision in the lower uterine segment to accommodate two fingers and then the incision is stretched manually with the surgeon and assistant in the opposite direction
- Uterus is exteriorized after the delivery of fetus and placenta
- Single-layer nonlocking uterine closure with synthetic absorbable suture
- Parietal and visceral peritoneum layers are not sutured
- Abdominal wall is closed in two layers (rectus sheath and skin).

COMPLICATIONS OF CESAREAN SECTION

It can be classified into short-term, long-term and those that present risks to future pregnancies. Also, complications to the newborn can arise from the procedure. The risk of complication depends to a great extent on the clinical conditions presented at the time of CS, i.e., the risk may not be same for a planned CS in an average weight woman and those done in emergency in morbidly obese patients with additional factors, like placenta previa.

Short-term Complications

- Hemorrhage: blood loss during CS may result from the laceration of uterine vessels which occurs due to the extension of uterine incision. In general, the blood loss at CS is 5–10 times that of a vaginal delivery. Sometimes, lacerations may extend into the vagina leading to significant bleeding. These may require blood transfusion at times and such risk is more in unplanned CSs with patients in labor and those with increasing number of previous cesarean deliveries[19,20]
- Infection: with the introduction of prophylactic antibiotics, this complication has been significantly brought down with regards to postpartum endometritis and wound infection[21]
- Thromboembolism: one of the causes of maternal mortality arising from CS is deep vein thrombosis resulting in pulmonary embolism and the risk is more than in vaginal delivery[22]
- Iatrogenic injury during surgery: the most common organ injured is the bladder. Others that may be affected includes ureter and bowel[23]
- Pain: it is observed more in CS than in vaginal deliveries. But with the application of newer technique, it has reduced significantly.[24]

Long-term Complications

- Adhesion formation: it is a major long-term consequence of any laparotomy. Although the incidence is comparatively less in pregnant patient due to higher amount of circulating steroid hormones compared to nonpregnant, adhesions are observed in patients who have undergone CS. It may contribute to the risk of ectopic pregnancy and chronic abdominal pain in women with prior cesarean deliveries[25]
- Pain: women have undergone cesarean deliveries are likely to complain of pain in the first 2 months after the surgery with around 25% reporting of incisional pain[26]
- Subfertility: it was found hard to conceive again for more than a year in patients who had undergone prior CS.[27]

Newborn Complications

- Respiratory difficulties: transient tachypnea of the newborn (TTN) is more common after elective cesarean delivery than after vaginal delivery[28]
- Asthma: children born out of planned or unplanned cesarean deliveries are more likely to be admitted in the hospital during their childhood for asthma.[29]
- Trauma: surgical cuts can occur to the fetus during emergency CS
- Failure to breastfeed: babies born by CS whether elective or unplanned have been observed to less likely to breastfeed than those born vaginally.[30]

RISKS TO FUTURE PREGNANCIES

- Uterine rupture: even though the risk is dependent on the route of delivery in future pregnancy, those undergoing elective CS is at increased risk of uterine perforation.[31]
- Abnormal placentation: women with prior cesarean deliveries are at risk of developing abnormal and morbidly adherent placenta in later pregnancies. Also, they are more likely to have placental abruption.[32-34]
- Hysterectomy: the risk of hysterectomy increases as the number of prior CS rises.[20]

RECENT ADVANCES

In view of the increasing trend in CS rates, certain areas need to be addressed while performing the procedure to minimize maternal morbidity and mortality. Recently, US Preventive Services Task Force (USPSTF) and National Institute for Health and Care Excellence (NICE) have evaluated evidence-based recommendations for each step of cesarean delivery. Some of the steps, which ought to be considered while performing the procedure are mentioned below.

Preoperative Prophylactic Antibiotics

There have been several randomized controlled trials (RCTs) regarding prophylactic use of antibiotics in CS to reduce postpartum endometritis. Various combinations have been tried, such as ampicillin/sulbactam,[35] triple antibiotics (ampicillin, gentamicin, and metronidazole),[36] penicillin and cephalothin.[37] But, studies do not demonstrate improved outcomes compared with single agent first-generation cephalosporins. Current consensus is the use of a single dose of ampicillin or first-generation cephalosporins, such as cefazolin as a preoperative prophylaxis in all women undergoing cesarean delivery.[38] Few concerns were raised about possible transfer of antibiotics into the neonate with the 1-hour prior injection, and there have been suggestions that injection may be given once the cord has been clamped. However, the general practice is to administer the injection 1-hour prior to skin incision.[39]

Thromboprophylaxis

Studies have indicated that there is an increased risk of thromboembolic events (pulmonary embolism and deep vein thrombosis) in women who underwent CS than those who had vaginal deliveries.[22] Various method of prophylaxis, such as graduated stockings, hydration, early mobilization, and low-molecular-weight heparin have been evaluated and should be considered in cesarean delivery taking into account risk of thromboembolic diseases.[40]

Preoperative Vaginal Preparation

Evidences have shown that vaginal cleaning with antiseptic solutions like povidone iodine solution in addition to the standard abdominal painting in women undergoing CS, especially with ruptured membranes have a lower incidence of postoperative endometritis. However, there are no reports of decrease in postoperative fever or wound infection.[41-43]

Indwelling Bladder Catheterization

Recently, there have been studies comparing "indwelling catheter", "intraoperative catheter only" and "no catheter" during cesarean deliveries. It has been observed that the group with indwelling catheter voided spontaneously on removal whereas the later needed recatheterization in some cases. This is explained by the fact that the anesthetic block, especially regional anesthesia, interferes with the normal bladder function.[44-46] However, there is a decrease in the incidence of urinary tract infection in nonindwelling group with no difference in urinary retention in either group.[47]

Intraoperative Techniques

Skin Incision Type

Studies comparing Misgav-Ladach technique with Pfannenstiel have shown improved operating times and possible cost savings in the former with minimal difference in maternal morbidity.[48-51] Also in Joel-Cohen method, certain advantages in terms of less blood loss, less fever, and lower duration of postoperative pain were observed.[52,53] For the above reasons, Joel-Cohen technique is mostly preferred.

Bladder Flap

Recently, studies have indicated that routine creation of bladder flap and closure of visceral peritoneum during CS do not appear to provide any immediate advantage, rather there has been concerns regarding the risk of adhesion formation and bladder injury during subsequent surgery due to pulling up of the bladder.[54,55] So, now-a-days most surgeons avoid bladder flap creation.

Expansion of Uterine Incision

When lower uterine segment is well formed, blunt up and down (cephalad-caudad) expansion is usually preferred to sharp expansion of uterine incisions as there are reports that suggest decreased maternal morbidity as measured by estimated blood loss and decrease in hemoglobin.[56,57] However, further larger trials are needed to support the above finding.

Delivery of the Head

In cephalic presentation, the fingers are passed below the head and the head is lifted up. Simultaneously the assistant presses the fundus for a downward pressure, resulting in forward and downward passage of the baby through the scar. The floating head may pose problems in delivery of the fetus. The first thing is to establish contractions—by giving intravenous (IV) oxytocin as well as by allowing the liquor drainage leading to reduced intrauterine bulk inducing a contraction. Elective forceps or a vacuum application may be used for controlled delivery. Specially designed forceps and vacuum cups are now available for CS. A deeply engaged head may also create difficulty in delivery. Few maneuvers may help:

- Filling up the bladder may disimpact the head
- Single shot of injection nitroglycerine 0.5 mL IV will relax the uterus to allow passage of fingers below the head
- Patwardhan maneuver: Delivery by pulling on to the foot first, followed by the buttocks, the torso and the head at the end, if the chest is in front. If back is in the front,

doubling the baby to deliver both the shoulders, followed by the chest, abdomen, buttocks and the feet and lastly the head.

Prevention of Postpartum Hemorrhage

Oxytocin infusion (10–40 IU in 1 L crystalloid over 4–8 hours) is currently being used for prevention of atonic bleeding. Oxytocin bolus has been tried but with limited effectiveness.[58] Misoprostol, also has not shown to be superior to oxytocin for atonic uterus in addition to side effects, like maternal shivering, diarrhea and pyrexia.[59] Tranexamic acid, 10 mg/kg IV given prior to incision in cesarean deliveries has been found to decrease intraoperative and postpartum blood loss (100–200 mL).[60]

Placental Drainage

It is the act of allowing fetal blood to egress both passively and actively by milking the umbilical cord before the cord is clamped and cut. Many recent studies have suggested certain benefits, like decrease in neonatal anemia, better systemic and pulmonary perfusion and better breastfeeding outcomes. In fact, the WHO has also started propagating delayed cord clamping in even preterm neonates. This contrast with previous observations that this may possibly harm the fetus due to polycythemia, hyperviscosity, hyperbilirubinemia, TTN, and maternal fetal transfusion in Rh-negative women.[61]

Uterine Exteriorization

Uterine exteriorization has been propagated for isolation of the uterine scar and reduced blood loss due to angulation of uterine vessels. Concerns are raised for a possible vasovagal effect due to stretching of ovarian pedicle.[62]

- Cervical dilation: till date, many perform cervical dilation after placental removal if the cervical internal os is closed in elective CS, for the concerns of postoperative hematometra and subsequent infection. However, recent studies have discouraged cervical dilation after placental removal either manually or via the use of surgical instruments[63]
- Closure of the uterine incision: traditionally, uterus is closed in two layers either with locking or unlocking continuous sutures. However, recent studies have pointed that there does not appear to be any benefit of a two-layer uterine closure in women with undesired future pregnancy.[64] There are mixed data regarding the incidence of scar dehiscence in subsequent pregnancy. Many surgeons continue to close uterine scar in double layers with this worry. However, Cochrane reviews have not been conclusive about this. But studies have shown that locking the stitch during continuous uterine closure is deleterious for good healing and may lead to dehiscence during future pregnancy and should be abandoned[65-67]
- Intra-abdominal irrigation: intra-abdominal irrigation with normal saline before abdominal closure has been evaluated in a study.[68] The rate of intraoperative nausea was significantly increased in the intra-abdominal irrigation group with no difference in estimated blood loss, operating time, intrapartum complications, hospital stay, return of gastrointestinal function, or infectious complications. Similar study with use of antibiotics showed no significant difference[69-71]
- Peritoneal closure: conventionally both, the visceral as well as parietal peritoneum openings were closed by sutures to restore anatomy and to reduce infection by forming an anatomical barrier. A few small studies suggest that parietal peritoneal closure may decrease the risk of future adhesion formation.[72,73] But large-scale studies have confirmed that nonclosure of the peritoneum leads to less postoperative fever, less operating time and reduced hospital stay. So, many guidelines favor nonclosure of both the peritoneum during CS[74-76]
- Subcutaneous closure versus drain: the general consensus is that subcutaneous closure should not be preformed routinely in CS as studies have shown no difference in wound infection or separation regardless of closure or nonclosure of subcutaneous layer. However, subcutaneous tissue should be closed if the thickness is of 2 cm or greater. Also, the subcutaneous drain placement, regardless of tissue thickness, does not appear to offer any additional benefit in reducing wound infection or hematoma[77-79]
- Skin closure: a recent analysis has observed that the wound complications and cosmetic outcomes are similar among subcutaneous sutures and Stapler groups. The concern in other studies using stapler is regarding cosmetic effect and more postoperative pain. As of today the best option is subcuticular absorbable sutures for skin closure.[80-82]

Some Special Situations in Cesarean Delivery

Prevention of Vertical Transmission of HIV Infection

An important advance in this regard was the demonstration that treatment of the mother with zidovudine (ZDV) during pregnancy and labor and of the neonate for the first 6 weeks after birth could reduce the transmission rate from 25% to 8%.[83]

Following points which need to be considered are:

- Patients should be counseled that in the absence of antiretroviral therapy, the risk of vertical transmission is approximately 25%. With ZDV therapy, the risk is reduced to 5–8%. A similar risk of 2% or less is seen among women with viral loads of less than 1,000 copies/mL, even without the systematic use of elective cesarean delivery
- Women infected with HIV, whose viral loads are greater than 1,000 copies/mL, should be counseled regarding the

potential benefit of elective cesarean delivery to further reduce the risk of vertical transmission of HIV beyond that achievable with antiretroviral therapy alone[84]
- There is no data to suggest reduction in the transmission rate if cesarean delivery is performed after the onset of labor or rupture of membranes[85]
- Patients receiving antiretroviral chemotherapy during pregnancy should not interrupted around the time of cesarean delivery
- The American Congress of Obstetricians and Gynecologists generally recommends that elective cesarean deliveries are not performed before 39 completed weeks of gestation. In women with HIV infection, however, delivery at 38 completed weeks of gestation is recommended to reduce the likelihood of onset of labor or rupture of membranes before delivery
- Amniocentesis to determine fetal lung maturity in pregnant women infected with HIV should be avoided whenever possible
- Current recommendations for adults indicate that plasma viral load should be determined at baseline and then every 3 months or following changes in therapy[86]
- Recently, NICE has come up with the latest recommendation for the prevention of vertical transmission of HIV infection in cesarean deliveries. It has suggested that CS should not be offered to HIV-infected pregnant women who are on highly active antiretroviral therapy (HAART) with a viral load of less than 400 copies/mL or on any antiretroviral therapy with a load of less than 50 copies/mL. It should be offered to those who are not on antiretroviral therapy or whose viral load is 400 copies/mL or more, even if they are on antiretroviral therapy to prevent vertical transmission.

Hepatitis B Infection

Mother-to-child transmission of hepatitis B can be reduced if the baby receives immunoglobulin and vaccination. In these situations, pregnant women with hepatitis B should not be offered a planned CS because there is insufficient evidence that this reduces mother-to-child transmission of hepatitis B virus (NICE 2004).

Hepatitis C Infection

Women who are infected with hepatitis C should not be offered a planned CS because this does not reduce mother-to-child transmission of the virus (NICE 2004). However, pregnant women who are coinfected with hepatitis C virus and HIV should be offered planned CS because it reduces mother-to-child transmission of both hepatitis C virus and HIV (NICE 2004).

Morbidly Obese Patient

Obesity (body mass index ≥30 kg/m^2) is a significant independent risk factor for many gestational complications, including cesarean delivery. Studies have indicated that a decreased cervical dilation rate, an increased induction rate, the presence of comorbid conditions, concern about shoulder dystocia, and weight gain in excess of recommendations during pregnancy, all may contribute to the high rate of cesarean delivery in obese women. Recent studies have failed to show increased risks from a prolonged course of labor with vaginal delivery in obese women including neonatal respiratory morbidity. Considering the increased anesthetic risks, wound complications, venous thromboembolism (VTE), etc. and failure of VBAC associated with cesarean delivery, a longer trial of labor in obese women without comorbid conditions is desirable.[87]

Preterm Birth

Preterm birth is the most common cause of neonatal mortality (47% of neonatal deaths are due to immaturity).[88] However, the effect of elective cesarean delivery in improving these neonatal outcomes remains uncertain and therefore CS should not routinely be offered outside a research context (NICE 2004). More RCTs are needed to evaluate the impact of CS on the benefits and risks to mothers and babies born preterm (NICE 2011).

Morbidly Adherent Placenta

Placenta previa is common in women with associated factors, like prior cesarean delivery, pregnancy termination, intrauterine surgery, smoking, multifetal gestation, increasing parity and maternal age. The risk of morbidly adherent placenta is increased with each increasing number of CSs with around 35–67% in women diagnosed with placenta previa, who had undergone three or more CS. Due to this, CS is the preferred mode of delivery. Therefore, accurate diagnosis is very essential.

Once the diagnosis is confirmed, certain things need to be kept in mind when performing a CS:
- Consultant obstetrician and a consultant anesthetist are present
- Experienced pediatrician is present
- Senior hematologist is available for advice
- Critical care bed is available
- Sufficient cross-matched blood and blood products are readily available (NICE 2011).

In a stable patient, cesarean delivery can be performed at 36–37 weeks of gestation after demonstration of fetal lung maturity by amniocentesis or else at 38 weeks. If future pregnancy is not desired, the therapeutic approach is usually cesarean delivery followed by hysterectomy. There is almost universal consensus that attempt should not be made to detach the placenta from the uterine wall. Also, the edges of the uterine incision should be oversewn for hemostasis before performing hysterectomy. Most surgeons are of the opinion that a vertical incision in the uterus allows delivery of the infant while avoiding the placenta. If future fertility is for consideration, then certain procedures such as embolization of the internal iliac vessels, treatment with methotrexate, resection of the affected segment of the uterus, uterine compression sutures and oversewing of the placental bed in addition to the no-touch technique of the placenta can be employed. However, further studies are required to identify the real candidates for conservative approach besides identifying risk factors associated with this management.[89]

CONCLUSION

With the introduction of CS as a means of delivering babies and its transformation over the years has contributed significantly in reducing both the maternal and neonatal morbidity and mortality. But, the worry is the alarming rate at which it is being performed by the overzealous obstetricians. Some fear that the art of vaginal delivery is fading day-by-day, others are concerned about its impact on the economic burden all over the world. As a procedure which is lifesaving to the mother and baby, the state-of-the-art should continue to progress as long as it is used judiciously. All said and done, the "cesarean delivery" has not only survived from an operation to be performed only on a dead woman, but has thrived to be entrenched as a very frequent mode of delivery and is slated to triumph over all other forms of deliveries and become an option for all deliveries in future.

REFERENCES

1. US National Library of Medicine. (NIH). (1998). Cesarean Section - a Brief History. [online]. Available from www.nlm.nih.gov/exhibition/cesarean/part1.html. [Accessed June, 2015].
2. Felkin RW. Notes on labour in Central Africa. Edinburgh Med J. 1884;20:922-30.
3. Boley JP. The history of caesarean section. 1935. CMAJ. 1991;145(4):319-22.
4. Gabert HA, Bey M. History and development of cesarean operation. Obstet Gynecol Clin North Am. 1988;15(4):591-605.
5. Lurie S, Glezerman M. The history of cesarean technique. Am J Obstet Gynecol. 2003;189(6):1803-6.
6. Ghosh S, James KS. Levels and trends in caesarean births: cause for concern? Econ Pol Week. 2010;45(5):18-22.
7. Sufang G, Padmadas SS, Fengmin Z, Brown JJ, Stones RW. Delivery settings and caesarean section rates in China. Bull World Health Organ. 2007;85(10):755-62.
8. World Health Organization (WHO). Global Health Observatory (GHO): World Health Statistics 2013. [online] Available from www.who.int/gho/publications/world_health_statistics/2013/en/. [Accessed June, 2015].
9. Baskett TF, Calder AA, Arulkumaran S. Caesarean section. In: Munro Kerr's Operative Obstetrics, 12th edition. Philadelphia, PA, USA: Elsevier; 2008. pp. 151-6.
10. Misra R. Caesarean section. In: Ian Donald's Practical Obstetric Problems, 7th edition. Boca Raton, Florida, USA: CRC Press; 2012. pp. 547-60.
11. Bucklin BA, Hawkins JL, Anderson JR, Ullrich FA. Obstetric anesthesia workforce survey: twenty-year update. Anesthesiology. 2005;103(3):645-53.
12. Banks A, Levy D. General anaesthesia for operative obstetrics. Anaes Int Care Med. 2007;8:317-9.
13. Munnur UB, de Boisblanc B, Suresh MS. Airway problems in pregnancy. Crit Care Med. 2005;33(10 Suppl):S259-68.
14. McGlennan A, Mustafa A. General anaesthesia for caesarean section. CEPD Rev. 2009;9:148-51.
15. Levy DM. Anaesthesia for caesarean section. CEPD Rev. 2001;1:171-6.
16. Sharp LM, Levy DM. Rapid sequence induction in obstetrics revisited. Curr Opin Anaesthesiol. 2009;22(3):357-61.
17. Levy DM. Traditional rapid sequence induction is an outmoded technique for caesarean section and should be modified. Int J Obstet Anesth. 2006;15(3):227-9.
18. Purva M, Russell IF, Kinsella M. Caesarean section anaesthesia: technique and failure rate. In: Colvin JR, Peden CJ (Eds). Raising the Standard: A Compendium of Audit Recipes for Continuous Quality Improvement in Anaesthesia, 3rd edition. London, United Kingdom: The Royal college of Anaesthetists; 2012. pp. 166-7.
19. Allen VM, O'Connell CM, Liston RM, Baskett TF. Maternal morbidity associated with cesarean delivery without labor compared with spontaneous onset of labor at term. Obstet Gynecol. 2003;102(3):477-82.
20. Silver RM, MFMU Network of NICHD. The MFMU cesarean section registry: maternal morbidity associated with multiple repeat cesarean delivery. Am J Obstet Gynecol. 2004;191:s17.
21. Hopkins L, Smaill F. Antibiotic prophylaxis regimens and drugs for cesarean section. Cochrane Database Syst Rev. 2000;(2):CD001136.
22. Simpson EL, Lawrenson RA, Nightingale AL, Farmer RD. Venous thromboembolism in pregnancy and the puerperium: incidence and additional risk factors from a London perinatal database. BJOG. 2001;108(1):56-60.
23. Phipps MG, Watabe B, Clemons JL, Weitzen S, Myers DL. Risk factors for bladder injury during cesarean delivery. Obstet Gynecol. 2005;105(1):156-60.
24. Fisher J, Astbury J, Smith A. Adverse psychological impact of operative obstetric interventions: a prospective longitudinal study. Aust N Z J Psychiatry. 1997;31(5):728-38.
25. Hemminki E. Impact of caesarean section on future pregnancy--a review of cohort studies. Paediatr Perinat Epidemiol. 1996;10(4):366-79.
26. Declercq ER, Sakala C, Corry MP, Applebaum S, Risher P. (2002). Listening to Mothers: Report of the First National U.S. Survey of Women's Childbearing Experiences. [online] Available from www.childbirthconnection.org/pdfs/LtMreport.pdf. [Accessed June, 2015].
27. Murphy DJ, Stirrat GM, Heron J; ALSPAC Study team. The relationship between Caesarean section and subfertility in a population-based sample of 14,541 pregnancies. Hum Reprod. 2002;17(7):1914-7.
28. Levine EM, Ghai V, Barton JJ, Strom CM. Mode of delivery and risk of respiratory diseases in newborns. Obstet Gynecol. 2001;97(3):439-42.
29. Håkansson S, Källén K. Caesarean section increases the risk of hospital care in childhood for asthma and gastroenteritis. Clin Exp Allergy. 2003;33(6):757-64.
30. DiMatteo MR, Morton SC, Lepper HS, Damush TM, Carney MF, Pearson M, et al. Cesarean childbirth and psychological outcomes: a meta-analysis. Health Psychol. 1996;15(4):303-14.

31. Rageth JC, Juzi C, Grossenbacher H. Delivery after previous cesarean: a risk evaluation. Swiss Working Group of Obstetric and Gynecologic Institutions. Obstet Gynecol. 1999;93(3):332-7.
32. Ananth CV, Smulian JC, Vintzileos AM. The association of placenta previa with history of cesarean delivery and abortion: a meta-analysis. Am J Obstet Gynecol. 1997;177(5):1071-8.
33. Clark SL, Koonings PP, Phelan JP. Placenta previa/accreta and prior cesarean section. Obstet Gynecol. 1985;966(1):89-92.
34. Miller DA, Chollet JA, Goodwin TM. Clinical risk factors for placenta previa-placenta accreta. Am J Obstet Gynecol. 1997;177(1):210-4.
35. Ziogos E, Tsiodras S, Matalliotakis I, Giamarellou H, Kanellakopoulou K. Ampicillin/sulbactam versus cefuroxime as antimicrobial prophylaxis for cesarean delivery: a randomized study. BMC Infect Dis. 2010;10:341.
36. Alekwe LO, Kuti O, Orji EO, Ogunniyi SO. Comparison of ceftriaxone versus triple drug regimen in the prevention of cesarean section infectious morbidities. J Matern Fetal Neonatal Med. 2008;21(9):638-42.
37. Rudge MV, Atallah AN, Peraçoli JC, Tristão Ada R, Mendonça Neto M. Randomized controlled trial on prevention of postcesarean infection using penicillin and cephalothin in Brazil. Acta Obstet Gynecol Scand. 2006;85(8):945-8.
38. Alfirevic Z, Gyte GM, Dou L. Different classes of antibiotics given to women routinely for preventing infection at caesarean section. Cochrane Database Syst Rev. 2010;(10):CD008726.
39. Costantine MM, Rahman M, Ghulmiyah L, Byers BD, Longo M, Wen T, et al. Timing of perioperative antibiotics for cesarean delivery: a meta-analysis. Am J Obstet Gynecol. 2008;199(3):301.e1-6.
40. Scottish Intercollegiate Guidelines Network (SIGN): Part of NHS Quality Improvement Scotland. Prophylaxis of venous thromboembolism: A National Clinical Guideline. SIGN Guideline No. 62. Edinburgh, United Kingdom: SIGN; 2002.
41. Starr RV, Zurawski J, Ismail M. Preoperative vaginal preparation with povidone-iodine and the risk of postcesarean endometritis. Obstet Gynecol. 2005;105(5 Pt 1):1024-9.
42. Haas DM, Pazouki F, Smith RR, Fry AM, Podzielinski I, Al-Darei SM, et al. vaginal cleansing before cesarean delivery to reduce postoperative infectious morbidity: a randomized, controlled trial. Am J Obstet Gynecol. 2010;202(3):310.e1-6.
43. Haas DM, Morgan Al Darei S, Contreras K. Vaginal preparation with antiseptic solution before cesarean section for preventing postoperative infections. Cochrane Database Syst Rev. 2010;(3):CD007892.
44. Tully L, Gates S, Brocklehurst P, McKenzie-McHarg K, Ayers S. Surgical techniques used during caesarean section operations: results of a national survey of practice in the UK. Eur J Obstet Gynecol Reprod Biol. 2002;102(2):120-6.
45. Kerr-Wilson RH, McNally S. Bladder drainage for caesarean section under epidural analgesia. Br J Obstet Gynaecol. 1986;93(1):28-30.
46. Ghoreishi J. Indwelling urinary catheters in cesarean delivery. Int J Gynaecol Obstet. 2003;83(3):267-270.
47. Li L, Wen J, Wang L, Li YP, Li Y. Is routine indwelling catheterisation of the bladder for caesarean section necessary? A systematic review. BJOG. 2011;118(4):400-9.
48. Naki MM, Api O, Celik H, Kars B, Yasar E, Unal O. Comparative study of Misgav-Ladach and Pfannenstiel-Kerr cesarean techniques: a randomized controlled trial. J Matern Fetal Neonatal Med. 2011;24(2):239-44.
49. Gedikbasi A, Akyol A, Ulker V, Yildirim D, Arslan O, Karaman E, et al. Cesarean techniques in cases with one previous cesarean delivery: comparison of modified Misgav-Ladach and Pfannenstiel-Kerr. Arch Gynecol Obstet. 2011;283(4):711-6.
50. Belci D, Kos M, Zorici D, Kuhari L, Slivar A, Begi -Razem E, et al. Comparative study of the "Misgav Ladach" and traditional Pfannenstiel surgical techniques for cesarean section. Minerva Ginecol. 2007;59(3):231-40.
51. Xavier P, Ayres-De-Campos D, Reynolds A, Guimarães M, Costa-Santos C, Patrício B. The modified Misgav-Ladach versus the Pfannenstiel-Kerr technique for cesarean section: a randomized trial. Acta Obstet Gynecol Scand. 2005;84(9):878-82.
52. Mathai M, Hofmeyr GJ. Abdominal surgical incisions for caesarean section. Cochrane Database Syst Rev. 2007;(1):CD004453.
53. Hofmeyr JG, Novikova N, Mathai M, Shah A. Techniques for cesarean section. Am J Obstet Gynecol. 2009;201(5):431-44.
54. Tuuli MG, Odibo AO, Fogertey P, Roehl K, Stamilio D, Macones GA. Utility of the bladder flap at cesarean delivery: a randomized controlled trial. Obstet Gynecol. 2012;119(4):815-21.
55. Malvasi A, Tinelli A, Guido M, Cavallotti C, Dell'Edera D, Zizza A, et al. Effect of avoiding bladder flap formation in caesarean section on repeat caesarean delivery. Eur J Obstet Gynecol Reprod Biol. 2011;159(2):300-4.
56. Sekhavat L, Dehghani Firouzabadi R, Mojiri P. Effect of expansion technique of uterine incision on maternal blood loss in cesarean section. Arch Gynecol Obstet. 2010;282(5):475-9.
57. Magann EF, Chauhan SP, Bufkin L, Field K, Roberts WE, Martin JN. Intra-operative haemorrhage by blunt versus sharp expansion of the uterine incision at caesarean delivery: a randomised clinical trial. BJOG. 2002;109(4):448-52.
58. Sheehan SR, Montgomery AA, Carey M, McAuliffe FM, Eogan M, Gleeson R, et al. Oxytocin bolus versus oxytocin bolus and infusion for control of blood loss at elective caesarean section: double blind, placebo controlled, randomised trial. BMJ. 2011;343:d4661.
59. Chaudhuri P, Banerjee GB, Mandal A. Rectally administered misoprostol versus intravenous oxytocin infusion during cesarean delivery to reduce intraoperative and postoperative blood loss. Int J Gynaecol Obstet. 2010;109:25-9.
60. Movafegh A, Eslamian L, Dorabadi A. Effect of intravenous tranexamic acid administration on blood loss during and after cesarean delivery. Int J Gynaecol Obstet. 2011;115(3):224-6.
61. Mercer JS. Current best evidence: a review of the literature on umbilical cord clamping. J Midwifery Womens Health. 2001;46(6):402-14.
62. Wahab MA, Karantzis P, Eccersley PS, Russell IF, Thompson JW, Lindow SW. A randomised, controlled study of uterine exteriorisation and repair at caesarean section. Br J Obstet Gynaecol. 1999;106(9):913-6.
63. Liabsuetrakul T, Peeyananjarassri K. Mechanical dilatation of the cervix at non-labour caesarean section for reducing postoperative morbidity. Cochrane Database Syst Rev. 2011;(11):CD008019.
64. Roberge S, Chaillet N, Boutin A, Moore L, Jastrow N, Brassard N, et al. Single- versus double-layer closure of the hysterotomy incision during cesarean delivery and risk of uterine rupture. Int J Gynaecol Obstet. 2011;115(1):5-10.
65. Enkin MW, Wilkinson, C. WITHDRAWN: Single versus two layer suturing for closing the uterine incision at Caesarean section. Cochrane Database Syst Rev. 2007;(3):CD000192.
66. Lal K, Tsomo P. Comparative study of single layer and conventional closure of uterine incision in cesarean section. Int J Obstet Gynaecol Obstet. 1988;27(3):349-52.
67. Bujold E, Bujold C, Hamilton EF, Harel F, Gauthier RJ. The impact of a single-layer or double-layer closure on the uterine rupture. Am J Obstet Gynecol. 2002;186(6):1326-30.
68. Viney R, Isaacs C, Chelmow D. Intra-abdominal irrigation at cesarean delivery: a randomized controlled trial. Obstet Gynecol. 2012;119(6):1106-11.

69. Harrigill KM, Miller HS, Haynes DE. The effect of intra-abdominal irrigation at cesarean delivery on maternal morbidity: a randomized trial. Obstet Gynecol. 2003;101(1):80-5.
70. Lewis DF, Otterson WN, Dunnihoo DR. Antibiotic prophylactic uterine lavage in cesarean section: a double-blind comparison of saline, ticarcillin, and cefoxitin irrigation in indigent patients. South Med J. 1990;83(3):274-6.
71. Magann EF, Dodson MK, Ray MA, Harris RL, Martin JN, Morrison JC. Preoperative skin preparation and intraoperative pelvic irrigation: impact on post-cesarean endometritis and wound infection. Obstet Gynecol. 1993;81(6):922-5.
72. Shi Z, Ma L, Yang Y, Wang H, Schreiber A, Li X, et al. Adhesion formation after previous caesarean section-a meta-analysis and systematic review. BJOG. 2011;118(4):410-22.
73. Cheong YC, Premkumar G, Metwally M, Peacock JL, Li TC. To close or not to close? A systematic review and a meta-analysis of peritoneal non-closure and adhesion formation after caesarean section. Eur J Obstet Gynecol Reprod Biol. 2009;147(1):3-8.
74. Wilkinson CS, Enkin MW. Peritoneal non-closure at caesarean section. Cochrane Database Syst Rev. 2000;(2):CD000163.
75. Højberg KE, Aagaard J, Laursen H, Diab L, Secher NJ. Closure versus non-closure of peritoneum at cesarean section--evaluation of pain. A randomized study. Acta Obstet Gynecol Scand. 1998;77(7):741-5.
76. Grundsell HS, Rizk DE, Kumar RM. Randomized study of non-closure of peritoneum in lower segment cesarean section. Acta Obstet Gynecol Scand. 1998;77(1):110-5.
77. Ramsey PS, White AM, Guinn DA, Lu GC, Ramin SM, Davies JK, et al. Subcutaneous tissue reapproximation, alone or in combination with drain, in obese women undergoing cesarean delivery. Obstet Gynecol. 2005;105(5 Pt 1):967-73.
78. Chelmow D, Huang E, Strohbehn K. Closure of the subcutaneous dead space and wound disruption after Cesarean delivery. J Matern Fetal Neonatal Med. 2002;11(6):403-8.
79. Allaire AD, Fisch J, McMahon MJ. Subcutaneous drain vs. suture in obese women undergoing cesarean delivery. A prospective, randomized trial. J Reprod Med. 2000;45(4):327-31.
80. Clay FS, Walsh CA, Walsh SR. Staples vs subcuticular sutures for skin closure at cesarean delivery: a meta-analysis of randomized controlled trials. Am J Obstet Gynecol. 2011;204(5):378-83.
81. Alderdice F, McKenna D, Dornan J. Techniques and materials for skin closure in caesarean section. Cochrane Database Syst Rev. 2003;(2):CD0003577.
82. Frishman GN, Schwartz T, Hogan JW. Closure of Pfannenstiel skin incisions. Staples vs. subcuticular suture. J Reprod Med. 1997;42(10):627-30.
83. Connor EM, Sperling RS, Gelber R, Kiselev P, Scott G, O'Sullivan MJ, et al. Reduction of maternal-infant transmission of human immunodeficiency virus type 1 with zidovudine treatment. Pediatric AIDS Clinical Trials Group Protocol 076 Study Group. N Engl J Med. 1994;331(18):1173-80.
84. Anderson BL, Cu-Uvin S. Pregnancy and optimal care of HIV-infected patients. Clin Infect Dis. 2009;48(4):449-55.
85. The mode of delivery and the risk of vertical transmission of human immunodeficiency virus type 1--a meta-analysis of 15 prospective cohort studies. The International Perinatal HIV Group. N Engl J Med. 1999;340(13):977-98.
86. Report of the NIH Panel to define principles of therapy of HIV infection. MMWR Recomm Rep. 1998;47(RR-5):1-41.
87. Wispelwey BP, Sheiner E. Cesarean delivery in obese women: a comprehensive review. J Mat Fetal Neonatal Med. 2013;26(6):547-51.
88. National Institute for Health and Care Excellence (NICE). (2012). National Collaborating Centre for Women's and Children's Health: Caesarean section. [online] Available from www.nice.org.uk/guidance/CG74. [Accessed June, 2015].
89. Oyelese Y, Smulian JC. Placenta previa, placenta accreta, and vasa previa. Obstet Gynecol. 2006;107(4):927-41.

CHAPTER 22

Vaginal Delivery after Cesarean

Kavita Mandrelle, Kanupriya Jain

INTRODUCTION

In the early part of 20th century, cesarean delivery was associated with a very high maternal mortality and therefore, was performed in extremely rare circumstances. As this procedure became more and more safe, slowly the rate of cesarean deliveries increased and it became the most commonly performed major surgical procedure in the world.

The rising trend continued and there was a huge rise in the rate of cesarean section, especially in the developed countries, towards the latter half of 20th century. The increased rate of cesarean delivery was attributed to electronic fetal monitoring during labor, a decrease in vaginal breech deliveries, decrease in forceps and ventouse deliveries, and many-a-times due to legal aspects involved. As a consequence, the number of women with previous cesarean deliveries increased and its resultant complications also increased in subsequent pregnancies. Incidence of placenta previa, morbidly adherent placenta, and obstetric hysterectomy also increased leading to a rise in the maternal mortality.

The notion "once a cesarean, always a cesarean" was followed which led to a rise in rate of second, third, and higher-order cesarean sections. In an attempt to check the rising rates, this ideology was challenged and encouragement given to "trial of labor after cesarean (TOLAC)" for the fulfillment of the goal of "vaginal birth after cesarean (VBAC)". This approach suffered a major setback when uterine ruptures and perinatal deaths were reported from all over the world during trial of labor (TOL).

Though there are many clinical uncertainties with regard to VBAC, yet evidence shows that TOL is a reasonable option for many women with a previously scarred uterus.

TERMINOLOGY

The following terms are recommended and adapted from the National Institutes of Health Consensus Statement (2010):[1]

- Trial of labor: This refers to a planned attempt to vaginal birth in a woman who has had a previous cesarean section. This is also sometimes called a "trial of vaginal birth after cesarean"
- Vaginal birth after cesarean: This refers to vaginal birth following a TOL
- Elective repeat cesarean section: This refers to planned cesarean section in a woman who has had one or more prior cesarean sections, whether or not cesarean section occurred at a scheduled time. It may also be termed as" elective repeat cesarean delivery (ERCD)"
- Unsuccessful TOL: Delivery by cesarean section of a woman who has had a TOL is referred as unsuccessful TOL.

RISKS AND BENEFITS OF TRIAL OF LABOR AFTER CESAREAN AND ELECTIVE REPEAT CESAREAN DELIVERY

The decision to undergo TOL in a previous cesarean section is not an easy one. There are three possible outcomes for a lady with previous cesarean delivery:

1. Successful TOL resulting in a vaginal delivery
2. Failed TOL and emergency repeat cesarean delivery
3. ERCD.

A successful TOLAC is associated with the lowest morbidity of all three possibilities and a failed TOLAC is associated with the highest morbidity. TOLAC is beneficial if it results in a vaginal delivery. There are risks involved with TOLAC which at times may be catastrophic for the mother and the baby.

Maternal Risks during Trial of Labor after Cesarean versus Elective Repeat Cesarean Delivery

Uterine Rupture

It is a life-threatening complication that can occur during labor. Scar rupture is a complete disruption of all the layers of uterus including the serosa and is associated with maternal hemorrhage and perinatal morbidity and mortality. Scar dehiscence is an incomplete or partial scar separation where the serosa remains intact. The risk of a scar rupture varies between 0.2 and 1.5% for a previous low-transverse incision, to 4–9% for a classical incision[2] (Table 1). With an elective lower segment cesarean section risk of rupture is 1 in 4,000.[3]

Infection

The incidence of postpartum pelvic infection is more in a failed TOLAC as compared to a successful VBAC and ERCD though this difference is not significant.

Peripartum Hysterectomy

Hysterectomy may be required for a uterine rupture in a patient undergoing TOLAC and also for placenta accreta in a repeat cesarean section.

Blood Transfusion

Risk of hemorrhage and subsequent need for transfusion is present with both TOLAC and ERCD.

Failed Trial of Labor after Cesarean

Maternal morbidity is the highest if TOLAC fails and an emergency cesarean section is performed. There are more chances of wound complications, infection, hemorrhage, hysterectomy, and blood transfusion.

Maternal Benefits with Vaginal Birth after Cesarean

If VBAC occurs, it is the best possible outcome. There is a shorter hospital stay, fewer postpartum complications and quick return to normal activities. Overall risk of maternal death is lower for TOLAC, but it may not be true for developing countries like India where women with previous cesarean delivery may deliver in grossly suboptimal conditions.

Maternal Benefits with Elective Repeat Cesarean Delivery

Elective repeat cesarean delivery is conveniently planned by the doctor and patient and sterilization can also be considered simultaneously.

Maternal Risks with Elective Repeat Cesarean Delivery

Immediate Complications

Each successive cesarean delivery is associated with a higher risk of injury to urinary bladder, ureter, and bowel due to presence of intra-abdominal adhesions. The risk of hemorrhage is also increased.

Long-term Complications

The incidence of placenta previa increases with the number of previous cesarean deliveries (Table 2). Hence, the risk of placenta accreta and risk of cesarean hysterectomy for placenta previa increases many fold with each cesarean delivery (Table 3).

Perinatal Risks

Mortality

The absolute risk of mortality to the fetus or the neonate is very low, but it is significantly more in TOLAC as compared to ERCD.

TABLE 1: Risk of uterine rupture according to the type of uterine incision[2]

Prior uterine incision	Risk of rupture (%)
Classical incision	4–9
T-shaped incision	4–9
Low-vertical incision	1–7
Low-transverse incision	0.2–0.5

TABLE 2: Incidence of placenta previa with successive cesarean deliveries[2]

Number of previous cesarean deliveries	Incidence of placenta previa (%)
Unscarred uterus	0.33
1	1
2	2
3	4

TABLE 3: Incidence of placenta accreta with successive cesarean deliveries[1]

Number of cesarean delivery	Incidence of placenta accreta (%)
1	0.24
2	0.31
3	0.57
4	2.10
5	2.30
6 or more	6.70

Hypoxic Ischemic Encephalopathy

The risk to the fetus is more in TOLAC as compared to almost nil in ERCD. The risk of uterine rupture leading to fetal death or major morbidity is 1 per 1,000.[4]

Other Neonatal Morbidities

The neonates born after ERCD have more respiratory problems which are mostly in the form of transient tachypnea of newborn. There is no difference in neonatal admissions when babies born after TOLAC are compared to those with ERCD, but the risk of sepsis and rate of intubation for meconium stained amniotic fluid is more for TOLAC.

CHOOSING THE ROUTE OF DELIVERY

Current recommendations by the American College of Obstetricians and Gynecologists (ACOGs) are that the patient should be informed of all the risks and benefits and decision making is a shared process where the patient and family's preference should be honored.[5] Patient counseling regarding route of delivery should preferably be started preconceptionally and reevaluated at each visit as certain factors may arise during the course of pregnancy which may alter the decision. A final decision to the route of delivery should be completed by 36 weeks of gestation.[6]

PREDICTION OF SUCCESSFUL TRIAL OF LABOR AFTER CESAREAN

We do not have any definitive data to predict maternal and fetal outcome after TOLAC. Though a number of predictive models have been developed to identify women with a previous cesarean delivery who will have successful TOLAC, but none of these have proven to be clinically useful. Some of these screening tools involve use of maternal demographics, such as age, body mass index (BMI), race, ethnicity, indications for previous cesarean delivery, number of previous vaginal deliveries, type and number of previous uterine incisions, and cervical favorability or bishop scoring at the time of admission. None of these screening tools have been able to consistently predict a successful outcome.

Use of imaging techniques, such as ultrasound measurement of anterior uterine wall and size of uterine scar defect to identify women at risk of uterine rupture or scar dehiscence has also been studied. But, at present, it has not been proven to be useful and has not given consistent results.

Candidates for Trial of Labor after Cesarean

The ACOG had issued a new practice bulletin in 2010 that states that attempting a VBAC is a safe and appropriate option for most women who have had a prior cesarean delivery.[5]

Appropriate Candidates

- One prior lower segment transverse cesarean section: Evidence suggests a success rate of 60–70% TOLAC in patients with one prior lower segment transverse cesarean section and even higher in patients with additional favorable characteristics[3]
- Previous successful vaginal delivery before or after the cesarean delivery: Success rate for these patients is close to 80%
- Spontaneous labor: The likelihood of a VBAC is almost 80% if the lady presents in labor before 40 weeks and who have a favorable bishop score at admission
- Nonrecurrent indication for prior cesarean delivery: Nonrecurrent indications have a higher probability of a successful TOLAC. The rate of success depends upon the indication for prior cesarean delivery which is 75% for fetal malpresentation, 60% for nonreassuring fetal heart rate pattern, and 54% for failure to progress or cephalopelvic disproportion[3,7]
- Demographic factors: The favorable factors for a VBAC are maternal age less than 35 years, education more than 12 years, non-Hispanic white race. Obese women (BMI <30 kg/m^2) are less likely to have a TOLAC
- Interdelivery interval: Interdelivery intervals of 18 months or less were associated with a threefold risk of uterine rupture compared with more than 18 months. So, an interdelivery interval of more than 18 months is desirable[8]
- Absence of pre-existing maternal medical disease, such as hypertension, diabetes, asthma, heart and renal diseases increases the likelihood of a TOLAC, but the evidence is still inconclusive
- Fetal weight: Success rates are higher in women with average-sized babies. A fetal weight of more than 4,000 g reduces the rate of VBAC to half.

Possibly Appropriate Candidates

In the following situations, an individualized risk assessment is required before the patients are considered for TOLAC as the evidence is not very consistent:

- Prior low vertical uterine incision: There is conflicting evidence for the risk of uterine rupture during TOLAC for women with prior low vertical incision. The Eunice Kennedy Shriver National Institute of Child Health and Human Development maternal-fetal medicine units network study found a significant difference in the rates of uterine rupture during TOLAC by the type of previous uterine incision. The rate of rupture for low transverse in this study is 0.7%, low vertical (2%), unknown (0.5%), and 1.9% in women who had a prior classical, inverted T- or J-shaped incision. Hence, many centers do not offer TOLAC to women with a prior low vertical uterine incision[9]
- Multiple prior low transverse uterine incisions: The rate of rupture is significantly higher for two prior uterine scars, so TOLAC is usually not offered. ACOG recommends that selected patients with a previous vaginal birth can be given an option of TOLAC[5]
- Unknown type of uterine incision: The incidence of rupture with unknown uterine incision is same as for previous one low transverse incision. The decision for TOLAC is individualized based on indication for prior delivery which may suggest the possibility of a low vertical incision
- Pregnancy more than 40 weeks: The possibility of a successful VBAC decreases after 40 weeks due to bigger baby, higher rate of labor induction, and higher risk of scar rupture (2–3%). Labor should be induced only if the cervix is favorable[10]
- Twin pregnancy: ACOG opinion is that women with twin pregnancy with one previous low transverse cesarean delivery can undergo TOLAC if there is no contraindication to vaginal birth.[5]

Inappropriate Candidates

A TOLAC is not advisable in these patients as the risk to mother and fetus is too high:

- High-risk uterine scars: The high-risk incisions are classical, T-shaped, J-shaped, transfundal as well as myomectomy incisions which enter the cavity. They are associated with a high-risk of scar rupture (1.9%).[9] A previous inadvertent uterine extension could also lead to high risk of rupture in a subsequent pregnancy
- Previous uterine rupture: These patients should undergo ERCD at 37 weeks as the possibility of rupture is as high as 32% (prior upper segment rupture).[11] Rarely, rupture may occur before 37 weeks, therefore close monitoring and intervention may be required early in some patients
- Previous uterine dehiscence: There is no consensus over management of these patients as data is scarce; therefore, TOLAC is not offered in these cases
- Patients in whom vaginal delivery is not advisable should not undergo TOLAC, e.g., placenta previa, breech presentation, contracted pelvis, twins with first fetus in noncephalic presentation, etc.
- Lack of a proper facility: TOLAC should not be offered in a place where electronic monitoring, round the clock anesthesia personnel, obstetrician, surgeon, pediatric staff, and blood bank facilities are not available.

MANAGEMENT OF LABOR AND DELIVERY

In addition to the routine care given to any woman during labor, a patient with previous cesarean delivery needs to be under extra vigilance for signs and symptoms of scar dehiscence and rupture, especially those who are augmented with oxytocin.

Prerequisites for Performing Trial of Labor after Cesarean

Appropriate Facility

Trial of labor after cesarean should be attempted in institutions and hospitals where there is immediate availability of personnel and equipment for performing an emergency cesarean delivery. Facility for obstetric anesthesia, an obstetrician capable of performing an emergency cesarean delivery, personnel and equipment for neonatal resuscitation, and blood bank facilities should be readily available round the clock.

If appropriate facilities are not available, it is important to discuss with the patient and referral to another hospital which has appropriate resources should be done so as to facilitate optimum maternal and fetal outcome. In case the patient elects to proceed with TOL in spite of lack of facilities, she should be well informed about the risk and implications.

Monitoring of Labor

Labor should be monitored by continuous tocography. Labor patterns and progress is similar in women with and without previous cesarean section delivery. Since the risk of uterine rupture is more in women with previous cesarean delivery, these patients need to be monitored by continuous monitoring of uterine activity and fetal heart rate. Internal pressure monitoring has not been shown to be a sensitive method for uterine rupture so, it is not preferred over external monitoring.

The Royal College of Obstetricians and Gynecologists states that an abnormal cardiotocograph is the most consistent finding in uterine rupture and is present in 55–87% of such cases.[6]

Monitoring of Patients

The following should be monitored closely during TOLAC:

- Pulse rate
- Blood pressure
- Temperature
- Uterine contractions: Frequency, intensity, duration
- Uterine contour
- Scar tenderness
- Per vaginal bleeding
- Color of urine
- Continuous electronic fetal heart monitoring.

Induction and Augmentation of Labor

Neither induction nor augmentation is strongly contraindicated in women undergoing TOLAC, but a cautious approach is suggested. Though there is no conclusive evidence, observational studies have suggested that uterotonic drugs in women with a prior cesarean delivery increases the risk of uterine rupture. If the cervix is favorable, an amniotomy is the preferred method to induce labor. According to the ACOG practice bulletin (2010), misoprostol (prostaglandin E_1) should not be used for cervical ripening or labor induction in the third trimester. ACOG also discourages use of other prostaglandins for labor induction and have recognized oxytocin or mechanical method as options for women undergoing TOLAC. These methods have a lower risk of uterine rupture than prostaglandin.[5] Consensus opinion according to the guidelines for clinical practice from the French College of Gynecologists and Obstetricians recommends against induction of labor in previous two cesarean deliveries.[12]

The ACOG supports use of oxytocin for augmentation of labor in women with previous cesarean delivery.[5] There is conflicting data regarding risk of uterine rupture with oxytocin augmentation of labor during TOLAC. The dose limit of oxytocin during TOLAC has not been evaluated.

Analgesia and anesthesia

Epidural analgesia can be given for pain relief during labor and it does not appear to mask the signs and symptoms of uterine rupture because the most common sign of rupture is fetal heart tracing abnormality. It is also seen that epidural analgesia does not decrease the likelihood of VBAC.[5]

Uterine exploration after delivery

Routine uterine exploration is followed by many clinicians though there is no sufficient data of its value to identify asymptomatic uterine dehiscence. Excessive vaginal bleeding or signs of hypovolemia should prompt complete exploration of the genital tract.[5]

External Cephalic Version

Limited data suggests that external cephalic version is not contraindicated in a woman who is at low risk of adverse maternal or neonatal outcome. Chance of successful external cephalic version has been found to be similar in women with and without previous cesarean delivery.

Intrauterine Fetal Demise

Some women with prior cesarean delivery may present with intrauterine fetal demise. Since there are no fetal risks during TOLAC in these circumstances, TOL is encouraged after weighing the risk and benefits in such cases.

Second trimester delivery of an intrauterine fetal demise can be accomplished using prostaglandins and oxytocin including misoprostol since the rate of rupture with labor induction has been found to be less than 1% in such cases.[5]

Those who present after 28 weeks with intrauterine fetal demise, cervical ripening can be achieved with a transcervical Foley's catheter. Uterine rupture rate using this method has been found to be comparable to those with spontaneous labor.[5]

Uterine Rupture

Uterine rupture is often sudden. There is no single pathognomonic feature, but acute onset of any of the following should prompt an immediate cesarean delivery or laparotomy.

Acute Signs and Symptoms

- Fetal bradycardia
- Severe abdominal pain, especially if persisting between contractions
- Chest pain or shoulder tip pain, acute onset of shortness of breath
- Acute onset scar tenderness
- Loss of previously efficient uterine activity
- Increased uterine contractions
- Vaginal bleeding, hematuria
- Maternal tachycardia, hypotension or shock
- Loss of fetal station
- New onset of intense uterine pain.

The final diagnosis is confirmed at laparotomy. The most common sign is fetal heart rate abnormality which is associated with 70% of cases.[6]

Even when a risk factor for uterine rupture is found, it is only a risk factor and not a true predictor. The vast majority of women with that risk factor will not experience a rupture even if they labor.

Coming up with a reasonable way to manage risk in women with a prior cesarean delivery is one of the greatest dilemma of obstetrics today. The best solution is to prevent the first cesarean whenever possible. Failing primary prevention, the best course is to offer fully informed consent about risk and benefit of each choice and then let the woman choose which option to pursue.

CONCLUSION

Any pregnant woman with a single previous cesarean delivery with a low transverse incision with no contraindications to vaginal delivery should be counseled for TOLAC, its attendant risks and benefits. The pregnant lady should choose between TOLAC and ERCD after an informed discussion.

The ACOG recommends that any lady with no more than one prior low transverse cesarean delivery, with a clinically adequate pelvis and no other uterine scar can undergo TOLAC in a facility with physician available for monitoring and performing cesarean section. Anesthesia and other personnel needed for a cesarean delivery should be available.

Women with previous two low transverse cesarean deliveries may be considered for TOLAC if a vaginal delivery has occurred in the past. Twin pregnancies with no other contraindication to vaginal delivery may be offered TOLAC. External cephalic version for breech can be tried in low-risk patients with previous one low transverse incision.

Induction of labor is an option but prostaglandins, especially misoprostol, are contraindicated with a previous cesarean delivery. High-risk patients with a prior classical cesarean delivery, fundal uterine scar, placenta previa or any other contraindication to vaginal delivery generally are not candidates for TOLAC. Possibility of a successful TOLAC is the maximum in patients with at least one prior vaginal delivery before or after a prior cesarean section or those who come in spontaneous labor with a favorable Bishop score, before 40 weeks of gestation and have an average-sized baby.

REFERENCES

1. Royal Australian and New Zealand College of Obstetricians and Gynecologists (RANZCOG). (2010). RANZCOG college statement C-OBS 38: Planned vaginal birth after caesarean section (Trial of Labour). [online] Available from www.ranzcog.edu.au/doc/planned-vbac.html. [Accessed June, 2015].
2. Cunningham FG, Leveno KJ, Bloom SL, Hauth JC, Gilstrap LC, Wenstrom KD (Eds). Williams Obstetrics, 22nd edition. Philadelphia, PA, USA: McGraw-Hill Professional; 2005.
3. Guise JM, Eden K, Emeis C, Denman MA, Marshall N, Fu R, et al. Vaginal birth after cesarean: new insights. Evid Rep Technol Assess (Full Rep). 2010;(191):1-397.
4. Chauhan SP, Martin JN, Henrichs CE, Morrison JC, Magann EF. Maternal and perinatal complications with uterine rupture in 142,075 patients who attempted vaginal birth after cesarean delivery: A review of literature. Am J Obstet Gynecol. 2003;189(2):408-17.
5. American College of Obstetricians and Gynecologists (ACOG). ACOG Practice bulletin no. 115: Vaginal birth after previous cesarean delivery. Obstet Gynecol. 2010;116(2 Pt 1):450-63.
6. Royal College of Obstetricians and Gynaecologists (RCOG). (2007). Birth after previous caesarean birth. Green-Top Guideline No. 45. [online] Available from www.rcog.org.uk/globalassets/documents/guidelines/gtg4511022011.pdf. [Accessed June, 2015].
7. Landon MB, Leindecker S, Spong CY, Hauth JC, Bloom S, Varner MW, et al. The MFMU Cesarean Registry: factors affecting the success of trial of labor after previous cesarean delivery. Am J Obstet Gynecol. 2005;193(3 Pt 2):1016-23.
8. Shipp TD, Zelop CM, Repke JT, Cohen A, Lieberman E. Interdelivery interval and risk of symptomatic uterine rupture. Obstet Gynecol. 2001;97(2):175-7.
9. Landon MB, Hauth JC, Leveno KJ, Spong CY, Leindecker S, Varner MW, et al. Maternal and perinatal outcomes associated with a trial of labor after prior cesarean delivery. N Engl J Med. 2004;351(25):2581-9.
10. Kiran TS, Chui YK, Bethel J, Bhal PS. Is gestational age an independent variable affecting uterine scar rupture rates? Eur J Obstet Gynecol Reprod Biol. 2006;126(1):68-71.
11. Ritchie EH. Pregnancy after rupture of the pregnant uterus. A report of 32 pregnancies and a study of cases reported since 1932. J Obstet Gynaecol Br Commonw. 1971;78(7):642-8.
12. Sentilhes L, Vayssiere C, Beucher G, Deneux-Tharaux C, Deruelle P, Diemunsch P, et al. Delivery for women with a previous cesarean: guidelines for clinical practice from the French College of Gynecologists and Obstetricians (CNGOF). Eur J Obstet Gynecol Reprod Biol. 2013;170(1):25-32.

Section 4

Postpartum

CHAPTER 23

Postpartum Hemorrhage

Sadhana Gupta

INTRODUCTION

Postpartum hemorrhage (PPH), that is, bleeding after childbirth, is the cause of around 25% of total maternal mortality [World Health Organization (WHO), 2007], reaching as high as 60% in some countries. Major PPH requiring blood transfusion and/or surgery is one of the criteria of severe acute maternal morbidity. It can be a cause of long-term morbidity, approximately 12% of women who survive PPH will have severe anemia and also significantly higher risk of dying in the year following PPH.[1,2]

Postpartum hemorrhage can occur in 10.5% of deliveries. A significant proportion of death from PPH is preventable. Prevention, early diagnosis and prompt aggressive treatment are the key to management of PPH.

DEFINITION

Postpartum hemorrhage has been defined in many ways. Few some of the relevant definitions are as follows:

- The most common and traditional definition of PPH is the estimated blood loss in excess of 500 mL after a vaginal delivery and 1,000 mL after cesarean delivery within 24 hours of delivery. The clinical inadequacy of this definition lies in the fact that assessed blood loss is usually 400–600 mL in vaginal delivery and 1,000 mL in cesarean delivery, so due to narrow margin of quantification between normal and potentially harmful blood loss, the clinicians are more likely to underestimate volume of blood loss and detect PPH.
- Another definition is any amount of blood loss after the delivery which is significant to cause symptoms of hypovolemia, or 10% drop in blood hematocrit or requiring blood products transfusion.[3] Such blood loss occurs in approximately 4% of vaginal deliveries and 6% of cesarean section.[4]
- Hemorrhage within first 24 hours is regarded as primary PPH, whereas hemorrhage after 24 hours and within 12 weeks of delivery is called secondary PPH.

RELEVANT PHYSIOLOGY

Systemic Physiology

The maternal blood volume expands by 40–50% during pregnancy because of rise in plasma volume and red cell mass, which amounts to 1–2 L in average size women. This increased blood volume protects the woman to some extent from the consequence of hemorrhage during and following delivery. However, in volume contracted state like pre-eclampsia, woman is more vulnerable to blood loss.[5] Besides this, the blood coagulation system is activated which reduces the risk of extensive blood loss during the delivery.[6]

Uterine Changes in Third Stage of Labor

Blood flow to gravid uterus at term is 800–1,000 mL/min. After delivery of placenta, the uterine muscle contracts as well as retracts, which occlude the blood vessels preventing blood loss. Inability to contraction of uterine muscle causes atonic PPH, which constitutes majority of PPH. Adherent placental piece or blood clot also prevents effective contraction of uterus muscle and causes PPH.[6] If the uterus muscles are well contracted and hemorrhage occurs, the cause of bleeding is more likely the genital tract laceration.

RISK FACTORS

Risk factors for postpartum hemorrhage are summarized in Box 1.

It should also be emphasized that prediction of PPH cannot be done only on risk factors as two-thirds of women who have PPH have no risk factors. Therefore, all obstetric patients are considered at risk of having PPH, and universal preventive measures of PPH must be incorporated in the management of third stage of labor.

ETIOLOGY

The causes of PPH are classically categorized as follows:
- Uterine atony—Tonus
- Retained clots or placental debris—Tissue
- Genital tract laceration—Trauma
- Disorders of coagulation—Thrombin

Uterine Atony

Uterine atony alone accounts for 60% of all cases of PPH. The predisposing factors are overdistension of uterus, myometrial laxity associated with malfunctioning, prolonged labor, use of tocolytic, use of oxytocic for prolonged time and use of general anesthesia.

Genital Tract Trauma

Trauma can be in lower genital tract such as bleeding from episiotomy, vulvar or vaginal hematoma and cervical tears. Upper genital tract trauma can be caused by dehiscence of uterine scar or bleeding from direct uterine or vascular injuries at the time of cesarean section.

Box 1: Risk factors of postpartum hemorrhage

• History of PPH	• Grand multiparity
• Prolonged labor	• Prolonged oxytocic and tocolytic use
• Instrumental delivery	• Fetal macrosomia
• Multifetal pregnancy	• Fibroid
• Polyhydramnios	• Prior cesarean delivery
• Fetal demise	• Placenta previa and accreta
• Abruptio placenta	• Chorioamnionitis
• Advanced maternal age	• Use of general anesthesia

Retained Tissue

5–10% of cases of PPH are caused by retained placental tissue, membranes or large blood clot. It can occur in placenta accreta, unrecognized succenturiate lobe of placenta or inappropriate management of third stage of labor.

Coagulation Defect

Coagulation defect can occur in several obstetric disorders like abruption placenta, excess thromboplastin from retained dead fetus, severe pre-eclampsia and sepsis. These coagulopathy may present as hypofibrinogenemia, thrombocytopenia and disseminated intravascular coagulation. Besides, women can have primary problems like use of anticoagulant drugs or coagulopathy.[6]

PREVENTION

Antenatal Care

- Anemia prevention in all reproductive age women is an important measure to ensure the patients against all possible effect of hemorrhage
- High-risk cases should be identified and they should be delivered in institutions, which have facility to manage obstetric hemorrhage
- Adherent placenta should be diagnosed antenatally

Intranatal Care

- First Stage of Labor
    - All patients admitted for labor must have IV line with 18 G cannula
    - All obstetric patients should have blood hemoglobin and group screened on admission. In high-risk cases blood type and crossmatching should be done
    - Prolonged labor should be avoided
    - Injudicious use of oxytocin in labor should be avoided
    - Anticoagulant drugs should be stopped before onset of labor
- Second Stage of labor
    - Judicious decision for assisted vaginal delivery should be taken. Difficult vaginal or instrumental delivery should be avoided
    - Practice of fundal pressure and bearing down before second stage of labor should be abandoned in labor room
    - Good perineal support should be provided
- Third Stage of Labor
    - Active management of third stage of labor (AMTSL) should be universal and strictly adhered in all obstetric facilities.[7,8] The WHO new guidelines for prevention of PPH are as follows:

- All women giving birth should be offered uterotonic drug during third stage of labor
- Oxytocin 10 unit IM within one minute of delivery after excluding another fetus is the uterotonic drug of first choice. Other uterotonic recommended are methylergometrine, syntometrine, prostaglandin F2-alpha and misoprostol as alternative only in situations where oxytocin is not available
- Controlled cord traction, only in settings where skilled birth attendant is present
- Surveillance of uterine tonus through abdominal palpation is recommended in all the women for early identification of uterine atony.[9,10]

The guidelines development group has combined use of uterotonic within one minute of childbirth as the main and most important intervention within AMTSL. In this context, use of misoprostol for prevention of PPH by community health worker is being supported in settings where skilled birth attendant is not available.[11,12]

MANAGEMENT

- Diagnosis and Recognition: prompt recognition of excessive bleeding after delivery is crucial. In PPH, diagnosis is based on symptoms and signs with laboratory test helping the diagnosis. The initial finding is a very modest increase in pulse rate. By the time her blood pressure is dropped appreciably, the woman has already lost 25–30% of her blood volume. However amount of hemorrhage making a patient symptomatic, e.g., developing pallor, lightheadedness, weakness, palpitation, confusion, diaphoresis, air hunger, syncope; the patient is immediately diagnosed having moderate to severe hemorrhage. Hypoxia, tachycardia, tachypnea, oliguria and low oxygen saturation are the signs of hypovolemic shock

  Underestimation of visible bleeding is the frequent cause of delayed intervention.[13] At larger volume, the tendency to underestimate is more pronounced.[14] The visual aid of estimating blood loss has been found to improve provider accuracy.[15,16]

  It can be said for practical purpose if pad or cloth soaked in 5 minute, full soakage of five pads, passage of big clot, or continuous trickling of blood, there is a need for prompt intervention. Figures 1A and B show the visual aid pocket card with images of measured volume of artificial blood. Likewise, Debdas bag which can be inserted after delivery of the baby under maternal buttock not only collects the whole blood lost but also marks the alert, and action line, which can guide clearly to healthcare provider for diagnosis of PPH (Figs 1A and B).

  Vaginal bleeding is usually noted, but in cases of intra-abdominal bleeding from cesarean delivery or silent uterine rupture, vaginal bleeding may be absent. In such a situation, signs of hypovolemia and tenderness, and increasing girth of abdomen give the clue. Exploration of uterine cavity is required if clinical findings suggest retained blood clot or placental piece.

  To summarize, the diagnosis of PPH includes:
  - Estimation of blood loss
  - Pulse rate and blood pressure measurement applying Benedetti classification (Table 1) and rule of 30 (Fig. 2)
  - Hematocrit estimation
  - Clotting factors in blood
  - Ultrasound in some situations

  A timely and accurate etiology based and quantitative diagnosis of PPH is crucial in order to initialize appropriate intervention as PPH can cause death in short span of 1–2 hours.[17]
- Initial general management: initial management irrespective of the cause of PPH plays a crucial role in saving the women from being critical; prompt resuscitative measures include:

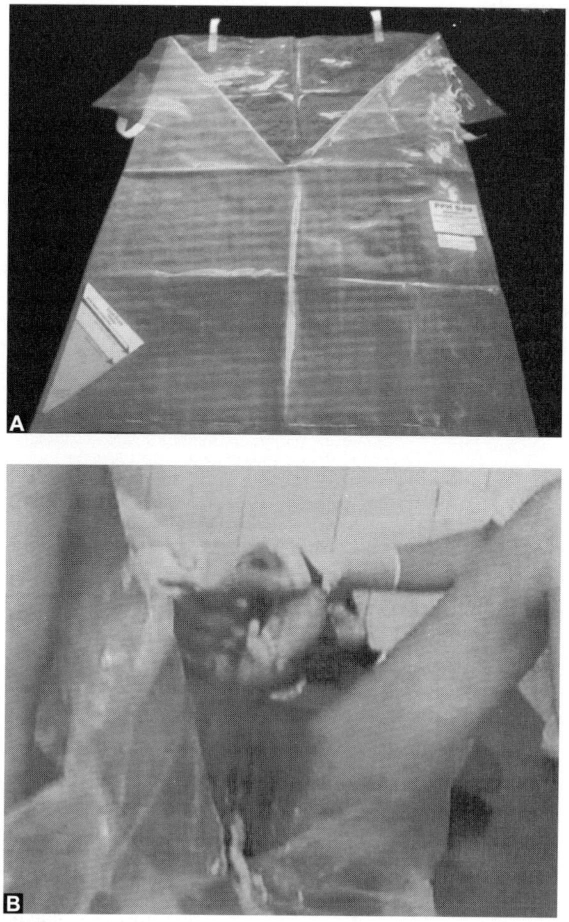

FIGS 1A AND B: **A,** Debdas Bag; **B,** Application of Debdas Bag *(For color version, see Plate 3).*

TABLE 1: Benedetti classification of postpartum hemorrhage

Clinical signs	Class 1 PPH	Class 2 PPH	Class 3 PPH	Class 4 PPH
Amount of blood loss (Volume loss)	500–1000 mL (<15%)	1000–1500 mL (15–30%)	1500–2000 mL (30–40%)	>2000 mL (>40%)
Pulse (beats/minute)	Normal/<100 (mild tachycardia)	>100	>120	>140
Systolic blood pressure (mmHg)	Normal	Normal	60–80	<60
Tissue perfusion indicators	Postural hypotension	Peripheral vasoconstriction (cold clammy)	Pallor, restlessness	Collapse, air hunger
Urinary output (mL/hour)	Normal	20–30	5–15 (Oliguria)	Anuria
Capillary refill	Normal	May be delayed	Delayed	Delayed

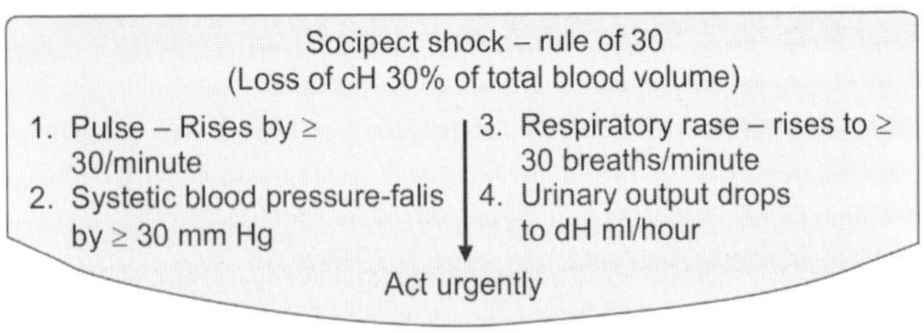

FIG. 2: Rule of 30 for assessment of postpartum hemorrhage.

  - Rapid infusion of crystalloid that is 1.5-2.5 L of Ringer's lactate or normal saline, followed by colloid and blood product if need arises
  - Foley catheterization to look for urine output, hematuria and making bladder empty for uterine tone and meassage
  - Oxygen inhalation and basic life-support, if needed
  - Call for help for member of the team, which should include anesthetist, senior obstetrician, OT nurse and running nurse

  Golden hour is the first hour after beginning of PPH when the resuscitative measures, if provided, give the maximum probability of maternal revival. Aggressive, prompt and focused initial resuscitative measures in golden hour play crucial role in survival of the mother
- Early decision for the corrective operative measures should be taken by a senior obstetrician before irreversible shock or dilutional coagulopathy sets in
- Medical management of PPH: medical management of PPH comprises of two main categories: (i) uterotonic, (ii) medication, which promotes coagulation or correct abnormalities of coagulation
  - Uterotonic
    - Oxytocin: it is the first-line oxytocic agent to prevent and treat PPH. It can be administered IM or IV. For AMTSL, 10 unit IM is given within one minute of delivery of child if there is no other baby. For therapeutic purpose, 20–40 unit in 500 mL of crystalloid infusion is given at 10–40 drop per minute. It is a nonapeptide and has biological similarity to antidiuretic hormone (ADH) so the large dosage can cause oliguria and water toxicity
    - Ergot alkaloid: ergot alkaloids such as methylergonovine and methylergometrine cause strong titanic uterine contraction. For PPH, IM dosage of 0.25 mg is usually given. It can cause significant rapid rise of blood pressure, so it is contraindicated in pre-eclampsia, hypertension and cardiac disease
    - Prostaglandin: 15-methylated prostaglandin F2-alpha is a potent uterotonic agent that has a long duration of action of 4–6 hours. It is usually given 250 microgram IM or local in uterine muscle up to a maximum of eight dosages. Prostaglandin agent may cause bronchospasm and rise of blood pressure so relative contraindications are bronchial asthma and hypertensive disorder. It can cause gastrointestinal side effect like vomiting, diarrhea and fever

  Misoprostol is prostaglandin E analog which can be used for prevention and treatment of PPH where oxytocin and prostaglandin F2-alpha are not available or storage facility are not feasible. Misoprostol is inexpensive, has good shelf-life at room temperature and does not need parenteral administration. It can be given orally, vaginally, rectally and sublingually. Usual dosages are 400–1,000 microgram for PPH. Diarrhea and fever are few side effects.
  - Hemostatics: the antifibrinolytic agent, tranexamic acid, prevents binding of plasminogen and plasmin to fibrin, may have a role in control of PPH in situation where coagulation is compromised and/or there is oozing from uterine surface. The use of recombinant factor as a hemostatic agent has been reported in some cases of PPH in dosage of 60–120 μg/kg. However, its use as a general practice guideline is not recommended

Table 2 contains the salient features of all uterotonic drugs.

TABLE 2: Salient features of uterotonic drugs used in prevention and treatment of postpartum hemorrhage

Drugs	Dose and route	Duration of action	Adverse effects	Contraindication
Oxytocin	5 units IV; 10 units IM; 20 units in 500 mL infusion	15–50 minutes	Insignificant hypotension and flushing, water intoxication in high doses (>200 units)	None
Ergometrine	0.2–0.25 mg IV or IM	1–2 hours	Nausea, vomiting, hypertension, vasospasm	Pre-eclampsia/ hypertension, cardiovascular disease
Syntometrine® (5 units oxytocin, 0.5 mg ergometrine)	1 ampoule IM	1–2 hours	Nausea, vomiting, hypertension, vasospasm	Pre-eclampsia/ hypertension, cardiovascular disease
15 methyl $PGF_{2\alpha}$	0.25 mg IM or IMM 0.25 mg in 500 mL infusion	4–6 hours	Vomiting, diarrhea, flushing, shivering, vasospasm, bronchospasm	Cardiovascular disease, asthma
Misoprostol	600 μg oral, sublingual 800–1000 μg, sublingual or rectal	1–2 hours	Nausea, diarrhea, shivering, pyrexia	None
Carbetocin	100 μg IM or IV	1–2 hours	Flushing	None

IM, intramuscular; IMM, intramyometrial; IV, intravenous.

Adapted with permission from Baskett TF. Essential management of obstetric emergencies. 4th edn. Bristol: Clinical Press, 2004.

SURGICAL MANAGEMENT

Surgical therapy for PPH can be as follows:
1. Method to reduce blood supply to uterus
2. Hysterectomy
3. Compression sutures to cause uterine contraction
4. Tamponade.

Method to Reduce Blood Supply to Uterus

Selective stepwise devascularization: these procedures can be done by any competent obstetric surgeon. The steps of it can be as follows:

- Uterine artery ligation: in this, an absorbable ligature is placed 2-3 cm medial to uterine artery with a large round body needle anterior to posterior through the myometrium approximately 1-2 cm medial to broad ligament. The suture is then directed posterior to anterior through clean avascular space in broad ligament close to lateral border of uterus and tied. The suture is placed at the junction of corpus and lower uterine segment. The technique is of mass ligature, and there is no need to dissect or mobilize uterine artery. It is effective in 75% of cases[18]
- Ovarian artery ligation: the anastomosis of ovarian vessel with uterine vessel can be ligated near the insertion of utero-ovarian ligament. A suture is placed on ovarian artery near the uterine cornua
- Internal iliac ligation: this should be attempted only by experienced surgeon who is well-versed in pelvic anatomy and retroperitoneal course of ureter. At present, it is performed less frequently because of availability of good uterotonic and procedure being time consuming and complicated. If it fails, it is important to proceed quickly for more definitive therapy like hysterectomy.[19] The technique of internal iliac ligation is to open peritoneum over common iliac artery by incising between infundibulopelvic ligament and round ligament. The ureter is identified at the site of branching of common iliac artery. The internal iliac artery is grasped with Babcock clamp and gently elevated. Then a long nonabsorbable silk suture is passed beneath the artery 2-3 cm distal to bifurcation where anterior division of internal iliac artery is located. Only a blunt tipped instrument as Mixter clamp should be used. The tip of clamp should be passed in a medial to lateral direction to reduce the chance of vessel injury. Pulsation of external iliac artery must be checked before tying the ligature. By bilateral ligature of anterior division of internal iliac artery, there is 85% reduction in pulse pressure distal to ligature, thus turning an arterial pressure approaching to venous circulation. It leads to hemostasis via clot formation. Risks of procedure are accidental injury to ureter, external iliac ligature and injury to internal iliac vein. Figure 3 explains complex pelvic vasculature system and sites of selective devascularization
- Definitive surgery: hysterectomy is required in approximately 1 in 1,000 deliveries for PPH.[20] On failure of medical and conservative surgical therapy, the decision of obstetric hysterectomy should be made in time. In cases of placenta accreta, hysterectomy should be the primary

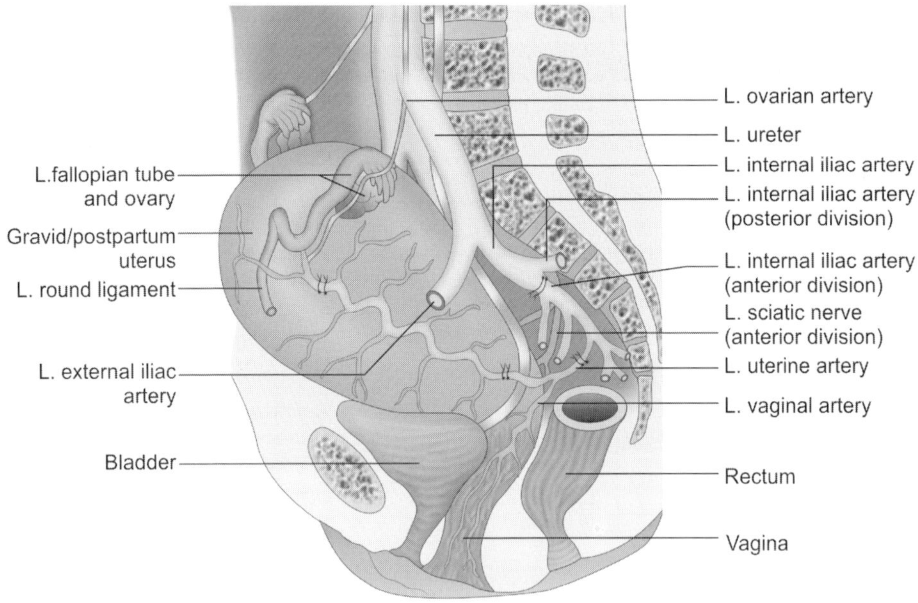

FIG. 3: The complex vascular distribution to the pelvic organs.

and planned procedure especially if the woman does not wish for future fertility. The technique of obstetric hysterectomy is similar to gynecological hysterectomy, but the following points should be considered while performing obstetric hysterectomy:

- The blood flow to the uterus is tremendous at term pregnancy and minimal error in dissection may lead to life-threatening situation
- There are more chances for injury to adjacent structure especially ureter and bladder
- Usually the patient is already compromised and hemodynamically unstable, so speed is important consideration
- Engorged and edematous tissue in pregnancy is liable to slippage of ligature.

In the hemodynamically unstable patient, the quick clamp, cut and drop technique should be used as rapidly as possible and the uterus is removed. When hemostasis is secured, the pedicles are tied. If the patient is relatively stable, it is good practice to keep pedicle small, and pedicles are carefully cut and doubly ligated. Total hysterectomy is generally the procedure of choice as lower uterine segment and cervix are frequently the site of bleeding. However, subtotal hysterectomy can be considered if bleeding is caused by atonic uterus, and patient is hemodynamically unstable. Urinary injury can complicate 5–22% of cesarean hysterectomy. Urinary bladder injury is most common, and, if suspected, should be confirmed on operation table by injecting methylene dye through Foley catheter. If confirmed, they should be repaired in the two layers by fine delayed absorbable suture like vicryl 3-0/2-0 with indwelling catheterization for 14 days. If ureteric injury is suspected, urologist opinion should be taken. Injection of indigo carmine 5–10 mL IV is given and passage of dye is visualized. Cystoscopy can be done to confirm urine passing through both ureteric orifices.

It is important to have multidisciplinary team for obstetric hysterectomy, as maternal mortality associated with emergency obstetric hysterectomy can be as high as 5%.[21]

Compression Suture

Compression suture involves suture around the uterus to oppose the anterior and posterior wall of the uterus. Compression sutures are tied only if uterine compression effectively controls bleeding. Following types of compression sutures are described:

- B-lynch suture: it was first described by Christopher B Lynch. It is vertical brace suture around the uterus. In this, uterus must be opened either during cesarean section or laparotomy after vaginal delivery. Steps of B-lynch suture is summarized in Figure 4
- Modified B-lynch: in this, two separate sutures are used, one for each side
- Hayman suture: in this, uterine cavity is not opened and explored. It is quicker and simpler in technique (Fig. 5A)
- Cho multiple square technique: in this, multiple full thickness square suture applied. There is risk of uterine synechiae and pyometra due to restriction in drainage of uterine cavity (Fig. 5B).

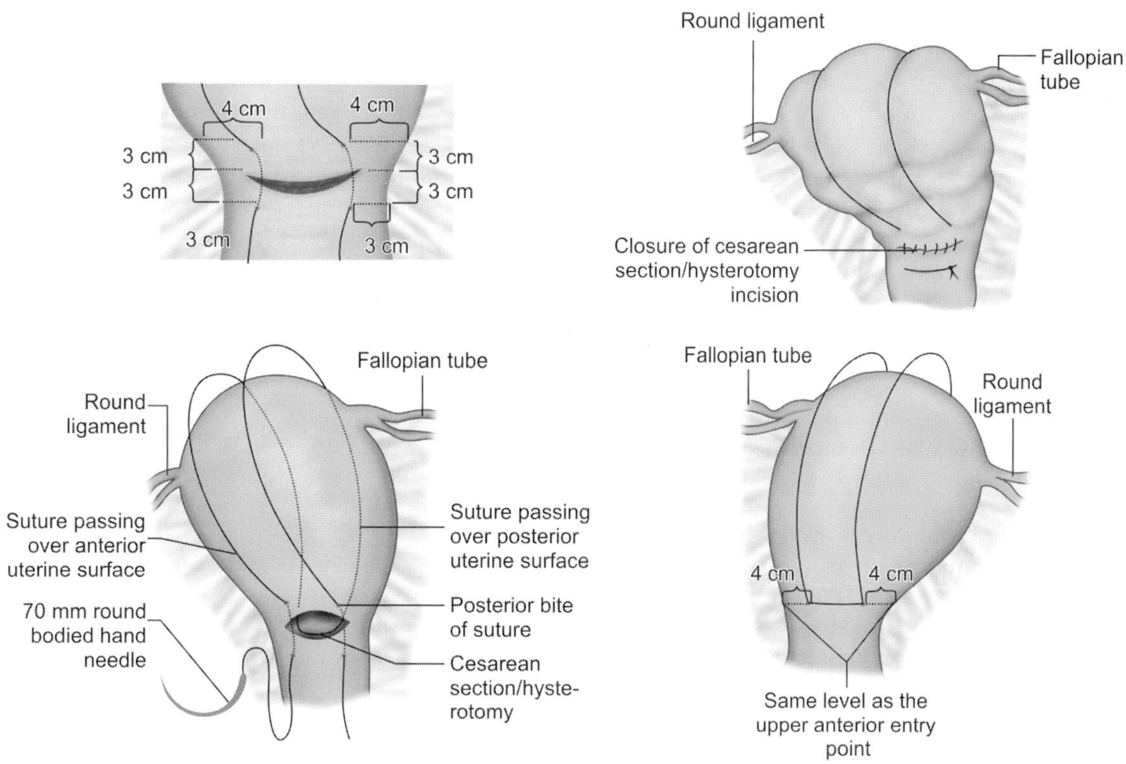

FIG. 4: Steps of B-Lynch compression suture.

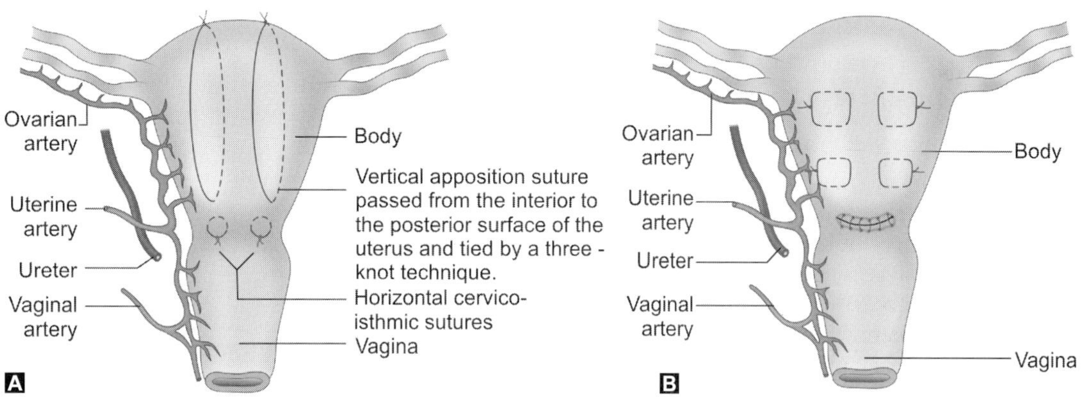

FIGS 5A AND B: **A,** Hayman suture; **B,** Cho multiple square suture.

Uterine Tamponade

A variety of techniques have been used to tamponade uterine cavity in the management of PPH, especially when there is oozing from uterine surface. Tamponade test is useful test to determine whether an intrauterine balloon will be effective or not.[22] Balloon tamponade is the least invasive and simple approach especially in PPH following vaginal delivery. It can be done by:

- Sengstaken-Blakemore esophageal catheter
- Bakri balloon catheter
- Foley catheter
- Condom or surgical glove catheter.

In the process, catheter is inserted in uterine cavity, outer end of catheter is connected to warmed normal saline. About 150–200 mL saline is infused to inflate balloon or condom till the balloon is palpable per abdominally or visible at cervical lumen (Fig. 6). The hydrostatic pressure of fluid acts as tamponade. The tamponade is fixed at inner thigh of the woman. Intravenous oxytocin infusion is continued, antibiotic given and vitals are monitored carefully.

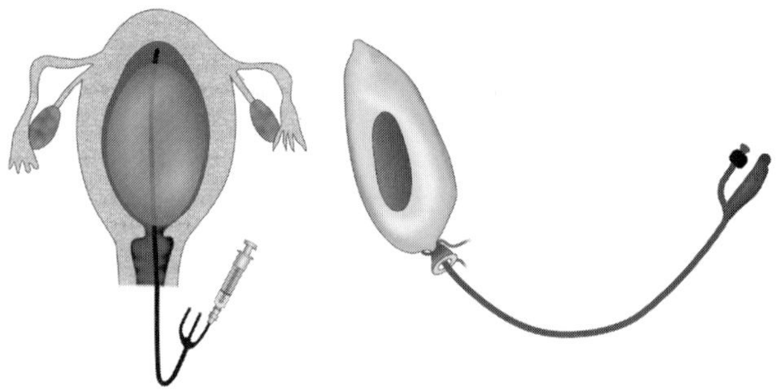

FIG. 6: Balloon uterine tamponade with Bakri balloon. Condom tied to Foley catheter.

Tamponade is considered successful if bleeding stops in 10–20 minutes. Tamponade is kept for 12–24 hours and then gradually removed.

It is a lifesaving procedure especially in low resource settings and during transport of patient to higher health facility with reported success rate of 60–71%.[23,24]

Uterine packing with 10 cm gauge has been used for controlling PPH, but now very infrequently used due to risk of infection and concealed hemorrhage. Recently, there has been renewed interest in this method as a method of emergency uterine tamponade. To make it easier and faster, the sterile plastic bag is first introduced in uterus and the bag is then packed with a 5 metres long strip of 8 cm wide gauze, which is folded twice. The gauze could be soaked in antiseptic cream.[25]

Embolization of Uterine Artery and Internal Iliac Artery

Radiographic embolization of uterine artery and internal iliac artery has come as an alternative modality for PPH management at tertiary care centers.[26] The catheter in vessels can be placed prophylactically in the radiology department in patient with risk of severe PPH like placenta accreta or also can be done as emergency procedure. Embolization is performed only after delivery of the baby. However, this procedure can be done in relatively hemodynamically stable patient. If women get pregnant, there is a risk of IUGR and recurrence of PPH in future pregnancy.

Management of Genital Tract Laceration

In case of traumatic PPH, the genital tract should be explained under good light, anesthetic with good equipment and an assistant. Genital tract should be visualized methodically from below upward. Hematomas are evacuated and packed for 12–24 hours. Cervical and vaginal tear are meticulously stitched. Patient is kept under observation for further bleeding and vitals. Intravenous fluid and blood product are given as per the clinical and laboratory values.

Management of Retained Placenta

If placenta is not expelled within 15 minute of delivery of baby, the manual removal of placenta should be considered without delay. In the absence of bleeding, the time frame of 30 minute is advocated, while in case of bleeding; immediate management of retained placenta is mandatory. Management of retained placenta should be done under general anesthesia with full aseptic precautions. Prior catheterization is a must. Uterus is stabilized by grasping fundus by abdominal hand; the other hand is introduced in vagina following the cord. When placental margin is located, placenta is peeled off the uterine wall like motion of separating leaves of a book. When placenta is completely separated, the placenta is withdrawn. Placenta is seen for completeness, if not a uterine cavity is again explored to take out remaining piece of placenta or membrane. Oxytocic is continued at the end of separation of placenta. Uterus contraction is assured, and the patient is kept under observation.

HAEMOSTASIS Algorithm

A systematic and stepwise management of PPH can be achieved with the use of the mnemonic "HAEMOSTASIS" following each step in rapid succession. The mnemonic is conveniently divided into two parts: medical and surgical.

General Medical Management

H: Ask for help
A: Assess (vital parameters, blood loss and resuscitate)
E: Establish etiology, ecbolic, ensure availability of blood
Establish etiology: 'four Ts'—tone, tissue, trauma, thrombin
Ecbolics (syntometrine, ergometrine, bolus syntocinon)
Ensure availability of blood and blood products
M: Massage the uterus
O: Oxytocin infusion, prostaglandins (intravenous, rectal, intramuscular, intramyometrial)

Specific Surgical Management

S: Shift to operating theater
Bimanual compression
Anti-shock garment, especially if transfer is required
T: Tissue and trauma to be excluded and proceed to tamponade balloon uterine packing
A: Apply compression sutures
S: Systematic pelvic devascularization (uterine, ovarian, quadruple, internal iliac)
I: Interventional radiology, uterine artery embolization
S: Subtotal or total abdominal hysterectomy

The Golden Hour

Severe hemorrhage can lead to cardiovascular failure. As the severity depends on body weight, hemoglobin levels, and body metabolism, emergency measures should be initiated if the estimated blood loss is more than one-third of the woman's blood volume. Blood volume [mL] = weight [kg] × 80) or more than 1000 mL or a change in hemodynamic status. As more time elapses between the onset of severe shock and resuscitation, the changes of survival decrease because metabolic acidosis sets in. The "golden hour" is the time at which resuscitation must be commenced to ensure the best chance of survival. The probability of survival decreases sharply after the first hour if the patient is not effectively resuscitated.[27]

For the general acute management of PPH, a "rule of 30" has been proposed. If the patient's systolic blood pressure (SBP) falls by 30 mmHg, heart rate (HR) rises by 30 beats/min, respiratory rate increases to more than 30 breaths/min and hemoglobin or hematocrit drop by 30%, and/or her urinary output is less than 30 mL/h, then the patient is most likely to have lost at least 30% of her blood volume and is in moderate shock leading to severe shock.[28]

The use of "Shock Index" (SI) may also be valuable in the monitoring and general management of women with PPH. It refers to HR divided by the SBP. The normal value is 0.5–0.7; however, with significant hemorrhage, it increases to 0.9–1.1.[31] The change in SI of an individual patient appears to be better correlate in identifying early acute blood loss than the HR, SBP, or diastolic blood pressure used in isolation.[29]

SPECIAL SITUATIONS IN POSTPARTUM HEMORRHAGE

Magnesium Sulfate

Women, who have received prolonged magnesium sulfate for seizure prophylaxis in pre-eclampsia, are at increased risk of atonic PPH.

Uterine Inversion

Uterine inversion occurs in 1 in 2,000 deliveries and causes severe hemorrhagic shock. Besid aggressive fluid and blood transfusion, uterine replacement is promptly requires. The techniques are manual replacement and use of hydrostatic pressure.[6]

Morbid Adherent Placenta

Morbid adherent placenta as cause of severe PPH is on the rise due to alarmingly increasing rates of primary cesarean section. A multidisciplinary approach is required for the management of these cases. Antenatal diagnosis and preoperative planning for obstetric hysterectomy or radiographic embolization and availability of blood product gives the good outcome.

CONCLUSION

The PPH remains one of the major obstetric complications and causes of maternal morbidity and mortality. The incidence of PPH can be reduced drastically by good antenatal care, identification of risk patient, and most importantly, the strict and universal adherence to AMTSL. PPH management and outcome, test the efficiency and adequacy of any obstetric healthcare system. Early recognition, aggressive and appropriate management with good teamwork can reduce morbidity and mortality in large number of cases. Availability of good choice of uterotonic, blood component therapy, and choice of conservative surgeries and method has changed the prognosis of PPH favorably. It is essential to fill in the gaps in obstetric care health system by imparting knowledge and skills to every level of healthcare providers.

REFERENCES

1. Khan KS, Wojdyra D, Say L, Gülmezoglu AM, Van Look PF. WHO analysis of cause of maternal death: a systematic review. Lancet. 2006,367:1066-74.
2. AbouZahr C. Global burden of maternal death and disability. Br Med Bull. 2003:67:1-11
3. American College of Obstetricians and Gynecologists. Practice Bulletin: Clinical Management guidelines for Obstetrician-Gynecologists, Number 76, October 2006: postpartum hemorrhage. Obstet Gynecol. 2006:108:1039-47.
4. Combs CA, Murphy EL, Larvs RK Jr. Factors associated with postpartum hemorrhage with vaginal birth. Obstet Gynecol. 1997:77:69-76.
5. Oyelese Y, Scorza WE, Mastrolia R, Smulian JC. Postpartum hemorrhage. Obstet Gynecol Clin North Am. 2007;34(3):421-41, x.
6. Sadhana Gupta; A Comprehensive Text Book of Obstetrics and Gynecology. New Delhi, India: Jaypee Brothers; 2011. pp. 540-9.
7. International Federation of midwives; International Federation of Gynecology & Obstetrics; Joint State Management of 3rd stage of labor to prevent postpartum hemorrhage; London: FIGO; 2003.
8. World Health Organization. WHO new guidelines for prevention and treatment of postpartum haemorrhage. Geneva: WHO; 2012.
9. Hema Diwakar, Azay Dhawle. AMTSL, WHO recommendation and global scenario. FOGSI Safe Motherhood Bulletin. 2013;4(1):20-4.
10. Revathy Janakiram. Prevention of postpartum hemorrhage in society and hospital. FOGSI Safe Motherhood Bulletin. 2013; 4(1):17-21.
11. Mobeen N, Durochar J, Zeberi N, Jahan N, Blum J, Wasim S, et al. Administration of misoprostol by trained traditional birth attendant to prevent PPH in home birth in Pakistan – A randomized placebo controlled trial. BJOG. 2011;118:353-61.
12. Rajbhandari S, Hodkins S, Sanghvi H, McPherson R, Pradhan YV, Baqui AH, et al. Expanding uterotonic protection following childbirth through community based distribution of misoprostol: operational research study in Nepal. Int J Gynecol Obstet. 2010;10813:282-8.
13. Young W, Karavolos S, Damodaram M, Madgwick K, Milestone N, Al-Habib A, et al. Observational accuracy and reproducibility of visual estimation of

blood volume in obstetrics: how accurate and consistent are health care professional; Arch Gynecol Obstet. 2010;281:207-13.
14. Maslovitz S, Barkai G, Lessing JB, Ziv A, Many A. Recurrent obstetric management mistake identification by simulator. Obs Gynecol. 2007;109:1295-1300.
15. Zuckerwise LC, Pettker CM, Illuzzi J, Raab CR, Lipkind HS. Use of novel visual aid to improve estimation of obstetric blood loss. Obstet Gynecol. 2014;123(5):982-6.
16. Debdas AK. Debdas postpartum hemorrhage bag. FOGSI Safe Motherhood Bulletin; 2013;4(1):15-6.
17. Rajat Ray. Defining and diagnosis of postpartum hemorrhage. FOGSI Safe Motherhood Bulletin. 2013;4(1)14.
18. Leary JA. Uterine artery ligation in control of postpartum hemorrhage. J. Reprod Med. 1995;40:189-93.
19. Evas C, Mc Shaw P. The efficacy of Internal Iliac Ligation in obstet haemorrhage. Surg Gyn Obste. 1985;160:200-3.
20. Habeek D, Be Carebic R. Emergency peripartum hysterectomy in a tertiary obstetric center 8-year evaluation. Fetal Diag Ther. 2007;22:139-42.
21. Kwee A, Bots ML, Visser GH, Bruinse HW. Emergency peripartum hysterectomy: a prospective study in Netherland. Eur J Obstet Gyne Reprod Biol. 2006;124:187-92.
22. Condous GS, Arulkumaran S, Synands I, Chapman R, Sinha A, Razvi K. The "Tampanode Test" in management of massive postpartum hemorrhage. Obstet Gynecol. 2002:101:767-72.
23. Seror J, Allouche C, Elhaik S. Use of Sengstaken-Blakemore tube in massive postpartum hemorrhage: a series of 17 cases. Acta Obstet Gynecol Scand. 2005;84(7):660-4.
24. Bakri YN, Amri A, Abdul Jabbar F. Tamponade-balloon for obstetrical bleeding. Int J Gynaecol Obstet. 2001;74(2):139-42.
25. Arul Kumaran S, Vikram S Talaulikar. Role of uterine and pelvic tamponade in management of postpartum hemorrhage. FOGSI Safe Motherhood Bulletin. 2013;4(1):39-42.
26. Soncini E, Pelicelli A, Larini P, Marcato C, Monaco D, Grignaffini A. Uterine artery embolization in treatment and prevention of postpartum hemorrhage. Int J Gynaecol Obstet. 2007;96(3):181-5.
27. Kakibde A, Daviss BA, Acosta A, Herschderfer K. Postpartum hemorrhage today; ICM/FIGO initiative 2004-2006. Int J Gynaecol Obstet. 2006;94:243-53.
28. Chandraharan E, Arulkumaran S. Massive postpartum haemorrhage and management of coagulopathy. Obstet Gynaecol Reprod Med. 2007;17:119-22.
29. Birkhahn RH, Gaeta TJ, Terry D, Bove JJ, Tloczkowski J. Shock index in diagnosing early acute hypovolemia. Am J Emerg Med. 2005;23(3):323-6.

CHAPTER 24

Birth Injuries

Charu Mittal

INTRODUCTION

In all cultures, the process of childbirth is an eagerly awaited and welcome event, expected to bring joy to the family. However occasionally, this dynamic and often unpredictable event can become a difficult and traumatic one for the mother or baby or both. Traumatic complications can occur in the form of birth injuries. Such birth injuries can be either maternal or neonatal. These injuries usually result from lack of care and precautions during difficult vaginal delivery with big baby, shoulder dystocia, breech delivery or instrumental delivery, especially incorrectly applied forceps.

If undiagnosed and not managed promptly, they can cause significant morbidity and occasionally, mortality. Awareness of such traumatic conditions and taking few precautions during delivery can help to reduce the risk as well as maintaining a keen postnatal evaluation and vigilance can allow early detection and management in most cases.

MATERNAL INJURIES

These can range from relatively minor, localized types, such as perineal or cervical lacerations, and tears up to the more severe visceral ones, such as bladder damage or rupture uterus. As per their location, they can be described as follows:

- Puerperal hematomas: vulvar, paravaginal, pelvic hematomas
- Tears: perineal tears, cervical tears, vaginal tears, colporrhexis
- Visceral injuries: urethral, bladder, and rectal injuries which may result in urethrovaginal fistula (UVF), vesicovaginal fistula (VVF) or rectovaginal fistula (RVF)
- Rupture uterus.

Puerperal Hematomas

Vulval, Paravaginal, and Pelvic Hematomas

Incidence

Puerperal hematomas occur in 1:300–1:1,500 deliveries, and rarely, are a potentially life-threatening complication of childbirth. They can occur after either a spontaneous or operative vaginal delivery.[1]

Risk factors

These include instrumental delivery (vacuum or forceps), nulliparity, preeclampsia, coagulation disorders, multiple gestation, trauma during infiltration for pudendal or paracervical block, and improper surgical repair of an episiotomy.

Mechanism

The mechanism of puerperal hematoma formation in the anterior and posterior triangles involves rupture of branches of the internal pudendal and inferior rectal arteries, respectively. Rupture of descending branches of the uterine artery can cause paravaginal hematoma formation. Rupture of any vessel of the perineal venous plexus may also result in a hematoma. Trauma to the above mentioned vessels may also occur as a result of a compound presentation, rapid descent, lacerations from an operative vaginal delivery including unrecognized tissue caught in the vacuum cup. Vessel rupture can occur without laceration of the superficial tissue due to shearing effect. Since the subcutaneous tissue in the vagina is quite pliable, hematomas can achieve massive dimensions before expansion ceases.

Symptoms and signs

The patient usually complains of pain or an inability to void depending on the size and location of the hematoma. On examination, there may be a visible bulge over the perineum, paravaginal hematoma may be felt on lateral vaginal wall or in case of pelvic hematomas there could be increasing pallor and hemodynamic instability. Thus, vital signs and symptoms of hypovolemia should be monitored more frequently in situations where concealed bleeding is suspected because failure to recognize ongoing retroperitoneal bleeding can be fatal.

Diagnosis

The diagnosis of puerperal hematomas is generally obvious but should prompt a thorough vaginal examination to determine the extent of the lesion. The hematoma may be located at the vulva (Fig. 1), may track into the vagina (Fig. 2) or may expand into the retroperitoneal space or abdominal cavity. In the latter case, blood loss can be concealed leading to hemodynamic instability if not recognized and addressed promptly. Clot formation can cause pressure necrosis and skin rupture resulting in life-threatening hemorrhage.

Imaging studies, like ultrasound and magnetic resonance imaging, can help define the dimensions of the paravaginal or pelvic hematomas in situations where physical examination is inconclusive.

Management

This depends on prompt recognition and the clinical acumen of the patient-care team. In some situations, the clot may provide sufficient pressure to tamponade bleeding vessels. If the hematoma is of average size and not acutely expanding, conservative measures, such as icepacks, observation, pain management, and bladder drainage, may be all that is necessary. In situations where there is an acutely expanding hematoma or a concealed hemorrhage is suspected, more aggressive management is required. The patient's input and output should be closely monitored, intravenous access should be maintained in case fluid resuscitation and/or blood transfusion is a possibility, and the other members of the healthcare team, such as operation theater staff and anesthesiologist should be notified. Surgical management includes prophylactic antibiotic administration, evacuation of the hematoma, identification and ligation of the bleeding vessel(s), and repair of the dead space or cavitary defect left from the evacuated hematoma. Artery embolization has been used successfully to manage ongoing hemorrhage in situations where bleeding is not controlled with conventional surgical techniques.

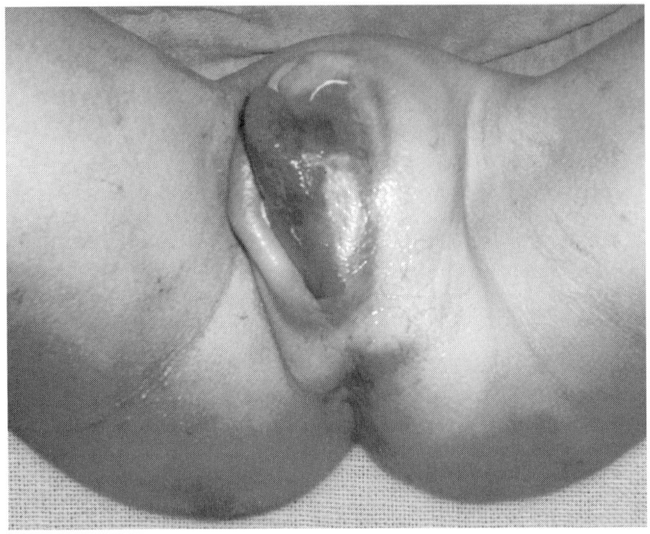

FIG. 1: Vulval hematoma *(For color version, see Plate 3).*

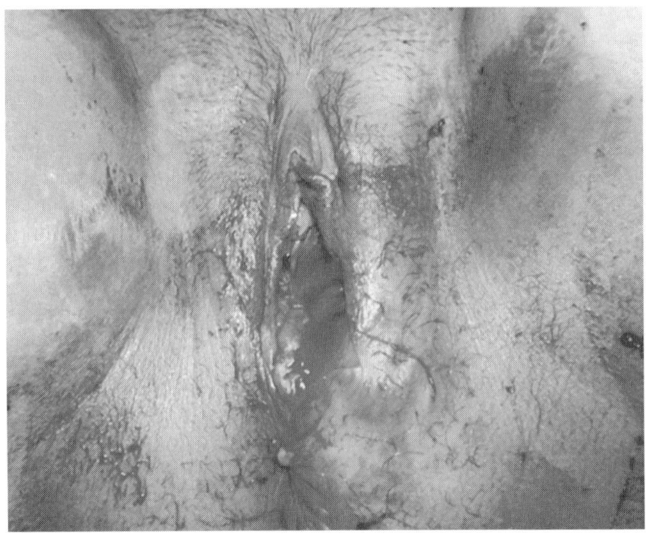

FIG. 2: Paravaginal hematoma *(For color version, see Plate 3).*

Tears

Perineal Tears

The perineum needs to be inspected after every delivery for timely detection and repair of any perineal tears which may range from minor ones involving only perineal skin or vaginal mucosa up to the major ones involving disruption of anal sphincter and anal mucosa.

Classification

There are various classifications of perineal tears. The following classification, described by Sultan, has been adopted by the International Consultation on Incontinence and the Royal College of Obstetricians and Gynecologists:[2]

- First-degree perineal tears: injury to perineal skin only
- Second-degree perineal tears: injury to perineum involving perineal muscles, but not involving the anal sphincter

- Third-degree perineal tears: injury to perineum involving the anal sphincter complex:
  - 3a: less than 50% of external anal sphincter (EAS) thickness torn
  - 3b: more than 50% of EAS thickness torn
  - 3c: both EAS and internal anal sphincter (IAS) torn
- Fourth-degree perineal tears: injury to perineum involving the anal sphincter complex (EAS and IAS) and anal epithelium.

Risk factors for third-degree tears have been identified in a number of retrospective studies.[3] With an overall risk of 1% of vaginal deliveries, the following factors are associated with an increased risk of a third-degree tear:

- Forceps delivery (up to 7%)
- Nulliparity (up to 4%)
- Second stage longer than 1 hour (up to 4%)
- Shoulder dystocia (up to 4%)
- Midline episiotomy (up to 3%)
- Persistent occipitoposterior position (up to 3%)
- Birth weight over 4 kg (up to 2%)
- Induction of labor (up to 2%)
- Epidural analgesia (up to 2%).

Identification of women at risk may facilitate the use, or avoidance, of certain obstetric interventions to minimize the occurrence of childbirth-associated perineal trauma. In a study by Groutz et al., primiparity, younger maternal age, Asian ethnicity, longer duration of second stage of labor, forceps or vacuum-assisted delivery, and heavier newborn birth weight were significantly more common among women who had third- or fourth-degree perineal tears.[4]

Management

As a good practice point, it is recommended that if there is any doubt about the grade of third-degree tear, it is advisable to classify it to the higher degree rather than lower degree.

Lacerations must be repaired immediately after delivery if possible and preferably within 24 hours. First- and second-degree tears can be easily repaired in layered manner from within outwards with chromic catgut and/or delayed absorbable suture material like polyglactin.

Principles of repair are aseptic precautions, adequate lighting and exposure with retraction by trained assistants, ensuring hemostasis, obliterating dead spaces, and correct tissue approximation.

The overall risk of obstetric anal sphincter injury is 1% of all vaginal deliveries. With increased awareness and training, there appears to be an increase in detection of anal sphincter injury. Obstetricians who are appropriately trained are more likely to provide a consistent, high standard of anal sphincter repair and contribute to reducing the extent of morbidity and litigation associated with anal sphincter injury.

Obstetric anal sphincter injury encompasses both third- and fourth-degree perineal tears.

A third-degree perineal tear is defined as a partial or complete disruption of the anal sphincter muscles, which may involve either or both the EAS and IAS muscles.

A fourth-degree tear is defined as a disruption of the anal sphincter muscles with a breach of the rectal mucosa. The IAS plays a role in the maintenance of continence. One study has reported that the incidence of anal incontinence is increased in women who had both IAS and EAS damage compared with those who had EAS damage alone. Inclusion of the IAS in the classification below would allow differentiation between future incontinence related to IAS injury rather than EAS alone. It is, however, recognized that in acute obstetric trauma, identification of the IAS may not be possible but a record of the degree of EAS damage (> or <50%) should be possible in all cases.

Technique of surgical repair

- For repair of the EAS, either an overlapping or end-to-end (approximation) method can be used, with equivalent outcome. When repair of the EAS muscle is being performed, either monofilament sutures such as polydioxanone (PDS) or modern braided sutures, such as polyglactin can be used with equivalent outcome
- Where the IAS can be identified, it is advisable to repair separately with interrupted sutures. When repair of the IAS muscle is being performed, fine suture size, such as 3-0 PDS and 2-0 polyglactin, may cause less irritation and discomfort
- When obstetric anal sphincter repairs are being performed, burying of surgical knots beneath the superficial perineal muscles is recommended to prevent knot migration to the skin. Women should be warned of the possibility of knot migration to the perineal surface, with long-acting and nonabsorbable suture materials.

Postoperative management

The use of broad-spectrum antibiotics is recommended following obstetric anal sphincter repair to reduce the incidence of postoperative infections and wound dehiscence. The use of postoperative laxatives is recommended to reduce the incidence of postoperative wound dehiscence. All women should be offered physiotherapy and pelvic-floor exercises for 6–12 weeks after obstetric anal sphincter repair. Women who have had obstetric anal sphincter repair should be reviewed 6–12 weeks postpartum by a consultant obstetrician and gynecologist. If a woman is experiencing incontinence or pain at follow-up, referral to a specialist gynecologist or colorectal surgeon for endoanal ultrasonography and anorectal manometry should be considered. A small number of women may require referral to a colorectal surgeon for consideration of secondary sphincter repair.

Cervical Tears

Cervical tears are usually directed longitudinally, commonly with lateral occurrence. Often they are small but can be long enough to reach up to vaginal vault or rarely open into the base of the broad ligament. Rarely, annular, circumferential or bucket handle tears (Fig. 3) can occur along the circumference of the cervix usually detaching the cervix from the vagina partially or completely.

Predisposing factors[5]

- Powerful uterine contractions against an unyielding cervical os (annular detachment)
- Scarred cervix: old tears, conization, amputation
- Delivery of large babies
- Manual cervical dilatation
- Forceps application before full dilatation
- After-coming head of breech.

Diagnosis

Excessive vaginal bleeding occurring with a palpably well contracted uterus can suggest a cervical tear and should prompt a thorough and adequate visual inspection of the cervical rim with adequate lighting and vaginal wall retraction using speculum and three ring forceps/sponge holders applied constantly on cervical rim at 12 o'clock position with the other two forceps being applied sequentially in a clockwise or anticlockwise manner. Slight fundal pressure by assistant can aid in exposing the cervix. Always examine complete cervical rim at first inspection and then suture any tear(s). As a routine precaution, cervix should be inspected after every difficult or instrumental delivery. If cervix is not actively bleeding and is too thinned out for efficient suturing, it is practically advisable to wait for 24–48 hours when cervix would have retracted and be in a thicker condition for suturing.

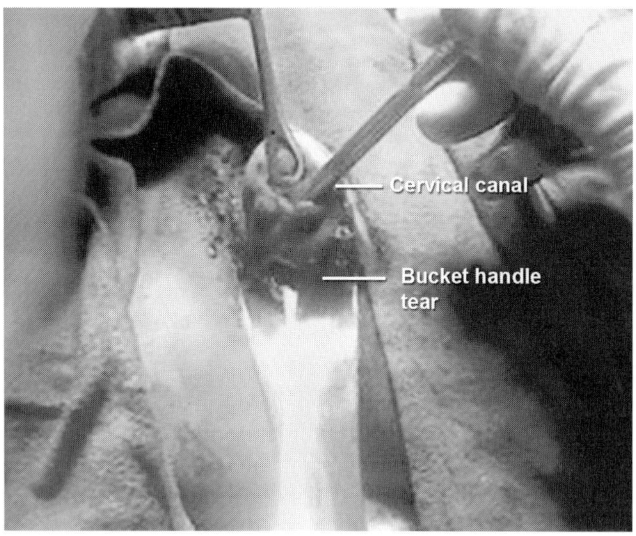

FIG. 3: Bucket handle tear *(For color version, see Plate 4)*.

Technique of repair

- Visualize the apex by holding anterior and posterior margins of the tear with ring forceps. Bucket handle tears must be sutured transversely for apposition
- Confirm the depth since any suspicion of extending upwards into lower uterine segment or broad ligament would require an exploratory laparotomy
- Once apex is visualized, gentle traction helps to reach 1 cm beyond the apex to start suturing with chromic catgut or delayed absorbable suture, like polyglactin, preferably with interrupted mattress sutures or continuous interlocking sutures
- Even though visualized, if one cannot reach beyond apex of a deep cervical tear with the first stitch, a practical tip is to apply the first suture at a lower accessible area and then give slight traction to bringer higher cervical tissue into visual field for securing apex
- Care must be taken to avoid needle prick injury of vaginal walls lying in proximity to the tear, which if undetected, can itself cause further bleeding or hematoma formation.

Sequel

Deep tears if undiagnosed and unrepaired can be fatal and even if not bleeding actively may lead to cervical incompetence. Small tears due to widening of cervical opening or ectropion can occasionally cause discomfort in the form of excessive vaginal discharge. Overenthusiastic suturing can rarely lead to narrowing or cervical stenosis.

Vaginal Tears

Vaginal tears during childbirth are also called perineal lacerations or tears as described earlier. Specific type of vaginal tear called colporrhexis is mentioned further in the text.

Colporrhexis

This condition is also called as rupture of the vaginal vault.[6] This can occur with deep cervical tears which have extended into the paracervical tissue or lower part of the broad ligament.

Symptoms and signs

They may not give rise to any symptoms unless the upper end reaches upwards into lower segment and the uterine vessels are damaged where there would be severe hemorrhage. Even if asymptomatic, infection can occur in such tears leading to pelvic thrombophlebitis and cellulitis while cervical incompetence can be a later sequel.

Predisposing factors

This form of rupture of vaginal vault can occur if forceps or vacuum is applied with an incompletely dilated cervix or during a difficult breech extraction.

Management

It is important to identify this injury because prompt diagnosis can help to avoid hysterectomy in such cases. Management involves suturing of anterior and posterior lips of cervix by pulling them down with ring forceps. Controlling hemorrhage in case of active bleeding where uterine vessels are torn, may require laparotomy if apex cannot be visualized from below. During laparotomy, ligation of anterior division of internal iliac artery can help in easy identification by reducing bleeding followed by repair.

Visceral Injuries

Urethral Injury

These injuries, though rare, can be encountered after difficult instrumental deliveries. The procedure of symphysiotomy, which was practiced earlier, can also be occasionally associated with urethral injury. Usually injuries in this region often heal spontaneously and indwelling catheterization for 7–10 days is advisable. If undetected and severe, urethral injury can result in UVF. Distal fistulae may be asymptomatic or there may be complaints of spraying of urine or an abnormal urinary stream. Midurethral fistulae can be asymptomatic or may present with stress incontinence or recurrent cystitis. Proximal fistulae involving urethra and bladder neck can mimic VVF.

Repair of UVF can be more difficult than VVF due to extensive urethral loss and lack of viable tissue. Usual success rate of repair is 50%.[6] Tissue interposition in the form of Martius flap is useful in most cases with higher success rates.

Bladder Injury

Bladder injury can range from temporary paralysis up to direct injury to bladder wall during cesarean section or difficult forceps delivery, while delayed presentation in cases of avascular necrosis due to obstructed labor can present as VVF.

Temporary paralysis: loss of tone of bladder due to overdistension during labor can be avoided by instruction for frequent voiding rarely resorting to drainage by intermittent catheterization during labor. Treatment is by indwelling catheterization for a short duration of 2–3 days.

Stress urinary incontinence: this can also be a sequel of vaginal delivery. This can be associated with a cystocele which is usually caused by overstretching of supports of anterior vaginal wall in region of bladder neck. It can occur if a fold of anterior vaginal wall is pushed down in front of the presenting head or pulled down during forceps extraction. If persistent and significant, stress urinary incontinence would require appropriate repair.

Vesicovaginal fistula: VVF was earlier a common sequel to be neglected, prolonged, obstructed labor with gross pelvic disproportion. It can have a delayed presentation after some days due to avascular necrosis from compression of maternal tissues between fetal head and pubic bones or rarely occurs immediately due to misjudged, difficult instrumentation in cases with pelvic disproportion leading to rupture of vesicovaginal septum.

Diagnosis

It may be obvious in large defects with constant leakage of urine while methylene blue dye two swab tests with instillation of dye into the bladder may be needed to identify small defects. Leakage through the fistula must be distinguished from stress incontinence where urine will be seen to come through urethral opening only when patient coughs.

Injury during cesarean section can rarely result in vesicocervical or vesicouterine fistulae where in the latter type, cyclical hematuria at the time of menstruation may be noted (Youssef's syndrome). Very rarely, extensive injury leading to ureteric damage can result in ureterovaginal fistula where ureter may open into the lateral fornix and urine may be seen coming in tell-tale spurts with no staining of the urine with methylene blue instilled in the bladder.

Management

Continuous drainage of bladder can help in closure of very small VVF while larger defects need layered closure. Repair of such fistulae are usually performed only after infection is treated and adequate healing and scarring of involved tissue has occurred to avoid apposing devitalized tissue. This may require a period of up to 3 months. Choice of vaginal route of repair versus abdominal route depends on the location, size, availability of surrounding healthy tissue for apposition, proximity of ureteric openings to defect, previous attempt at repair, operator experience and skills, etc.

Rectal Injury

This may be associated with unrecognized or improperly repaired complete perineal tear, especially at the apex, rarely central rupture of the perineum with rectal damage or rupture of posterior wall of vagina where fetal part, like foot can present through the anal canal.[7] Ischemic necrosis can occur in anterior wall of middle part of the rectum where it is compressed for a prolonged time against the flat sacrum in contracted midpelvis. Correct and timely diagnosis with adequate repair of tissues in a layered manner can prevent the development of RVF.

Rupture Uterus

This catastrophic event is an obstetrician's nightmare and an important cause of maternal morbidity and mortality. Though the incidence of rupture uterus due to neglected labor is steadily decreasing as institutional deliveries are being encouraged, the risk of rupture uterus in scarred uterus is constantly present while conducting a trial of vaginal birth after cesarean section (VBAC). The detection of rupture uterus would usually be an ante- or intrapartum events while rarely late, silent rupture during expulsion of baby in second stage may be detected postnatally due to signs of developing hypovolemia. Routine palpation of lower segment is not advocated nor is it practically helpful in detecting such late rupture of lower segment.

Risk Factors

Risk factors include previous cesarean section, misuse of oxytocic drugs, multiparity, cervical scarring, difficult forceps delivery, manual removal of placenta (MRP), internal podalic version.

Sudden deterioration of general condition with signs of hypovolemia with or without externally visible hemorrhage following difficult vaginal delivery can indicate possibility of rupture. Rarely, there may be shortening of the cord due to extrusion of placenta through site of rupture into peritoneal cavity. Treatment involves exploration and repair or hysterectomy, if unrepairable.

Nerve Injuries[8]

Nerve injuries sustained by the obstetric patient are generally short-lived, but can be a cause of significant short-term and more rarely, long-term morbidity. Lower extremity neuropathies can occur in association with labor and delivery, but upper extremity injuries can be sustained as well. Neurologic injury can occur during labor, spontaneous vaginal delivery, operative vaginal delivery, or cesarean section. Acute nerve injury may occur as a result of transection, traction, compression, or vascular injury. Compression or traction on a nerve can result in compromised perineural blood flow and resulting ischemia. This can cause focal demyelination and conduction block, which generally resolves quickly via remyelination. In more serious injuries, there can be axonal damage, which resolves more slowly, and can cause permanent impairment of nerve function.

Lumbosacral Plexus

Lumbosacral plexus or trunk injury can cause foot drop, and other neurologic symptoms consistent with peripheral mononeuropathies (single or multiple) of the nerves that branch from the plexus. Risk factors for lumbosacral plexus or trunk injuries include fetal macrosomia, malpresentations (occiput posterior or brow presentation), and certain pelvic features like platypelloid pelvis, shallow anterior sacral ala, and flattened sacral promontory.

Lateral Femoral Cutaneous Nerve

Injury to the lateral femoral cutaneous nerve causes burning, pain, or numbness of the anterolateral thigh and known as meralgia paresthetica syndrome. The lateral femoral cutaneous nerve is at risk of injury during prolonged pushing with hip flexion as the nerve is compressed under the inguinal ligament. A wide Pfannenstiel incision at cesarean section may lead to transection of the lateral femoral cutaneous nerve.

Femoral Nerve

Injury to the femoral nerve can result in quadriceps weakness and/or sensory symptoms of the anteromedial thigh. Motor compromise can cause significant functional impairment. Compression of the femoral nerve under the inguinal ligament can occur with prolonged pushing in extreme hip flexion.

Common Peroneal Nerve

Injury to the common peroneal nerve can result in paresthesias on the dorsa of the feet and lateral calves, as well as foot drop. There have been several cases of peroneal nerve palsy related to prolonged squatting during childbirth, hyperflexion of the knees during delivery,[6] and direct compression of the nerve over the fibular head by the patient holding her own legs with fingers placed over the anterior tibia and palms over the fibular head.

Sciatic Nerve

There is a possibility of sciatic nerve stretch injury in high lithotomy position with prolonged hip hyperflexion and excessive external rotation.

Obturator Nerve

The lithotomy position causes angulation of the obturator nerve as it leaves the obturator foramen. Pudendal nerve blocks have also been known to cause hematomas and entrapment of the obturator nerve.

Upper Extremity Nerves

For the patient undergoing cesarean section under general anesthesia, the usual arm positioning risks apply. The brachial plexus can be injured by improper arm positioning including hyperabduction or positioning of the armboards below the level of the operating table. Inadequate or improper padding over the bony prominences of the elbow may result in ulnar nerve injury.

Nerve injury in the obstetrical patient must be a consideration by obstetricians. It is important to prevent these injuries by avoiding prolonged hyperflexion and abduction of the hips during birth. This may be accomplished by allowing for passive descent of the fetal head into the pelvis before pushing begins. However, this technique may not be successful in preventing nerve injuries related to compression of nerves in the pelvis by the fetal head.

NEONATAL INJURIES

Neonatal birth injury is an important cause of perinatal morbidity and mortality in developing countries with inadequate delivery facilities and unskilled birth attendants.[9] The superficial injuries may be apparent at birth while the internal trauma may manifest later in some cases. They can be described on the basis of location.

Injury to Scalp/Head

Bruises/Lacerations

These can be iatrogenic, affecting the scalp, face, and other soft parts. They can occur due to abrasion by forceps or vacuum, fetal scalp electrodes, incised wound during cesarean section or episiotomy. Buttocks in breech delivery and eyelids, face or nose in face presentation may be swollen and congested. In case of active bleeding, injuries may require to be sutured and dressing applied. Though they appear alarming to parents, usually they do not have long-term sequelae unless pyogenic infection occurs.

Caput Succedaneum

This soft, edematous swelling of the superficial tissues forms over the presenting part usually after the membranes have ruptured, especially where presenting part comes in contact with cervical rim (cervical caput). Pelvic caput occurs in severe cephalopelvic disproportion where rim of contact is fetal head and pelvic brim. It can also form after application of ventouse for delivering the fetal head in second stage. It is usually harmless and self-limiting and resolves within a few days.

Cephalohematoma

This is a collection of blood under the pericranium. It can be differentiated from caput by the fact that it appears some hours after delivery, is limited to particular bones due to attachment of periosteum and commonly develops in rapid labor. Differentiated from meningocele by the fact that meningocele always lies over a suture line and there will be impulse on coughing. Commonly occurs over parietal bone, occasionally over frontal or occipital bones. It is a soft, circumscribed, fluctuant, and incompressible swelling. Later, edges become hard due to organization of blood. It can occur following forceps delivery or occasionally following normal delivery. Prognosis is good with spontaneous resorption of blood occurring over a course of 6–8 weeks. Precautions are avoidance of trauma and prevention of infection, hence drainage is not advisable.

Indentation/Depression of Skull

This is rarely seen. Injury is situated on parietal or frontal bone near the anterior fontanelle. It occurs due to flattening of maternal pelvis. It can occur spontaneously due to head being pressed against the projecting sacral promontory by uterine contractions or during application of suprapubic pressure for delivery of after-coming head in breech. In forceps delivery, it is due to pressure of head against promontory rather than from blades of the forceps. Slight degree of depression may be asymptomatic and requires no intervention. Spontaneous restoration occurs within first year of life. However, if symptomatic with slow heart beat and slow respiration, it may be associated with subdural hematoma requiring intervention.

Skull Fracture

These can be produced due to malapplication of forceps blades, especially where child's head is grasped obliquely when occipital and frontal bones can be damaged due to pressure. Fracture may be associated with cephalohematoma, extradural or subdural hemorrhage or hematoma. A fissure fracture may be asymptomatic while a depressed fracture can produce pressure effects. Associated subdural hematoma in symptomatic cases requires surgical decompression. Separation of condyloid of occipital bone can occur due to severe difficulty in extracting an after-coming head of breech. In such a case, death can result from intracranial hemorrhage or direct injury to medulla.

Injury to Nervous System (Brain/Spinal Cord/ Peripheral Nerves)

Intracranial Hemorrhage

This can occur due to excessive molding of fetal head, difficult forceps deliveries with wrong application of blades, sudden compression and decompression of head in precipitate labor or during delivery of the after-coming head in breech delivery. It may be extradural or subdural in location. Baby may be delivered still born if the hemorrhage is fatal while there may be severe birth asphyxia or respiratory depression in other cases. During recovery phase, signs of cerebral irritation can appear like high-pitched cry, convulsions, restlessness, jitteriness, neck retraction, incoordinate ocular movements, bulging fontanelle, etc. Cerebral depression can manifest as shallow respiratory movements, depresses reflexes, apathy, and refusal to suckle. Those infants who make a rapid recovery with no residual symptoms, like abnormal neurological signs or convulsions, usually develop normally while the prognosis for others is guarded.

Spinal cord: it may be damaged during extreme traction on trunk during difficult breech delivery or delivery of impacted shoulders due to fracture of odontoid process or fracture dislocation of cervical vertebrae where instantaneous death can occur due to compression of medulla or there can be injury to vertebral arteries or their branches leading to ischemic damage to grey matter in cervical cord. Slight injuries to lower cervical, dorsal or lumbar regions may lead to complete paralysis of the legs or arms and legs.

Facial Nerve Palsy

Facial nerve can be injured at site of its exit from stylomastoid foramen due to pressure of forceps blades, or occasionally during normal deliveries. Injury becomes apparent during crying when mouth gets drawn to unaffected side while there is failure to close eyelid on affected side. Sucking is not affected. It is usually unilateral and self-limiting. Treatment involves protection of eye with antiseptic ointment while baby sleeps.[10]

Brachial Plexus Injury (Erb's Palsy and Klumpke's Paralysis)

Injury to brachial plexus can occur due to stretching of the roots or trunks of the plexus during breech delivery or shoulder dystocia. The injury results from the head being pulled sideways to one or the other side, away from shoulder. Erb's palsy results from damage to upper roots, i.e., 5th and 6th cervical nerve roots. Arm on affected side lies limply with elbow extended, forearm pronated, and wrist flexed. External splinting is advised with external rotation and abduction at right angle. Passive movements and massaging of the arm are advised. Complete recovery can take several weeks. Occasionally, permanent damage may persist. Klumpke's paralysis is caused by an injury to the brachial plexus in which the first thoracic nerve (T1) and the eighth cervical nerve (C8) are injured before or after they have joined to form the lower trunk. This type of injury usually occurs during difficult vaginal deliveries, especially in situations where the mother is small and the baby has a large birth weight. The prevalence of all brachial plexus injuries, including Klumpke's palsy, is 0.2–2.5/1,000 births.

Injury to Viscera

Abdominal and Thoracic Organs

Injury to liver, kidneys, adrenals or lungs can occur during breech delivery. The most common result of injury can be hemorrhage which may be fatal, if severe. The treatment is to correct the hypovolemia and anemia. Specific surgical treatment may be required as indicated for the injured organs.

Injury to Musculoskeletal System

Sternomastoid

Damage to fibers and blood vessels of sternomastoid muscle can lead to hemorrhage and hematoma formation followed by contracture. It can result from excessive lateral flexion of the neck, difficult breech delivery or vigorous attempts at delivery following shoulder dystocia. The swelling appears after about 7–10 days after delivery and there is transient torticollis which should not be massaged. Gentle movements with stretching of neck muscles are helpful and swelling usually subsides by 6 months of age.

Fracture of Bones

The bones most likely to fracture in a difficult vaginal delivery are clavicle, humerus, and femur.

Clavicle

Fracture of clavicle usually causes no discomfort, there is usually no difficulty in movement of arm and injury may be overlooked.

Humerus

Separation of upper epiphysis of humerus may occur resulting in a varying degree of deformity. In severe injury hand may be paralyzed.

Femur

This can be fractured during breech delivery due to excessive traction on lower limbs.

Fractures are usually of the greenstick type but may occasionally be complete. Nature remarkably shapes the broken bones of a newborn child and rapid healing is common with callus formation. Deformity rarely occurs even with bone ends not being well aligned.

PREVENTION OF INJURIES

Proper antenatal care can help in detection of high-risk pregnancy, like short stature, malpresentations, big baby, pelvic deformity or inadequacy, uterocervical prolapse, history of previous cesarean section, myomectomy or cervical amputation, and repair of complete perineal tear after previous delivery. Such women would be at higher risk of injury during delivery and require appropriate intrapartum management to reduce the risk of maternal and neonatal injuries.

Maternal Injury

- Judicious selection of patients for trial of vaginal delivery
- Close monitoring of labor to detect problems with descent and cervical dilatation to prevent risks of obstruction and prolonged compression of maternal tissues due to cephalopelvic disproportion
- Judicious use of oxytocin infusion only when indicated with close monitoring to avoid uterine hyperstimulation. It should never be administered intramuscularly before delivery
- Avoid difficult forceps application with preference for cesarean section in such cases
- Avoid forceps application and breech delivery through an incompletely dilated cervix
- Timely and adequate episiotomy in rigid perineum, instrumental delivery, breech delivery
- Destructive operations when indicated to be performed only by experienced personnel
- Careful removal of adherent placenta during MRP
- Proper examination of maternal tissues after delivery to assess need for repair
- Trial of VBAC after proper selection with close monitoring of vital signs only in appropriate institution with facilities for fetal monitoring and immediate cesarean section
- During cesarean section:
  - Open visceral peritoneum in upper part of incision after palpation to avoid injury to underlying structures, like bladder and bowel
  - Avoid low incision on lower uterine segment which might damage bladder
- Close vigilance for early detection and management of injuries.

Neonatal Injury

- Elective cesarean section for contracted pelvis, cephalopelvic disproportion, breech, transverse lie can reduce the risk of traumatic delivery
- Place two fingers between head and maternal tissues for protection of fetal scalp/buttocks during episiotomy or incision on lower uterine segment during cesarean section
- Avoid undue stretching and lateral flexion of neck during delivery of head
- Apply ventouse cup over fetal scalp for short duration only
- Avoid incorrect application of forceps. Forceps blades when applied should be in correct biparietal plane
- Precautions and care with gentleness during breech delivery: Deliver after-coming head patiently without undue haste to avoid sudden compression and decompression, forceps may be applied for after-coming head, avoid acute extension of cervical spine, trunk should not be pulled too much to either side, limbs must be delivered gently without excessive pressure, rotation of trunk by grasping thoracic cage and not abdomen, performing Lovset's maneuver with hands on pelvic girdle.

CONCLUSION

While conducting delivery, whether by normal or operative routes, every maternal healthcare provider must be aware of the potential situations which can result in birth injury. Appropriate preventive and corrective measures for tackling such situations can reduce the risk for maternal and neonatal damage to a large extent and provide improved quality of life instead of resulting in prolonged suffering and disability.

REFERENCES

1. Barrett T. (2012). Hematoma after a vacuum delivery. In: Pearls of Exxcellence. [online] Available from www.exxcellence.org/pearls.php?id=53 [Accessed June, 2015].
2. Sultan AH. Editorial: Obstetric perineal injury and anal incontinence. Clin Risk. 1999;5(5):193-6.
3. The Royal College of Obstetricians and Gynaecologists (RCOGs). (2015). Third- and Fourth-degree Perineal Tears, Management (Green-top Guideline No. 29) [online] Available from www.rcog.org.uk/en/guidelines-research-services/guidelines/gtg29/. [Accessed June, 2015].
4. Groutz A, Cohen A, Gold R, Hasson J, Wengier A, Lessing JB, et al. Risk factors for severe perineal injury during childbirth: a case-control study of 60 consecutive cases. Colorectal Dis. 2011;13(8):e216-9.
5. Kriplani A, Sumana G. Repair of tears: vaginal, perineal and cervical. In: Puri R, Malhotra N (Eds). Operative Obstetrics and Gynecology, 2nd edition. New Delhi, India: Jaypee Brothers Medical publishers; 2014. pp. 202-9.
6. Thompson JD. Vesicovaginal and urethrovaginal fistulas. In: Rock JA, Thompson JD (Eds). Telinde's Operative Gynecology, 8th edition. Philadelphia, PA, USA: Lippincott-Raven Publishers; 1997.
7. Myerscough PR. Maternal injuries. In: Baskett TF, Calder AA, Arulkumaran S (Eds). Munro Kerr's Operative Obstetrics, 12th edition. New Delhi, India: AITBS Publishers; 2014.
8. McDonald A, Natale R. Obstetrical nerve injury. Partner. 2008;31:1-3.
9. Myerscough PR. Neonatal asphyxia, birth injury, handicap. In: Baskett TF, Calder AA, Arulkumaran S (Eds). Munro Kerr's Operative Obstetrics, 10th edition. New Delhi, India: AITBS Publishers; 1995.
10. Daftary SN (Ed). The newborn. In: Holland and Brews Manual of Obstetrics, 16th edition. New Delhi, India: BI Churchill Livingstone; 1998.

CHAPTER 25

Inversion of Uterus

Kapil Malhotra

INTRODUCTION

Uterine inversion is a potentially fatal childbirth complication with a maternal survival rate of about 85%. It occurs when the placenta fails to detach from the uterus as it exits, pulls on the inside surface, and turns the organ inside out. It is very rare.

Uterine inversion is a rare complication of vaginal delivery in which the uterus partially or completely turns inside out. Complete inversion occurs when the uterus is turned completely inside out, with the very top of the uterus protruding through the cervix. The entire uterus rarely prolapses out of the vagina.

The immediate problem with uterine inversion is postpartum hemorrhage. Bleeding can be massive and patients may go into shock. Though this condition can be fatal, it can be successfully treated with rapid recognition, intravenous fluids, and blood transfusion.

DISCUSSION

Uterine inversion is classified not only by the degree of inversion but by the time of onset as well. The uterine fundus that has inverted and lies within the endometrial cavity without extending beyond the external os is called an incomplete inversion. Complete inversion describes an inverted fundus that extends beyond the external os.[1] A prolapsed inversion is one in which the inverted uterine fundus extends beyond the vaginal introitus.[2] A total inversion, usually nonpuerperal and tumor related, results in inversion of the uterus and vaginal wall as well.[1] In terms of onset of the inversion, acute describes the event occurring before cervical ring contraction. If the cervical ring has contracted, a subacute inversion has occurred. The inversion is classified as chronic if 4 weeks have elapsed before the event.[1,3,4]

BACKGROUND INFORMATION

The incidence of uterine inversion varies according to geographical location and ranges from 1:2,500 to 1:20,000.[5-7]

Classification According to Severity of Uterine Inversion[1]

- First degree: the fundus reaches the internal os. The inverted fundus extends to but not through the cervix (Fig. 1)
- Second degree: the body or corpus of the uterus is inverted to the internal os. The inverted fundus extends through cervix but remains in the vagina (Fig. 2)
- Third degree: the uterus, cervix and vagina are inverted and are visible. The inverted fundus coming out from vagina (Fig. 3).

Classification According to Timing of the Event[6,7]

- Acute: occurs within 24 hours of birth

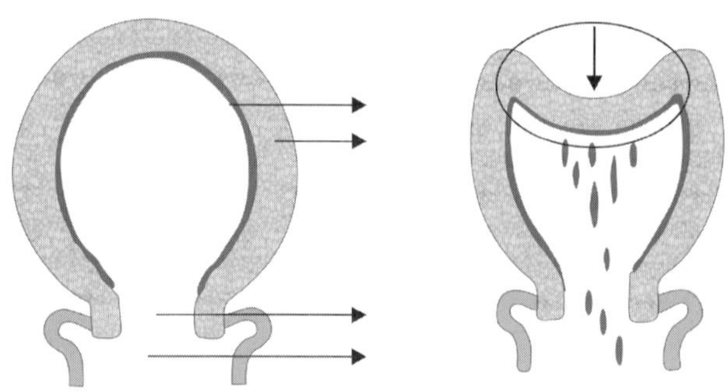

FIG. 1: First degree uterine inversion.

- Subacute: occurs after 24 hours, within 4 weeks
- Chronic: occurs after 4 weeks, rare.

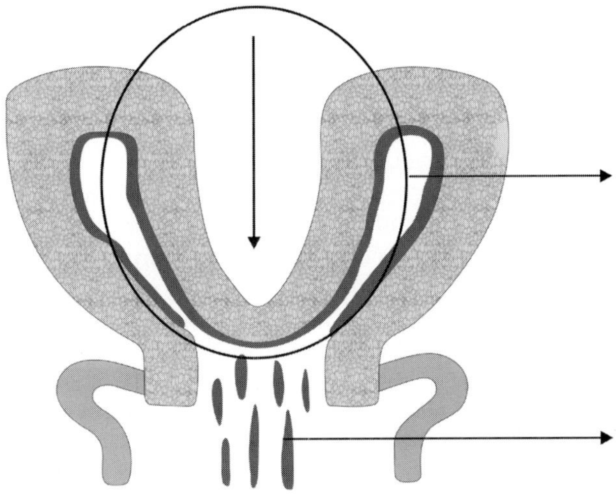

FIG. 2: Second degree uterine inversion.

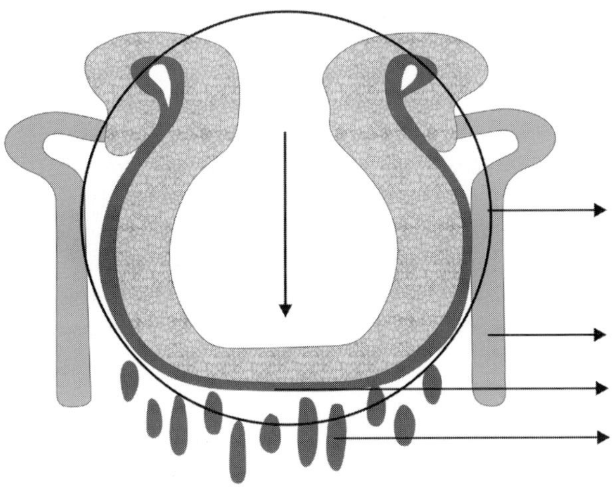

FIG. 3: Third degree uterine inversion.

CAUSES AND RISK FACTORS

These include:

- Mismanagement of the third stage, e.g. premature or excessive cord traction during active management of the third stage,[6-8] a combination of fundal pressure and cord traction to deliver the placenta, or use of fundal pressure when the uterus is atonic during placental delivery[7]
- Abnormally adherent placenta[6-8] (Fig. 4)
- Short umbilical cord[7,8]
- Spontaneous inversion of unknown etiology[7]
- Sudden emptying of a distended uterus[7]
- Nulliparity[6,8]
- Fundal placement of the placenta[6,7] (Fig. 5)
- Antepartum use of magnesium sulfate.[9]

SIGNS AND SYMPTOMS OF A UTERINE INVERSION

Signs and symptoms of uterine inversion may include:

- Postpartum hemorrhage[6,9]
- Shock[5,8] thought to be due to the parasympathetic effect caused by traction of the ligaments supporting the uterus, and hypotension with inadequate tissue perfusion[9]
- Severe abdominal pain[7]
- Physical examination can reveal first- or second-degree uterine inversion[7]

MANAGEMENT

Key points

- Concurrent maternal resuscitation with manual uterine replacement is the first line of management.
- If the placenta is still adherent following uterine inversion, leave in place to reduce blood loss.[4]
- Uterine rupture should be excluded prior to performing hydrostatic reduction of the uterus.

Principles of management are to treat the shock and replace the uterus. The patient should be moved rapidly to

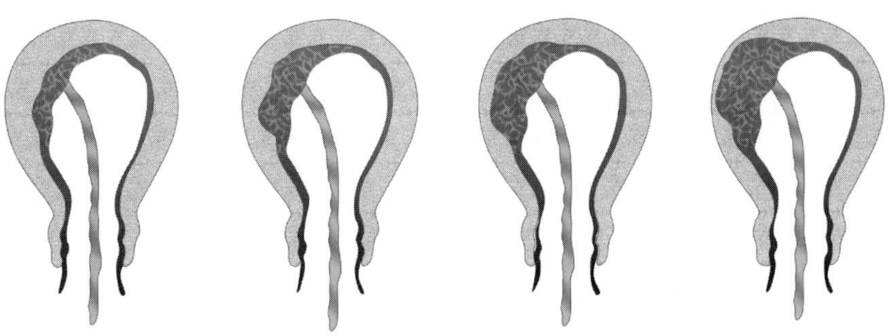

FIG. 4: Abnormally adherent placenta.

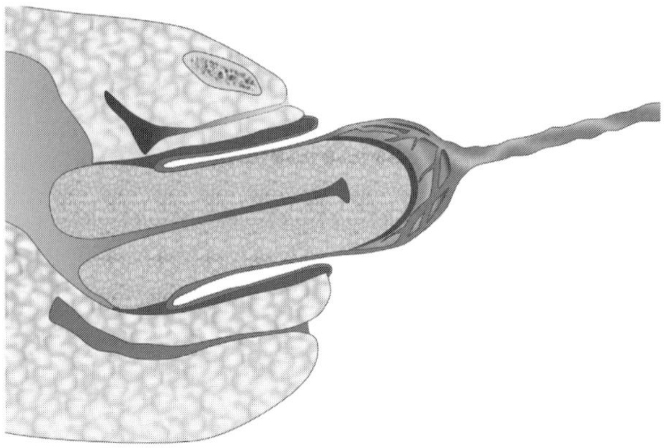

FIG. 5: Fundal placement of the placenta.

the operating room to facilitate anesthesia monitoring during this procedure. Usually this complication is only recognized after delivery of the placenta, wherein oxytocin has already been started, which just exacerbates the problem. The uterus clamps down around the inversion making it very difficult to perform a replacement. This is a true obstetrical emergency, so additional doctors, nurses, anesthesiologists should be summoned to the room to assist. The oxytocin should be turned off immediately. Giving tocolytics such as terbutaline or magnesium sulfate have a lower success rate. Halothane and nitroglycerine (100–200 µg intravenously) have a higher success rate. Once you have achieved uterine relaxation, place your fist into the vagina. Find the biggest part of the inversion and push with your fist cephalad to replace the uterus. This takes firm steady force, so keep your fist in the vagina if you need to rest your hand. Then continue more force toward the fundus to replace the uterus. You can use your left hand on the outside of the abdomen to help you feel where the fundus should be replaced. This helps to guide the angle of your fist in replacing the uterus. Once it is replaced, give the patient, misoprostol 1,000 µg rectally to help with increasing uterine tone. Other medications such as methergine and carboprost 250 µg can be used. If heavy bleeding, consider inserting a Bakri balloon into the uterine cavity to tamponade the bleeding.[8]

These patients have usually sustained heavy blood loss, and should be monitored in the intensive care unit postoperatively. If you have given nitroglycerine, they must have cardiac monitoring postoperatively. Other personnel should be monitoring vital signs, ordering blood products, assisting the anesthesiologist, drawing laboratory, and stabilizing the patient. Remember that nitroglycerine can cause hypotension, which can be reversed with ephedrine. If external replacement fails, a laparotomy may be required, in which the uterus is gently pulled the right way round using forceps.

Note:
- Maternal resuscitation while attempting uterine replacement should be initiated simultaneously.
- If the placenta is still in situ, leave in place until uterine replacement is complete.
- Attempt manual replacement of the uterus by re-inverting it, and keeping the hand in the uterus until firm contraction of the uterus is felt.[1]

If uterine replacement is unsuccessful:
- Insert two 16 gauge intravenous cannulae. Group and cross-match four units of blood and order a full blood picture.[10] Consider performing coagulation studies.[10,11]
- Commence intravenous fluids, if the woman has blood loss more than 1,000 mL and continues to bleed or show signs of clinical shock.[11] In consultation with the anesthetist, the volume and rate of fluids is adjusted according to the clinical situation. Warming of the solution may be required.
- If not already administered, withhold the oxytocic until uterine replacement is complete.[6]
- Assess vital signs—blood pressure, pulse, respirations, and oxygen saturation levels at 15-minute intervals (more frequently if maternal conditions necessitates). Monitor vital signs continuously as soon as practical with access to continuous monitoring equipment.
- Administer oxygen via a facemask.
- Insert an indwelling catheter. Monitor urine output.
- If the uterus is successfully replaced, commence an oxytocic infusion (30 IU oxytocin in 500 mL Hartmann's solution commencing at 240 mL/hour) as per PPH therapeutic infusion regimen.
- If the replacement of the uterus is not possible, resuscitate the woman and transfer her to operation theater immediately.

In Operation Theater:
- Stabilize the woman and obtain effective anesthesia.
- Relax the uterus with either:
  - Glyceryl trinitrate 600 µg—sublingual
  - Terbutaline 250 µg—subcutaneous
- Replace the uterus
- Administer prophylactic antibiotics:
  - Cefazolin 2 g intravenous—one dose only
  - Metronidazole 500 mg intravenous—one dose only

Commence oxytocin therapy following uterine replacement.

METHODS OF UTERINE REPOSITIONING

Manual Replacement (Johnson Maneuver)[10] (Fig. 6)

The uterus may require relaxation prior to manual replacement.

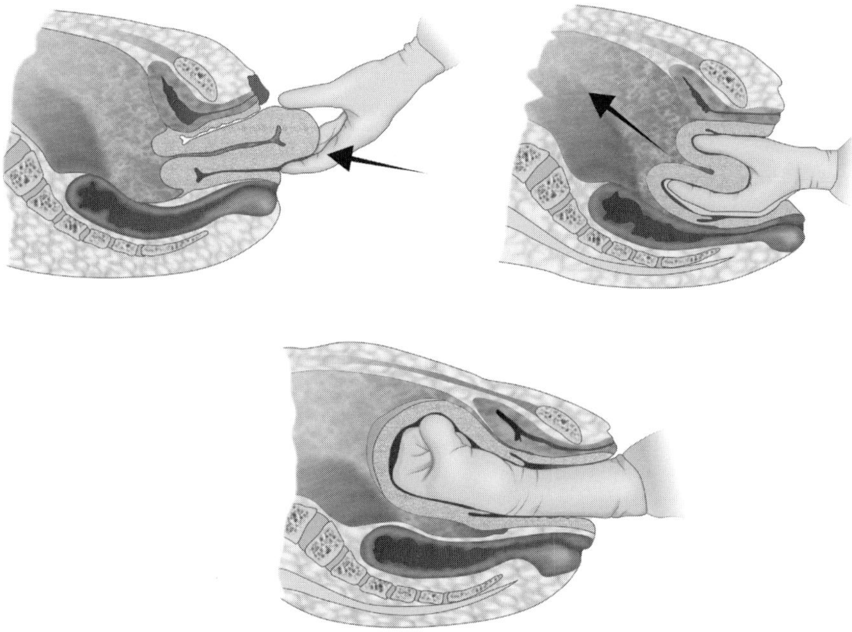

FIG. 6: Manual replacement (Johnson maneuver).

- Using the palm of the hand, push the fundus of the uterus along the direction of the vagina toward the posterior fornix[7]
- Then lift the uterus toward the umbilicus and return to its normal position[7]
- Maintain the hand in situ until a firm contraction is palpated.

Oxytocin therapy should be administered to initiate and maintain contraction of the uterus.

Hydrostatic Reduction (O'Sullivan's Technique)[10] (Fig. 7)

- Hydrostatic reduction is a method of reinverting the uterus by infusing warm saline into the vagina.

Note: Uterine rupture should be excluded prior to performing the procedure.[10]

- The women may be placed in the reverse Trendelenburg position[12] to assist gravity and reduce traction on the infundibulopelvic ligaments, round ligaments, and the ovaries.[13]

Method One

- Attach a 2 × 1 liter bag of warmed saline to a Y-cystoscopy giving set. Additional fluids may be required
- Insert the hand into the vagina with the open end of the tubing near the posterior fornix. Obtain a seal at the vaginal entrance by enclosing the labia around the wrist/hand to prevent fluid leakage.[13]

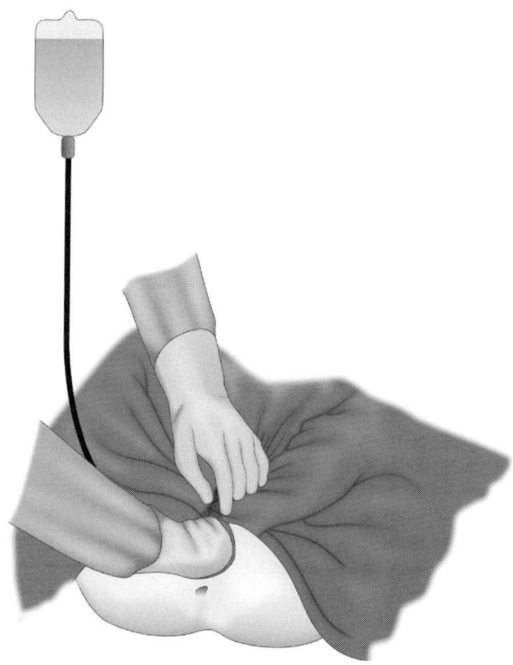

FIG. 7: Hydrostatic reduction (O'Sullivan's technique).

- Infuse warmed fluid under gravity. Several liters of fluid may be required.

Method Two

- Attach a 2 × 1 liter bag of warmed saline to a Y-cystoscopy giving set.

- Gently push the inverted uterus into the vagina[12]
- Insert a 6 cm (or appropriate sized) silastic ventouse cup into the lower vagina. Avoid pushing the cup deep into the vagina. Attach tubing to a container with warmed saline tubing or the giving set and then place it 1 meter above the patient[12-14]
- If leaking occurs at the introitus, gently withdraw the cup until it fits against the inner aspect of the introitus.

Following the procedure, the uterus should be digitally explored. The hand should be kept in the uterus until the oxytocic therapy produces a contracted uterus.[10-12]

New Technique (Ogueh and Ayida)[14]

Attaching the intravenous tubing to silicone cup used in vacuum extraction. By placing the cup in the vagina, an excellent seal is created (Fig. 8).

AFTER REPOSITIONING

- Discontinue uterine relaxant/general anesthesia
- Start infusion of oxytocin or ergot alkaloids
- Continue fluid and blood replacement
- Bimanual uterine compression and massage are maintained until the uterus is well-contracted and hemorrhage is ceased (Fig. 9)
- Remove placenta if retained following replacement of the inverted uterus
- Careful manual exploration to rule out the possibility of genital tract trauma
- Antibiotics
- Adequate analgesics
- Oxytocics ergot are continued for at least 24 hours
- Monitor closely after replacement to avoid reinversion.

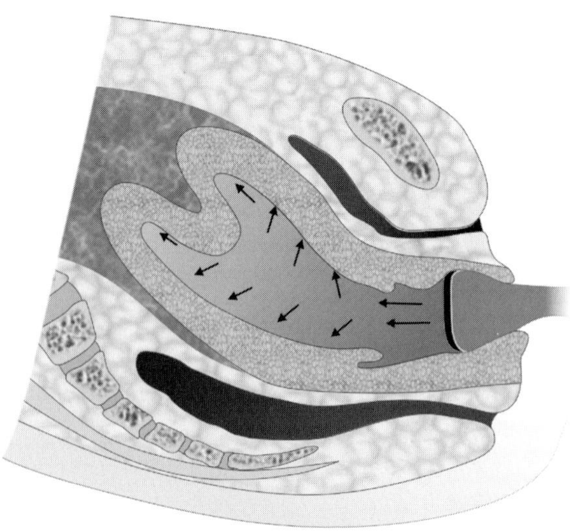

FIG. 8: New Technique (Ogueh and Ayida).

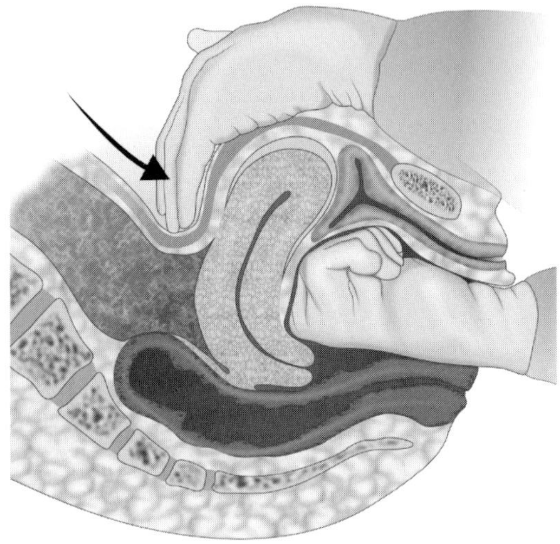

FIG. 9: Bimanual uterine compression.

MANAGEMENT OF CHRONIC UTERINE INVERSION

Surgical Management

- Abdominal route:
  - Huntington's procedure (Fig. 10)
    - Locate the cup of the uterus formed by the inversion
    - Dilate the constricting cervical ring digitally
    - Stepwise traction on the funnel of the inverted uterus or the round ligament is given with Allis forceps
    - Reapplied progressively as fundus emerges
  - Haultain's procedure (Fig. 11): incision is made in uterine wall posteriorly through the cervix, relieving cervical constriction to increase the size of the ring and allowing traction on the round ligament for the replacement of uterus with subsequent repair of incision from inside the abdomen
- Vaginal route
  - Spinelli's method: anterior colpotomy is done and incision on the constricting cervical ring is given for the replacement of uterus
  - Kustner's method: posterior colpotomy is done and incision of the cervix similar to that of Spinelli's method
  - Hysterectomy
    - Failure of conservative surgery
    - Family is completed
    - Sepsis.

PREVENTION

Many cases of acute uterine inversion result from mismanagement of the third stage of labor in women who

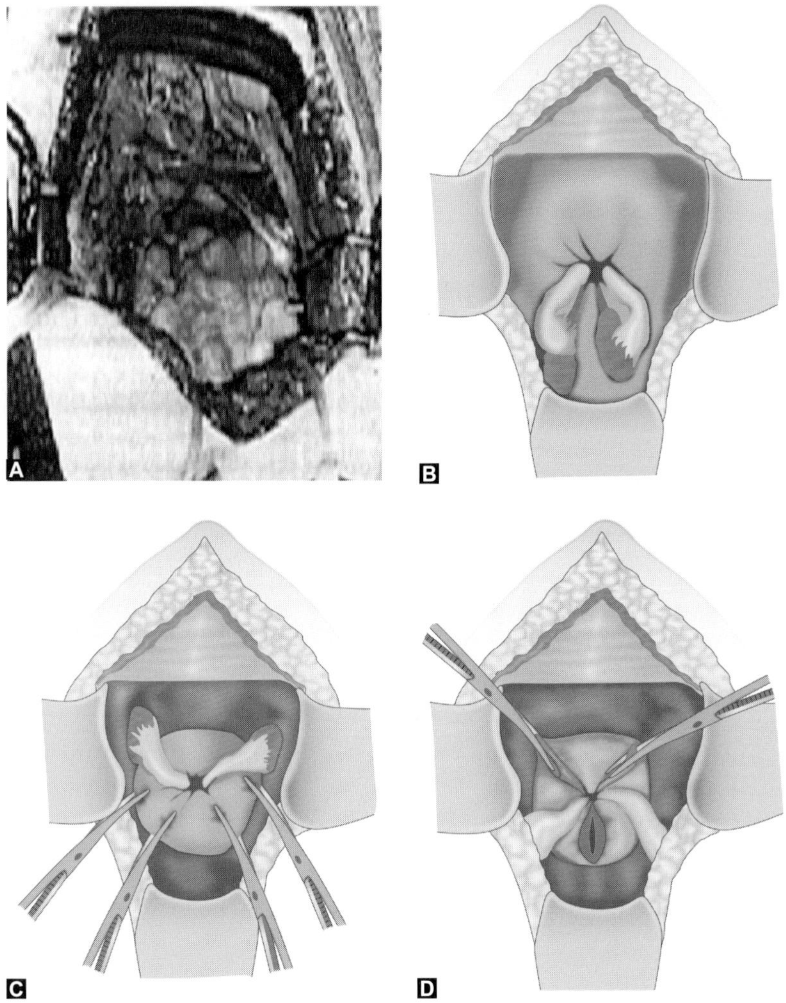

FIG. 10: Huntington's procedure.

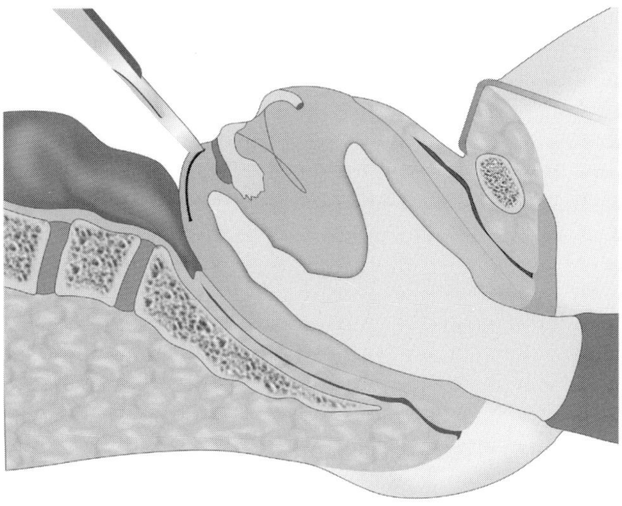

FIG. 11: Haultain's procedure.

are already at risk. Education and training of traditional birth attendants: lady health visitor (LHV), lady health worker (LHW), community midwives (CMW), junior doctors regarding active management of third stage of labor.

Maneuvers are to be avoided:

- Excessive traction on the umbilical cord
- Excessive fundal pressure
- Excessive intra-abdominal pressure
- Excessively vigorous manual removal of placenta.

CONCLUSION

In summary, uterine inversion can be a life-threatening obstetric complication. Although uncommon, if unrecognized, severe hemorrhage and shock will lead to maternal death. Manual manipulation aided by tocolytic or halogenated anesthetic agents is often successful in correcting the inversion. In the most resistant of inversions, surgical correction through the abdomen might be needed. In any case, the best prognosis is achieved by prompt recognition of the condition and immediate attempts to correct the inversion. Thus, it is important that physicians providing obstetric care be aware of the common signs of inversion so that the diagnosis can be determined and treatment initiated immediately.

REFERENCES

1. Salomon CG, Patel SK. Computed tomography of chronic nonpuerperal uterine inversion. J Comput Assist Tomogr. 1990;14:1024-6.
2. Lewin JS, Bryan PJ. MR imaging of uterine inversion. J Comput Assist Tomogr. 1989;13:357-9.
3. Momani AW, Hassan A. Treatment of puerperal uterine inversion by the hydrostatic method: reports of five cases. Eur J Obstet Gynecol Reprod Biol. 1989;32:281-5.
4. Zahn CM, Yeomans ER. Postpartum hemorrhage: placenta accreta, uterine inversion, and puerperal hematomas. Clin Obstet Gynecol. 1990;33:422-31.
5. You WB, Zahn CM. Postpartum hemorrhage: abnormally adherent placenta, uterine inversion, and puerperal hematomas. Clin Obstet Gynecol. 2006;49(1):184-97.
6. Mirza FG, Gaddipati S. Obstetric Emergencies. Sem Perinatol. 2009;33:97-103.
7. Coates T. Midwifery and obstetric emergencies. In: Fraser DM, MA C, (Eds). Myles Textbook for Midwives. 15th edition. London: Churchill Livingstone; 2009. pp. 625-47.
8. Majd HS, Pilsniak A, Reginald PW. Recurrent uterine inversion: a novel treatment approach using SOS Baki balloon. BJOG. 2009;116:999-1001.
9. Beringer RM, Patteril M. Puerperal uterine inversion and shock. Br J Anaes. 2004;92(3):439-41.
10. Grady K, Howell C, Cox C, (Eds). The Moet Course Manual. Managing Obstetric Emergencies and Trauma. 2nd edition. London: RCOG Press; 2007.
11. Royal College of Obstetricians and Gynaecologists. Prevention and Management of Postpartum Haemorrhage. Green-Top Guideline No. 52. London: RCOG; 2009.
12. Tan KH, Luddin NSY. Hydrostatic reduction of acute uterine inversion. Int J Gynecol Obstet. 2005;91:63-4.
13. Baskett TF. Essential Management of Obstetric Emergencies 170. 4th edition. Bristol: Clinical Press Limited; 2004.
14. Ogueh O, Ayida G. Acute uterine inversion: a new technique of hydrostatic replacement. Br J Obstet Gynaecol. 1997;104:951-2.

CHAPTER 26

Postpartum Collapse

Chanderdeep Sharma, Kewal A Mistry

INTRODUCTION

Maternal death is a very distressing condition for family and society as a whole. It is a direct indicator of level of health care of a nation. The importance of this unfortunate event was highlighted by the inclusion of this parameter (reduction of maternal mortality) in Millennium Development Goals set up by World Health Organization.

Postpartum maternal collapse is a catastrophic event, which directly contribute to maternal death. Even though exact data on maternal collapse is limited; however, a fairly accurate assessment of the same can be made from leading causes of maternal deaths (Fig. 1), i.e., hemorrhage, sepsis, and hypertension which are also leading causes of maternal collapse.[1]

Majority (75%) of obstetric patients admitted to intensive care unit (ICU) are postpartum, with hemorrhage and hypertension as the leading causes.[2]

DEFINITION

Maternal collapse is defined as an acute event involving the cardiorespiratory systems and/or brain, resulting in a reduced or absent conscious level (and potentially death), at any stage in pregnancy and up to 6 weeks after delivery.[3]

RISK FACTORS

Postpartum maternal collapse is a sudden dramatic catastrophic event which may occur in the absence of any significant risk factor. Nonetheless some of the predisposing risk factors are severe anemia, severe hypertensive disorder of pregnancy, coagulation abnormalities, sepsis, prolonged labor, previous cesarean section, morbid adherent placenta, poor socioeconomic status, pre-existing medical or surgical disorders with pregnancy (chronic hypertension, diabetes mellitus, cardiac disease, epilepsy, chronic liver or renal disease, etc.).

There are many causes of postpartum collapse. Table 1 enumerates the common causes of postpartum maternal collapse.

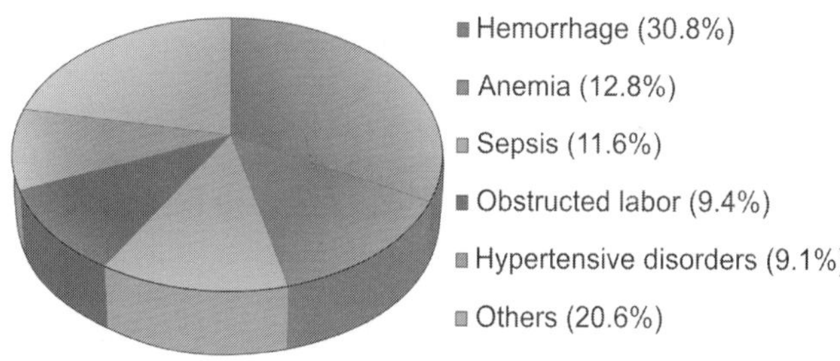

FIG. 1: Leading causes of maternal deaths in Asia ***(For color version, see Plate 4)***.[1]

OBSTETRIC CAUSES

Hemorrhagic Causes

Postpartum Hemorrhage

Incidence

The most common cause of maternal death in India is hemorrhage. Postpartum hemorrhage (PPH) is estimated to occur in as high as 10% of all deliveries, even though all

TABLE 1: Causes of postpartum maternal collapse

Obstetric causes	
Hemorrhagic causes	• Postpartum hemorrhage (PPH) • Rupture uterus
Nonhemorrhagic causes	• Sepsis • Eclampsia • Acute uterine inversion • Amniotic fluid embolism • Pulmonary thromboembolism • Air embolism • Mendelson's syndrome
Nonobstetric causes	
Neurological causes	• Intracranial hemorrhage • Epilepsy • Subarachnoid hemorrhage • Cerebral venous sinus thrombosis
Cardiac causes	• Myocardial infarction • Cardiac arrhythmias • Infective endocarditis • Cardiomyopathy
Pulmonary	• Thromboembolism
Metabolic	• Hypoglycemia
Anaphylaxis	• Anaphylactic shock
Drug overdose	• Magnesium sulfate • Lignocaine

of them may not have postpartum collapse. It is directly responsible for 38% of all maternal deaths in India.[4]

Etiology and risk factors

Four basic causes of PPH are four T's, which are as follows:

1. Tone (poor uterine contractions after delivery)
2. Tissue (retained products of conception or blood clots)
3. Trauma (to the genital tract) and
4. Tthrombin (coagulation abnormalities).

Overdistended uterus (multiple pregnancy, polyhydramnios), anemia, prolonged labor, mismanaged third stage of labor, precipitate labor, operative vaginal delivery, placenta previa, and antepartum hemorrhage, can also predispose to this complication.

Clinical presentation

In majority of cases, vaginal bleeding is visible except for vulvovaginal hematomas or PPH after cesarean section. Atonic PPH is apparently painless; however, in cases of vulvovaginal hematomas and abdominal collection, perineal/abdominal pain can be very severe.

Typical signs of hypovolemia are seen, i.e., tachycardia, hypotension, oliguria, and in advanced cases, renal failure, shock, cardiac arrest, and cardiovascular failure leading to maternal death.

Definitive management

Golden hour is the first hour of initial insult by which management or resuscitative efforts must be started to have best chances of survival. Mainstay of the treatment is early diagnosis of the cause of PPH and adequate blood replacement. Table 2 shows an algorithm showing both general and specific management of PPH.

Rupture Uterus

Incidence

Rupture of pregnant uterus is a very rare presentation with an estimated incidence of 1 per 5–10,000 deliveries. However, due to recent spurt in incidence of cesarean deliveries, this rare complication is becoming fairly common (0.5–1.0%), especially in women with previous cesarean delivery.

Causes

History of previous cesarean delivery is a major risk factor with 90–95% of all uterine ruptures occurring in these women (Table 3). However, other relatively less common risk factors are injudicious and excessive use of oxytocics in labor, induction of labor with prostaglandins (misoprostol or dinoprostone), previous uterine surgery (myomectomy, uterine perforation, etc.), and obstructed labor. In developing countries, cesarean delivery by unskilled staff (paramedical staff or even quacks) with unknown uterine incision (extension of low segment uterine incision, T-shaped or even classical cesarean), is a significant causative factor (Fig. 2).

TABLE 2: Typical management algorithm includes HAEMOSTASIS[5]

General medical management	
H	• Ask for help
A	• Assess (vital parameters, blood loss)
E	• Etiology (four T's; trauma, tissue, tone, and thrombin) • Ecbolics • Ensure availability of blood
M	• Massage the uterus
O	• Oxytocin infusion
Specific surgical management	
S	• Shift to operation theater (bimanual compression)
T	• Uterine tamponade (balloon or uterine packing)
A	• Apply compression sutures
S	• Systematic pelvic devascularization (uterine, ovarian, quadruple, internal iliac)
I	• Intervention radiology and uterine artery embolization
S	• Subtotal or total abdominal hysterectomy

TABLE 3: Risk of uterine rupture with type of uterine incision*

Prior incision	Estimated risk of uterine rupture (%)
One lower segment cesarean section	0.2–0.9
≥two lower segment cesarean section	0.9–1.8
Low-vertical cesarean section	1–7
T-shaped uterine incision	4–9
Classical cesarean section	2–9
Previous uterine rupture: • Lower segment • Upper segment	 • 2–6 • 9–32

*The American College of Obstetricians and Gynecologists guidelines 2013a.

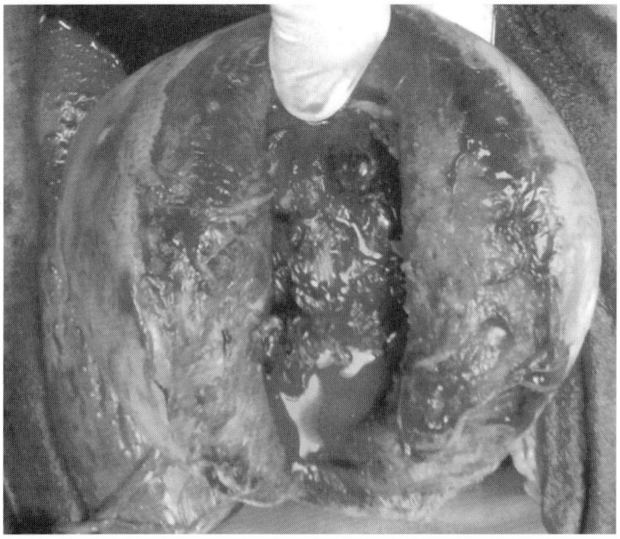

FIG. 2: Uterine rupture in a woman with classical cesarean diagnosed intraoperatively (type of uterine incision was unknown beforehand; a relatively common occurrence in developing countries) ***(For color version, see Plate 4)***.

Types

It is broadly classified into two types:

1. Complete uterine rupture, i.e., full thickness of uterine wall is disrupted
2. Incomplete uterine rupture or uterine dehiscence, i.e., when uterine wall rupture but visceral peritoneum remains intact.

Clinical presentation

The clinical presentation primarily depends upon type of uterine rupture, whereas complete rupture may present as a dramatic emergency threatening maternal and fetal life, on contrast incomplete rupture may be asymptomatic. The most common presentation during labor is fetal heart rate (FHR) abnormalities in a woman with previous cesarean delivery. Hence, according to American College of Obstetricians and Gynecologists guidelines, all women with previous cesarean delivery should be under continuous electronic fetal heart surveillance in labor. In addition, use of oxytocics for induction or augmentation of labor is associated with higher incidence of uterine rupture. The classical triad of FHR abnormalities, pain, and vaginal bleeding is uncommon. A very high index of suspicion is required in high-risk women. Complete rupture may be dramatic and catastrophic with constant lower abdominal pain, cesarean scar tenderness, vaginal bleeding, shock out of proportion to bleeding, hematuria, and loss of uterine contour. Operative vaginal delivery is an independent risk factor for uterine rupture. Very rarely, omentum or gut may be seen protruding per vaginum after vaginal delivery in women with scarred uterus which necessitates emergency laparotomy. Prelabor uterine rupture should be suspected in any women with previous cesarean with intrauterine fetal death with shock (out of proportion to bleeding). Rarely, blunt trauma abdomen (fall on abdomen or violence) may lead to uterine rupture.

Definitive management

Early diagnosis and prompt maternal resuscitation and surgical intervention are mainstay of management. Urgent laparotomy after maternal stabilization is required for definite diagnosis. If fetus or placenta is already expelled, neonatal survival is very poor. After delivery of fetus and placenta, hemorrhage control is done either by repair of uterine rent or peripartum hysterectomy as deemed essential for optimal maternal outcome. Decision for sterilization should be planned before hand and is inadvisable intraoperatively.

Nonhemorrhagic Causes

Sepsis

Incidence

The second most common cause of maternal death in India (after hemorrhage) is sepsis.[4] Table 4 shows the definitions related to sepsis.

Puerperal sepsis

This refers to infection of the genital tract occurring at any time between the rupture of membranes or labor and the 42nd day postpartum, of which two or more of the following are present:

- Pelvic pain
- Fever 38.5°C or more
- Abnormal vaginal discharge/smell of discharge
- Delay in reduction of size of uterus (<2 cm a day during the first 8 days).

Risk factors

Risk factors are given as follows:

- History of group B streptococcal infection or vaginal discharge or pelvic infection, prolonged spontaneous

TABLE 4: Definitions related to sepsis

SIRS (any two of these four)	• Temperature >38°C (100.4°F) or <36°C (96.8°F) • Heart rate >90 beats/min • Respiratory rate >20 breaths/min or $PaCO_2$ <32 mmHg • WBC count >12,000/µL or <4,000/µL
Sepsis	• SIRS with proven or suspected microbiological etiology
Septicemia	• Presence of microbes or their toxins in blood
Severe sepsis (≥ one of these)	• CVS; SBP <90 mmHg or MAP <70 mmHg (responds to intravenous fluids) • Renal; oliguria <0.5 mL/kg/h (at least 1 h after adequate fluid replacement) • Respiratory; PaO_2/FiO_2 ≤250 • Hematological; platelets <80,000/mm^3 • Unexplained metabolic acidosis; pH <7.3 or base deficit <5 mEq/L • PAWP ≥12 mmHg or CVP ≥8 mmHg despite adequate fluid resuscitation
Septic shock	• Sepsis with hypotension (SBP <90 mmHg or 40 mmHg < patient's normal BP) for at least 1 h after adequate fluid replacement OR • Need for vasopressors to maintain SBP >90 mmHg or MAP >70 mmHg
MODS	• Disruption of ≥ one organ system to maintain homeostasis

SIRS, systemic inflammatory response syndrome; $PaCO_2$, partial pressure of arterial carbon dioxide; WBC, white blood cell; CVS, cardiovascular system; SBP, systolic blood pressure; MAP, mean arterial pressure; PaO_2, partial pressure of oxygen; FiO_2, fraction of inspired oxygen; PAWP, pulmonary arterial wedge pressure; CVP, central venous pressure; BP, blood pressure; MODS, multiple organ dysfunction syndrome.

*American College of Chest Physicians/Society of Critical Care Medicine

rupture of membranes, amniocentesis and other invasive procedures, cervical encirclage, cesarean section, vaginal trauma, wound hematoma, multiple pregnancies, assisted reproduction.[6,7]

- Table 5 shows care bundle management of septic shock.

Clinical presentation

Clinical features are given as follows:

- Fever or rigors, diarrhea or vomiting [may indicate exotoxin production (early-toxic shock)], rash (generalized streptococcal maculopapular rash or purpura fulminans), abdominal/pelvic pain and tenderness, offensive vaginal discharge (smelly suggests anaerobes; serosanguineous suggests streptococcal infection).

Definitive management

Diagnosis is mainly clinical. High index of suspicion and early treatment is cornerstone of management. Intravenous (IV) immunoglobulin may be of some use in severe sepsis. Table 6 shows various indications in which the patient is to be shifted to ICU and table 7 enumerates antibiotics to be used in sepsis.

Eclampsia

Incidence

It is highly variable ranging from 1:30 to 1:500 in rural India.[8]

Risk factors

Major risk factors are age, primigravida, multiple pregnancies, family history, past history, obesity, hyperhomocystinuria, metabolic syndrome, etc.

TABLE 5: Septic shock care bundle management[6,7]

Serum lactate	Measure serum lactate
Culture profile	• Blood cultures and culture swabs before antibiotic administration
Antibiotics	• Administer broad-spectrum antibiotics within the first hour of recognition of severe sepsis and septic shock according to local protocol
Hypotension or lactate >4 mmol/L	• Deliver an initial minimum of 20 mL/kg of crystalloid or colloid • Once adequate volume replacement has been achieved, a vasopressor (e.g., norepinephrine, epinephrine), inotrope (e.g., dobutamine), or both
Septic shock	• Achieve central venous pressure >8 mmHg (or >12 mmHg mechanically ventilated) • Consider steroids • Maintain oxygen saturation with facial oxygen • Consider transfusion if hemoglobin is below 7 g/dL

TABLE 6: Indications for transfer to intensive care unit[6,7]

System	Indications
Cardiovascular system	• Hypotension or raised lactate levels (despite adequate fluid resuscitation) • Need for inotropes
Respiratory system	• Pulmonary edema • Mechanical ventilation
Renal system	• Renal dialysis
Neurological system	• Altered sensorium
Miscellaneous	• Multiorgan failure • Uncorrected acidosis • Hypothermia

TABLE 7: Antibiotics to be used in sepsis[6,7]

Co-amoxiclav	• Do not cover MRSA *Pseudomonas*
Metronidazole	• Only active against anaerobes
Clindamycin	• For *Staphylococcus/Streptococcus* and MRSA • Decreases exotoxin production • Significant reduction in mortality • Not nephrotoxic
Piperacillin-tazobactam	• Covers most organisms, except MRSA • Not nephrotoxic
Gentamicin	• Renal function tests required for prolonged use

MRSA, methicillin-resistant Staphylococcus aureus

Clinical presentation

It is marked by sudden and dramatic onset of seizures. In majority of women (80%), eclampsia is preceded by preeclampsia. Premonitory symptoms, i.e., headache, blurring of vision or epigastric pain may represent impending eclampsia.

Definitive management

Delivery is the mainstay of treatment. Magnesium sulfate (4–6 g IV loading dose; 5 g intramuscular in each buttock, repeatedly 4 hourly if patellar reflex present, respiratory rate more than 12 breaths/min and urine output more than 100 mL/4 h), is the drug of choice.

Acute blood pressure (BP) control (hydralazine, labetalol, nifedipine or α-methyldopa), is also required simultaneously to prevent major organ damage.

Acute Uterine Inversion

Incidence

Acute uterine inversion is a rare, but life-threatening complication of third stage of labor with an estimated incidence of 1:2,000–1:50,000.[9]

Types

- Incomplete: fundus of uterus inverted, but not descended through the cervix
- Complete: fundus of uterus inverted and lying in the vagina or outside introitus.

Risk factors

Risk factors for acute uterine inversion include following:

- Mismanagement of third stage of labor (undue fiddling or pulling the umbilical cord prematurely in a relaxed uterus after delivery)
- Abnormally short umbilical cord
- Morbid adherent fundal implantation of placenta
- Sudden rise in intra-abdominal pressure (coughing, vomiting or straining) in fundal attachment of placenta with relaxed uterus
- Manual removal of placenta
- Connective tissue disorders.

Clinical presentation

It is marked by large boggy mass appearing at introitus (Fig. 3), severe and sustained hypogastric pain, shock out of proportion of blood loss (vasovagal stimulus due to stretching of infundibulopelvic ligaments, round ligaments, ovaries and associated nerves), sudden bradycardia, hypotension, and cardiac arrest. It is usually also associated with marked hemorrhage and hypovolemic shock. Uterus may not be palpable per abdomen, inverted uterine fundus seen at introitus or on per vaginal examination.

Definitive management

Immediate manual reversion of inverted fundus, if diagnosed on the spot. Within minutes increasing congestion, edema and contraction of inverted fundus, makes reversion of inverted uterus extremely painful and difficult to achieve without anesthesia. If placenta still attached, do not attempt to remove it. Immediately shift to operation theater. General anesthesia is preferred for relaxation of uterus. Time is of essence, as quickly as the maneuver is undertaken so are the chances of success. After adequate anesthesia and tocolysis (IV nitroglycerin drip titrated to achieve desired effect), manual reposition is attempted. Fundus of uterus is cupped in palm of hand; fingers and thumb are extended to feel the uterocervical junction. Lift the uterus, gradually reducing the inversion, maintain the pressure for 3–5 minutes and after correction, immediately stop tocolysis and start uterotonics. The part inverted first is usually last to be corrected. If manual reposition fails, hydrostatic replacement by O'Sullivan's

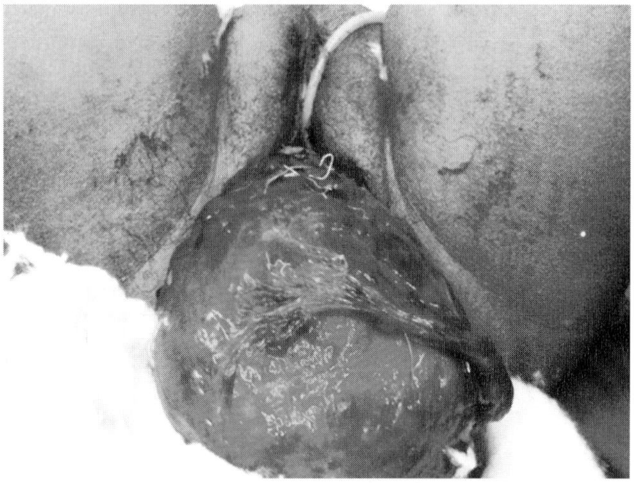

FIG. 3: Acute uterine inversion (complete) ***(For color version, see Plate 4)***.

technique can be done, by infusing 3–5 L of fluid into the upper vagina (only after ensuring there are no vaginal or cervical lacerations), seal the introitus by hand or vacuum cup to achieve desired result. Rarely, when reposition fails, surgical replacement requires laparotomy with Huntington's operation (stretch the cervical ring, gradually pull the myometrium just inside the uterine dimple and revert the inversion) or Haultain's repair (incision of posterior cervical ring and gradual repositioning of uterine fundus). Very rarely, hysterectomy is the last resort in management of recurrent inversion. Uterotonics should be continued for at least 8 hours, broad-spectrum antibiotics should be given and beforehand preparation for hemorrhagic shock should be done.

"Prevention is better than cure"; this dictum holds true for this scenario, with acute uterine inversion being completely preventable with proper management of third stage of labor.

Amniotic Fluid Embolism

Incidence

It is extremely rare with an incidence of 2–3/100,000 deliveries. Despite its rarity, it has very high fatality rate (20–35%).

Risk factors

Risk factors are induction of labor, multiple pregnancies, increasing age, cesarean section.

Clinical presentation

Sudden acute respiratory distress and cardiovascular collapse in a woman in labor or immediately after delivery is usual presentation. Triggering event can be amniotomy or cesarean section. It is a diagnosis of exclusion. Acute maternal collapse (excluding maternal hemorrhage) with either of following: acute fetal compromise, cardiac arrest or arrhythmias, coagulopathy, convulsions, hypotension, shortness of breath, premonitory symptoms (restlessness, numbness, agitation, tingling). Diagnosis is confirmed after finding fetal squames or hairs in maternal lungs at autopsy.

Definitive management

Cardiopulmonary resuscitation (CPR) is mainstay of treatment and preventing death. If initial event is survived, overall chances of survival are excellent. Specialist assistance of anesthetist, intensive care or hematology is vital. Perimortem cesarean section should be considered to improve effectiveness of CPR. Intubation, ventilation, ionotropic support, and correction of coagulopathy may be required. Permanent neurological damage may occur if there is delay in institution of initial resuscitative measures. Emergency hysterectomy may offer the only treatment for acute hemorrhage. Fetal prognosis is extremely poor unless delivered within 5–10 minutes of acute insult.

Pulmonary Thromboembolism

Incidence

It is very rare with an incidence of 13/100,000 deliveries.

Risk factors

All pregnant women are at increased risk of thromboembolism. Venous stasis, expanded venous volume, and increase in fibrinogen and coagulation factors are the factors that predispose to thromboembolism during pregnancy. Immobility in a pregnant patient further increases this risk. Increased maternal age, multiparity, prolonged labor, preeclampsia, cesarean section, sepsis or thrombophilias are additional risk factors.

Clinical presentation

Sudden onset severe pleuritic chest pain, followed by collapse, dyspnea, cyanosis, confusion may be there due to hypoxia. Large emboli may lead to pulmonary hypertension, right ventricular failure, and cardiac arrest. Figure 4 shows contrast-enhanced computed tomography scan of pulmonary thromboembolism.

Definitive management

Typical electrocardiogram (ECG) findings of S1Q3T3 may be present. Urgent lung scan, i.e., ventilation-perfusion scan or a computed tomography pulmonary angiogram is required for confirmation of diagnosis in absence of typical ECG changes. Treatment is symptomatic with resuscitation with fluid and oxygen. If hypotension persists, thrombolysis may be considered but postpartum, it is associated with serious genital tract bleeding. Surgical embolectomy may

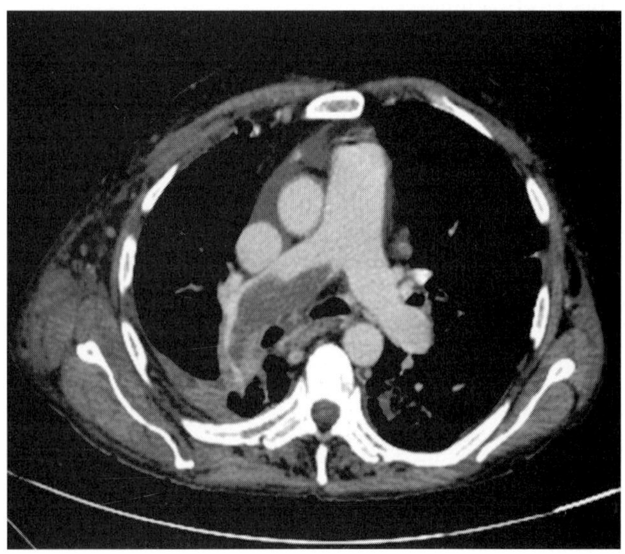

FIG. 4: Contrast-enhanced computed tomography scan image showing pulmonary thromboembolism.

be considered in women with massive life-threatening pulmonary embolus.

Air Embolism

Incidence

Air embolism is characterized by air in the vascular system. It can be arterial or venous air embolism (VAE). Its exact incidence is not known. VAE is a predominantly iatrogenic complication and is associated with 1% of all maternal deaths.

Risk factors

Traditionally, it has been estimated that more than 5 mL/kg of air displaced into the IV space is required for significant injury (shock or cardiac arrest) to occur. However, complications have been reported with as little as 20 mL of air (the length of IV infusion tubing) injected intravenously, 2–3 mL of air into the cerebral circulation and 0.5 mL of air in the left anterior descending coronary artery can be fatal.

Cesarean delivery carries a relatively higher risk for VAE of more than 50%. The risk factors for VAE during cesarean delivery are surgery in the Trendelenburg's position, abruptio placentae, placenta previa, exteriorization of the uterus, manual extraction of the placenta, severe preeclampsia, antepartum hemorrhage, and hypovolemia.

In addition, other invasive therapeutic and/or diagnostic procedures associated with VAE are central venous catheterization, lumbar puncture, high-pressure infusion of medications, blood products, and/or IV contrast agents, patients on positive pressure ventilation. Peripartum/postpartum orogenital sexual intercourse (air may enter veins of the myometrium) can also be reason for VAE.

Clinical presentation

Many cases of VAE are subclinical with no adverse outcome and thus go unreported. Usually, when symptoms are present, they are nonspecific, and a high index of clinical suspicion is required.

Main signs and symptoms are dyspnea, continuous cough, "gasp" reflex (a classic gasp at times reported when a bolus of air enters the pulmonary circulation and causes acute hypoxemia), dizziness/lightheadedness/vertigo, nausea, substernal chest pain, agitation/disorientation/sense of impending doom, dysrhythmias (tachyarrhythmias/bradycardias), hypotension, myocardial ischemia, nonspecific ST-segment, T-wave changes and/or evidence of right heart strain, circulatory shock/cardiovascular collapse, pulmonary edema, apnea, seizure, loss of consciousness, collapse, and coma.

Definitive management

The goals of management when severe VAE is manifested are prevention of further gas entry, removal of entrained gas, and maintenance of hemodynamic stability. Management is mainly symptomatic (100% oxygen, left lateral and reverse Trendelenburg's position, supportive care, fluid resuscitation, hyperbaric oxygen may be required).

Mendelson's Syndrome

Incidence

Mendelson's syndrome or aspiration pneumonitis occurs following aspiration of gastric contents when laryngeal reflexes are abolished, e.g., during general anesthesia or coma. With recent advances and widespread use of regional anesthesia, its incidence is very rare (1 in 200,000 surgical procedures). Nonetheless, once it occurs it is a catastrophic event with significant maternal morbidity and mortality.

Risk factors

Increased risk has been observed in women with difficult intubation, especially with preeclampsia or eclampsia syndrome (especially after seizures), obesity, protracted vomiting, nasogastric intubation and delayed gastric emptying time, e.g., with gestational diabetes. Historically, residual gastric volume of greater than 25 mL, with pH less than 2.5, was considered a significant risk factor.

Clinical presentation

The main clinical features are signs of general hypoxia (30–60 min after aspiration). Such features may include cyanosis, dyspnea, tachycardia, pulmonary edema, bronchospasm, hypotension, and hypovolemia. Pulmonary edema can cause sudden death or death may occur later from pulmonary complications. Chest X-ray may show consolidation within the first 2 days (Fig. 5).

Definitive management

Prevention is better than cure. Administration of H_2 blockers is a routine practice before cesarean delivery and has drastically reduced the incidence of this catastrophe. Recent Cochrane review also emphasizes this therapeutic intervention, especially in women for cesarean delivery under general anesthesia. Symptomatic management in the form of 100% oxygen, nasogastric decompression of gastric contents and adequate fluid management is done. Intermittent positive pressure ventilation may be required. Role of corticosteroids and antibiotics is controversial.

Differential diagnosis

Amniotic fluid embolism, pulmonary embolus, other causes of shock and circulatory collapse (abruptio placentae, heart disease, pulmonary causes, e.g., asthma, pneumothorax, subarachnoid hemorrhage), are some of the common differential diagnosis.

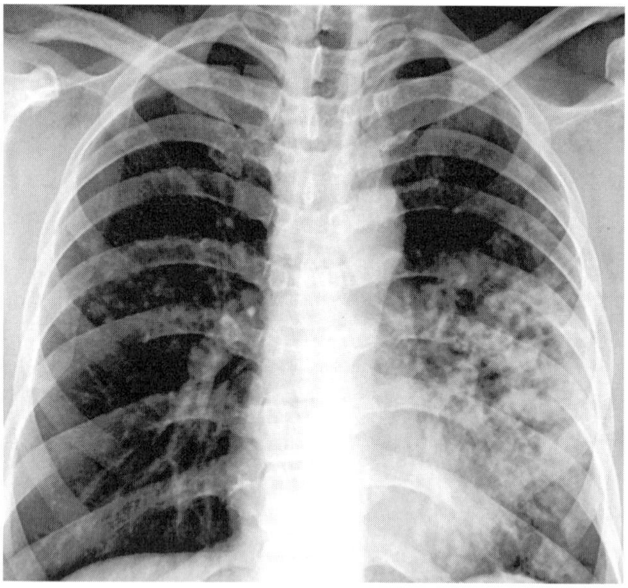

FIG. 5: Chest X-ray showing patchy consolidations in left lower lobe (post aspiration).

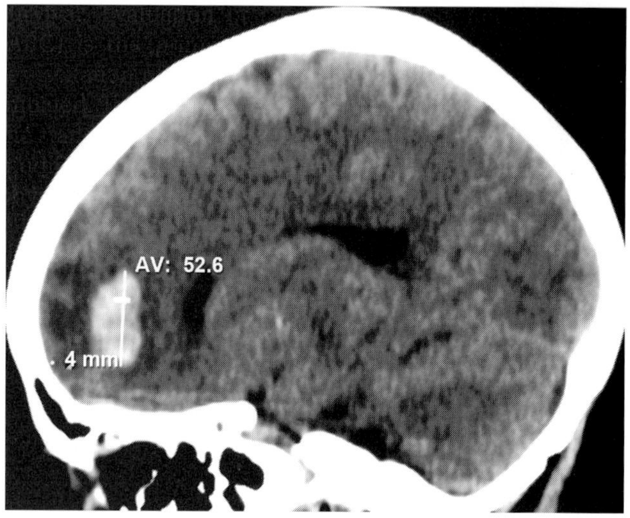

FIG. 6: Computed tomography scan image showing intracranial hemorrhage.

NONOBSTETRIC CAUSES

Neurological Cause

Intracranial Hemorrhage

Incidence

It is very rare with an incidence of 6/100,000 deliveries. Mortality rates of 20% are observed.

Risk factors

Pre-existing hypertension or pregnancy-induced hypertension is a major risk factor, especially with coagulopathy.

Clinical presentation

Altered sensorium, headache, vomiting or seizures may be there. The clinical findings of focal neurological deficit or anisocoria mandates urgent computed tomography or magnetic resonance imaging scanning (Fig. 6).

Definitive management

Respiratory support, intubation, and hypertension control are the basic principles guiding the treatment. Opinion of neurosurgeon for surgical evacuation must be sought.

Cardiac Cause

Sudden Cardiac Arrest

Incidence

Cardiopulmonary arrest in pregnancy is rare occurring in 1 in 30,000 pregnancies.

TABLE 8: Main causes of cardiac arrest in pregnancy

Obstetric causes	Nonobstetric causes
Hemorrhage	Pulmonary embolism
Pregnancy-induced hypertension	Sepsis
Peripartum cardiomyopathy	Stroke
Anesthesia complications	Myocardial infarction
Amniotic fluid embolism	Trauma

Causes

The main causes of cardiac arrest in pregnancy are enumerated in Table 8.

Clinical presentation

Usually the presentation is dramatic with sudden collapse of patient, typically characterized by shock. In few cases, few premonitory symptoms in terms of sudden onset of breathlessness, fear of impending doom or gasping may be present.

Definitive management

Timing of resuscitative efforts is main factor in determining survival. Evaluation of airway, breathing, and circulation (ABC) is the primary focus. The first priority should be resuscitation of the mother, before evaluation of the fetus is initiated. The American Heart Association recommends that the standard resuscitation algorithm be followed, with a few modifications to compensate for the altered anatomy and physiology of pregnancy. The primary ABC survey requires no modification to the assessment of airway or breathing for the maternal patient. Tilting the patient 15–30° to the left or having someone pull the gravid uterus to the left, will relieve compression on the inferior vena cava and allow for optimal cardiac return. No modifications are needed in positioning or dosage for defibrillation. Defibrillation does not carry any increased risk for the fetus, but the fetal monitor should be removed prior to defibrillation and 100% oxygen should be started immediately. Maintain a low threshold for intubation. Securing the airway promotes proper oxygenation and reduces the risk of aspiration. Immediately following maternal stabilization, fetus should be assessed. Verification of fetal heart sounds is the first step in fetal evaluation. In the absence of fetal heart sounds upon presentation to the emergency department, the chance of fetal resuscitation is poor. In this situation, focus full attention on the mother and treatment of her condition, regardless of gestational age. If fetal heart sounds are present, and the mother is stable, fetal evaluation should be continued. For a patient requiring CPR not responding after 5 minutes of resuscitation, perimortem cesarean section should be performed for maternal indication.

Drug Overdose

Magnesium Sulfate Toxicity

Magnesium sulfate is treatment of choice for eclampsia/impending eclampsia. It is a drug with narrow therapeutic index (4–7 mEq/L). Toxicity starts at levels more than 8 mEq/L:

- Patellar reflex disappears if serum magnesium is more than or equal to 10 mEq/L
- Breathing depressed at levels more than or equal to 10 mEq/L
- Respiratory paralysis and arrest at levels more than or equal to 12 mEq/L.

Magnesium sulfate is excreted mainly by kidneys. Toxicity is unlikely if glomerular filtration rate is normal (usually associated with normal urine output). However, serum creatinine levels must be done to detect glomerular filtration rate. Initial loading dose (4 g IV and 5 g intramuscular in each buttock) need not to be altered even if renal functions are abnormal. However, if serum creatinine levels are more than 1 mg/mL, serum magnesium levels are measured to guide the infusion rate.

Clinical features

Prominent clinical features are absent deep tendon reflexes, drowsiness, lethargy, respiratory depression, respiratory and cardiac arrest.

Treatment

Withhold further magnesium sulfate and calcium gluconate (10% of 10 mL) or calcium chloride 1 g intravenously will usually reverse mild-to-moderate respiratory depression. In severe cases, prompt tracheal intubation and mechanical ventilation is lifesaving.

RESUSCITATION GUIDELINES

- Multidisciplinary team, including senior obstetrician and senior obstetric anesthetist/intensivist, should manage women with postpartum collapse
- High-risk women should be identified early (especially those with known medical/surgical disorders). They should be managed by respective medical/surgical specialists to achieve optimum disease control before the catastrophe
- Immediately ensure "basic life support" (Flowchart 1):
  - Airway: intubation as soon as possible
  - Breathing: immediately start supplemental oxygen and bag-mask ventilation till intubation is done
  - Circulation: in absence of breathing, immediately start chest compressions
  - Two large bore cannula to be secured
  - Aggressive approach to volume replacement

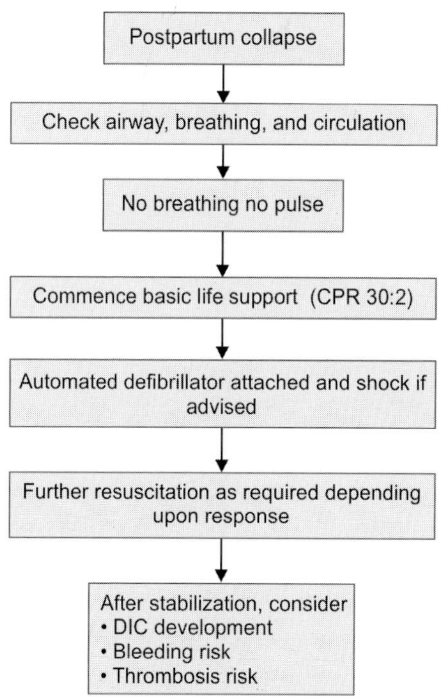

CPR, cardiopulmonary resuscitation; DIC, disseminated intravascular coagulation.

FLOWCHART 1: Resuscitation algorithm for postpartum collapse.

- Urgent abdominal ultrasonography to rule out concealed hemorrhage
- Same defibrillation energy as in nonpregnant
- No alteration in algorithm of drugs or their doses
- Shift to ICU as soon as possible

- Identify the cause and manage accordingly:
  - Hemorrhage: Adequate blood and blood products replacement
  - Eclampsia: Magnesium sulfate and BP control
  - Sepsis: Early institute broad-spectrum antibiotics
  - Amniotic fluid embolism: Supportive management
  - Cardiac disease: Early involvement of cardiologist
  - After stabilization, consider the risk of disseminated intravascular coagulation, bleeding, and thrombosis.

CONCLUSION

Maternal collapse is a sudden and dramatic events associated with severe maternal and fetal mortality and morbidity. About 75% of obstetric patients admitted to the ICU are postpartum. Hemorrhage and hypertension are two leading causes of admission to ICU in obstetric patients. Early administration of basic life support and identifying the cause of collapse are key to successful outcome. Meticulous record keeping of resuscitation (whether or not successful) and audit of these events can be helpful in proper management of such emergencies in long-term basis.

REFERENCES

1. Khan KS, Wojdyla D, Say L, Gülmezoglu AM, Van Look PF. WHO analysis of causes of maternal death: a systematic review. Lancet. 2006;367(9516):1066-74.
2. American College of Obstetricians and Gynecologists. ACOG Practice Bulletin No. 100: Critical care in pregnancy. Obstet Gynecol. 2009;113(2 Pt 1):443-50.
3. Royal College of Obstetricians and Gynaecologists (RCOGs). (2011). Maternal Collapse in Pregnancy and the Puerperium (Green-top Guideline No. 56). [online] Available from www.rcog.org.uk/en/guidelines-research-services/guidelines/gtg56/. [Accessed June, 2015].
4. Park K. Preventive medicine in obstetrics, pediatrics and geriatrics. In: Park JE. Park's Textbook of Preventive and Social Medicine, 21st edition. Jabalpur, Madhya Pradesh, India: Banarsidas Bhanot Publishers; 2011. p. 482.
5. Doumouchtsis SK, Arulkumaran S. Postpartum haemorrhage: changing practices. In: Ledger W, Dunlop W (Eds). Recent Advances in Obstetrics and Gynecology, 24th edition. London, UK: Royal Society of Medicine Press; 2008. p. 93.
6. Royal College of Obstetricians and Gynaecologists (RCOGs). (2012). Sepsis in Pregnancy, Bacterial (Green-top guideline No. 64a). [online] Available from: www.rcog.org.uk/en/guidelines-research-services/guidelines/gtg64a/. [Accessed June, 2015].
7. Royal College of Obstetricians and Gynaecologists (RCOGs). (2012). Sepsis following Pregnancy, Bacterial (Green-top guideline No. 64b). [online] Available from www.rcog.org.uk/en/guidelines-research-services/guidelines/gtg64b/. [Accessed June, 2015].
8. Dutta DC. Hypertensive disorders in pregnancy. In: Konar HL (Ed). DC Dutta's Textbook of Obstetrics, 8th edition. New Delhi, India: Jaypee Brothers Medical Publishers; 2015. pp. 255-81.
9. Baskett T, Calder A, Arulkumaran S (Eds). Acute uterine inversion. In: Munro Kerr's Operative Obstetrics, 12th edition. Philadelphia, PA, USA: Elsevier-Saunders; 2014. p. 211.

CHAPTER 27

Massive Obstetric Hemorrhage and Disseminated Intravascular Coagulation

Arti Luthra, Manishi Mittal, Daizy Pathak

INTRODUCTION

Massive obstetric hemorrhage and disseminated intravascular coagulation (DIC) are two of the major causes for maternal mortality in India. Early recognition and proactive management of both is a necessity for reduction of both maternal mortality and morbidity.

MASSIVE OBSTETRIC HEMORRHAGE

Hemorrhage may occur as antepartum hemorrhage (APH), intrapartum hemorrhage (IPH), or postpartum hemorrhage (PPH). A drop in the hemodynamic status of the mother indicates clinically significant hemorrhage. Massive obstetric hemorrhage is labeled when there is a 30–40% (>2 L) loss of the patient's blood volume,[1] or transfusion of 5 units of blood or treatment for coagulopathy.

Epidemiology

Hemorrhage is the single most important cause of maternal death worldwide responsible for around 25–30% of all maternal deaths. Postpartum hemorrhage complicates around 4% of vaginal and 6% of cesarean deliveries. According to World Health Organization (WHO) estimates, PPH accounts for around 30% maternal deaths worldwide.[2] However, due to difference in opinion for the definition of hemorrhage incidence is variable.

Mortality

Mortality occurs due to rapid cardiovascular decompensation and coagulopathy. Figure 1 shows the levels of different delays in seeking, reaching and receiving appropriate health care. It shows that a patient suffering from massive obstetric hemorrhage dies when there is a delay in: seeking medical care, reaching health-care facility, or receiving appropriate health care in the hospital.

Etiology

- Early pregnancy:
  - Ruptured ectopic pregnancy
  - Incomplete abortion
  - Placental abruption.
- Antepartum hemorrhage:
  - Placenta previa
  - Severe chorioamnionitis or septicemia

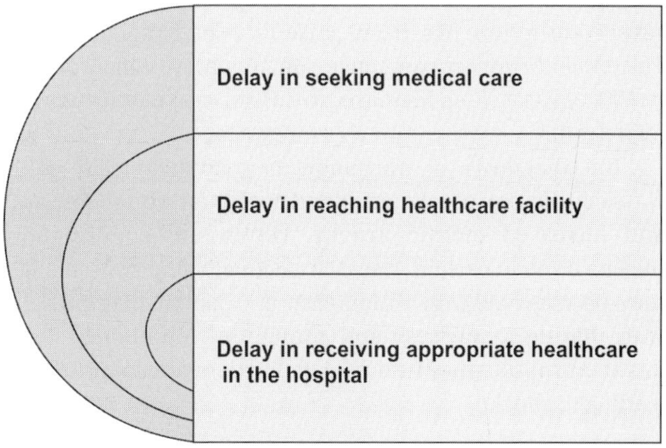

FIG. 1: Levels of different delays in seeking, reaching, and receiving appropriate healthcare.

    - Severe pre-eclampsia (hepatic rupture)
    - Retained intrauterine dead fetus
- Intrapartum hemorrhage:
    - Placental abruption
    - Rupture uterus
    - Amniotic fluid embolism
    - Complications of cesarean: Angular or broad ligament tears
- Postpartum hemorrhage:
    - Tone: atonic uterus
    - Tissue: retained products of conception (RPOC)
    - Trauma: trauma to upper or lower genital tract
    - Thrombin: coagulopathy, DIC
    - Secondary PPH (>24 hours to 6 weeks after delivery):
        - Infection
        - Gestational trophoblastic disease
        - Rarely, uterine arteriovenous (AV) malformation.

Antepartum and Intrapartum Hemorrhage

Antepartum hemorrhage is defined as bleeding from the genital tract after 24 weeks of gestation. The incidence is 2–5% of all pregnancies beyond 24 weeks. The incidence of placenta previa is around 4–5 per 1,000 pregnancies while of abruptio placentae is about 0.6–1.0% of all births.[3]

Placental abruption

This complication is seen in about 1% of pregnancies and is the leading cause of vaginal bleeding in the latter half of pregnancy. Various risk factors for abruptio placentae include hypertension, pre-eclampsia, advanced maternal age, multiparity, maternal/paternal tobacco use, cocaine use, trauma, premature rupture of membranes, chorioamnionitis, inherited and acquired thrombophilias, external trauma, uterine leiomyomas, and prior abruption. Recurrence of severe abruption has been seen in 1 in 8 pregnancies.[4] Placental abruption can cause coagulopathy, which occurs in 10% of cases. Rate increases to 50% in case of intrauterine fetal death.[5]

The diagnosis of abruption is made clinically with classical picture of vaginal blood loss, uterine tenderness, and increased uterine activity. Ultrasound confirmation may be done in certain cases. Occasionally, the hemorrhage may be concealed, in which case the patient may present with uterine tenderness and sometimes intrauterine fetal death. Abruption may be associated with severe hemorrhage leading to shock.

Management: in case of massive hemorrhage due to abruption (Fig. 2), the mother's condition needs to be stabilized first of all with the help of crystalloid infusion, oxygen inhalation, blood transfusion, and immediate delivery.

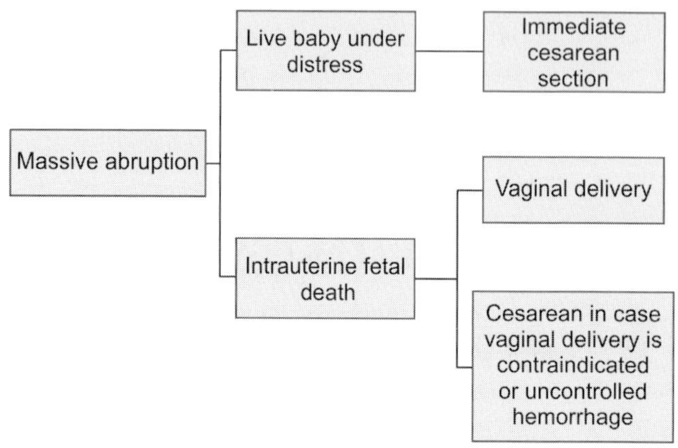

FIG. 2: Management of massive abruption.

Placenta previa

Placenta previa is the condition in which the placenta is implanted in the lower uterine segment. It may be partial or complete. The incidence of placenta previa is 0.5% of all pregnancies.[5] It is seen in conditions associated with prior uterine trauma, i.e., multiparity, advanced maternal age, previous cesarean section (CS) or other uterine surgery, and prior placenta previa.

Placenta previa presents classically with painless vaginal bleeding during the 2nd or 3rd trimester. Diagnosis is confirmed by ultrasound.

Management: in case of massive hemorrhage due to placenta previa, there is a need for immediate delivery. The most commonly followed method of delivery is by CS. Early delivery of the fetus is important during the cesarean as blood flow to fetus may be compromised when placenta is cut. Usually transverse incision is given.

There is a high risk of PPH due to the poorly contractile nature of the lower uterine segment.

Vasa previa

This is a condition in which the umbilical cord is the presenting part. Hemorrhage in this case is dangerous for the fetus.

Abnormally adherent placenta

As a result of the increasing rate of CS, the incidence of placenta accreta is increasing. The combination of a placenta previa and a previous uterine scar increases the risk significantly.

Placenta accreta is defined as an abnormally adherent placenta, without invasion in the myometrium. Placenta increta invades the myometrium and placenta percreta perforates the uterine muscle and invades the serosa or the surrounding pelvic structures, usually the bladder.

Diagnosis is made by ultrasound in suspected cases and confirmed by magnetic resonance imaging (MRI). Antepartum haemorrhage occurs when placenta accreta is associated with placenta previa. Usually, it causes PPH.

Uterine rupture

Previous CS is the major risk factor for uterine rupture. The incidence of rupture is around 0.2% in females with previous cesarean, whereas it is 10 times less in women with an unscarred uterus.[6] Prior uterine surgery, such as myomectomy, also causes uterine scarring, hence increasing risk of uterine rupture. Causes for rupture in an unscarred uterus include uterine anomalies, dystocia, use of uterotonic drugs, and abnormal placentation.

Bleeding is classically more severe in rupture of unscarred uterus rather than a scarred uterus. Clinical presentation can vary from subtle findings, such as subsidence of labor pains, uterine tenderness, and nonreassuring fetal heart patterns, to severe localized abdominal pain and a rapid onset of maternal hypovolemic shock.

Management: uterine rupture has a high incidence of perinatal and maternal mortality. Hence, early recognition is necessary, so that prompt surgical intervention may help to save the patient's life.

Amniotic fluid embolism

Peripartum hemorrhage results from rapid and dire coagulopathy. Amniotic fluid embolism is now thought to be more common than previously believed because of undiagnosed "moderate" forms.

Coagulopathy may present soon after the initial presenting symptoms or may be the only symptom.

Postpartum Hemorrhage

Postpartum hemorrhage remains one of the leading causes of maternal morbidity and mortality throughout the world. It complicates in about 1–5% of all deliveries.[7]

Primary PPH occurs during the first 24 hours after delivery and is more likely to result in maternal morbidity and mortality while secondary hemorrhage refers to hemorrhage 24 hours to 6 weeks after delivery (Table 1). Postpartum hemorrhage can further be categorized in terms of the amount of blood loss as:

- Minor PPH (500–1,000 mL)
- Major PPH (>1,000 mL).

Table 2 shows various risk factors for PPH. Even though mothers with these factors need to be monitored, but every parturient should be considered at risk and thus every maternity unit needs to be prepared to deal with PPH.

Uterine atony is the most common cause of PPH, defined as the lack of efficient uterine contractility after placental separation. Risk factors for uterine atony include conditions causing uterus to be:

- Overdistended (polyhydramnios, multiple gestation, and macrosomia)
- Fatigued (prolonged labor, chorioamnionitis)
- Unable to contract (due to tocolytics or general anesthesia).

Atonic uterus presents as painless continuous bleeding, often progressing slowly. Blood may get concealed in the uterus and is not obvious until external compression of the uterine fundus is performed. Classically, it is suspected by abdominal palpation of a soft and oversized uterus.

Retained placenta is the second most important etiology of PPH (approximately 20–30% of cases), but it must be systematically investigated first, because uterine atony is frequently associated.[5]

Vaginal, perineal, or cervical lacerations are responsible for around 10% of cases,[5] and it is more likely to occur after instrumental delivery, fetal macrosomia, precipitate labor, delivery before full cervical dilation, nulliparity, episiotomy, advanced maternal age, breech presentation, and multiple gestations. Diagnosis is suggested when retained placenta and uterine atony have been discarded. The common

TABLE 1: Etiology of postpartum hemorrhage

Primary PPH	Secondary PPH

• Uterine atony
• Trauma:
  ○ Upper and lower genital tract
  ○ Uterine rupture
• Abnormally adherent placenta
• RPOC
• Uterine inversion
• Coagulopathy
	• Infection
	• Retained products of conception (RPOC)
	• Placental site bleeding
	• Coagulopathy

PPH, postpartum hemorrhage

TABLE 2: Risk factors for postpartum hemorrhage

Preconception	• Age > 40 years • Asian ethnicity • Body mass index > 35 kg/m^2
During pregnancy	• Anemia • Placenta previa • Placental abruption • Multiple pregnancy • Preeclampsia • Induction of labor
At delivery	• Operative vaginal delivery • Cesarean section • Prolonged labor • Big baby • Retained placenta • Pyrexia in labor

presenting signs and symptoms are based on the location of the injury and include a rectal or vaginal mass, discoloration, and perineal pain or pressure.

The possibility of an inherited bleeding disorder has to be considered in case of unexplained and recurrent hemorrhage, e.g., von Willebrand's disease, hemolysis, elevated liver enzymes, and low platelet count (HELLP) syndrome, DIC or anticoagulation therapy.

Prevention

By recognizing the risk factors for hemorrhage and initiating a treatment, the clinician can minimize blood loss. Prevention can be done by active management of the third stage of labor, as follows:

- Controlled cord traction after separation of placenta. However, there is no evidence that, in an uncomplicated delivery without bleeding, interventions to accelerate delivery of the placenta before 30–45 minutes reduces the risk of PPH
- Uterine massage
- Use of a uterotonic agent:[8]
  - Oxytocin (5–10 IU), administered intramuscularly (IM) after the delivery of anterior shoulder, is the preferred in low-risk vaginal deliveries
  - Intravenous (IV) infusion of oxytocin (20–40 IU in 1000 mL, 150 mL/hour)
  - Ergonovine (0.2 mg IM or IV after delivery of anterior shoulder) is considered second choice to oxytocin due to higher maternal adverse effects and the need for manual removal of a retained placenta. It is contraindicated in hypertensive patients
  - Carbetocin, 100 µg given as an IV bolus over 1 minute, should be used instead of continuous oxytocin infusion in elective CS
  - Misoprostol, 600–800 µg given by the oral, sublingual, or rectal route, is another choice.

The Royal College of Obstetricians and Gynecologists (RCOG) recommends the use of oxytocics routinely in the management of the third stage of labor in all women, as their use reduces the risk of PPH by about 60%. Misoprostol should be made available at the community level as it is stable without refrigeration and no syringes or needles are required for its administration.

Implications

Immediate Implications

- Hypovolemic shock and cardiac arrest
- Problems associated with blood transfusion: Allergic reaction, infection transmission, or transfusion associated lung injury
- Acute renal failure
- Pulmonary edema
- Coagulopathy
- Operative management
- Intensive care unit requirement.

Long-term Implications

- Psychological: postpartum depression, post-traumatic stress disorder
- Sheehan's syndrome (postpartum pituitary necrosis)
- Secondary infertility
- Anemia.

Management

Early recognition is necessary to ensure maternal hemodynamic stability, identification, and treatment of the underlying cause. The pregnant patient is able to adapt to hemorrhage more effectively than her nonpregnant counterparts due to the hemodynamic changes occurring in pregnancy. Hence, these physiological changes may become deceptive for obstetricians as a pregnant lady can tolerate large blood losses without a marked change in vital signs. These compensatory mechanisms get exhausted only if the loss is very significant and patient suddenly develops features of hemorrhagic shock. The obstetrician therefore is left with very less time for therapeutic intervention. This narrow timeframe is often referred to as the "GOLDEN HOUR", which refers to the time in which resuscitation must begin to ensure the best chances of survival.

Important Steps for Initial Management

- Organization of a multidisciplinary team
- Large bore access with fluid and blood replacement
- Correction of defective coagulation with blood products and factors
- Hemodynamic and laboratory assessments
- Correction of the underlying cause of the bleeding.

A multidisciplinary approach is necessary involving the obstetrician, anesthesiologist, hematologist, nursing staff, and theater staff.

An initial assessment regarding the degree of blood loss and the severity of the hemodynamic instability is vital and it is always better to overestimate the blood loss and to anticipate the possibility of further bleeding. Obstetric hemorrhage may present with varying degrees of shock. Table 3 shows classification of shock based upon total blood volume with various parameters to be looked when examining a patient with massive hemorrhage.

Various pointers towards massive hemorrhage are:

- Visible blood loss more than 2 L
- Ongoing bleeding more than 150 mL/minutes
- Rule of 30: if the patient's systolic blood pressure falls by 30 mmHg, heart rate rises by 30 beats/minutes, respiratory rate increases to more than 30 breaths/minutes,

TABLE 3: Classification of shock[1]

Parameters	Stages			
	I (compensated)	II (mild)	III (moderate)	IV (severe)
Blood loss	<15%; 750–1,000 mL	15–30%; 1,000–1,500 mL	30–40%; 1,500–2,000 mL	>40%; ≥2,000 mL
Heart rate (beats/minutes)	<100	>100	>120	>140
Arterial pressure	Normal; vasoconstriction redistributes blood flow, slight increase in diastolic pressure	Orthostatic changes in arterial pressure, vasoconstriction intensifies in noncritical organs (skin, muscle, gut)	Markedly decreased (systolic arterial pressure <90 mmHg); vasoconstriction decreases perfusion to abdominal organs	Profoundly decreased (systolic arterial pressure <80 mmHg); decreased perfusion to vital organs (brain, heart)
Respiration	Normal	Mild increase	Moderate tachypnea	Marked tachypnea—respiratory failure
Mental status	Normal, slightly anxious	Mildly anxious, agitated	Confused, agitated	Obtunded
Urine output (mL/hour)	>30	20–30	<20	None (anuria)
Capillary refill	Normal (<2 seconds)	>2 seconds; clammy skin	Usually >3 seconds; cool, pale skin	>3 seconds; cold and mottled skin

hemoglobin or hematocrit drop by 30% and/or urinary output is less than 30 mL/hour, then the patient is most likely to have lost at least 30% of her blood volume, and is in moderate shock leading to severe shock[9]

- Shock index (pulse rate/systolic blood pressure) more than 0.9. Normal: 0.5–0.7
- Concealed hemorrhage in placental abruption (tense tender abdomen with intrauterine death).

At this stage, baseline laboratory evaluation of hemoglobin, hematocrit, platelet count, fibrinogen, prothrombin time (PT), and activated partial thromboplastin time (aPTT) should be taken. Figure 3 shows the stepwise management of PPH by following the pneumonic "HAEMOSTASIS".[10]

Resuscitation

It involves maintenance of airway, breathing, and circulation.

- Left lateral tilt (if antepartum) to relieve venacaval compression
- High flow oxygen by face mask
- Assess airway and respiration
- Two large bore IV cannulae
- Investigations: Hemogram, cross match, renal function tests, electrolytes, coagulopathy screen
- Intravenous crystalloids [0.9% normal saline (NS) or Hartmann's solution]. Use of colloids has recently been found to interfere with cross-matching and platelet function and hence it has been widely condemned. If used, the maximum dosage is 1,500 mL/24 hours
- Catheterize and measure hourly urine output
- Blood transfusion (O negative or matched blood):
  - Signs of inadequate oxygen-carrying capacity
  - Hemoglobin of less than 7 g/dL, or when blood loss is ongoing, the hemoglobin is around 7 g/dL

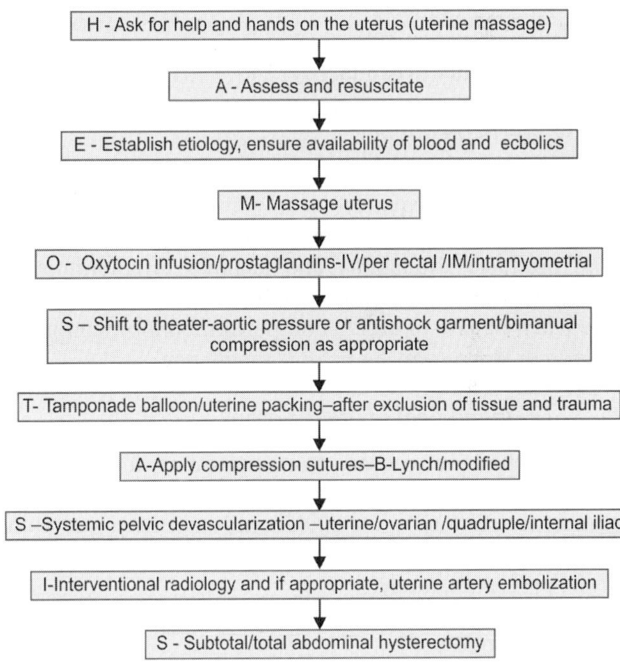

PPH, postpartum hemorrhage; PG, prostaglandins; IV, intravenous; IM, intramuscular.

FIG. 3: Stepwise management of postpartum hemorrhage is done easily by following the pneumonic "HAEMOSTASIS".

- Replacement of clotting factors:
  - Fresh-frozen plasma (FFP) 4 units for every 6 units of blood
  - Cryoprecipitate
  - Recombinant activated factor VII (rFVIIa): Synthetic vitamin K-dependent glycoprotein that has been

administered for hemorrhage unresponsive to conventional blood product resuscitation
  - Transfusion of platelet concentrates is recommended to treat active bleeding associated with thrombocytopenia
  - However, there is no current uniform consensus on the optimal ratio of blood products to transfuse into severely bleeding patients and prior recommendations for FFP: red blood cell (RBC) and platelets: RBC transfusion ratios range from 1:10 to 2:3 and 6:10 to 12:10, respectively
- Assess need for central venous line and ICU care
- Broad-spectrum antibiotic prophylaxis is added to resuscitation measures to reduce the high infectious risk associated with massive bleeding management.

Principles of Management

- Empty the uterus:
  - Termination of pregnancy in case of antepartum
  - Removal of RPOC
- Treat uterine atony (physically, medically, and surgically)
- Repair of injury to genital tract.

Termination of pregnancy

In case of massive obstetric hemorrhage, pregnancy has to be terminated immediately, usually by CS. But care has to be taken to perform the procedure at a place with adequate blood products' availability and facilities for monitoring. Written informed consent has to be taken. Same care has to be taken in case of evacuation performed for incomplete abortion or laparotomy for ectopic pregnancy.

Physical management of uterine atony

These methods are used to supplement the medical management, and include uterine massage and bimanual compression. Emptying the bladder aids uterine contraction and bimanual pelvic examination. Manual pressure on aorta may be performed rarely.

Medical management

Various drugs are used to treat atonic PPH. Table 4 shows different drugs with their doses to treat atonic PPH.

When atony is due to tocolytic therapy, an IV push of 1 ampoule of calcium gluconate is effective in improving uterine tone.

Surgical management

Uterine balloon tamponade or packing

There are occasions when uterine atony does not respond to administration of uterotonic agents. In that case, next step is to proceed to uterine tamponade using packing with gauze, a Foley's catheter with 30 cc balloon (Fig. 4), a Sengstaken-Blakemore tube, a Surgical Obstetric Silicone (SOS)-Bakri tamponade balloon or a condom with open end closely tied around a 16-size rubber catheter which can be inflated with water.

Uterine packing with gauze requires careful layering of the material back and forth from one cornu to the other using a sponge holder, and packing back and forth ending in cervical os. However, due to their potential traumatic placement and concern for concealed ongoing hemorrhage, the use of balloon tamponade has been favored.

The SOS-Bakri tamponade balloon is inserted through the cervix into the endometrial cavity, with a sponge holding forceps. After steadying the tube the balloon is distended using 300–400 mL of warm saline or sterile water, until it becomes visible in the cervical canal. If little or no bleeding is observed via the cervix or through the lumen of the catheter, the tamponade test is considered positive and laparotomy is avoided. An overall success rate of 84% has been reported with this technique.[11] It has the advantage of being easy to use and requiring minimal analgesia for both insertion and removal, and it preserves fertility. The balloon may be removed after 6–8 hours, if the uterine fundus remains at the same level and there is no active bleeding.

TABLE 4: Different drugs with their doses to manage atonic postpartum hemorrhage

Drug	Dose
Oxytocin	10 units intramuscularly (IM), infusion 20–40 units/L
Methergine	0.1–0.2 mg IM; maximum 5 doses
15-methyl PGF2α (carboprost)	250 μg IM every 15 minutes; maximum 2 mg
Misoprostol	800–1,000 μg rectally
PGE2 (dinoprostone)	20 mg rectally

PG, prostaglandin.

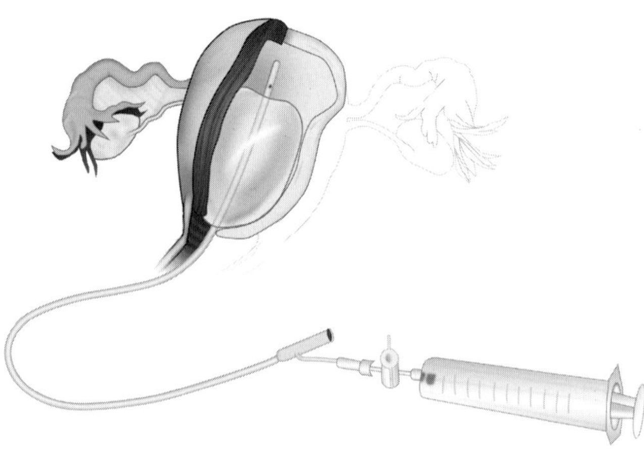

FIG. 4: Uterine balloon tamponade.

When bleeding continues despite conservative therapy, surgical management via laparotomy must be considered. Interventions include uterine compression sutures, arterial ligation, and hysterectomy.

Direct uterine massage

It involves rubbing the myometrium between the surgeon's hands to stimulate contractions and may be tried initially. This is an extension of bimanual compression as laparotomy enables direct myometrial compression. Intramyometrial injection of prostaglandins (PGs) may be tried at this stage.

Uterine compression sutures

They are most useful in cases of refractory uterine atony, but have also been used in cases of retained placenta and coagulopathy. Advantages include a high success rate, ease of placement at the time of laparotomy, and fertility preservation. Disadvantages include the need for laparotomy and reported complications including uterine wall erosion, uterine necrosis, and pyometra.

Techniques commonly employed include B-Lynch, Hayman, and Cho sutures. The B-Lynch technique is a suture that envelops and compresses the uterus and decreases bleeding. The B-Lynch suture, first described in 1997, has been used worldwide (Figs 5A and B).

The operation requires minimal training, conserves the uterus, is less technically challenging, and is associated with less blood loss than hysterectomy.

The Hayman technique uses two separate vertical compression sutures instead of one to increase the tension applied and hence, the compression force. It has the advantage of allowing blood to flow out from the uterine cavity and possibility of two or three additional cervical sutures medial to the first two sutures. Horizontal full thickness compression sutures have also been tried, especially to control the bleeding from the placental site in placenta previa at the time of CS.

A combination of multiple vertical compression sutures may be needed in some cases to arrest hemorrhage. Cho et al. described a "multiple square" suturing technique, which approximates anterior and posterior uterine walls at various points, virtually obliterating the uterine cavity.[12]

It is recommended that a tamponade balloon be placed with suture placement to ensure adequate hemorrhage control. They can help junior obstetric trainees to arrest or reduce hemorrhage while awaiting senior's help.

Stepwise devascularization

If the compression sutures fail to achieve homeostasis, ligation of blood vessels supplying the uterus could be tried in a systematic manner. It includes five steps to be used in case of uncontrolled hemorrhage:

1. Unilateral uterine vessel ligation
2. Bilateral uterine vessel ligation
3. Low uterine vessel ligation
4. Unilateral ovarian vessel ligation
5. Bilateral ovarian vessel ligation (quadruple ligation).

Large, curved needle is passed through the lower uterine myometrium, about 2 cm from the lateral margin, and then tied, on the other side. If the bleeding continues, tubal branches of both ovarian arteries can be tied medial to the ovarian ligament.

However, ligation techniques are technically challenging and time-consuming requiring both surgical expertise and a hemodynamically stable patient.

Bakri has described a bilateral looped uterine suture technique that compresses the uterine vessels against the entire thickness of the lateral uterine wall.

Internal iliac artery ligation

This requires an experienced surgeon who is familiar with the anatomy of the lateral pelvic wall.

The internal iliac artery should be then traced from above downwards until it divides into the anterior and posterior divisions. The anterior division should be ligated with black silk or linen (permanent suture material). Bilateral internal iliac artery ligation has been shown to reduce the pelvic

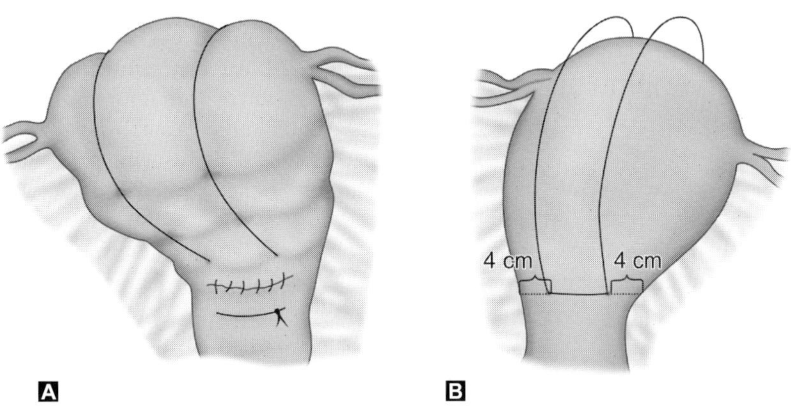

A B

FIG. 5: Application of B-Lynch sutures on atonic uterus to prevent postpartum hemorrhage.

blood flow by 49% and pulse pressure by 85% in arteries distal to the ligation. A success rate of 84% has been described.[13] Risks associated with ligation of the internal iliac artery include postischemic lower motor neuron damage, acute intestinal obstruction, claudication like pain, and peripheral nerve ischemia.

Uterine artery embolization

Embolization requires fluoroscopic guidance and the expertise of an interventional radiologist. Using angiography, the radiologist can identify the vessels responsible for the bleeding and embolizes them. The procedure involves placement of the arterial catheter under a fluoroscopic guidance and injection of an embolus. Embolic materials available for vascular occlusion include: gel foam (gelatin), polyvinyl alcohol particles, steel coils and *n*-butyl-2-cyanoacrylate glue. The success rate may be as high as 85–95%.[14] The patient must be stable enough for transfer to a radiological suite and should be monitored at all times with the ability to proceed to surgical intervention should the patient become unstable.

Reported complications of this procedure include fever, vascular perforation, lower extremity ischemia, bladder, and rectal wall necrosis. Flow through the vessels return over time, preserving both the uterus and fertility. Embolization therapy is unlikely to be successful after arterial ligation.

Embolization can be used for bleeding that continues after hysterectomy. Although the procedure has the potential of preserving future fertility, the need for specialized equipment and the availability of experienced interventional radiologist and resources, preclude its widespread use.

Hysterectomy

Hysterectomy is a radical surgical option to save life when all other conservative measures have failed, or if the patient is hemodynamically very unstable. Peripartum hysterectomy is estimated to occur in around 0.8 per 1,000 deliveries.[15] If alternative interventions fail, hysterectomy should not be delayed in patients who continue to bleed. Prompt control of uterine hemorrhage is vital to decrease morbidity and prevent death, as continued blood loss can lead to DIC.

Indications for hysterectomy

- Abnormal placentation
- Persistent uterine atony
- Uterine trauma after obstetric manipulations
- Lateral extension of the lower uterine segment incision into the uterine artery
- Sepsis.

Complications of hysterectomy include operative site infection, bladder and ureteral injuries, further intra-abdominal hemorrhage, and injury to other organs.

The decision to perform hysterectomy to control PPH is difficult. Emergency peripartum hysterectomy is an unequivocal marker of severe maternal morbidity and "near miss" mortality.

Current Concepts and New Developments

Antishock Garment

It reverses the effect of shock on the body's blood distribution by applying external counter pressure to the legs and abdomen. Vital organs like brain, heart and lungs suffer hypoxia in a person in shock. Anti-shock garment (ASG) stabilizes blood pressure until a patient can be shifted to a tertiary center.

Tamponade Test

Uterine tamponade works by exerting a counterpressure on placental bed. It can also be used as a diagnostic test. An inflated Sengstaken-Blakemore balloon catheter creates tamponade and identifies those who will or will not need surgery. If the bleeding gets arrested after uterine tamponade, 87.5% patients do not require a laparotomy.[16]

Recombinant Activated Factor VII (NovoSeven®)

Recombinant activated factor VII (rFVIIa) (NovoSeven®) is a synthetic vitamin K-dependent glycoprotein that has recently been tried to control PPH that did not respond to conventional measures. It works by activating the extrinsic coagulation pathway leading to increased formation of thrombin and a stable fibrin plug at the site of injury. It has been seen to be effective at stopping or reducing the bleeding when conventional treatments failed. Success rate of 80% has been reported in a study with minimal side effects.[17] The dosage used in various studies lies between 20 μg/kg and 120 μg/kg, but no proper dose-response relationship has been established.[18] The use, dosage, and timing of rFVIIa are still controversial. Reported side-effect is an increased risk of thromboembolism.[19] High cost precludes its widespread use for control of massive obstetric hemorrhage.

Recent European guidelines state that "rFVIIa may be considered as treatment for life-threatening PPH, but should not be considered as a substitute for, nor should it delay, the performance of a lifesaving procedure such as embolization or surgery, nor the transfer to a referring center".[17]

DISSEMINATED INTRAVASCULAR COAGULATION

Disseminated intravascular coagulation is a clinical scenario, which is characterized by accelerated formation of fibrin clots with simultaneous breakdown of these same clots. It is a consumptive coagulopathy, wherein there is rapid consumption of clotting factors. Normally our body is in a constant balance between fibrin generation and fibrinolysis. When this delicate balance is disturbed, the coagulation cascade and fibrinolytic system goes unchecked, DIC results. Pregnancy is already a hypercoagulable state, therefore, increasing the risk of DIC with any intercurrent pathology.

Disseminated intravascular coagulation arises from massive activation of the coagulation system that overwhelms the endogenous control mechanism. It may be initiated by exposure of blood to tissue factor which triggers activation of the extrinsic clotting system. This may result due to trauma or endotoxins damaging tissue or proteolytic enzyme release occurring in abruptio placentae.

Disseminated intravascular coagulation is typically characterized by the simultaneous thrombosis in vessels throughout the body, hence affecting blood supply to some organs, causing organ failure.

Causes

- Common causes:
  - Massive hemorrhage, especially with inadequate fluid replacement
  - Placental abruption and placenta previa
  - Severe pre-eclampsia/HELLP syndrome
- Rare causes:
  - Sepsis (septic abortion and intrauterine infection)
  - Intrauterine fetal demise (after 1 month)
  - Amniotic fluid embolism
  - Adult respiratory distress syndrome
  - Autoimmune disease
  - Acute fatty liver of pregnancy.

Diagnosis

Clinical Features

- Bleeding from venipuncture sites, incision sites and mucous membranes
- Profuse vaginal bleeding (postpartum with firm uterus)
- Associated shock (may be out of proportion to observed blood loss).

Laboratory Studies (Table 5)

- Decreased fibrinogen
- Increased fibrin degradation products
- Increased D-dimer
- Prolonged PT/international normalized ratio
- Prolonged aPTT (occasionally)
- Decreased antithrombin III
- Falling hemoglobin/hematocrit
- Rising lactate dehydrogenase (LDH)
- Rising bilirubin.

TABLE 5: Laboratory studies of disseminated intravascular coagulation

Test	Normal results
Fibrinogen	150–600 mg/dL
Prothrombin time	11–16 seconds
Activated partial thromboplastin time	22–37 seconds
Platelet count	1,200–350,000/mm^3
D-dimer	<0.5 mg/dL
Fibrin degradation products	<10 ng/dL

It is important to remember that concentration of fibrinogen is usually greatly increased in pregnancy. Hence, a normally labeled value for a pregnant lady may actually be very low. Falling fibrinogen is the hallmark of DIC.

Treatment

Treatment of DIC involves reversing the inciting events and simultaneous blood component therapy. Treat inciting event:

- Massive hemorrhage:
  - Treat cause (uterotonic agents, repair lacerations)
- Placental abruption:
  - Delivery
  - Attempt vaginal delivery if fetus and mother stable
- Pre-eclampsia/HELLP syndrome:
  - Delivery
  - Control of blood pressure
- Acute fatty liver:
  - Delivery
- Amniotic fluid embolism:
  - Cardiovascular support
  - Steroids
- Sepsis:
  - Broad spectrum IV antibiotics
- Adult respiratory distress syndrome:
  - Ventilator support
  - Cardiovascular support
- Retained dead fetus:
  - Delivery.

Blood Component Therapy

- Fresh-frozen plasma (volume = 250 cc): it is used to correct PT, aPTT, and fibrinogen levels. It is usually used as 4 units initially and then more if needed. Each unit of FFP increases the circulatory fibrinogen by 5–10 mg/dL
- Cryoprecipitate (volume = 35–40 cc): it is rich in fibrinogen and used to raise fibrinogen utilizing less volume than FFP. Each unit of cryoprecipitate increases the circulatory fibrinogen by 5–10 mg/dL

- Platelets: each pack of pooled platelets increases the platelet counts by 7,000–10,000/mm^3. However, in DIC, transfused platelets are consumed rapidly
- Packed RBCs: these increase the oxygen-carrying capacity (a primary priority). They have to be transfused rapidly to keep up with clinical bleeding, and try to keep hematocrit more than 25%.

CONCLUSION

Obstetric hemorrhage is the leading cause of maternal morbidity and mortality. Identification of risk factors is helpful, but massive obstetric hemorrhage is unpredictable. A multidisciplinary approach is required for proper resuscitation, restoration of circulating blood volume, and identification of cause of bleeding. Protocols for prevention and management of obstetric hemorrhage should be in place in every maternity unit.

REFERENCES

1. Nama V, Chandraharan E. Massive obstetric haemorrhage. In: Chandraharan E, Arulkumaran S (Eds). Obstetric and Intrapartum Emergencies: A Practical Guide to Management, 1st edition. Cambridge, USA: Cambridge University Press; 2012. pp. 33-40.
2. World Health Organization (WHO). The World Health Report 2005: Make Every Mother and Child Count. Geneva, Switzerland: WHO Press; 2005.
3. Calleja-Agius J, Custo R, Brincat M, et al. Placental abruption and placenta praevia. Eur Clin Obstet Gynaecol. 2006;2:121-7.
4. Pritchard JA, Mason R, Corley M, Pritchard S. Genesis of severe placental abruption. Am J Obstet Gynecol. 1970;108(1):22-7.
5. Mercier FJ, Van de Velde M. Major obstetric hemorrhage. Anesthesiol Clin. 2008;26(1):53-66.
6. Ofir K, Sheiner E, Levy A, Katz M, Mazor M. Uterine rupture: differences between a scarred and an unscarred uterus. Am J Obstet Gynecol. 2004;191(2):425-9.
7. American College of Obstetricians and Gynecologists. ACOG Practice Bulletin: Clinical Management Guidelines for Obstetrician-Gynecologist Number 76, October 2006: Postpartum hemorrhage. Obstet Gynecol. 2006;108(4):1039-47.
8. Leduc D, Senikas V, Lalonde AB, Ballerman C, Biringer A, Delaney M, et al. Active management of the third stage of labour: prevention and treatment of postpartum hemorrhage. J Obstet Gynaecol Can. 2009;31(10):980-93.
9. Mukherjee S, Arulkumaran S. Post-partum haemorrhage. Obstet Gynaecol Reprod Med. 2009;19(5):121-6.
10. Varatharajan L, Chandraharan E, Sutton J, Lowe V, Arulkumaran S. Outcome of the management of massive postpartum hemorrhage using the algorithm "HEMOSTASIS". Int J Gynaecol Obstet. 2011;113(2):152-4.
11. Dabelea VG, Schultze PM, McDuffie RS. Intrauterine balloon tamponade in the management of postpartum hemorrhage. Am J Perinatol. 2007;24(6):359-64.
12. Cho JH, Jun HS, Lee CN. Hemostatic suturing technique for uterine bleeding during cesarean delivery. Obstet Gynecol. 2000;96(1):129-31.
13. Doumouchtsis SK, Papageorghiou AT, Arulkumaran S. Systematic review of conservative management of postpartum hemorrhage: what to do when medical treatment fails? Obstet Gynecol Surv. 2007;62(8):540-7.
14. Mayer DC, Smith KA. Antepartum and postpartum hemorrhage. In: Chestnut DH, Wong CA, Tsen LC, Ngan Kee WD, Beilin Y, Mhyre J (Eds). Chestnut's Obstetric Anesthesia: Principles and Practice, 5th edition. Philadelphia, PA, USA: Saunders; 2014. pp. 825-30.
15. Glaze S, Ekwalanga P, Roberts G, Lange I, Birch C, Rosengarten A, et al. Peripartum hysterectomy: 1999 to 2006. Obstet Gynecol. 2008;111(3):732-8.
16. Condous GS, Arulkumaran S, Symonds I, Chapman R, Sinha A, Razvi K. The "tamponade test" in the management of massive postpartum hemorrhage. Obstet Gynecol. 2003;101(4):767-72.
17. Vincent JL, Rossaint R, Riou B, Ozier Y, Zideman D, Spahn DR. Recommendations on the use of recombinant activated factor VII as an adjunctive treatment for massive bleeding--a European perspective. Crit Care. 2006;10(4):R120.
18. Ahonen J, Jokela R. Recombinant factor VIIa for life-threatening post-partum haemorrhage. Br J Anaesth. 2005;94(5):592-5.
19. Welsh A, McLintock C, Gatt S, Somerset D, Popham P, Ogle R. Guidelines for the use of recombinant activated factor VII in massive obstetric haemorrhage. Aust N Z J Obstet Gynaecol 2008;48(1):12-6.

CHAPTER 28

Normal Puerperium

Susheela Rani, Charmila Ayyavoo

INTRODUCTION

The period following the delivery of baby and placenta up to 6 weeks is the puerperium. In the Ayurveda, this period of seclusion and confinement is up to 40 days. This period is very important as it determines the well-being and future of both the mother and the infant. The changes which have occurred during pregnancy revert to normal as much as possible during this period.

This period is also termed as "postnatal" and "postpartum". The World Health Organization[1] has defined "postnatal" as issues pertaining to the baby and "postpartum" as issues pertaining to the mother. According to the National Institute for Health and Care Excellence guidelines,[2] this period can be divided into three phases:

- The initial phase—within 24 hours of birth
- The second phase—from 2 to 7 days
- The final phase—from 8 to 42 days.

Lyon[3] has divided this period as the "acute" phase—lasting for 6–12 hours postpartum, "subacute" phase—lasting for 2–6 weeks, and "delayed" phase—which may last for 6 months.

The changes, which occur in this period, are mainly in the reproductive system, breasts, urinary tract, cardiovascular system, etc.

REPRODUCTIVE SYSTEM

Uterine Changes

At birth, the uterus weighs about 1 kg and this does not include placenta, fluids, etc. After 6 weeks, it weighs about 50–100 g. Maximum reduction in size and weight is in the first 2 weeks and then the reduction is gradual. The reduction in size of the uterus is due to decrease in size of individual myometrial cells. The return of the uterus to a nonpregnant state after birth is called "involution." At the end of 6 weeks, it would have shrunk to prepregnant levels, but the overall size is bigger than prior to gestation. This is because the increase in the amount of connective tissue, elastin in the myometrium and blood vessels, and the increase in the number of cells are permanent to some extent.

Afterpains

These are pains due to uterine contractions experienced by the woman after delivery. They are more common in multiparous women in whom the uterus contracts intermittently, especially during breastfeeding. Infant suckling causes oxytocin release and thereby uterine contractions. Often well tolerated, and decreasing in intensity by the third day, afterpains may necessitate analgesic administration in some women.

Very low levels of estrogen and progesterone in the puerperium may reduce the size of uterus to even slightly smaller than normal. According to Negishi et al.,[4] more than 80% of breastfeeding mothers had smaller uteri at 3 months compared to nonlactating mothers.

Height of Uterus

Immediately after the delivery, the uterus is 2 cm below the umbilicus with the fundus resting on the promontory. Within

12 hours, the fundus may rise 1 cm above the umbilicus. In 24 hours it is about the size of a 20 weeks gestational uterus. By the sixth postpartum day, it is halfway between the umbilicus and pubic symphysis. After that it descends about 1 fingerbreadth every 24 hours. After the 10th day of delivery, the uterus is not palpable in the abdomen.

Endometrium

By seventh day, endometrial glands are evident. At 16th day, the endometrium is restored throughout the uterus except at the placental site.[5]

Placental Site

After delivery of the placenta, there is arterial smooth muscle contraction and compression of the blood vessels at the placental site, which is now reduced to an irregular nodular and elevated area. The endometrium grows upward and covers the sloughed area of the placental site. Thus the placental site heals without formation of scar. This enables the endometrium to resume its cyclical changes and allows implantation and placentation in future pregnancies.

Lochia

Discharge from the uterus after birth is called lochia. It is the unique ability of the uterus to rid itself of the debris remaining after delivery. It consists of blood, tissue, and mucus, and can last up to 6 weeks following delivery. A lochial pattern of bleeding may persist much longer in some women; however, the median in a Philippines study[6] of breastfeeding women was found to be 27 days. The color and nature of the lochial discharge varies and is named accordingly.

- Lochia rubra is a red, blood-tinged flow which lasts for 2–4 days
- Lochia serosa is pinkish brown and watery which lasts up to the 10th day
- Lochia alba is thin, yellowish to white, and usually lasts up to 5 weeks.

Lochial discharge can be scant in women receiving oxytocic medication. Following cesarean section, lochia can be significantly lesser than a vaginal delivery. It can be slightly heavy after breastfeeding due to release of oxytocin. Lochial discharge has a menstrual odor and a foul smelling lochia is indicative of infection, typically endometritis.

Cervix

Cervix is initially soft and edematous with little tone. It regains its shape by the end of first week and becomes firm and thick. Cervical os which had dilated to 10 cm during labor slowly reduces its opening. It might admit 2 fingerbreadth by 6 days postpartum. However, by the end of 2 weeks, it is almost closed but the shape is that of a transverse slit (like a fish mouth) instead of circular opening seen in nulliparous women.

Vagina

Post vaginal delivery, the vagina is swollen and has poor tone. Resolution of vascularity and edema occurs by 3 weeks and rugae appear if not breastfeeding. Vaginal rugae are completely restored by 6–10 weeks. Reappearance of rugae is delayed in breastfeeding women because estrogen levels are persistently reduced.

Perineum

In vaginal delivery, swollen and bruised perineum heals in 1–2 weeks. The muscle tone is regained in 6 weeks and further improves in the following months. The extent of injury determines the degree of muscle tone regained. A study conducted by Christianson et al.,[7] which evaluated risk factors for perineal injury, found that an episiotomy produced more loss of perineal muscle performance after birth than that produced by a second-degree perineal injury. Even if the perineal muscle tone recovered, it took longer for its function to recover. This was evident in a study by Handa et al.,[8] who showed that pudendal nerve terminal motor latency recovers after 2 months but functional disturbances in the pelvic floor persists for at least 6 months.

Abdominal Wall

After birth, the abdominal wall remains soft and relatively poorly toned for many weeks. The tone is regained gradually over a period of time. However, the extent of muscle tone that is regain depends on the maternal exercises. Women who lack exercise have poorly toned abdominal muscles.

Ovaries

The return of normal ovarian function depends on breastfeeding. If breastfeeding is not established, ovulation can happen as early as 27 days. The mean time to first menstruation is approximately 55–60 days,[9] and in many women, menstruation is resumed by 12 weeks. If breastfeeding is established, there is a delay in return of menstruation. This is because ovulation is suppressed by high prolactin levels. Gonadotropin-releasing hormone pulsatility is affected by prolactin, which affects pituitary release of gonadotropins. Most women who breastfeed will begin menstruation within 36 weeks of delivery.

URINARY SYSTEM

Renal anatomic changes, like dilated ureters, persist for 5 days postpartum.[10] Renal function, i.e., plasma flow and glomerular filtration rate reach prepregnant levels by 6 weeks postpartum.[11]

Immediately after delivery, bladder mucosa shows varying degrees of edema and hyperemia. Bladder tone is also diminished due to pudendal nerve trauma during delivery. Decreased sensation even with increasing pressure causes overdistension with overflow incontinence and incomplete emptying of bladder. With adequate bladder emptying, the tone is usually restored within 5–7 days. Some of the bladder symptoms triggered during pregnancy, such as urgency, frequency, and nocturia, tend to disappear in the late-postpartum period regardless of method of delivery.[12] Stress incontinence tends to persist in late-postpartum period after vaginal delivery.

Mood Changes

The falling levels of estrogen and progesterone are thought to play a role in the mood changes of the puerperium.[13] Activity levels, sleep pattern, and emotional stress also contribute to mood changes.

Sexual Function

Sexual intercourse can be resumed when the lochia ceases, the vagina and vulva are healed, and the woman is physically comfortable and emotionally ready. Physical readiness usually takes about 3–5 weeks, but the woman may not feel ready for sexual intercourse for a longer period and she should not be forced to accept it. Women with major trauma have greater fears regarding sexuality than women with minor trauma during delivery.[14]

CARDIOVASCULAR SYSTEM

The hemodynamic changes that take place in the postpartum period can be summarized as follows:
- Blood volume decreases and the magnitude of this decline is about 10% with vaginal deliveries and about 5–30% with cesarean sections
- Cardiac output increases by as much as 60–80% immediately postpartum. This is due to a massive volume shift due to elimination of placental site leading to increased venous return.[15] This increase in blood volume is responsible for the profound diuresis in early puerperium and a fall in hematocrit. It then drops to levels slightly higher than nonpregnant state, and it may remain at this level for a few weeks postpartum
- Stroke volume increases
- Heart rate decreases, which can be from 4 to 17 beats per minutes
- Blood pressure can be variable depending on the blood loss and other hemodynamic parameters. Peripheral vascular resistance is usually increased or it may remain unchanged.

Most of the cardiac parameters will recover in the first 2 weeks postpartum, with more gradual shifts continuing over the next 4–5 months.[16]

Hematocrit

There is a fall in hematocrit due to the increased blood volume and also due to the blood loss during delivery. The hematocrit rises by third to seventh postpartum day.

BREASTS

Lactation

The second stage of lactogenesis occurs in the puerperium; the first stage occurs during pregnancy. Lactation occurs with the help of two hormones—prolactin and oxytocin.

Prolactin stimulates mammary glandular ductal growth and epithelial cell proliferation and induces milk protein synthesis. Oxytocin is involved in the milk ejection or letdown reflex. The infant's suckling creates afferent impulses that stimulate the posterior pituitary gland. Oxytocin causes the contraction of the myoepithelial cells that line the ducts of the breast and aid milk ejection. Milk synthesis remains remarkably constant at approximately 800 mL/day. Milk production is responsive to maternal states of well-being. Thus, stress and fatigue adversely affect a woman's milk supply by dopamine, norepinephrine, or both, which inhibit prolactin synthesis. Relaxation is a key for successful lactation.

Human milk, in addition to its numerous nutrients that make it an ideal food source for the growing term infant, is a bioactive fluid that evolves from colostrum to mature milk as the infant matures.

HEMOSTATIC CHANGES

There is increase in clotting factors I, II, VII, VIII, IX, and XII. There is a decrease in protein S and inhibition of fibrinolysis. There is also a significant fall in the activity of activated protein C, an important anticoagulant. These physiological changes, which are important for minimizing intrapartum blood loss, also entail an increased risk for thromboembolism in the postpartum period.[17]

TABLE 1: Physiological changes in the puerperium

Reproductive system	• Placenta: separates within 15–30 min • Uterine involution: ischemia retraction of muscles, autolysis of enzymes decrease cell size, phagocytosis (fibrosis tissue removed) • Endometrium: superficial layer sloughed off as lochia • Placental site takes 6–7 weeks to heal and heals from the center to margins
Hematological changes	• Hemoglobin increases in the immediate postpartum and then decreases • Leukocytosis immediately after delivery followed by return to nonpregnant levels by 4 weeks • Platelet count increases in reaction to and as a compensation for increased platelet consumption during the process of delivery
Cardiovascular system	• Blood volume decreases, 10% with vaginal deliveries and about 5–30% with cesarean deliveries • Cardiac output increases by as much as 60–80% immediately postpartum. It then drops to levels slightly higher than nonpregnant state, and it may remain at this level for a few weeks postpartum • Stroke volume increases • Heart rate decreases, which can be from 4 to 17 beats per minutes • Blood pressure can be variable depending on the blood loss and other hemodynamic parameters
Lactation	• Placenta delivery: decrease estrogen, progesterone • Anterior pituitary: release prolactin, level increases with each breastfeeding session • Oxytocin is released for "letdown reflex"
Return to ovulation	• Breastfeeding mothers: ovulation delays up to 3 months due to prolactin surges • Non-breastfeeding mothers Ovulation usually returns between 6 and 12 weeks
Bone density	• No long-term bone loss
Sexual function	• Physical readiness usually takes about 3–5 weeks

HEMATOLOGICAL CHANGES[18]

Red Blood Cell

Post pregnancy, plasma volume decreases as a result of diuresis, and the blood volume returns to nonpregnant values. Hemoglobin and hematocrit increase consequently. Plasma volume increases again 2–5 days later, possibly because of a rise in aldosterone secretion. Later, it again decreases. Significant elevation has been documented between measurements of hemoglobin taken at 6–8 weeks postpartum and those taken at 4–6 months postpartum, indicating that it takes at least 4–6 months postpregnancy to restore the physiological dip in hemoglobin to the nonpregnant values.

White Blood Cell

The stress of delivery may itself lead to brisk leukocytosis. Few hours after delivery, healthy women have been documented as having a white blood cell (WBC) count varying from 9,000 to 25,000/mm^3. By 4 weeks postdelivery, typical WBC ranges are similar to those in healthy nonpregnant women.

Platelets

Post delivery, platelet count increases in reaction to and as a compensation for increased platelet consumption during the process of delivery.

BONE DENSITY

Bone density can decrease during pregnancy, probably because of calcium mobilization from maternal skeleton to fetus. Some studies have shown continued loss during breastfeeding. Exact time taken for maternal bone remineralization is not clear but there is no long-term loss of bone mineral density associated with pregnancy.[19]

Weight Changes

Weight changes are uneven in the puerperium with average weight loss being maximum in the first 2–3 weeks. Emptying of the uterus, uterine involution, and diuresis contributes to weight loss in the puerperium. Though most women are expected to return to their prepregnancy weight by 6 months after delivery, many retain 1.4 kg on an average.[20] Epidemiologic studies[21] that measure weight before and after pregnancy in primiparous have consistently found that primiparity is associated with higher weight gain among women already overweight before pregnancy. Furthermore, these findings consistently show that weight gain after delivery does not differ across racial and ethnic groups.

PSYCHOLOGICAL CHANGES

Since motherhood is typically viewed as a "happy time" and childbirth is seen as an event from which a woman should "bounce back" within a few days, many women experience a lack of understanding and/or support from those around them. Mothers need significant coping skills to deal with so many new challenges.[22] The sudden drop in estrogen, progesterone, endorphins, and other hormones may trigger depression; the same way, moodiness may be triggered by premenstrual changes in these hormones.

Many women feel exhausted after labor and delivery and may need a long time to fully recover. Cesarean births require an even longer recovery.

Hypothyroidism may occur for the first time after birth and the symptoms of thyroid deficiency may mimic depression.

CONCLUSION

In the words of Deborah S Lyon, "After a woman has safely negotiated the physiologic hardships of pregnancy and three stages of labor, the attention of virtually everyone (family, friends, and caregivers) often turns to the infant. The enormous physical and emotional changes required to return from the status of term pregnancy to the nonpregnant state are underappreciated and often underevaluated."[3] A good understanding of the normal physiology of the puerperium will help the healthcare provider to provide the right kind of support that is so very much needed in this period and also to identify and treat problems at the earliest.

REFERENCES

1. World Health Organization (WHO). (2010). Maternal, newborn, child and adolescent health. WHO Technical Consultation on Postpartum and Postnatal care. [online] Available from: www.who.int/maternal_child_adolescent/documents/WHO_MPS_10_03/en/. [Accessed June, 2015].
2. Demott K, Bick D, Norman R, Ritchie G, Turnbull N, Adams C, et al. Postnatal care: Routine Postnatal Care of Women and Their Babies. NICE Clinical Guidelines, No. 37. London, United Kingdom: National Collaborating Centre for Primary Care and Royal College of General Practitioners; 2006.
3. Lyon DS. (2008). Postpartum care. [online] Available from: www.glowm.com/section_view/heading/Postpartum%20Care/item/143. [Accessed June, 2015].
4. Negishi H, Kishida T, Yamada H, Hirayama E, Mikini M, Fujimoto S. Changes in uterine size after vaginal delivery and cesarean section determined by vaginal sonography in the puerperium. Arch Gynecol Obstet. 1999;263(1-2):13-6.
5. Sharman A. Post-partum regeneration of the human endometrium. J Anat. 1953;87(1):1-10.
6. Visness CM, Kennedy KI, Ramos R. The duration and character of postpartum bleeding among breast-feeding women. Obstet Gynecol. 1997;89(2):159-63.
7. Christianson LM, Bovbjerg VE, McDavitt EC, Hullfish KL. Risk factors for perineal injury during delivery. Am J Obstet Gynecol. 2003;189(1):255-60.
8. Handa VL, Harvey L, Fox HE, Kjerulff KH. Parity and route of delivery: does cesarean delivery reduce bladder symptoms late in life? Am J Obstet Gynecol. 2004;191(2):463-9.
9. Perez A. Lactational amenorrhea and natural family planning. In: Hafez ESE, editor. Human Ovulation: Mechanisms, Prediction, Detection, and Induction. 1st edition. Amsterdam, USA: Elsevier/North-Holland Biomedical Press; 1979. pp. 501-13.
10. Bailey RR, Rolleston GL. Kidney length and ureteral dilatation in the puerperium. J Obstet Gynaecol Br Commonw. 1971;78(1):55-61.
11. Sims EA, Krantz KE. Serial studies of renal function during pregnancy and the puerperium in normal women. J Clin Invest. 1958;37(12):1764-74.
12. Botelho S, da Silva JM, Palma P, Herrmann V, Riccetto C. Can the delivery method influence lower urinary tract symptoms triggered by the first pregnancy? Int Braz J Urol. 2012;38(2):267-76.
13. Halbreich U, Kahn LS. Role of estrogen in the aetiology and treatment of mood disorders. CNS Drugs. 2001;15(10):797-817.
14. Hicks TL, Goodall SF, Quattrone EM, Lydon-Rochelle MT. Postpartum sexual functioning and method of delivery: summary of the evidence. J Midwifery Womens Health. 2004;49(5):430-6.
15. Van Oppen AC, Van der Tweel I, Alsbach GP, Heethaar RM, Bruinse HW. A longitudinal study of maternal hemodynamics during normal pregnancy. Obstet Gynecol. 1996;88(1):40-6.
16. Robson SC, Hunter S, Moore M, Dunlop W. Haemodynamic changes during the puerperium: a Doppler and M-mode echocardiographic study. Br J Obstet Gynaecol. 1987;94(11):1028-39.
17. Bremme KA. Haemostatic changes in pregnancy. Best Pract Res Clin Haematol. 2003;16(2):153-68.
18. Chandra S, Tripathi AK, Mishra S, Amzarul M, Vaish AK. Physiological changes in hematological parameters during pregnancy. Indian J Hematol Blood Transfus. 2012;28(3):144-6.
19. Ensom MH, Liu PY, Stephenson MD. Effect of pregnancy on bone mineral density in healthy women. Obstet Gynecol Surv. 2002;57(2):99-111.
20. Greene GW, Smiciklas-Wright H, Scholl TO, Karp RJ. Postpartum weight change: how much of the weight gained in pregnancy will be lost after delivery? Obstet Gynecol. 1988;71(5):701-7.
21. Gunderson EP. Childbearing and obesity in women: weight before, during, and after pregnancy. Obstet Gynecol Clin North Am. 2009;36(2):317-32, ix.
22. Hibbert CG. Postpartum Mood Disorders: An Informational Guide for Couples. [online] Available from: psychotherapy.com/mom.html. [Accessed June, 2015].

CHAPTER 29

Abnormal Puerperium and Its Management

Rubina Sohail, Saima Iqbal

INTRODUCTION

Puerperium is the 6 weeks period following the birth of a child during which the physiological and anatomical changes that had occurred during pregnancy return back to normal. These changes take place rapidly during the first 2 weeks and then slow down and are completed by 6 weeks postpartum.

CHANGES OF PUERPERIUM: THE NORMAL PUERPERIUM

In puerperium, changes take place not only in the genital system and breasts, but also in blood, cardiovascular system, respiratory system, and renal system. In the genital tract, involution of uterus takes place so that within 1 week after delivery, the uterus becomes a pelvic organ and is not palpable. There is gradual reduction in the size of the vagina and rugae reappear at 3–4 weeks. Lochia appears as frank blood and remains red (lochia rubra) for the first couple of days, later it changes to brown pink in color (lochia serosa), and eventually yellowish white (lochia alba).

The plasma volume reduces by 20%, red cell mass returns to normal within 24 hours and erythrocyte sedimentation rate level becomes normal within 4 weeks. Heart rate, heart sounds, cardiac output, and blood pressure come to normal in 2 weeks' time. Lung volume, capacity volume, and tidal volume revert to normal in 2–6 weeks. The size of the kidneys, the dilatation of the upper urinary tract, and bladder function come to normal in 2–6 weeks.

For the first 2–3 days postnatal, the breasts secrete only colostrum. The milk secretion gradually increases and by the sixth day, around 500 mL is produced every 24 hours. After lactation is established, on an average 800 mL of milk is secreted every 24 hours. Exclusive breastfeeding is recommended for the first 6 months to reduce the chances of conception to as low as 1–5%. Ovulation generally resumes around 28 days postpartum, therefore, either the woman should be exclusively breastfeeding or some other form of contraception should be started to avoid an unplanned pregnancy.[1,2]

IMPORTANCE OF PUERPERIUM

Puerperium is an important time for the woman and her child for multiple reasons. Basically, it is the time when the physiological changes of pregnancy revert back to normal, but it is also the time when complications like puerperal sepsis and secondary postpartum hemorrhage (PPH) can also happen, which are potential causes of maternal death. At this juncture, the women need help and training for care of baby and breasts during lactation, and she has to be made aware of the importance of hygiene. Due to her new responsibility and increasing demands of the baby, the patient is advised adequate periods of rest, preferably 8 hours a day. Puerperium is also the time when fertility resumes and unless proper birth-spacing practices are adopted, there is likelihood of pregnancy. Therefore, advise on contraception and helping the couple choose an appropriate method is an important part of puerperium management.

Keeping in mind the importance of puerperium, the World Health Organization recommends that the woman should be discharged from the facility after 24 hours and at least three postnatal visits are recommended on day 3, day 7–14, and 6 weeks after birth. At each visit, the child is evaluated for growth, breastfeeding, cord care, and immunization and the mother for urinary and bowel symptoms, wound, breast pain, uterine tenderness, lochia, and any psychological dysfunction.

SITUATION IN SOUTH ASIA

According to the current data, maternal mortality is high in South Asia. It is believed that there are certain common factors in almost all the countries of South Asia.

- Literacy rate is low in almost all the countries
- The antenatal coverage is poor and there are only a small percentage of booked patients
- Quality of antenatal services is not up to the minimal standard
- Even less postnatal coverage and quality is also deficient
- Women rarely seek postnatal care and only 10–15% women present for postnatal visit. During the visit, the quality of care that they receive is substandard
- There is lack of emphasis on contraception
- There is lack of emphasis on breastfeeding.

Various causes of abnormal puerperium are given in table 1.

EVALUATION OF PATIENT WITH ABNORMAL PUERPERIUM

History

Fever, malaise, vaginal discharge, foul smell, painful micturition, breast lump, breast pain, lack of control over feces, lack of energy, noncommunicative, lack of interest towards baby or aggression towards baby

Examination

- General physical examination to assess pallor, pulse, temperature, blood pressure, and state of hydration
- Examination of calf muscles legs for tenderness and edema to look for deep vein thrombosis
- Auscultation of the chest
- Breast examination to look for hard lumpy breast and tenderness
- Abdominal examination for fundal height and abdominal tenderness
- Pelvic examination for color and smell of lochia, inspection of episiotomy, size of uterus, and fullness in adnexa.[3]

Investigations

Important investigations will include complete blood count, high-vaginal swab, urine routine investigation, culture and sensitivity on midstream specimen and pelvic ultrasound for uterus, products of conception, adnexa, tubo-ovarian mass, or pelvic abscess. Other relevant investigations include X-ray of chest, blood urea, and serum electrolytes. In seriously ill patients with features of septicemia, clotting profile and arterial blood gases should be performed for detection of hypoxia or acidosis. General investigations may be needed if not already performed. These include grouping and Rh factor, hepatitis B surface antigen, anti-hepatitis C virus, and blood sugar random.

Diagnosis

After review of history, examination, and investigations, the diagnosis will be established.

AIMS OF MANAGEMENT

- To diagnose and treat the cause of abnormal puerperium
- To establish infant feeding
- Provide emotional support
- Information and decision making on contraception.

TABLE 1: Causes of abnormal puerperium[2]

Minor causes		
Voiding difficulty and overdistension of bladder	• Urinary stress incontinence	• Perineal discomfort
Constipation	• Anal incontinence	• Baby blues
Breast engorgement	• Painful/cracked nipples	• Mastitis
Major causes		
Puerperal pyrexia	• Genital tract infection • Urinary tract infection • Mastitis and breast abscess • Wound infection following C-section and perineal infection following episiotomy • Thrombophlebitis and deep vein thrombosis • Other infections, such as chest infection	
Psychiatric disorders	• Postnatal depression • Postpartum psychosis	
Secondary postpartum hemorrhage	• It is bleeding from the genital tract between 24 h and 6 weeks after delivery	

Management of Abnormal Puerperium

Counseling

The couple will be explained about the current condition, discuss the management options, likely prognosis, and outcome. Counseling of the family members is also relevant.

General Care

It includes hydration, correction of anemia, improvement of general health, focusing on personal hygiene, taking appropriate nutrition, effective analgesia, care of the breasts and nipples, bladder and bowel care, psychological support, physiotherapy, and mobilization. Pelvic floor exercises are encouraged. Myths and misconceptions related to puerperium are identified and dealt with.

Minor Issues

Many a times, minor issues occur during puerperium. These include bladder dysfunction, such as voiding difficulty, overdistension, urinary retention, stress incontinence; bowel dysfunction, such as constipation and anal incontinence, perineal discomfort (~80%), breast engorgement, painful or cracked nipples, tiredness, sleep disorders, and postpartum blues. Most of these conditions can be managed by simple measures, such as counseling, advise on self-care, and minor medication. The general guidance to women during puerperium is to eat well (high-roughage diet), drink at least 8 glasses of water daily, and have plenty of sleep—at least 8 hours a day. Postnatal exercises as Kegel exercise can significantly benefit the urinary symptoms. But the specific management of both minor and major issues during postnatal period is given in tables 2 and 3.

TABLE 2: Specific management: minor issues

Minor issues	Outline of management
Voiding difficulty and overdistension	This can happen in the immediate postnatal period due to decreased tone and less sensitivity of the urinary bladder. It may need catheterization for a short time
Urinary stress incontinence	Kegel exercises are helpful, starting in the early postnatal period
Constipation	High-fiber diet, increased water intake and laxatives
Anal incontinence	Look for third- or fourth-degree perineal tear; immediate surgical correction or at 3 months
Perineal discomfort	This can be helped by use of cold pack or the traditional "sitz bath"
Mastitis	Care of nipples, analgesia, and antibiotic if needed
Baby blues	Family support for care of baby, psychological support, family counseling, and medication if needed

TABLE 3: Specific management: major issues[2]

Major causes	Disease	Outline of management
Puerperal pyrexia	• Genital tract infection	• Antibiotics is the mainstay but may need removal of products of conception or surgical treatment for tubo-ovarian mass or drainage of pelvic abscess
	• Mastitis	• Simple analgesic as paracetamol, care of nipples, and antibiotics if needed • *Staphylococcus aureus* is the main organism and 3 out of 65 infections progress to breast abscess[4]
	• Abscess	• Incision drainage and suppression of breast-feeding by bromocriptine mesylate, 2.5 mg twice a day for 10 days[5]
	• Perineal infections	• Perineal wash, keeping perineum dry, analgesia, antibiotics, use of magnesium sulfate paste, and in certain cases resuturing of the episiotomy
	• Urinary tract infection	• Increased water intake and antibiotics
	• Deep vein thrombosis	• Heparin is the mainstay of treatment
Psychiatric disorders	• Postpartum depression • Puerperal psychosis	• Psychological support and medication • Psychological support, medication, family counseling, and home help
Secondary postpartum hemorrhage	• Could be due to retention of placental tissue or membranes. Treated by evacuation of the contents of the uterus by suction, dilatation and curettage or manual vacuum aspiration. After giving the loading dose of antibiotic, there should be no delay in emptying the uterus	

Specific Measures

Specific measures will entail treating the cause effectively.

Review of specific conditions: three issues will be discussed in detail. These include puerperal pyrexia, psychiatric disorders, and breast disorders in the puerperium.

PUERPERAL PYREXIA

After delivery, the woman is prone to infections due to various reasons. These include the raw placental site, tissue trauma during delivery, lacerations of the genital tract, low resistance due to anemia or hemorrhage, and prolonged labor. The infections can result in cellulitis, septicemia, or peritonitis. The predisposition to infection increases with multiple pelvic examinations and inadequate attention to antisepsis and disinfection. The severity of the illness depends on the virulence of the infecting organism, the resistance of the invaded tissues, and the general health of the woman.

Puerperal pyrexia, also known as "childbed fever", is defined as temperature of 38°C (100.4°F) or higher on any 2 of the first 10 days postpartum, exclusive of the first 24 hours. Pyrexia is quite common following delivery and can be secondary to the breast problems (18%). Puerperal sepsis causes puerperal pyrexia, pelvic pain, abnormal or foul smelling lochia, and delayed involution. Puerperal infection includes not only infections of the genital tract, but also many extragenital and incidental infections. Common causes are urinary tract infection, genital tract infection, mastitis, wound infection following C-section and episiotomy, thrombophlebitis, deep vein thrombosis, and other infections including chest and throat infections.

Organisms commonly producing this infection are *Streptococcus pyogenes*; *Staphylococci* (inhabitants of skin and pimples, carbuncles, and many other pustular eruptions); the anaerobic streptococci, which flourish in devitalized tissues, such as may be present after long and injurious labor and unskilled instrumental delivery; *Escherichia coli* and *Clostridium welchii* (inhabitants of the lower bowel); and *C. tetani*.[6]

Causes of Puerperal Fever (Pyrexia)

- Puerperal sepsis (uterine infection)
- Postsurgical wound infection
- Infections of perineum, vagina, and cervix
- Breast infection: mastitis
- Infective pelvic and femoral venous thrombophlebitis
- Urinary tract infections
- Pulmonary complications, like atelectasis
- Meningitis following spinal or epidural analgesia
- Other incidental infections:
  - Tuberculosis
  - Malaria
  - Typhoid
  - Chest infections, e.g., pneumonia, bronchitis
  - Human immunodeficiency virus/acquired immunodeficiency syndrome
- Unknown origin.

Incriminating Organisms

The major pathogens causing sepsis in the puerperium are:
- *Streptococcus pyogenes*, which is a Gram-positive bacterium and also called group A β-hemolytic streptococcus (GABHS). Typically produces large zones of β-hemolysis with disruption of erythrocytes and release of hemoglobin.[7] The number of maternal deaths from GABHS infection has been increasing over past 10 years. Group A streptococcus is typically community-based and 5–30% of populations are asymptomatic carriers on skin or in throat. Antenatal education should raise awareness of this and the importance of good personal hygiene and washing hands before and after using the lavatory or changing sanitary towels[8]
- Staphylococci are normal inhabitants of the skin and can result in infections such as carbuncles or pimples. Typically produce a localized infection
- *Peptostreptococcus* is anaerobic Gram-positive spore-forming bacteria. It is slow growing and has increasing resistance to antimicrobial drugs. It is a normal commensal of skin, mouth, gastrointestinal tract, urinary tract, vagina and can become pathogenic and also cause septicemia in traumatic or immunosuppressed conditions. It can cause abscess in the breast, brain, liver, and also cause necrotizing soft-tissue infections. It flourishes in devitalized tissues, which may be present after long and injurious labor and unskilled instrumental delivery. It is susceptible to β-lactam antibiotics
- *Escherichia coli* are Gram-negative, facultative anaerobic bacteria commonly found in the lower intestines. Mostly harmless but can cause food contamination
- *Clostridium perfringens,* previously called *Clostridium welchii,* is a Gram-positive, anaerobic spore-forming bacteria commonly found in the lower intestines. Also found in the gastrointestinal tract of humans. Infections due to *Clostridium perfringens* show evidence of tissue necrosis, bacteremia, and gas gangrene or myonecrosis
- Methicillin-resistant *Staphylococcus aureus* (MRSA) is responsible for difficult-to-treat infections and has resistance to β-lactam antibiotics which include penicillins, methicillin, oxacillin, and cephalosporins. MRSA began as a hospital-acquired infection (nosocomial infection) but has developed limited endemic status.[9]

Prevention

- Preventing and treating anemia in the antenatal period and taking care of nutrition. Screening all women

for β-hemolytic streptococci is practiced in Western countries but not in India
- Maintaining a partogram to manage labor, detecting slow labor early, and taking timely action, like augmentation of labor, are important preventive measures
- Use of aseptic techniques, like handwashing, minimizing number of vaginal examinations in labor, avoidance of tissue trauma, and blood loss during delivery
- Any laceration in vagina, perineum, or cervix should be repaired immediately
- Prophylactic antibiotics should be given for high-risk cases. Perioperative antimicrobial prophylaxis reduces rate of pelvic infections by 70–80% in all types of cesarean deliveries (Level IA Evidence)
- Gross-inspection of the placenta and membranes for their completeness in all deliveries is essential.

Urinary Tract Infection

Urinary tract infection is a common infection following delivery. It is commonly caused by Gram-negative *E. coli.* It may be due to frequent or prolonged use of indwelling catheter during labor. The patient may present with fever, dysuria, or burning micturition. The presence of leukocytes, proteins, or blood in the midstream specimen of urine support the diagnoses of urinary tract infection. Urine culture should be sent.

Genital Tract Infection

Despite the improvement of medical facilities and use of broad-spectrum antibiotics, genital tract infection and sepsis remain a very common cause of maternal death. This mounts to around 10 deaths per year in the UK. The situation is even worse in the developing countries. Severe sepsis and acute organ dysfunction has a mortality rate of 20–40% rising to around 50%, if septic shock develops. Puerperal infection is usually polymicrobial and involves contaminants from the bowel that colonize the lower genital tract and the perineum.[9]

After delivery, the natural barriers to infection are temporarily removed and therefore organisms with pathogenic potential can ascend from the lower genital tract to the pelvic organs. Separation of placenta exposes a large raw area; retained product of conception and blood clots within the uterus provide good culture media for polypathogens to prosper.

Symptoms of genital tract infection

- Fever with chills and rigors (persistent spiking temperature suggests abscess)
- Abdominal discomfort, vomiting, and diarrhea
- Offensive vaginal discharge.

Signs of genital tract infection

- Tachycardia
- Pyrexia
- Abdominal or pelvic tenderness
- Delay in uterine involution
- Uterus: boggy, tender, enlarged
- Bogginess: pelvic abscess
- Infected wounds: C-section/perineal
- Paralytic ileus.

Investigations

Patient will be investigated as follows:
- Full blood count: for diagnosis of low hemoglobin, leukocytosis, and thrombocytopenia
- Urea and serum electrolyte: to detect fluid and electrolyte imbalance
- High-vaginal swab: for diagnosis of infection
- Blood culture: for diagnosis of septicemia
- Pelvic ultrasound: for retained products or pelvic abscess
- Clotting profile: to diagnose disseminated intravascular coagulation
- Arterial blood gas: to detect hypoxia and acidosis.

Management

Early treatment should be started with suitable antibiotic. Mild-to-moderate infections can be treated with broad-spectrum antibiotics such as co-amoxicillin 1 g twice a day for 7 days or a cephalosporin's such as cephalexin 400 mg once a day for 7 days plus metronidazole, or 500 mg 8 hourly for 5 days. The choice of route for the antibiotic whether oral or parenteral, may be crucial in determining the outcome. Abdominal pain, fever (>38°C) and tachycardia (>90 beats per minutes) are indications for admission for intravenous antibiotics. Depending on the severity, the first few doses should be given intravenously. The speed of onset or deterioration in symptoms and signs is important. The focus of infection should be sought and dealt with. This may be done by uterine evacuation or by drainage of a breast abscess, wound or pelvic abscess. Broad-spectrum antibiotics should be given to cover these procedures.[9]

Use of Injectable Antibiotics in Puerperal Pyrexia

Administration of intravenous broad-spectrum antibiotics within 1 hour of suspicion of severe sepsis with/without septic shock is recommended. In principal, the antibiotic therapy should be guided by the Gram-stain of any aspirate or biopsy; however, in actual clinical practice, the patient is usually so sick that there is no time to wait; hence initial empirical prescribing of broad-spectrum antibiotics is essential. Intravenous broad-spectrum antibiotics should be given within 1 hour of suspicion of severe sepsis (Royal College of Obstetricians and Gynaecologists guidelines).[10]

Antibiotics should be commenced after taking specimens and should not be delayed until the results are available. Broad-spectrum coverage must be initiated immediately after collection of cultures.[11] Giving amoxicillin or ampicillin 500–1,000 mg intravenous with gentamycin 80 mg intramuscular 8 hourly and metronidazole 500 mg intravenous 8 hourly provides the broadest coverage. If improvement occurs continue intravenous antibiotics for 3 days and then follow with oral antibiotics for 7 days. Group A streptococcus is exquisitely sensitive to β-lactams. Amoxiclav 1.2 g intravenous 8 hourly with or without gentamycin is better than ampicillin or amoxicillin alone.

If response is poor, a combination of either piperacillin/tazobactam 3.375 g intravenous every 6 hours or a carbapenem 500 mg, 8 hourly intravenous plus clindamycin 450–900 mg intravenous every 8 hours provides one of the broadest ranges of treatment. In deranged renal functions, dosage of carbapenem and clindamycin has to be adjusted according to the renal functions. MRSA may be resistant to clindamycin; hence if the woman is or is highly likely to be MRSA positive, vancomycin 15 mg/kg body weight, intravenous, 8 hourly or teicoplanin 400 mg 12 hourly for 3 doses followed by 400 mg once a day, intravenous, may be added until sensitivity is known. Teicoplanin should be given with caution in breastfeeding mothers.

Breastfeeding limits the use of antimicrobials; hence the advice of a consultant microbiologist should be sought at an early stage. Intravenous immunoglobulin is recommended for severe invasive streptococcal or staphylococcal infection if other therapies have failed. If fever is prolonged then treatment with heparin should also be considered.[10,12]

PSYCHIATRIC DISORDERS IN PUERPERIUM

Psychiatric problems in puerperium usually remain undetected, mainly because newborn is the focus of attention for the couple and the family. Moreover there is limited awareness both of family and the attending doctor about such disorders. In South Asia, most of the women do not present for even a single postnatal visit, therefore, any opportunity to diagnose the disorders is lost.

Depression affects a significant proportion of the women in the postnatal period. Sometimes the emotional changes of the postnatal period closely mimic depression, making the diagnosis difficult to make. The prevalence of postnatal depression ranges from 4.5 to 28%. The risk of depression is increased by threefold in the first 5 postnatal weeks. Precipitating factors of depression can be physical exhaustion of the mother, difficulty in establishing breastfeeding, sleep deprivation, loss of normal figure due to weight gain, stretch marks, and social deprivation such as loss of employment, limited income, confinement to home, and boredom.

Postpartum psychiatric disorders can be divided into three broad groups:
1. Postpartum anxiety/blues
3. Postpartum depression
4. Postpartum psychosis.

Postpartum Anxiety/Blues

These are also called as "maternity blues" or "baby blues". It is a very common problem occurring in 50–80% women. The symptoms occur typically after the third postpartum day, peak at the fifth day, and resolve spontaneously by the tenth postpartum day. The symptoms are generally transient and accompanied with rapid mood changes. The symptoms include tearfulness, irritability, anxiety, insomnia, lack of energy, loss of appetite, and feeling of being overwhelmed. Postpartum blues should be differentiated from postpartum psychosis, which will have more symptoms of confusion, agitation, paranoid delusions, and somatic symptoms. About 75% of these patients will recover spontaneously and 25% will end up with postpartum depression. Usually no treatment is required except for psychotherapy and monitoring for progression to postpartum depression.[13]

Postpartum Depression

This occurs in 10–20% of women in the postpartum period (Box 1). The condition generally starts as postpartum blues on the third postpartum day but become prolonged. Causes of postpartum depression include a history of previous depression or antepartum depression, adverse social conditions, difficult relationship, burden of childbearing, and some evidence of association with C-section, miscarriage, and menstrual disorders. Symptoms include low mood, decreased appetite and sleep, decreased interest in daily activities (unable to do household chores), decreased concentration, child neglect, irritability and aggression, impatience, social withdrawal, anxiety, anger, death wish, or suicidal ideas. Treatment starts with the diagnosis as

Box 1: Women at risk of postpartum depression

- If Personal history of depression
- Family history of depression
- History of depression in previous pregnancy
- Stress during pregnancy or early puerperium
- Women with sleep deprivation and exhaustion
- Adolescent mother
- Difficulty in breast-feeding
- Lack of social support
- Being socially disadvantaged
- Poor marital relationship
- Adverse early life experience

many of the women do not accept that they are ill and do not seek care. Effective screening tool is Edinburgh Postnatal Depression Scale. The patient is identified by screening; should have a detailed interview regarding the symptoms and cause of disease, similar history in previous life, problems in pregnancy, relationship with husband, family, and other children. Psychotherapy and medications are the mainstay of treatment. Many patients require antidepressant drugs and few require electroconvulsive therapy. Selective serotonin reuptake inhibitors have been shown to be effective. Treatment should be started with half of the recommended starting dose: 25 mg of sertraline per day or 10 mg paroxetine per day for 4 days and then increased by smaller increments till symptoms are controlled. If the symptoms are controlled with these drugs in 6 weeks, then the treatment should be continued for 6 months after control of symptoms to prevent a relapse. If the symptoms are not controlled in 6 weeks or the patient has a relapse after control of symptoms, than referral to a psychiatrist is a good option. Psychotherapy and prophylactic antidepressants can be given to the women with previous history of severe or prolonged postpartum depression.

Selective serotonin reuptake inhibitor is the drug of choice, especially for women with prior history of depression and is also used to relieve severe anxiety and depression.[13,14]

Postpartum Psychosis

Postpartum psychosis is the most severe form of postpartum psychiatric disorders. It is rare condition, affecting 0.1–0.2% of postpartum 1 in 500 to 1 in 1,000 women. It usually occurs in women with bipolar disorders (maniac depressive variety) and those with history of bipolar disorders in the family. It starts 2–14 days after delivery. Mania is severe with delusions and hallucinations. Risk factors include a personal or family history of postpartum psychosis or bipolar affective disorder. Typically, the mother rapidly develops psychotic symptoms with disorganized behavior and cognitive impairment. About 28–35% of women describe delusions about their infant like the child is not her child, or is a son of a devil, or going to spread evil in the world, or she is a virgin. About 9% have infanticidal thoughts with 4% actually committing infanticide. Of the women who develop early postpartum psychosis, 72–88% have bipolar affective disorder (manic depressive), and the remaining 12% have schizophrenia.[15,16]

Before the advent of modern therapy, it lasted for about 6 months but with modern treatments (electroconvulsive therapy) and neurotropic medication it is reduced to a few weeks. Recurrence occurs in 20–25% of subsequent pregnancies. Complications of the mother include poor marital and social relationships, decreased work output. About 7% of the mothers who experience this and are not treated, end their lives by committing suicide. Effects on child include lowered intelligence quotient in adolescence and impaired language development and developmental delay.

Electroconvulsive therapy is highly effective in all types of puerperal psychosis. Neurotropic medications, e.g., phenothiazines and chlorpromazine are effective. Dosage of chlorpromazine is 30–75 mg/day into divided doses, 6–12 hourly initially, followed by a maintenance dose of 200 mg/day. Breastfeeding is not contraindicated but monotherapy is advised. Because of high incidence of mania in postpartum psychosis, antipsychotic medication may be needed. Lithium is effective and may have adverse effects on breast-feeding infants, therefore, breastfeeding is contraindicated as it is excreted by infant's kidney. The use of valproic acid (initiate therapy at 10–15 mg/kg/day, dosage should be increased by 5–10 mg/kg/week to achieve optimal clinical response) and carbamazepine (200 mg twice a day and can be increased) as mood stabilizers is safer in lactating mothers who insist on breastfeeding but infant should be monitored by clinical symptoms, liver function tests, and platelet count. The patient should be kept on medication for at least 6 months after resolution of symptoms and minimal doses of drugs should be used. Various studies have supported the role of psychotherapy for these patients. One study examined outcomes in 120 postpartum women. In these women, psychotherapy was effective in relieving symptoms of postpartum depression. In another study, psychotherapy and fluoxetine had similar outcome in postpartum depression as with fluoxetine alone. Electroconvulsive therapy treatment in these women requires referral to a psychiatrist. There is a place for prophylactic treatment with psychotropic medication in women with bipolar disorder.[15,16]

Selective serotonin reuptake inhibitor is the drug of choice, especially for women with prior history of depression. Its treatment is not recommended if there is a history of seizure disorder or mania including bipolar disorder as these conditions can be made worse by an selective serotonin reuptake inhibitors.[15,16]

Table 4 summarizes the presentation of postpartum blues, depression, and psychosis in postnatal women.

BREAST DISORDERS DURING PUERPERIUM

Inverted Nipple

Symptoms of inverted nipple include difficulty in feeding, with the finding of inverted nipples or nipple retraction on examination. Management includes manual squeezing and use of breast shield.

Breast Engorgement

Breast engorgement is unpleasant distressing condition affecting many women in puerperium, which may inhibit development of successful breastfeeding. This usually

TABLE 4: Presentation: postpartum blues, depression, and psychosis

Blues	Depression	Psychosis
• Tearfulness • Lack of energy • Irritability • Loss of appetite • Anxiety • Overwhelmed • Insomnia	• Low mood • Anger • Social withdrawal • Irritability • Child neglect • Loss of appetite • Aggression • Anxiety • Lack of concentration • Insomnia • Impatience	• Severe mania • Social withdrawal • Hallucinations • Loss of appetite • Delusions • Infanticidal and suicidal thoughts

occurs on the third day after delivery. This presents with feeding difficulty, painful swollen breasts, and fever. On examination, the breasts are swollen, tender, veins visible, and fever is present. Counseling, analgesics, antipyretics, and cold fomentation form the mainstay of treatment supported by hot fomentation, expression of milk (manual or breast pump), and encouragement of breastfeeding. The role of counseling is absolutely vital, the patient has to be explained that it will resolve with time.[17]

Cracked Nipples

It is a painful and distressing condition, which predisposes to breast infection. It can occur due to dryness of nipples and unhygienic habits. Most of the time faulty suckling of baby is the main cause (baby leaves the nipple too frequently if his nose is obstructed or position of baby during suckling is not proper). Leaving the baby too long on the breast or feeding very frequently can also be one of the causes of cracked nipples. Patients of cracked nipples, present with painful and sometimes bleeding nipples and feeding difficulty. These cracks on the nipples can lead to engorgement of breast. These women need counseling about the correct method of breastfeeding, in addition to analgesics and cold fomentation. The use of breast shield is encouraged. If feeding is too painful then milk expression is recommended. After feeding, salt water rinse is advisable. The local application of lanolin ointment is of great help but antibiotic ointment can also be used in case of infection.

Mastitis and Breast Abscess

The incidence of mastitis is 2–3%. The causative organism in this case is *Staphylococcus aureus* and cracked nipples are the predisposing factor. Mastitis if not treated in time with antibiotics can lead to breast abscess. It presents with painful area in breast and high-grade fever. On examination, there may be redness and presence of a tender area on the breast; if abscess is present, than a tender smooth area may be present. Axillary glands may be tender. Cloxacillin (500 mg orally every 6 hours for 7 days) is the agent of choice but in case of abscess has to be accompanied with incision and drainage. The pus has to be sent for culture and sensitivity. Simple analgesics, such as paracetamol, may be used to relieve pain.[18]

SUBINVOLUTION OF UTERUS

The slow and defective involution of uterus after delivery is defined as subinvolution. It is more common than complete absence of involution (noninvolution).

Etiology

Antepartum Factors

- Maternal malnutrition and anemia
- Elderly gravidas and grand multiparas
- Uterine overdistension as in polyhydramnios or multiple pregnancy
- Leiomyoma uterus.

Intrapartum Factors

Essentially any deviation from normal delivery can cause it.
- Prolonged labor
- Obstructed labor
- Uterine overdistension as in polyhydramnios or multiple pregnancy
- Cesarean delivery
- Repeated vaginal examinations, e.g., by traditional birth attendant.

Postpartum Factors

- Retained bits of placenta
- Puerperal sepsis.

Clinical Features

- Some women may be asymptomatic
- Abnormal and unhealthy lochia discharge
- Abnormal uterine bleeding
- Fever
- Abdominal cramps.

Examination

- Tachycardia
- Pyrexia
- The uterine height is more than normal for that day of puerperium
- Pelvic and abdominal examination may clinch the diagnosis.

Treatment

- Only slight subinvolution may not require any treatment unless associated with abnormal lochia or infection
- Management is by treatment of the primary cause of subinvolution like treatment of endometritis and puerperal sepsis with adequate hydration and appropriate antibiotics
- Evacuation of uterus under antibiotic cover is done in presence of retained bits of placenta
- Ring pessary may be used for genital prolapse
- Ergometrine and methylergometrine are popular for their use but are of no proven benefit.

SECONDARY POSTPARTUM HEMORRHAGE

Secondary PPH occurs after 24 hours of delivery. It is due to infection (retained products, etc.) and is managed with antibiotic treatment and removal of retained products of conception (placental bits or membranes).

Urinary Problems in Puerperium

Urinary Retention

Retention of urine is more common after operative and instrumental deliveries. Vaginal and perineal tears, especially paraurethral tears, can also cause urinary retention due to reflex action.

Treatment

The woman should be given adequate hydration. Her mind should be deviated towards running tap and lukewarm water can be sprinkled over lower abdomen and perineum. These simple measures can help her to pass urine. If these measures fail, then Foley's catheter should be placed for at least 48 hours. It helps in evacuating the bladder and gives rest to the tissues. Antibiotics are given for a week for urinary tract infection. Drugs like flavoxate or tolterodine given for few days may help.

Urinary Tract Infections

Both cystitis and pyelonephritis can occur in puerperium manifesting as fever with chills, malaise, and suprapubic tenderness. Treatment is by antibiotics.

Urinary Incontinence

Urinary incontinence can occur in puerperium and can be due to overflow incontinence as discussed above.

Stress urinary incontinence (SUI) or true incontinence: SUI is treated by perineal floor exercises and duloxetine (20 mg twice daily for few weeks) and rarely surgery for persistent incontinence. True incontinence needs surgery after 3 months.

Immediate Postpartum

This period is extremely important to ensure that the woman remains stable, has a quick recovery, and learns to nurse the newborn. Pulse rate and blood pressure should be monitored frequently for the first 4 hours, which is the most critical period for PPH. Amount of vaginal bleeding is noted and uterine fundus palpated to ensure that it is well contracted. If uterus is found to be relaxed, ensure that the bladder is not full which can cause uterine relaxation. In case the bleeding is excessive, uterus is massaged to rub up a contraction and oxytocics administered.

Care of Vulva

The vulva is usually little sore after a vaginal delivery, particularly if a perineal tear or an episiotomy has been sutured. If the pain is severe, a vulval hematoma should be ruled out on inspection and if required by gentle vaginal examination. Vulva is cleansed always from above downwards, moving towards the anus. In women with episiotomy, immediate icepacks are applied for first 24 hours to reduce edema and discomfort. Thereafter "sitz baths" can be taken for the next few days. Pain medications are helpful both as systemic nonsteroidal anti-inflammatory drugs and local anesthetic spray to perineum.

Bladder Care

Bladder sensation is reduced postpartum either because of epidural analgesia or reflex spasm due to episiotomy and vaginal lacerations. Keeping these in mind, patient must be encouraged to void within 4 hours of delivery. If difficulty is encountered a local hematoma is ruled out and bladder is catheterized for 24 hours.

Early Ambulation

Women are now encouraged to be out of bed within a few hours after vaginal delivery. Early ambulation reduces the incidence of deep vein thrombosis.[19]

Bowel Care

Constipation may occur in the early puerperium because of decreased food intake during labor. It is also common in presence of episiotomy or painful hemorrhoids. Hemorrhoids often resolve spontaneously as the perineum recovers so only symptomatic relief is advocated.

Diet

The nutritional requirements of lactating women increase, particularly in terms of calories, proteins, and calcium.

Contraception

During the hospital stay, the various contraceptive methods suitable for the patient, depending on whether she wishes to breastfeed or not, should be discussed. Lactating mothers can benefit from the contraceptive effect of lactational amenorrhea. Breastfeeding women who are not using any additional contraceptive have been less than 2% risk of pregnancy in the first 6 months after delivery, provided they are fully or nearly fully breastfeeding and amenorrhoeic.[20] Alternative contraceptive methods include the progestin-only pills, depot medroxyprogesterone acetate injections, intrauterine device, or barrier methods such as a diaphragm or condoms. Combined oral contraceptive pills are not recommended in the first 6 months after delivery as they affect lactation.

Time of Discharge

Hospital stay beyond 48 hours is not required for women with uncomplicated vaginal delivery. After C-section, woman can be discharged after 72–96 hours if there are no postoperative complications.[21] At the time of discharge, women should be counselled regarding the following:
- Anticipated normal physiological changes
- Lochia patterns
- Dietary advice
- Care of vulva, abdominal wound if any
- Importance of breastfeeding
- Infant care and immunization
- To report if febrile, excessive bleeding or unhealthy discharge per vagina, swelling and/or pain in the leg
- Contraception
- Postnatal exercises
- Postnatal checkup schedule.

Resumption of Coitus

There is no definite timeframe which can be recommended for coitus to be resumed. Sexual activity can be resumed when all lochial discharge has cleared and the women feel fully recovered and comfortable to have intercourse, which often takes 6 weeks or longer. A number of factors may influence recovery like the duration of labor, the mode of delivery, any perineal lacerations or episiotomy, and individual physical and mental health. Resumption too soon may be unpleasant due to vaginal lacerations. According to a survey in 1,075 postpartum women, it found that 70% had intercourse within 8 weeks of delivery. The medium interval between delivery and intercourse was 5 weeks with a range of 1–12 weeks.[22]

REFERENCES

1. Cunningham FG, Gant NF, Leveno KJ, Gilstrap LC, Huth JC, Wenstrom KD. In: William's Obstetrics, 21st edition. New York, USA: McGraw-Hill Medical Publication Division; 2001. pp. 672-85.
2. Baker Philip N, Louise K. Obstetrics by Ten Teacher, 19th edition. London, United Kingdom: Holder Arnold; 2011. pp. 262-5.
3. Lewis G (Ed). The Confidential Enquiry into Maternal and Child Health (CEMACH). Saving Mothers' Lives: Reviewing Maternal Deaths to Make Motherhood Safer 2003-2005. The Seventh Report on Confidential Enquiries into Maternal Deaths in the United Kingdom. London, United Kingdom: CEMACH; 2007.
4. Marshall BR, Hepper JK, Zirbel CC. Sporadic puerperal mastitis. An infection that need not interrupt lactation. JAMA. 1975;233(13):1377-9.
5. Almedia OD, Kitay DZ. Lactation suppression and puerperal fever. Am J Obstet Gynecol. 1986;154(4):940-1.
6. Maharaj D. Puerperal pyrexia: a review. Part I. Obstet Gynecol Surv. 2007;62(6):393-9.
7. Maternal sepsis (puerperal fever) due to group A streptococcus, Jun 25, 2012, Ministry of Health.
8. Centre for Maternal and Child Enquiries (CMACE). Saving Mothers' Lives: reviewing maternal deaths to make motherhood safer: 2006-08. The Eighth Report on Confidential Enquiries into Maternal Deaths in the United Kingdom. BJOG. 2011;118(Suppl 1):1-203.
9. Miller A. Review of bacteriology of puerperal sepsis in resource poor settings, 2006; Centre for International Health, Burnet Institute. [online] Available from www.wchnowledgehub.com.au/sites/default/.../WP_Miller_Nove.12.pdf. [Accessed June, 2015].
10. Royal College of Obstetricians and Gynaecologists. (2012). Sepsis following pregnancy, bacterial.
11. Dellinger RP, Levy MM, Carlet JM, Bion J, Parker MM, Jaeschke R, et al. Surviving Sepsis Campaign: International Guidelines for Management of Severe Sepsis and Septic Shock: 2008. Crit Care Med. 2008;36(1):296-327; [Erratum in Crit Care Med. 2008;36(4):1394-6].
12. Management of Puerperal Sepsis---SLCOG National Guidelines. Available from: www. gfmer.ch/--.
13. Wisner KL, Parry BL, Piontek CM. Clinical practice, postpartum depression. N Eng J Med. 2002:347:194.
14. Gayness BN, Ganin N, Meltzer-brody S, Lohr KN, Swinson T. Perinatal depression: Prevalence, screening accuracy and screening outcomes. Evid Rep Technol Assess. 2005;119:1.
15. Gelder G, Lopez JJ, Ibor, Andreasen NC. New Oxford Textbook of Psychiatry. Oxford, United Kingdom: Oxford University Press; 2006. pp. 1202-6.
16. Sadock PJ, Sadock VA, Kaplan PR. Saduk's Comprehensive Textbook of Psychiatry, 9th edition. Lippincott Willaims & Wilkins; 2009. pp. 2552-8.
17. Academy of Breast-feeding Medicine Engorgement (2009).
18. Lloyd CW. What is breast abscess. Last Annual Review. Aug 23, 2013. Available from: www.Localhealth.com/article. May 2, 2011.
19. Toglia MR, Weg JG. Venous thromboembolism in pregnancy. N Eng J Med. 1996;335:108.
20. Postpartum care of the mother and newborn: a practical guide. Department of Reproductive health and Research. World Health Organization. 1998.
21. American Academy Pediatrics and the American College of Obstetricians and Gynecologists: Guidelines for Perinatal Care, 4th edition. Washington, DC, 1997.
22. Glazener CM. Sexual function after childbirth. Women's experiences, persistent morbidity and lack of professional recognition. Br J Obstet Gynaecol. 1997;104-330.

CHAPTER 30

Breast-feeding

Nidhika Chhabra

INTRODUCTION

Lactation is a physiological process which is common to all mammals. Despite its central place in the natural reproductive cycle, many women find breast-feeding a difficult skill to learn and the human species is the only one in which lactation has been widely replaced by artificial feeding. The American Academy of Pediatrics (AAP) recommends exclusive breast-feeding for about 6 months, followed by continued breast-feeding for 1 year or longer.[1]

Infants normally thrive on their mother's milk. The period of neonatal life and early infancy is characterized by rapid growth so that the average baby at 4 months of life weighs twice as much as at birth and three times as much when 12 months old. The nutrients required to sustain such a rapid growth are all supplied by breast milk alone in the first 6 months of life, in all infants. Hospital routines to encourage and support the initiation and sustaining of exclusive breast-feeding should be based on the AAP endorsed by the World Health Organization (WHO)/United Nations Children's Fund (UNICEF) "Ten Steps to Successful Breast-feeding".[2]

This chapter will consider how knowledge of the anatomy and the physiology of lactation can underpin an understanding of the maternal adaptations to breast-feeding and its substantial effects on infant health; in addition, some of the steps that can be taken to promote effective breast-feeding will also be discussed.

ANATOMY OF BREAST AND ITS DEVELOPMENT

The breast extends from the second to the sixth rib and from the sternum to the midaxillary line with a tail extending into each axilla, the tail of Spence. It overlies the pectoralis major, serratus anterior, and external oblique muscles.

The main constituents of the breast are the glandular cells with their associated ducts, a very variable quantity of adipose tissue, connective tissue, blood vessels, nerves, and lymphatics (Fig. 1). The lactiferous ducts lead to the nipple and dilate to form sinuses immediately below the surface of the areola (Fig. 2). The nipple is surrounded by the areola, a pigmented area of varying size which darkens during pregnancy. The areola contains sebaceous glands which hypertrophy and become prominent during pregnancy, called Montgomery's tubercles. These glands secrete lubricating and anti-infective substances immunoglobulin A (IgA) that protect the nipples and areola during nursing. The areola is richly supplied with sensory nerves, which are important during suckling. Throughout pregnancy, the areola

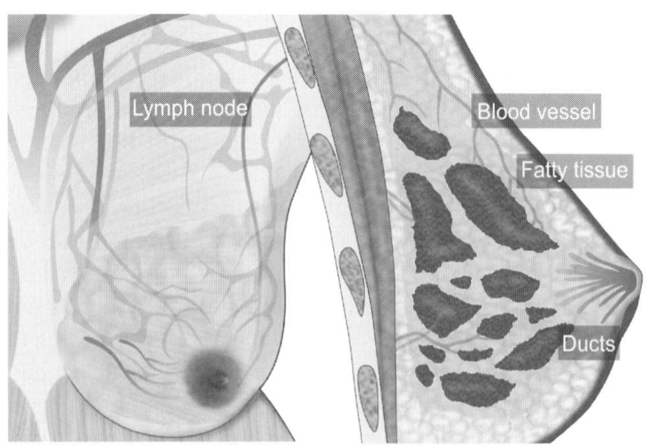

FIG. 1: Constituents of breast.

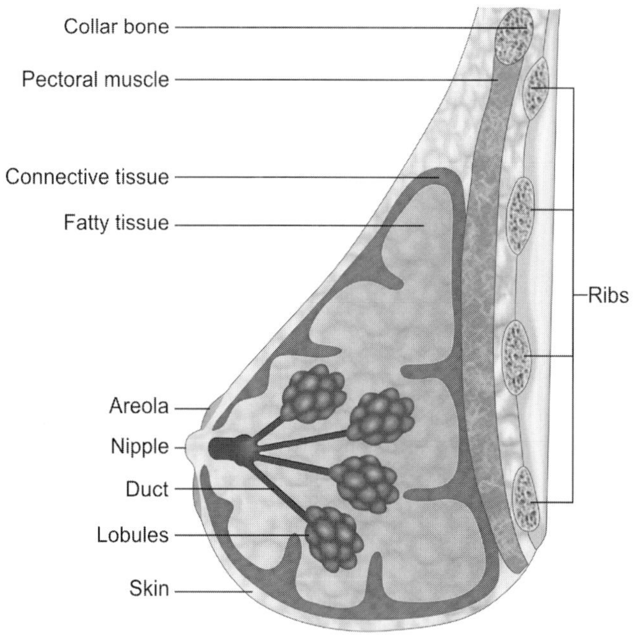

FIG. 2: Anatomy of breast.

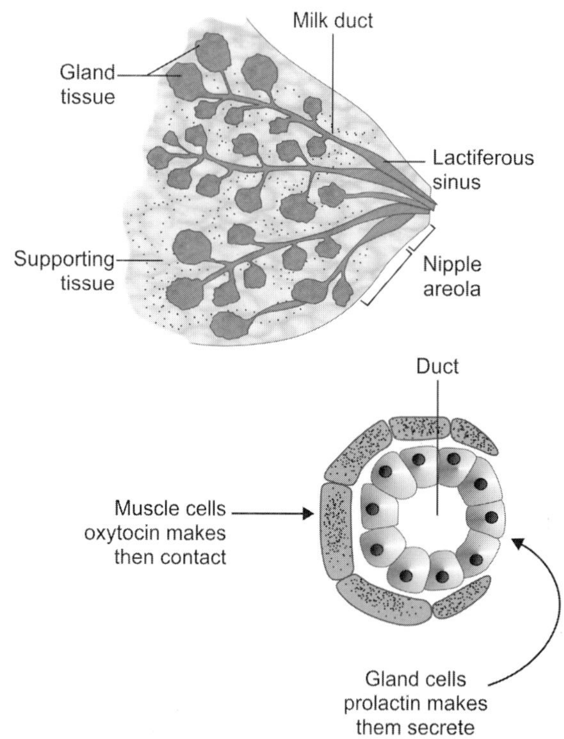

FIG. 3: Ductal-lobular-alveolar system of breast.

is relatively insensitive to touch but sensitivity increases greatly immediately after delivery. This change ensures that the suckling of the infant sends a stream of afferent neural impulses to the hypothalamus to control not only the process of lactation itself but also other important maternal adaptations, which are discussed later.

The glandular tissue of the breast is derived from the ectoderm and is arranged in 15–20 ductal-lobular-alveolar systems (Fig. 3). The alveolar or secreting cells are grouped in grape-like bunches around the ductules, which join to form the main ducts leading to the nipple. The alveolar cells are cuboidal in the resting breast, which develop full secretory features during lactation. They are surrounded by contractile myoepithelial cells, which play an important part in milk ejection.

The alveolar cells produce milk under the influence of prolactin. The myoepithelial cells eject the milk produced into the lactiferous ducts under the influence of oxytocin.

There are several anatomical facts which are to be borne in mind while giving surgical incisions on the breast. Because of the radial projection of lactiferous ducts, incisions deep into the breast parenchyma are usually made radially to avoid cutting them. On the contrary, superficial skin incisions parallel to the circumareolar line, have better cosmetic healing. A circumareolar incision deep into the breast parenchyma can also injure the lateral cutaneous branch of the fourth intercostal nerve which is vital to the production, and ejection of breast milk.[3]

The breast develops from an ectodermal thickening called the mammary ridge. The ridge extends from the axilla to the groin. In humans it disappears over most of its extent persisting only in the pectoral region which later on canalizes to form breast. Hypermastia (accessory breast) occurs in 2–6% of women; the most common site being the axilla. Accessory breast tissue may cause painful axillary enlargements presenting in the immediate postpartum period. Cold compresses and symptomatic pain relief for 2–3 days usually suffices.

PHYSIOLOGY OF LACTATION (FLOWCHART 1)

Lactogenesis

Following parturition, there is a progressive rise in the volume of milk secreted in the breast; this is maintained in mothers who suckle their infants. During the first 30 hours after parturition, the early milk or colostrum has high concentration of lactose. During the next 3 days, the concentrations of lactose increase sharply under the influence of prolactin stimulation and, in order to maintain ionic equilibrium, water is drawn into the breast causing an increase in milk volume. After this phase of transitional milk formation, a relatively stable phase of mature milk production is reached at about day 5, after which there is a slow but steady increase in milk volume to a peak around 3 weeks postpartum.

Galactopoiesis

Mothers who do not suckle their infants secrete some milk and this may persist for 3–4 weeks postpartum. In the absence

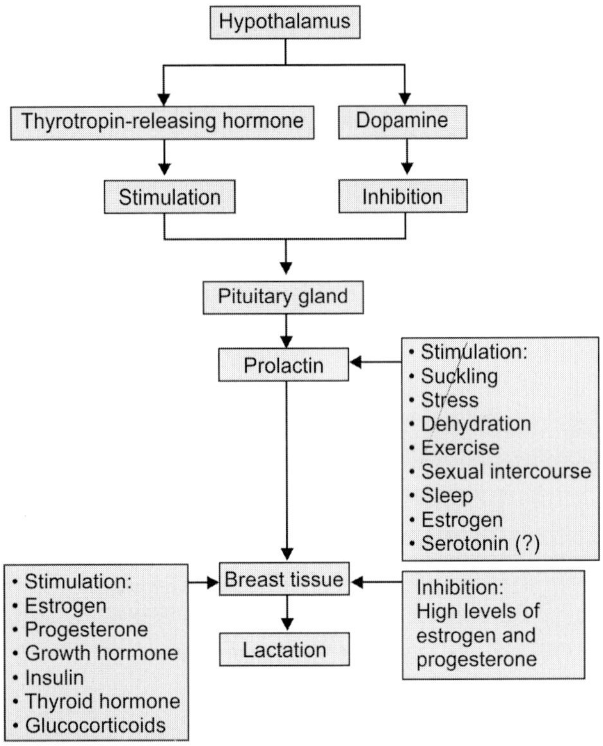

FLOWCHART 1: Physiology of lactation.

of breast milk transfer to the infant, the intraductal presence[4] and lactation inhibitory factor[5] initiate autolytic degradation of the secretory epithelial cells. This leads to decrease in the milk production by the alveolar cells.[6,7]

The suckling stimulus, which releases both prolactin and oxytocin, is essential for the maintenance of lactation. Provided that the breast is emptied regularly by sucking, lactation can be maintained for long periods. Average daily volume of milk production in a healthy well-nourished mother is of the order of 750–800 mL/day.

Prolactin and Milk Production

Prolactin is a long-chain polypeptide hormone which is secreted from the anterior pituitary gland in response to suckling and it is essential for successful lactation (Fig. 4).

The suckling stimulus of the baby sends afferent impulses to the hypothalamus, leading to a surge of prolactin release. Prolactin release is controlled by prolactin inhibitory factors secreted into the pituitary portal blood system; dopamine is generally considered to be the most important.

In response to suckling, prolactin levels rise quickly to reach a peak about 30 minutes after the baby is put to the breast and then progressively decline to reach presuckling levels after about 120 minutes. Basal prolactin levels are high in the immediate postpartum period and progressively decline after the 6th postpartum week at a rate that is dependent upon suckling frequency and duration. The peak levels of prolactin achieved in response to suckling also decline progressively over time.

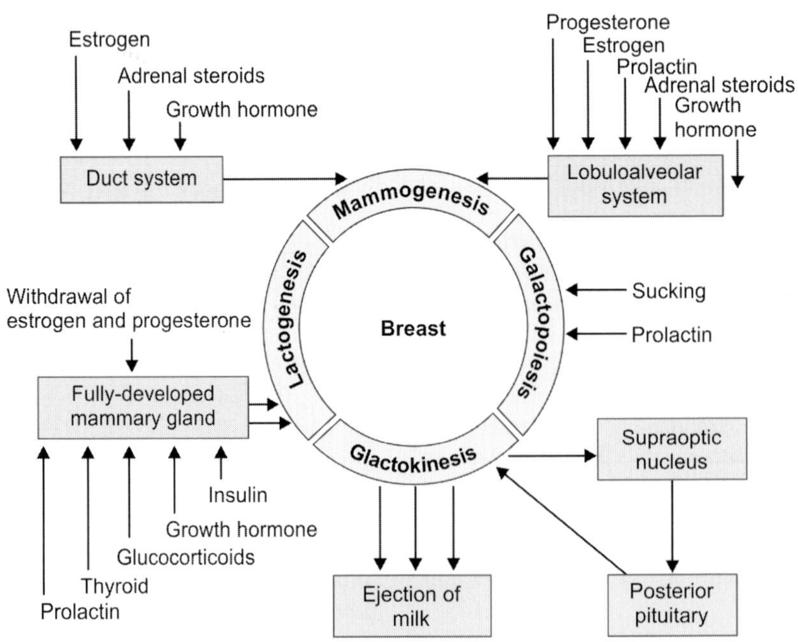

FIG. 4: Endocrine glands in relation to lactation.

Prolactin has a diurnal variation, being higher during hours of sleep, and it has been shown that prolactin responses to suckling are higher in the evening hours compared with those achieved earlier in the same day. These considerations suggest that prolactin production is increased by frequent suckling at regular intervals throughout the 24 hours including the night-time, and that feeding practices that encourage such suckling patterns will produce optimal milk volumes.

The action of prolactin is to bind to receptors on the alveolar milk-secreting cells of the breast. Prolactin appears to act at multiple sites to stimulate the synthesis of several milk components including casein, lactalbumin (which may regulate lactose synthesis), fatty acids, and other constituents. Prolactin interaction with the plasma membrane of the alveolar cells sets in motion a series of intracellular events that lead to the synthesis and secretion of all milk components.[8-12]

Oxytocin and the Milk Ejection Reflex (Galactokinesis)

The milk ejection reflex is responsible for transferring milk from the secreting glands of the breast to the baby. This reflex is mediated by the hormone oxytocin, an octapeptide synthesized in specialized magnocellular neurons in the supraoptic and paraventricular nuclei of the hypothalamus. The neuroendocrine reflex leading to oxytocin release can be initiated not just by the sucking of the infant, but also by the mother handling the baby, hearing its cry or even just thinking of feeding.

In contrast to prolactin, oxytocin is released in short bursts lasting less than a minute, and frequently the largest release of oxytocin occurs in response to the cry of the baby before feeding begins. This prefeeding release of oxytocin in part explains why rooming-in of mother and baby is associated with successful breast-feeding.[13,14]

The action of oxytocin is to bind to specific receptors on the myoepithelial cells of the breast, thereby causing them to contract. When the milk ejection reflex occurs, the contraction of the myoepithelial cells around the alveoli expels the milk into the ducts. When the milk-ejection reflex is well established, a mother may be aware of milk being spontaneously ejected from the breast while she suckles her baby on the other.

The milk-ejection reflex is very sensitive to emotional stress and the adverse effects of threatening or discouraging remarks to the nursing mother may act in this way. Inhibition of oxytocin release may occur, and catecholamines released by stress may cause constriction of the mammary vessels and prevent oxytocin access to the myoepithelial cells.

Milk Transfer

In addition to milk secretion and ejection by the mother, effective suckling by the infant is also an important part of successful breast-feeding. It is now clear that effective removal of milk during suckling is a very important stimulus for the maintenance of milk production. In contrast to bottle-feeding, where the baby obtains the milk by negative pressure, breast-feeding involves milking of the cisterns of the breast, which lie deep to the nipple. To do this, the baby must take the whole nipple into its mouth and place its tongue under the adjacent areola (Fig. 5). A baby properly fixed in this way will milk the cisterns with its tongue and, aided by the milk-ejection reflex, will establish a good milk flow. One of the most important aspects in the clinical management of breast-feeding is to ensure that the baby is properly fixed. This can be assisted by encouraging the rooting reflex of the baby with the smell and feel of the nipple round its mouth. This makes the baby open its mouth widely and fix properly on the breast.

Proper fixing of the baby's mouth on the areola enables successful breast-feeding by stimulating the following:

- Effective sucking movements from the baby
- Frequent neural impulses to the maternal anterior and posterior pituitary glands
- Prolactin secretion to promote milk production
- Oxytocin release to induce milk let-down
- Efficient milk flow from mother to baby
- Reduced risk of cracked and painful nipples.

Detailed observation of babies during breast-feeding has shown two distinct sucking patterns, which have been described as nutritive and non-nutritive sucking. Nutritive sucking is characterized by a continuous stream of strong, slow suckles, while non-nutritive sucking shows an alteration of rapid shallow bursts of sucking with rests. Nutritive

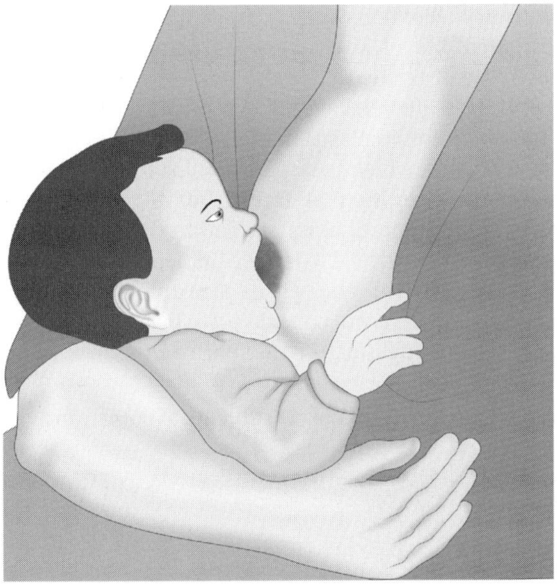

FIG. 5: Suckling in good position. Baby is unwrapped; is close to the mother; chin touches the breast; mouth is wide open; lower lip is everted; and much of the areola is in the mouth. Baby takes slow deep sucks and causes no pain to the mother.

sucking occurs predominantly at the beginning of the feed and is increasingly replaced by nonnutritive sucking as the feed progresses.

As a result of the changing suckling pattern the greatest proportion of milk transfer occurs in the early part of the feed. The fat rich and calorie dense hind milk is obtained in the remainder of the time sucking at each breast.[15]

BREAST MILK: THE GOLD STANDARD

Constituents

The composition of milk varies greatly among species, suggesting that evolution has developed specific milks suited to the needs of the young of each species. Studies of human milk composition also show that the concentrations of the various constituents are not constant. The constituents vary from one mother to another and, in any one mother, the milk content varies between one feed and another on the same day and even between the beginning and the end of the same feed. Probably the most important variable is the length of time postpartum, suggesting that the milk content adapts to meet the needs of the infant at any particular stage of development.

The composition of mature human milk is used as a guide for the preparation of artificial feeds; the recommended figures for some of the major constituents are shown in Table 1.

Carbohydrates

Human milk contains one of the highest concentrations of carbohydrate of any mammal, mainly in the form of lactose. The dramatic rise in the synthesis of lactose in the first few days after delivery is one of the main features of the transition from colostrum to mature milk. The intestinal enzyme lactase, which is responsible for the hydrolysis and subsequent absorption of lactose, develops late in fetal life so that any intestinal inflammation that interferes with lactase function will lead to lactose intolerance and diarrhea. When lactose is digested, it yields a mixture of galactose and glucose, so lactose is not considered to be an essential sugar. The reason for high-lactose content in human milk is not clear, but it may be important in controlling stool acidity and the characteristics of intestinal flora.

TABLE 1: Comparison of the constituents of human and cow's milk

Constituents	Human milk	Cow's milk
Energy (kcal/100 mL)	75	66
Protein (g/100 mL)	1.1	3.5
Fat (g/100 mL)	4.5	3.7
Lactose (g/100 mL)	6.8	4.9
Sodium (mEq/L)	7	22

Protein

The total protein content of human milk is much lower than that of cow's milk, and about 40% is in the form of casein. This means that the curds formed in human milk are much softer, more flocculent, and more easily digestible for the intestinal tract. The remaining proteins are called whey proteins; they represent a mixture of soluble proteins left after the casein curd has formed. Many of these soluble proteins, such as the immunoglobulins, lactoferrins, and lysozyme, are important for the anti-infective qualities of human milk and these are discussed below.

Human milk contains high concentrations of alpha-lactalbumin and, although it has been proposed as a regulator of lactose synthesis, a direct correlation between lactose and alpha-lactalbumin levels has yet to be established.

Fat

Lipid, which appears mainly as triglycerides, is the most variable constituent of human milk, the highest concentrations appearing in the hindmilk as milk-fat globules. Fat is the major source of energy in human milk. The fat content of the human milk is also important as a carrier of the fat-soluble vitamins A, D, E, and K and of the essential fatty acids. Deficiency of vitamin D can lead to rickets, while that of vitamin K may lead to hemorrhagic disease of the newborn.

Minerals

Compared with cow's milk, human milk has low concentrations of sodium, chloride, iron, and some other minerals. The low levels of sodium and chloride are advantageous in infants with diarrhea because milks with a high-solute load can aggravate dehydration. The concentration of iron is low (0.5 μmol/mL) in human milk and some clinicians advise iron supplements in breast-fed babies. There is a much higher absorption of iron from breast milk (>75%) compared with cow's milk (30%) or iron-supplemented infant formula (10%) and, although the reason for the greater bioavailability of iron from breast milk is not known, its binding to lactoferrin in human milk may be responsible.

MAMMARY FUNCTION DURING WEANING

Breast milk contains a natural inhibitor so that, if her milk is not being removed on a regular basis, the mother will lose secretory activity from her breasts. Thus, during this process of weaning, when there is a reduction in suckling the milk supply will progressively decline. When weaning is abrupt the concentrations of potassium, glucose, and lactose decrease, while those of sodium, chloride, and protein increase. During gradual weaning the changes are similar but they occur over a longer period of time. If conception occurs during lactation, the rising levels of placental steroids inhibit milk secretion and this overrides the positive stimulus of the infant's sucking.

Following the cessation of regular sucking, the mammary gland quickly ceases secretory activity and enters a phase of regression. The milk in the ducts and alveoli is resorbed and although there is a decrease in parenchyma elements, the breast does not return to its prenatal state as many alveoli persist.

ANTI-INFECTIVE PROPERTIES

Breast milk contains a number of proteins with antimicrobial activity. The anti-infective properties of breast milk are an important protection for the breast-feeding infant and the antimicrobial proteins may also protect the breasts against infection and abscess formation.

Lactoferrin

Lactoferrin is an iron-binding glycoprotein that inhibits bacterial growth nonspecifically. *Escherichia coli* have a high requirement for free iron; lactoferrin, with its high affinity for iron, may restrict the growth of pathogenic iron-dependent bacteria. The action of lactoferrin may be low in the stomach as little iron is protein-bound in an acidic environment. In the proximal duodenum, however, bicarbonate secretion will favor the binding of iron to lactoferrin and enhance its bacteriostatic action in the intestinal tract.

Lysozyme

Lysozyme is a cationic protein that is present in concentrations of 30–40 mg/100 mL of human milk. Its bactericidal activity is mediated by its ability to cleave proteoglycans in the cell walls of a number of Gram-positive and Gram-negative bacteria. The activity is promoted by other milk components, especially IgA.

Immunoglobulins

The major immunoglobulin in breast milk is IgA, with smaller amounts of immunoglobulin M (IgM) and immunoglobulin G (IgG). The concentration of IgA is particularly high in colostrum and, although its concentration falls to about 2 mg/mL in mature milk, the daily yield remains relatively constant. The IgA in breast milk is poorly absorbed and persists in the infant's gastrointestinal tract to protect against infection. The high concentration of IgA in colostrum enables it to enter the proteoglycan lining of the gastrointestinal tract and this may provide initial surface protection.

Specific IgA antibodies, mostly against gastrointestinal pathogens, are also present in human milk. It is suggested that if the mother meets a potential pathogen in her own gastrointestinal tract, the antigen is taken up by the gut-associated lymphoid tissue in the Peyer's patches of her terminal ileum. Plasma cells are formed which migrate to the breast where specific IgA is secreted into the breast milk. In this way, the mother is able to give her baby specific protection against pathogens endemic in her environment. This remarkable interaction between mother and baby is, of course, a mechanism that cannot be replicated by artificial feeds.

Other Anti-infective Factors

Human milk contains a growth factor for *Lactobacillus bifidus* which facilitates colonization with this organism, which competes with intestinal pathogens. Breast milk also contains cells in the form of macrophages and leukocytes, small amounts of complement, and lactoperoxidases.

ROLE OF THE HEALTHCARE PROVIDER

The healthcare provider plays a primary role in the initiation of breast-feeding.[16] Breasts examination should be done routinely during the family planning visits. During the third trimester visits, the healthcare provider should teach the mother regarding simple concepts of breast-feeding physiology and technique. Also the fact that "no supplementation unless directed by a pediatrician" should be impressed upon.

In 1989, the essential "ten steps" in "Protecting, Promoting and Supporting Breast-feeding" were published in a joint statement by the WHO/UNICEF.[2] These have become institutionalized in the Baby-Friendly Hospital Initiative (BFHI) and accreditation process. These steps are well founded on evidence-based medicine that demonstrates improvement in breast-feeding success.[17-19]

1. Have a written policy to support breast-feeding
2. Train all healthcare providers
3. Inform all pregnant women about the benefits of management of breast-feeding
4. Initiate breast-feeding within 1 hour after birth
5. Show mothers how to breast-feed and maintain lactation even if they are separated from their infants
6. Give newborn infants no food or drink other than breast milk, unless medically indicated
7. Allow mothers and infants to remain together 24 hours a day (i.e., rooming in)
8. Encourage breast-feeding on demand
9. Give no artificial teats and pacifiers
10. Foster the establishment of breast-feeding support groups and refer mothers to them on discharge from the hospital or clinic.

ANATOMICAL ABNORMALITIES OF BREAST

Although congenital abnormalities of the breasts are rare, the most significant defect is glandular hypoplasia which means no or abnormal development of one or both breasts during sexual maturation. There can be issues regarding lactational failure in these ladies; however, the final evaluation must await the expected growth of breasts during pregnancy. Massage of the perialveolar tissue is recommended if nipple tethering is present.

Severe congenital tethering of the nipple to the underlying fascia is manifested by an inverted nipple. Gentle nipple pulling in the antenatal period might help. A breast pump can be used at low settings to draw the teat out and the infant is immediately offered that breast. Alternatively, a 10 mL or 20 mL plastic syringe can be cut with a sharp blade at the end where the needle attaches (Fig. 6). The plunger is inserted from the cut end and the nipple is placed in the smooth, plunger end of the syringe. The mother gently pulls the plunger until the nipple everts.

To prevent cracking of nipples during lactation, the alveolar skin can be toughened by wearing a nursing brassiere with the flaps open. Application of breast cream or expression of colostrum has not shown any significant reduction in the incidence of nipple sensitivity and trauma when compared with untreated nipples.

Past history of breast surgery may have a role to play in patients who experience lactational insufficiency.[20] Breast augmentation, reduction mammoplasty, and circumareolar incisions are associated with lactational failure.[21]

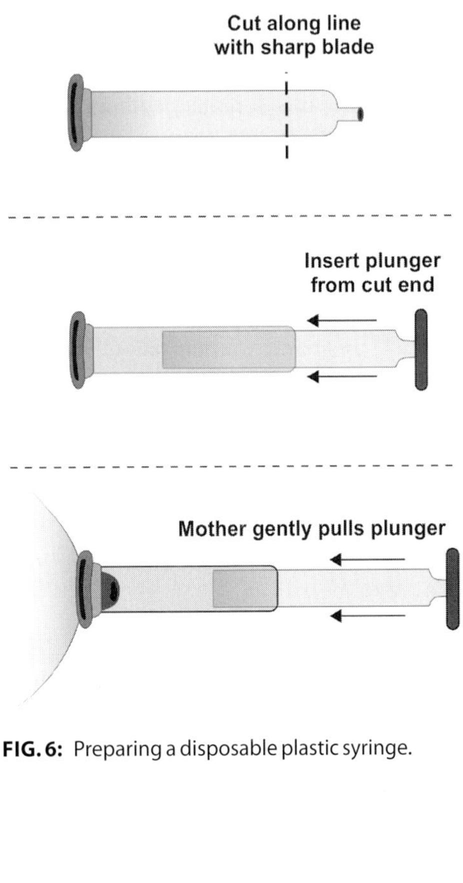

FIG. 6: Preparing a disposable plastic syringe.

EARLY DAYS OF LACTATION

The early days establish the trend for lactation. With a good start breast-feeding is likely to remain trouble-free and mutually satisfying to both mother and infant. The establishment of successful lactation is a process which is dependent upon the constitutional, physiological, and personality characteristic of the mother and the baby. Putting the baby to the breast soon after the delivery is desirable. Prelacteal feeds using a bottle are not indicated.

After all full-term normal births the modern practice is to offer the baby to the mother as soon as possible, ensuring skin-to-skin and eye-to-eye contacts. Putting the baby to breast at this time helps to establish lactation, by initiating the let-down reflex, and promotes bonding.

For the first few days most babies feed at intervals of 2–4 hours. This period of frequent feeding is a physiological response of the baby to the initial weight loss, which is on an average 5% of birth weight.[22] As the milk comes in and the baby begins to regain his birth weight, the feeds space out to intervals of 3–4 hours.

There is no hard and fast rule about the frequency of feeding. However, after the early days, feeds which are too frequent (<1 hour apart) might indicate that feeding technique is faulty.[23,24] It is likely that the hind milk is not getting to the baby in sufficient amounts. At each feed, the mother should be encouraged to let the baby completely empty one breast before transferring to the other side. Breast emptying regulates supply and maximizes milk quality in particular the fat concentration of the milk which in turn triggers satiety in the infant.

In the initial stages, many mothers need to be explained how to hold the baby during a feed. The baby should be held in the crook of the arm so that the head is free to move about and the back is supported. The nipple should be pointed at the baby's nose at the time of beginning a feed. The baby should be held close enough for his chin to touch the breast. In such a position, the nipple is more likely to reach the top of his mouth, which is ideal for establishing feeding behavior.

BREAST ENGORGEMENT

Breast engorgement may cause breast or nipple pain which is the most frequent complaint of lactating mother.[25-28] When secretion of milk is in excess of the infant's requirements, breast engorgement occurs.[26] As milk accumulates in the duct system, it causes back pressure so that circulation in the veins and lymphatics becomes sluggish leading to edema and mastalgia. The best way of handling such a situation is to empty the breasts of milk by suggesting more frequent feeds, or by means of a breast pump or by manual expression. Sore nipple due to cracks and fissures, may be the first sign of breast engorgement. Because of the engorged breast the infant finds a small nipple on which he cannot take a firm grip and the chewing action which ensues traumatizes the nipple and causes cracks or fissures. Management consists of manually expressing a small amount of milk at the commencement of a feed and then putting the child to the breast as this will reduce the tension in the milk ducts and restore the concavity between the nipple and the areola.

MASTITIS

Infectious process of the breast characterized by high-grade fever, localized erythema, induration, and tenderness is defined as mastitis.[29] It occurs most commonly in the first 2–4 weeks postpartum. *Staphylococcus aureus, S. epidermidis, Streptococci* and occasionally Gram-negative rods are commonly associated with mastitis. Management includes proper breast support, assessment of nursing technique, proper emptying of breasts (either by nursing the child or using a breast pump), analgesics, and antibiotics. Dicloxacillin, 250 mg 4 times a day or erythromycin should be continued for a period of 7–10 days.

Once a breast abscess is formed, drainage of the abscess is indicated. Skin incision should be made on the most fluctuant area. All loculi should be reduced bluntly and the cavity should be irrigated with normal saline. The wound should be packed as secondary closure ensues.[30]

GALACTOGOGUES

Agents, which increase prolactin production, and therefore improve milk secretion, are known as galactogogues. The commonly used galactogogues include metoclopramide, sulpiride, and nasal oxytocin which have been shown to be quite efficacious in clinical trials.

Metoclopramide increases the basal prolactin levels multifold. Usual starting dose is 10–15 mg, 3 times a day and it is usually tapered over 4 weeks. Domperidone blocks the dopamine receptors in the gut and the brainstem and leads to a dose-dependent increase in milk secretion when used in doses of 10–20 mg, 3–4 times a day. Intranasal oxytocin contracts the myoepithelial cells and overcomes an inhibited let-down reflex. Because oxytocin is destroyed by the gastrointestinal enzymes, it is not given orally.

CLINICAL EFFECTS OF BREAST-FEEDING

There has been a recent surge in the amount of research investigating the short- and long-term effects of infant feeding on health and development.

Effects on Infant Mortality

In nonindustrialized countries, breast-feeding is a matter of life and death for newborn babies and infants. The WHO estimates that 1.5 million deaths per annum could be prevented if women were encouraged to breast-feed their infants exclusively for 6 months and partially until 2 years of age. The benefits are greatest in those settings where clean water supplies cannot be guaranteed and adequate supplies of infant formula cannot be provided.

Gastrointestinal Infection

Even in industrialized countries, there is now strong evidence that breast-feeding has a protective effect against infantile gastrointestinal illness. Studies have shown that babies who were bottle-fed from birth or weaned at an early stage had gastrointestinal illness rates of 5–8 times greater than those who were fully or partially breast-fed for 13 weeks. The clearest benefits have been shown against *Escherichia coli, Giardia, Salmonella,* and *Campylobacter* but less clearly against rotavirus diarrhea.

Nongastrointestinal Infections

Respiratory infections are the most common cause of morbidity amongst infants. Evidence suggests that breast-feeding has a protective action against lower rather than upper respiratory tract infections.

In respect of acute and chronic otitis media, there is consistent evidence of protection with extended duration of breast-feeding. Other infections, which are reduced by breast-feeding, include *Haemophilus influenzae type B meningitis,* neonatal sepsis, and urinary tract infection.

Human Immunodeficiency Virus Infection

There is now clear evidence that human immunodeficiency virus (HIV) infection can be transferred from mother to child through breast milk. Mothers who are known to be HIV positive should be advised to bottle-feed in developed countries where infant formula can be given as a safe alternative to breast milk. However, in poor resource countries where the infant mortality due to diarrheal diseases is high, breast-feeding by HIV positive mothers may be permitted.

Allergic Disease

Although there is a widespread belief that breast-feeding protects against asthma, eczema, and allergy, the evidence to support this is inconsistent. It is clear that family history of allergic disorders is crucially important. Babies who are breast-fed are less likely to be given solid food at an early stage, and avoiding early solids may be more important than breast-feeding itself in reducing the risk of allergy.

Necrotizing Enterocolitis

This condition occurs in premature babies and there is good evidence that breast milk helps to reduce its incidence and severity.

Insulin-dependent Diabetes Mellitus

Recent evidence has suggested that exposure to bovine human albumin through infant feeding could trigger the autoimmune process leading to juvenile-onset diabetes. Some studies have shown an association between formula feeding and insulin-dependent diabetes mellitus.

Hemorrhagic Disease of Newborn

Breast-fed babies are at a greater risk of this disorder because vitamin K is absent in breast milk. But it can be prevented by the appropriate use of vitamin K supplementation.

Neoplastic Disease

There have been some reports that breast-feeding is associated with reduced levels of childhood cancer, particularly lymphoma. There is, however, considerable evidence to show that breast-feeding is associated with a small, but important, reduction in premenopausal breast-cancer among lactating mothers. The protection increases with duration of breast-feeding, but it does not extend to offer any protection against the more common postmenopausal breast-cancer.

REFERENCES

1. Breastfeeding and the use of human milk. American Academy of Pediatrics. Work Group on Breastfeeding. Pediatrics. 1997;100(6):1035-9.
2. World Health Organization (WHO)/United Nations Children's Fund (UNICEF). Ten steps to successful breast-feeding. In: Protecting, Promoting and Supporting Breast-feeding: The Special Role of Maternity Services. A Joint WHO/UNICEF Statement. Geneva, Switzerland: World Health Organization; 1989. p. iv.
3. Neifert M, DeMarzo S, Seacat J, Young D, Leff M, Orleans M. The influence of breast surgery, breast appearance, and pregnancy-induced breast changes on lactation sufficiency as measured by infant weight gain. Birth. 1990;17(1):31-8.
4. Peaker M. The effect of raised intramammary pressure on mammary function in the goat in relation to the cessation of lactation. J Physiol. 1980;310:415-28.
5. Wilde CJ, Addey CV, Boddy LM, Peaker M. Autocrine regulation of milk secretion by a protein in milk. Biochem J. 1995;305(Pt 1):51-8.
6. Lund LR, Rømer J, Thomasset N, Solberg H, Pyke C, Bissell MJ, et al. Two distinct phases of apoptosis in mammary gland involution: proteinase-independent and -dependent pathways. Development. 1996;122(1):181-93.
7. Prentice A, Addey CV, Wilde CJ. Evidence for local feedback control of human milk secretion. Biochem Soc Trans. 1989;16:122.
8. Neville MC. Physiology of lactation. Clin Perinatol. 1999;26(2):251-79.
9. Hall B. Changing composition of human milk and early development of an appetite control. Lancet. 1975;1(7910):779-81.
10. Neville MC, Keller R, Seacat J, Lutes V, Neifert M, Casey C, et al. Studies in human lactation: milk volumes in lactating women during the onset of lactation and full lactation. Am J Clin Nutr. 1988;48(6):1375-86.
11. Neville MC, Keller RP, Seacat J, Casey CE, Allen JC, Archer P. Studies on human lactation. I. Within-feed and between-breast variation in selected components of human milk. Am J Clin Nutr. 1984;40(3):635-46.
12. Hartmann PE, Cregan MD, Ramsay DT, Simmer K, Kent JC. Physiology of lactation in preterm mothers: initiation and maintenance. Pediatr Ann. 2003;32(5):351-5.
13. Uvnäs-Moberg K. Oxytocin linked antistress effects--the relaxation and growth response. Acta Physiol Scand Suppl. 1997;640:38-42.
14. Moore ER, Anderson GC, Bergman N. Early skin-to-skin contact for mothers and their healthy newborn infants. Cochrane Database Sys Rev. 2007;(3):CD003519.
15. Lucas A, Lucas PJ, Baum JD. Differences in the pattern of milk intake between breast and bottle fed infants. Early Hum Dev. 1981;5(2):195-9.
16. Dettwyler KA. A time to wean: the hominid blueprint for the natural age of weaning in modern human populations. In: Stuart-MacAdam P, Dettwyler KA (Eds). Breastfeeding: Biocultural Perspectives. New York, NY, USA: Aldine de Gruyter; 1995. pp. 39-60.
17. Cadwell K, Turner-Maffei C. Continuity of Care in Breastfeeding: Best Practices in the Maternity Setting. Sudbury, MA, USA: Jones & Bartlett Publishers; 2009.
18. DiGirolamo AM, Grummer-Strawn LM, Fein SB. Effect of maternity-care practices on breastfeeding. Pediatrics. 2008;122(Suppl 2):s43-9.
19. Cramton R, Zain-Ul-Abideen M, Whalen B. Optimizing successful breastfeeding in the newborn. Curr Opin Pediatr. 2009;21(3):386-96.
20. Hurst NM. Lactation after augmentation mammoplasty. Obstet Gynecol. 1996;87(1):30-4.
21. Kjøller K, McLaughlin JK, Friis S, Blot WJ, Mellemkjaer L, Høgsted C, et al. Health outcomes in offspring of mothers with breast implants. Pediatrics. 1998;102(5):1112-5.
22. Egli GE, Egli NS, Newton M. The influence of the number of breast feedings on milk production. Pediatrics. 1961;27:314-7.
23. Howard C, Howard F, Lawrence R, Andresen E, DeBlieck E, Weitzman M. Office prenatal formula advertising and its effect on breast-feeding patterns. Obstet Gynecol. 2000;95(2):296-303.
24. Howard FM, Howard CR, Weitzman ML. The physician as advertiser: the unintentional discouragement of breast-feeding. Obstet Gynecol. 1993;81(6):1048-51.
25. Mass S. Breast pain: engorgement, nipple pain and mastitis. Clin Obstet Gynecol. 2004;47(3):676-82.
26. Hill PD, Humenick SS. The occurrence of breast engorgement. J Hum Lact. 1994;10(2):79-86.
27. Livingstone V, Stringer LJ. The treatment of Staphylococcus aureus infected sore nipples: a randomized comparative study. J Hum Lact. 1999;15(3):241-6.
28. Morland-Schultz K, Hill PD. Prevention of and therapies for nipple pain: a systematic review. J Obstet Gynecol Neonatal Nurs. 2005;34(4):428-37.
29. Academy of Breastfeeding Medicine Protocol Committee. ABM clinical protocol #4: mastitis. Revision, May 2008. Breastfeed Med. 2008;3(3):177-80.
30. Dener C, Inan A. Breast abscesses in lactating women. World J Surg. 2003;27(2):130-3.

CHAPTER 31

Contraception

Shashwat K Jani, Anu Namgyal

INTRODUCTION

Fast-growing population is a major concern worldwide. Awareness about contraception is the only solution. Slow and constant growth of population will save natural resources, increase standard of living and health status of individual and family.

It is important to understand few terms before we move forward:

- Contraception: these are the methods which prevent pregnancy
- Interception: these are the methods which intercept the embryo before its implantation in the uterus. These prevent implantation and results in expulsion of the embryo. Examples of interceptives are:
    - Progestogens to make uterine endometrium not receptive to embryo (mini pills, injections, and implants)
    - High doses of estrogens or progestogens just after sexual intercourse (emergency contraception)
    - Intrauterine device that prevents nidation
- Contragestives: these are the methods which lead to loss of barely implanted embryo. Contragestive techniques are always and exclusively abortive. Examples of contragestives are:
    - Antiprogesterones such as RU 486 followed by misoprostol
    - Methotrexate that leads to death of the cells of trophoblasts and causes implanted embryo to detach
    - Antihuman chorionic gonadotropin (Anti-HCG) vaccines.

COUNSELING

Counseling is sitting with a couple in a personal space and discussing various options of family planning methods which are available, which is also known as the "cafeteria approach". In a cafeteria approach, the patient or a couple is given all the available options with the advantages and disadvantages, and the patient or the couple decides what method best suits them.

Counseling is done in six steps. They can be remembered as "Gather" approach.

G: Greet clients. Give full attention and assure confidentiality.
A: Ask clients about their family-planning wishes, concerns and current reproductive health experiences.
T: Tell them about all possible options on the basis of their requirement.
H: Help clients to choose from the different options, they are provided.
E: Explain in detail about the method which they finalize.
R: Return visit should be encouraged.
Clients should be informed about follow-up.

Criteria for Ideal Contraceptive Methods

- Widely acceptable
- Inexpensive
- Easy to use
- Safe
- Highly effective
- Requires minimal motivation, maintenance and supervision.

The effectiveness of birth-control methods is critically important for reducing the risk of unintended pregnancy. Effectiveness can be measured during "perfect use", when the method is used correctly and consistently as directed, or during "typical use", which is how effective the method is during actual use (including inconsistent and incorrect use).

PEARL INDEX

The Pearl index of contraceptive failure was first introduced by Raymond Pearl in 1932.[1]
Pregnancy rate per hundred women year

$$= \frac{\text{Total accidental pregnancies} \times 1200}{\text{Total months of exposure to unintended pregnancies}}$$

[Factor 1200 is number of months in 100 years.
Total months of exposure = the months in which contraception was not possible (10 months deducted for a pregnancy and 4 months for an abortion)].

METHODS (FIG. 1)

- Behavioral
    - Fertility awareness
    - Withdrawal
    - Abstinence
    - Lactation
- Barrier
- Hormonal
- Intrauterine devices
- Emergency
- Sterilization
- Dual protection

Behavioral

Behavioral methods involve regulating the timing or method of intercourse to prevent introduction of sperm into the female reproductive tract, either altogether or when an egg may be present. If used perfectly, the first-year failure rate may be around 3.4%, however if used poorly first-year failure rates may approach 85%.

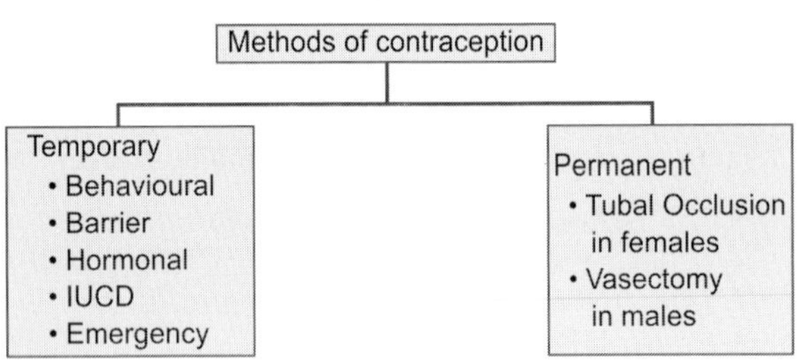

FIG. 1: Methods of contraception.

Fertility Awareness

Fertility awareness methods involve determining the most fertile days of the menstrual cycle and avoiding unprotected intercourse. Techniques for determining fertility include monitoring basal body temperature, cervical secretions, or the day of the cycle. They have typical first-year failure rates of 24%; perfect use first-year failure rates depend on which method is used and range from 0.4–5%.

If based on both basal body temperature and another primary sign, the method is referred to as symptothermal. Overall, first-year failure rates of less than 2–20% have been reported in clinical studies of the symptothermal method.

- Calendar (rhythm) method (Knaus Ogino method): after recording last few months of menstrual cycles the next ovulation time is determined. Ovulation usually occurs on day 14 of the periods (11th–16th day). The fertile days start 5 days before ovulation and end on the day of ovulation. This method works, if your menstrual cycle is regular, but very few women have regular 28-day cycles. Even women who have regular cycles can have irregular periods from time to time. So the calendar method alone is not the most effective method
- Standard days method (SDM): the SDM works best for women who have cycles between 26 days and 32 days long. A special colored string of beads (cycle beads) is used to keep track of a cycle. The red bead is the first day (day 1) of the period. Each day is counted as one bead. A dark brown bead marks day 26 and the last brown bead before the red bead is day 32. If a lady has more than one cycle in one year that is shorter than 26 days or longer than 32 days, she may need to use another method to avoid pregnancy
- Basal body temperature (BBT) method: a woman's hormone levels during her menstrual cycle naturally cause her BBT to fall 1–2 days before ovulation and then rise 1–2 days after ovulation. Female thermogenesis results from hormonal changes. Rise in basal body temperature is thought to be secondary to progesterone changes in the cycling female, but the primary reason for this temperature increase at ovulation is the increase in production and secretion of norepinephrine, which is a thermogenic neural hormone. World health organization research findings led to its definition of changes in basal body temperature which states that a shift in basal body temperature to the hyperthermic phase of the cycle should occur within a period of 24 hours or less; 3 consecutive daily basal body temperatures should be at least 0.2 degrees centigrade higher than the previous 6 daily temperatures to indirectly assume ovulation had occurred. However, a monophasic basal body temperature does not necessarily mean that ovulation did not occur

- Cervical mucus method (Billings method): the amount, texture, and look of cervical mucus changes during the menstrual cycle
    - Right after the menstrual period cervical mucus is thick, cloudy, and sticky
    - Just before and during ovulation, cervical mucus is thin, clear, and stringy.

  Creighton model (CrM), also called NaProTechnology, is more standardized in the way secretions are characterized, using pictures and precise words to describe them. The male partner is responsible for charting and interpreting the data, a step supporters believe encourages sharing responsibility for family planning and facilitates communication and relationship building.

  The Two Days Method (TDM) is a simpler method that can be taught during a routine office visit. The woman is taught to identify cervical secretions of any type regardless of their characteristics. She then is instructed to ask herself, "Did I notice any cervical secretions today?" If the answer is no, she then asks, "Did I notice any cervical secretions yesterday?" If the answer is no, then intercourse is unlikely to result in pregnancy. If the answer to either of the 2 questions is "yes," then intercourse has a high probability of resulting in a pregnancy. The same preovulatory cervical secretion check rules described above apply. There are no restrictions on coitus when cervical secretions meet the 2-day rule after peak fertility and until the onset of the next menstruation.
- Hormone monitoring: home ovulation kits can be used to check the level of luteinizing hormone (LH) in urine. A dipstick or test strip is dipped in urine, and the level on the strip is checked or the strip is put in a small computer unit that shows the level of LH. The computer can tell the most fertile days
- Combined (symptothermal) method: basal body temperature, changes in cervical mucus, and a hormone test, and signs of ovulation (such as breast tenderness, belly pain, and mood changes) can be checked.

Withdrawal

The withdrawal method (also known as coitus interruptus) is the practice of ending intercourse ("pulling out") before ejaculation. The main risk of the withdrawal method is that the man may not perform the maneuver correctly or in a timely manner. First-year failure rates vary from 4% with perfect usage to 22% with typical usage.[2] The withdrawal method is used as birth control by about 3% of couples.

Abstinence

Though some groups advocate total sexual abstinence, by which they mean the avoidance of all sexual activity, in the context of birth control the term usually means abstinence from vaginal intercourse. Abstinence is 100% effective in preventing pregnancy; however, not everyone who intends to be abstinent refrains from all sexual activity.

Lactational Amenorrhea

The lactational amenorrhea method involves the use of a woman's natural postpartum infertility which occurs after delivery and may be extended by breastfeeding. This usually requires the presence of no periods, exclusively breastfeeding the infant, and a child younger than 6 months. The World Health Organization states that if breastfeeding is the infant's only source of nutrition, the failure rate is 2% in the 6 months following delivery.[3,4] Failure rates increase to 4–7% at 1 year and 13% at 2 years. Feeding formula, pumping instead of nursing, the use of a pacifier, and feeding solids all increase its failure rate. In those who are exclusively breastfeeding, about 10% begin having periods before 3 months and 20% before 6 months. In those who are not breastfeeding, fertility may return 4 weeks after delivery.[5]

Barrier Methods

These prevent sperm from entering the uterus. Types of barrier methods include:

- Male condoms: this condom is a thin sheath that covers the penis to collect sperm and prevent it from entering the woman's body. Male condoms are generally made of latex or polyurethane. Latex or polyurethane condoms reduce the risk of spreading sexually transmitted diseases (STDs)[6,7]
- Female condoms: these are thin, flexible plastic pouches. A portion of the condom is inserted into a woman's vagina before intercourse to prevent sperm from entering the uterus. The female condom also reduces the risk of STDs. Female condoms are disposed of after a single use. The female condom was invented by AVK Reddy, Lasse Hessel, and Max Frieberg. It was approved by US Food and Drug Administration (USFDA) in 1993 at the height of the acquired immunodeficiency syndrome (AIDS) epidemic. It is made of polyurethane, is tougher than the male condom, and can be used with oil-based lubricant. It is impermeable to HIV and other organisms causing sexually transmitted infections (STI)[8]
- Diaphragms: each diaphragm is a shallow, flexible cup made of latex or soft rubber that is inserted into the vagina before intercourse, blocking sperm from entering the uterus. The diaphragm should remain in place for 6–8 hours after intercourse to prevent pregnancy, but it should be removed within 24 hours. The diaphragm is held in place between the pubic bond and the posterior fornix by a spring in its rim. Since this distance is variable, the diaphragm must be fitted by a health worker and

correctly sized. A spermicide is placed inside the dome before insertion, which increases its effectiveness[9]

- Cervical caps: these are similar to diaphragms, but smaller, more rigid, and less noticeable. The cervical cap is a thin silicone cup that is inserted into the vagina before intercourse to block sperm from entering the uterus. The cervical cap should be used with spermicidal cream or jelly. The cap must remain in place for 6–8 hours after intercourse to prevent pregnancy, but it should be removed within 48 hours. Currently, FemCap is the only cervical cap approved by the FDA. The FemCap is the only device that is currently available in the USA and was approved by USFDA in March 2003. It is also available in France, Austria, Netherlands and Switzerland. In the United Kingdom (UK), it is supplied free of cost through the family planning clinics of the National Health Service. The size selection of FemCap is determined by obstetrical history. A removal strap was added to the device in 2005. It can be used with a spermicide. It may be inserted 48 hours prior to intercourse; hence, it does not disrupt the act. It provides a microbicide reservoir on the vaginal side for protection from STI. It may offer similar protection as the diaphragm but further studies are needed[10,11]
- Contraceptive sponges: these are soft, disposable, spermicide-filled foam sponges. One is inserted into the vagina before intercourse. The sponge blocks sperm from entering the uterus, and the spermicide also kills the sperm cells. The sponge should be left in place for at least 6 hours after intercourse and then removed within 30 hours after intercourse. Currently, the "Today" Vaginal Contraceptive Sponge is the only sponge approved by the FDA[12]
- Spermicides: a spermicide destroys sperm. A spermicide can be used alone or in combination with a diaphragm or cervical cap. The most common spermicidal agent is a chemical called nonoxynol-9 (N-9). It is available in several concentrations and forms, including foam, jelly, cream, suppository, and film. A spermicide should be inserted into the vagina close to the uterus no more than 30 minutes prior to intercourse and left in place 6–8 hours after intercourse to prevent pregnancy. Spermicides do not prevent the transmission of STDs and may cause allergic reactions or vaginitis.[13]

Hormonal Methods

Hormonal methods of birth control use hormones to regulate or stop ovulation and prevent pregnancy. Hormones can be introduced into the body through various methods, including pills, injections, skin patches, transdermal gels, vaginal rings, intrauterine systems, and implantable rods.

Oral Contraceptives

- Combined oral contraceptives (COCs): it contains different combinations of the synthetic estrogens and progestins and are given to interfere with ovulation. A woman takes one pill daily, preferably at the same time each day.[14]

The formulations of oral contraceptive pills have changed dramatically over the years. High doses of norethynodrel (progestin) and mestranol (estrogen) were used initially. It contained norethynodrel—one of the first-generation progestins called "estranes". This class includes the current agents norethindrone, norethindrone acetate, and ethynodiol diacetate.

Levonorgestrel, a more potent, second-generation progestin, was developed in about 1970. Over the past several decades, the dose of the estrogen component of oral contraceptive pills has decreased from the original 150–50 µg and then to 20–35 µg. These changes were made to lower the risk of thromboembolic complications associated with the use of oral contraceptive pills.

The third-generation progestins from the gonane class were incorporated into oral contraceptive pill formulations to reduce the androgenic and metabolic side effects that occur with older agents. These new progestins include desogestrel, gestodene (not available in the United States), and norgestimate.

Originally, most combination oral contraceptive pill formulations were monophasic, with each active tablet containing a fixed dose of estrogen and progestin throughout the cycle. Multiphasic preparations (biphasic and triphasic) were developed in the 1980s to reduce the total dosage of progestin throughout the cycle without increasing the risk of breakthrough bleeding.

The noncontraceptive benefits (and favorable side-effect profiles) of oral contraceptive pills are important. Labeled and unlabeled indications for oral contraceptive pills include acne, dysmenorrhea, premenstrual syndrome (PMS), and endometriosis.

Noncontraceptive benefits of oral contraceptive pills:

- Dysmenorrhea
- Dysfunctional uterine bleeding
- Premenstrual syndrome
- Functional ovarian cysts
- Endometriosis
- Benign breast diseases
- Hirsutism
- Acne
- Prevention of ovarian and endometrial cancer.

According to WHO various contraindications for the use of oral contraceptives are listed as below (Tables 1):

- Progestin-only pills (POPs or mini pills): these type of pills do not contain estrogen, so they do not suppress lactation and thus can be used by postpartum women irrespective of breast feeding status. Although minimum amount of progestin secreted in breast-milk has not shown any adverse effect on infant growth or development, but because of theoretical concern about effect of sex

TABLE 1: Various contraindications for the use of oral contraceptives

Category 1 (No restriction)	Category 2 (Advantages outweigh risks)
• Postpartum >21 days • Postabortion • Varicose veins • Mild headaches • Irregular vaginal bleeding without anemia • Past,current or recent h/o PID • Current or recent h/o STD • Vaginitis without purulent cervicitis • Increased risk of STD • Family h/o breast/ovarian/ endometrial cancer • Obesity • Thyroid conditions • Cervical ectropion • Viral hepatitis carrier • HIV positive	• Severe headaches after initiation of OCPs • Diabetes mellitus • Major surgery without prolonged immobilization • Sickle cell disease • Hypertension • Undiagnosed breast mass • Cervical cancer • Age >50 years • Conditions leading to noncompliance • Family h/o lipid disorders or premature myocardial infarction
Category 3 (Exercise caution)	**Category 4 (Refrain from use)**
• Postpartum <21 days • Lactation (6 weeks–6 months) • Undiagnosed vaginal or uterine bleeding • Age >35 years and smokes <20 cigarettes per day • H/o breast cancer but no recurrence in past 5 years • Interacting drugs • Gall bladder disease	• Venous thromboembolism • Cerebrovascular or coronary artery disease • Structural heart disease • Diabetes with complication • Breast cancer • Pregnancy • Lactation (<6 weeks postpartum) • Liver disease • Severe hypertension • Major surgery with prolonged immobilization • Age >35 years with >20 cigarettes per day • Headaches with focal neurological symptoms

OCPs, oral contraceptive pills; PID, pelvic inflammatory disease; STD, sexually transmitted disease; h/o, history of; HIV, human immunodeficiency virus.

steroids on the neonate the commencement of POP is recommended after 3 weeks postpartum. Progestin-only pills can be started within first 5 days of menses. It must be taken at same time of the day. Progestin-only pills alter the normal cyclical changes in the uterine lining and may result in unscheduled or breakthrough bleeding. These hormones do not appear to be associated with an increased risk of blood clots (Fig. 2).[15,16]

Compositions used are

- Norethindrone 0.350 mg
- Levonorgesterol 0.075 mg

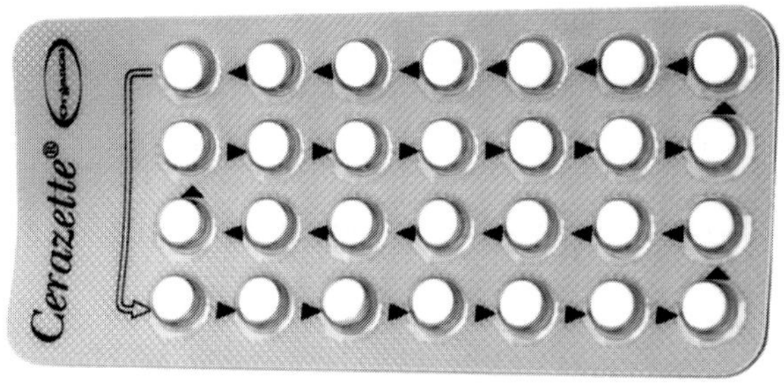

FIG. 2: Progestin-only pills.

- Norgesterol 0.030 mg
- Ethynodial diacetate 0.500 mg
- Desogestrel 0.075 mg

Mechanism of action

- Thickening of cervical mucus
- Suppression of ovulation
- Involution of endometrium

  → 99.95% effective with correct and consistent use.

  Failure rate only 0.5% in first year in breast-feeding women.

Instructions on the use of oral contraceptive pills

- Start the pill from day 1 of menstrual cycle
- First Sunday after menstrual cycle begins
- Immediately if she is not pregnant and has not had sexual intercourse since her last menstrual period
- If it has been less than 24 hours since the last pill was taken, the patient takes a pill right away and then returns to normal pill-taking routine
- If it has been 24 hours since the last pill was taken, the patient takes both the missed pill and the next scheduled pill at the same time
- If it has been more than 24 hours since the last pill was taken (i.e., two or more missed pills), the patient takes the last pill that was missed, throws out the other missed pills and takes the next pill on time. Additional contraception is used for the remainder of the cycle
- The patient uses an additional contraceptive method for the first 7 days after initially starting oral contraceptive pills
- The patient uses an additional contraceptive method for 7 days if she is more than 12 hours late in taking an oral contraceptive pill
- The patient uses an additional contraceptive method while she is taking an interacting drug and for 7 days thereafter.
- Contraceptive patch: this is a thin, plastic patch that sticks to the skin and releases hormones through the skin into the bloodstream. The patch is placed on the lower abdomen, buttocks, outer arm, or upper body. A

new patch is applied once a week for 3 weeks, and no patch is used on the fourth week to enable menstruation. Currently, Ortho Evra is the only patch that is FDA approved
- Injectable birth control: this method involves injection of a progestin, Depo-Provera (DMPA—depo medroxyprogesterone acetate), given in the arm or buttocks in a dose of 150 mg, once every 3 months. This method of birth control can cause a temporary loss of bone density, particularly in adolescents. However, this bone loss is generally regained after discontinuing use of DMPA.[17,18]
    - Depot medroxyprogesterone acetate: available as Depo-Provera, a 1 mL, injectable containing 150 mg of depot medroxyprogesterone acetate (DMPA) provides contraceptive effect for 12–14 weeks.
    - Noretbisterone enantbate: a 1 mL injectable containing 200 mg of norethisterone enanthate (NET-EN/Noristerate) is effective as contraceptive for 8–9 weeks.

Administration of Injectable Contraceptives

- Depot medroxyprogesterone acetate, an aqueous microcrystalline suspension, is administered by intramuscular injection in every 90 days (3 months) and NET-EN, an oily preparation, is administered as an intramuscular injection at 8-weekly intervals (2 months)
- Aseptic techniques should be maintained when administering injectable contraceptives
- Disposable syringes are advisable though not essential. Reusable glass syringes are also equally good if sterilized properly. Reusable glass syringes should be steam sterilized at 121°C for 20 minutes or autoclaved. It should be stored in sterile container. Needles and syringes should be sterilized separately
- First injection: it should be given during the first 7 days of a menstrual cycle in order to minimize the risk of administering the first injection in the presence of an undiagnosed pregnancy. However, if a woman requests the injectable or any other time during the cycle, it should be provided only after the possibility of a pregnancy is ruled out
- Ideally, breast-feeding women should not use the injectable earlier than 6 weeks postpartum
- It can be provided immediately or within 7 days after medical termination of pregnancy or spontaneous miscarriage
- Vaginal rings: the ring is thin, flexible, and approximately 2 inches in diameter. It delivers a combination of a synthetic estrogen (ethinyl estradiol) and a progestin. The ring is inserted into the vagina, where it continually releases hormones for 3 weeks. The woman removes it for the fourth week and reinserts a new ring 7 days later. Currently, the NuvaRing is the only FDA-approved vaginal ring. A new contraceptive vaginal ring that can be used for 13 cycles is under clinical development
- Implantable rods: implant is a long-acting reversible contraceptive (LARC) method. The advantage of this form of contraception is that it provides effective long-term contraception that does not depend on the recipients daily compliance. It was in the year 1990, levonorgestrel contraceptive implant received USFDA approval. Norplant consists of 6 silicone rods each measuring 34 mm long and 2.4 mm in diameter. Each rod contains 36 mg of levonorgestrel and releases approximately 80 ug of levonorgestrel per 24 hours during the first year of use, achieving effective serum level of 04–0.45 ng/mL within first 24 hours. In later years of use, the rate of release decreases to an average of 30 ug/day. It provides contraception for 5 years and the contraceptive protection begins within 24 hours of insertion
    - A single-rod implant (Implanon)[19] is a thin flexible plastic rod, measuring 40 mm in length and 2 mm in diameter. It is a progestin-only implant which is inserted just under the skin on the inner side of upper arm. This method provides pregnancy protection for about 3 years and can be removed any time before 3 years if required. This implant received FDA approval in July 2006. Local anesthesia is required before its insertion and the method takes a few minutes only. This single-rod implant does not contain latex or silicone and will not dissolve, so it must be removed
    - Implanon consists of a single rod made of ethylene vinylacetate copolymer that is 4 cm long and 2 mm in diameter. It is similar to a matchstick in size. The rod contains 68 mg of etonogestrel (3-keto-destrogestrel). Each rod is matchstick-sized, flexible, and plastic. It is surgically inserted under the skin of upper arm, inner side, 8–10 cm (3–4 inches) above the medial epicondyle of the humerus to prevent neural and vascular injuries. The rods can remain implanted for up to 3 years (Fig. 3)
    - A two-rod method, Jadelle (Norplant II), developed by the population council, consists of two small (2.5 mm × 43 mm) silicone rods each containing 75 mg of levonorgestrel in a polymer matrix, instead of six capsules (as in Norplant I) which is FDA approved is also available. Norplant is implanted under the skin in the upper arm, by creating a small incision and inserting the capsules in a fanlike shape. Once inserted, the contraceptive works within 24 hours and lasts up to 5 years (Fig. 4).
    - A new levonorgestrel-releasing, two-rod method, Sino Implant, is in clinical development.

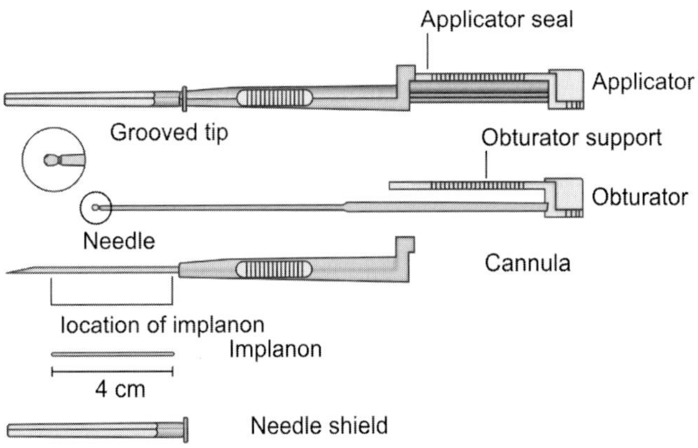

FIG. 3: Single-rod implant (Implanon).

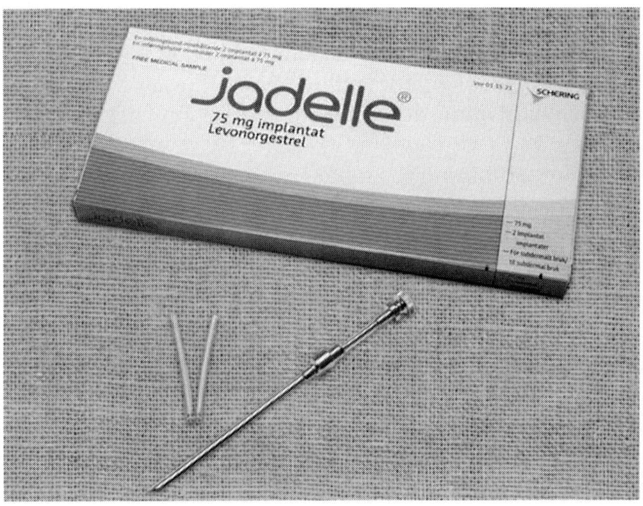

FIG. 4: Two-rod implant, Jadelle (Norplant II).

Intrauterine Contraceptive Devices (Fig. 5)

An intrauterine contraceptive devices (IUCD) is a small, T-shaped device that is inserted into the uterus to prevent pregnancy An IUCD can remain and function effectively for many years at a time. Two types of IUCDs are available nowadays:

- Copper containing
- Progesterone containing
- A copper IUD releases a small amount of copper into the uterus, causing an inflammatory reaction that generally prevents sperm from reaching and fertilizing the egg. If fertilization of the egg does occur, the physical presence of the device prevents the fertilized egg from implanting into the lining of the uterus. A copper IUCD is not recommended for women who may be pregnant, have pelvic infections, or had uterine perforations during previous IUCD insertions. It also is not recommended for women who have cervical cancer or cancer of the uterus, unexplained vaginal bleeding, or pelvic tuberculosis.

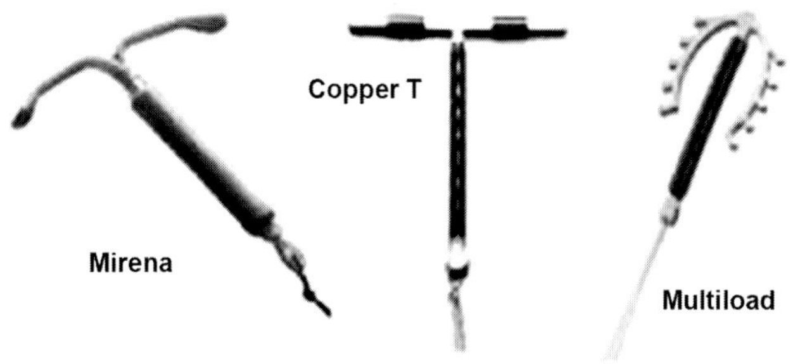

FIG. 5: Intrauterine contraceptive device.

Usual Timings for Insertion

- Immediate Postpartum:
  - Postplacental: insertion within 10 minutes after expulsion of the placenta following a vaginal delivery on the same delivery table
  - Intracesarean: insertion that takes place during a cesarean delivery, after removal of the placenta and before closure of the uterine incision
  - Within 48 hours after delivery: insertion within 48 hours of delivery and prior to discharge from the postpartum ward
- Postabortion: insertion following an abortion, if there is no infection, bleeding or any other contraindications
- Extended postpartum/interval: insertion any time after 6 weeks postpartum.

The IUCD should not be inserted from 48 hours–6 weeks following delivery because there is an increased risk of infection and expulsion.

Postpartum Intrauterine Contraceptive Device

Copper T 380A (CuT-380A) or Copper U 375 (Cu-375) IUCD inserted in the postpartum period within 48 hours after a childbirth is called postpartum intrauterine contraceptive device (PPIUCD).

Intrauterine contraceptive device is a reliable, effective, long-term and reversible contraceptive method for spacing or limiting pregnancies. Inserting IUCD during this new time of postpartum period helps in providing an additional time for the option of IUCD use by a woman who has just given birth and who either does not want a baby in the near future or never. This is a convenient time for the woman and the provider if the woman is at the health facility for her labor, delivery and postpartum period for at least 2 days.

Medical Eligibility Criteria and Client Assessment for Ppiucd

Client assessment

First client assessment should be done during antenatal care to exclude known contraindications like:
- Distorted uterine cavity
- Acute purulent discharge
- Current/risk of gonorrhea or chlamydia
- Malignant or benign trophoblastic disease
- HIV/acquired immunodeficiency syndrom (AIDS) and neither clinically well nor on antiretroviral therapy

Second-client assessment should be done immediately prior to insertion to ensure that the process of labor has not created a clinical situation in which IUCD may not be an appropriate option, such as:
- Chorioamnionitis
- Postpartum endometritis, metritis
- Puerperal sepsis
- More than 18 hours from rupture of membranes to delivery
- Unresolved postpartum hemorrhage (PPH)
- Extensive genital trauma

If IUCD is unsuitable for the woman, she should be offered other methods of postpartum family planning (PPFP). IUCD should be inserted prior to starting the repair of multiple lacerations or episiotomy if they are not bleeding heavily.[20]

Postpartum hemorrhage or unresolved postpartum bleeding is an emergency and must be attended to on priority. Once it is controlled, and woman is still willing for PPIUCD, she can be provided with the services after excluding active infection. IUCD may be provided in category three conditions when there is availability of sound clinical judgment and facilities for investigations are present and if other appropriate contraceptive methods are either not available or not acceptable to the client or couple.

Mirena

- A hormonal IUCD releases levonorgestrel (LNG) into the uterus. The released hormone causes thickening of the cervical mucus, inhibits sperm from reaching or fertilizing the egg, thins the uterine lining, and also may prevent the ovaries from releasing eggs. It is a modern LNG containing IUD containing 40–60 mg of LNG and releasing 20 mcg per day[21]
- It is effective for 5 years
- Failure rate is 0.1–0.4 per 100 women in the first year.

Dual Protection

Dual protection is the use of methods that prevent both sexually transmitted infections and pregnancy. This can be with condoms either alone or along with another birth control method or by the avoidance of penetrative sex. If pregnancy is a high concern, using two methods at the same time is reasonable, and two forms of birth control is recommended in those taking the antiacne drug isotretinoin, due to the high risk of birth defects if taken during pregnancy.

Sterilization

Surgical sterilization is available in the form of tubal ligation for women and vasectomy for men. There are no significant long-term side effects, and tubal ligation decreases the risk of ovarian cancer.

Female sterilization using laparoscopic technique is the most commonly used permanent method of birth control in industrialized countries. It is one of the safest operative gynecological procedures with complications occurring in less than 1% of the cases.[22]

Male sterilization is a mere 1.8% of all sterilizations done in the country. Vasectomy is a safe, simple and effective method even when compared to tubectomy and is the only established long-term method available for men. There are two methods of approach to vas. Incisional and no scalpel vasectomy (NSV) was introduced in China by Li Shung Qiang in 1974.[23] This does not require a scrotal incision or stitch and is done under local anesthesia. NSV was introduced in India in 1992.

Research

Females: improvements of existing birth control methods are needed, as around half of those who get pregnant unintentionally are using birth control at the time. A number of alterations of existing contraceptive methods are being studied, including a better female condom, an improved diaphragm, a patch containing only progestin, and a vaginal ring containing long-acting progesterone. This vaginal ring appears to be effective for three or four months and is currently available in some areas of the world. For women who rarely have sex, the taking of the hormonal birth control levonorgestrel around the time of sex looks promising.

A number of methods to perform sterilization via the cervix are being studied. One involves putting quinacrine in the uterus which causes scarring and infertility. While the procedure is inexpensive and does not require surgical skills, there are concerns regarding long-term side effects. Another substance, polidocanol, which functions in the same manner is being looked at. A device called Essure, which expands when placed in the fallopian tubes and blocks them, was approved in the United States in 2002.

Males: a number of hormonal and nonhormonal methods are in trials, and there is some research looking at the possibility of contraceptive vaccines.

A reversible surgical method under investigation is reversible inhibition of sperm under guidance (RISUG) which consists of injecting a polymer gel, styrene maleic anhydride in dimethyl sulfoxide, into the vas deferens. An injection with sodium bicarbonate washes out the substance and restores fertility.

Another is an intravas device which involves putting a urethane plug into the vas deferens to block it. A combination of an androgen and a progestin seems promising, as do selective androgen receptor modulators. Ultrasound and methods to heat the testicles have undergone preliminary studies.

REFERENCES

1. Pearl, John, Potts Malcom. Textbook of Contraceptive Practice, Cambridge University Press; 1970.
2. Hawkins DF, Elder MG. Human Fertility Control: Theory and Practice, Butterworth, London. 1979.
3. McCann MF, Liskin LS, Piottow PT, Rinehart W, and Fox G. Breastfeeding, fertility, and family planning. Population Reports, series. 1981;J-24:525-75.
4. Jain AK, Bongaarts. Breastfeeding patterns, correlates and fertility effects. Studies in Family Planning. 1981;12:79.
5. ICMR Bulletin, December 1983.
6. Dalsimer IA, Piottrow PT, Dumm JJ. Population report. barrier methods, Series H, No. 1, H2, Department of Medical and Public Affairs. USA: The George Washington University Medical Center; 1973.
7. Sherris JD. (Ed). Barrier Methods, Population Report Series H:6. 1982.
8. Holmes KK, Levine R, Weaver M. Effectiveness of condoms in preventing sexually transmitted infections. Bull Health Organ. 2004;82:454-61.
9. Allen RE, Diaphragm fitting. Am Fam Physician. 2004;69:97-100, 103, 105-106.
10. Mauck CK, Weiner DH, Creinin MD, Archer DF, Schwartz JL, Pymar HC, et al. FemCap with removal strap: ease of removal, safety and acceptability. Contraception. 2006;73:59-64.
11. Shihata A. New FDA-approved woman-controlled, latex- free barrier contraceptive device "Fem Cap. In: Daya S. Gunby J, Pierson R, (Eds). Research Papers in Fertility and Rep5roductive Medicine: Proceedings of the 18th World Congress on Fertility and Sterility (IFFS 2004) held in Montreal Canada, between 23 and 28 May (2004), Ist Edition (Internal Congress. Toronto, Canada; Elsevier Science; 2004. pp. 303-6.
12. Skerine R. The Practitioner. 1984;229:441-6.
13. Belsky Raymond (Ed). Barrier Methods George Washington University Medical Centre (Population Report Series B 3), Washington DC. 1975.
14. Wynn V, Adams PW, Godsland I, Melrose J, Niththyananthan R, Oakley NW, et al. Comparison of effects of different combined oral contraceptive formulations on carbohydrate and lipid metabolism. Lancet. 1979;1(8125):1045-9.
15. Spellacy WN. A perspective on progestogens in oral contraceptives. Am J Obstet Gynecol. 1982;142:717.
16. McEwan J. The Practitioner. 1985;229:415-23.
17. Scholes D, LaCroix AZ, Ichikawa LE, Barlow WE, Ott SM. Injectable hormone contraception and bone density: results from a prospective study. Epidemiology. 2002;13:581-7.
18. Contraception Report. DMPA and bone density loss. Contraception Rep. 1999;10:4-10.
19. Levine JP, Senofsky FE, Christ MF. Implanon US study Group. Assessment of Implanon insertion and removal contraception. 2008;78:409-17.
20. Family Planning Division, Ministry of Health and Family Welfare. Government of India. (2010). Postpartum IUCD Reference Manual (Online) Available from pdf. Usaid. Gov/pdf-docs/PNADW 249. Pdf. [Accessed May, 2014].
21. Thiery M. Intrauterine contraception: From silver ring to intrauterine implant. Dur J Obstet Gynecol Reprod Biol. 2000;90:145-52.
22. Kuller R, Boulvain M, Walker D, Candolle G, Campana A. Minilaparotomy and endoscopic techniques for tubal sterilization. Cochrane Database Syst Rev. 2004;(3):CD001328.
23. Li SQ. Vasal sterilization techniques Teaching material for the National Standard Workshop, Chongqing, People's Republic of China: Scientific and Technical Literature Press; 1988. pp. 176.

Section 5

Neonate

CHAPTER 32

Examination of Newborn

Jiya Lal

INTRODUCTION

Examination of the newborn is slightly different from that of an adult. It needs meticulous and careful observations. Eliciting signs is difficult in neonatal age-group. The components of assessment include history taking (Table 1) and physical examination. The physical examination should be done at birth, after 24 hours, and before discharge from the nursery.[1] At birth examination is done to assess the successful transition from intra-uterine to extra-uterine environments and to detect congenital malformations (CMFs).[2] First-day examination is directed to record measurements, look for CMFs, screening systemic illnesses, and to assess feeding.

EXAMINATION AT BIRTH

The first routine examination reveals more information, if done appropriately.

Prerequisites

Room should be warm; baby completely undressed; use flat surface for placing the baby; examine under natural source of light; and examiner's hands should be clean and warm. Before doing physical examination, it is essential to take detailed history about conception, antenatal events, and maternal medical and obstetrical history, mode of delivery, any instruments applied, and resuscitation details (Table 2).

History

Important maternal conditions and their implications for the newborn have been described in Table 2.

TABLE 1: History in newborn examination

Important maternal and perinatal history	
Family history	• Especially ask for inherited disorders in the family, e.g., hemophilia, cystic fibrosis, perinatal adverse events, and congenital malformations (CMFs). History of (H/o) consanguinity must be inquired
Maternal history	• Particularly important are: maternal age at conception, blood group, chronic maternal illness, like diabetes, hypertension, renal disorders, cardiac illnesses, and bleeding disorders. H/o recent infections, like urinary tract infection (UTI), foul smelling liquor, lower abdominal pain, and fever is of paramount importance
Previous pregnancy outcome	• Abortions, prematurity, malformations, early neonatal deaths, jaundice, apnea, and respiratory distress should be asked for
Antenatal events	• Bleeding per vaginum, infections, chest X-ray exposure, oligohydramnios or polyhydramnios, Doppler ultrasonography revealing: absent end-diastolic flow (AEDF)/reduced end-diastolic flow (REDF), abnormal biophysical profile, etc., use of antenatal corticosteroids, drug intake, especially antithyroid and antiepileptic drugs should be asked in detail. Use of iron, folic acid, calcium supplements, and tetanus prophylaxis should be asked for
Perinatal events	• Presentation, onset and duration of labor, duration of rupture of membranes, instrumentation, induction of labor, maternal fever, liquor (foul smelling, meconium or blood stained), APGAR (Appearance, Pulse, Grimace, Activity, Respiration) score, and details of resuscitation

TABLE 2: Maternal conditions and implications for the newborn[3]

Maternal conditions	Implications for the newborn
Pregnancy-induced hypertension	Intrauterine growth retardation (IUGR), birth asphyxia, thrombocytopenia
Use of beta-blocker	Hypoglycemia
Use of magnesium sulfate	Neonatal respiratory depression
Diabetes mellitus (DM)	Congenital malformation (CMF)
hypothyroidism/ hyperthyroidism	IUGR, prematurity, intrauterine death (IUD), birth asphyxia
Severe anemia	IUGR, prematurity, hemoglobinopathy
Antiphospholipid antibodies	Thrombocytopenia
Systemic lupus erythematosus	Thrombocytopenia, heart blocks, hydrops fetalis, asphyxia
Rheumatic heart disease	IUGR, prematurity, IUD
Coronary heart disease	IUGR, recurrence risk
Hemolysis, Elevated Liver enzymes Low-Platelet count (HELLP) syndrome	Cautious interpretation of neonatal renal function tests
Poor antenatal supervision	IUGR
Primi delivered by lower-segment cesarean section	Hypoglycemia
Malpresentation	Instrumental delivery
Precipitate labor	Birth trauma
Rh negative/O blood group	Isoimmunization
Multiple pregnancy	Prematurity, birth asphyxia, CMF, malpresentation
Polyhydramnios	Prematurity, neural tube defects, atresia of gastrointestinal tract
Oligohydramnios	Birth asphyxia, Potter phenotype, pulmonary hypoplasia
Cholestasis of pregnancy	IUD
Acute fatty liver	IUD
Advance maternal age	Chromosomal anomalies
Malnutrition	IUGR
Short stature	Birth trauma, asphyxia
Smoking	IUGR, IUD, prematurity
Alcohol intake	Fetal alcohol syndrome, IUD
Radiation exposure	CMF
Chorioamnionitis	Early-onset neonatal sepsis (EOS), prematurity, periventricular leukomalacia (PVL)
Urinary tract infection, diarrhea, systemic infection	EOS, prematurity
Toxoplasmosis, rubella, cytomegalovirus, herpes simplex (TORCH) infection	Congenital/perinatal TORCH infection
Human immunodeficiency virus	Perinatal transmission
Hepatitis B	Perinatal transmission, need for hepatitis B immunoglobulin vaccine
Previous baby affected by significant hyperbilirubinemia	Recurrence

Physical Examination

Examination at birth should be directed to detect CMFs. congenital malformations represent defects in morphogenesis during early fetal life and account for 8–15% of perinatal deaths and 13–16% of neonatal deaths in India. The proportion of perinatal deaths due to CMFs is increasing as a result of reduction of mortality due to other causes owing to the improvement in perinatal and neonatal cares.[4]

Birth Weight and Gestation

Preterm and symmetric intrauterine growth retardation (IUGR) babies are more frequently associated with CMFs;[5] therefore, these babies should be screened thoroughly.

Orifice Counting

The CMFs should be looked around the orifices. Examine oral cavity to rule out cleft lip, cleft palate, and rule out esophageal atresia by passing nasogastric (NG) tube through mouth. Look for anal patency.

Midline Defects

Examine back and spine to rule out meningocele, meningomyelocele, spina bifida, and ambiguous genitalia.

Single Umbilical Artery

Single umbilical artery is associated with CMFs, especially esophageal atresia, and genitourinary anomalies. Umbilical cord should be examined to note the number of umbilical vessels.

General examination: it should be done to look for normal transition to extrauterine life. Vitals including temperature, heart rate, respiratory rate, capillary refill time, and oxygen saturation (SpO_2) should be recorded. Under no circumstances hypothermia should be allowed to set in. Keep baby warm and examine under radiant warmer.

Systemic examination: look for signs of respiratory distress—tachypnea, chest wall retractions, nasal flaring, head bobbing, and grunting. Cardiovascular system is examined for any cyanosis and heart murmur.

Subsequent Examination

Examination should be done in warm environment while the baby is under radiant warmer and at least 1 hour post-feed time with clean and warm hands. Remove clothes from one part of the body before examination and put them back before next part is examined to avoid hypothermia. Mother should be informed about the examination.

General Examination

It includes noticing the babies' activity, spontaneous movements, color, and state-to-state variability.

Color

Normal color of the infant is pink. Skin color is the most important index of cardiorespiratory function in a newborn.

- Bluishness or cyanosis: it is usually present in the hands, feet and occasionally on the lips (acrocyanosis). If there is central cyanosis, it is indicative of poor ventilation or cyanotic heart disease. Look for bluishness in lips and oral mucosa
- Pallor: paleness is indicative of anemia. In neonate, usual causes are: frequent bloodletting, twin-to-twin transfusion syndrome, abruption placenta or placenta previa, and hemolytic anemia
- Icterus: it is assessed by blanching the skin on forehead, chest, palms, and soles with gentle digital pressure and noticing the color. Yellowish tinge of the skin suggests jaundice.

Vitals

Assessment of vitals includes measurement of temperature, heart rate, respiratory rate, blood pressure (BP), capillary refill time, and SpO_2.

- Temperature: this is the first vital sign to be recorded in neonates. It is measured with thermometer, kept in the roof of axilla for complete 5 minutes as per World Health Organization (WHO) guidelines.[6] The normal temperature of the neonate is 36.5–37.5°C. The temperature between 36.4°C and 36°C is called mild hypothermia or cold stress. Temperature between 35.9°C and 32°C is called moderate hypothermia and temperature less than 32°C is termed as severe hypothermia. Temperature assessment can be done by touching the baby with dorsum of hand (in community) also. If central and acral parts are warm to touch baby is said to be in euthermia. If the peripheries are cold and central body parts are warm, it is cold stress. In hypothermia, both central and acral parts are cold to touch
- Heart rate: it should be counted for full 1 minute. Normal heart rate in neonate is 110-160 beats/min. It varies with changes in the activity, like it increases during crying or activity of the baby. Any irregularity in rhythm or rate should alert the pediatrician for an underlying heart disease
- Respiratory rate: the normal respiratory rate in neonate is 40–60 breaths/minute. All infants are periodic breathers. Therefore, babies breathe at a regular rate for a brief period (usually 15–20 seconds) and then have a short period of apnea (5–10 seconds). This period of apnea is not associated with change in heart rate or cyanosis. Presence of respiratory distress indicates affection of respiratory, cardiovascular, metabolic, or neurological system
- Blood pressure: blood pressure in the neonate is taken with neonatal cuff. The normal BP at birth is 60–76 mmHg/30–45 mmHg. The BP measured should be plotted on Zubrow's chart[7] and interpretation done accordingly. Shows expected systolic blood pressure (BP) and diastolic BP according to age (Table 3).[8]

  Blood pressure should be measured in all four limbs to rule out coarctation of aorta. In infants with coarctation, pulses are weak in the lower limbs and BP high in upper limb (>10 mmHg compared to lower limb)[9]
- Capillary refill time: it is used to assess the peripheral perfusion. The pressure with finger is applied on skin to blanch it on forehead or sternum and watch for refilling and color change. If the area becomes pink after 3 seconds, it is called prolonged capillary refill and is a marker of poor peripheral perfusion
- Oxygen saturation: it is called as fifth vital sign. It is measured with pulse oximeter applied on fingers or toes. Care should be taken to take reading, while the waveform is regular and the heart rate of the meter is matching with that of baby. Routine pulse oximetry performed on asymptomatic newborns after 24 hours of life, but before hospital discharge, may detect congenital cyanotic heart disease (CCHD).[10] Deoxygenated hemoglobin absorbs light in the red band (600–750 nm), whereas oxygenated hemoglobin absorbs light in the infrared band (850–1,000 nm).[11] The ratio of light absorbance at these 2 wavelengths correlates with the saturation of hemoglobin

TABLE 3: Expected systolic blood pressure (BP) and diastolic BP according to age[8]

Age	Systolic blood pressure (BP) (mmHg)	Diastolic BP (mmHg)
1 day	60–76	30–45
2–4 days	67–84	35–53
4 days to 1 month	73–94	36–56
1–3 months	78–103	44–65

in the capillaries.[12] Falsely low-oximetry readings in the newborn population are known to be associated with low-peripheral perfusion and motion artifact, probe placement site and partial probe detachment and hyperbilirubinemia or dyshemoglobinemias.[13] Normal SpO_2 in term neonates is 87–93%. When neonates are having hypoxemia (SpO_2 <95%), it is necessary to evaluate them for congenital heart disease.

Head-to-toe Examination

Look for CMFs. The incidence of congenital anomalies is higher among the stillbirths than among the live-born babies.[14]

Head and Neck

Always look for shape and size of head and any visible swelling (caput succedaneum, cephalohematoma, subgaleal bleed, and encephalocele). Look for any puncture wounds, lacerations, edema or bruising of scalp which may result due to forceps or ventouse application. Caput succedaneum is a boggy area of edema present at the presenting part of head; seen at birth. It crosses suture lines, and disappears within a few days. Cephalohematoma is seen in 1–2% of newborn. It is subperiosteal collection of blood and does not cross the midline. It subsides in 4–6 weeks' time. Palpation of skull should be done to look for suture overriding or separation. Fontanels should be checked when the baby is quite and in sitting position. Craniotabes (softening of skull bone, ping-pong-like sensation) is normally seen in preterm babies.

Face

Look for facial dimorphism, retrognathia (which may suggest Pierre-Robin sequence), and potter faces. Neonates keep their eyes closed. The eyes can be made to open by holding the baby upright and rocking back and forward in diffuse light. The size, orientation, and position of the eyes should be noted. Upward slanting of the palpebral fissure is seen in trisomy 21 patients.

Ears

Deformities of pinna are sometimes encountered. One must look for preauricular skin tags or fistulae, patency of external auditory canal and low set ears (defined as placement of superior aspect pinna attached to cranium is below the line joining the inner canthi), which are found in Down syndrome.

Mouth

Prenatal teeth, if found, may be indicative of Ellis-van Creveld or Hallermann-Streiff syndrome. Soft and hard palate should be inspected and palpated for a complete or submucosal cleft. Other abnormalities that may be found are: high-arched palate, bifid uvula, and Epstein pearls (on the hard palate on either side of the raphe). These are accumulations of epithelial cells. Micrognathia is seen in Pierre-Robin sequence.

Chest

Abnormal chest shapes should be noticed like shield-shaped chest, pectus excavatum, and pectus carinatum. Nipple abnormalities, viz., widely placed nipples, supernumerary nipples, etc. should be looked for.

Genitals

Special attention should be directed to look for genital ambiguity, hypospadias or epispadias, and anal opening (anal atresia, anorectal malformations).

- Male: look for size of penis, scrotum, and position of external urethral meatus. The stretched penile length should be more than 2.5 cm in term neonate. Testes are bilaterally descended in term neonate. Palpate inguinal regions to locate the undescended testes. Look for any obvious swelling in the inguinoscrotal region, its reducibility and relation to crying or straining (congenital inguinal hernia)
- Female: in term neonate, the labia majora covers the labia minora and clitoris, whereas these structures are prominent in preterm babies. Look for any vaginal tags and labial adhesions. Presence of palpable mass in the inguinal region should alert the physician to hernia or ectopic gonads (testes or ovaries). Presence of clitoromegaly, labioscrotal fusion and hyperpigmentation of genitalia are indicators of virilization and possibility of congenital adrenal hyperplasia should be born in mind.[15]

Anus

Look for anal position and patency. Presence of imperforate anus is a surgical condition and may have vertebral, anal, cardiac, tracheoesophageal, renal, and limb anomalies (VACTERL) or vertebral anomalies, anal atresia, tracheoesophageal fistula, and renal dysplasia (VATER) associations.

Extremities

One should look for limb asymmetry, digital abnormalities (polydactyly, syndactyly, and hypoplasia), congenital talipes equinovarus (CTEV), Erb's palsy, etc. Presence of these finding may point towards dysmorphic syndrome.

Hip

It is mandatory to rule-out developmental dysplasia of hip (DDH) by Barlow and Ortolani maneuvers. Developmental dysplasia of hip is usually seen with breach presentation and in female neonates. On examination, there may be asymmetry of skin folds around the hip and shortening of the affected leg.

- Barlow test: it is performed by putting the baby in supine position and holding the hip by hand with thumb facing the crease of groin and fingers on the greater trochanter. Adduct the hip gently and apply pressure posteriorly to push the femur head out of acetabular cavity if there is displacement of 5 mm or more the joint is said to be dislocatable. Care must be taken not to lift the pelvis from the surface while performing the test
- Ortolani test: it is reverse of previously described test. In this test the hip is hold in similar fashion and the hip is abducted, with this movement the head of the femur goes inside the acetabulum and clunk is heard, if the joint is dislocated. Developmental dysplasia of hip if suspected on above tests and ultrasonography (USG) of hip joint and orthopedic consultation should be sought immediately.[16]

Skin Examination

The stratum corneum of preterm neonate is thin and it matures over 1–2 weeks' time. Look for stork bites, nevus, and Mongolian spots. Special attention should be paid to skin where saturation probe or thermistor is placed, cannula site and nappy area. Newborn has benign lesions. These conditions are very common and almost expected in newborns.[17] The attending physician should be well versed with these physiological skin findings.

- Vernix caseosa: the fetus is covered by protective membrane called as vernix caseosa. It is composed of dead epithelial cells, lanugo hairs, and sebaceous secretions. It provides mechanical barrier to skin. It is known to have antibacterial and antifungal properties[18]
- Erythema toxicum: it is seen in 75% of term neonates. These are small erythematous macules usually associated with papules located on face, trunk, and extremities. The lesions subjected to microscopic examination reveal eosinophils. Eosinophilia in peripheral blood film may also be seen. It is a benign condition usually subsides in 4 weeks spontaneously[19]
- Transient neonatal pustular dermatosis: it occurs in 0.2–4% of neonates. These lesions are more common in forehead and mandibular region. These are pustular lesion, without any surrounding edema. Microscopic examination of the lesion shows abundance of neutrophils. It resolves in few days; however, hyperpigmentation may take place and it takes several weeks to months to disappear[20]
- Mongolian spot: it is blue-grey or blue-green macular patch which is located over sacral and gluteal regions. Histological examination shows presence of melanocytes in deep dermis with collagen fibers. Typically, the irregular patch increases in size and intensity over the first year of life and then fades in early childhood[21]
- Salmon patch: it is a pale-pink patch usually seen on forehead or nape of neck. When it is located on the nape of neck, it is called as stork bite. Most of these lesions disappear in infancy or early childhood[22]
- Milia: it is seen in 40–50% of newborns with no racial or gender tendency. Presents in term neonates after 4–5 days and can be delayed from days to weeks in preterm infants. These are 1–2 mm pearly-white lesions present on chin, nose, forehead, and cheeks.[23] Known as Epstein pearls if located on the soft or hard palate. These lesions resolve within 1–2 months. No treatment is required
- Seborrheic dermatitis (cradle cap): these are greasy, scaling with patchy redness, fissuring, and occasional weeping lesions mostly seen on scalp, but can also appear on the face, ears, forehead, eyebrows, trunks, and flexural areas; occurs due to inflammatory process related to maternal androgens. It is benign, self-limited condition. Treatment of scalp with shampoo (such as Selsun blue) to soften the greasy scale followed with gentle combing with a fine-toothed comb to remove them is sufficient. It resolves by 8–12 months of age.

Spine

Look for deformities of the spine, tuft of hair or dimple at lumbosacral region, out-pouching of skin or meninges (i.e., meningocele, meningomyelocele). Pay attention to presence of sinus, lipoma, hemangioma, or abnormal curvatures of the spine.

Anthropometric Assessment (Table 4)

It includes assessment of weight, length, and head circumference.

- Weight: it should be preferably done within 24 hours of birth, in minimum clothing in an electronic digital weighing scale with a minimum scale of 5 g. Weight thus measured should be plotted on the nomogram chart. Following charts are used of this purpose: WHO charts, Fenton's charts, Ehrenkranz's charts [for very low-birth-weight (VLBW) babies]. Lubchencho's charts are obsolete now-a-days. According to the weight, baby is classified as AGA (appropriate-for-gestational age) if weight lies between 10th centiles and 90th centiles, weight more than 90th centiles is leveled as LGA (large-for-gestational

TABLE 4: Desired gain in anthropometric parameters in neonates

Parameters	Preterm	Term
Weight	15–20 g/kg/day	20–30 g/day
Length	0.7–1.0 cm/week	2 cm/month
Occipitofrontal circumference	0.7–1.0 cm/week	0.5 cm/week

age) and for weight less than 10th centiles, small-for-gestational age (SGA). Depending on the weight, neonates are termed as low-birth-weight (LBW; weight <2,500 g), VLBW, (<1,500 g) and extremely LBW (ELBW <1,000 g)

- Length: it is measured with infantometer where head end is fixed and the foot plate is adjustable. The infant should be laid supine with head fixed with hand and knees are kept straight. Indian term infants have average length of 50 cm at birth. It varies between 47 cm and 50 cm in term neonate
- Head circumference: it should be measured with the help of a nonstretchable fibrotic tape measuring the maximum circumference of head. It is 33–37 cm at birth in term neonate. Microcephaly is said to be present if occipitofrontal circumference (OFC) is more than 3SD (standard deviation) below the mean.

Gestational Age Assessment (Figure 1 and Tables 5–8)

Gestational age is assessed by physical and neurological maturity scoring of the baby. Gestational age assessment can be done from last menstrual period and USG. New Ballard scoring is done by assessing physical and neurologic maturity of the newborn.[24] Score of physical maturity signs and score of neuromuscular maturity that is assigned to a neonate after physical examination is added and gestational age is achieved as per table 7 as depicted against respective total scores.

The expanded new Ballard scoring has accuracy of 1 week. This scoring is to be done within 7 days of postnatal life.[25]

Systemic Examination

All systems must be examined thoroughly. Systemic examination includes assessment of cardiovascular, respiratory, gastrointestinal tract (GIT) and neurological systems.

Respiratory System

The respiratory system examination includes:

- Inspection: look for size, shape, symmetry, and bony abnormalities. Absence of pectoral muscles is seen in Poland syndrome. Pectus excavatum (funnel chest) and carinatum (pigeon breast) should be looked for. Watch for signs of respiratory distress
- Palpation: feel for any swelling or tenderness
- Percussion: it has limited role in respiratory system examination in neonates
- Auscultation: attention should be paid to air entry, quality of breath sounds, and adventitious sounds.

Cardiovascular System

- Inspection: one should watch for precordial activity, apical impulse, and any abnormality of precardium. Presence of cyanosis in the absence of respiratory distress is suggestive of CCHD
- Palpation: palpation of the femoral pulses should be carried out. Weak femoral pulses are seen in coarctation of aorta. Palpate for apex beat and its location and character
- Auscultation: identification of abnormal heart sounds is difficult owing to fast heart beats in neonates. Look for any heart murmur. However, heart defects are known to exist

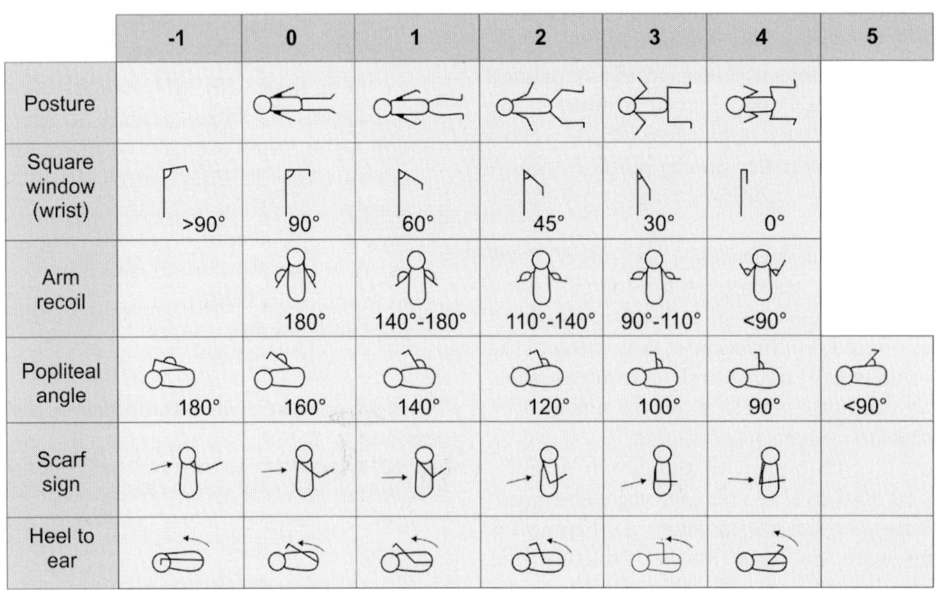

FIG. 1: Neuromuscular maturity.

TABLE 5: Assessment of neuromuscular maturity

Posture	Observe the unrestrained infant in the supine position
Square window	• Flex the wrist and measure the minimal angle between the ventral surface of the forearm and the palm
Arm recoil	• With the infant supine and the head midline, hold the forearm against the arm for 5 seconds, then fully extend and release the arm. Note the time it takes the infant to resume a flexed posture
Popliteal angle	• Flex the hips with the thighs on the abdomen. Then, without lifting the hips from the bed surface, extend the knee as far as possible until resistance is met. (One may overestimate the extent of extension if one attempts to continue extending the knee beyond the point where resistance is first met.)
Scarf sign	• Keeping the head in the midline, pull the hand across the chest to encircle the neck as a scarf and note the position of the elbow relative to the midline
Heel to ear	• With the infant supine and the pelvis kept on the examining surface, the feet are brought back as far as possible toward the head, allowing the knees to be positioned alongside the abdomen

TABLE 6: Physical maturity parameters

Physical maturity sign	Score						
	–1	0	1	2	3	4	5
Skin	Sticky, friable, transparent	Gelatinous, red, translucent	Smooth, pink, visible veins	Superficial peeling and/or rash, few veins	Cracking pale areas, rare veins	Parchment, deep cracking, no vessels	Leathery, cracked, wrinkled
Lanugo	None	Sparse	Abundant	Thinning	Bald areas	Mostly bald	
Plantar surface	Heel-toe: 40–50 mm: –1 <40 mm: –2	>50 mm; no crease	Faint-red marks	Anterior transverse crease only stippled		Creases over entire sole	
Breast	Imperceptible	Barely perceptible	Flat areola, no buds	Areola 1–2 mm bud well curved	Raised areola 3–4 mm bud formed and firm	Full areola 5–10 mm bud	
Eye/ear	Lids fused Loosely: –1 Tightly: –2	Lids open, Pinna flat	lightly-curved pinna; soft; slow recoil	pinna; soft but ready recoil	Instant recoil	Thick cartilage, ear stiff	
Genitals, male	Scrotum flat, smooth	Scrotum empty, faint rugae	Testes in upper canal, rare rugae	Testes descending, few rugae	Testes down, good rugae	Testes pendulous, deep rugae	
Genitals, female	Clitoris prominent, labia flat	Prominent clitoris, small labia minora	Prominent clitoris, enlarging minora	Majora and minora equally prominent	Majora large, minora small	Minora small, majora covers clitoris and minora	

in the absence of murmur. If heart murmur is identified, the cardiovascular system should be further evaluated by chest X-ray (CXR) and echocardiography. Murmurs if detected during diastole, loud in intensity (i.e., more than grade 3) and pan systolic in nature is usually pathological.

Abdomen

- Inspection: majority of the infants have rounded abdomen on inspection. Congenital diaphragmatic hernia should be suspected if the shape of abdomen is scaphoid. Look for position of umbilicus, abdominal wall defects, like omphaloceles and gastroschisis
- Palpation: palpation is done with clean and warm hands. The liver is usually palpable 1-2 cm below the right costal margin, and the left lobe extends across the midline. The liver is normally smooth and its edge is soft and rounded. Umbilical cord has two arteries and a vein. Spleen is not palpable. Spleen palpable more than 1 cm below costal margin is pathological. Look for any palpable mass. Palpation of kidneys due to hydronephrosis and cystic disease is the most common abdominal mass felt per abdomen in neonates. Tenderness, if present, should also be noted
- Percussion: percussion has limited role in newborn examination

- Auscultation: bowel sounds are heard during auscultation. Absent or reduced bowel sounds are indicative of hypokalemia, necrotizing enterocolitis or septic ileus.

Hernial sites and perineal area should be checked before the abdominal examination findings are concluded.

Neurological Examination

Examination of neurological system consists of assessment of higher-mental function, cranial nerves, motor system, sensory system, and neonatal reflexes. The neurological examination can be a challenging part of a newborn's full evaluation. The Dubowitz assessment is a standardized approach to the neonatal neurological examination designed for use by pediatricians in routine practice.[26]

TABLE 7: Maturity rating

Score	Gestational age
– 10	20
– 5	22
0	24
5	26
10	28
15	30
20	32
25	34
30	36
35	38
40	40
45	42
50	44

Higher-mental function

Neurological system should be examined when the baby is in state 3 or 4. There are five neurobehavioral states:

1. State 1: This is deep sleep with regular respiration
2. State 2: The baby is in rapid eye movement sleep, heart and respiratory rates may be irregular and eye ball movements are present
3. State 3: Awake, eyes are open with no gross movements
4. State 4: Awake, but gross body movements are present
5. State 5: Crying and gross movements are present, eyes may be open or closed.

Highermental functions include:

- Level of alertness, i.e., state: mention should be made of state-to-state variability, predominant state, maximum state achieved, and the state in which examination was done
- Habituation: it is assessed by putting gentle finger taps on the glabella. 3–5 taps are given and response of the baby is seen. Similarly habituation to light can be tested. In normal situation, baby habituates in 3–4 stimuli
- Consolability and cuddliness: it is assessed by patting, rocking the baby in arms and holding the baby in the crook of arm. It is willingness of the baby to be handled. Irritable and inconsolable baby usually has neurological insult
- Cry: assess volume, quality, and quantity of cry
- Orientation: response to visual or auditory stimuli is checked
- Defence reaction: a small clean and sterile paper or napkin is placed on the face of baby and she/he tries to pull it away or turns the face to other side. Preserved higher mental functions are indicative of intact cerebral cortex.

TABLE 8: Physical maturity assessment

Skin	• With maturation, the skin becomes thicker, less translucent and, eventually, dry and peeling
Lanugo	• This fine, nonpigmented hair is evenly distributed over the body and is most prominent at 27–28 weeks' gestation, then it gradually disappears, usually first from the lower back. Although present over the entire body, the lanugo over the back is used for gestational-age assessment
Plantar surface	• As with the hands, the presence of creases in the foot is a reflection of intrauterine activity as well as maturation. The absence of creases may indicate an underlying neurologic problem as well as immaturity
Breast	• The areola development is not dependent on adequacy of intrauterine nutrition. There is no difference in male or female infants
Ear cartilage	• With maturation, the ear cartilage becomes increasingly stiff and the auricle thickens. Fold the top of the ear and assess the recoil. Eyelid opening: Dr. Ballard included the degree of fusion of the lids as a new assessment tool. She defined "tightly fused" as both lids being inseparable by gentle traction, and "loosely fused" as either lid being able to be partly separated by gentle traction. Tightly fused lids were observed in 20% of infants born at 26 weeks' gestation, and only 5% of babies delivered at 27 weeks.
External genitalia, male	• Palpate for level of testicular descent and observe the degree of rugation
External genitalia, female	• The labia minora and clitoris are prominent in the immature newborn, at/with maturation, the labia majora becomes fat-filled and therefore prominent

Cranial nerve examination

- First cranial nerve is tested by seeing the response of the baby to smell of milk. Usually not tested
- Second nerve is checked by looking response to light. Visual fixation and attention should be seen by using red dangling ring held at 8–10 inches away. Red reflex is seen on fundus examination
- Third, fourth, and sixth nerves are checked by noticing the eyeball movements by gentle rocking the baby
- Fifth nerve: rooting, response to touch on face
- Seventh nerve: facial asymmetry, deviation of face on crying or sucking, ptosis
- Eighth nerve is assessed by noticing startle response, change in activity, blinking or change in heart rate in response to sound. A bell is used for this purpose and a sound stimulus of 500–1,000 cycles/sec is given. Bell is held at a distance of 30 cm from the ear
- Ninth and tenth nerves are checked by swallowing, nasal regurgitation
- Eleventh nerve: look for bulk of sternocleidomastoid after extending the neck and turning it laterally
- Twelfth nerve: tongue atrophy, deviation, and inability to make a seal while sucking.

Motor system

- Bulk: note the bulk of muscles and compare it with other side
- Movements: look for spontaneous movements. Newborns exhibit rich variety of movements. Poor movements are indicative of central nervous system (CNS) damage or neuromuscular disorder
- Tone: the tone of the muscle progresses in cephalocaudal directions.
    - Passive tone: Head should be kept in midline. It is assessed by:
        - Posture: baby is kept supine and position of arms and legs is noted
        - Popliteal angle: knees are fixed on to the abdomen and legs are extended gently with index finger behind the ankle and angle at the knee is noted. Each angle is tested separately
        - Heel to ear: with baby in supine position the foot is brought near to the head as close as it can go gently. Observe the extension of knee
        - Arm recoil: both hands are taken and arms are extended quickly parallel to the body and then released. The back movement of the arm to original position is noted
        - Scarf sign: arm of the baby is taken across the chest like a scarf while the baby is supine and head in midline. Position of the elbow in relation to midline is noted
        - Ventral flexion and dorsal extension: both the legs are hold and trunk flexed. In dorsal extension trunk is held in one hand and legs in other with the baby on its side and the trunk is extended
        - Resistance to passive movements is checked.
    - Active tone:
        - Baby is grasped by shoulder and raised to sitting position, head is allowed to fall forward and ability of the infant to extend the neck. In second phase, the head is allowed to fall backward and ability of the baby to flex the neck is noted
        - Ventral suspension: Infant is hold in ventral position and curvature of the back, flexion of the limbs and position of the head in relation to trunk is noted.

Sensory system

It is assessed by looking the response to tactile stimulation.

Reflexes (Table 9)

- Deep tendon reflexes: they are tested with appropriate-sized hammer. Knee, ankle, and biceps reflexes can be elicited in newborn
- Superficial reflexes: plantar reflex.

Primitive reflexes

Newborns have primitive reflexes. These reflexes are brainstem-mediated automatic responses. They are rooting and sucking reflex; palmer and plantar grasp; Moro's reflex; asymmetric tonic reflex; and crossed extensor response.

- Moro's reflex: it is checked by supporting the baby with arm and dropping the head by 15–30° in relation to rest of the body. The response has two components. First component is extension of the arms and opening of the hands followed by adduction of arms, may be associated with cry. The hand opening is present by 28 weeks, adduction and abduction by 32 weeks and anterior

TABLE 9: Time of appearance and disappearance of neonatal reflexes[29]

Reflex	Time of appearance	Fully mature	Age of disappearance
Palmer grasp	28 weeks of gestation	32 weeks of gestation	2–3 months
Rooting	32 weeks of gestation	36 weeks of gestation	Less prominent after 1 month
Moro's reflex	28–32 weeks of gestation	37 weeks of gestation	5–6 months
Tonic neck	35 weeks of gestation	1 month of age	6–7 months
Parachute	7–8 months of age	10–11 months of age	Remains throughout life

flexion by 37 weeks. Asymmetric Moro's is seen in Erb's palsy, fracture of the clavicle and humerus.[27] The Moro's reflex disappears by 3-6 months in normal infants. Hung up Moro's is seen in kernicterus

- Palmer grasp: it is checked by stroking the ulnar aspect of hand with finger. The baby in response holds the stroking finger tightly
- Rooting and sucking reflex: stimulation of angle of mouth or lip initiates rooting and sucking. The pulp of the finger should be upwards. Note of sucking frequency and strength be made. It persists for 3-months postnatally
- Asymmetric tonic neck reflex: when babies head is turned to one side the ipsilateral leg and arm gets extended and the contralateral limbs are flexed. The standard neurological examination of the newborn and infant includes the elicitation of the tonic neck reflex. Normally present, its persistence is suggestive of neurologic dysfunction and a prognostic marker highly suggestive of an adverse outcome.[28]

Infants with cerebral palsy have been known to manifest persistence or delay in the disappearance of primitive reflexes and pathologic or absent postural reactions.[30]

ROOMING-IN

This model of maternity care places newborns in their mothers' rooms instead of central nurseries. Termed rooming-in, this approach first appeared in Hospitals in the United States in the early 1940s.[31] Rooming-in stems from a trend to make all phases of childbearing as natural as possible and to foster mother-child relationships at an early date. By 24 hours, the mother is generally fully ambulatory. Thereafter, with rooming-in, she can usually provide routine care for herself and her newborn. An obvious advantage is her increased ability to assume full care of the infant when she arrives home.

HOSPITAL DISCHARGE

Traditionally, the newborn is discharged with its mother, and in most cases, maternal stay has determined that of the neonate. From 1970 to the mid-1990, the average maternal postpartum length of stay declined steadily, and many mothers were discharged in under 48 hours. This is not true uniformly that not every time most of the newborns can be discharged safely within 48 hours. It is only after the proper examination of the newborn.

REFERENCES

1. Singh M (Ed). Examination of the baby. In: Care of the Newborn, 6th edition. New Delhi, India: Sagar Publications; 2004. pp. 117-30.
2. Johnson L, Cochran WD. Assessment of the newborn history and physical examination of the newborn. Manual of Neonatal Care. 7th ed. Philadelphia: Lippincott Williams and Wilkins; 2012. pp. 91-110.
3. Dutta S, Kumar P (Eds). Pregnant mothers from neonatal perspective. In: The PGI NICU Handbook of Protocols, 4th edition. Chandigarh, India: The New Heart Trust; 2010. pp. 9-16.
4. Jangra B, Singh M, Rattan KN, Kadian YS, Kaur A. Congenital anomalies in paediatric surgery in North India. Afr J Paediatr Surg. 2014;11(1):39-43.
5. Wolke D, Dave S, Hayer J, Townsend J, Tomlin M. Routine examination of the newborn and maternal satisfaction: a randomized controlled trial. Arch Dis Child Fetal Neonatal Ed. 2002;86(3):F155-60.
6. World Health Organization (WHO), Maternal and Newborn Health/Safe Motherhood. (1997). Thermal Protection of the Newborn: A Practical Guide. [online] Available from www.who.int/maternal_child_adolescent/documents/ws42097th/en/. [Accessed September, 2015].
7. Dutta S, Kumar P (Eds). Normograms (N14.1); Zubrow's Charts for BP recording to GA (gestational age). The PGI NICU Handbook of Protocols, 4th edition. Chandigarh: The New Heart Trust; 2010. pp. 507-509.
8. National Institute of Health, National Heart, Lung, and Blood Institute (NHLBI). (2005). The Fourth Report on the Diagnosis, Evaluation, and Treatment of High Blood Pressure in Children and Adolescents. [online]. Available from www.nhlbi.nih.gov/files/docs/resources/heart/hbp_ped.pdf. [Accessed September, 2015].
9. Mahle WT, Newburger JW, Matherne GP, Smith FC, Hoke TR, Koppel R, et al. Role of pulse oximetry in examining newborns for congenital heart disease: a scientific statement from the AHA and AAP. Pediatrics. 2009;124(2):823-36.
10. Liske MR, Greeley CS, Law DJ, Reich JD, Morrow WR, Baldwin HS, et al. Report of the Tennessee Task Force on Screening Newborn Infants for Critical Congenital Heart Disease. Pediatrics. 2006;118(4):e1250-6.
11. Salyer JW. Neonatal and pediatric pulse oximetry. Respir Care. 2003;48(4):386-96.
12. Clayton DG, Webb RK, Ralston AC, Duthie D, Runciman WB. Pulse oximeter probes. A comparison between finger, nose, ear and forehead probes under conditions of poor perfusion. Anaesthesia. 1991;46(4):260-5.
13. Mishra PC, Baveja R. Congenital malformations in the newborn--a prospective study. Indian Pediatr. 1989;26(1):32-5.
14. Swain S, Agrawal A, Bhatia BD. Congenital malformations at birth. Indian Pediatr. 1994;31(10):1187-91.
15. Hughes IA, Houk C, Ahmed SF, Lee PA; LWPES Consensus Group; ESPE Consensus Group. Consensus statement on management of intersex disorders. Arch Dis Child. 2006;91(7):554-63.
16. Clarke NM. Diagnosing congenital dislocation of the hip. BMJ. 1992;305(6851):435-6.
17. Chang MW, Orlow SJ. Noenatal, pediatric and adolescent dermatology. In: Freedberg IM, Eisen AZ, Wolff K, Austen KF, Goldsmith LA, Katz SI (Eds). Fitzpatrick's Dermatology in Medicine, 6th edition. New York, USA: McGraw-Hill Company; 2003. pp. 1366-86.
18. Tüzün Y, Zahmacıoğlu Z. Yenidoğanda geçici deri belirtileri. In: Tüzün Y, Kotoğyan A, Serdaroğlu S, Çokuğraş H, Tüzün B, Mat MC (Eds). Pediyatrik Dermatoloji, 1st edition. İstanbul, Turkey: Nobel Kitabevi; 2005. pp. 43-52.
19. Atherton DJ, Gennery AR, Cant AJ. The Neonate. In: Burns T, Breathnach S, Cox N, Griffiths C (Eds). Rook's Textbook of Dermatology, 7th edition. Oxford, UK: Oxford Blackwell Publishers; 2004. pp. 14.1-86.
20. Mallory SB, Bree A, Chern P. Illustrated Manual of Pediatric Dermatology: Diagnosis and Management, 1st edition. Abingdon, Oxon, UK: Taylor and Francis Group; 2005. pp. 9-33.

21. Yaşar ŞP, Mansur T. [Yenidoğan dönemindeki fizyolojik deri bulguları]. Türkiye Klinikleri J Pediatr. 2005;14:184-92.
22. Serdaroğl S, Çakıl B. Physiologic skin findings of newborn. J Turk Acad Dermatol. 2008;2(4):8240.
23. O'connor NR, McLaughlin MR, Ham P. Newborn skin: part I. Common rashes. Am Fam Physician. 2008;77(1):47-52.
24. Ballard JL, Khoury JC, Wedig K, Wang L, Eilers-Walsman BL, Lipp R. New Ballard Score, expanded to include extremely premature infants. J Pediatr. 1991;119(3):417-23.
25. Aggarwal R, Paul VK, Deorari AK. Newborn Infants. In: Paul VK, Bagga A (Eds). Ghai Essential Pediatrics, 8th edition. New Delhi, India: CBS Publishers & Distributors Private Limited; 2013. pp. 124-83.
26. Wusthoff CJ. How to use: the neonatal neurological examination. Arch Dis Child Educ Pract Ed. 2013;98(4):148-53.
27. Avery GB, MacDonald MG, Seshia MK, Mullett MD (Eds). Neurological and neuromuscular disorders. In: Avery's Neonatology: Pathophysiology & Management of the Newborn, 6th edition. Philadelphia, PA, USA: Lippincott Williams & Wilkins; 2005. pp. 1384-407.
28. Shevell M. The tripartite origins of the tonic neck reflex: Gesell, Gerstmann, and Magnus. Neurology. 2009;72(9):850-3.
29. Robert M, Haslam A. Neurologic evaluation. In: Richard E, Behrmann M, Robert M, Kliegman M, Hal B, Jenson M (Eds). Nelson's Textbook of Pediatrics, 19th edition. Philadelphia, PA, USA: WB Saunders; 2011. pp. 1979-82.
30. Zafeiriou DI. Primitive reflexes and postural reactions in the neurodevelopmental examination. Pediatr Neurol. 2004;31(1):1-8.
31. Temkin E. Rooming-in: redesigning hospitals and motherhood in cold war America. Bull Hist Med. 2002;76(2):271-98.

CHAPTER 33

Neonatal Resuscitation

Ashwani Kumar K Sood, Naveen Bajaj

INTRODUCTION

Background

Neonatal resuscitation skills are essential for all health-care providers who are involved in the delivery of newborns.

The transition of fetus from intrauterine to extrauterine life is accompanied by rapid and complex physiological changes, yet in 90% of the deliveries, the birth process is usually accomplished with relative ease. Approximately 10% of newborns require some assistance to initiate spontaneous respirations at birth. More intensive resuscitation, including positive-pressure ventilation (PPV), is required by 1% of newly born infants, and extensive resuscitation requiring chest compressions and/or drug therapy is only required in 1–2 per 1,000 live births. Perinatal asphyxia and extreme prematurity are the two complications of pregnancy that most frequently necessitate complex resuscitation by skilled personnel. However, only 60% of asphyxiated newborns can be predicted antepartum. The remaining newborns are not identified until the time of birth. Additionally, approximately 80% of low-birth-weight infants require resuscitation and stabilization at delivery.

Anticipation, adequate preparation, accurate evaluation, and prompt intervention are critical for successful resuscitation of these depressed newborns.

Response to Asphyxia

A fetus newborn that is subjected to asphyxia initiates a "diving reflex" (so termed because of certain similarities to the physiology of diving seals) in an attempt to maintain perfusion and oxygen delivery to vital organs. Hypoxia and acidosis lead to pulmonary arteriolar vasoconstriction. Pulmonary vascular resistance increases, leading to decreased pulmonary blood flow and increased blood flow directly to the left atrium (Flowchart 1).

Systemic cardiac output is redistributed, with increased flow to the heart, brain, and adrenal glands and decreased flow to the rest of the body. Early in the course of asphyxia, systemic blood pressure (BP) increases. With ongoing hypoxia and acidosis, however, the myocardium fails and bradycardia occurs; this causes a decrease in BP and tissue perfusion, leading to eventual tissue ischemia and hypoxia.[1]

Infants who are undergoing asphyxia exhibit an altered respiratory pattern. Initially, they have rapid respirations. These respiratory efforts eventually cease with continued

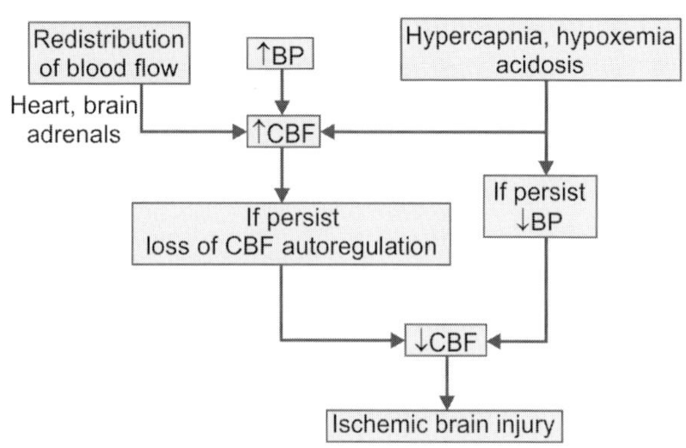

BP, blood pressure; CBF, cerebral blood flow.

FLOWCHART 1: Fetal response to asphyxia illustrating initial redistribution of blood flow to vital organs. With prolonged asphyxial insult and failure of compensatory mechanisms, cerebral blood flow falls, leading to ischemic brain injury.

asphyxia (primary apnea). During primary apnea, the infant responds to stimulation with reinstitution of breathing. However, if the asphyxia continues, the infant then begins irregular gasping efforts, which slowly decrease in frequency and eventually cease (secondary apnea).

Infants who experience secondary apnea do not respond to tactile or noxious stimulation and require PPV to restore ventilation. Primary and secondary apnea cannot be clinically distinguished. Therefore, if an infant does not readily respond to stimulation, PPV should be instituted as outlined in the Neonatal Resuscitation Program (NRP) guidelines.

If an infant is experiencing primary apnea, the stimulation of the ventilatory efforts causes the infant to resume breathing. If the infant is in secondary apnea, PPV is required for a longer period. The longer the infant undergoes asphyxia, the longer the onset of spontaneous respirations is delayed after the initiation of effective ventilation through the use of PPV.

ANTICIPATING AND PREPARATION OF RESUSCITATION

Anticipating the Need for Resuscitation

The goals of resuscitation are to assist with the initiation and maintenance of adequate ventilation and oxygenation, adequate cardiac output and tissue perfusion, and normal core temperature and serum glucose. These goals may be attained more readily when risk factors are identified early, neonatal problems are anticipated, equipment is available, personnel are qualified and available, and a care plan is formulated.

A large number of antepartum and intrapartum maternal conditions carry an increased risk for intrapartum asphyxia and a detailed review of these problems is beyond the scope of this chapter.[2,3]

Risk Factors

Often but not always the following maternal, fetal, and intrapartum circumstances help in predicting the need for resuscitation in the delivery room (Table 1).

TABLE 1: Risk factors for neonatal resuscitation

Risk factors	
Maternal	• Prolonged rupture of membranes (>18 hours) • Bleeding in 2nd or 3rd trimester • Pregnancy-induced hypertension • Chronic hypertension • Substance abuse • Drug therapy (e.g., lithium, magnesium, adrenergic-blocking agents, narcotics) • Diabetes mellitus • Chronic illness (e.g., anemia, cyanotic congenital heart disease) • Maternal pyrexia • Maternal infection • Chorioamnionitis • Heavy sedation • Previous fetal or neonatal death • No prenatal care
Fetal	• Multiple gestation (e.g., twins, triplets) • Preterm gestation (especially <35 weeks) • Post-term gestation (<41 weeks) • Large for dates • Fetal growth restriction • Alloimmune hemolytic disease (e.g., anti-D, anti-Kell, especially if fetal anemia or hydrops fetalis present) • Polyhydramnios and oligohydramnios • Reduced fetal movement before onset of labor • Congenital abnormalities which may affect breathing, cardiovascular function or other aspects of perinatal transition • Intrauterine infection • Hydrops fetalis
Intrapartum	• Nonreassuring fetal heart rate patterns on cardiotocograph • Abnormal presentation • Prolapsed cord • Prolonged labor (or prolonged second stage of labor) • Precipitate labor • Antepartum hemorrhage (e.g., abruption, placenta previa, vasa previa) • Meconium in the amniotic fluid • Narcotic administration to mother within 4 hours of birth • Forceps birth • Vacuum-assisted (ventouse) birth • Maternal general anesthesia

Trained Personal

Every delivery should be attended by at least one person dedicated for the newborn and being capable of initiating resuscitation, including administration of PPV and chest compressions. Either this person or someone else who is promptly available should have the skills required to perform a complete resuscitation, including endotracheal intubation and administration of medications. In the presence of risk factors when need for resuscitation is anticipated, additional skilled personnel should be recruited. All personnel should work as team with a defined leader and required to have efficient communication and behavioral skills (Table 2).

TABLE 2: Key behavioral skills of neonatal resuscitation team

• Know your environment • Anticipate and plan • Assume the leadership role • Communicate effectively • Delegate workload optimally	• Allocate attention wisely • Use all available information • Use all available resources • Call for help when needed • Maintain professional behavior

Thermoregulation

Preventing heat loss during resuscitation is essential. Intrauterine thermoregulation is passive, with no use of calories or oxygen by the fetus. This passive thermoregulation process allows the fetus to achieve maximal intrauterine growth without having to expend energy on thermal homeostasis. Brown fat storage begins during the 3rd trimester and it may be used for heat production in the newborn period.

Several factors lead to increased heat losses in the newborn. Neonates have a high ratio of skin surface area to body weight, which increases heat loss and evaporative fluid loss. The fluid loss from the skin (due not to sweating but to direct transdermal water loss) results in massive heat loss. The thin fetal skin, with blood vessels that are near the surface, provides poor insulation, which leads to further heat loss.

The American Heart Association (AHA) and the American Academy of Pediatrics (AAP) have stated that the goal (of the first temperature) should be an axillary temperature of 36.5°C. The aim is to achieve normothermia and avoid hyperthermia, which is associated with progressive cerebral injury.

Equipment

Resuscitation should be performed under aseptic conditions, which includes sterile equipments and asepsis measures by the resuscitation team. All the equipment necessary for resuscitation must be in the delivery room and operational. Equipments should be checked before delivery in the same order as they are used in resuscitation flow diagram. Neonatal resuscitation program preresuscitation equipment checklist is provided in Table 3.

Assessment Before Birth

Ask the following questions:
- Gestational age
- Amniotic fluid clear or not
- Singleton or multiple pregnancies
- Any other obstetrical or medical risk factors.

TABLE 3: Neonatal Resuscitation Program preresuscitation equipment checklist

Warm	• Preheated radiant warmer or other heat source with firm padded resuscitation surface • Sterile towels/sheets/blankets
Clear airway	• Suction catheters sizes: 5-F, 6-F, 10-F, 12-F, and 14-F • Suction apparatus: Wall/foot operated suction set at 80–100 mm Hg, Dee Lee mucus trap • Meconium aspirator
Auscultate	• Stethoscope
Oxygenate	• Gas flow 5–10 L/min • Oxygen source and methods to administer free-flow oxygen: tubing, mask, flow-inflating bag or T-piece • Compressed air source and blender, if available • Pulse oximeter and neonatal probe, if available
Ventilate	• Positive-pressure ventilation (PPV) device (bag and mask equipment): Self-inflating bag, flow-inflating bag, T-piece with facemask for term and preterm babies • Manometer if available • 8-F feeding tube and 20 mL syringe
Intubate	• Laryngoscope with straight blades of No. 0 (preterm) and No. 1 (term) • Endotracheal tube (ETT) sizes: 2.5 mm, 3.0 mm, 3.5 mm, and 4.0 mm • Stylets (optional) • Tapes for ETT fixation
Medicate	• Epinephrine 1: 10,000: In India, it is available in 1: 1,000 concentrations. Dilute 1 mL of 1: 1,000 with 9 mL of normal saline to get 10 mL of 1: 10,000 epinephrine solution • Normal saline 100 mL, 250 mL, and 500 mL • Ringer's lactate • Dextrose 10% • Syringes 2 mL, 5 mL, 10 mL, 20 mL, and 50 mL • Needle 23-G, 24-G
Umbilical vessel catheterization	• Gloves, scissor, blade • Antiseptic solution: chlorhexidine, spirit solution • Umbilical catheters 3.5-F, 5-F, and 6-F • Three-way stopcock • Umbilical tape, Tegaderm
Thermoregulate	• Food-grade plastic bag or plastic wrap • Warming pad, if available
Miscellaneous	• Gloves appropriate sizes • Gown, mask • Clock with seconds hand

Resuscitation Steps (Flowchart 2)

Assessment of Need for Resuscitation[4]

The need for resuscitation is determined on the basis of only one question:
"Breathing or crying"

If answer to the above question is "yes", then provide routine care:

- Provide warmth
- Clear airway, if necessary
- Dry and stimulate
- Ongoing evaluation of breathing, activity, and color while the baby stays with the mother.

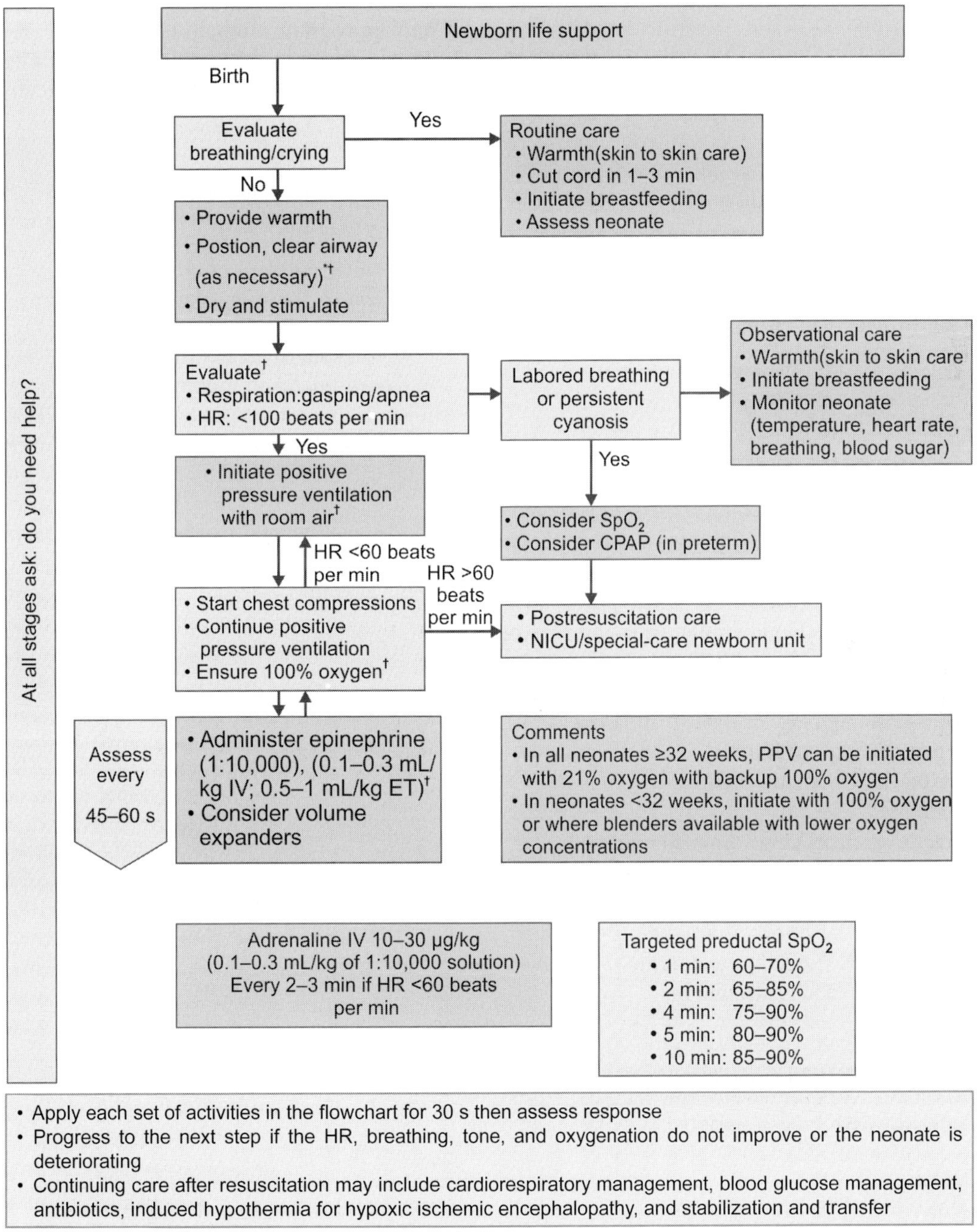

SpO_2, arterial oxygen saturation; HR, heart rate; IV, intravenous; PPV, positive-pressure ventilation; CPAP, continuous positive airway pressure; NICU, neonatal intensive care unit; ETT, endotracheal tube.

*In meconium-stained depressed neonates after oral suction, endotracheal suction may be considered.

†Endotracheal intubation may be considered at several steps.

FLOWCHART 2: Indian Academy of Pediatrics National Neonatology Forum resuscitation algorithm.

If answer to the above questions is "no", baby needs one or more of the four categories of action in sequence:
1. Initial steps
2. Ventilation
3. Chest compressions
4. Medications.

Approximately 60 seconds are allotted for completing the initial steps, re-evaluating, and beginning ventilation, if required and termed as "The Golden Minute". The progression to next resuscitation step following initial steps is by simultaneous assessment of two vital signs:
1. Respiration
2. Heart rate (HR).

If available, assess the level of oxygenation also by pulse oximeter. The auscultation of the heart over the precordium is the preferred technique to evaluate the HR. When pulse is detectable, palpation of umbilical pulse provides rapid estimate of HR and is more reliable than palpation at other sites. Progression to next step occurs only after successful completion of the preceding step.

Use of Pulse Oximeter

Cyanosis is not a reliable sign of assessment of oxygenation or efficacy of the resuscitation as the color of the skin is a poor indicator of oxygen saturation (SpO_2) during the immediate neonatal period. Hence, whenever feasible, pulse oximeter should be used to assess the oxygenation. The percentage of inspired oxygen concentration is titrated so as to achieve the target SpO_2 values as mentioned in Box 1 if hypoxemia persists.

If available, use pulse oximetry for both term and preterm in:
- Anticipated need for resuscitation
- Need for PPV for more than few breaths
- Persistent cyanosis
- Supplementary oxygen is being administered.

Apply neonatal probe to right hand or wrist (measure pre-ductal saturations) of the baby before connecting it to machine, reliable reading can be obtained within 1-2 minute. Pulse oximeter with signal extraction technique (SET) gives quicker reading, is preferred in resuscitation:

Box 1: Acceptable preductal oxygen saturation (SpO_2)
- Acceptable preductal SpO_2 ranges (same for both term and preterm):
  - 1 min: 60–65%
  - 2 min: 65–70%
  - 3 min: 75–80%
  - 5 min: 80–85%
  - 10 min: 85–90%.

Initial Steps

- Provide warmth
- Dry: The baby should be immediately dried with dry, pre-warmed towels
- Position on the back with neck slightly extended using shoulder roll, clear airway if necessary
- Stimulate: Gentle rubbing or slapping the soles and, or rubbing the back, trunk, and the extremities are the safe and appropriate methods to provide tactile stimulation
- No routine suction. Suction is recommended only if, there is obvious obstruction to spontaneous breathing or need for PPV.

Positive-pressure Ventilation (Table 4)

Indication (any 1 out of 3)

- Apnea or gasping respiration or
- Heart rate is less than 100 beats/minute or
- Has persistent central cyanosis or SpO_2 below target values despite 100% free-flow oxygen (if facilities exist).

Use manometer to monitor inflation pressure wherever feasible. Positive end-expiratory pressure (PEEP) is beneficial for initial stabilization of apneic preterm infants requiring PPV and can be delivered by T-piece or flow-inflating bags.

Initial oxygen concentration for resuscitation with PPV: oxygen blender is required to titrate an oxygen concentration between 21% and 100%. If available, it is desirable to use oxygen blender during resuscitation of all babies, especially preterm babies (Table 3):

TABLE 4: Positive-pressure ventilation (PPV) strategies

Aspect	Consideration
Indications	• After stimulation commence positive-pressure ventilation (PPV) if: ○ The newborn remains apneic and ○ Newborn's heart rate (HR) is <100 beats/min even with breathing and/or ○ Breathing is inadequate, gasping is not adequate breathing or ○ Has persistent central cyanosis or low oxygen saturation (SpO_2), despite free-flow oxygen increased to 100%.
Technique	• Ensuring the jaw is supported; keep the neck slightly extended in the "sniffing position" with the use of shoulder roll
Rate	• 40–60 breaths/min
Pressures	• For most newborns, ventilation can be accomplished with progressively lower pressures and rates as resuscitation proceeds

Continued

Continued

Aspect	Consideration
Assessment of effectiveness	• Ventilation effectiveness is confirmed by observing: ○ Slight rise of chest and upper abdomen with each inflation ○ HR increasing to >100 beats/min ○ Improving oxygenation (preferably assessed using pulse oximetry) • Reassess technique if: ○ Chest and abdomen do not rise with each inflation ○ HR does not rise >100 beats/min ○ Oxygenation does not improve. • Consider tracheal intubation if facemask ventilation remains ineffective despite corrective intervention
Positive end expiratory pressure (PEEP) during resuscitation	• If suitable equipment is available, PEEP (at least 5 cm H_2O) should be used during resuscitation to: ○ Assist lung expansion ○ Help establish a functional residual capacity ○ Improve oxygenation
Continuous positive airway pressure (CPAP)	• A trial of CPAP is reasonable for: ○ Spontaneously breathing newborns who have labored breathing/respiratory distress ○ Newborns who are breathing, but whose saturations are not meeting targets.

- Term infants and preterm more than or equal to 32 weeks: The standard recommendation is to begin with room air rather than 100% O_2. If despite effective ventilation there is no rise in HR or if oxygenation as being monitored by pulse oximetry remains below target value, use increased oxygen concentration of up to 100%
- Preterm less than 32 weeks: If blender is available, begin with O_2 concentration of 30% or 90% and then titrate it up or down to achieve target SpO_2. In case, blender is not available, initiate with 100% oxygen.

Ensure adequate ventilation before initiating chest compressions. Remember pneumonic: "MR SOPA" (Box 2).

Reassessment of heart rate: heart rate is assessed after 30 seconds of effective PPV.

Continuous positive airway pressure during resuscitation (CPAP): in preterms, CPAP is beneficial if the newborn is breathing spontaneously with HR more than 100 beats/min, but has labored respirations, persistent cyanosis or a low SpO_2. Spontaneously breathing preterm infants who have respiratory distress may be supported with CPAP or intubation and mechanical ventilation as guided by local expertise. No evidence to support or refute the use of CPAP in the term baby.

Box 2: Ventilation corrective steps

- M: Reapply mask
- R: Reposition airway
- S: Suction mouth and nose
- O: Open mouth
- P: Pressure increase
- A: Airway alternative.

Chest Compression

Indications: heart rate less than 60 beats/min despite 30 seconds of effective PPV.

Chest compression to ventilation ratio: chest compression to ventilation ratio is 3: 1. If arrest is due to a clear cardiac etiology, especially in babies who are beyond immediate newborn period, higher ratio (e.g., 15: 2) may be used.

Technique: thumb technique is preferred over the two-finger technique:

- Site for chest compression: Lower one-third of sternum
- Depth of chest compression: One-third of anteroposterior diameter of chest.

Reassessment of heart rate: heart rate is assessed after 45-60 seconds of well-coordinated chest compressions and ventilation as return of coronary perfusion pressure and spontaneous circulation may take 45 seconds or longer.

Drugs and Fluids

Drugs and fluids are rarely indicated for resuscitation of newborns. Bradycardia is usually caused by hypoxia and inadequate ventilation and apnea by insufficient oxygenation of the brainstem. Establishing adequate ventilation is the most important step to improve HR. Administration of drugs should not detract from the efficiency and continuity of ventilation and chest compressions.

Epinephrine

Indication: heart rate less than 60 beats/minute after at least another 45-60 seconds of coordinated chest compressions and effective ventilation.

Dose: 0.1-0.3 mL/kg of 1: 10,000 intravenous (IV) as a rapid bolus followed by 0.5-1.0 mL of normal saline flush to make sure that the drug reaches in the blood. If HR does not rise more than 60 beats/minute after first dose, the same dose can be repeated every 3-5 minute.

Volume expansion: consider when blood loss is suspected and baby appears to be in shock and is not responding to resuscitation. The preferred solution is normal saline in a dose of 10 mL/kg over 5–10 minute through umbilical vein. Ringer's lactate or O-negative blood can also be used.

Naloxone: the focus is on effective ventilation and administration of naloxone is not necessary as long as the baby can be adequately ventilated. It may be considered in a baby with continued respiratory depression when there is a history of maternal narcotic administration within the preceding 4 hours.

Administration routes: preferred vascular access is via the umbilical vein. Alternative access is via an endotracheal tube (ETT), peripheral vein, or intraosseous lines (Table 5).

Endotracheal Intubation

Indications

- Tracheal suctioning of nonvigorous meconium-stained amniotic fluid (MSAF) babies
- Ineffective or prolonged bag-mask ventilation
- When chest compressions are performed
- special circumstances, such as congenital diaphragmatic hernia or extremely low-birth-weight (ELBW; <1,000 g) babies

Choose the appropriate-sized endotracheal tube (ETT) (Table 6). The intubation procedure should be completed within 30 seconds. In case of delay, reoxygenate the baby with bag and mask ventilation and attempt again.

TABLE 5: Drug administration routes during resuscitation

Route	Considerations
Umbilical vein	• The umbilical vein is the most rapidly accessible intravascular route for adrenaline and an umbilical venous catheter (UVC) can also be used for fluid administration • A three-way tap should be attached to the UVC and both primed with normal saline before use • A UVC can provide continued vascular access until an alternative route is establishe • Blood gases from the UVC may be useful in guiding treatment
Endotracheal tube (ETT)	• Give only adrenaline via the ETT • ETT administration of adrenaline is acceptable when the heart rate is <60 beats/min despite adequate ventilation and chest compressions and when there is no intravenous (IV) access • Administration of ETT adrenaline should not delay attempts to obtain vascular access for administration of IV adrenaline
Peripheral vein	• Access can be difficult • Access may take too long
Intraosseous lines	• Not commonly used in newborns • Can be used if umbilical or venous access is not available • Consider if the resuscitator has greater experience with inserting intraosseous lines

TABLE 6: Endotracheal tube sizes

Weight (g)	Gestational age (weeks)	Tube size (internal diameter in mm)	ETT measurement at lip (cm)
<1,000	<28	2.5	7
1,000–2,000	28–34	3.0	8
2,000–3,000	34–38	3.5	9
>3,000	>38	3.5–4.0	10

ETT, endotracheal tube

Special Circumstances

Thermoregulation in Preterm Babies

- Delivery room temperatures should be at least 26°C.
- Preterms less than or equal to 28-weeks gestation should be completely covered in a polythene wrap or bag up to their necks without drying immediately after birth and then placed under a radiant heater.

Neonates Born Through Meconium-stained Amniotic Fluid (Flowcharts 2 and 3):

- Vigorous baby:
  - No intrapartum suction
  - Use large bore suction catheter (12–14 F) to clear secretions and meconium from the mouth and nose as needed. The baby stays with his mother and receives routine care and ongoing evaluation.
- Nonvigorous baby:
  - Endotracheal suctioning

It is important to record and document for the meticulous and stepwise action initiated during resuscitation (Box 3).

Postresuscitation management

Levels of Care

- Routine care: Babies who are breathing spontaneously or crying at birth qualify for routine care. Components are:
  - Provide warmth, skin-to-skin contact
  - Cut the cord within 1–3 minute
  - Initiate breast-feeding
  - Assessment of breathing, HR, activity, and color while the baby stays with the mother.
- Observational care:
  - Babies requiring initial steps and brief PPV of less than 1 minute are monitored frequently
  - Assess temperature, breathing, HR, color, and SpO_2 by pulse oximetry (if possible) for at least 2 hours,

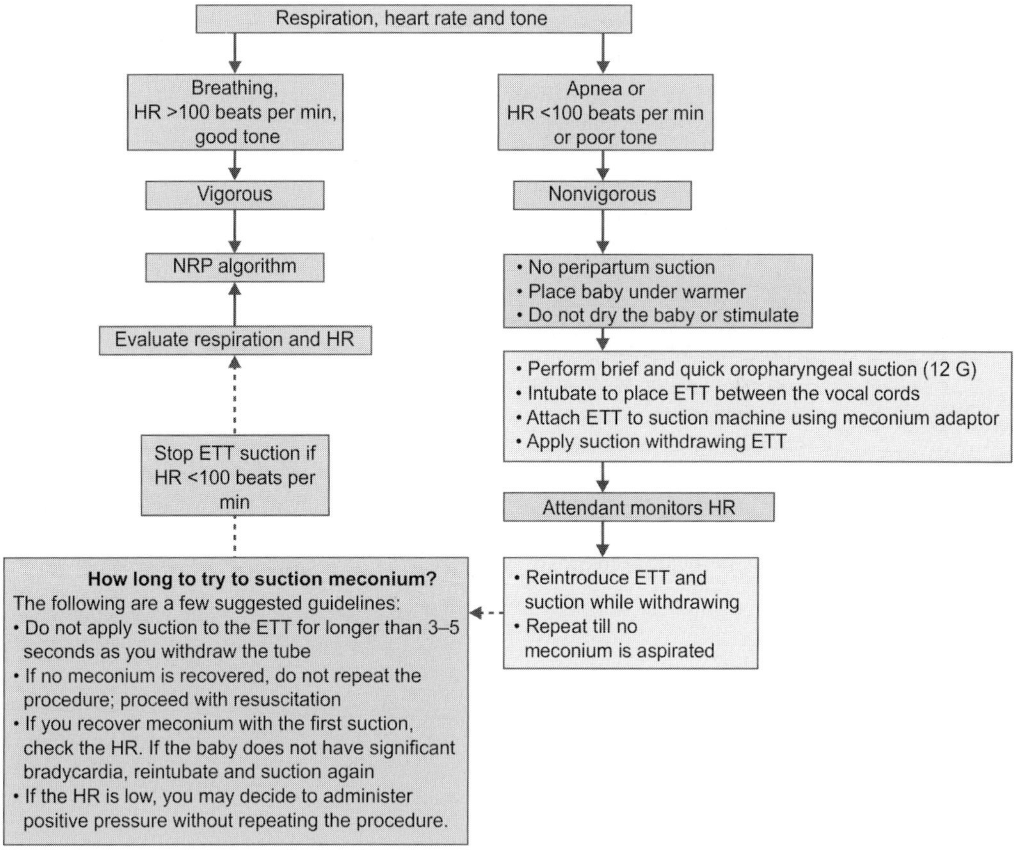

HR, heart rate; ETT, endotracheal tube; NRP, Neonatal Resuscitation Program.

FLOWCHART 3: Algorithm for meconium-stained liquor.

Box 3: Documentation

- Comprehensive and contemporaneous
- When possible, one person should be appointed to document, the time, interventions, and newborn's response during resuscitation
- Use of a standardized neonatal resuscitation record is recommended

then accordingly shift the baby to routine care or postresuscitation care

- Postresuscitation care: babies requiring prolonged resuscitation or having labored breathing, cyanosis and/or low SpO_2 requiring CPAP in the delivery room should be shifted to nursery/neonatal intensive care unit (NICU) for further evaluation and monitoring.

Glucose

Intravenous glucose infusion should be considered as soon as feasible after resuscitation, with the goal of avoiding hypoglycemia.

Therapeutic Hypothermia

If the expertise and facilities exist for providing therapeutic hypothermia, it should be considered in infants more than or equal to 36 weeks gestation with evolving moderate-to-severe hypoxic-ischemic encephalopathy and should be used but only after taking appropriate informed consent from parents as per protocols used for research interventions.

TIMING OF CORD CLAMPING

Delayed cord clamping for 1 minute or more is safe in both term and preterm babies not requiring resuscitation at birth. In preterm babies, it aids in maintaining adequacy of circulation during the first day of life and also reduces the need for blood transfusions.

Guidelines for Withholding and Discontinuation of Resuscitation

The decision of when not to resuscitate, or how long to resuscitate, is complex. Such decisions are best made considering local neonatal data and ethical issues, including

TABLE 7: Ethical issues

Issue	Consideration
Initiating resuscitation	• Where unexpected anomalies are present, offer full resuscitation, ongoing care can be discussed with parent(s) after assessment of the neonate's condition. Examples of exceptions include neonates with: ○ Anencephaly ○ Extreme prematurity for whom there is very little possibility of intact survival
Discontinuing resuscitation	• Consider discontinuing resuscitation, if the heart rate (HR) is undetectable and remains so for 10 min in a new-born baby • The decision to continue resuscitation beyond 10 min when there is no or very low HR may be influenced by: ○ Presumed diagnosis ○ Gestation of neonate ○ Presence or absence of complications ○ Parent(s) previously expressed views regarding acceptable risk of morbidity • When withdrawing or withholding resuscitation, care should be focused on the neonate's comfort and dignity • Autopsy may be appropriate after failed resuscitation (refer to guideline)

the rights of the newborn and the parents. Ideally, healthcare team and family should sit and discuss together to make the best possible decision.[5]

Major Criteria to Withhold Resuscitation

- Gestational age less than 23 weeks
- Birth weight less than 400 g
- Major chromosomal anomalies (e.g., trisomy 13)
- Anencephaly.

Discontinuation

If no detectable HR after 10 min of complete and adequate resuscitation, decision to continue resuscitation beyond 10 min with no HR should be an informed decision and never be taken in haste. In case of dilemma, continue with the process of resuscitation.

Ethical Issues

The birth of extremely premature neonates and those with severe congenital anomalies raise questions with parent(s) and among clinicians about initiation of resuscitation (Table 7).

REFERENCES

1. Kattwinkel J, Perlman JM, Aziz K, Colby C, Fairchild K, Gallagher J, et al. Neonatal resuscitation: 2010 American Heart Association Guidelines for Cardiopulmonary Resuscitation and Emergency Cardiovascular Care. Pediatrics. 2010;126(5):e1400-13.
2. Perlman JM, Wyllie J, Kattwinkel J, Atkins DL, Chameides L, Goldsmith JP, et al. Part 11: Neonatal resuscitation: 2010 International Consensus on Cardiopulmonary Resuscitation and Emergency Cardiovascular Care Science with Treatment Recommendations. Circulation. 2010;122(Suppl 2):S516-38.
3. American Academy of Pediatrics, American Heart Association; Kattwinkel J (Eds). (2011). NRP Neonatal Resuscitation Textbook, 6th edition. [Online]. Available from ebooks.aappublications.org/content/nrp-neonatal-resuscitation-textbook-6th-edition-english-version. [Accessed October, 2015].
4. World Health Organization (WHO). (2012). Guidelines on Basic Newborn Resuscitation 2012. [Online]. Available from apps.who.int/iris/bitstream/10665/75157/1/9789241503693_eng.pdf. [Accessed October, 2015].
5. New Zealand and Australian Resuscitation Councils. (2014). Standards for Resuscitation: Clinical Practice and Education. A Resource for Healthcare. Neonatal Guidelines 2010. [Online]. Available from www.nzrc.org.nz/assets/Uploads/Guidelines/Standards-for-Resuscitation-Clinical-Practice-and-Education.pdf. [Accessed October, 2015].

CHAPTER 34

Diseases of Fetus and Newborn

Ram K Kaushal

INTRODUCTION

About 27 million babies are born annually in India and about 1.2 million of them die during neonatal period, accounting for two-third of infant mortality and half of under-five mortality. In order to contain this early loss of precious lives, the essential newborn care should be made available at all healthcare levels.[1]

DEFINITIONS

Some of the commonly used definitions in relation to newborn are given below.[1]

Neonate/newborn: infant up to first 28 days of life is called newborn or neonate.

Newly born: newborn baby up to few hours of birth.

Term or full term baby: baby born at gestational age of 37–41 + 6/7 weeks (259–293 days).

Preterm (premature): baby born at less than 37 weeks (<259 days) of gestation.

Postterm (postmature): baby born at or more than 42 weeks (294 days) of gestation.

Late preterm: infant born between 34 and 36 + 6/7 weeks of gestation, (i.e., 239–259 days).

Early term: infant born between 37 and 38 + 6/7 weeks (259–272 days) of gestation.

Low birth weight (LBW) babies: babies with a birth weight of less than 2,500 g (≤2,499 g) irrespective of period of gestation.

Birth weight: it is the first weight of a live or still born baby recorded without clothes preferably soon after birth or latest by 24 hours of birth.

Very low birth weight (VLBW) babies: infants with a birth weight of less than 1,500 g (≤1,499 g) irrespective of period of gestation.

Extremely low birth weight (ELBW) babies: infant with a birth weight of less than 1,000 g (≤999 g) irrespective of period of gestation.

Appropriate for gestational age or date: neonates with birth weight between 10th and 90th percentile for their period of gestation on the intrauterine growth chart.

Small for gestational age or date: babies with a birth weight of less than 10th percentile for their period of gestation on the intrauterine growth chart. This is also referred to as intrauterine growth retardation (IUGR).

Large for gestational age or dates: babies with a birth weight of more than 90th percentile for their period of gestation on the intrauterine growth charts.

Perinatal period: it is defined as period extending from 28 weeks of gestation to 7th day of life.

Neonatal mortality rate: it is defined as number of neonatal deaths (up to 28 days of life) per 1,000 live births.

Perinatal mortality rate (PMR): it is defined as late fetal plus early neonatal (up to 7 days of life) deaths per 1,000 total births.

$$\text{PMR} = \text{Number of still births after 28 weeks of gestation} + \frac{\text{Deaths during first week of life in a year}}{\text{Total number of births (still + alive) in year}} \times 1{,}000$$

Still or live birth:
- Birth weight ≥1,000 g or
- Gestation ≥28 weeks or
- Birth length ≥35 cm.

ESSENTIAL POSTNATAL CARE OF NORMAL NEWBORN

Baby should be given a thorough physical examination in the postnatal ward to ascertain the adaptation of the baby to the extrauterine environment by recording the baseline anthropometry, vitals, gestation, and search for any injury or congenital anomalies. Mother is advised about prevention of hypothermia, infection, and initiation of breastfeeding. She is also explained about certain danger symptoms or signs which warrant immediate attention of the doctor.

Prevention of Hypothermia

The baby and mother should be kept on the same bed (bedding-in). It not only prevents hypothermia, but also promotes emotional bonding of baby and mother, initiation, and establishment of breastfeeding. Baby needs proper clothes; a vest, full sleeve shirt or frock, a cap, and socks are required even in summer months. In winter, two- to three additional layers of woolen clothes are necessary. Baby should be wrapped in double layer of cotton sheets in summer and woolen blanket in winter. Clothes of natural fabric are preferred. The room should be kept warm. Warm and pink extremities indicate baby's thermal comfort. Baby bath should be delayed until 2nd or 3rd day after birth when the temperature has stabilized. Wet napkins should be changed promptly.

Breastfeeding

The preparation and motivation for breastfeeding should begin in the antenatal period. The breast milk is species and baby specific and it is most suitable to meet the physiological, biochemical, immunological, and emotional needs of the baby. Baby should be put to the breast within 0.5–1 hour of birth in normal delivery and usually within 4 hours after cesarean section. Mother can feed the baby in any position which is comfortable to both but ensure proper attachment of the baby to the breast. Appropriate attachment is characterized by baby's chin touching the breast, wide open mouth, most of the areola inside the mouth with more of it visible above than below the mouth, and lower lip turned outwards with rounded cheeks. Prelacteal feeds should be discouraged as it can introduce infection and also delays establishment of breast-feeding. Colostrum, a concentrated form of breast milk secreted in the first 2–3 days, which though small in quantity but is adequate for the needs of the baby. It is extremely rich in immunoglobulins. Apart from meeting the nutritional needs of the baby it also serves as the first vaccine. Baby should be fed every 2–3 hours on a semi-demand schedule but ensure at least 8 feeds in 24 hours. The act of sucking will stimulate prolactin and oxytocin reflexes which regulate adequate secretion and availability of milk as per the nutritional needs of the baby. The baby should be allowed to empty one breast completely before putting on to the other and offer alternate breast at each feed so that the baby gets fore as well as hind milk. To prevent regurgitation due to swallowed air, baby should be burped at the end of each feed by holding the baby upright against the shoulder. Baby should be exclusively breastfed up to 6 months of age. The baby does not need water even during summer months.

Care of the Umbilical Stump

The umbilical stump should be inspected for any bleeding which may occur due to accidental slipping of ligature, disposable clamp, or band. The stump should be kept dry. Avoid application of ghee, turmeric, cow dung, etc. on the stump. Also avoid dip bath till the cord is shed, which takes about 7–10 days. Observe for any induration or discharge.

Care of the Skin and Eyes

While giving bath, special care should be observed to clean scalp, skin creases around neck, axillae, groins, and diaper area. Massage with any vegetable oil before bath is relaxing, improves circulation, and tone of the muscles. Mustard oil should be avoided as it is an irritant to the delicate skin of the baby. Some oil or moisturizer should also be applied to the skin after the bath to prevent dryness.

Eyes need no special care, may just be cleaned with normal saline or boiled water. No *kajal/surma* should be applied which may cause infection or other harmful effects like lead poisoning. Observe for any watering, stickiness, or discharge.

Prevention of Infection

Handwashing before handling the baby and after diaper change is most effective intervention in prevention of infection. Barrier nursing should be observed even at home.

Prevention of Vitamin K Deficiency Bleeding

Newborn baby is prone to bleeding due to vitamin K deficiency (VKD) in the 1st week of life. It is attributed to poor transfer of vitamin K across placenta, breast milk being poor source of vitamin K and lack of development of gut flora (source of vitamin K) in the first few days after birth. Hence to prevent vitamin K deficiency bleeding (VKDB), all babies delivered in the institutions are routinely administered vitamin K, 0.5 and 1 mg in babies with birth weight of less than 1,500 g and more than 1,500 g, respectively.

TABLE 1: National immunization schedule[1]

Age	Vaccine
Birth to 48 h	Hepatitis B_1
0–7 days	Bacillus Calmette-Guérin and zero-dose OPV
6 weeks	Hepatitis B_2, DPT_1, OPV_1
10 weeks	DPT_2, OPV_2
14 weeks	DPT_3, OPV_3
6 months	Hepatitis B_3
9 months	Measles
18 months	DPT, OPV (booster 1)
4–5 years	DPT, OPV (booster 2)
10 years and 16 years	Tetanus toxoid

OPV, oral polio vaccine; DPT, diphtheria-pertussis-tetanus.

Immunization

To prevent vertical transmission of hepatitis B, vaccination with hepatitis B vaccine should be given as early as possible, preferably within 48 hours of birth. Bacillus Calmette-Guérin and zero dose of oral polio vaccine (OPV) should be administered before discharge. The mother is advised to get the baby vaccinated subsequently as per the National Immunization Schedule (Table 1) from the nearest health facility.

Early Identification of Disease

While in the hospital and after discharge, the baby should be observed for certain symptoms/signs which are indicators of possible serious problem and need immediate attention of the doctor, these are labeled as danger signs.

Danger signs

Appearance of jaundice within 24 hours of birth, passing yellow urine or whitish stools, failure to pass meconium within 24 hours and urine within 48 hours of birth, excessive lethargy or crying, poor feeding, drooling of saliva or choking during feeds, persistent vomiting, diarrhea, abdominal distension, respiratory difficulty, cyanosis, sudden rise or fall of temperature, bleeding from any site, seizures, umbilical sepsis, and conjunctivitis.

Discharge and Follow up

There are no uniform discharge criteria, but it is important to ensure that both mother and baby are well, baby is taking breastfeeds, maintaining vitals, and has passed urine and stool. Mother is advised regarding exclusive breastfeeding till 6 months, prevention of hypothermia and infection, immunization, early recognition, and reporting of danger signs at the nearest health facility. Importance of monitoring growth and development once a month till 6 months and 2–3 monthly thereafter should be emphasized.

DEVELOPMENTAL PECULIARITIES AND MINOR PHYSICAL PROBLEMS OF NORMAL NEONATES

There are many minor physical and normal developmental peculiarities pertaining to this age, which are of no serious consequences but could be cause of significant worry in the mother.[1]

Bladder and Bowel Movement

Almost all babies void urine within 48 hours of birth and frequency varies from 6 times to even 20 times per day. Some babies may cry before passing urine (unpleasant sensation of full bladder) and even after the act due to wet napkin. However, crying during act of micturition may be an indication to look for urinary tract infection. All healthy newborns pass meconium within 24 hours of birth. After having passed black, tarry meconium on first 2 days, stool becomes greenish-yellow for the next 2–3 days with a frequency of 4–8 stools per day (transitional stools). It is then followed by soft-to-little loose golden-yellow, 4–8 stools per day or even passage of small amount of stool after each breastfeed due to prominent gastrocolic reflex. On the contrary, some babies may pass a soft stool once in 4–6 days. If the baby is comfortable, has no dehydration or abdominal distension, feeds well, and gains weight, mother simply needs to be reassured.

Vomiting or Regurgitation of Feeds

All babies swallow some air (aerophagy) during the act of feeding, and as the air is expelled, many of them regurgitate small amount of curdy milk after the feed. It is nonprojectile, baby sleeps well after the feed, and continues to gain adequate weight. It responds well to burping after each feed. Hiccup after the feed is another normal phenomenon and a cause of worry for some mothers. It simply indicates that baby has taken enough milk to distend the stomach which irritates the diaphragm. Persistent or projectile vomiting, abdominal distension, or failure to thrive needs evaluation.

Weight Loss

All babies usually lose 5–7% of their birth weight during the first 2–3 days of life; then remains stable for the next 2–3 days and regain the birth weight by 7–10 days. Subsequently, the average daily weight gain is around 30 g, 20 g, 15 g, and 12 g in the 1st, 2nd, 3rd, and 4th 3-month period, respectively, in the first year of life. There is no need to monitor early weight changes in healthy newborns to avoid unnecessary maternal anxiety.

Physiological Jaundice

About 70–80% of normal newborns develop jaundice on 2nd or 3rd day of life mainly due to relatively large red blood cell (RBC) mass, lower lifespan of fetal RBCs, relative immaturity of hepatic bilirubin conjugation mechanism, and increased enterohepatic circulation of deconjugated bilirubin from the poorly colonized gut in the first few days of life. It peaks around 5th day and disappears by 7–10 days. Deep yellow staining of skin, staining of palms and soles, appearance of jaundice within 24 hours of birth and persistence beyond 7–10 days in term babies, and passage of whitish stool or yellow urine in a sick baby warrants further evaluation for pathological jaundice.

Effects of Maternal Hormones

Due to transplacental transfer of maternal progesterone and estrogens, term babies of either sex may develop non-inflammatory breast enlargement in the 1st week of life. This self-limiting hypertrophy may last for few days to weeks. Any massage, fomentation, or squeezing milk may lead to complications.

Baby girls may develop grayish-white, slimy, mucoid, nonpurulent, nonfoul smelling vaginal discharge due to these maternal sex hormones. Some may develop menstruation-like withdrawal vaginal bleeding, which is mild and may last for 2–4 days. Apart from local hygiene, no other intervention is needed. Maternal androgens may cause typical acne-like lesions over the forehead, nose, and cheeks (acne neonatorum). Being self-limiting, it needs no treatment.

Skin Changes

Erythema toxicum is a self-limiting, idiopathic erythematous rash with central pallor. It spreads in cephalocaudal direction and disappears spontaneously within 2–3 days after appearance. Harlequin color change is an episodic transient sharply demarcated erythema of the dependent half of body in lateral decubitus position. It indicates some unexplained, harmless vasomotor phenomenon. Milia are yellowish-white self-limiting spots on the nose due to retained sebum, seen in most of the newborns. Discrete pinkish gray, sparse capillary hemangioma are frequently seen over nape of neck, upper eyelids, forehead, and root of the nose. They blanch on pressure and become prominent on crying. They tend to disappear in few weeks to months. Mongolian spots are irregular blue patches of skin pigmentation often seen over the sacral and buttock region. They usually disappear by late infancy. Sacral dimple in midline over sacrococcygeal area should not be confused with pilonidal sinus.[1,2]

Prominent xiphisternum: prominent xiphisternal cartilage in some babies is of no consequence.

Umbilical Hernia

Umbilical hernia may manifest after the umbilical stump has been shed. If there are no associated signs or symptoms suggestive of some systemic disease like hypothyroidism, it should be left alone as it usually disappears by 6 months to 1 year of age. Surgical closure is indicated if it is greater than 2.5 cm in size.

Umbilical Granuloma

It is seen as a small flesh-like a raspberry at the base of umbilicus with persistent discharge. It responds well to application of common salt crystals till the base is dry. Topical antibiotic application is indicated if there is local sepsis.

Cradle Cap

Seborrheic crusting over the scalp is known as cradle cap. It responds to repeated overnight application of coconut oil over the scalp followed by scalp wash with cetrimide or cetavlon shampoo.

Caput Succedaneum

It is a boggy, diffuse, edematous swelling of scalp over the presenting part in vertex deliveries. It is present at birth and its size is related to the duration of labor. It is pitting, nonfluctuant, and not limited by the suture lines (unlike cephalohematoma). It disappears over the next 2–3 days.

Nonretractable Prepuce

The prepuce is attached to the glans and not retractable in the newborn. It becomes retractable in about 40% of children by 1 year, 90% by 4 years, and 99% by 15 years of age. Urethral opening is small and there is some ballooning of foreskin during micturition. If the urinary stream is good, forceful, and uninterrupted, it should be left alone.

Epstein Pearls

These are whitish spots on either side of median raphe of hard palate, which are possibly epithelial inclusion cysts and of no consequence.

Sucking Callosity

This is a button-like cornified plaque over the center of upper lip as a result of sucking the breast. It may be present even at birth indicating *in utero* sucking efforts of the baby.

Natal Teeth

These are supernumerary lower incisors present at birth. They may become loose and interfere with breastfeeding or pose risk of dislodgment and aspiration. Sometimes they may cause ulceration of mandibular surface of tongue. Extraction is indicated if they are loose or interfering with breastfeeding.

Dehydration Fever

Some healthy neonates may develop fever on the 2nd or 3rd day of life due to poor physiologic initial lactation period or poor heat dissipation mechanism in high environmental temperature (summer months, over-clothing, overheated room). The baby is otherwise active, alert, and feeds well. Hydrotherapy (tepid sponging), lowering of environmental temperature, and continuing to feed is all that is required.

Evening Colic and Crying at Night

In the first 2–3 months of life, most of the babies sleep well during the day, are awake, noisy, and cry at night. It is related to the baby adopting his/her own diurnal and circadian rhythms as opposed to the intrauterine maternal rhythms enjoyed by the baby in the amniotic fluid sac. It takes about 8–12 weeks for the baby to establish the routine of sleeping more at night. Evening colic occurs as bouts of unexplained crying spells in the evening after few days of birth. It possibly occurs due to intestinal colic as indicated by excessive gurgling or peristaltic sounds on palpation or auscultation of abdomen and often relieved by effective release of wind from above or below. Rhythmic calming techniques like swinging back and forth, putting the baby on side or stomach, swaddling with allowance for flexion of hips, making "shhh" sound near the baby's ear, and let the baby suck on breast or clean finger are effective in calming the colicky babies.

Watering from the Eyes

Watering or persistent wetness of one or both eyes without redness indicates obstruction in the nasolacrimal duct often due to epithelial debris. Massaging the nasolacrimal sac (between eye and nose) and nasolacrimal duct along the lateral margins of the nose from above downwards, 15–20 times in a day, may restore the patency by 4–6 months of age. If it fails, probing and syringing through the punctum is indicated.

CARE OF LOW BIRTH WEIGHT BABIES

In India, 30% babies are born LBW.[1] Baby can be LBW due to prematurity or IUGR or combination of both. Fetal weight and size are directly linked to gestation and thus those born prematurely are likely to be LBW. In IUGR, baby is undernourished and/or undersized. Such a baby is also called small for gestational age or small for gestational date baby. If the growth retardation sets in early pregnancy, the baby is undersized (symmetrical IUGR); whereas in late-onset growth restriction, the baby is thin and undernourished (asymmetrical IUGR) with loose skinfolds, particularly around buttocks and thighs. Preterm LBW babies have fuzzy or wooly scalp hair, soft ear pinna which does not recoil promptly on release after being folded, scrotum lacks rugae and testes are not descended into the scrotum in male babies; in females the clitoris is prominent and the labia majora are widely separated not covering the labia minora. The deep sole creases are either absent or present only on the anterior one-third of the sole.

Causes of Low Birth Weight

- Maternal undernutrition before and during pregnancy (weight <40 kg, height <145 cm)
- Maternal illness like hypertension, chronic cardiac, renal, respiratory, and liver diseases
- Complications of pregnancy like preeclampsia, multiple pregnancy, multiparity, postmaturity, and antepartum hemorrhage
- Maternal smoking and drug abuse
- Low-inherent growth potential of fetus as in chromosomal anomalies and early intrauterine infections
- Prematurity is mostly idiopathic (45–50%), but may also be iatrogenic as in Rh isoimmunization and diabetes mellitus.

Handicaps of Low Birth Weight

Premature Low Birth Weight

- These babies basically have nutrient deprivation and developmental immaturity of organ systems
- Birth asphyxia and hyaline membrane disease due to lung immaturity
- Apneic spells due to poor respiratory control mechanism
- Hypothermia due to lack of brown fat and inability to limit heat loss by adopting flexed posture
- Infections due to inefficient humoral, cellular, and mucosal immune mechanisms; also requiring more handling and interventions in the setting of a contaminated environment
- Regurgitation of feeds due to immature and lax gastroesophageal junction and small stomach capacity
- Inability to feed and risk of aspiration because of lack of sucking and swallowing coordination below 35 weeks of gestation
- Risk of necrotizing enterocolitis
- Osteopenia and limited renal function
- Intracranial bleeds, particularly intraventricular hemorrhage due to immature vascular bed around the ventricular system
- Hypoglycemia and hyperbilirubinemia
- Retinopathy of prematurity due to oxygen toxicity.

Small for Gestational Date (Intrauterine Growth Retardation) Low Birth Weight

- Here, the basic underlying problem is *in utero* undernutrition
- Meconium passage *in utero* with resultant birth asphyxia and meconium aspiration
- Hypothermia due to inadequate subcutaneous and brown fat in addition to requiring more handling and interventions
- Hypoglycemia due to poor glycogen stores
- Infections due to adverse effects of chronic intrauterine stress on the immune system
- Feeding difficulty due to small size and vigor
- Higher incidence of congenital malformations.

Management of Low Birth Weight

Ideally, mother anticipating to deliver a LBW baby should be referred to an institution well equipped to take care of a baby of that particular gestation and weight (*in utero* transportation).

At Home Care

Low birth weight babies with birth weight more than 1,800 g, gestation more than or equal to 34 weeks and otherwise well can be managed at home similar to full-term normal babies.

Indications for Hospitalization

- Birth weight less than 1,800 g
- Gestation less than 34 weeks
- Unable to feed from breast or spoon and katori
- Sick baby irrespective of weight and gestation.

Low birth weight babies requiring hospitalization should be managed under the care of a neonatologist/pediatrician. Before transfer, the baby should be stabilized with particular attention to prevent hypothermia and infection, administration of vitamin K, initiate enteral feeding or parenteral fluids appropriate for gestational and chronological age. Ideally, a doctor or nurse should accompany the baby with a referral slip bearing note of antenatal and perinatal details.

Prevention of Hypothermia Before and During Transportation

Provision of warmth to prevent hypothermia is of utmost importance in neonatal care. Mother should accompany the baby as she herself is a source of warmth for the baby. Providing kangaroo mother care (mothering-in) or nursing the well-clothed baby close to the mother (bedding-in) in a warm room (28–30°C) prevents hypothermia. In a rural set up, hot water bottle filled with lukewarm water (39°C) tightly capped and wrapped in double layer of cloth can be used to keep the baby warm. Extreme caution should be taken to prevent accidental burn/scalding of the baby while using hot water bottle. In the hospital, overhead radiant warmer or open care system or incubator may be used as per availability.

Feeding and Fluids

Breast milk of the biological mother of the baby is the ideal food for LBW baby as it contains appropriate proteins, calories, and is uniquely suitable to provide optimum nutrition. The ultimate goal is to establish direct and exclusive breastfeeding. To begin with birth weight, gestation, vigor, and presence or absence of any sickness determines the mode and type of feed or parenteral fluids. The broad outline is depicted in table 2.

The daily fluid requirement of LBW babies is shown in table 3.

Extra fluids amounting to 20–30 mL/kg/day and 15 mL/kg/day are added to above requirement in case the baby is under radiant warmer and phototherapy, respectively.

Schedule and Guidelines for Gavage Feeding of Low Birth Weight Babies

The amount of expressed breast milk (EBM) to be fed per feed, interval between the feeds, acceptable residual before next feed, and time taken to reach full feeds is broadly outlined in table 4.

The feeding of every baby should be individualized, only the broad guidelines are shown in table 4. Extremely low birth weight and VLBW babies will need intravenous (IV) fluids initially. For the first 2 days of life, IV fluid should consist of

TABLE 2: Guidelines for initiating feeding of low birth weight babies[1]

Age	Category of neonate		
	Birth weight ≤1,200 g (gestation ≤30 weeks)	Birth weight = 1,200–1,800 g (gestation 30–34 weeks)	Birth weight >1,800 g (gestation ≥34 weeks)
Initial (1st day)	Intravenous fluids; gavage feed may be tried if baby is not sick	Gavage [expressed breast milk (EBM)]	Try direct breastfeed if unsatisfactory add katori-spoon (EBM)
2–7 days	Gavage (EBM)	Katorispoon (EBM)	Direct breastfeed
1–3 weeks	Katorispoon (EBM)	Direct breastfeed	Direct breastfeed
≥4 weeks	Direct breastfeed	Direct breastfeed	Direct breastfeed

10% glucose; subsequently, sodium and potassium, 3-5 mEq/kg/day and 2-3 mEq/kg/day, respectively should be added to dextrose. Enteral feeds are added gradually by gavage as the acute problems become passive. In due course, the baby should be gradually shifted to katorispoon at around 30-32 weeks of gestation. It acts as a bridge between gavage and direct breastfeeding. All LBW babies on gavage or katorispoon feeds should be put on breasts before each feed for 5–10 minutes in order to promote lactation and enable the baby to learn sucking.

Care should be exercised while giving gavage feeds. At the time of feeding, the outer end of the feeding tube is attached to 10 mL syringe containing milk without plunger; the milk is allowed to trickle by gravity. After the feed, the baby is placed in the right lateral position to avoid regurgitation. There is no need to burp a gavage fed baby. Check abdominal girth and prefeed aspirate for amount and character. Prefeed aspirate more than 25% of the previous feed, green or bloody color and increase of abdominal girth by more than 2 cm from the baseline needs evaluation.

TABLE 3: Fluid requirement of low birth weight neonates (mL/kg/day)[3]

Days of life	Birth weight		
	<1,000 g	1,000–1,500 g	>1,500 g
1	100	80	60
2	115	95	75
3	130	110	90
4	145	125	105
5	160	140	120
6	175	155	135
≥7	190	170	150

Vitamin and Mineral Supplementation

Breast milk does not fully meet the requirements of certain micronutrients in LBW babies. Table 5 shows the minerals and vitamins to be supplemented in these babies.

Growth Monitoring

Adequacy of feeding should be assessed by growth monitoring. All nutritional supplements and fluids should be administered by birth weight till the baby regains birth weight after initial weight loss. Subsequently, all the requirements should be met as per current weight.

After initial physiological weight loss of 8–10% of birth weight, the daily weight gain is around 15 g/day till the weight reaches 2 kg and thereafter the daily weight gain is aimed at 20–30 g.

Causes of Inadequate Weight Gain

- Inadequate calories (provided/consumed)
- Cold stress

TABLE 4: Guidelines for gavage feeding of low birth weight neonates[1]

Parameter	Birth weight			
	<1,000 g	1,000–1,500 g	1,500–2,000 g	>2,000 g
First feed (mL) (within 1 h)	1	2	3	10
Interval (h)	1–2	2	2–3	3
2nd to 4th feed (mL)	2	3	4	10
Increment on alternate feed (mL)	1	1	2	5
Final maximum (full) feed (mL)	10–15	20–30	Ad lib	Ad lib
Acceptable residual (mL)	1–2	2–3	3–4	4–5
Total time taken to full feed (days)	10–14	7–10	5–7	3–5

TABLE 5: Micronutrient supplementation in low birth weight babies[1]

Micronutrients	Daily dose	Duration of supplementation
Vitamin K	1 mg IM stat	Given once at birth. Repeat weekly if enteral feeding not established or on prolonged systemic antibiotics
Vitamin A	1,000 IU	Till 6 months of age or 4.5 kg weight
Vitamin D	400 IU	
Iron	3–4 mg/kg (elemental)	Start at 4–6 weeks in LBW and 2 weeks in VLBW, given till 6 months to 1 year of age
Calcium (elemental)	150–240 mg/kg (elemental)	Till corrected age of term (37–40 weeks) or weight 3–3.5 kg
Phosphorus	75–120 mg/kg	

IM, intramuscularly; LBW, low birth weight; VLBW, very low birth weight.

TABLE 6: Approximate composition of lactodex-human milk fortifier 2 g[4]

Components	Approximate composition
Protein	0.2 g
Fat	0.1 g
Carbohydrate	1.46 g
Calcium	50 mg
Phosphorus	25 mg
Sodium	1.75 mg
Zinc	0.1 mg
Vitamin A	730 IU
Vitamin D	250 IU
Energy	7.5 kcal

- Underlying systemic disease
- Late metabolic acidosis.

Inadequate weight gain in spite of optimum amount of EBM intake and other causes of poor weight gain having been excluded; the human milk fortifier (HMF) may be used. It is available as lactodex-HMF 2 g sachet, to be added to 50 mL of EBM in preterm babies with birth weight below 1,500 g. It is stopped once the baby reaches corrected gestational age of term or weight of 2–2.5 kg (Table 6).

Vaccination, Discharge, and Follow up

Vaccination should be initiated once the baby is stable and all acute problems have become passive. The schedule is same as in normal newborn described earlier. Baby is ready for discharge when there are no signs of any illness, is stable, gaining weight on katorispoon or direct breastfeeding, and maintaining color and temperature. Mother should be explained the danger signs to recognize serious illness at the earliest. The baby should initially be called within 7–10 days of discharge to check whether the baby and parents have adjusted in home environment. Subsequently, the baby is reviewed every month to monitor growth, development, vaccination, feeding, and detection of any abnormality.

NEONATAL JAUNDICE

Jaundice is the most common abnormality seen in neonates. About 60–80% of babies develop physiologic jaundice in the first week of life.[5]

Bilirubin Metabolism

Bilirubin is derived from breakdown of hemeproteins present in hemoglobin, myoglobin, and certain enzymes like cytochrome and catalase. One gram hemoglobin is catabolized to give 35 mg of bilirubin. It is then transported as bilirubin-albumin complex to the liver where it is taken up by ligandins in the hepatocyte. It is then conjugated with glucuronic acid in the presence of uridine 5'-diphospho-glucuronyltransferase enzyme (UGT1A1) to mono- and diglucuronides. This conjugated bilirubin is water soluble and is excreted in the bile. In the gut, the bacteria reduce it to urobilinogen which is excreted in the urine and stool.

Why Newborns Develop Physiologic Jaundice?

- Increased bilirubin production: 1 g of hemoglobin gives rise to 35 mg bilirubin and normal newborn produces on an average 8–10 mg/kg bilirubin daily, which is more than twice that of normal daily bilirubin production in an adult. It is attributed to higher RBC mass, lower RBC survival, increased ineffective erythropoiesis, and enterohepatic circulation
- Decreased clearance of bilirubin from the plasma: relatively deficient ligandins and UGT1A1 enzyme in the hepatocytes during the first week of life results in decreased clearance of bilirubin load presented to the liver. In LBW babies, low serum albumin further adds to the load of unconjugated bilirubin. Though not rate limiting, excretion of conjugated bilirubin into the bile is impaired.

Features of Physiologic Jaundice

All neonates have total serum bilirubin (TSB) more than or equal to 1 mg/dL (upper limit of normal in adult) in the first week of life. Icterus becomes clinically evident at TSB level of more than or equal to 5 mg/dL. The jaundice in a healthy term baby becomes visible on the 2nd or 3rd day, peaks on 5th day (TSB ≤12.9 mg/dL), and decreases to normal by the 7th day. In preterm, babies onset is similar but it peaks around 6th day (TSB ≤15 mg/dL) and subsides by about 2 weeks of life. Since it is due to raised unconjugated bilirubin, the urine remains colorless and stool is yellow. The diagnosis of physiologic jaundice can be established only by excluding known causes of jaundice. It does not need any therapy but must be watched closely for progression.

In preterm/LBW infant, TSB of even 8–10 mg/dL may cause neurologic damage. Hence the term "physiologic" or "nonphysiologic" jaundice in LBW infants is no longer relevant and hyperbilirubinemia in these infants is invariably treated at levels far below that previously defined as "nonphysiologic".[6]

Pathologic Jaundice

Jaundice is considered pathologic if time of appearance, severity, duration, pattern, and type of raised bilirubin monitored serially vary significantly from that of physiologic

jaundice. In the presence of any of the following, the jaundice must be investigated:
- Clinical jaundice appearing within 24 hours of birth
- TSB ≥12.9 mg/dL and 15 mg/dL in term and preterm baby, respectively
- Persistent jaundice beyond 1 week and 2 weeks in term and preterm baby, respectively
- Rate of rise of serum bilirubin more than 5 mg/dL/day
- High-colored urine and or clay-colored stools are suggestive of conjugated/obstructive type of jaundice
- Icterus involving palms and soles indicating TSB more than 15 mg/dL
- Jaundiced baby with any other sign/symptom of sickness.

However, it is important to remember that absence of above features of pathologic jaundice does not imply that the jaundice is physiologic.

Known Common Etiological Factors of Pathologic Jaundice in India

Even after extensive investigations, the cause of jaundice may remain elusive in more than 30% of cases. Common known causes are listed below.
- Blood group incompatibilities
- Glucose-6-phosphate dehydrogenase deficiency (G6PD)
- Intrauterine and postnatal infections
- Extravasations of blood like bruising, cephalohematoma, and intracranial bleed
- Breast milk and breastfeeding jaundice.

Breastfeeding and Jaundice

Breastfed infants are 3–6 times more likely to develop TSB levels more than 12–15 mg/dL compared to formula-fed infants. "Breastfeeding jaundice syndrome" or "breastfeeding associated jaundice" or "starvation jaundice" appears in first 2–4 days in exclusively breastfed infants and calorie deprivation appears to be a major cause in genesis of this entity. Calorie deprivation leads to increase in enterohepatic circulation of unconjugated bilirubin. These infants are likely to have excessive weight loss, i.e., more than or equal to 4% by 24 hours, more than or equal to 8% by 48 hours, and more than or equal to 10% by 72 hours.

Another group of breastfed babies have "breast milk jaundice syndrome" which appears later at around 4–7 days of age and persists for 2–6 weeks, and even up to 3 months in some babies. There is considerable overlap between these two entities. Usually, the infants in the second category are the same infants who had higher bilirubin in the first week of life. However in some of these infants with breast milk jaundice syndrome, mutation of UGT1A1 gene and some substances which inhibit the hepatic conjugation play a role in its pathogenesis.[6]

Assessment of a Jaundiced Baby

In assessment of a baby with jaundice, it is important to consider postnatal age in hours, gestation, weight, maternal, and perinatal history for predisposing factors like jaundice in previous babies, oxytocin use, traumatic delivery, blood group incompatibility, birth asphyxia, passage of meconium, adequacy of breastfeeding, and color of urine and stool. Conduct physical examination of the baby for extent/severity of jaundice, extravasated blood, clues to congenital intrauterine, and postnatal infection. Since the important concern of unconjugated hyperbilirubinemia is bilirubin encephalopathy (kernicterus); deeply jaundiced baby should also be evaluated for its presence or absence by lethargy, poor feeding, seizures, opisthotonus, and poor or absent neonatal reflexes.

Clinical Assessment of Extent of Jaundice

Jaundice in the neonate develops first on the face and has cephalocaudal progression which is related to the thickness of the skin at various parts of the body; being thinnest on the face and thickest over palms and soles. Sclera is not the right place to look for icterus due to physiological photophobia. Icterus should be looked for in the skin in good day light. It can be better appreciated by blanching the skin lightly to mask the physiologic plethora and reveal underlying yellowish staining of the subcutaneous tissue. By experience, one can learn to make an assessment of likely levels of TSB in a neonate who has not yet received phototherapy. With increasing levels of bilirubin and extent of skin staining, the body has been divided into five zones:
1. Zone 1 (head and neck): 6 mg/dL
2. Zone 2 (up to umbilicus): 9 mg/dL
3. Zone 3 (up to knees): 12 mg/dL
4. Zone 4 (up to ankles): 15 mg/dL
5. Zone 5 (palms and soles): >15 mg/dL.

Investigations

Total serum bilirubin, direct or indirect reacting bilirubin, blood groups of mother and baby, hematocrit, reticulocyte count, and peripheral smear for RBC morphology gives enough clue to the diagnosis in many cases. If necessary, other relevant investigations like G6PD, sepsis screen, thyroid function tests, or screening for congenital intrauterine infections may be required.

Treatment

The treatment in neonatal jaundice is aimed to lower the indirect bilirubin levels to prevent bilirubin encephalopathy (kernicterus). Two main modalities of treatment are:
1. Phototherapy
2. Exchange transfusion.

The decision to treat depends upon the gestation, postnatal age in hours, birth weight, TSB level, cause of jaundice, presence or absence of risk factors like asphyxia, sepsis, and acidosis.

The general guide (rule of thumb) is to start phototherapy or do exchange transfusion when the TSB is 0.75% and 1% of the birth weight (in grams), respectively. Phototherapy is to be stopped when TSB is persistently within 5 mg below the starting level.

Prevention of Unconjugated Hyperbilirubinemia

- Rh hemolytic disease of newborn: obstetricians play an important role in prevention of Rh hemolytic disease of newborn by administering anti-D to nonsensitized mother giving birth to Rh positive product of conception. Fetomaternal hemorrhages keep occurring in normal pregnancy but most of it occurs at the time of parturition to an extent of 5–30 mL:[1]
  - It is recommended to administer 300–500 μg of anti-D to a Rh negative nonsensitized mother within 72 hours of delivery or abortion if the baby/fetus is Rh positive
  - Dose of anti-D is doubled in multiple gestations
  - Anti-D is also recommended in Rh negative pregnant mother undergoing podalic version, chorionic villous sampling, and manual removal of placenta.
- Prevention of hyperbilirubinemia in high-risk babies: certain groups of babies are at risk of developing high levels of TSB and need more attention to prevent hyperbilirubinemia:[5]
  - High but safe TSB before discharge
  - Babies born at 35–37 weeks of gestation (late preterm)
  - Breastfeeding not going well (weight loss >8–10%)
  - Jaundice appearing within 24 h of birth
  - Lot of bruising/cephalohematoma
  - History of a parent or sibling who had high TSB requiring phototherapy.

Indications for Prophylactic Phototherapy

- Rhisoimmunization
- ELBW (<1,000 g)
- Severely bruised babies.

Period of greatest risk of high TSB is 72–96 hours of life. So, babies who have been discharged before this period must be reviewed for jaundice within 2 days of discharge.

Conjugated Hyperbilirubinemia

Definition

If the TSB is at or below 5 mg/dL (85 μmol/L), a direct or conjugated bilirubin of more than 1 mg/dL (17.1 μmol/L) and for TSB more than 5 mg/dL a direct bilirubin of more than 20% of TSB is defined as conjugated hyperbilirubinemia.[5,7] It is always pathological. There is no risk of kernicterus but needs evaluation for etiology and appropriate management.

Causes of Conjugated Hyperbilirubinemia

- Neonatal hepatitis
- Biliary atresia
- Choledochal cyst
- Inspissated bile syndrome
- Intrauterine infection—Toxoplasmosis, Other infections, Rubella, Cytomegalovirus infection, and Herpes simplex (TORCH)
- Sepsis
- Metabolic disorders: galactosemia, α_1-antitrypsin deficiency, tyrosinemia, hereditary fructose intolerance
- Hypothyroidism
- Total parenteral nutrition (TPN).

Early recognition and prompt evaluation for identification of the cause is essential for a favorable outcome. To ensure recognition of biliary atresia and its referral to tertiary care center at the earliest (latest by 60 days of age) for optimum surgical treatment, it is essential that pediatricians, obstetricians, and primary care physicians are well sensitized for evaluation of conjugated hyperbilirubinemia in neonates.

NEONATAL SEPSIS

Neonatal sepsis is one of the most important causes of neonatal morbidity and mortality.[1] Depending upon the site/extent of involvement and age of onset of symptoms, it is classified as:

- Septicemia or systemic infection
- Superficial infection
- Early-onset sepsis (EOS)
- Late-onset sepsis (LOS).

Septicemia or Systemic Infection

It is defined as clinical syndrome of bacteremia with systemic symptoms and signs of infection in the first 28 days of life. In simple terms, an unwell neonate with bacteremia is labeled as septicemic.

When the pathogenic organism gains access into bloodstream, it may cause overwhelming infection without identifiable localization or may get predominantly localized to one or more systems like lungs (pneumonia), meninges (meningitis), or skeletal system (osteomyelitis).

Superficial Infections

The organism does not invade the bloodstream and cause symptoms pertaining to the involved superficial site like conjunctivitis, pyoderma, and umbilical sepsis.

Early-onset Sepsis

Sepsis is considered early onset when the symptoms appear within 72 hours of birth. It is caused by organisms prevalent in the maternal genital tract or in the immediate birth area (labor room, operation theater). Often it presents as pneumonia and less commonly as septicemia or meningitis.

Predisposing Factors for Early-onset Sepsis

- LBW
- Birth asphyxia
- Foul smelling liquor
- Single unclean or multiple (>3) per vaginal examinations during labor
- Maternal fever
- Prolonged labor (>24 h)
- Prolonged rupture of membranes (>12 h)
- Meconium aspiration.

Late-onset Sepsis

Here, the onset of symptoms is beyond 72 hours of birth. It is caused by organisms in the environment of the baby at home or hospital. The infection is often transmitted through the hands of care providers. It usually presents as septicemia, pneumonia, or meningitis.

Predisposing Factors for Late-onset Sepsis

- Local or superficial infections
- Aspiration of feeds
- Venous sampling/IV catheters and other invasive procedures.

Causative Organisms

Any microorganism can cause sepsis at any age, but there is general pattern which varies from place to place and also over the time at the same place. Gram-negative enteric bacilli, particularly *Escherichia coli*, *Klebsiella*, and *Enterobacter* species predominate in EOS; whereas in LOS, in addition, Gram-positive bacteria including coagulase positive and negative staphylococci are important causative agents.

Clinical Features

The manifestations of neonatal septicemia are often vague and need high index of suspicion for early diagnosis. Very sensitive early indictors of sepsis are changes in affect, peripheral perfusion, and respiratory status. In LOS, infection may localize and cause symptoms of meningitis, pneumonia, urinary tract infection, septic arthritis, and soft-tissue infection. Varied clinical features are enlisted in box 1.

Box 1: Clinical features of neonatal sepsis[1]

- Lethargy
- Poor feeding
- Poor cry
- Diarrhea
- Abdominal distension
- Vomiting
- Hypothermia/fever
- Prolonged capillary refill time/shock
- Bleeding
- Oliguria/anuria
- Tachypnea*
- Tachycardia*
- Apnea/gasping*
- Grunting*
- Cyanosis*
- Seizures†
- High-pitched cry†
- Irritability†
- Neck retraction,† bulging anterior fontanel†

*Suggestive of pneumonia.
†Suggestive of meningitis.

Diagnosis

Isolation of microorganism from blood or normally sterile body fluids is diagnostic. Positive blood culture is the only definitive or gold standard measure to establish the diagnosis. Most of other available indirect laboratory tests when considered alone are unable to provide reliable and early diagnosis. In order to circumvent this problem, a panel of screening tests (sepsis screen) has been devised; which apart from having a reasonable positive predictive value (39%) also have remarkable negative predictive value (99%). This sepsis screen is suggestive of sepsis if more than or equal to 2 of the following are present:[8]

- Total leucocyte count <5,000/mm^3
- Immature to total neutrophil ratio (I:T ratio) ≥0.2
- Latex C-reactive protein more than 1 mg/dL
- Neutropenia (absolute neutrophil count <1,800/mm^3)
- Microerythrocyte sedimentation rate ≥15 mm at 1 hours.

Other tests include X-ray of chest and lumbar puncture as and when indicated.

Treatment

Early recognition and initiation of empiric effective antibacterial agents with optimal supportive care is crucial for favorable outcome. No investigation is needed as a prerequisite to start treatment in a clinically obvious case as waiting for the test reports will lose precious time (Table 7).

TABLE 7: Guidelines for empiric antibiotic therapy in neonatal sepsis[8]

Clinical setting	First-line antibiotic regimen	Alternative regimen
Early-onset sepsis	Ampicillin + gentamycin	Ampicillin + cefotaxime
Community-acquired late-onset sepsis (LOS)	Ampicillin + cefotaxime	Ampicillin + gentamycin + cefotaxime
Hospital-acquired LOS (no intravenous catheters *in situ*)	Ampicillin + gentamycin	Ampicillin + cefotaxime
Hospital-acquired LOS (intravenous catheters *in situ*)	Vancomycin + gentamycin	Vancomycin + cefotaxime

Principles of Antibiotics Selection

- To cover usual causative agents in a particular community/nursery
- Combination of two or more antibiotics which effectively cover the spectrum of pathogens in that area/nursery. It should be based on monitoring of the bacterial flora of the neonatal intensive care unit and the antibiotic sensitivity pattern of pathogens, as the bacterial flora is dynamic, different from one place to the other and it changes in the same place over a period of time. Antibiotic sensitivity pattern also changes over time depending upon frequently used regimens
- Pharmacokinetic properties of antibiotic in newborn infant in relation to gestational and postnatal age.

Continuation of Antibiotic Therapy after Culture Reports

Once the causative agent is known, a single appropriate antibiotic as per sensitivity is usually satisfactory.

Duration of the Therapy

A period of 10–14 days is sufficient for septicemia, whereas for Gram-negative skeletal infection and meningitis it should be 21 days. Dose, route, and frequency of administration of different antibiotics are shown in table 8.

Supportive Care

The purpose of supportive care is to normalize temperature and cardiorespiratory function, prevent and correct hypoglycemia, provide optimum nutrition and fluid management, prevent and treat any bleeding by administering vitamin K, and if needed fresh blood transfusion.

TABLE 8: Dose, route, and frequency of administration of antibiotics[8]

Antibiotic	Dose (mg/kg/dose)		Frequency (h)		Route
			Age		
	Septicemia	Meningitis	<7 days	>7 days	
Ampicillin	50	100	12	8	IV
Cloxacillin	50	100	12	8	IV
Gentamycin	2.5	2.5	12	8	IV
Amikacin	7.5	7.5	12	12	IV
Cefotaxime	50	50	12	8	IV
Vancomycin	15	15	12	8	IV

IV, intravenous.

Superficial Infections

Superficial infections occur in the form of pyoderma, purulent conjunctivitis, oral thrush, and umbilical sepsis. These can be easily treated by local application of antimicrobial agents. Pustules can be punctured with sterile needle and cleaned with spirit or betadine. If the pustules are large or numerous, systemic erythromycin 25–40 mg/kg/day in two divided doses for 5–7 days is effective. Purulent conjunctivitis should be treated by repeated cleaning of eyes with cool boiled water/normal saline and local instillation of antibiotic drops. Oral thrush responds to cleaning with 7.5% sodium bicarbonate followed by local application of clotrimazole in between the feeds. Umbilical sepsis responds well to local cleaning with spirit and application of antibiotic powder or cream.

Prevention of Infection

- Good antenatal care
- Tetanus toxoid to all mothers in antenatal period
- Early and exclusive breastfeeding
- No prelacteal feeds
- Care of the umbilical cord
- Avoid unnecessary interventions/instrumentation
- Strict hand hygiene
- Barrier nursing
- Aseptic management of IV lines/catheters.

RESPIRATORY DISTRESS IN NEWBORN

Normal healthy newborn, usually breaths 40–50 times/min and respiratory rate above 60 breaths/min is considered tachypnea. Tachypnea in association with increased work of breathing denotes distress. So, if the respiratory rate is more than 60 breaths/min and is associated with inspiratory costal recessions or expiratory grunt in a quiet state, it is labeled as respiratory distress.[6] There are numerous causes of respiratory distress enumerated in table 9.

Clinical Recognition of Respiratory Distress

Tachypnea is the most frequent and easily recognized sign. It may be followed later by apnea due to accumulation of carbon dioxide or muscular exhaustion. Inspiratory retractions of intercostal spaces, infra- and suprasternal notches and xiphoid region indicate respiratory distress. It is an attempt of increased effort by way of decreasing the pleural pressure to expand the noncompliant lung, resulting in indrawing of very complaint neonatal rib cage. The degree of retraction correlates well with severity of the disease. Flaring of alae nasi is also an attempt to lower/upper airway resistance in the presence of hypoxia.

Grunting is very common in infants with hyaline membrane disease (HMD). It is produced by passage of exhaled air through a narrowed glottis with an attempt to elevate intra-alveolar pressure in order to prevent alveolar collapse at the end of expiration. Clinical cyanosis indicates arterial partial pressure (PO_2) less than 40 mmHg.[6]

Downe's scoring system (Table 10) is a simple clinical method which does not need access to blood gas analysis and acts as a guide for treatment as well as prognosis.

TABLE 9: Causes of respiratory distress in neonates[3]

Pulmonary causes	• Congenital anomalies: ○ Lung cysts ○ Congenital cystic adenomatoid malformation ○ Lobar emphysema ○ Hypoplasia and aplasia of lung ○ Congenital pulmonary lymphangiectasis ○ Congenital diaphragmatic hernia • Acquired disorders: ○ Respiratory distress syndrome (hyaline membrane disease) ○ Meconium aspiration syndrome ○ Transient tachypnea of newborn ○ Pneumonia ○ Pulmonary hemorrhage ○ Pneumothorax/ pneumomediastinum ○ Bronchopulmonary dysplasia
Airway obstruction	• Congenital anomalies: ○ Choanal atresia ○ Laryngeal webs ○ Laryngomalacia ○ Tracheal stenosis ○ Tracheoesophageal fistula • Extrinsic airway compression: ○ Vascular rings ○ Cysts
Non-respiratory causes	• Heat failure • Intracranial (IC) pathology like IC bleed • Metabolic acidosis
Miscellaneous causes	• Phrenic nerve palsy • Chest wall deformities (pectus excavatum) • Muscular disorders

Common Clinical Conditions Causing Respiratory Distress in Newborn[6]

Respiratory distress syndrome (RDS) also called HMD is the most common cause of respiratory distress in preterm babies. Its incidence is inversely related to gestational age at birth. In India, its incidence is 1.2 and 6.4% in intra- and extramural deliveries. Male gender, prenatal asphyxia, lower segment cesarean section without trial of labor, and chorioamnionitis are important predisposing factors. A constant feature of RDS is early onset of respiratory distress within 6 hours of birth. Typical X-ray of chest findings are bilateral reticulogranular pattern (due to scattered atelectasis), ground glass appearance (due to confluent reticulogranular shadows), air bronchogram (translucent air-filled bronchi against airless, solid, atelectatic lungs), complete white out lungs (loss of delineation of heart margins due to global atelectasis), normal or slightly increased heart size), and large thymic silhouette. Lecithin to sphingomyelin ratio (L:S ratio) of more than 2 predicts absence of RDS in 98% neonates. Positive bubble or shake test performed on the bedside; showing complete ring of bubbles at the meniscus in 1:2 dilution of amniotic fluid is rarely associated with RDS.

Treatment

It comprises of general supportive measures supplemented with early surfactant therapy and assisted ventilation.

TABLE 10: Downe's clinical respiratory distress scoring system[3,9]

Parameter	Score		
	0	1	2
Respiratory rate/min	<60	60–80	>80 or apnea
Cyanosis	None in room air	In 40% O_2	≥40% O_2
Retractions	None	Mild	Moderate to severe
Grunting	None	Audible with stethoscope	Audible without stethoscope
Air entry	Good	Decreased	Barely audible or absent

Score: Normal infant = 0; impending respiratory failure ≥6 and severe respiratory distress = 10.

Meconium Aspiration Syndrome

Meconium aspiration syndrome (MAS) occurs when the neonate aspirates amniotic fluid containing meconium into lungs *in utero* or during and/or immediately after birth. It is defined as respiratory distress in an infant born through meconium-stained amniotic fluid (MSAF) in whom other causes of distress have been ruled out. MSAF occurs in 10–15% of all deliveries and 5% of these develop MAS. There may be green staining of skin, nails, and umbilical cord. Meconium aspiration causes respiratory distress by several mechanisms, viz., mechanical airway obstruction, chemical injury or pneumonitis, surfactant dysfunction, and persistent pulmonary hypertension (PPHN). Distress usually develops within 4–6 hours of birth. X-ray of chest shows patchy atelectasis and scattered infiltrates in the lung fields. There may be hyperinflation of both lungs with flattened/pushed down diaphragms. In 25% cases, there may be air leaks. Echocardiogram identifies PPHN and its severity.

Transient Tachypnea of Newborn

Transient tachypnea of newborn is a benign condition, usually seen in term babies born by cesarean or precipitate delivery. It is also called "wet lung syndrome" as it may be due to failure of fluid drainage through lymphatics or airways occurring as a result of squeezing effect of normal vaginal delivery. It is also called type 2 RDS as it may represent a mild equivalent of HMD. These babies are well and have only tachypnea with rates as high as 80–100/min without significant chest retractions. Management is simply supportive.

Neonatal Pneumonia

It has been described under sepsis in the heading "Neonate".

Management of Neonates with Respiratory Distress

The principal problem in these neonates is poor oxygenation and increasing respiratory difficulty. Therapeutic goals therefore, include oxygen administration to maintain oxygen saturation (SpO_2)/partial arterial pressure of oxygen (PaO_2) within acceptable range. The second aspect is supportive therapy; to minimize work of breathing, maintain temperature, and to provide adequate fluid and calories. Antibiotics should be started in all infants who present with respiratory distress at or soon after birth after obtaining blood culture and sepsis screen. Discontinue antibiotics after 3–5 days if blood culture is negative.

Indications for Respiratory Support

Continuous Positive Airway Pressure

- Fraction of inspired oxygen (FiO_2) more than 0.4–0.5 (by oxygen hood) in preterms with RDS
- Frequent apnea with documented hypoxemia
- Significant chest retraction after recent extubation from mechanical ventilation.

Mechanical Ventilation

- Prolonged apnea
- $APaO_2$ <50 mmHg or FiO_2 >0.8 (except in congenital cyanotic heart disease)
- Partial arterial pressure of carbon dioxide ($PaCO_2$) more than 60 mmHg with persistent acidosis
- Failure of continuous positive airway pressure (CPAP) at FiO_2 more than 0.6–0.7
- To relieve the "work of breathing" with increasing respiratory distress.

Prevention of Respiratory Distress[1]

Respiratory distress syndrome: when induction of premature labor is unavoidable, antenatal glucocorticoids are recommended to achieve pharmacologic maturity of lungs.

Indication: 24–34 weeks of gestation at high risk of delivery within next 7 days.

Timing: at least 24 hours to 7 days prior to anticipated delivery.

Drugs and schedule:
- Betamethasone: 12 mg intramuscularly, 2 doses, 24 h apart
- Dexamethasone: 6 mg intramuscularly, 4 doses, 12 h apart.

Contraindication: chorioamnionitis.

Prophylactic surfactant: preterm infants born at less than or equal to 30 weeks of gestation benefit from prophylactic surfactant in terms of reduction of incidence, severity, and complications of RDS. A prophylactic or preventive surfactant strategy is defined as surfactant administration within 10–30 minutes of birth to preterm infant at very high risk of developing RDS, before the onset of symptoms. But its cost and availability at all places is a major constraint.

Meconium aspiration syndrome: appropriate peripartum management of nonvigorous babies born through MSAF lowers the risk and severity of MAS. Nonvigorous babies at birth as indicated by poor or no respiratory effort, limpness and bradycardia (heart rate <100 beats/min) should be intubated and tracheal suction of meconium under direct visualization should be carried out.

HYPOGLYCEMIA IN NEWBORN

Glucose serves as the predominant brain fuel. Glucose accounts for more than 90% of the brain energy utilization. Because of higher brain to body size ratio, glucose requirement of 6–8 mg/kg/min of a neonate far exceeds that of 1–2 mg/kg/min in adults.

Definition

It is defined as blood glucose (BG) level of less than 40 mg/dL (2.2 mmol/L), irrespective of gestation on any day up to 28 days of life, associated with symptoms of hypoglycemia or confirmed on repeat analysis in asymptomatic babies.[3,6]

GLUCOSE HOMEOSTASIS AT BIRTH

The infant is born with BG concentration of 60–70% of the maternal BG level and it falls at the rate of 0.77%/min. The lowest value reaches at 3 hours of age. The acute interruption of maternal glucose transfer to the fetus at delivery imposes an immediate need to mobilize endogenous glucose. Hypoglycemia represents a defect in one or several complex interactions that normally integrate glucose homeostasis during fasting. The elements of fasting homeostasis are:
- Glycogenolysis
- Gluconeogenesis
- Fatty acid oxidation (FAO).
- Ketogenesis.

These elements of glucose homeostasis are controlled by insulin. Insulin suppresses, whereas counterregulatory hormones namely glucagon, cortisol, epinephrine, and growth hormone act redundantly to stimulate the fasting systems.

In the initial phase of fasting, insulin secretion is suppressed and there is three- to fivefold abrupt increase in glucagon concentrations and dramatic surge in spontaneous catecholamines and other counterregulatory hormones. After the glycogen stores get depleted, a transition to fat utilization occurs to prevent the consumption of all muscle stores. Lipolysis provides substrate for muscle FAO and hepatic ketogenesis. The former allows diversion of glucose away from the muscles to brain, while the later provides an alternate fuel to the brain. Gluconeogenesis remains constant. Gluconeogenesis and ketogenesis are not so well developed at birth and may take 2–7 days to be fully mature. So hypoglycemia ensues when glycogen stores are depleted, resulting in no glycemic response to glucagon. In hyperinsulinemic states, there is no acidemia, low or absent free-fatty acids (FAs), and ketones. Elevated free-FAs, suppressed ketones and no acidemia suggest disorders of FAO and ketogenesis.

Causes of Hypoglycemia[3]

- Diminished stores of substrate (glycogen, lipid) and impaired fuel generation (gluconeogenesis, ketogenesis):
  - IUGR
  - Prematurity
  - Polycythemia
  - Inborn errors of metabolism
  - Endocrinal abnormalities
  - FAO disorders
- Hyperinsulinism:
  - Insulin-dependent diabetes mellitus (IDM), infants of gestational diabetic mothers (IGDM)
  - Large for gestational dates babies
  - Erythroblastosis fetalis
  - Islet cell adenomas
  - Beckwith-Wiedemann syndrome
  - Rapid tapering of high strength glucose infusion
  - Congenital hyperinsulinism
- Increased metabolic needs:
  - RDS
  - Septicemia
  - Cardiac failure
  - Birth asphyxia.

Clinical Features

Classical signs of hypoglycemia are related to sympathetic adrenergic activation and central nervous system (CNS) impairment as listed below:
- Jitteriness
- Tremors
- Episodes of cyanosis
- Convulsions
- Intermittent apneic spells
- Tachypnea
- Weak or high-pitched cry
- Limpness/lethargy
- Feeding difficulty
- Eye rolling
- Episodes of sweating, sudden pallor, hypothermia, and cardiac arrest.

Since these clinical features are nonspecific and may result from various other causes, it is critical to measure BG in such babies and reversal of symptoms by raising blood sugar confirms the diagnosis. Presence of midline defects like cleft lip/palate and micropenis in a male infant suggests hypopituitarism.

Anticipation of Hypoglycemia and Monitoring

Following infants are at high risk of developing hypoglycemia and need monitoring of BG:
- Insulin-dependent diabetes mellitus and IGDM

- Small for gestational date
- Prematurity
- Rh isoimmunization
- Asphyxia, hypothermia, polycythemia, septicemia, or any other sickness
- Any baby on IV fluids or TPN.

Frequency of Monitoring

- Insulin-dependent diabetes mellitus/IGDM: cord blood, 1 h, 2 h, 3 h, and 6 h of age, and then 6 hourly × 48 h
- Low birth weight: 1 h, 2 h, 3 h, and 6 h of age, and then 6 hourly × 72 h
- Other high-risk categories: 6 hourly
- After exchange transfusion with citrate-phosphate dextrose blood: 2 h after the procedure.

In babies who are on enteral feeds, the BG should be measured just before the feed.

Diagnosis of the Underlying Cause of Hypoglycemia

Etiology of hypoglycemia may be identified by combination of clinical examination, timing of hypoglycemic episode, and response of circulating fuels and hormones at the time of hypoglycemia. Sample of blood is obtained at the time of hypoglycemic episode to measure BG, bicarbonate, lactate, free-FAs, ketones, insulin, cortisol, and growth hormone. This is termed as "critical sample". Frequent episodes of hypoglycemia within short period of feeding, suggests hyperinsulinism. Hypoglycemia after a long gap between feeds is more consistent with gluconeogenic or FAO defect.

Management

Asymptomatic hypoglycemia without seizures is treated with IV bolus of 10% dextrose, 2 mL/kg (200 mg/kg). Those with seizures, bolus of 10% dextrose, 4 mL/kg (400 mg/kg) is given. After the bolus, maintain dextrose infusion at the rate of 8 mg/kg/min. Assess BG 2 hourly, once normal, then 6 hourly till BG remains normal and baby is asymptomatic for 24–48 hours. Then start enteral feeds and taper glucose infusion by 2 mg/kg/min every 12 hour, till the BG is maintained in the normal range at glucose infusion rate (GIR) of 4 mg/kg/min for 24 hours. GIR should be titrated by close monitoring to maintain BG level above 60 mg/dL preferably within optimal range of 75–100 mg/dL.

Intractable Hypoglycemia

When GIR of more than 12 mg/kg/min is required to maintain BG, it is labeled as intractable hypoglycemia. Congenital hyperinsulinism is the most common cause followed by pituitary deficiency. Glucagon, 300 µg/kg (maximum 1 mg) IM or IV may help transiently by mobilizing glycogen stores. Diazoxide, 10–15 mg/kg/day, 8–12 hourly is helpful in hyperinsulinism by suppressing insulin secretion.

These babies with congenital hyperinsulinism may ultimately need surgical resection of focal lesion or 90% pancreatectomy. Glucocorticoids, as a nonspecific therapy should be avoided when the underlying cause has not been identified. However, such cases need thorough investigations to find out the cause so that specific treatment is instituted at the earliest. For GIR of more than 10 mg/kg/min, infusion should be administered through central vein. The desired strength of dextrose can be prepared by mixing appropriate amount of 5 and 25% dextrose which can be calculated by the following formula:

Formula: 5A – 25 = mL of 25% dextrose to be added to 5% dextrose to make 100 mL of desired strength. Where "A" denotes the desired strength of dextrose to be prepared.

Example: to make 13% dextrose, 5 × 13 – 25 = 40, i.e., add 40 mL of 25% dextrose to 60 mL of 5% dextrose to make 100 mL of 13% dextrose.

Prevention of Hypoglycemia

Since any newborn can develop hypoglycemia, first feed should not be delayed beyond 1 hour. Those at increased risk should be monitored by assessment of BG as described in the text. If enteral feeds are contraindicated or poorly tolerated, 10% dextrose to maintain GIR of 6–8 mg/kg/min should be given as IV infusion. Avoid abrupt or rapid tapering of glucose infusion.

SEIZURE DISORDERS IN NEWBORN

Seizure is the most common clinical manifestation of CNS dysfunction in the neonates. Neonates are more prone to seizures in comparison to all other age groups. It is related to unique neurobiology of the immature brain, with an abundance of excitatory circuits and sparse inhibitory circuits.[3]

Definition of Seizure

It is the occurrence of a paroxysmal, synchronous electrical discharge of a group of neurons in the brain manifesting clinically as abnormal neurologic function which includes motor, sensory, behavior, and/or autonomic function with/without loss of consciousness.

If abnormal electrical discharge is represented in the concomitant electroencephalogram (EEG), it is called epileptic seizure. If the EEG shows abnormality without clinical correlates, it is called EEG seizure. At times, clinical seizures occur without concomitant EEG abnormality and it is labeled as nonepileptic seizures such as subtle or generalized tonic seizures. Because the neocortical network is not so well developed at birth, many neonatal seizures are mediated by brainstem and subcortical structures, which may not be picked up by surface EEG monitoring.

Types of Seizures

Neonatal seizures can be clinically classified as:
- Subtle seizures
- Clonic seizures: focal or multifocal
- Tonic seizures
- Myoclonic seizures.

Subtle Seizures

These are predominant type of seizures and account for 50% of all seizures in neonates. It manifests as ocular movements, lip smacking, bicycling movements, and apnea. Apnea as a seizure manifestation is associated with either normal HR or tachycardia and other subtle manifestations such as eye or mouth movements (apnea due to prematurity per se and other causes is accompanied with bradycardia and no other subtle movement).

Clonic Seizures

It is characterized by rhythmic movements of muscle groups with a slow and a fast component. These can either be focal or multifocal and invariably associated with surface EEG abnormality.

Tonic Seizures

It is sustained, generalized, or focal extension of axial or appendicular muscle groups manifesting as stereotyped, abrupt, or slower tonic posturing of limbs and/or trunk or eyes, often accompanied with apnea, flushing, or mild cyanosis. EEG usually has no abnormality.

Myoclonic Seizures

These are characterized by focal or multifocal, lightning, and fast jerks of upper and lower limbs with predilection for flexor muscles. EEG abnormality may or may not be associated.

What is Jitteriness?

Jitter is a movement disorder and should not be mistaken as a seizure. It is characterized by tremulous, pendular, and stimulus sensitive movement lacking fast and slow components. It ceases with passive flexion or holding of the limb, not accompanied by any abnormality of gaze or eye movement. EEG is normal. It may occur due to hypoglycemia, hypocalcemia or hypoxic-ischemic encephalopathy.

Causes of Seizures

- Hypoxic-ischemic encephalopathy
- CNS infection:
  - Congenital intrauterine infections (TORCH)
  - Acquired bacterial infections (meningitis)
- IC hemorrhage
- Metabolic derangements:
  - Hypoglycemia
  - Hypocalcemia
  - Hypomagnesemia
  - Hypo- and hypernatremia
  - Inborn errors of metabolism:
    - Aminoacidurias
    - Urea cycle defects
    - Biotinidase deficiency
    - Organic acidopathies
    - Peroxisomal disorders
    - Pyridoxine dependency
- Developmental malformations of the brain:
  - Cerebral dysgenesis
  - Neuronal migration defects
- Benign neonatal seizures:
  - Benign familial neonatal convulsions
  - Benign idiopathic neonatal convulsions (5th day fits)
  - Benign neonatal sleep myoclonus
- Neonatal epileptic syndromes:
  - Early myoclonic encephalopathy
  - Early infantile epileptic encephalopathy
- Idiopathic.

Diagnostic Work Up

The investigation should be tailored as per clinical suspicion:
- BG
- Serum calcium, magnesium, and other electrolytes
- Sepsis screen, cerebrospinal fluid (CSF)
- Maternal and neonatal titers for TORCH infection
- Neuroimaging of the brain
- EEG (in intractable cases with pyridoxine infusion).

Screening for Inborn Errors of Metabolism

- Blood lactate, ammonia, and pyruvate
- Biotinidase level
- Quantitative amino acids and very long chain FAs
- Urine for organic acids
- CSF glucose (with concomitant BG), pyruvate, lactate, and amino acids.

Treatment

The aim of treatment is to:
- Identify the cause
- To treat the cause and seizure activity to minimize physiologic and metabolic derangement

- Continuous EEG monitoring is advised to identify EEG abnormality or EEG seizure without clinical correlates, quantify and demonstrate the efficacy of treatment.
- To prevent recurrences of seizure
- Nurse the baby in thermoneutral environment
- Ensure airway patency, breathing, and circulation
- Obtain IV access and collect blood sample for BG, serum calcium, magnesium, and other relevant investigations
- If BG less than 40 mg/dL, administer 2–4 mL/kg of 10% dextrose IV followed by 10% dextrose infusion at GIR of 8 mg/kg/min
- If serum calcium is less than 7 mg/dL, administer 10% calcium gluconate, 1–2 mL/kg diluted in equal volume of distilled water, IV slowly over 5–10 minutes under cardiac monitoring
- If seizure is not controlled, suspect hypomagnesemia and administer IM 0.2 mL/kg of 50% magnesium sulfate.

If baby still has seizures give anticonvulsants as follows:

- Phenobarbitone 20 mg/kg IV over 20 minutes, if response is nil or poor, additional doses of phenobarbitone are repeated at the rate of 5 mg/kg/dose every 15 min till a total cumulative dose of 40 mg/kg inclusive of loading dose is reached
- If convulsions are still not controlled, give phenytoin 20 mg/kg at the rate of 1 mg/kg/min, diluted in normal saline
- Maintenance doses of phenobarbitone and phenytoin are begun 12 h after the loading dose, at the rate of 5 mg/kg/day in two divided doses
- If seizures persist, consider pyridoxine dependency, try pyridoxine, 100 mg stat followed by 50–100 mg/day
- If seizures still not controlled administer 5% paraldehyde 200–400 mg/kg IV diluted in 5% dextrose or it may also be given per rectum diluted in double the volume of olive oil or coconut oil
- If seizures are still intractable, try the following:
  - Lorazepam 50 μg/kg IV slowly over 2–5 min or
  - Clonazepam 100–200 μg/kg IV slowly over 30 sec or
  - Lidocaine 2 mg/kg/IV bolus, followed by IV infusion at the rate of 6 mg/kg/hour or
  - Sodium valproate 20 mg/kg IV or oral followed by 10 mg/kg 12 hourly.

For How Long to Continue Anticonvulsants?

- Duration of anticonvulsant therapy is guided by control of seizures, neurological status, cause of seizures, and EEG
- Once the seizure is controlled, stop all anticonvulsants except phenobarbitone
- If neurological examination is normal, stop phenobarbitone at discharge
- If neurological examination is abnormal, discharge on phenobarbitone and review after 1 month. If neurological examination still abnormal, obtain EEG; if EEG shows no abnormality, taper off phenobarbitone
- If EEG is abnormal, continue the anticonvulsant and follow up every 3 months with repetition of EEG. Stop anticonvulsant once the EEG shows no abnormality.

VITAMIN K DEFICIENCY BLEEDING OF NEWBORN

The original term, hemorrhagic disease of newborn has been replaced with VKDB, because the former included infants with bleeding due to other causes as well.[6]

The coagulopathy of VKD is one of the most frequent causes of bleeding in otherwise well infants. Vitamin K is required for synthesis of coagulation factors II, VII, IX, and X. Neonates are predisposed to VKDB because transplacental transfer of vitamin K is minimal and its storage in liver is also limited. Breast milk is a poor source of vitamin K (5 μg/L) and is insufficient to meet the minimum daily need of 12 μg. It is further compounded by delayed and poor colonization of gut by flora known to synthesis vitamin K endogenously. Neonatal VKDB syndromes differ in time of onset and predominant etiology of VKD. Clinical presentation of VKDB can be classified into three patterns, viz., early, classic, and late.[3]

Early vitamin K deficiency bleeding: it manifests in the first 24 hours of life and is almost exclusively linked to maternal use of specific medications interfering with vitamin K stores or function. These medications include anticonvulsants, antibiotics, antitubercular drugs, and vitamin K antagonists. Common sites of bleeding are IC, intrathoracic, and intra-abdominal.

Classic vitamin K deficiency bleeding: it is the most common pattern of bleeding due to VKD in the exclusively breastfed neonates. It usually manifests on 2nd or 3rd day (range 1–7 days) after birth; infant usually bleeds from umbilical stump, gastrointestinal tract (GIT), nose, after surgical procedure or puncture sites for sampling.

Late vitamin K deficiency bleeding: bleeding manifests between 2 weeks and 8 weeks, and rarely up to 16 weeks in almost exclusively breastfed infants. Infants with hepatobiliary disease, cystic fibrosis, or those on prolonged broad-spectrum antibiotics are more predisposed to VKDB. Bleeding sites include IC vessels, GIT, skin, and mucus membranes.

Diagnosis

Association of predisposing factors, age of onset of bleeding, and well looking child are some clinical clues to the diagnosis. Coagulation tests reveal a substantial prolongation of prothrombin time and partial thromboplastin time.

Fibrinogen, D-dimer, and platelet counts are normal. An immunologic test for noncarboxylated prothrombin called PIVKA-II test (protein-induced vitamin K absence) is positive. This test is rarely required to diagnose VKDB, but because it remains positive for up to 3 days following treatment with vitamin K, it can be valuable to confirm the diagnosis in case the treatment has been instituted prior to the diagnostic tests. Rapid correction of coagulation parameters within 0.5–2 hours of parenteral vitamin K administration is also diagnostic of VKD.

Treatment

Administer 1–2 mg of vitamin K, IV or subcutaneously (no IM injections due to risk of hematoma formation). In life-threatening hemorrhage, vitamin K should be followed with 10–20 mL/kg of fresh-frozen plasma. In case of shock, whole blood should be transfused.

Prevention

American Academy of Pediatrics recommends 1 mg vitamin K to all neonates at birth for prevention of VKDB. In preterm and LBW babies, the dose is 0.5 mg. Mothers of babies at risk for early VKDB should be given 10 mg vitamin K and such babies should receive 2 mg vitamin K prophylaxis at birth. Infants at risk of late VKDB should be given periodic vitamin K prophylaxis; weekly in babies on TPN and prolonged antibiotics; and monthly in those with malabsorption and hepatobiliary disease.[6]

PERINATAL TRAUMA OR BIRTH INJURIES

Definition

It is define as avoidable or unavoidable injury occurring *in utero*, intrapartum, or during resuscitation, resulting in an impairment of the body structure or function in a newly born baby.[3]

Types of Birth Injury

- Head and neck injuries
- CNS and peripheral nervous system injuries
- Birth fractures
- Visceral injuries.

Predisposing Factors

- Intrapartum asphyxia
- Short stature of mother
- Cephalopelvic disproportion
- Prolonged or precipitate labor
- Oligohydramnios
- Malpresentation
- Instrumentation
- Macrosomia
- Prematurity
- Congenital malformations
- Inexperienced obstetrician
- Osteoporosis in the fetus (for birth fractures).

Head and Neck Injuries

- Abrasions, lacerations, and incisional injuries: these injuries occur due to malpositioned fetal monitoring electrode, fetal blood sampling, forceps or vacuum-assisted deliveries, or accidental incisions in cesarean section. Increased venous congestion and pressure during delivery can cause petechiae, bruising, retinal, and subconjunctival hemorrhages
- Extracranial hemorrhages: these include caput succedaneum, cephalohematoma, and subgaleal or subaponeurotic bleed
  - Caput succedaneum is formed over the presenting part of the head as a result of subcutaneous fluid collection and some extraperiosteal blood. It has poorly defined margins, crosses suture lines and resolves in 2–3 days after birth
  - Cephalohematoma is a subperiosteal hematoma, appears after birth, is limited by suture lines, and may have underlying skull fracture in 5–20% cases. It resolves in 8–12 weeks and may get calcified. Large size cephalohematoma predisposes to neonatal hyperbilirubinemia
  - Subgaleal hematoma is a bleed under the aponeurosis of the scalp, may cover the whole scalp from orbital ridges to the nape of neck resulting in massive blood loss and shock. Hyperbilirubinemia may be a later complication
- Intracranial bleeds: these occur in the form of subdural and intracerebral hemorrhages. Usually present as irritability, cerebral depression, circulatory instability due to hypovolemia, or its effects on the autonomic nervous system and bulging anterior fontanel. It can be diagnosed with ultrasonography
- Sternomastoid tumor: it is also called congenital or muscular torticollis. It is noted as firm, 1–2 cm mass in the midportion of the sternomastoid muscle with torticollis of the neck on the affected side. It is due to presence of hematoma as a result of trauma (hyperextension and rupture of some muscle fibers) which may subsequently lead to fibrosis and shortening. Mother should be advised to stretch the muscle several times a day by turning the baby's head with lateral flexion towards opposite, i.e., normal side. Surgical correction is required if it persists beyond 6–12 months.

Central Nervous System and Peripheral Nervous System Injuries

Central nervous system injury usually occurs as IC bleed described above. Rarely spinal cord transaction may occur following difficulty breech extraction and may be associated with cervical spine fracture. It presents as flaccid paraplegia, respiratory failure, urinary retention with overflow, and dull or absent sensations below the site of lesion. Facial nerve palsy of lower motor neuron type is the most common cranial nerve injury secondary to birth trauma. It may or may not be related to forceps application. It is commonly injured at its exit from stylomastoid foramen due to compression by forceps or pressure on the nerve against the sacral promontory of the mother. It presents as facial asymmetry on crying. It usually resolves after about a week. Care of the eye on the affected side is important to avoid exposure keratitis. Phrenic nerve injury can occur in breech and difficult forceps deliveries due to stretching as a result of hyperextension. It results in paralysis of ipsilateral diaphragm with persistent tachypnea, respiratory distress, and decreased breath sounds at the lung base. X-ray of chest reveals elevated diaphragm on the affected side.[3]

Brachial plexus injuries occur due to excessive traction on head, neck, and shoulder. Cervical dystocia, breech presentation, and macrosomia are important predisposing factors. The nerves are compressed within the nerve sheath due to hemorrhage and edema. In severe cases, there may be avulsion of nerve from the spinal cord. It is mostly unilateral and 2 times more common on the right side. Most frequent of brachial plexus injuries involve upper trunk (C5, 6 ± 7) and it is called Erb-Duchenne palsy. Weakness of the deltoid, biceps, brachioradialis, and supinator muscles result in classical posture of the limb as tight adduction and internal rotation at shoulder, extension and pronation at elbow and if C7 is also involved it will in addition have exaggerated flexion of wrist and fingers (policeman taking bribe). Next common is global plexus paralysis involving entire brachial plexus (C5-T1), resulting in complete paralysis and flaccid upper limb. The mororesponse is asymmetrical in these injuries. Finally, the least common isolated brachial plexus injury is Klumpke paralysis (C8, T1) presenting as flaccid hand with absent grasp reflex. It may also be a manifestation of residual global plexus injury.[6]

The early treatment of brachial plexus injury is conservative and consists of physiotherapy to prevent contractures. The arm should be kept in natural position avoiding over immobilization. Passive exercises should be started after swelling has subsided (usually 5–7 days). Gentle handling of the limb is important to avoid additional injury to the plexus. Prognosis depends upon the severity of injury. Complete recovery usually occurs in neurapraxia over several weeks. When there is neurotmesis or complete avulsion, no recovery takes place. Electromyogram and nerve conduction may be required to differentiate the two at a later date, if the recovery is poor or nil. Prognosis is poor in Klumpke and global plexus injuries. Complete recovery is almost unlikely if the biceps function recovers later than 3 months. Neuroplasty is indicated if paralysis does not recover by 3 months.

Birth Fractures

Birth fractures most commonly involve the clavicle, followed by humerus and femur. Fractures of clavicle and humerus are due to arm extension, often required in shoulder dystocia and breech deliveries. The obstetrician who hears or feels a snap when the diaphysis breaks while the baby is being extracted can generally make the diagnosis. Crepitus, bony irregularity, and pseudoparalysis of the limb are presenting features. Radiographs confirm the diagnosis. Ultrasound examination to detect the proximal humeral physeal separation is indicated if the X-ray of the upper limb is normal. The natural history of isolated birth fractures of the extremities is that of uneventful rapid healing without untoward sequelae. The fractures of clavicle (displaced) and humerus are treated by strapping the arm to the chest with a soft padding in between the two. Elbow is kept flexed at 90°. Strapping is kept for 8–10 days after which the callus is sufficient for immobilization to be discontinued. Fractures of femoral shaft can be held with a posterior splint which extends below the knee to the waist and is held in place with an elastic bandage for 10–14 days.[9]

Visceral Injuries

Liver and spleen are common viscera which get injured during birth or overenthusiastic chest compression during resuscitation. These may present as abdominal distension, upper abdomen lump, discoloration and even shock at birth or within few days of birth. Early clinical recognition and confirmation on ultrasound abdomen is crucial for appropriate management and favorable outcome.

REFERENCES

1. Singh M. Care of the Newborn. 7th ed. New Delhi: Sagar Publications; 2010.
2. Dhar S. Colour Atlas of Pediatric Dermatology. 2nd ed. New Delhi: Jaypee Brothers Medical Publishers; 2007.
3. Gupte S. Textbook of Neonatal Emergencies. 1st ed. New Delhi: Peepee Publishers and Distributors; 2006.
4. Gupte S. Recent Advances in Pediatrics: Pediatric Hematology (Special Volume 20). 1st ed. New Delhi: Jaypee Brothers Medical Publishers; 2009.
5. American Academy of Pediatrics. Pediatric Clinical Practice Guidelines, 13th ed. (reprint). New Delhi: Jaypee Brothers Medical Publishers; 2013.

6. MacDonald MG, Seshia MMK, Mullett MD. Avery's neonatology: Pathophysiology and management of the newborn. 6th ed. New Delhi: Wolters Kluwer (India) Pvt. Ltd; 2005 (Indian reprint 2014).
7. Bhatia V, Bavdekar A, Matthai J, Waikar Y, Sibal A. Management of neonatal cholestasis: consensus statement of the Pediatric Gastroenterology Chapter of Indian Academy of Pediatrics. Indian Pediatr. 2014;51(3):203-10.
8. Gupte S. Recent advances in pediatrics: nutrition, growth and development (Special Volume 21). 1st ed. New Delhi: Jaypee Brothers Medical Publishers; 2011.
9. Taeuschm HW, Ballard RA, Gleason CA. Avery's diseases of the newborn. 8th ed. New Delhi: Elsevier; 2005.

Section 6

Obstetrical Complications

CHAPTER 35

Preterm Labor

Parikshit D Tank

INTRODUCTION

The definition of spontaneous preterm labor is labor resulting in birth before 37 completed weeks (259 days) of gestational age. Signs of immaturity at birth and shorter than average gestational length have an unusually high incidence in *Homo sapiens* when compared with other mammals. This has been attributed to the development of a narrow pelvis, following the evolution to a bipedal gait, coupled with the more recent development of a large brain and head associated with the acquisition of language and social skills.[1] This combination results in a relatively high incidence of obstructed labor, which favors an evolutionary trend towards earlier birth.

DEFINITION

Preterm delivery is defined as delivery between 20 weeks and 37 weeks of pregnancy. This period has been further divided to stratify risk and management decisions. This is presented in table 1.

A woman is said to be in preterm labor based on clinical criteria of regular uterine contractions accompanied by a change in cervical status (dilation, effacement, or both) or initial presentation with regular contractions and cervical dilation of at least 2 cm. Less than 10% of women with the clinical diagnosis of preterm labor actually give birth within 7 days of presentation.[2] This reflects the low threshold at which preterm labor is diagnosed in clinical settings.

TABLE 1: Preterm birth terminology by gestational age

Gestational age	Terminology
Before 24 completed weeks	Previable birth or abortion
25–28 weeks	Extreme preterm birth
29–32 weeks	Very preterm birth
33–37 weeks	Late preterm births

MAGNITUDE OF THE PROBLEM

The main burden of preterm birth exists in developing countries. There are no accurate recent worldwide data, but estimates of preterm birth rates range from 5% in developed countries to 18% in developing countries.[2] India has the largest number of preterm births in the world. In 2010, this was estimated at about 3.5 million preterm births per year.[3] Even in developed countries, where the rate of preterm labor and delivery is below 10%, they account for a disproportionately high 75% of neonatal deaths. The greatest etiological factor worldwide is infection, mainly due to malaria and human immunodeficiency virus.[4] In developed countries, iatrogenic delivery is responsible for almost half of the births between 28 and 35 weeks and hypertension is a major contributor to these decisions. This chapter explores the essential etiopathology, clinical dilemmas, and evidence that guide management of preterm labor in contemporary obstetrics. This chapter will exclude extreme preterm labor before 24 weeks since it falls outside the purview of the third trimester.

ETIOPATHOLOGY

Labor is believed to be a result of biochemical, endocrine, and anatomical changes working towards a common pathway. Preterm labor represents a pathological activation of this pathway. The chief underlying factors responsible for the initiation of preterm labor are:

Infections of the Genital Tract

Bacterial vaginosis is seen in 10–40% of pregnant women. About 45% of them will have upper genital tract colonization as well. Clinical and more commonly subclinical chorioamnionitis activates the preterm delivery pathway. This usually occurs in preterm births before 32 weeks of gestation. In support of this hypothesis, there is evidence that infection screening and treatment programs in pregnant women may reduce preterm birth and preterm low-birth-weights.[5]

Inflammation

This results in the activation of a number of cytokines and chemokines which, in turn, may trigger preterm contractions, cervical ripening, labor, and rupture of the membranes, especially at early gestation (<30 weeks). More than 50 cytokines and chemokines have been studied, of which interleukin (IL)-6 and IL-8 are significantly associated with preterm births. Though the usual site of initiation the inflammatory response is the cervicovaginal tract, inflammation anywhere in the body has the potential to trigger preterm labor. This has been demonstrated in the correlation with systemic infection and inflammation such as malaria[4] and focal infection such as periodontal disease.[6]

Alterations in the Fetal Membranes

Changes in the structure and extracellular matrix homeostasis can cause weakness of the membranes and rupture before term. Preterm prelabor rupture of membranes is responsible for 30% of spontaneous preterm births. A mechanism involving the activation of matrix metalloproteinases-9, a 92-kDa type IV collagenase, as an essential mediator of tissue damage is under investigation. It is probably mediated by bacterial products, cytokines and other para- and autocrine signals.[7]

Changes in Cervical Competence

Before labor (term or preterm begins), there is a remodeling of the cervical structure, by reorientation and changes in the integrity of collagen fibers. This is a result of alteration in the content of water, proteoglycans, and hyaluronic acid. These morphological changes are exaggerated and early in onset when the cervix is anatomically deficient or the changes have been initiated by infective and inflammatory events.[8] Preterm labor has been thought to be a continuum of an incompetent cervix.

Genetic Factors

Several lines of evidence support a genetic predisposition to spontaneous preterm labor and preterm birth. A leading risk factor for spontaneous preterm labor and preterm birth is a personal or family history. Women who are themselves born preterm are at the highest risk for giving preterm births. This predisposition is not seen with fathers who are born preterm. The frequent association of spontaneous preterm labor and preterm birth with histological infection/inflammation and elevated body fluid concentrations of inflammatory cytokines has focused investigations on single gene polymorphisms of these cytokines in both mother and fetus. The polymorphisms tumor necrosis factor-α-308, IL-1H þ 3953/3954 and IL-6-174 have been most consistently associated with spontaneous preterm labor and preterm birth. Maternal and fetal polymorphisms of the toll-like receptor-4 gene have also been implicated in this mechanism.[9]

PREDICTION OF PRETERM LABOR

The primary predictors for spontaneous labor and preterm birth currently used are based on either risk factors (e.g., socioeconomic, history, lifestyle) or clinical information that becomes available during the course of pregnancy (e.g., digital cervical examination, uterine contractions, bleeding). The benefits of considering these factors in prenatal surveillance have not yet been demonstrated. In recent years, new markers for the risk of preterm birth have been proposed as primary predictors in low-risk populations. These biological markers include cervical ultrasound, fetal fibronectin, salivary estriol, and others. They may be more relevant than standard markers and thereby improve the efficacy of our management of spontaneous preterm labor by enabling more precise and earlier diagnosis.

Standard Predictors of Preterm Labor

Traditionally, a number of scoring systems comprising of demographic, socioeconomic, psychological characteristics, and pregnancy events have been proposed.[10] Results with these systems have been equivocal, and in general, their use is cumbersome. Certain features are more useful than others in predicting preterm labor. The most important one seems to be a prior preterm birth. The other parameters are summarized in table 2.[11] In an American study assessing the value of risk factors in predicting preterm labor, 2,929 women from the general population were studied. After analysis of more than 100 parameters, the criteria retained in the model were race, history of preterm birth, low body mass index, uterine contractions in the past 2 weeks, vaginal bleeding during pregnancy, and a high Bishop's score. Unfortunately, this score still identifies only a minority of the women who will give birth preterm. The sensitivity was 24.2% for nulliparae and 18.2% for multiparae, with positive predictive values of 28.6% and 33.3%, respectively.[12]

Newer Predictors of Preterm Labor

In pursuit of better predictors of preterm labor, a number of biological phenomena (structural and biochemical) which

TABLE 2: Risk factors for preterm labor and possibility of prevention[11]

	Association with SPB	Possibility of intervention
Demographic risk factors		
Black	+	No
Young age (<19 years)	+	Yes
Lives alone	+	No
Domestic violence	++	Yes
Low socioeconomic class	++	?
Stress, depression, life events	++	Yes
Hard work (>42 h/week, >6 h standing/day)	++	Yes
No/inadequate antenatal care	++	Yes
Smoking/cocaine use	+	Yes
Short stature, low body mass index before pregnancy	+	No
Weight gain during pregnancy	–	–
Alcohol use	–	–
Risk factors on reproductive health history		
PTD or second trimester pregnancy loss	++++	Yes
Family history of PTD (maternal)	++	No
Previous cone biopsy of the cervix	?+	–
Müllerian anomalies	+	Yes
Parity	–	–
Short interval between pregnancies	–	–
Risk factors in present pregnancy		
ART conception	++	No
Twins	++	?
High-order multiple pregnancies	++++	Yes
Placenta previa	++	No
Bleeding in two trimesters	++	No
Cervicovaginal infection	++	Yes
Uterine contractions	+	Yes
Cervical dilatation and effacement	++	Yes

SPB, spontaneous preterm birth; PTD, preterm delivery; ART, assisted reproductive technique.

precede preterm labor have been studied. Their performance has been outlined in table 3.

Cervical Ultrasound

There is a gradual relationship between the length of the cervix and the risk of preterm birth. The relative risk of birth before 35 weeks of gestation is 14-fold higher if the cervical length (CL) is below the 1st percentile and ninefold higher if it is below the 5th percentile.[13] Digital cervical examination is not reproducible or standardized compared to ultrasound assessment. The cervix should be assessed by transvaginal ultrasound rather than transabdominal imaging. The CL, internal os diameter and shape of the junction of the uterus and internal os (T, V, U, or Y-shaped) should be assessed. Optimal cutoff values for CL varied between individual studies and ranged between 25 and 35 mm. Earlier screening has been sought in order to improve the success of a cerclage procedure.[14]

Fetal Fibronectin

Fetal fibronectin (FFN) is an extracellular glycoprotein located on the decidua and the fetal membranes, secreted at the maternal-fetal interface by the trophoblast. Once the membranes fuse at 22 weeks, FFN is not normally released in vaginal mucus except when the membranes are disrupted. FFN is found in cervicovaginal secretions of women in preterm labor either by the separation of chorion from deciduae or by secretion in the cervical canal as a result of inflammation. FFN-based tests are quantitative or qualitative. The qualitative tests are bedside and give an instant result which is more in keeping with clinical needs. The main value seems to be the negative predictive value in LR symptomatic women.[15] A negative test is reassuring and could prevent unnecessary hospitalization, tocolysis, and other interventions.

Salivary Estriol

Estriol is essentially a fetal product. Its plasma concentration rises throughout pregnancy. Plasma and salivary estriol levels peak 3–5 weeks before the onset of preterm or term labor. The estriol concentration in saliva very precisely reflects the free-estriol concentration in plasma. The advantages of saliva are

TABLE 3: Performance of new primary predictors of preterm labor in low-risk women

References	Preterm delivery (%)	Number of patients	Sensitivity	Specificity	LR (+)	LR (+)
Iams[13] (24 weeks)						
CL ≤25 mm	4.3	2,195	37	92	4.6	0.7
CL ≤30 mm			54	76	2.3	0.6
Protrusion			25	94	4.2	0.8

LR (+), likelihood ratio for positive test result; LR (–), likelihood ratio for negative test result; CL, cervical length; FFN, fetal fibronectin.

the ease and noninvasiveness of its collection, the stability of the concentration during transport and a reliable and reproducible assay technique.[16]

Other Biological Markers

A number of new biological markers such as corticotrophin-releasing hormone (CRH), IL-6 assay from the blood and cervicovaginal secretions, β-human chorionic gonadotropin, α-fetoprotein, and glycoproteins, such as activin, inhibin, and relaxin, are being studied. Their role is not well defined at present and further research is required to identify clinically relevant markers. Ambulatory uterine contraction monitoring has not shown to be effective in predicting preterm labor.

Use of Multiple Markers

As the current evidence stands, no marker has yet been shown to fulfill the requirements of an ideal screening test for preterm labor. Hence, multiple marker tests based on combinations of several independent markers have been proposed. Cervical ultrasound and FFN have a potentially additive effect as markers and should be studied in combination. Crane et al. assessed 140 LR women between 20 and 24 weeks.[17] A preterm birth risk score includes previous preterm delivery, multiple gestation, suspected preterm labor, bleeding after 12 weeks, cervical dilatation more than 1 cm, and CL less than 1 cm. The preterm birth score was combined with FFN. Similarly, the value of a combination of cervical ultrasound and FFN has been studied in order to predict preterm birth at different gestational ages.[18] The results of this study are presented in tables 4 and 5.

PREVENTION TOOLS

The ideal goal to prevent preterm births is to prevent preterm labor. Though a number of interventions have been proposed, there is no consensus on their utility or rationale. General measures, such as smoking and tobacco cessation and modifying hard physical activity including long durations of standing, are part of routine antenatal care. Also, the management of infections, such as malaria and acquired immunodeficiency syndrome reduces the risk of preterm birth.[4] This advice should be uniform for all pregnant women irrespective of risk stratification of preterm birth.

TABLE 4: Cervical length, fetal fibronectin, and the risk of preterm delivery in nulliparous women[18]

	Delivery <32 weeks (%)	Delivery <35 weeks (%)	Delivery <37 weeks (%)
Both tests negative	0.6	1.7	6
CL ≤25 mm	3.7	9.2	18.4
FFN positive	3.9	5.8	11.5
Both tests positive	35.3	58.8	64.7

CL, Cervical Length; FFN, Fetal Fibronectin.

TABLE 5: Cervical length, fetal fibronectin, and the risk of preterm delivery in multiparous women with or without previous spontaneous preterm birth[18]

	Delivery <32 weeks (%)	Delivery <35 weeks (%)	Delivery <37 weeks (%)
All markers negative	0.5	1.5	7.3
Previous SPB alone	1.8	8.6	17.6
Previous SPB and CL ≤25 mm	8.3	29.2	35.4
Previous SPB and FFN positive	24	40	48
All markers positive	50	60	60

SPB, spontaneous preterm birth; CL, cervical length; FFN, fetal fibronectin.

Bed rest

One of the most commonly prescribed prophylactic and/or therapeutic interventions in obstetrics is bed rest. This is true for preterm labor as well. However, as in other conditions, the value of bed rest is questionable. There is no evidence-based comparison for this intervention. In four randomized trials of hospitalization and bed rest for the prevention and/or treatment of preterm delivery in twin pregnancies, two found no benefit and two found an increased risk of preterm births.[19] It is prudent to advise limitation of physical activity and sexual intercourse. However, there is no benefit from bed rest.

Antibiotics

Empiric therapy with antibiotics prescribed systemically or vaginally is not likely to be of benefit in preventing preterm labor or preterm births. It may of use for a select population with symptoms of vaginal discharge, examination findings suggestive of mixed vaginitis, a previous history of midtrimester loss or early preterm labor and births.[5] Vaginal administration of clindamycin and oral metronidazole are recommended.

Cervical Cerclage

The critical factor in determining the effectiveness of cervical cerclage as an intervention to prevent preterm births hinges on patient selection. Its overuse is common. A well selected, deserving population has much to gain by a cervical cerclage. At present, the most objective tool to assess women is a transvaginal ultrasound. A meta-analysis of four randomized trials involving over 600 women found that for women carrying a singleton and a previous preterm birth showed that cervical cerclage was an effective intervention when CL was less than 25 mm.[20] The Royal College of Obstetricians and Gynecologists has recommendations along similar lines.[21]

Progesterone

One of the most ubiquitously prescribed molecules in obstetric practice is progesterone in some form or the other. The rationale for progesterone as an agent for prevention arises from its role in maintaining uterine quiescence, the theory of progesterone withdrawal leading to onset of labor and the use of anti-progesterones to induce labor. For the prevention of preterm birth, the current evidence suggests that it is effective in women with a previous preterm birth or have a short CL (<25 mm). Even in this well selected population, the number needed to treat is 10 to prevent one preterm birth. It should be started in the early second trimester and should be continued till 34–36 weeks. Progesterone may be administered as a weekly injection of 250 mg of 17-α-hydroxyprogesterone caproate or a daily application of 90 mg of vaginal gel of progesterone. It is not effective as a tocolytic agent once preterm labor has begun or as a follow-up therapy.[22]

DIAGNOSIS OF THREATENED OR ESTABLISHED PRETERM LABOR

The diagnosis of preterm labor is challenging. Less than half the women who are admitted with established preterm labor and only 10% of those admitted with suspected or threatened preterm labor actually have a preterm birth.[2] The criteria to diagnose and treat women are difficult to establish because of a low threshold for diagnosis and intervention and low rate of eventual outcomes (preterm birth). As such, in clinical practice, symptomatology (pain, contractions, vaginal discharge, and show) and obstetric examination findings (palpable contractions, cervical dilatation, and effacement) are used to make the diagnosis. Some clinicians prefer a speculum examination to a digital vaginal examination. This is especially of note in women who have ruptured membranes. Even though latency may be reduced by digital examination, it should be performed when there is doubt. One or two digital examinations undertaken in an aseptic manner in the course of the expectant management even in the presence of ruptured membranes do not worsen the maternal or neonatal outcome.[23]

Initial Evaluation and Laboratory Tests in Preterm Labor

The priorities in evaluating a woman and her fetus with preterm labor in the third trimester are:

- Establish the gestational age and/or fetal maturity: gestational age should be established as per the menstrual dates and an early ultrasound date. Fetal maturity testing is generally not advised when the gestational age is established. There is no greater predictive value of measuring the lecithin to sphingomyelin ratio (L:S) or the lamellar body count in predicting fetal lung maturity.[24] If the gestational age is not established and there is doubt about maturity, it would be prudent to assume that the fetus is not mature and manage conservatively
- Evaluate maternal and fetal wellbeing: the initial evaluation is done by a clinical examination and electronic fetal monitoring. Acute complications, such as abruption placentae, intrauterine infection, cord compression, or prolapse, would require urgent intervention. Rupture of membranes should be ruled out since this is commonly associated with preterm labor and changes the interventions to be offered. In other women, further assessment based on a complete blood count, C-reactive protein, and ultrasound should be done. Ultrasound measurements should be compared to previous growth parameters if available to look for intrauterine growth restriction (IUGR). There is an association between IUGR and preterm delivery based on risk factors and epidemiological evidence.[25] If growth restriction is identified, it should be further evaluated using color Doppler of the utero- and fetoplacental circulations.

DECISION MAKING IN PRETERM LABOR–MANAGEMENT ISSUES

Preterm labor presents the clinician with a number of medical, infrastructure, and social issues which all weigh into the ultimate decision-making process. In general, the reasons to wait and prolong the pregnancy and enhance fetal maturity, allow corticosteroids and antibiotics to act and allow *in utero* transfer where indicated. Early intervention and proceeding to delivery is more rational when the fetus is nearly mature, labor is so far advanced that intervention would not be of use to stop labor from progressing and to prevent fetal complications. The medical decision to intervene with tocolytics and corticosteroids should be taken judiciously. In some situations, it may be beneficial to allow delivery rather than conserve the pregnancy. These are outlined in table 6. Interventions are thought to be unnecessary or counterproductive if the gestational age is more than 34 weeks or less than 24 weeks. In addition, contraindications to particular tocolytics or steroids should also be considered.

It is also necessary to consider the available obstetric, surgical, and neonatal facilities in managing these women. If the gestational age is lower than what can be managed at the existing care setting, it is necessary to consider an *in utero* transfer. It is safer for the neonate to be transported in the mother before delivery, rather than *ex utero*. The feasibility of an *in utero* transfer would depend on the distance to the tertiary-care facility, available transport, and state of labor.

TABLE 6: Contraindications to conservative management in preterm labor

Maternal indicators	Chorioamnionitis diagnosed clinically by fever >100.4 in addition to two other criteria such as: • Uterine tenderness • Maternal or fetal tachycardia • Foul/purulent amniotic fluid • Leukocytosis
Obstetric indicators	• >34 weeks or <24 weeks • Severe preeclampsia • Placental abruption • Cord prolapse • Malpresentation
Abnormal fetal wellbeing tests	• Fetal demise or lethal anomaly • Nonreactive nonstress test (persistent fetal tachycardia, variable decelerations) • Low biophysical profile score • Severe oligohydramnios

Tocolysis

An editorial in the *British Medical Journal* had very appropriately summarized the role of tocolysis in obstetric practice. It said that the use of tocolytics in preterm labor was frequently unnecessary, often ineffective, and occasionally harmful.[26] Even though the editorial is from 1969, it rings true today. Tocolysis, even after years of empiric use has not shown to clearly reduce perinatal or neonatal mortality or serious neonatal morbidity. The number of women who deliver preterm is not remarkably different whether tocolysis is used or not. The main effect of tocolytic drugs is to reduce the numbers who deliver within 48 hours or 7 days of commencing the drug. Data on long-term outcome are limited. Therefore, it is probable that the benefits of tocolysis are essentially limited to women who need the action of corticosteroids for fetal maturity or *in utero* transfer.[27] However, even these benefits have not been formally evaluated in randomized trials.

There is no particular tocolytic agent which is better than another. The main classes and their salient features are outlined in table 7.[19,28] Betamimetic agents are the most popular in clinical settings. However, the choice, based on safety profile, is to use calcium-channel blockers or atosiban. At the time of writing, the latter is not marketed in India.

There is no role for maintenance therapy with tocolytic agents. Their prolonged use does not reduce the number of preterm births or associated neonatal morbidity. This has been shown in a meta-analysis comparing magnesium sulfate versus β-mimetics or placebo.[29] Atosiban may have some role in maintenance therapy. A study showed benefits in comparison to placebo in terms of prolonging pregnancy.[30] However, availability and cost remain concerns.

Antenatal Corticosteroids

The singlemost useful intervention in preterm labor is the administration of corticosteroids to the mother. It is universally endorsed as an intervention to reduce neonatal morbidity and mortality in preterm births.[28,31] Corticosteroids should be given for gestations between 24 weeks and 34 weeks. Women who are at risk for delivery in the next 7 days should be given a course of corticosteroids. The corticosteroids are to be administered irrespective of membrane status. There are very few contraindications and barring chorioamnionitis, systemic sepsis and wide spread tuberculosis, they can be used safely in all clinical settings. Betamethasone and dexamethasone can be used. Other corticosteroids, such as cortisone and prednisolone, do not cross the placenta adequately and are not used. Parenteral route is associated with fewer systemic side effects and is preferred over the oral route. Either betamethasone or dexamethasone is administered as two doses of 12 mg intramuscularly 24 hours apart or four 6 mg doses given every 12 hours. In the past, there was a practice of repeating the course every week. However, this is no longer recommended. Only one course of steroids is sufficient. Recently, some data is emerging that a rescue dose of steroids may be considered for women whose pregnancies continue for more than a week after the initial course and are less than 34 weeks when delivery becomes subsequently imminent.[32] Corticosteroids have immense benefits in reducing neonatal mortality. Neonates whose mothers have received a course of corticosteroids have significantly lower frequency and severity of respiratory distress syndrome, intracranial hemorrhage, necrotizing enterocolitis, and death. There is also some benefit in reducing the risk of retinopathy of prematurity and platelet dysfunction. Betamethasone may be marginally better than dexamethasone in reducing the risk of periventricular leukomalacia.[33] The efficacy of corticosteroids may be reduced in neonates of diabetic mothers, twins, and those who are hydropic. However, administration is still advised. Despite the well-established efficacy and recommendations, the use of this intervention is not optimal. Only about half the women who are eligible to receive them are given corticosteroids. Implementation research and contextualized health policies are needed to improve drug availability and increase compliance with best obstetric practice.[34]

Antibiotics

Bacterial infection and inflammation is believed to play an important role in the etiopathogenesis in the initiation of preterm labor, especially at early gestations (<32 weeks). This was the rationale for antibiotic therapy as a measure to prolong latency in women with preterm labor. However, a meta-analysis of eight randomized trials has shown that antibiotic is not better than placebo in increasing latency and

TABLE 7: Tocolytic agents for preterm labor–an overview

Class and mechanism	Agent and initial dose	Contraindications	Maternal side effects	Fetal side effects	Comment
β-mimetic agents	• Terbutaline 10 µg/min IV • Ritodrine 50 µg/min IV • Isoxsuprine 200 µg/min IV	• Tachycardia-sensitive maternal conditions (severe anemia, heart disease, hyperthyroidism), diabetes mellitus	• Tachycardia, hypotension, palpitations, tremors, shortness of breath, chest discomfort, pulmonary edema, hypokalemia, hyperglycemia	• Tachycardia	• Administer by infusion pump • Monitor fluid and electrolyte balance and cardiac rhythm
Calcium-channel blocker	• Nifedipine 10–20 mg oral followed by doses every 2–4 hourly	• Hypotension, preload-dependent maternal cardiac lesions such as aortic stenosis	• Dizziness, flushing, bradycardia, hypotension, raised hepatic enzymes	• Not known	• Monitor blood pressure; caution advised when combined with magnesium sulfate
Calcium antagonist	• Magnesium sulfate 4 g loading dose IM followed by 1 g/h	• Muscle weakness, myasthenia gravis	• Flushing, diaphoresis, nausea, loss of deep tendon reflexes, respiratory depression, cardiac arrest	• Neonatal depression	• Monitor blood pressure, urine output, deep tendon reflexes and respiratory rate
NSAIDs	• Indomethacin 50 mg oral followed by 25 mg 6 hourly	• Asthma, gastritis, renal or hepatic dysfunction, low platelet count, bleeding disorders	• Nausea, emesis, gastritis, reflux, platelet dysfunction	• *In utero* constriction of the ductus and patent ductus arteriosus in the neonate, oligohydramnios, necrotizing enterocolitis	• Avoid after 32 weeks or for more than 48 hour; may be considered when polyhydramnios is associated
Oxytocin antagonist	• Atosiban initial IV bolus of 6.75 mg followed by 300 µg/min	• Known hypersensitivity	• Nausea, vomiting, flushing, tachycardia, pruritus	• Not known	• Limited availability, experience

NSAIDs, non-steroidal anti-inflammatory drugs; IV, intravenous; IM, intramuscularly.

delaying preterm birth. There is no reduction in respiratory distress, necrotizing enterocolitis, or neonatal sepsis. There was a small nonstatistically significant benefit towards fewer maternal infections.[35] Antibiotics are not recommended in preterm labor with intact membranes. This is distinct from the recommendations for their use in women with ruptured membranes or documented group B streptococcus infection. In these women, erythromycin, ampicillin, or a cephalosporin may be used.

Magnesium Sulfate for Neuroprotection

There is growing evidence that the administration of magnesium sulfate reduces the risk of adverse neurological outcomes in the neonate. The early observations arose from the studies where magnesium sulfate was used as a tocolytic agent or as an anticonvulsant in preeclampsia/eclampsia. Subsequently, randomized trials have been conducted with the intent to study its neuroprotective effect in preterm births. The most commonly used regimen is to give a loading dose of 4 g slow intravenous followed by an infusion of 1 g/h for a period of 24 hours. Shorter regimens using only the loading dose or infusion for 12 hours are also effective. There is a reduction in intraventricular hemorrhage, stillbirths, neonatal deaths, and cerebral palsy at follow up of 2 years. The maximum benefit was found for neonates who were delivered before 32 weeks of gestation. Maternal side effects such as local reactions were noted, serious problems such as cardiac arrest or respiratory depression were not seen.[36] Further studies are required to confirm these beneficial effects in larger populations and to establish the optimum protocol for its use.

Labor and Delivery in Preterm Gestation

The greatest improvements in neonatal outcomes of preterm births have occurred because of developments in neonatal care. The delivery should be conducted in the presence of an experienced and trained neonatologist. Resuscitation equipment should be readily available and checked before birth. The neonatal care facility should be in close proximity to the site of delivery.

The route of delivery does not have a major impact on neonatal outcomes in preterm birth. A meta-analysis of six studies including 122 women compared outcomes in women who were allocated to immediate cesarean section or planned vaginal delivery in preterm labor. There was no difference in neonatal outcomes such as Apgar score less than 7 at 5 minutes, birth asphyxia, hypoxic ischemic encephalopathy, birth trauma, or neonatal seizures. Maternal outcomes were better in the group which was planned for vaginal delivery with a significantly lower risk of serious postpartum complications, admission to intensive care, and puerperal pyrexia.[37]

In labor, the aim is to optimize maternal and neonatal condition at birth. Epidural analgesia can be offered. Augmentation of labor with oxytocin should be judicious since the fetal reserves and tolerance to strong uterine contractions is less as compared to a term fetus. Continuous electronic fetal monitoring should ideally be available and offered. Fetal scalp electrodes should be avoided. A timely episiotomy can cut short the second stage. If instrumentation is required, forceps delivery is preferred over a ventouse. The ventouse may add to the risk of scalp hemorrhage, hematomas, and intraventricular hemorrhage.[19]

For fetuses in breech presentation, there seems to be benefit from a cesarean delivery. A systematic review of non-randomized studies involving a total of 3,557 women, found the weighted risk of neonatal mortality to be 3.8% in the cesarean group and 11.5% in the vaginal delivery group.[38] This difference could be ascribed to delivery of the fetus at less than 32 weeks gestation. A breech presentation at this time is likely to be a non-frank breech and therefore would have a higher risk of cord accidents, poor progress, manipulation, birth trauma, and head entrapment. As such, the route of delivery should be an individualized obstetric decision. However, with diminishing expertise of breech delivery available on the labor ward, it seems appropriate to offer a cesarean section as a preferred mode of delivery for a preterm viable breech presentation. A cesarean section may also be indicated for other abnormal presentations, acute complications or nonprogress of labor. Cesarean section may be difficult at very preterm gestations. The lower segment is not formed. There is a risk of neonatal and maternal trauma. Extensions may have to be made surgically or may occur accidentally. Lateral extensions could cause injuries to the uterine vessels and broad ligament hematomas. A combination of the thick lower segment, extensions, uterine manipulation, and possibility of sepsis could contribute to a higher postpartum hemorrhage risk. Appropriate preparations should be made and precautions taken to counter this.

CONCLUSION

Preterm labor and birth are a relatively frequent complication in obstetric practice. Preterm birth contributes disproportionately to neonatal morbidity and mortality. A number of etiopathological factors have been described, chiefly focusing on infection and inflammation, especially at early gestations. The standard predictive tools are epidemiological and clinical. Improvements in accuracy of prediction through ultrasound and FFN are useful in directing prophylactic measures. Preventive strategies on a population basis are the treatment of infections and smoking cessation. Specifically for women at risk, cerclage, and progesterone are useful interventions. The diagnosis of suspected or established preterm labor is clinical. The initial evaluation should establish correct gestational age and rule out acute complications. Interventions to prolong pregnancy should be weighed. Tocolytic therapy should be used in the acute phase when action of steroids is awaited or *in utero* transfer is planned. Nifedipine and atosiban are the preferred tocolytics. Antenatal corticosteroids are useful and proven in reducing neonatal morbidity and mortality. Magnesium sulfate can offer preterm fetuses neuroprotection. Labor and delivery should be managed vigilantly. There may be benefit from a cesarean delivery for the preterm breech fetus. High-quality neonatal care should be available and in attendance at every preterm birth.

REFERENCES

1. Rosenberg K, Trevethan W. Bipedalism and human birth: the obstetrical dilemma revisited. Evol Anthropol. 1995;4(5):161-8.
2. Steer P. The epidemiology of preterm labor. BJOG. 2005;112(Suppl 1):1-3.
3. Blencowe H, Cousens S, Oestergaard M, Chou D, Moller AB, Narwal R, et al. National, regional, and worldwide estimates of preterm birth rates in the year 2010 with time trends since 1990 for selected countries: a systematic analysis and implications. Lancet. 2012;379(9832):2162-72.
4. Ticconi C, Mapfumo M, Dorrucci M, Naha N, Tarira E, Pietropolli A, et al. Effect of maternal HIV and malaria infection on pregnancy and perinatal outcome in Zimbabwe. J Acquir Immune Defic Syndr. 2003;34(3):289-94.
5. Sangkomkamhang US, Lumbiganon P, Prasertcharoensuk W, Laopaiboon M. Antenatal lower genital tract infection screening and treatment programs for preventing preterm delivery. Cochrane Database Syst Rev. 2015;2:CD006178.
6. Polyzos NP, Polyzos IP, Mauri D, Tzioras S, Tsappi M, Cortinovis I, et al. Effect of periodontal disease treatment during pregnancy on preterm birth incidence: a meta-analysis of randomized trials. Am J Obstet Gynecol. 2009;200(3):225-32.
7. Vadillo-Ortega F, Sadowsky DW, Haluska GJ, Hernandez-Guerrero C, Guevara-Silva R, Gravett MG, et al. Identification of matrix metralloproteinase-9 in amniotic fluid and amniochorion in spontaneous labor and after experimental intrauterine infection or interleukin-1 beta infusion in pregnant rhesus monkeys. Am J Obstet Gynecol. 2002;186(1):128-38.
8. Lotgering FK. Clinical aspects of cervical insufficiency. BMC Pregnancy Childbirth. 2007;7(Suppl 1):S17-21.

9. Varner MW, Esplin MS. Current understanding of genetic factors in preterm birth. BJOG. 2005;112(Suppl 1):28-31.
10. Papiernik E, Kaminski M. Multifactorial study of the risk of prematurity at 32 weeks of gestation. I. A study of the frequency of 30 predictive characteristics. J Perinat Med. 1974;2(1):30-6.
11. Goffinet F. Primary predictors of preterm labor. BJOG. 2005;112(Suppl 1):38-47.
12. Mercer BM, Goldenberg RL, Das A, Moawad AH, Iams JD, Meis PJ, et al. The preterm prediction study: a clinical risk assessment system. Am J Obstet Gynecol. 1996;174(6):1885-93.
13. Iams JD, Goldenberg RL, Meis PJ, Mercer BM, Moawad A, Das A, et al. The length of the cervix and the risk of spontaneous premature delivery. National Institute of Child Health and Human Development Maternal Fetal Medicine Unit Network. N Engl J Med. 1996;334(9):562-72.
14. Honest H, Bachmann LM, Coomarasamy A, Gupta JK, Kleijnen J, Khan KS. Accuracy of cervical transvaginal sonography in predicting preterm birth: a systematic review. Ultrasound Obstet Gynecol. 2003;22(3):305-22.
15. Faron G, Boulvain M, Irion O, Bernard PM, Fraser WD. Prediction of preterm delivery by fetal fibronectin: a meta-analysis. Obstet Gynecol. 1998;92(1):153-8.
16. McGregor JA, Jackson GM, Lachelin GC, Goodwin TM, Artal R, Hastings C, et al. Salivary estriol as risk assessment for preterm labor: a prospective trial. Am J Obstet Gynecol. 1995;173(4):1337-42.
17. Crane JM, Armson BA, Dodds L, Feinberg RF, Kennedy W, Kirkland SA. Risk scoring, fetal fibronectin, and bacterial vaginosis to predict preterm delivery. Obstet Gynecol. 1999;93(4):517-22.
18. Goldenberg RL, Iams JD, Mercer BM, Meis PJ, Moawad AH, Copper RL, et al. The preterm prediction study: the value of new vs. standard risk factors in predicting early and all spontaneous preterm births. NICHD MFMU Network. Am J Public Health. 1998;88(2):233-8.
19. Goldenberg RL. The management of preterm labor. Obstet Gynecol. 2002;100(5 Pt 1):1020-37.
20. Berghella V, Keeler SM, To MS, Althuisius SM, Rust OA. Effectiveness of cerclage according to severity of cervical length shortening: a meta-analysis. Ultrasound Obstet Gynecol. 2010;35(4):468-73.
21. Royal College of Obstetricians and Gynaecologists. (2011). Cervical cerclage. Green-Top Guideline No. 60. [online]. Available from: www.rcog.org.uk/globalassets/documents/guidelines/gtg_60.pdf. [Accessed October, 2015].
22. Farine D, Mundle WR, Dodd J, Basso M, Delisle MF, Farine D, et al. [The use of progesterone for prevention of preterm birth]. J Obstet Gynaecol Can. 2008;30(1):67-77.
23. Alexander JM, Mercer BM, Miodovnik M, Thurnau GR, Goldenberg RL, Das AF, et al. The impact of digital cervical examination on expectantly managed preterm rupture of membranes. Am J Obstet Gynecol. 2000;183(4):1003-7.
24. Wijnberger LD, de Kleine M, Voorbij HA, Arabin B, Engel H, Bruinse HW, et al. Comparison of vaginal and transabdominal collection of amniotic fluid for fetal lung maturity tests. J Matern Fetal Neonatal Med. 2010;23(7):613-6.
25. Lackman F, Capewell V, Richardson B, daSilva O, Gagnon R. The risks of spontaneous preterm delivery and neonatal mortality in relation to size at birth according to fetal versus neonatal growth standards. Am J Obstet Gynecol. 2001;184(5):946-53.
26. Drugs in threatened preterm labour. Br Med J. 1979;1(6156):71.
27. Royal College of Obstetricians and Gynaecologists. (2011). Tocolysis for women in preterm labour. Green-top Guideline No. 1b. [online] Available from: www.rcog.org.uk/globalassets/documents/guidelines/gtg1b26072011.pdf. [Accessed October, 2015].
28. American College of Obstetricians and Gynecologists; Committee on Practice Bulletins–Obstetrics. ACOG practice bulletin no. 127: Management of preterm labor. Obstet Gynecol. 2012;119(6):1308-17.
29. Han S, Crowther CA, Moore V. Magnesium maintenance therapy for preventing preterm birth after threatened preterm labour. Cochrane Database Syst Rev. 2010;(7):CD000940.
30. Valenzuela GJ, Sanchez-Ramos L, Romero R, Silver HM, Koltun WD, Millar L, et al. Maintenance treatment of preterm labor with the oxytocin antagonist atosiban. The Atosiban PTL-098 Study Group. Am J Obstet Gynecol. 2000;182(5):1184-90.
31. Royal College of Obstetricians and Gynaecologists. (2010). Antenatal corticosteroids to reduce neonatal morbidity and mortality. Green-Top Guideline No. 7. [online] Available from: www.rcog.org.uk/globalassets/documents/guidelines/gtg_7.pdf. [Accessed October, 2015].
32. Crowther CA, McKinlay CJ, Middleton P, Harding JE. Repeat doses of prenatal corticosteroids for women at risk of preterm birth for improving neonatal health outcomes. Cochrane Database Syst Rev. 2011;(6):CD003935.
33. Roberts D, Dalziel SR. Antenatal corticosteroids for accelerating fetal lung maturation for women at risk of preterm birth. Cochrane Database Syst Rev. 2006;(3):CD004454.
34. Vogel JP, Souza JP, Gülmezoglu AM, Mori R, Lumbiganon P, Qureshi Z, et al. Use of antenatal corticosteroids and tocolytic drugs in preterm births in 29 countries: an analysis of the WHO Multicountry Survey on Maternal and Newborn Health. Lancet. 2014;384(9957):1869-77.
35. Flenady V, Hawley G, Stock OM, Kenyon S, Badawi N. Prophylactic antibiotics for inhibiting preterm labour with intact membranes. Cochrane Database Syst Rev. 2013;12:CD000246.
36. American College of Obstetricians and Gynecologists Committee on Obstetric Practice; Society for Maternal-Fetal Medicine. Committee Opinion No. 455: Magnesium sulfate before anticipated preterm birth for neuroprotection. Obstet Gynecol. 2010;115(3):669-71.
37. Alfirevic Z, Milan SJ, Livio S. Caesarean section versus vaginal delivery for preterm birth in singletons. Cochrane Database Syst Rev. 2013;9:CD000078.
38. Bergenhenegouwen LA, Meertens LJ, Schaaf J, Nijhuis JG, Mol BW, Kok M, et al. Vaginal delivery versus caesarean section in preterm breech delivery: a systematic review. Eur J Obstet Gynecol Reprod Biol. 2014;172:1-6.

CHAPTER 36

Premature Rupture of Membranes

Kumud B Gupta, Neerja Jamwal

INTRODUCTION

The term premature rupture of membranes (PROM) can be defined as the spontaneous rupture of membranes prior to the onset of labor.[1,2] Premature rupture of membranes occurs in 5-15% of pregnancies. Of these, majority of cases (10%) occur at term and 2-3.5% occur before term.[3] Prelabor rupture of membranes is a common variant of normal pregnancy in term babies. Previable premature rupture of membranes can be defined as the rupture of membranes at or less than 24 week gestation.[4] It complicates about 1 in 1,000 births and is responsible for increased perinatal mortality. Out of all the births, 3% account for preterm premature rupture of membranes (PPROM) and lead to 30% neonatal morbidity and mortality in preterm infants. It is termed prolonged rupture of membrane if it persists for more than 24 hours prior to the onset of labor [5]. Indian studies report an incidence of PROM in 7-12% of all labors.[6] Incidence of PROM was 8.09% in a study conducted by Jolly and Gunwant (2012).[7] It complicates around 2-4% of all singleton and 7-20% of twin pregnancies.[7]

ETIOPATHOGENESIS

The membranes around the amniotic cavity are composed of the amnion and the chorion .These are closely adherent layers consisting of several cell types, including epithelial cells, mesenchymal cells, and trophoblast cells, and are embedded in a collagenous matrix. They store amniotic fluid, secrete substances into the amniotic fluid and act as a guard for the fetus against infection ascending from the reproductive tract. The membranes normally rupture during labor. Traditionally, rupture of the membranes has been attributed to physical stress, particularly which is associated with labor. However, recent evidence also suggests that rupture is also related to biochemical processes, including disruption of collagen within the extracellular matrix of the amnion and the chorion and programed death of cells (apoptosis) in the fetal membranes. The fetal membranes and the maternal uterine lining (decidua) respond to stimuli like membrane stretching and infection of the reproductive tract, and by producing mediators, like prostaglandins, cytokines, and protein hormones, which govern the activities of matrix degrading enzymes. The changes in the membranes, like decreased collagen content, alteration of collagen structure, and increased collagenolytic activity, are all risk factors for PROM.[8] Connective tissue disorders lead to weakening of the fetal membranes and thus increase the incidence of PPROM. The deficiency of copper and ascorbic acid contributes to an abnormal structure of fetal membrane collagen in smokers. An association between reduced collagen crosslinking (dietary deficiencies or behavioral activities) and predisposition to PROM has been found in women. Inappropriate degradation of extracellular matrices of membranes may also lead to PROM. This may occur because of disturbed activities of matrix metalloproteinase and the tissue inhibitors. Genetic association between increased activity of matrix metalloproteinase and PROM has been found. These women may also present with periodontitis and preterm labor. Bacterial infection of the genital tract with pathological microorganisms like group B streptococci (GBS), *Chlamydia trachomatis, Neisseria gonorrhea*, vaginal anaerobes, *Gardnerella vaginalis*, *Mobiluncus* species, and genital mycoplasmas has an increased risk of PPROM. Many of them produce collagenase and phospholipase which have a weakening effect on membrane structure and integrity. There is significant association between maternal genital tract colonization of GBS and occurrence of PROM.

Box 1: Factors contributing to preterm premature rupture of membranes[8–14]

- Intra-amniotic infection
- Low socioeconomic status
- Smoking
- Low body mass index (<19.8)
- Prior history of PROM
- Cervical insufficiency
- History of subchorionic bleeding/hematoma
- Urinary tract infection
- Lower genital tract, sexually transmitted infections
- Asymptomatic bacteriuria
- Presence of circlage
- Invasive uterine procedures (e.g., amniocentesis, cordocentesis, chorionic villus sampling, cervical cerclage)
- Abnormal placentation
- Multiparity
- Hydramnios
- History of preterm labor or PROM in previous pregnancy

PROM, premature rupture of membranes.

Programed cell death, or apoptosis, has also been implicated in the remodeling of various tissues, including those of the uterus and cervix. Human amnion and chorion obtained at term after PROM have many apoptotic cells in areas adjacent to the rupture site and fewer apoptotic cells in other areas of the membranes. Box 1 shows the factors contributing to PPROM.

COMPLICATIONS

One of the most common complications of PPROM is preterm delivery. The latent period, which is the time from membrane rupture until delivery, generally is inversely proportional to the gestational age at which PROM occurs. When PROM occurs too early, the neonates may develop complications of prematurity such as hyaline membrane disease, low birth weight, necrotizing enterocolitis, intraventricular hemorrhage, etc.[15] Malpresentation, cord compression, cord prolapse, nonreassuring fetal heart rate patterns, and placental separation can occur due to decreased liquor in both term and preterm cases. Neurologic impairment, cerebral palsy, and retinopathy can occur as delayed complications. When rupture of membranes occurs remote from term, pulmonary hypoplasia and fetal deformities of face and skeleton can occur due to severe prolonged oligohydramnios. Neonatal sepsis is the most feared complication in both term and preterm rupture of membranes (Box 2). Complications of PROM in mother include acute or subclinical chorioamnionitis, placental separation, and postpartum endometritis. Above all, parents have to bear the economic burden of the premature child (Box 3).

Box 2: Neonatal complications of premature rupture of membranes

- Preterm delivery
- Respiratory distress syndrome
- Cord compression
- Chorioamnionitis
- Abruptio placentae
- Antepartum fetal death
- Facial and limb deformities

Box 3: Maternal complications of premature rupture of membranes

- Acute chorioamnionitis
- Subclinical chorioamnionitis
- Placental abruption
- Postpartum endometritis
- Stress anxiety

DIAGNOSIS

The diagnosis of spontaneous rupture of the membranes is best achieved by maternal history followed by a sterile speculum examination (Fig. 1). History of duration of rupture of membranes is important as it is directly proportional to risk of chorioamnionitis and neonatal sepsis. Patients often report a sudden gush of fluid with continued leakage with absence of active labor. Always ask whether the patient is having labor pains, bleeding per vaginum, or has had an intercourse recently, or has a fever. Differential diagnosis includes cervical mucus or show, physiological vaginal discharge, incontinence of urine, and bacterial infection.

It is important to verify the patient's estimated due date because this information will direct subsequent treatment. A sterile speculum examination without any lubricating jelly will also evaluate, if any cervical dilation and effacement and cord prolapsed are present.

The presence of a pool of fluid in the vagina at sterile speculum examination is highly suggestive of rupture of

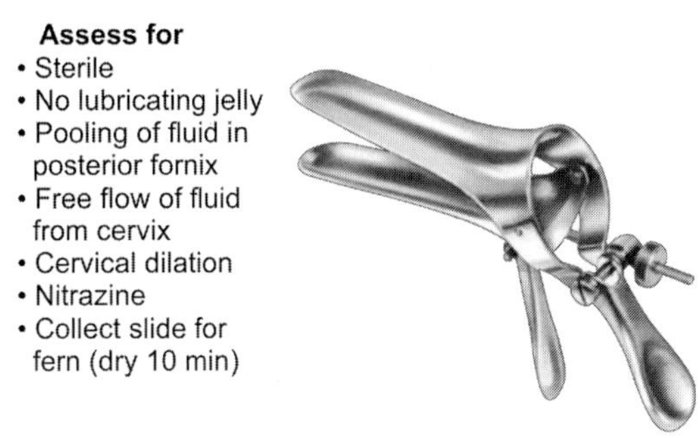

FIG.1: Sterile speculum examination in premature rupture of membranes.

membranes. Liquor flows freely from the cervix. Flecks of vernix or meconium may be additional symptoms. Cervical changes can also be looked simultaneously. Sample can also be collected for nitrazine test and for ferning on a clean slide. The number of vaginal examinations should be minimum to decrease chorioamnionitis. The size of uterus may be reduced and fetus may be prominently palpable

Many bedside tests[16] have been used to confirm membrane rupture. The most widely used has been the nitrazine test, which detects pH change.[17,18] The normal vagina has pH between 4.5 and 6.0. Amniotic fluid is more alkaline, and has a pH of 7.1–7.3. Nitrazine paper turns blue when the pH is above 6.0, remains yellow or changes to olive yellow if membranes are intact. However, the presence of contaminating substances (e.g., blood, semen, alkaline antiseptics, urine) may also cause nitrazine paper to turn blue, giving a false positive result. Bacterial vaginosis and trichomoniasis may give a similar result (Figs 2 and 3).

Microscopic examination of the vaginal fluid for the characteristic ferning of the crystalline pattern of dried amniotic fluid owing to its sodium chloride and protein structure, (arborization) can also be used for diagnosis[19] (Fig. 4).

Examination for lanugo hair in amniotic fluid and fetal epithelial cells stained with nile blue can also be used.[21]

The best results are obtained with nitrazine and ferning tests. Both are around 90% sensitive. Contamination with urine, blood, or semen may lead to false positive test reports. The false positivity for nitrazine paper and fern test is 17 and 6%, respectively. A clinical history of rapid passage of clear fluid from vagina also has the similar sensitivity and false positive rate.

Ultrasound examination[22,23] demonstrating oligohydramnios is also useful to help confirm the diagnosis of spontaneous rupture of the membranes. If a normal amniotic fluid index is seen on ultrasound, it does not exclude the diagnosis of PPROM, even when ultrasonography is not necessary to confirm PROM, it may help determine the gestational age, position of the fetus, estimated fetal weight, placental location, and presence of congenital anomalies.

AmniSure is a rapid immunoassay, and has been shown to be accurate in the diagnosis of ruptured membranes with a sensitivity and specificity of 98.9 and 100%, respectively.[24] In doubtful cases where diagnosis cannot be made, AmniSure is very useful.

Do not do a digital vaginal examination unless the woman is in labor. While doing digital examination, the microorganisms from the vagina may get transported to the cervix. This can lead to the release of prostaglandins and preterm labor and also intra-uterine infection. This also shortens the latency period between onset of rupture of membranes and time of delivery.[25] Hence, a sterile speculum examination is preferred over digital vaginal examination.[26]

- Visualization of amniotic fluid pooling in the vagina
- Fluid leaking from the cervical os when the patient is asked to cough or when fundal pressure is applied
- Soakage of vulval pad.

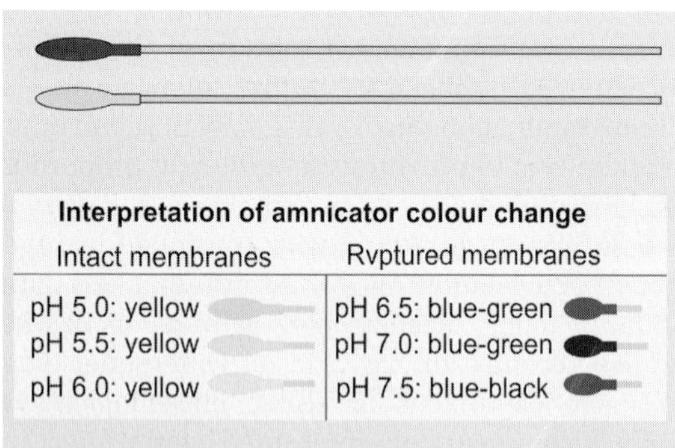

FIG. 2: Color change in amnicator test on premature rupture of membrane *(For color version, see Plate 4)*.

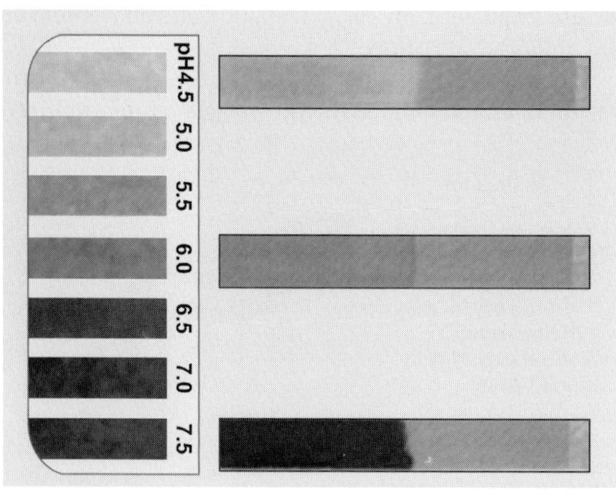

FIG. 3: Nitrazine paper test. Blue color indicates presence of amniotic fluid *(For color version, see Plate 4)*.

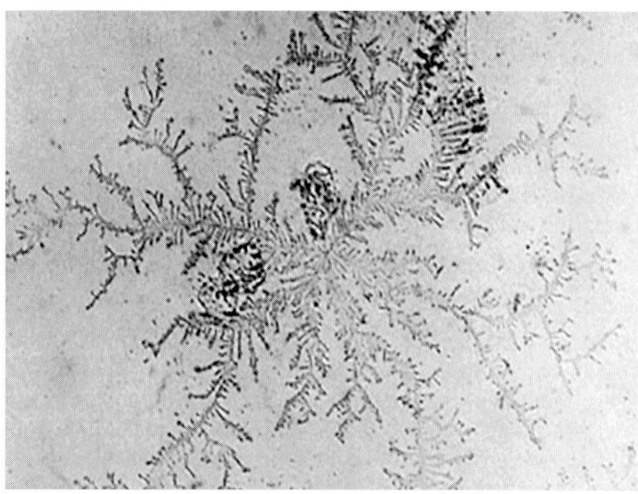

FIG. 4: Arborization pattern seen under microscope.[20]

Women with cervical infections are seven times more prone to PROM. Hence, when doing the sterile speculum examination, cervical cultures should be obtained. A vaginal and anal or perianal swab for GBS screening should also be obtained.

In cases of conflicting history and clinical findings, (history is highly suspicious for ruptured membranes but with a normal fern test and nitrazine test), or when contemplating transport to a tertiary care facility where a precise diagnosis is a must, amniocentesis may help to determine whether the membranes are ruptured. The test is done by instillation of 1 mL of indigo carmine dye mixed in 9 mL of sterile saline into amniotic cavity. If the membranes are ruptured, the blue dye will be seen on the vaginal pad within 30 minutes of instillation. Methylene blue dye should not be used because it has been associated with hyperbilirubinemia and hemolytic anemia in infants. Fetal fibronectin in amniotic fluid can be detected in the endocervix in patients with PROM.

MANAGEMENT

A woman with history of ruptured membranes confirmed on examination or tests should be admitted to the hospital. Initial management includes confirmation of diagnosis and determination of gestational age. Identification of women who need to be delivered is of utmost importance. Digital vaginal examination must be avoided as it increases risk of infection and decreases latency period. Abdominal palpation for fetal lie and presentation and uterine tenderness should be done. Women should be observed for signs of clinical chorioamnionitis. A high vaginal swab and maternal full blood count should be considered. A bedside ultrasound for estimation of gestational age, measurement of amniotic fluid volume, fetal parameters and weight, fetal position, and measurement of cervical length should be undertaken. Fetal monitoring using cardiotocography should be considered where regular fetal surveillance is required. Women should be commenced on broad spectrum antibiotics.

The criteria for the diagnosis of clinical chorioamnionitis include:

- Maternal fever
- Tachycardia
- Leukocytosis
- Uterine tenderness
- Offensive vaginal discharge
- Fetal tachycardia

The maternal temperature, pulse, and fetal heart rate auscultation should be done between every 4–8 hours. Leukocytosis has a sensitivity of 29–47% in predicting clinical chorioamnionitis with a false positive rate of 5–18%.[27,28] Following corticosteroids administration, there is usually a transient rise in white blood cell count for 48 hours. The specificity of C-reactive protein (CRP) is 38–55%. However, the presence of leukocytosis may be useful clinically, if doubt about the diagnosis of chorioamnionitis arises.

The noninvasive tests to detect fetuses at risk and need to be delivered include biophysical profile (BPP), Doppler velocimetry of placental and fetal circulation, and cardiotocography.[29] Though they cannot differentiate between infected and noninfected fetuses, they are useful in antepartum monitoring.

Noninvasive tests in predicting clinical chorioamnionitis.[30,31]

- Abnormal BPP
- Increased systolic to diastolic (S/D) ratio in umbilical artery
- Fetal tachycardia in cardiotocograms
- False positive rate 2–9%
- True positive rate 30–80%.

WHAT IS THE ROLE OF AMNIOCENTESIS?

A documented association between subclinical intra-uterine infection and adverse neonatal outcome is there. Still, the role of amniocentesis in improving outcome is not clear. There is insufficient evidence to recommend the use of amniocentesis in the diagnosis of intra-uterine infection. Intra-uterine infection, as identified by positive amniotic fluid cultures, is found in 36% of women with PPROM. Mostly, the infections are subclinical with no obvious signs of chorioamnionitis. If the amniotic fluid cultures are positive, the risks of preterm delivery, neonatal sepsis, respiratory distress syndrome (RDS), chronic lung disease, periventricular leukomalacia, intraventricular hemorrhage, cerebral palsy, and endometritis are markedly increased.

Rapid tests[32-34] can be performed on amniotic fluid such as Gram stain and of cytokines assay of interleukins 6, 18, 36, 38, and 39 which indicate intra-uterine infection. Prophylactic antibiotic therapy in cases of PPROM has been shown to have benefits. Still, treatment should be targeted to appropriate women because a potential adverse effect of prolonged antibiotic therapy in PPROM includes superinfection with virulent organisms. It remains to be determined in future studies whether amniocentesis[35] improves outcomes. Also, amniocentesis should be performed in specialized units. The role of amniocentesis in improving outcome remains to be determined but is not recommended as a routine in these cases.

WHO NEEDS TO BE DELIVERED REGARDLESS OF GESTATIONAL AGE?

There are both maternal and fetal indications for immediate delivery. These women need to be identified to prevent neonatal and maternal complications.

- Advanced preterm labor
- Acute chorioamnionitis
- Women at high risk for severe infection
- Fetus >34 weeks
- Nonreassuring fetal heart rate

- Acute cord complications
- Severe oligohydramnios
- Lethal abnormalities in fetus
- Placental abruption

ROLE OF CORTICOSTEROIDS

Corticosteroids help in bringing down perinatal morbidity and mortality rates after PPROM. Women with PROM between 23 and 34 weeks gestation should receive a single course of antenatal corticosteroids. Although the beneficial effect of steroids at 32–33 weeks in the setting of PROM are weak, but administration has its potential benefits as seen in the setting of intact membranes and this has been recently recommended by American College of Obstetricians and Gynecologists (ACOG).[36] To sum up, antenatal corticosteroids should be given to all women with PROM less than 34 weeks. The most widely used and recommended regimens include intramuscular betamethasone [12 mg every 24 hours for 2 days, or intramuscular dexamethasone (Decadron) 6 mg every 12 hours for 2 days]. After 34 weeks' gestation, corticosteroids are not recommended unless there is evidence of fetal lung immaturity by amniocentesis. Multiple courses are not recommended because studies have shown that two or more courses can result in decreased infant birth weight, head circumference, and body length. Neonatal mortality is reduced by approximately 40%, RDS by 30%, and cerebroventricular hemorrhage by 50% in infants of women who are given antenatal corticosteroids within 24 hours of previable premature rupture of membrane.[37,38] Administration of antenatal steroids in the setting of PPROM does not increase the likelihood of fetal death, maternal death, maternal fever, chorioamnionitis, or puerperal sepsis.

MAGNESIUM SULFATE FOR NEUROPROTECTION

Women with PPROM before 32 weeks who are thought to be at risk of imminent delivery should be considered candidates for fetal neuroprotective treatment with intravenous magnesium sulfate (ACOG, 2013). Intravenous infusion of magnesium sulfate in a loading dose of 6 g over 20–30 minutes, followed by a maintenance dose of infusion of 2 g/h is given. Infusion may be discontinued if delivery does not occur in 12 hours and another loading dose may be given, if delivery is again considered to be imminent.

ROLE OF ANTIBIOTICS

Antibiotics in patients with PPROM reduce neonatal infections, maternal infections, and prolong the latency period.[39] It decreases the occurrence of postpartum endometritis, chorioamnionitis, neonatal sepsis, neonatal pneumonia, and intraventricular hemorrhage. There is an approximate 40% reduction in chorioamnionitis, a 30% reduction in neonatal infection, and a 20% reduction in intraventricular hemorrhage.[40,41] Prolongation of latency period also helps corticosteroids to take effect. Several antibiotics have been used in different trials and the results with different antibiotic regimes have been similar. The key elements are; (1) a broad spectrum β-lactam type antibiotic with Gram-negative coverage and (2) a macrolide antibiotic with coverage for atypical organisms. Latency antibiotics should be continued until the onset of labor or until 10 days of therapy have been completed. Group B streptococci prophylaxis should be provided during labor unless a recent culture documented negative results regardless of latency antibiotics. In cases of chorioamnionitis or maternal sepsis, broad spectrum intravenous antibiotics should be commenced.[42,43] Later on, treatment can be guided based upon culture sensitivity reports. Delivery is indicated in the management of chorioamnionitis. Amoxicillin-clavulanate is not recommended as it has been found to increase the rate of neonatal necrotizing enterocolitis.

TOCOLYTICS IN PRETERM PREMATURE RUPTURE OF MEMBRANES

Prophylactic tocolysis in women with PPROM without uterine activity is usually not recommended. Women who require intra-uterine transfer to a tertiary care center or antenatal corticosteroids may be candidates for a short course of tocolysis. The decision needs to be considered in light of the possibility of pre-existing intra-uterine infection, the only clinical feature of which might be labor pains. Tocolysis is not recommended, if chorioamnionitis is suspected. There is no clear evidence that tocolysis improves neonatal outcome following PPROM, hence it is reasonable not to use them.[44-46] Tocolysis in labor with ruptured membranes may have adverse effects, like delaying delivery from an infected environment, due to an association between intra-uterine infection, prostaglandin and cytokine release, and delivery. It would seem wise to consider tocolysis for transfer of women and administration of antenatal steroids (use should be limited to 48 h), depending on clinical circumstances.

MANAGEMENT BASED ON GESTATIONAL AGE

37 Weeks or More (Term Preterm Premature Rupture of Membranes)

Around 60–80% of cases of PROM occur at term. These cases account for 10% of inductions of labor and around 1–2% of cesarean rates. The latency period of term rupture of membranes is usually short and 75% of these patients go in labor spontaneously. Without induction of labor, 75% deliver in 24 hours, 90% in 48 hours, and around 95% in 72 hours. There has been a long debate regarding expectant management versus induction of labor in PROM more than 37 weeks. A woman with rupture of membranes over 37 weeks should be given a choice of early induction of labor or expectant management till onset of labor pains. She may change her opinion and come for induction in between. The contraindications to expectant management include cord prolapsed, meconium stained liquor, vaginal bleeding, maternal pyrexia ,pregnancy with previous cesarean section, multiple pregnancy, noncephalic presentation, and infection with GBS. Though the rate of instrumental delivery and cesarean section is not different in the two groups, expectant management definitely carries some risks. Fetal risks include neonatal sepsis, cord compression, meconium aspiration, and cord prolapsed. Although the risk of neonatal sepsis with broad spectrum antibiotics is less expectant management is associated with prolonged hospital stay in neonates. Maternal risks include endometritis in the postnatal period. The risk of complications increases in cases of prolonged rupture of membranes, prolonged labor, and cesarean deliveries. The number of vaginal examinations is directly proportional to maternal and neonatal sepsis and hence, should be minimum. Antibiotics with broad spectrum coverage should be started.

Induction of labor can be done by the usual methods. Oxytocin is preferred as it has the least chances of chorioamnionitis. However, if the bishop score is poor, induction with prostaglandins can be done. Cesarian is done for obstetric indications. Partographic management of labor should be done. Minimum number of vaginal examinations should be done. Neonates should be watched for sepsis in the form of meconium aspiration, poor Apgar score, lethargy, poor feeding, seizure, tachypnea, and tachycardia.

34–37 Weeks

In PPROM occuring at 34–37 weeks' gestation, labor induction clearly is beneficial as fetuses will have adequate lung maturity and latency period is short. Both the risks and benefits of expectant management should be explained to the parents.[47] Conservative management between 34 and 36 weeks' gestational age has benefits of decreased risk of prematurity, respiratory problems, and neonatal jaundice but results in an increased risk of chorioamnionitis, neonatal sepsis, and lower Apgar scores. Also, there is no neonatal advantage after 34 weeks' gestation and it may lead to prolonged hospital stay of both mother and neonate and more prolonged antibiotic therapy in neonates. Corticosteroids are not indicated after 34 weeks' gestation. However, if fetal lung maturity is a concern, there is no harm in giving steroids.

If parents opt for expectant management, woman should be hospitalized. Broad spectrum antibiotics should be initiated and maternal and fetal surveillance should be done. Expectant management should be stopped if chorioamnionitis supervenes, patient goes in active labor, nonreassuring fetal heart rate appears, bleeding per vaginum appears, leukocytosis and CRP increase, and ultrasound shows severe oligohydramnios with largest amniotic fluid pocket less than 2 cm or cord prolapsed occurs. Appropriate antibiotics for GBS prophylaxis should be considered during labor.

Maternal transport to a skilled center in caring for premature neonates should be undertaken, if possible. Oxytocin induction can be used as PPROM is not a contraindication for vaginal delivery. Cesarian section should be done for obstetric indications.

24–33 Weeks

Delivery before 34 weeks' gestation can lead to severe neonatal morbidity and mortality. If intra-amniotic infection is not there, every attempt should be made to prolong the gestation until 34 weeks' gestation. Contraindications to conservative therapy include chorioamnionitis, abruptio placentae, and nonreassuring fetal heart patterns. Prolongation of the latent phase, prevention of RDS, and intraventricular hemorrhage and prevention of sepsis—both maternal and neonatal is the aim. Hence, steroids, antibiotics, and short-term tocolysis include the management. Transport to a facility to care for preterm neonates should be done.

Maternal Surveillance
- Pulse
- Fever
- History of pain
- Uterine tenderness
- Foul smelling discharge or liquor
- Bleeding per vaginum
- Total leukocyte count
- C-reactive protein
- Vaginal swabs

Fetal Surveillance
- Daily fetal movement count
- Fetal heart rate auscultation
- Ultrasonography (confirm dates, fetal biometry, estimated weight, placental localization, fetal position, amniotic fluid)
- Fetal Doppler velocimetery
- Biophysical profile
- Cardiotocograms

Stop expectant management if:
- Active labor starts
- Chorioamnionitis
- Cord prolapsed
- Bleeding (abruption)
- Nonreassuring fetal status
- Severe oligohydramnios
- More than 34 weeks.

Women need to be inpatient with complete bed rest with bathroom privileges. A sterile vulval pad should be applied. Broad spectrum antibiotics should be started and a course of antenatal steroids should be given. A complete maternal blood count including total leukocyte count and CRP should be sought. An assessment of fetal well-being by fetal monitoring daily or ultrasonography weekly should be done. Intensive fetal and maternal surveillance should be done. Women should daily be asked to keep a track of baby movements. Umbilical cord compression is common (32–76%) with PPROM before 34 weeks' gestation; therefore, at least daily fetal monitoring in the form of fetal heart rate auscultation daily is indicated. Fetal tachycardia is a late sign of fetal infection. In addition, the woman should be observed closely for fetal or maternal tachycardia, temperature exceeding 100.4°F (38°C), foul smelling discharge, bleeding per vaginum, regular contractions, uterine tenderness, or leukocytosis, and increase in CRP which are possible indicators of amnionitis. The frequency of taking maternal pulse, temperature, and fetal heart rate should be 4–8 hourly.

A high vaginal swab, swab for GBS screening should be sent to guide antibiotic prophylaxis. Corticosteroid administration may lead to an elevated leukocyte count, if given within 5–7 days of PROM. Biophysical profile may show abnormalities in the form of decreased amniotic fluid, decreased fetal movements, decreased fetal breathing movements, and nonreactive nonstress test (NST) in infected fetuses. Fetal velocimetory may show increased S/D ratio in umbilical artery in infected fetuses. To start with, intravenous antibiotics are given for 48 hours followed by a course of oral antibiotics for 7–10 days, if the woman does not deliver. Prolonged latency may increase the risk of intra-amniotic infection and neonatal sepsis. Delivery is necessary for patients with evidence of amnionitis.

In cases where the diagnosis of an intra-uterine infection is suspected, amniocentesis can be performed to find out a decreased glucose level or a positive Gram stain and differential count can be performed. In patients who reach 32–33 weeks' gestation, amniocentesis can be done for fetal lung maturity and evidence of intra-amniotic infection.

Before 24 Weeks

The pulmonary canalicular development in the fetus occurs before 24 weeks. In previable rupture of membranes, mostly the women deliver in 1 week. In those who do not, the babies may have long-term neurological and developmental abnormalities, chronic lung problems, cerebral palsy[48], and hydrocephalus. These babies may have potter facies, pressure deformities of face and limbs, and pulmonary hypoplasia. The lesser the gestational age at which rupture of membranes occurs, more is the incidence of complications.

If PROM occurs less than 24 weeks, parents should be counseled about the risks of expectant management including fetal death and long-term sequelae if baby survives. Risk of maternal chorioamnionitis should also be explained. They should be offered termination of pregnancy to avoid morbidity. If a viable fetus is born, neonatologist should assess whether neonatal support is to be given. Consultation with a perinatologist or neonatologist can be done before induction. Transport to a tertiary facility for neonates should be done. Home management of patients with PPROM is controversial. Bed rest at home for stable patients may be acceptable with precise education of symptoms of infection and preterm labor. Readmission to the hospital should be considered for these patients after 24 weeks' gestation for close fetal and maternal monitoring.

OUTPATIENT MANAGEMENT

Inpatient management is preferred over outpatient in the management of PROM as both fetal and neonatal surveillance are to be carried out. A woman should be given outpatient treatment only if she has close accessibility to the hospital, is not in active labor, has no infection, and no fetal compromise is there. In stable patients not in labor requesting for home based care, it is reasonable that the woman is kept in hospital for at least 48 hours before she is sent home. She should be clearly given instructions to take regular temperature chartings at home. Warning signs like loss of fetal movements, fever, foul smelling liquor or discharge, pain, and bleeding per vaginum mandate hospital visit. Woman should be advised to avoid intercourse and maintain personal hygiene. She should change her vaginal pads frequently. She should visit hospital as assigned and perform regular tests.

NEW DEVELOPMENTS IN MANAGEMENT

Preterm premature rupture of membranes is a subject of continued research. Many genetic factors are being studied in the pathogenesis as it is evident that environmental factors plus genetic factors may be responsible for the etiology. Pleomorphisms in relaxin gene are upcoming subject of research. Similarly, assay for insulin-like growth factor binding protein-1 is done in Actim PROM test. This is also rapid, bedside, and compliments diagnosis.

AmniSure is a rapid bed side test to confirm rupture of membranes from vaginal fluid. It is an immunoassay detection of placental α-microglobulin-1 and is highly accurate.

- Insert vaginal swab 5–7 cm deep carefully into the vagina and withdraw the swab after 1 minute
- Place the tip of the polyester swab with patient sample into the labeled, prepared vial and rinse in the solvent by rotating for 1 minute
- Insert the dipstick into the solvent
- Interpret results after 5–10 minutes (Fig. 5).

Endoscopic visualization of the site of rupture is currently being used to seal the rent using fibrin glue (thrombin with cryoprecipitate)[49] amniopatch (successive intra-uterine

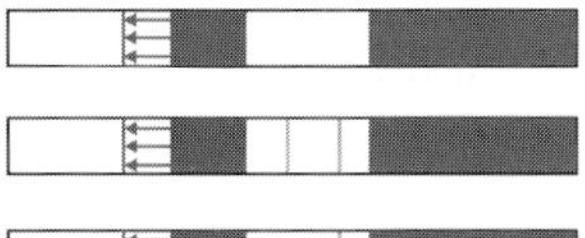

FIG. 5: Interpretation of results on AmniSure dipstick *(For color version, see Plate 5)*.

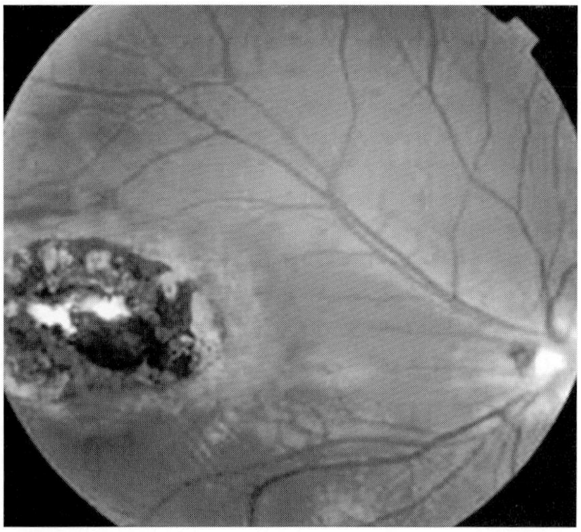

FIG. 6: Endoscopic view of the site of membrane rupture *(For color version, see Plate 5)*.

injections of platelets and cryoprecipitate) and amniograft. Gelatin sponge embolization is another technique under study. These approaches are more useful in traumatic rupture following amniocentesis or fetal surgery than in spontaneous rupture. Yet, they are in the experimental stages and need further treatments and case reportings for validity (Fig. 6).

CONCLUSION

Premature rupture of membranes is the leading cause of neonatal and maternal morbidity. The gold standard for diagnosis is maternal history and a sterile speculum examination. Ultrasound examination for liquor as well as fetal parameters should be done. Digital vaginal examination should be avoided. Observe for signs of clinical chorioamnionitis every 4–6 hours. A weekly high vaginal swab and a weekly maternal full blood count should be done. Fetal monitoring using cardiotocography for fetal surveillance. Oral antibiotics for 10 days following the diagnosis of PPROM from 20 weeks' gestation if there is no clinical evidence of chorioamnionitis or maternal sepsis. If clinical signs of chorioamnionitis start on broad spectrum intravenous antibiotics and delivery should be undertaken. Antenatal corticosteroids to be administered in women between 24 and 34 weeks' gestation. Prophylactic tocolysis without preterm labor is not recommended. If intra-uterine transfer to a higher center is required or antenatal corticosteroids need to be administered, short course of tocolysis may be given. If there is a significant suspicion of chorioamnionitis, then tocolysis is not recommended. Deliver after 34 weeks gestation. If on expectant plan beyond 34 weeks, deliver no later than 36 weeks and 6 days gestation. Outpatient management should be given only after a period of 48–72 hours of inpatient care. Women should be clearly explained the dos and don'ts and should come for regular follow-up. Premature rupture of membranes at or after 37 weeks, option for immediate delivery or expectant management should be given. Immediate induction is more useful. Induction with oxytocin has the least side effects. In unripe cervix, prostaglandins can be used. Antibiotics to be given to all.

REFERENCES

1. American College of Obstetrician and Gynecologists. Premature rupture of membranes (1989). Washington, DC: American College of Obstetrics and Gynecologists; 1989. ACOG Practice Bulletin No 1.
2. Caughey AB, Robinson JN, Norwitz ER. Contemporary Diagnosis and Management of Preterm Premature Rupture of Membranes. Reviews in Obstetrics & Gynecology. 2008;1(1):11-22.
3. Hernández Y Ballinas A, López Farán JA, Gámez Guevara C. Comparison of maternal and perinatal outcomes in the conservative treatment preterm premature membrane rupture between the use of erythromycin and clindamycin. [Article in Spanish]. Ginecol Obstet Mex. 2011;79(7):403-10.
4. Margato MF, Martins GL, Passini Júnior R, Nomura ML. Previable preterm rupture of membranes: gestational and neonatal outcomes. Arch Gynecol Obstet. 2012;285(6):1529-34.
5. Jazayeri A. Premature rupture of membrane. Medicine Clinical Reference; 2008;1-11.
6. Fernando Arias, Shirish N Daftary, Amarnath G Bhide. Premature rupture of membranes. 3rd edition. Practical Guide to High-Risk Pregnancy and Delivery–A South Asian perspective. Noida: Elsevier; 2009. pp. 240-58.
7. Jolly Vaishnav, Gunvant Vaishnav. Prelabour rupture of membranes (PROM) .Medicine Science. 2012;1(2):118-24.
8. Stuart EL, Evans GS, Lin YS, Powers HJ. Reduced collagen and ascorbic acid concentrations and increased proteolytic susceptibility with prelabor fetal membrane rupture in women. Biol Reprod. 2005;72:230-5.
9. American College of Obstetricians and Gynecologists. Premature rupture of membranes. Clinical management guidelines for obstetrician-gynecologists. ACOG practice bulletin no. 1. Int J Gynaecol Obstet. 1998;63:75-84.
10. Mercer BM. Preterm premature rupture of the membranes. Obstet Gynecol. 2003;101:178-93.
11. Smith CV, Greenspoon J, Phelan JP, Platt LD. Clinical utility of the nonstress test in the conservative management of women with preterm spontaneous premature rupture of the membranes. J Reprod Med. 1987;32:1-4.
12. Cox SM, Leveno KJ. Intentional delivery versus expectant management with preterm ruptured membranes at 30–34 weeks' gestation. Obstet Gynecol. 1995;86:875-9.
13. Ananth CV, Savitz DA, Williams MA. Placental abruption and its association with hypertension and prolonged rupture of membranes: a methodologic review and meta-analysis. Obstet Gynecol. 1996;88:309-18.

14. Gonen R, Hannah ME, Milligan JE. Does prolonged preterm premature rupture of the membranes predispose to abruptio placentae? Obstet Gynecol. 1989;74(3 pt 1):347-50.
15. The American College of Obstetricians and Gynecologists (2012).. Management of Preterm Labor Practice Bulletin 127. [Practice Bulletin No. 127].
16. Baptisti A. Chemical test for the determination of ruptured membranes. Am J Obstet Gynecol. 1938;35:688-90.
17. Abe T. The detection of rupture of the fetal membranes with the nitrazine indicator. Am J Obstet Gynecol. 1940;39:400-4.
18. Friedman ML, McElin TW. Diagnosis of ruptured fetal membranes. Clinical study and review of the literature. Am J Obstet Gynecol. 1969;104:544-50.
19. Paavola A. Methods based on the study of crystals and fat staining: use in diagnosing rupture of the membranes. Ann Chir Gynaecol Fenn. 1958;47:22-8.
20. Volet B, Morier-Genoud J. The crystallization test in amniotic fluid. Gynaecologia 1960;149:151-61.
21. Brosens I, Gordon H. The cytologic diagnosis of ruptured membranes using Nile Blue sulfate staining. J Obstet Gynecol Br Commonwealth. 1965;72:342-6.
22. Carroll SG, Papiaoannou S, Nicolaides KH. Assessment of fetal activity and amniotic fluid volume in the prediction of intrauterine infection in preterm prelabor amniorrhexis. Am J Obstet Gynecol. 1995;172:1427-35.
23. Vintzileos AM, Campbell WA, Nochimson DJ, Weinbaum PJ, Mirochnick MH, Escoto DT. Fetal biophysical profile score versus amniocentesis in predicting infection in preterm premature rupture of the membranes. Obstet Gynecol; 1986;68(4):488-94.
24. Cousins LM, Smok DP, Lovett SM, Poelter DM. AmniSure placental alpha microglobulin-1 rapid immunoassay versus standard diagnostic methods for detection of rupture of membranes.Am J Perinatol. 2005;22:317-20.
25. Carroll SG, VilleY, Greenough A, Gamsu H, Patel B, Philpott-Howard J, et al. Preterm prelabour amniorrhexis: intrauterineinfection and interval between membrane rupture and delivery. Arch Dis Child Fetal Neonatal Ed. 1995;72:F43-6.
26. Lewis DF, Major CA, Towers CV, Asrat T, Harding JA, GariteTJ. Effects of digital vaginal examination on latency period in preterm premature rupture of membranes. Obstet Gynecol. 1992;80:630-4.
27. Ismail MA, Zinaman MJ, Lowensohn RI, Moawad AH. The significance of C-reactive protein levels in women with premature rupture of membranes. Am J Obstet Gynecol. 1985151:5414.
28. Romem Y, Artal R. C-reactive protein as a predictor for chorioamnionitis in cases of premature rupture of the membranes. Am J Obstet Gynecol. 1984;150:546-50.
29. Carroll SG, Papiaoannou S, Nicolaides KH. Doppler studies of the placental and fetal circulation in pregnancies with preterm prelabour amniorrhexis. Ultrasound Obstet Gynecol. 1995;5:184-8.
30. Carroll SG, Papiaoannou S, Nicolaides KH. Assessment of fetal activity and amniotic fluid volume in pregnancies complicated by preterm prelabour amniorrhexis. Am J Obstet Gynecol. 1995;172:1427-35.
31. Goldstein I, Romero R, Merrill S, O'Connor WM, Mazor M, Hobbins JC. Fetal body and breathing movements as predictors of intraamniotic infection in preterm premature rupture of membranes. Am J Obstet Gynecol. 1988;159:363-8.
32. Jacobsson B, Holst RM, Mattsby-Baltzer I, Nikolaitchouk N, Wennerholm UB, Hagberg H. Interleukin-18 in cervical mucus and amniotic fluid: relationship to microbial invasion of the amniotic fluid, intra-amniotic inflammation and preterm delivery. BJOG. 2003;110:598-603.
33. Coultrip LL, Grossman JH. Evaluation of rapid diagnostic tests in the detection of microbial invasion of the amniotic cavity. Am J Obstet Gynecol. 1992;167:1231-42.
34. Yoon BH, Romero R, Jun JK, Park KH, Park JD, Ghezzi F, et al. Amniotic fluid cytokines (interleukin-6, tumor necrosis factor-alpha, interleukin-1 beta, and interleukin-8) and the risk for the development of bronchopulmonary dysplasia. Am J Obstet Gynecol. 1997;177:825-30.
35. Carroll SG, Sebire NJ, Nicolaides KH. 1996. Preterm Prelabour Amniorrhexis. Parthenon Publishing Group, UK.
36. The American College of Obstetricians and Gynecologists. (2013). Premature Rupture of Membranes Practice Bulletin #139. [ACOG Practice Bulletin #139].
37. Roberts D, Dalziel SR. Antenatal corticosteroids for accelerating fetal lung maturation for women at risk of preterm birth. Cochrane Database of Syst Rev. 2006, Issue 3:CD004454.
38. Vidaeff AC, Doyle NM, Gilstrap LC III. Antenatal corticosteroids for fetal maturation in women at risk for preterm delivery. Clin Perinatol. 2003;30:825-40,vii.
39. Kenyon S, Boulvain M, Neilson JP. Antibiotics for preterm rupture of membranes. Cochrane Database of Systematic Reviews. 2003, Issue 2. Art. No.: CD001058.
40. Kenyon S, Pike K, Jones DR, Brocklehurst P, Marlow N, Salt A, et al. Childhood outcomes after prescription of antibiotics to pregnant women with preterm rupture of the membranes: 7 year follow-up of the ORACLE 1 trial. Lancet. 2008;372(9646):1310-8.
41. Kenyon S, Boulvain M, Neilson J. (2010) Antibiotics for preterm rupture of membranes. The Cochrane Collaboration. Cochrane Library.
42. ACOG. (2013). Premature Rupture of Membranes Practice Bulletin #139. [ACOG Practice Bulletin #139]. The American College of Obstetricians and Gynecologists.
43. Kenyon S, Taylor DJ, Tarnow-Mordi W. Broad-spectrum antibiotics for preterm, prelabour rupture of fetal membranes: the ORACLE 1 randomised trial. ORACLE Collaborative Group. Lancet. 2001;357:979-88.
44. Combs CA, McCune M, Clark R, Fishman A. Aggressive tocolysis does not prolong pregnancy or reduce neonatal morbidity after preterm premature rupture of the membranes. Am J Obstet Gynecol. 2004;190:1723-8.
45. How HY, Cook CR, Cook VD, Miles DE, Spinnato JA. Preterm premature rupture of membranes: aggressive tocolysis versus expectant management. J Matern Fetal Med. 1998;7:8-12.
46. Jazayeri A, Jazayeri MK, Sutkin G. Tocolysis does not improve neonatal outcome in patients with preterm rupture of membranes. Am J Perinatol. 2003;20:189-93.
47. Carlan SJ, O'Brien WF, Parsons MT, Lense JJ. Preterm premature rupture of membranes: a randomised study of home versus hospital management. Obstet Gynecol. 1993;81:61-4.
48. Yoon BH, Park CW, Chaiorapongsa T. Intrauterine infection and the development of cerebral palsy. BJOG. 2003;110 Suppl 20:124-7.
49. Young BK, Roque H, Abdelhak YF, Poiolek D, Demopulos R, Lockwood CJ. Minimally invasive endoscopy in the treatment of preterm premature rupture of membranes by application of fibrin sealant. J Perinat Med. 2000;28:326-30.

CHAPTER 37

Post-term Pregnancy

Manishi Mittal

INTRODUCTION

The importance of defining "term gestation" lies in the fact that it provides guidance to clinicians and affects the public's perceptions about the optimal timing of delivery of a healthy baby. The International Classification of Diseases defines "term pregnancy" as delivery between 37 weeks 0 days and 41 weeks 6 days. However, this is an arbitrary limit and recent data shows that maternal and neonatal adverse outcome rates are not the same across this 6-week range. In fact, the frequency of adverse outcomes is U-shaped, with the nadir lying between 39 weeks 0 days and 40 weeks 6 days' gestation.[1] Table 1 shows the description and the recommended gestational age of preterm, term- and post-term pregnancies (PTP).

The terms "postdate" and "prolonged pregnancy" are ill-defined and best avoided.[3] Figure 1 shows the need to define PTP.

TABLE 1: Recommendations of the "defining term pregnancy" workgroup[2]

Description		Gestational age (weeks)
Preterm pregnancy		• <37
	• Late-preterm pregnancy	• 34 0/7 to 36 6/7
Term pregnancy		• 37 0/7 to 41 6/7
	• Early-term pregnancy • Full-term pregnancy • Late-term pregnancy	• 37 0/7 to 38 6/7 • 39 0/7 to 41 6/7 • 41 0/7 to 41 6/7
Post-term pregnancy		>42

HISTORY

The concept of an upper limit of human gestation period was developed after it was observed that perinatal mortality (PM) rises after pregnancy crosses the expected due date. The definition of post-term as after 42 weeks was most probably accepted after a report from Sweden in 1956 describing a dramatic increase in PM seen beyond this time.[4]

INCIDENCE

Studies from different settings suggest that the incidence of PTP varies between 3% and 14%, regardless of ethnicity.[5]

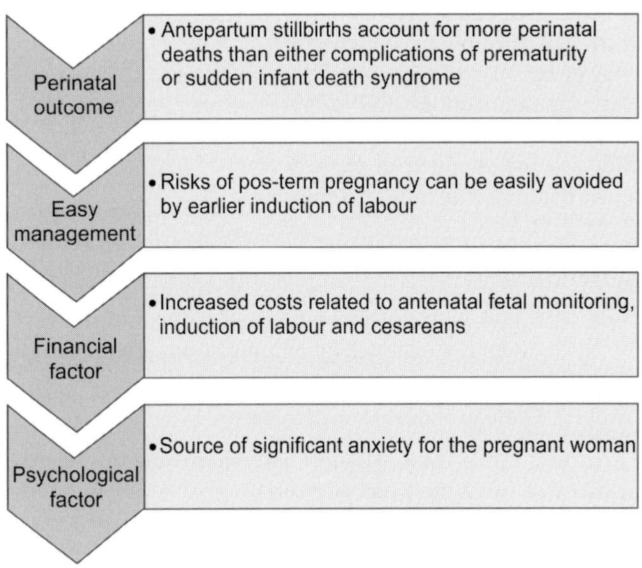

FIG. 1: Why definition of post-term pregnancy (PTP) is important?

Prevalence is affected by various population characteristics, such as the proportion of primigravidas in the population studied, the prevalence of obesity, previous history of PTP, and genetic predisposition. The percentage of females with pregnancy complications and the incidence of spontaneous preterm labor also affect the frequency of PTP. The significance of various maternal demographic factors, like parity, socioeconomic class and age, are not established.

Local management protocols, like scheduled induction of labor, ultrasound for pregnancy dating and elective cesarean section also influence the prevalence. Early ultrasound, if used for pregnancy dating, decreases significantly the incidence of PTP (from 12% to 3%).[6]

ETIOLOGY

There are many causes which lead to PTP. Some of them are enlisted in Table 2.

Around half of women with PTP may have recurrence in next pregnancy.[7] Other causes have been proposed. Use of non-steroidal anti-inflammatory drugs (NSAIDs) may prolong gestation as they inhibit synthesis of prostaglandins. Male sex and genetic predisposition have been associated with PTP.[8] Incidence of PTP is higher in women whose twin sister had PTP (more for monozygotic).[9]

A higher incidence of PTP has been reported in obese women.[10] Altered metabolic status and hormonal action of adipose tissue may affect the factors involved in labor initiation.

PATHOGENESIS

Production of corticotrophin-releasing hormone (CRH) by the placenta has been associated with the length of gestation. It rises exponentially with advancing pregnancy, peaking during parturition. In women with PTP, this rise is slow.[11] This may be because of gene polymorphisms on the physiological pathway connecting CRH to labor, or an altered response of maternal tissues to the routine hormonal signals during labor, as may happen in obese women.[12] Reduced cervical nitric oxide release may also contribute.[13]

COMPLICATIONS

Most PTP end with an uncomplicated labor and delivery, however, there is a high risk for complications. The common problems associated with PTP include fetal macrosomia, placental insufficiency, birth trauma and meconium aspiration.

Postmaturity Syndrome

Postmaturity, postmaturity syndrome and dysmaturity describe the clinical features of a neonate born after 42 weeks of gestation. These features are seen secondary to uteroplacental insufficiency seen in a PTP.[7]

This syndrome was described by Clifford in 1954, depicted by features like wrinkled, patchy, peeling skin and a long, thin body suggesting wasting. Infant is said to be of advanced maturity as baby is open-eyed, unusually alert, and appears old and worried-looking.[14] Skin wrinkling is usually more prominent on the palms and soles. The nails are typically quite long. Most such postmature infants are not growth restricted. But, severe growth restriction may occur which must have preceded completion of 42 weeks.

Clifford suggested that the skin changes of dysmaturity were due to loss of the protective effects of vernix caseosa as well as placental senescence. However, no significant morphological or quantitative evidence has been found to prove placental insufficiency.

Shime and colleagues described this syndrome in around 10% of pregnancies between 41 weeks and 43 weeks and about 33% at 44 weeks.[15] Vorherr et al. found that around 20% of infants born postterm have dysmaturity syndrome.[16] Intrauterine, these fetuses are at higher risk of umbilical cord compression, compression from oligohydramnios, meconium aspiration and nonreassuring fetal testing. Neonatal complications, like hypoglycemia, seizures, and respiratory insufficiency may occur.

Perinatal Mortality

Rate of intrauterine fetal death is higher beyond 42 weeks 0 days and before 38 weeks 0 days as compared to the period in between.[17] A higher neonatal mortality rate is reported in few studies, but not in others. This risk is primarily increased due to intrauterine growth restriction and major congenital malformations.[18] Rates of newborn morbidities, like respiratory distress, acidemia, meconium aspiration syndrome (MAS), clavicular fracture, Erb's palsy, ventilator use and neonatal intensive care unit admissions are lowest when born between 39 weeks 0 days and 40 weeks 6 days, while

TABLE 2: Etiology of post-term pregnancy

Perceived post-term	• Incorrect dates (most common cause) • Biological variability	
True post-term	• Maternal factors (most common identifiable risk factors) • Fetal factors • Placental factors	• Previous post-term pregnancy, primiparity • Congenital anomalies (adrenal hypoplasia, anencephaly) • X-linked recessive sulfatase deficiency

higher rates are seen both before and after.[19] Other neonatal complications in post-term babies include hypothermia due to poor subcutaneous fat, hypoglycemia and hypocalcemia.

The PM rate beyond 42 weeks is double of that at term (4–7 versus 2–3 deaths per 1,000 deliveries). It rises to six-times and more beyond 43 weeks.[20] Furthermore, recent epidemiologic studies propose that these calculations might underestimate the risk of stillbirth and early neonatal death, as these data used all pregnancies rather than ongoing pregnancies as the denominator. However, once the baby is delivered, it is no longer at risk of stillbirth.[21]

The common causes for high PM are uteroplacental insufficiency, MAS, asphyxia, and intrauterine infection. In addition, PTP is an independent risk factor for low umbilical artery pH levels at delivery and poor 5-minute Apgar scores.[22]

Meconium aspiration syndrome is a neonatal complication characterized by respiratory compromise with tachypnea, cyanosis, and decreased pulmonary compliance after exposure to meconium in-utero. It is primarily seen in infants born post-term. Meconium staining of amniotic fluid (AF) is found in almost 50% pregnancies at 42 weeks' gestation. The incidence of MAS decreased four-fold in the United States of America (USA) from 1990 to 1998, primarily due to a fall in the postterm delivery rate.[23]

Usually, postterm neonates are larger than term neonates and incidence of fetal macrosomia is higher (2.5–10% versus 0.8–1%).[7] Fetal macrosomia is associated with prolonged labor, cephalopelvic disproportion and shoulder dystocia with consequent problems of orthopedic or neurologic injury. Accuracy of ultrasound to detect macrosomia in PTP is relatively less. Hence, prophylactic cesarean is not advocated. Policy with either a 4 kg or 4.5 kg threshold would require more than 1,000 deliveries and very high financial burden to avert a single permanent brachial plexus injury. Such a policy would result in one maternal death for every 3.2 brachial plexus injuries prevented.[24]

Cord erythropoietin levels have been found to be significantly higher in pregnancies beyond 41 weeks, although Apgar scores and cord blood pH values were normal. Meconium staining of AF is seen with high erythropoietin at any gestational age.[25]

Few complications, like stillbirth, meconium aspiration, and neonatal acidemia, have been described as being more even at 40–41 weeks of gestation in comparison with 39 weeks gestation.[26] In addition, neonatal morbidities including birth injuries appear to nadir around 38 weeks and then rise in a continuous manner.[27] Hence, 42 weeks of gestation cannot be considered as a threshold beyond which fetal and maternal risks abruptly rise.

Few retrospective cohort studies have come out which have excluded complications with careful monitoring of maternal and fetal well-being.[28,29] They concluded that in uncomplicated PTP, PM is not high.

The risk of intrauterine fetal death is significantly higher than that of neonatal death at any time beyond 40+2 weeks gestation. Therefore, after this period, the fetus gets an unnecessary risk of demise without any benefit of fall in neonatal mortality with extended intrauterine stay.[7,30]

Infant Mortality and Morbidity

Infant mortality rate is higher in postterm babies. Some infant deaths are the result of peripartum complications (e.g., MAS), but most have no known cause. Post-term pregnancies is also an independent risk factor for neonatal encephalopathy.[31]

It is not proven if these infants are at risk of long-term neurologic sequelae. Shime et al. found no difference between term and post-term infants regarding general intelligence quotient, physical milestones, and frequency of intercurrent illnesses till 2 years age.[32]

Maternal Morbidity

Postterm pregnancy is associated with a higher rate of labor dystocia (9–12% versus 2–7% at term), severe perineal injury due to macrosomia (3.3% versus 2.6% at term), and twice the rate of cesarean delivery. Cesarean delivery in itself is related to complications, like endometritis, hemorrhage, and thromboembolic diseases. Importantly, prolonged gestation can be a source of substantial anxiety and frustration for the pregnant woman.[33,34]

Problems, like chorioamnionitis, severe perineal lacerations, cesarean delivery, operative vaginal deliveries, hemorrhage, and endomyometritis, have been documented to rise progressively after 39 weeks of gestation.[35]

Oligohydramnios

Oligohydramnios is increasingly seen with PTP, and it substantially increases the likelihood of postmaturity in the baby. For diagnosis, ultrasound finding (Fig. 2) of deepest vertical AF pocket less than 2 cm is preferable to AF index less than 5 cm.[36] Trimmer and colleagues found that the largest vertical pocket was less than or equal to 1 cm at 42 weeks and 88% of the neonates were postmature.[37] AF volume is thought to fall by 33% per week after 40 weeks' gestation.[38] If meconium is released into such reduced AF, it becomes thick and viscous that is implicated in MAS.

Studies with doppler found that fetal renal blood flow is decreased in PTP with oligohydramnios.[39] Adverse outcomes, like nonreassuring fetal heart rate, neonatal intensive care unit admission, and low Apgar score, are more common when oligohydramnios is present (Fig. 3).

MANAGEMENT

In short, management of PTP is shown in figure 4.

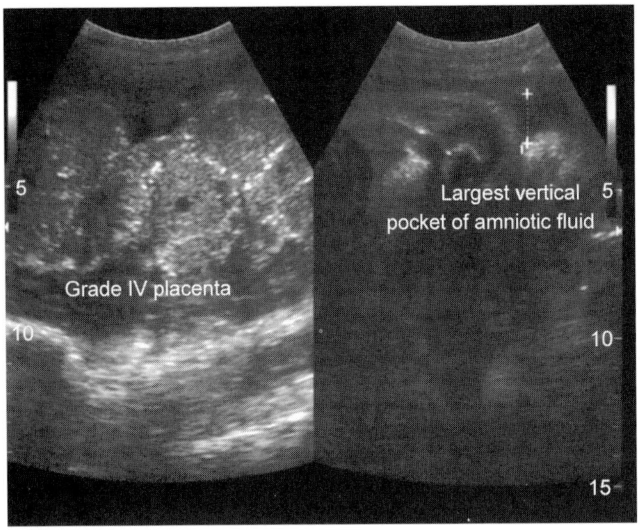

FIG. 2: Ultrasound showing mature placenta (grade IV) and oligohydramnios (vertical pocket <2 cm).

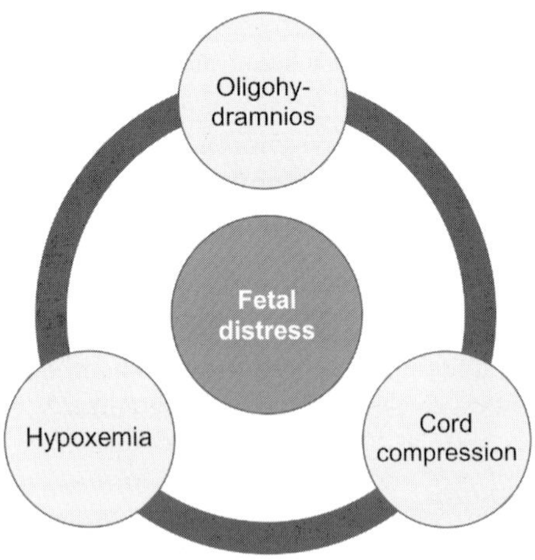

FIG. 3: Vicious circle associated with oligohydramnios.

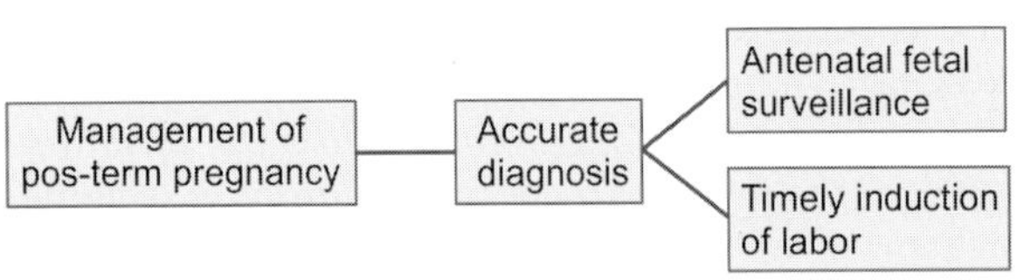

FIG. 4: Management of post-term pregnancy.

Accurate Gestational Age Assessment

Calculation of gestational age by last menstrual period (LMP) could be inaccurate due to cycle irregularity, recent use of hormonal contraception or bleeding early in pregnancy. In addition, follicular phase even in women with regular cycles is variable.

Blondel and colleagues[40] found that the proportion of births beyond 42 weeks was 6.4% according to the LMP alone, while it was 1.9% when based on ultrasound alone. When scan and LMP dates were compared with known dates in patients who had undergone assisted reproduction, it was shown that 95% confidence interval (CI) for scan dates was ±8.3 days and –9 to +27 days for menstrual dating.[41]

For more accuracy, dating should be done in early pregnancy. Routine ultrasound in early first trimester decreases the number of false-positive diagnoses and hence lowers rate of induction for postmturity.[42] unnecessary interventions are prevented. Still, a practice of routine ultrasonography for pregnancy dating is controversial and recommendations vary.

Variation in estimation of gestational age by ultrasound is ±7 days up to 20 weeks of gestation, ±14 days between 20 weeks and 30 weeks of gestation, and ±21 days beyond 30 weeks of gestation. If the period of gestation calculated from patient's LMP differs from that estimated by ultrasound by more than this range, then ultrasound calculation should be used.[3,43]

PREVENTION OF POST-TERM PREGNANCY

"Prevention is better than cure"; this idiom holds good even for PTP. Many minimally invasive procedures have been suggested for this, like membrane sweeping, unprotected sexual intercourse, nipple stimulation and acupuncture.

Membrane sweeping causes local release of prostaglandins and studies document decreased interval to spontaneous onset of labor, and consequently PTP. However, there is no consistent documentation that it decreases the rates of operative deliveries or maternal and neonatal complications.[44] It leads to problems, like bleeding and irregular contractions, and is uncomfortable for the patient.

Sexual intercourse has been popularly considered to facilitate initiation of labor. The mechanism of action may be a combination of factors, like the physical stimulation of the lower uterine segment, endogenous release of oxytocin and uterine activity (provoked by orgasm); or direct action of prostaglandins in semen. However, its role as a method of induction of labor is uncertain.[45]

Acupuncture is commonly used in few societies for labor initiation. No significant maternal or fetal complications have been seen. A cochrane review did not find any clear evidence for the efficacy of this method.[46]

Various studies have seen that breast stimulation appears useful in decreasing the number of women not in labor after 72 hours, and postpartum hemorrhage rates.[47] However, it should not be used in high-risk women or as a routine till safety concerns are fully addressed.

Antenatal Fetal Surveillance

Post-term Pregnancy is a universally accepted indication for fetal surveillance. However, the efficacy of antenatal fetal monitoring has not been established by prospective randomized trials. Moreover, because of ethical and medicolegal issues, no studies include a nonmonitored control group, and it is highly improbable that such a trial will be conducted.

Various methods available for assessing fetal well-being include nonstress test (NST) with or without AF volume assessment, biophysical profile, oxytocin challenge test, or a combination of these. Assessment of the fetal heart rate variability gives a reliable estimate of fetal hypoxemia and acidemia. No single method has been proven to be superior over the other.[48] Another easy method is testing for maternal ketonuria which has been associated with high risk of oligohydramnios, nonreactive NST and fetal heart rate decelarations.[49]

The American College of Obstetricians and Gynecologists (ACOG) recommends that antepartum fetal monitoring should be started by 41 weeks of gestation without a specific suggestion about the type of test or frequency. The most commonly advised frequency is twice-weekly testing with inclusion of assessment of AF volume, as AF may fall drastically within 24–48 hours.[36,48]

The diagnosis of small-for-gestational age fetuses is the most important risk factor for subsequent fetal and neonatal adverse outcomes in PTP. Ultrasound estimation of fetal size should not be performed at intervals less than 2 weeks.

Use of umbilical artery doppler velocimetry does not provide a better positive predictive value of fetal testing in PTP.[50]

The drawbacks of monitoring are that false-positive tests lead to unnecessary invasive procedures and no program of fetal surveillance has been proven to completely eliminate risk of stillbirth.

Indians may have a tendency toward early maturity. Therefore, antenatal surveillance is recommended to be started even before 40 completed weeks.[51]

Induction of Labor

The World Health Organization (WHO) recommends a policy of routine induction of labor at 41 completed weeks.[5] This would reduce the time of hospitalization, which is especially useful where women are admitted earlier in pregnancy as they would be unable to reach the hospital in an emergency. However, accurate estimation of gestational age is a prerequisite. There is a need for more powerful studies for PTP in settings where facilities for close fetal monitoring are not available.

Patients with high-risk pregnancies should not be allowed to progress beyond 42 weeks of gestation, as in these pregnancies delivery around 38–39 weeks gestation is preferred.

Whether to continue or terminate a low-risk post-term pregnancy depends on the following factors:

- Results of antepartum fetal assessment
- Favorability of the cervix for induction
- Gestational age
- Maternal preference.

Induction of labor is to be done if any evidence is found of fetal compromise or oligohydramnios during fetal surveillance (Box 1). Many methods have been assessed to predict the likelihood of successful induction, like Bishop's score, ultrasound assessment of cervical length and recent biochemical markers (estriol to estradiol ratio).

According to some studies, transvaginal ultrasound for estimation of cervical length is quite accurate for predicting the success of induction.[52,53] The best cut-off level in prediction of a successful induction was a cervical length of less than 28 mm.

The ongoing risk of stillbirth (although less) is higher as compared to the risk of failed induction leading to cesarean delivery in patient with a favorable cervical examination. Therefore, routine induction of labor at 41 weeks' is quite reasonable in women with favorable cervix.

Around 80% of women who reach 42 weeks gestation have an unfavorable cervix (Bishop's score ≤ 6). In these both fetal monitoring and labor induction are associated with low-complication rates in low-risk women. Still, induction of labor with cervical ripening agents at 41 weeks' gestation has a slightly better prognosis.[54] Cervical ripening before induction has resulted in lesser failed inductions, lesser fetal and maternal morbidity, earlier discharge from hospital, lower medical cost, and probably a lower rate of cesarean delivery.[55] Prostaglandin gel can be used safely in PTP. Several placebo-controlled trials have documented significant changes in Bishop score, shorter duration of labor, lower maximum doses of oxytocin, and a decreased incidence of cesarean delivery among postterm women who received prostaglandin E_2 (PGE_2) gel.[56,57] However, no standardized dose or dosing interval has been recommended. Overall, few side effects were reported. Higher doses of PG (especially PGE_1) may lead to uterine tachysystole and hyperstimulation leading to nonreassuring fetal testing.[58] Therefore, lower doses are preferable. Fetal heart rate monitoring should be a dictum.

Box 1: Conditions for which immediate delivery is advised in post-term pregnancy[38]

- Medical or obstetrical complications of pregnancy
- Favorable cervix
- Oligohydramnios
- Estimated fetal weight ≥4,500 g
- Suspected fetal compromise
- Fetal congenital anomalies
- Senescent placenta

Routine labor induction is reported to have no effect on the instrumental delivery rate, use of analgesia, or incidence of fetal heart rate abnormality.[59] The risk of meconium-stained AF is decreased; however, the risks of MAS and neonatal seizures remain unaffected. The actual risk of stillbirth during the 41st week of gestation is thought to be 1.04–1.27 per 1,000 undelivered women, which is lesser than 1.55–3.1 per 1,000 women seen at or beyond 42 weeks of gestation.[60]

A cochrane review of 19 trials suggested that routine induction of labor at 41 weeks of gestation has fetal benefit (lower PM: 1/2, 986 versus 9/2,953 in expectant management) without adding to the risk of a higher cesarean rate. As absolute risk is small, women should be counseled regarding both relative and absolute risks. In addition, women at 37–40 weeks were more likely to have a cesarean section with expectant management than with elective induction of labor.[54]

Current obstetric guidelines from Canada (British Columbia Reproductive 2005) and the United Kingdom (Royal College of Obstetricians and Gynaecologist (RCOG)/ National Institute for Health and Care Excellence 2001) recommend induction of labor after 41 completed weeks.[54]

For women with history of previous cesarean section who want a trial for vaginal delivery, failure to go into spontaneous labor by 41 weeks should prompt counseling for elective cesarean. There is limited data regarding the efficacy or safety of vaginal birth after cesarean after 42 weeks of gestation.

MULTIPLE PREGNANCIES

The average duration of gestation is 40 weeks in singletons, 36 weeks in twins, 33 weeks in triplets and 29 weeks in quadruplets.[61] The lowest PM was seen at 38 weeks in multiple pregnancies as opposed to 40 weeks in singleton (10.5 versus 9.7 deaths per 1,000 deliveries, respectively). Perinatal mortality rose after this gestation.[62] No consensus has been reached, but this study suggests that the normal length of gestation for twins should be considered as 38 weeks rather than 40 weeks. Furthermore, every effort should be made to deliver uncomplicated twins by 40 weeks' gestation (post-term for twins).

INTRAPARTUM MANAGEMENT

The postterm fetus is at high risk of intrapartum fetal distress. Therefore, continuous electronic fetal monitoring should be done during labor. Intrapartum spontaneous or induced fetal heart rate accelerations along with moderate fetal heart rate variability (category 1 tracings) are reliable signs of a non-acidotic fetus.

Artificial rupture of membranes causes further reduction in fluid volume increasing the possibility of cord compression. On the other hand, it aids diagnosis of thick meconium.

CONCLUSION

Post-term pregnancy is associated with fetal, neonatal, and maternal morbidity, along with higher PM. To prevent these, accurate dating of gestation is important. There is emerging evidence that fetal, neonatal, and maternal complications increase even before 42 weeks (from 38 weeks to 39 weeks onwards with an obvious rise after 41-weeks gestation). In the Indian setting, especially in low-resource areas, induction of labor at 41 weeks should be practiced as a routine rather than expectant management.

REFERENCES

1. Tita AT, Landon MB, Spong CY, Lai Y, Leveno KJ, Varner MW, et al. Timing of elective repeat cesarean delivery at term and neonatal outcomes. N Engl J Med. 2009;360(2):111-20.
2. Spong CY. Defining "term" pregnancy: recommendations from the Defining "Term" Pregnancy Workgroup. JAMA. 2013;309(23):2445-6.
3. ACOG Committee on Practice Bulletins-Obstetrics. ACOG Practice Bulletin. Clinical management guidelines for obstetricians-gynecologists. Number 55, September 2004 (replaces practice pattern number 6, October 1997). Management of Postterm Pregnancy. Obstet Gynecol. 2004;104(3):639-46.
4. Lindell A. Prolonged pregnancy. Acta Obstet Gynecol Scand. 1956;35(2):136-63.
5. Cuervo LG. (2015). Induction of labour for improving birth outcomes for women at or beyond term. RHL: The WHO Reproductive Health Library. [online] Available from apps.who.int/rhl/pregnancy_childbirth/complications/prolonged_pregnancy/lgccom/en/. [Accessed October, 2015].
6. Savitz DA, Terry JW, Dole N, Thorp JM, Siega-Riz AM, Herring AH. Comparison of pregnancy dating by last menstrual period, ultrasound scanning, and their combination. Am J Obstet Gynecol. 2002;187(6):1660-6.
7. Gabbe SG, Niebyl JR, Simpson JL, Galan HL, Jauniaux ERM, Landon MB, Simpson JL, Driscoll DA (Eds). Obstetrics: Normal and Problem Pregnancies, 6th edition. Philadelphia, PA, USA: Elsevier-Saunders; 2012.
8. Divon MY, Ferber A, Nisell H, Westgren M. Male gender predisposes to prolongation of pregnancy. Am J Obstet Gynecol. 2002;187(4):1081-3.
9. Laursen M, Bille C, Olesen AW, Hjelmborg J, Skytthe A, Christensen K. Genetic influence on prolonged gestation: a population-based Danish twin study. Am J Obstet Gynecol. 2004;190(2):489-94.
10. Usha Kiran TS, Hemmadi S, Bethel J, Evans J. Outcome of pregnancy in a woman with an increased body mass index. BJOG. 2005;112(6):768-72.
11. Torricelli M, Novembri R, Voltolini C, Conti N, Biliotti G, Piccolini E, et al. Biochemical and biophysical predictors of the response to the induction of labor in nulliparous postterm pregnancy. Am J Obstet Gynecol. 2011;204(1):39.e1-6.
12. Galal M, Symonds I, Murray H, Petraglia F, Smith R. Postterm pregnancy. Facts Views Vis Obgyn. 2012;4(3):175-87.
13. Cunningham F, Leveno K, Bloom S, Spong CY, Dashe J (Eds). Williams Obstetrics, 24th edition. New York, USA: McGraw-Hill Education/Medical Publishers; 2014.
14. Clifford SH. Postmaturity, with placental dysfunction; clinical syndrome and pathologic findings. J Pediatr. 1954;44(1):1-13.
15. Shime J, Gare DJ, Andrews J, Bertrand M, Salgado J, Whillans G. Prolonged pregnancy: surveillance of the fetus and the neonate and the course of labor and delivery. Am J Obstet Gynecol. 1984;148(5):547-52.

16. Vorherr H. Placental insufficiency in relation to postterm pregnancy and fetal postmaturity. Evaluation of fetoplacental function; management of the postterm gravida. Am J Obstet Gynecol. 1975;123(1):67-103.
17. MacDorman MF, Kirmeyer SE, Wilson EC. Fetal and perinatal mortality, United States, 2006. Natl Vital Stat Rep. 2012;60(8):1-22.
18. Mandruzzato G, Alfirevic Z, Chervenak F, Gruenebaum A, Heimstad R, Heinonen S, et al. Guidelines for the management of postterm pregnancy. J Perinat Med. 2010;38(2):111-9.
19. Oshiro BT, Henry E, Wilson J, Branch DW, Varner MW; Women and Newborn Clinical Integration Program. Decreasing elective deliveries before 39 weeks of gestation in an integrated health care system. Obstet Gynecol. 2009;113(4):804-11.
20. Hilder L, Costeloe K, Thilaganathan B. Prolonged pregnancy: evaluating gestation-specific risks of fetal and infant mortality. Br J Obstet Gynaecol. 1998;105(2):169-73.
21. Queenan JT, Spong CY, Lockwood CJ (Eds). Queenan's Management of High-Risk Pregnancy: An Evidence-Based Approach, 6th edition. Chichester, West Sussex, UK: Wiley-Blackwell; 2012.
22. Kitlinski ML, Kallen K, Marsal K, Olofsson P. Gestational age-dependent reference values for pH in umbilical cord arterial blood at term. Obstet Gynecol. 2003;102(2):338-45.
23. Yoder BA, Kirsch EA, Barth WH, Gordon MC. Changing obstetric practices associated with decreasing incidence of meconium aspiration syndrome. Obstet Gynecol. 2002;99(5 Pt 1):731-9.
24. Rouse DJ, Owen J. Prophylactic cesarean delivery for fetal macrosomia diagnosed by means of ultrasonography--A Faustian bargain? Am J Obstet Gynecol. 1999;181(2):332-8.
25. Manchanda R, Vora M, Gruslin A. Influence of postdatism and meconium on fetal erythropoietin. J Perinatol. 1999;19(7):479-82.
26. Caughey AB, Washington AE, Laros RK. Neonatal complications of term pregnancy: rates by gestational age increase in a continuous, not threshold, fashion. Am J Obstet Gynecol. 2005;192(1):185-90.
27. Nicholson JM, Kellar LC, Kellar GM. The impact of the interaction between increasing gestational age and obstetrical risk on birth outcomes: evidence of a varying optimal time of delivery. J Perinatol. 2006;26(7):392-402.
28. Weinstein D, Ezra Y, Picard R, Furman M, Elchalal U. Expectant management of post-term patients: observations and outcome. J Matern Fetal Med. 1996;5(5):293-7.
29. Abotalib ZM, Soltan MH, Chowdhury N, Adelusi B. Obstetric outcome in uncomplicated prolonged pregnancy. Int J Gynaecol Obstet. 1996;55(3):225-30.
30. Divon MY, Ferber A, Sanderson M, Nisell H, Westgren M. A functional definition of prolonged pregnancy based on daily fetal and neonatal mortality rates. Ultrasound Obstet Gynecol. 2004;23(5):423-6.
31. Badawi N, Kurinczuk JJ, Keogh JM, Alessandri LM, O'Sullivan F, Burton PR, et al. Antepartum risk factors for newborn encephalopathy: the Western Australian case-control study. BMJ. 1998;317(7172):1549-53.
32. Shime J, Librach CL, Gare DJ, Cook CJ. The influence of prolonged pregnancy on infant development at one and two years of age: a prospective controlled study. Am J Obstet Gynecol. 1986;154(2):341-5.
33. Alexander JM, McIntire DD, Leveno KJ. Forty weeks and beyond: pregnancy outcomes by week of gestation. Obstet Gynecol. 2000;96(2):291-4.
34. Treger M, Hallak M, Silberstein T, Friger M, Katz M, Mazor M. Post-term pregnancy: should induction of labor be considered before 42 weeks? J Matern Fetal Neonatal Med. 2002;11(1):50-3.
35. Caughey AB, Musci TJ. Complications of term pregnancies beyond 37 weeks of gestation. Obstet Gynecol. 2004;103(1):57-62.
36. American Congress of Obstetricians and Gynecologists. Practice Bulletin no. 146: Management of late-term and postterm pregnancies. Obstet Gynecol. 2014;124(2 Pt 1):390-6.
37. Trimmer KJ, Leveno KJ, Peters MT, Kelly MA. Observations on the cause of oligohydramnios in prolonged pregnancy. Am J Obstet Gynecol. 1990;163(6 Pt 1):1900-3.
38. Arias F, Bhide A, Arulkumaran S, Damania K, Daftary SN (Eds). Practical Guide to High Risk Pregnancy and Delivery: A South Asian Perspective, 3rd edition. New Delhi, India: Elsevier; 2008.
39. Oz AU, Holub B, Mendilcioglu I, Mari G, Bahado-Singh RO. Renal artery Doppler investigation of the etiology of oligohydramnios in postterm pregnancy. Obstet Gynecol. 2002;100(4):715-8.
40. Blondel B, Morin I, Platt RW, Kramer MS, Usher R, Bréart G. Algorithms for combining menstrual and ultrasound estimates of gestational age: consequences for rates of preterm and postterm birth. BJOG. 2002;109(6):718-20.
41. Mul T, Mongelli M, Gardosi J. A comparative analysis of second-trimester ultrasound dating formulae in pregnancies conceived with artificial reproductive techniques. Ultrasound Obstet Gynecol. 1996;8(6):397-402.
42. Whitworth M, Bricker L, Mullan C. Ultrasound for fetal assessment in early pregnancy. Cochrane Database Syst Rev. 2015;7:CD007058.
43. American Academy of Pediatrics (AAP) and American College of Obstetricians and Gynecologists (ACOG). Guidelines for Perinatal Care, 6th edition. Washington, DC, USA: AAP and ACOG; 2007.
44. Boulvain M, Stan C, Irion O. Membrane sweeping for induction of labour. Cochrane Database Syst Rev. 2005;(1):CD000451.
45. Kavanagh J, Kelly AJ, Thomas J. Sexual intercourse for cervical ripening and induction of labour. Cochrane database Syst Rev. 2001;(2):CD003093.
46. Smith CA, Crowther CA, Grant SJ. Acupuncture for induction of labour. Cochrane Database Syst Rev. 2013;8:CD002962.
47. Kavanagh J, Kelly AJ, Thomas J. Breast stimulation for cervical ripening and induction of labour. Cochrane Database Syst Rev. 2005;(3):CD003392.
48. Practice bulletin no. 145: antepartum fetal surveillance. Obstet Gynecol. 2014;124(1):182-92.
49. Onyeije CI, Divon MY. The impact of maternal ketonuria on fetal test results in the setting of postterm pregnancy. Am J Obstet Gynecol. 2001;184(4):713-8.
50. Stokes HJ, Roberts RV, Newnham JP. Doppler flow velocity waveform analysis in postdate pregnancies. Aust N Z J Obstet Gynaecol. 1991;31(1):27-30.
51. Tambyraja RL. Current concepts of the low birth weight Indian baby. In: Ratnam SS, Bhasker Rao K, Arulkumaran S (Eds). Obstetrics and Gynaecology for Postgraduates, 1st edition. Hyderabad, India: Orient Longman; 1992. p. 88.
52. Tan PC, Vallikkannu N, Suguna S, Quek KF, Hassan J. Transvaginal sonography of cervical length and Bishop score as predictors of successful induction of term labor: the effect of parity. Clin Exp Obstet Gynecol. 2009;36(1):35-9.
53. Uyar Y, Erbay G, Demir CS, Baytur Y. Comparison of the Bishop score, body mass index and transvaginal cervical length in predicting the success of labor induction. Arch Gynecol Obstet. 2009;280(3):357-62.
54. Gülmezoglu AM, Crowther CA, Middleton P, Heatley E. Induction of labour for improving birth outcomes for women at or beyond term. Cochrane Database Syst Rev. 2012;6:CD004945.
55. Poma PA. Cervical ripening. A review and recommendations for clinical practice. J Reprod Med. 1999;44(8):657-68.
56. Papageorgiou I, Tsionou C, Minaretzis D, Michalas S, Aravantinos D. Labor characteristics of uncomplicated prolonged pregnancies after induction

with intracervical prostaglandin E2 gel versus intravenous oxytocin. Gynecol Obstet Invest. 1992;34(2):92-6.

57. Sawai SK, O'Brien WF, Mastrogiannis DS, Krammer J, Mastry MG, Porter GW. Patient-administered outpatient intravaginal prostaglandin E2 suppositories in post-date pregnancies: a double-blind, randomized, placebo-controlled study. Obstet Gynecol. 1994;84:807-10.
58. Sanchez-Ramos L, Kaunitz AM, Delke I. Labor induction with 25 µg versus 50 µg intravaginal misoprostol: a systematic review. Obstet Gynecol. 2002;99(1):145-51.
59. Crowley P. Interventions for preventing or improving the outcome of delivery at or beyond term. Cochrane Database Syst Rev. 2000;2:CD000170.
60. Menticoglou SM, Hall PF. Routine induction of labour at 41 weeks gestation: nonsensus consensus. BJOG. 2002;109(5):485-91.
61. Kahn B, Lumey LH, Zybert PA, Lorenz JM, Cleary-Goldman J, D'Alton ME, et al. Prospective risk of fetal death in singleton, twin, and triplet gestations: implications for practice. Obstet Gynecol. 2003;102(4):685-92.
62. Minakami H, Sato I. Reestimating date of delivery in multifetal pregnancies. JAMA. 1996;275(18):1432-4.

CHAPTER 38

Placental Adhesive Disorders and Umbilical Cord Abnormalities

Sujata Misra, Saumya Nanda

PLACENTAL ADHESIVE DISORDERS

Introduction

Placental adhesive disorders encompass two pathologies: (1) placenta adherens/simple adherent placenta: placentae that are adherent to the uterine wall but easily separated manually and (2) placenta accreta/morbidly adherent placenta: the placentae invade the myometrium or serosa.

Of all the retained placentae, 53% are just trapped behind a closed cervix (trapped or incarcerated placentae), morbidly adherent placenta account for less than 0.25%.[1] The incidence of placenta accreta is less than 0.25%.[1]

Placenta Accreta

Definition

Placenta accreta represents the abnormal attachment of the placenta to the uterine lining due to an absence of the decidua basalis and an incomplete development of the fibrinoid layer.[2]

Depending on the extent of invasion of the placenta, the condition is further classified as placenta accreta (reaching the myometrium), placenta increta (into the myometrium) and placenta percreta (invading the serosa or beyond).[3] In the literature the term "placenta accreta" is often used interchangeably as a general term to describe all three conditions. Figure 1 shows the diagrammatic representation of various types of invasive placentations and Table 1 describes them.

Pathogenesis

The exact pathogenesis of placenta accreta is unknown. A proposed hypothesis includes a maldevelopment of decidua, excessive trophoblastic invasion, or a combination of both.[4] Morbidly adherent placenta is thought to be due to an absence or deficiency of Nitabuch's layer or the spongiosus layer of the decidua. Benirschke et al. suggested this to happen as a consequence of failure of reconstitution of the decidua basalis after repair of cesarean incision, thus resulting in absence of intervening decidual tissue

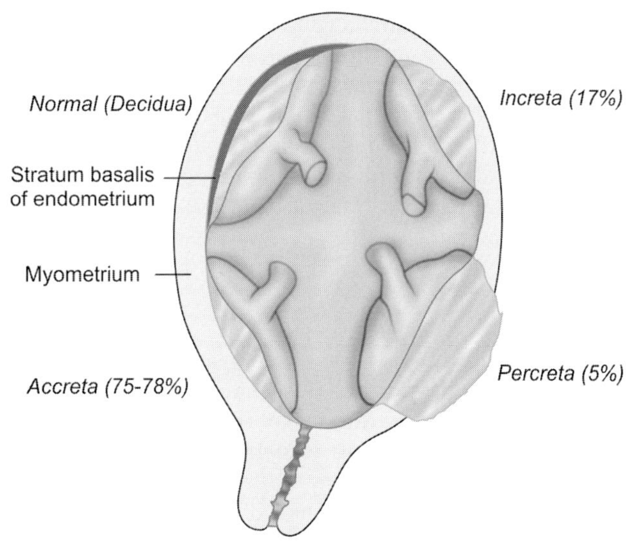

FIG. 1: Uteroplacental relationship found in invasive placentation.

TABLE 1: Types of morbidly invasive placenta

Type	Fraction	Description
Placenta accreta	75–78%	The placenta attaches strongly to the myometrium, but does not penetrate it. This form of the condition accounts for around 75% of all cases
Placenta increta	17%	Occurs when the placenta penetrates the myometrium
Placenta percreta	5–7%	The worst form of the condition is when the placenta penetrates the entire myometrium to the uterine serosa (invades through entire uterine wall). This variant can lead to the placenta attaching to other organs such as the rectum or bladder

between the invading trophoblast and the myometrium.[5] It has been proposed that the abnormality of the placental uterine interface leads to leakage of fetal alpha-fetoproteins into the maternal circulation resulting in elevated levels of maternal serum alpha-fetoproteins.[6,7] According to Chou and Tseng, abnormal expression of growth, angiogenesis and invasion-related factors in the trophoblast populations are the main factors responsible for the occurrence of placenta accreta.[8] Data from Tantbirojn et al. explained invasion of larger vessels in the outer myometrium and near the serosa to be determined by access rather than a pre-existing defect in trophoblastic growth that would produce uncontrolled invasion through the entire depth of the myometrium in cases of accreta.[9] Garmi et al. showed, *in vitro*, that an induced sharp decidual incision, imitating the *in vivo* process, i.e., cesarean section, increased significantly the invasion potential of the trophoblastic cells. Complete reapproximation of the incised edges of the decidua *in vitro* made the incised decidua to behave similarly to intact deciduas while restricting once again the extent of the invasiveness. Using the same cohort of trophoblast cells, while changing only the decidual anatomic characteristics, the invasion potential of trophoblastic cells *in vitro* changed accordingly emphasizing the role of decidua on the invasion potential.[10] The molecular basis of this disorder is still unexplored. Decidual maldevelopment may decrease production of tissue inhibitors of metalloprotease and transforming growth factor beta resulting in abnormal invasiveness.

Risk Factors

The vast majority of women with placenta accreta have an identifiable risk factor.[11] Placenta previa and previous cesarean deliveries are the major risk factors for placenta accreta. The risk increases with the number of previous cesarean sections[12-14] (Table 2). Myometrial trauma and scarring resulting from repeated dilatation and curettage, previous myomectomy, submucous leiomyomas, thermal ablation and uterine artery embolization (UAE) also contribute to the risk of developing abnormal placental adherence. Advanced maternal age has also been identified as an independent risk factor. Others include smoking, grand multiparity and recurrent miscarriages.[15-17] Female fetal

TABLE 2: Link between number of previous cesarean sections and risk of placenta accreta[14]

Number of previous cesarean section(s)	Chance of placenta accreta if placenta previa
0	3%
1	11%
2	40%
3	61%
4	67%
5	67%

gender is more common with invasive placentation.[18] In a review of 72 cases of placenta accreta treated conservatively, 15% had a subsequent pregnancy, 18% of whom developed a repeated placenta accreta, hence prior placenta accreta is probably a major risk factor.[19]

Incidence

The incidence of placenta accreta has been escalating, from a reported occurrence of one in 30,000 deliveries in 1950 to 1 in 2,500 deliveries (a 10-fold increase) in 1997.[11,14] Researchers have reported the incidence of placenta accreta as 1 in 533 pregnancies for the period of 1982-2002.[20] This marked increase has been attributed to the increase in cesarean section rates worldwide. Urinary bladder involvement commonly occurs in placenta percreta and is associated with substantial morbidity.

Diagnosis

A high degree of clinical suspicion coupled with ultrasonography (USG) and occasionally supplemented by magnetic resonance imaging (MRI) and cystoscopy helps in antenatal diagnosis. The value of making the diagnosis of placenta accreta before delivery is that it allows for multidisciplinary planning in an attempt to minimize potential maternal or neonatal morbidity and mortality.[21] Women who have had a previous cesarean section who also have either placenta previa or an anterior placenta underlying the old cesarean section scar at 32 weeks of gestation are at increased risk of placenta accreta and should be managed as if they have placenta accreta, with appropriate preparations for surgery made.

Shih et al.[22] compared the diagnostic performance of gray-scale, color Doppler and three-dimensional power Doppler in 170 women of whom 72 had had a previous cesarean section. 38 of the women with a previous cesarean section had placenta accreta identified at delivery. The diagnostic performance of different USG modalities have been summarized in Table 3 and it can be seen that three-dimensional power Doppler gives the best overall results when an isolated criterion is found.

Ultrasound Criteria for Diagnosis

- Gray-scale:
  - Loss of the retroplacental sonolucent zone
  - Thinning or disruption of the hyperechoic serosa-bladder interface
  - Presence of focal exophytic masses invading the urinary bladder
  - Abnormal placental lacunae
- Color Doppler:
  - Diffuse or focal lacunar flow
  - Vascular lakes with turbulent flow (peak systolic velocity over 15 cm/s)
  - Hypervascularity of serosa-bladder interface
  - Markedly dilated vessels over peripheral subplacental zone
- Three-Dimensional Power Doppler:
  - Numerous coherent vessels involving the whole uterine serosa-bladder junction (basal view)
  - Hypervascularity (lateral view)
  - Inseparable cotyledonal and intervillous circulations, chaotic branching, detour vessels (lateral view).

Comstock et al.[23] reported that of the four criteria for diagnosing placenta accreta using gray-scale ultrasonographic examination during the 2nd and 3rd trimesters, the presence of intraplacental lacunae was found to be the most reliable one, with 93% sensitivity and 93% positive-predictive value. Furthermore, they reported that intraplacental lacunae were first observed at about the 15th gestational week, thus they serve as useful indicators for the early diagnosis of placenta accreta at around 15–20 weeks' gestation, with a sensitivity of 79% and positive-predictive value of 92%. Intraplacental lacunae are graded as:

- Grade 0: When none was seen
- Grade 1^+: When 1–3 generally small lacunae were present
- Grade 2^+: When 4–6 larger or more irregular lacunae were present
- Grade 3^+: When there were many throughout the placenta, some appearing large and irregular in shape.[24]

Yang et al.[25] studied 51 patients with placenta previa totalis diagnosed by transvaginal sonography and with a history of cesarean section and when lacunae of more than or equal to Grade 2^+ were considered, the sensitivity, specificity, positive- and negative-predictive values of diagnosing placenta increta or percreta were 100%, 97.2%, 93.8% and 100%, respectively. The number of massive transfusions and intensive care unit admissions and cases of disseminated intravascular coagulopathy and cesarean hysterectomy were significantly greater in those with lacunae ($p < 0.0001$).

Magnetic Resonance Imaging

The role of MRI in diagnosing placenta accreta is still debated. It is considered an adjunctive modality and adds little to the diagnostic accuracy of USG.[21] The indications of MRI are:

- When ultrasound findings are ambiguous
- Posterior placenta accreta
- Lateral placenta accreta helps in confirmation of parametrial invasion and possible ureteral involvement.

The main MRI features of placenta accreta[26] include:

- Uterine bulging
- Heterogeneous signal intensity within the placenta
- Dark intraplacental bands on T_2-weighted imaging.

Biochemical Markers

Elevated levels of maternal α-fetoprotein and β-human chorionic gonadotropin (β-hCG) within the triple screening test have been reported to be associated with an increased risk of placenta accreta. Abnormality of the placental-uterine interface that may lead to leakage into the maternal circulation may explain this increase.[27,28]

At this time no antenatal diagnostic technique affords the clinician 100% assurance of either ruling in or ruling out the presence of placenta accreta.[4]

Histopathology

The definitive diagnosis of placenta accreta is usually made postpartum on hysterectomy specimens when an area of

TABLE 3: Diagnostic performance of different ultrasonography (USG) modalities[22]

Ultrasound criteria for diagnosis	Sensitivity (%)	Specificity (%)	Positive-predictive value (%)	Risk
Gray-scale	95	76	82	93
Color Doppler	92	68	76	89
Three-dimensional power Doppler	100	85	88	100

accretion shows chorionic villi in direct contact with the myometrium and absence of deciduas.[5,9]

Management

Generally, the recommended management of suspected placenta accreta is planned preterm cesarean hysterectomy with the placenta left *in situ* because removal of the placenta is associated with significant hemorrhagic morbidity. However, surgical management of placenta accreta may be individualized (Flowchart 1).

General Considerations

It is critically important that obstetricians and radiologists are familiar with the risk factors and diagnostic modalities for placenta accreta because of its potential emergent nature and life-threatening hemorrhage.[21] Delivery should be planned in tertiary health-care centers. Delivery planning may involve an anesthesiologist, obstetrician, pelvic surgeon, intensivist, maternal-fetal medicine specialists, neonatologist, urologist, hematologist and interventional radiologist to optimize the patient's outcome.[29]

Delivery Planning

The timing of delivery should be individualized and the decision should be made jointly by the patient, obstetrician and neonatologist.[21] Any woman with suspected placenta previa accreta should be reviewed by a consultant obstetrician in the antenatal period. The different risks and treatment options should have been discussed and a plan agreed, which should be reflected clearly in the consent form. This should include the anticipated skin and uterine incisions

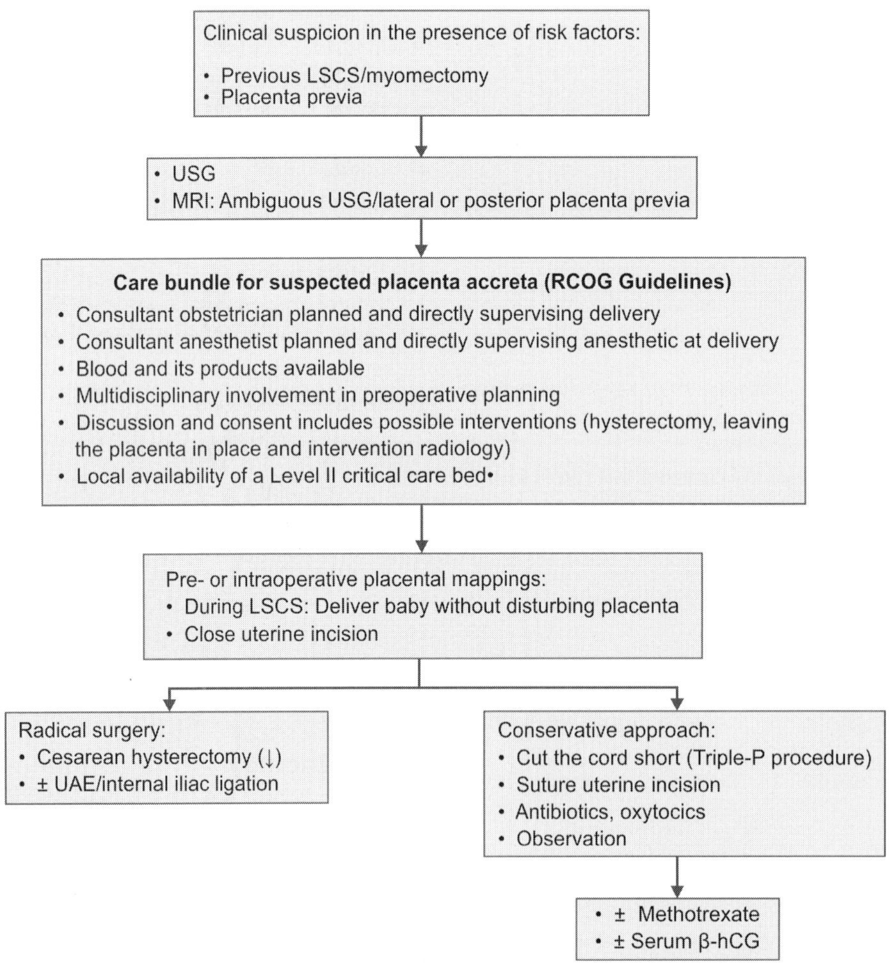

LSCS, lower segment cesarean section; USG, ultrasonography; MRI, magnetic resonance imaging; RCOG, Royal College of Obstetricians and Gynaecologists; UAE, uterine artery embolization; β-hCG, beta human chorionic gonadotropin.

FLOWCHART 1: Management of placenta accreta.

and whether conservative management of the placenta or proceeding straight to hysterectomy is preferred in the situation where accreta is confirmed at surgery. Additional possible interventions in the case of massive hemorrhage should also be discussed, including interventional radiology when available.[30]

The anticipation and planning of surgery for suspected placenta accreta enables logical and timely decisions to be made without the element of surprise and often without the urgency of massive hemorrhage.[31] Although a planned delivery is the goal, a contingency plan for emergency delivery should be developed for each patient.[21] Ideally, delivery should be elective at the gestational age of proven lung maturity. Often, however, bleeding will prompt earlier surgical intervention. It may be appropriate to consider elective cesarean hysterectomy at 34 weeks' gestation or even earlier, irrespective of fetal lung maturity, in patients with diffuse lacunar flow pattern in color-Doppler imaging, particularly associated with strong evidence of extensive placenta increta/percreta and episodes of antepartum hemorrhage, in order to decrease the risk of maternal morbidity and mortality associated with emergency surgery.[32] For patients with a focal lacunar flow pattern, uneventful cesarean hysterectomy can usually be performed at more advanced gestation (35–37 weeks' gestation). Further studies are necessary to support these suggestions. If color-Doppler imaging shows a diffuse lacunar flow pattern and bladder-uterine serosa interface hypervascularity, urologic assessment, including cystoscopy and pre- or intraoperative placements of a ureteral stent, should be considered. Blood bank should be intimated regarding the possibility of massive hemorrhage. Current recommendations for blood replacement in trauma situations suggest a 1:1 ratio of packed cells to fresh-frozen plasma.[21]

Surgical Technique

Surgeons delivering the baby by cesarean section in the presence of a suspected placenta previa accreta should consider opening the uterus at a site distant from the placenta, and delivering the baby without disturbing the placenta, in order to enable conservative management of the placenta or elective hysterectomy to be performed if the accreta is confirmed. Going straight through the placenta to achieve delivery is associated with more bleeding and a high chance of hysterectomy and should be avoided. Conservative management of placenta accreta when the woman is already bleeding is unlikely to be successful and risks wasting valuable time.[30]

Hysterectomy

The recommended management of suspected placenta accreta is planned cesarean hysterectomy with the placenta left *in situ*, except for women who have a strong desire for future fertility. A classical uterine incision may be necessary to avoid disturbing the placenta and delivering the baby. It is reasonable to wait for spontaneous separation of placenta to confirm placenta accreta clinically and attempts at manual removal of placenta should be avoided. Placenta is left *in situ*, uterine incision is closed and hysterectomy is performed. Prompt hysterectomy has led to a reduction of maternal mortality to less than 2%.[33]

Conservative Methods

Conservative approach includes cutting the cord short; leaving the placenta *in situ* and uterine incision is closed. Potential life-threatening complications include severe postpartum hemorrhage, disseminated intravascular coagulopathy and infection resistant to antimicrobial therapy that may require laparotomy and hysterectomy.[21] When placenta is left *in situ*, serial USG and serum β-hCG is performed. The placenta is left to resorb to expel spontaneously.

Role of methotrexate

Use of methotrexate for placenta percreta was first reported by Arulkumaran et al. in 1986.[34] Methotrexate, a folate antagonist, acts primarily against rapidly dividing cells, and therefore is effective against dividing trophoblast. Opponents argue that after delivery of the fetus, the placenta is no longer dividing and methotrexate is of no value.[35] Other studies have shown mixed results, failure of therapy and need for hysterectomy following postpartum hemorrhage. Currently there is no convincing data for the use of methotrexate for postpartum management of placenta accreta.[21]

The "Triple-P procedure" for percreta has been developed as a conservative surgical alternative to peripartum hysterectomy. Triple-P involves three steps: (1) preoperative or intraoperative placental localization using a transabdominal ultrasound scan to delineate the upper border of the placenta on the operation table and delivery of the fetus through a uterine incision placed above the upper border of the placenta; (2) pelvic devascularization immediately after delivery of the fetus by inflation of prepositioned uterine artery occlusion balloons to reduce blood supply to the myometrium and placental nonseparation and (3) myometrial excision (to avoid separation of the morbidly adherent placenta from the underlying myometrial bed) with reconstruction of the uterine wall. The line of placental infiltration into the bladder is left untouched as attempts at separation may result in perforation of the urinary bladder.[36] Triple-P procedure has the potential to be a very effective alternative to peripartum hysterectomy in anterior placenta percreta infiltrating a previous cesarean section scar. Technical difficulties may be faced with placenta infiltrating the cervix and the broad ligament where myometrial resection may not be possible. This procedure is also not possible for lateral placentae infiltrating the ureters.

Interventional Radiologic Procedures

Current evidence is insufficient to make a firm recommendation on the use of balloon catheter occlusion or embolization to reduce blood loss and improve surgical outcome, but individual situations may warrant their use.[21]

Placenta percreta involving the urinary bladder

Management of patients with bladder involvement requires careful preoperative planning and involvement of the urologist. Preoperative ureteric stenting aids in identifying the ureters, which will help reduce ureteric injuries. Care must be taken during surgery not to attempt to dissect the bladder off the lower uterine segment which results in torrential bleeding. Anterior bladder wall incision is particularly helpful in defining dissection planes and the location of the ureters.[37]

ABNORMALITIES OF THE UMBILICAL CORD

Introduction

The umbilical cord develops from the zygote by the 5th week of fetal development, replacing the yolk sac as the source of nutrients for the fetus. The cord joins the placenta, and transfers materials to and from the mother's blood without allowing direct mixing. The length of the umbilical cord is approximately equal to the crown-rump length of the fetus throughout pregnancy. The umbilical cord in a full-term neonate is usually about 50–55 cm long, about 1–2 cm in diameter and contains 11 helices.[38] The umbilical cord contains Wharton's jelly, a gelatinous substance made largely from mucopolysaccharides which protects the blood vessels inside. It contains one vein, which carries oxygenated, nutrient-rich blood to the fetus, and two arteries that carry deoxygenated, nutrient-depleted blood away. Abnormalities of the cord are numerous, few are harmless and others life-threatening to the fetus.

Cord Measurements

Cord Length

Cord length ranges from achordia (no cord) to 300 cm. Short cord is defined when the length is less than 35 cm and long cord when the length is more than 80 cm. It is determined by volume of amniotic fluid and fetal mobility. Short cord is associated with intrauterine growth restriction, congenital malformation, like fetal movement disorders, Down's syndrome, intrapartum distress, placental abruption and two-fold increased risk of death. Long cord is associated with cord entanglement, prolapse, fetal anomalies, distress, true knots and thrombi.

Diameter

Thin umbilical cords have been associated with fetal growth restriction and thick cords have been associated with macrosomia.[39]

Cord Coiling

Umbilical cords are helical in nature and most cords coil to the left.

$$\text{Umbilical coiling index} = \frac{\text{Number of complete coils}}{\text{Length of the cord (in cm)}}$$

Hypocoiling has been associated with fetal demise and hypercoiling with fetal growth restriction and intrapartum acidosis, but recent studies show that degree of coiling is not significant.[40]

Vessel Number

Single Umbilical Artery

The incidence is less than 1% in singleton pregnancies and around 3% in twins. It is believed to occur because of agenesis or atrophy of a previously normal artery. Usually the left artery is absent but associated fetal anomalies are more common when the right artery is absent. 20% or more of fetuses with single umbilical artery have associated congenital anomalies including cardiovascular, gastrointestinal, renal and vertebral defects and chromosomal anomalies, like trisomy 18.[41,42] The incidence is more in women with diabetes, epilepsy, pre-eclampsia, antepartum hemorrhage and oligohydramnios. Diagnosis can be made prenatally by USG and once diagnosed a detailed anomaly scan, fetal echocardiogram should be considered. Serial USG to rule out fetal growth retardation can be done. Perinatal mortality rate is 5–20% of which two-thirds occur antenatally and one-third occur postnatally.[43]

Cord Insertion

Battledore Placenta

The cord is attached to the margin of placenta. If associated with low lying placenta there is chance of cord compression during vaginal delivery, otherwise it has got little clinical significance.

Velamentous Insertion

In such cases, the umbilical cord inserts into the chorion away from the placental edge, and the vessels traverse varying distance to reach the placenta between the amnion and chorion. The incidence is around 1% in singleton pregnancies, 15% in monochorionic twins[44] and common in triplets and placenta previa. Mechanism: (1) when placental tissue grows laterally or (2) when the cord implants in the trophoblast anterior to the decidua capsularis instead of the trophoblastic tissue destined to become the placenta.[45] Diagnosis is possible antenatally by 2nd trimester USG.[46] High levels of maternal serum β-hCG and low levels of maternal serum alpha-fetoprotein have been associated with this condition. It is associated with low-birth weight, prematurity, abnormal fetal heart tracing in labor. If the velamentous insertion is in the lower segment elective cesarean section should be planned to prevent vasa previa rupture and fetal distress.[46]

Vasa Previa

In this condition, the fetal vessels traversing through the membranes lie below the presenting part of the fetus overlying the internal os. It may occur because of velamentous insertion of the cord or vessels running between the placenta and succenturiate lobe. According to Hasegawa et al., 2012[47] the incidence is as high as 1 in 365 pregnancies based on ultrasound diagnosis. The risk factors include 2nd trimester placenta previa, bilobate placenta or placenta with succenturiate lobes, multiple pregnancies and *in vitro* fertilization (IVF) pregnancies.

Antepartum diagnosis carries better fetal prognosis compared to intrapartum diagnosis. Cases diagnosed antenatally had 97% fetal survival rate compared to 48% in cases diagnosed intrapartum. Occasionally vasa previa may be palpated clinically. In gray-scale transvaginal USG, a series of gray lines in the vicinity of the internal os is visualized. Color-Doppler can be used to trace the course of vessels, and pulse Doppler can be used to confirm fetal origin.[45] During labor, a sinusoidal fetal heart pattern, fetal bradycardia or fetal heart rate decelerations may be suggestive of rupture of vasa previa. Apt test may be used to determine that bleeding is of fetal origin which is based on increased resistance of fetal hemoglobin to alkali denaturation compared to maternal. The risk of fetal exsanguination and fetal demise can occur in 50–75% cases if membranes rupture. Cesarean delivery is planned after lung maturity or urgent if significant bleeding occurs.

Cord Abnormalities Impeding Blood Flow

Cord Knots

False knots are focal protuberances of Wharton's jelly from cord surface with no clinical significance. True knots arise from fetal movements and affect 1% of pregnancies. Risk factors include monoamniotic twins, advanced maternal age, multiparity and long umbilical cord. This condition is associated with 5–10 times increased risk of fetal death.

Nuchal Cord

Cord loops may be present around different fetal parts and when present around the neck is termed nuchal cord. Single loop of cord may be present in 20% of cases and multiple loops in 5%.[47,48] Diagnosis can be made by color-Doppler. It is associated with prolonged 2nd stage of labor and fetal heart rate abnormalities. Rarely, it is a cause of fetal demise and is not an indication for cesarean section.

Cord Presentation

Rarely, the umbilical cord may be the fetal presenting part and is associated with malpresentation, long umbilical cord, polyhydramnios, prematurity and unengaged presenting part. Cord may be visualized by color-Doppler USG in front of the presenting part. It can be diagnosed clinically during labor and may resolve spontaneously or may be reduced by the presenting part during labor. Cord prolapse may occur after the membranes rupture which is an obstetric emergency and mandates immediate vaginal delivery or a cesarean section.

Cord Stricture

It is a focal narrowing or stricture of the cord associated with absence of Wharton's jelly, stenosis and obliteration of the cord. Antenatal diagnosis is not possible and most fetuses are stillborn.

REFERENCES

1. Rogers J, Wood J, McCandlish R, Ayers S, Truesdale A, Elbourne D. Active versus expectant management of third stage of labour: the Hinchingbrooke randomized control trial. Lancet. 1998;351(9104):693-9.
2. Francois KE, Michael RF. Antepartum and postpartum hemorrhage. In: Gabbe SG, Niebyl JR, Simpson JL (Eds). Obstetrics Normal and Problem Pregnancies, 6th edition. Philadelphia, PA, USA: Elsevier-Saunders; 2013. pp. 423-5.
3. Breen JL, Neubecker RT, Gregori CA, Franklin JE. Placenta accreta, increta, and percreta. A survey of 40 cases. Obstet Gynecol. 1977;49(1):43-7.
4. Garmi G, Salim R. Epidemiology, etiology, diagnosis, and management of placenta accreta. Obstet Gynecol Int. 2012;2012:873929.
5. Benirschke K, Kaufmann P, Baergen RN. In: Pathology of Human Placenta, 5th edition. New York, USA: Springer; 2006.
6. Zelop C, Nadel A, Frigoletto FD, Pauker S, MacMillan M, Benacerraf BR. Placenta accreta/percreta/increta: a cause of elevated maternal serum alpha-fetoprotein. Obstet Gynecol. 1992;80(4):693-4.
7. Kupferminc MJ, Tamura RK, Wigton TR, Glassenberg R, Socol ML. Placenta accreta is associated with elevated maternal serum alpha-fetoprotein. Obstet Gynecol. 1993;82(2):266-9.
8. Tseng JJ, Chou MM. Differential expression of growth-, angiogenesis- and invasion-related factors in the development of placenta accrete. Taiwan J Obstet Gynecol. 2006;45(2):100-6.
9. Tantbirojn P, Crum CP, Parast MM. Pathophysiology of placenta accreta: the role of decidua and extravillous trophoblast. Placenta. 2008;29(7):639-45.
10. Garmi G, Goldman S, Shalev E, Salim R. The effects of decidual injury on the invasion potential of trophoblastic cells. Obstet Gynecol. 2011;117(1):55-9.

11. Doumouchtsis SK, Arulkumaran S. The morbidly adherent placenta: an overview of management options. Acta Obstet Gynecol Scand. 2010;89(9):1126-33.
12. Clark SL, Koonings PP, Phelan JP. Placenta previa/accreta and prior cesarean section. Obstet Gynecol. 1985;66(1):89-92.
13. To WW, Leung WC. Placenta previa and previous cesarean section. Int J Gynaecol Obstet. 1995;51(1):25-31.
14. Silver RM, Landon MB, Rouse DJ, Leveno KJ, Spong CY, Thom EA, et al. Maternal morbidity associated with multiple repeat caesarean deliveries. Obstet Gynecol. 2006;107(6):1226-32.
15. Miller DA, Chollet JA, Goodwin TM. Clinical risk factors for placenta previa-placenta accreta. Am J Obstet Gynecol. 1997;177(1):210-4.
16. Esakoff TF, Sparks TN, Kaimal AJ, Kim LH, Feldstein VA, Goldstein RB, et al. Diagnosis and morbidity of placenta accreta. Ultrasound Obstet Gynecol. 2011;37(3):324-7.
17. Gielchinsky Y, Rojansky N, Fasouliotis SJ, Ezra Y. Placenta accreta--summary of 10 years: a survey of 310 cases. Placenta. 2002;23(2-3):210-4.
18. James WH. Sex ratios of offspring and the causes of placental pathology. Hum Reprod. 1995;10(6):1403-6.
19. Alanis M, Hurst BS, Marshburn PB, Matthews ML. Conservative management of placenta increta with selective arterial embolization preserves future fertility and results in a favorable outcome in subsequent pregnancies. Fertil Steril. 2006;86(5):1514.e3-7.
20. Wu S, Kocherginsky M, Hibbard JU. Abnormal placentation: twenty-year analysis. Am J Obstet Gynecol. 2005;192(5):1458-61.
21. Committee on Obstetric Practice. Committee opinion no. 529: Placenta accreta. Obstet Gynecol. 2012;120(1):207-11.
22. Shih JC, Palacios Jaraquemada JM, Su YN, Shyu MK, Lin CH, Lin SY, et al. Role of three-dimensional power Doppler in the antenatal diagnosis of placenta accreta: comparison with gray-scale and color Doppler techniques. Ultrasound Obstet Gynecol. 2009;33(2):193-203.
23. Comstock CH, Love JJ, Bronsteen RA, Lee W, Vettraino IM, Huang RR, et al. Sonographic detection of placenta accreta in the second and third trimesters of pregnancy. Am J Obstet Gynecol. 2004;190(4):1135-40.
24. Finberg HJ, Williams JW. Placenta accreta: prospective sonographic diagnosis in patients with placenta previa and prior cesarean section. J Ultrasound Med. 1992;11(7):333-43.
25. Yang JI, Lim YK, Kim HS, Chang KH, Lee JP, Ryu HS. Sonographic findings of placental lacunae and the prediction of adherent placenta in with placenta previa totalis and prior Cesarean section. Ultrasound Obstet Gynecol. 2006;28(2):178-82.
26. Lax A, Prince MR, Mennitt KW, Schwebach JR, Budorick NE. The value of specific MRI features in the evaluation of suspected placental invasion. Magn Reson Imaging. 2007;25(1):87-93.
27. Zelop C, Nadel A, Frigoletto FD, Pauker S, MacMillan M, Benacerraf BR. Placenta accreta/percreta/increta: a cause of elevated maternal serum alpha-fetoprotein. Obstet Gynecol. 1992;80(4):693-4.
28. Mazouni C, Gorincour G, Juhan V, Bretelle F. Placenta accreta: a review of current advances in prenatal diagnosis. Placenta. 2007;28(7):599-603.
29. Eller AG, Bennet MA, Sharshiner M, Masheter C, Soisson AP, Dodson M, et al. Maternal morbidity in cases of placenta accreta managed by a multidisciplinary care team compared with standard obstetric care. Obstet Gynecol. 2011;117(2 Pt 1):331-7.
30. Royal College of Obstetricians and Gynaecologists (RCOG). (2005). Placenta praevia, placenta praevia accreta and vasa praevia: diagnosis and management. Green-top Guideline No. 27. [online]. Available from www.rcog.org.uk/globalassets/documents/guidelines/gtg_27.pdf. [Accessed October, 2015].
31. Centre for Maternal and Child Enquiries (CMACE). (2011). Saving mothers' lives: reviewing maternal deaths to make motherhood safer: 2006-08. The Eighth Report of the Confidential Enquiries into Maternal Deaths in the United Kingdom. [online]. Available from www.cdph.ca.gov/data/statistics/Documents/MO-CAPAMR-CMACE-2006-08-BJOG-2011.pdf. [Accessed October, 2015].
32. Chou MM, Ho ES, Lee YH. Prenatal diagnosis of placenta previa accreta by transabdominal color Doppler ultrasound. Ultrasound Obstet Gynecol. 2000;15(1):28-35.
33. Khadra M, Obhrai M, Keriakos R, Johanson R. Placenta percreta revisited. J Obstet Gynaecol. 2002;22(6):689.
34. Arulkumaran S, Ng CS, Ingemarsson I, Ratnam SS. Medical treatment of placenta accreta with methotrexate. Acta Obstet Gynecol Scand. 1986;65(3):285-6.
35. Herath RP, Wijesinghe PS. Management of morbidly adherent placenta. Sri Lanka J Obstet Gynaecol. 2011;33:39-44.
36. Chandraharan E, Rao S, Belli AM, Arulkumaran S. The Triple-P procedure as a conservative surgical alternative to peripartum hysterectomy for placenta percreta. Int J Gynaecol Obstet. 2012;117(2):191-4.
37. Abbas F, Talati J, Wasti S, Akram S, Ghaffar S, Qureshi R. Placenta percreta with bladder invasion as a cause of life threatening hemorrhage. J Urol. 2000;164(4):1270-4.
38. Heifetz SA. The umbilical cord: obstetrically important lesions. Clin Obstet Gynecol. 1996;39(3):571-87.
39. Barbieri C, Cecatti JG, Krupa F, Marussi EF, Costa JV. Validation study of the capacity of the reference curves of ultrasonographic measurements of the umbilical cord to identify deviations in estimated fetal weight. Acta Obstet Gynecol Scand. 2008;87(3):286-91.
40. Jessop FA, Lees CC, Pathak S, Hook CE, Sebire NJ. Umbilical cord coiling: clinical outcomes in an unselected population and systematic review. Virchows Arch. 2014;464(1):105-12.
41. Thummala MR, Raju TN, Langenberg P. Isolated single umbilical artery anomaly and the risk for congenital malformations: a meta-analysis. J Pediatr Surg. 1998;33(4):580-5.
42. Martinez-Frias ML, Bermejo-Sanchez E, Rodriguez-Pinilla E, Prieto-Merino D; Grupo de Periférico del ECEMC. Characteristics of neonates with and without a single umbilical artery. Analysis of two consecutive series of neonates with and without congenital defects. Ann Pediatr (Barc). 2006;65(6):541-50.
43. Volpe G, Volpe P, Boscia FM, Volpe N, Buonadonna AL, Gentile M. "Isolated" single umbilical artery: incidence, cytogenetic abnormalities, malformation and perinatal outcome. Minerva Ginecol. 2005;57(2):189-98.
44. Lopriore E, Sueters M, Middeldorp JM, Oepkes D, Walther FJ, Vandenbussche FP. Velamentous cord insertion and unequal placental territories in monochorionic twins with and without twin-to-twin-transfusion syndrome. Am J Obstet Gynecol. 2007;196(2):159.e1-5.
45. Beall MH, Ross MG, Talavera F, Gaupp FB, Chelmow D. Umbilical Cord Complications. [online]. Available from emedicine.medscape.com/article/262470. [Accessed October, 2015].
46. Hasegawa J, Matsuoka R, Ichizuka K, Sekizawa A, Okai T. Velamentous cord insertion: significance of prenatal detection to predict perinatal complications. Taiwan J Obstet Gynecol. 2006;45(1):21-5.
47. Ogueh O, Al-Tarkait A, Vallerand D, Rouah F, Morin L, Benjamin A, et al. Obstetrical factors related to nuchal cord. Acta Obstet Gynecol Scand. 2006;85(7):810-4.
48. Schaffer L, Burkhardt T, Zimmermann R, Kurmanavicius J. Nuchal cords in term and postterm deliveries--do we need to know? Obstet Gynecol. 2005;106(1):23-8.

CHAPTER 39

Multiple Gestations

Reena J Wani, Madhuri Mehendale

INTRODUCTION

Multiple gestations include all gestations where more than one conceptus is formed. Twin pregnancy is the most commonly seen type of multiple pregnancies with two fetuses *in utero*. The incidence of twin pregnancy has risen 70% in last few years with the advent of assisted reproductive technology and twins now account for 3% of all births.[1]

Approximately 50% of twin pregnancies deliver preterm. Prematurity, low birth weight, congenital anomalies, twin-to-twin transfusion syndrome (TTTS), and intrauterine growth restriction (IUGR) are the main contributors to raised perinatal mortality and morbidity. These complications drive the perinatal mortality rate of twins to 7 times that of singletons. Intrapartum asphyxia and trauma are additional risks, with malpresentation of one or both twins being present in 60% of deliveries. Although delivery may take place due to iatrogenic or spontaneous etiologies—no matter what the indication—optimizing the route of delivery for twins is an important component of care that must be thoughtfully considered.

CLASSIFICATION

- Monozygous (identical or true twins):
  - 25% of all twins: derived from single zygote
  - Dichorionic diamniotic: cleavage at blastomere stage (day 2–3)
  - Monochorionic diamniotic: cleavage at blastocyst stage (day 4–6), inner cell mass divides
  - Monochorionic monoamniotic: cleavage at primitive germ disk stage (day 7–13)
  - Conjoined-monochorionic monoamniotic: after 14 days, incomplete separation occurs. They may be: thoracopagus (thorax), omphalopagus (umbilicus), pygopagus (sacrum), ischiopagus (buttocks), craniopagus (head)
- Dizygous (similar or fraternal twins): 75%, derived from two separate zygotes.

INCIDENCE

- Monozygous twins: 3–5 per 1,000 births
- Dizygous twins: affected by various factors:
  - Race: Blacks > Whites > Mongoloids genetically
  - Maternal age: increases with age (peak 35–40 years)
  - Parity: increase with parity
  - Ovulation induction and assisted reproductive technology.

EPIDEMIOLOGY

The incidence of monozygotic twins is constant worldwide (~4 per 1,000 births). Approximately two-thirds of twins are dizygotic. Birth rates of dizygotic twins vary by:

- Race: 10–40 per 1,000 in Blacks, 7–10 per 1,000 births in Whites, and approximately 3 per 1,000 in Asians
- Maternal age: increasing frequency with increasing maternal age less than or equal to 40 years
- Parity: increased incidence, especially from 5th gravida onwards
- Hereditary predisposition: likely to be more transmitted through maternal side

- Mode of fertilization: most artificially conceived twins are dizygotic; however, 6–10% are monozygotic.

In India, the incidence is about 1 in 80. According to Hellin's rule, incidence is twins 1 in 80, triplets 1 in 80^2, quadruplets 1 in 80^3 and so on.

Naturally occurring triplet births occur in approximately 1 per 7,000–10,000 births; naturally occurring quadruplet births occur in approximately 1 per 600,000 births.

DIAGNOSIS

History

Use of ovulation-inducing drugs, or family history of dizygotic twins should alert the possibility of a multifetal pregnancy.

Symptoms

Minor ailments of normal pregnancy are usually exaggerated due to excess of human chorionic gonadotropin hormone:
- Increased nausea and vomiting
- Tendency of swelling of legs, varicose veins, and hemorrhoids
- Cardiorespiratory symptoms, like palpitation, and shortness of breath
- Unusual rate of abdominal enlargement
- Excessive fetal movements.

CLINICAL FINDINGS

- Palpation of three fetal poles or two heads or two breeches
- Two fetal heart sound (FHS) auscultated by two observers simultaneously differing by 10 beats per minute.

Ultrasound

Ultrasound is an invaluable tool as it is used for:
- Early diagnosis in first trimester
- Establish chorionicity and determine zygosity
- Prenatal diagnosis: nuchal translucency at 10–13 weeks, structural anomalies and soft markers for chromosomal defects at 18–20 weeks
- Assess fetal growth and detect discordance
- Detect unique problems like TTTS, single fetal demise
- Guide procedures like chorionic villus sampling, amniocentesis or selective feticide in higher-order pregnancies
- Cervical length and internal os status
- Fetal wellbeing: biophysical profile (BPP), placental grade, liquor, amniotic fluid index
- Intrapartum: confirm lie, positions at term/onset of labor.

MATERNAL RISKS OF HIGHER-ORDER MULTIPLES[2,3]

- Preterm labor (75%)
- Pregnancy-induced hypertension (PIH): twins 9%, triplets 27%, quadruplets 44%
- Gestational diabetes: quadruplets 22%, triplets 13%
- Cesarean section: 90% of triplets
- Hemorrhage: antepartum hemorrhage, postpartum hemorrhage (PPH)
- Hyperemesis gravidarum
- Cholestasis of pregnancy (quadruplets 33%, triplets 17%)
- Acute fatty liver (triplets 7%)
- Six times higher chances of antenatal hospitalization
- Three times more risk of maternal mortality.

FETAL RISKS IN TWINS

More in second of twins:[2,3]
- Fetal demise of one twin: 5% (excluding early loss)
- Lower birth weight than singleton
- Increase malpresentations
- Four times increase mortality
- Increase prematurity: around 3 weeks earlier
- Two to three times malformation
- Cervical incompetence
- Prematurity
- Antepartum hemorrhage: abruption of second sac
- Monochorionic twin problems: TTTS, cord prolapse, cord entanglements, fetus papyraceous, intrauterine fetal demise (IUFD) of one or both.

ANTENATAL CARE[2,3]

- Like any high-risk pregnancy
- Early detection and treatment of anemia, PIH, diabetes, preterm labor
- Measure blood pressure and test urine for proteinuria to screen for hypertensive disorders at each antenatal appointment in twin and triplet pregnancies as in routine antenatal care.

  Women with twin and triplet pregnancies should be advised to take 75 mg of aspirin daily from 12 weeks until the birth of the babies if they have one or more of the following risk factors for hypertension:[2]
- First pregnancy
- Age 40 years or older
- Pregnancy interval of more than 10 years
- Body mass index of 35 kg/m^2 or more at first visit
- Family history of preeclampsia.
- Predicting the risk of preterm birth:[2]
  - Be aware that women with twin pregnancies have a higher risk of spontaneous preterm birth if they

have had a spontaneous preterm birth in a previous singleton pregnancy
  - Do not use fetal fibronectin (fFN) testing alone to predict the risk of spontaneous preterm birth in twin or triplet pregnancies
  - Do not use home uterine activity monitoring to predict the risk of spontaneous preterm birth in twin or triplet pregnancies
  - Do not use cervical length (with or without fFN) routinely to predict the risk of spontaneous preterm birth in twin or triplet pregnancies
- Preventing preterm birth: do not use the following interventions (alone or in combination) routinely to prevent spontaneous preterm birth in twin or triplet pregnancies:
  - Bed rest at home or in hospital
  - Intramuscular or vaginal progesterone
  - Cervical cerclage
  - Oral tocolytics
- Inform women with twin and triplet pregnancies of their increased risk of preterm birth and about the benefits of targeted corticosteroids
- Do not use single or multiple untargeted (routine) courses of corticosteroids in twin or triplet pregnancies
- Monitor fetal wellbeing [clinical, nonstress testing (NST), BPP], growth of each fetus.

FETAL ASSESSMENT

- First trimester:
  - Downs screening with nuchal thickness at 9–13 weeks
  - Determine chorionicity and amnionicity
- Second trimester:
  - Triple marker at 14–18 weeks may not be reliable in multiples, serum α-fetoprotein can be offered for neural tube defects screen
  - Level II ultrasonography to rule out fetal anomalies
- Third trimester:
  - Fetal growth and discordance
  - Placental localization
  - Color Doppler of umbilical arteries at 28 weeks, and 3 weekly after that weekly NST from 36 weeks.

TIMING OF BIRTH[2]

- Discuss with women with twin and triplet pregnancies the timing of birth and possible modes of delivery early in the third trimester
- About 60% of twin pregnancies result in spontaneous birth before 37 weeks and 75% of triplet pregnancies result in spontaneous birth before 35 weeks
- Inform women with uncomplicated monochorionic twin pregnancies that elective birth from 36 weeks and uncomplicated dichorionic twin pregnancies that elective birth from 37 weeks, does not appear to be associated with an increased risk of serious adverse outcomes, and that continuing uncomplicated twin pregnancies beyond 38 weeks increases the risk of fetal death
- Inform women with triplet pregnancies that continuing uncomplicated triplet pregnancies beyond 36 weeks increases the risk of fetal death
- For women who decline elective birth, offer weekly appointments with the specialist obstetrician. At each appointment offer an ultrasound scan, and perform weekly BPP assessments and fortnightly fetal growth scans.

ROUTE OF DELIVERY

- The American College of Obstetricians and Gynecologists suggest that individual obstetricians recommend the best route for their patients: "The route of delivery for twins should be determined by the position of the fetuses, the ease of fetal heart rate (FHR) monitoring and the maternal and fetal status"[4]
- The Canadian Guidelines in the Consensus Statement 20 reads: "Delivery of cephalic twin A/noncephalic twin B: Estimated weight 1,500–4,000 g. Vaginal delivery is indicated as long as the obstetrician is comfortable with, and skilled in, vaginal breech delivery"[5]
- Consensus Statement 21 in the same document addresses preterm twins as: "Delivery of cephalic twin A/noncephalic twin B: Estimated weight 500–1,500 g. In this weight range, the group acknowledged that there is no consistent evidence to support either cesarean section or the vaginal route for delivery"[5]
- The Cochrane Database reviewed the one randomized trial on mode of delivery for twins and concluded that cesarean delivery should not be universally adopted as the route of delivery for twins. Therefore, the question persists: Is there a preferred delivery method for twins?[6]

INTRAPARTUM MANAGEMENT OF TWIN PREGNANCY[7,8]

- A vertex B vertex: manage labor as singleton
- A nonvertex: elective lower segment cesarean section (LSCS).

A Vertex B Nonvertex

Manage labor as singleton, with preparation for twin B once twin A delivers:
- Twin B vertex: oxytocin, amniotomy, FHR monitor: vaginal delivery
- Twin B nonvertex: external version:
  - Failed: consider individual factors (available skill, weight discrepancy in A and B, weight extremes <1,500 g >3,500 g, age, parity, fertility) to decide LSCS or internal version and breech extraction

- Successful version to vertex: oxytocin, amniotomy, FHR monitor: vaginal delivery
- Successful version to breech: individual factors (available skill, weight discrepancy in A and B, weight extremes <1,500 g >3,500 g, age, parity, fertility) considered to decide LSCS or internal version and breech extraction or assisted breech delivery
- Nonreassuring FHS, intrapartum bleeding or cord prolapsed: accelerate labor and perform assisted vaginal delivery.

Eighty percent of second twin delivers within 30 minutes.

Third Stage of Labor

- Active management recommended to avoid PPH
- Perinatal outcome is perhaps the most important concern when choosing the preferred route of delivery for twin gestations:
    - The best method by which to deliver pregnancies in which only the presenting twin is cephalic remains controversial
    - Evidence supports a vaginal trial of labor in late preterm and term twins
    - Routes of delivery for preterm twins lighter than 1,500 g remains unclear, with compelling data for both planned cesarean and planned vaginal delivery
    - Obstetricians need to be prepared for, and skilled in, breech extraction of the second twin
    - Individualized patient counseling regarding mode of delivery is important when offering a vaginal trial of labor to women with a twin gestation.

Triplets and Higher-order Pregnancy

- Maternal mortality and morbidity is higher in triplets and higher-order pregnancies
- Viable triplet pregnancies are preferably delivered by elective cesarean section for a combination of reasons:
    - In one-third cases in triplets, presenting fetus is nonvertex
    - Chances of need of intrauterine manipulation for second and third fetus is high
    - Technically difficult to monitor three FHS simultaneously:
        - There is no proof that cesarean delivery brings better perinatal outcome
        - Individual hospitals will have to make their own decisions based on local facilities, personnel and experience.

MULTIFETAL PREGNANCY REDUCTION

Multifetal pregnancy reduction (MFPR) is a procedure used to reduce the number of fetuses in a multiple pregnancy, usually to two. When a pregnancy involves 3 or more fetuses (high-order pregnancy), the risks of miscarriage, stillbirth and lifelong disability increase with each additional fetus.

The goal of MFPR is to increase the chance of a successful, healthy pregnancy:

- Is usually done early in a pregnancy, between the 9th and 12th weeks
- Is most often done when there are four or more fetuses present
- Can be used to reduce triplets to twins
- Is known as "selective termination" when it involves a fetus with severe defects or one that is expected to die later in the pregnancy, which would threaten the life of the surviving fetus or fetuses.

Procedure

This procedure is generally carried out during the first trimester of pregnancy. The most common method is to inject potassium chloride into the fetus's heart; the heart stops and the fetus dies as a result. Generally, the fetal material is reabsorbed into the woman's body. While the procedure generally reduces the overall risk level for the remaining fetus or fetuses, reduction does have its own risks, including the possibility that one or more of the remaining fetuses will also die. Association with preterm premature rupture of membranes (pPROM) and preterm labor is also reported. Reduction from twins to singleton remains controversial.

COMPLICATIONS

Antepartum complications develop in over 80% of multiple pregnancies compared with approximately 25% of singleton gestations.[9]

- Maternal complications include: hyperemesis, anemia, preeclampsia (25%), gestational diabetes, preterm labor and birth, hydramnios, malpresentations, cesarean delivery, and acute fatty liver (very rare)
- Uteroplacental complications include: placenta previa, placental abruption, pPROM, cord entanglement, PPH
- Fetal complications include: spontaneous abortion, growth discordance, IUGR, intrauterine demise of one or both twins, congenital anomalies, TTTS, twin reversed arterial perfusion syndrome/sequence
- Specific complications are discussed below.

Specific Complications

Spontaneous Pregnancy Loss

Approximately 14% (range 8–36%) of multiple pregnancies will reduce spontaneously to a singleton by the end of first trimester.[10] Many of these events go unrecognized. The phenomenon of "vanishing twin" can occur before 14 weeks' gestation without any consequence for the remaining fetus and without any evidence of multiple gestations on subsequent antenatal evaluation.[5] The vanishing twin can cause problems in screening for neural tube defects and a discrepancy in karyotyping. Monochorionic greatly outnumber dichorionic abortuses with an 18:1 ratio, thus implicating monozygosity as the risk factor.

Intrauterine Fetal Demise

The twin infant death rate is fivefold higher than that of singletons (37 vs. 7 per 1,000 live births).[11] The causes of IUFD can be identified in only around 50% of cases. Pathologic examination of fetus and placenta/fetal membranes is the singlemost useful test. Early detection and appropriate management of underlying maternal disorders (diabetes, preeclampsia) may reduce the risk of IUFD.

Death of both twins

In general, the earlier the gestational age, the longer the latency period (the period from fetal demise to delivery). Management options include surgical dilation and evacuation or induction of labor with cervical ripening, if indicated. Around 20–25% of women who retain a dead fetus for longer than 3 weeks will develop disseminated intravascular coagulopathy (DIC). Therefore, delivery should be affected within this time period.

Death of a co-twin

The death of one twin confers an increased risk of major morbidity to the surviving twin, including IUFD, neurologic injury, multiorgan system failure, thrombosis, distal limb necrosis, placental abruption, and premature labor.[12] The prognosis for the surviving twin is dependent on the cause of death, gestational age, chorionicity, and time interval between death of the first twin and delivery of the second. In dizygous pregnancies, dead twin may be resorbed completely or become compressed (*fetus papyraceous*). DIC in the surviving fetus and/or mother is rare. It is therefore not necessary to monitor for maternal coagulopathy although a platelet count and fibrinogen level are desirable before delivery. On the other hand, if one fetus in monozygous twins dies, the co-twin has 20–40% risk of developing neurologic injury (multicystic encephalomalacia).[13] More recent reports suggest that the inciting event is immediate and profound hypotension in the surviving co-twin due to loss of blood into the dead twin resulting from a loss of vascular tone. Unfortunately, immediate cesarean delivery does not appear to protect the surviving twin from neurologic injury, and ultrasound and fetal testing may not be able to identify fetuses with multicystic encephalopathy.[14] Therefore, management of a surviving co-twin depends on chorionicity and gestational age. Fetal surveillance (kick charts, NST, BPP) should be instituted on a regular basis and delivery considered in the setting of nonreassuring fetal testing or at a favorable gestational age.

Intrauterine Growth Restriction

The growth rate of twins is not significantly different from that of singletons in the first and second trimesters. Most studies have described slower fetal growth after 30–32 weeks of gestation. This has been attributed to placental crowding and anomalous umbilical cord insertion. IUGR is a risk factor for increased perinatal morbidity and mortality in twin pregnancies. Bed rest and low-dose aspirin have not been shown to prevent IUGR. Principles of management include identification of women at risk, early antepartum diagnosis, attempts to identify etiology, regular (usually twice-weekly) fetal surveillance, and appropriate timing of delivery. Cesarean delivery should be reserved for the usual obstetric indications. However, up to 50–80% of IUGR fetuses will show evidence of nonreassuring fetal testing in labor requiring cesarean delivery.[15]

Fetal Growth Discordance

Fetal growth discordance typically defined as a more than or equal to 20% difference in estimated fetal weight between fetuses of same pregnancy. Other ultrasound criteria include: (i) an intra-pair difference in biparietal diameter of 5 mm or more and a fall in BPD below 2 standard deviation for gestational age on their normal twin curve and (ii) intra-pair difference in abdominal circumference of 2 cm or more. Significant risk factors for discordant growth include monochorionic placentation, preeclampsia, and antepartum bleeding. Fetal growth discordance is evident in 5–15% of twins and 30% of triplets, and is associated with a sixfold increase in perinatal morbidity and mortality.[16] In the absence of IUGR or nonreassuring fetal status, delivery is usually contemplated at term.

Preterm Premature Rupture of Membranes

Preterm premature rupture of membranes complicates 2–4% of singleton and 7–10% of twin pregnancies. It is associated with 30–40% of preterm births and 10% of all perinatal mortality. It typically occurs in the presenting sac, but can occur in the nonpresenting twin, especially after invasive procedures, such as amniocentesis. The management of pPROM should not differ significantly in twin as compared with singleton pregnancies.

Preterm Labor and Birth

Approximately 57% of twin pregnancies deliver before 37 weeks' gestation. A large multicenter study of cervical length in twin pregnancies found that a cervix shorter than 25 mm at 24 weeks of gestation was the best predictor of delivery before 32 weeks, 35 weeks, and 37 weeks of gestation.[17] Fetal fibronectin measured in the cervicovaginal discharge of women at 22 to 0/7 to 34 to 6/7 weeks' gestation is useful as a marker for preterm birth in singleton pregnancies. It may also have some predictive value in twin gestations. A number of interventions have been recommended in an attempt to prevent preterm birth. Randomized trials of hospitalization or bed rest have failed to show a prolongation of gestational age at delivery.[18] There are too little data to comment on the use of cervical cerclage in high-order multiple pregnancies. Use of tocolytic drugs is associated with pulmonary edema because of their higher blood volume and lower colloid osmotic pressure. As such, these drugs should be used with caution. Use of progesterone supplements may be appropriate in women with one or more prior spontaneous preterm deliveries. The National Institutes of Health recommends that all women in preterm labor who have no contraindications to steroid use be given one course of steroids, regardless of the number of fetuses.[19]

Twin-to-twin Transfusion Syndrome

Twin-to-twin transfusion syndrome complicates up to 15% of monochorionic twins and is believed to occur as the result of uncompensated arteriovenous anastomoses, which lead to greater net blood flow going to one twin at the expense of the other. The donor twin usually is anemic and growth restricted and appears "stuck" to one spot in uterus because the lack of amniotic fluid in its sac precludes movement; the recipient twin usually is plethoric and much larger, and hydramnios is evident. The syndrome usually becomes apparent in the second trimester and can rapidly lead to premature rupture of membranes, preterm labor, or early mortality because of heart failure in either of the fetuses.

Diagnosis is made *in utero* by ultrasound:

- Single placenta
- Same gender fetuses
- Significant weight discordance
- Significant amniotic fluid discordance (maximum vertical pocket <2 cm for donor twin and >8 cm for recipient twin).

Quintero-staging system[20]

- Stage I: oligohydramnios is evident, but donor twin's bladder is visible
- Stage II: bladder no longer visible
- Stage III: abnormal Doppler studies
- Stage IV: complicated by hydrops
- Stage V: one or both fetuses have died.

Serial therapeutic amniocenteses of the recipient twin's amniotic sac are most frequently used. This therapy is believed to work by favorably changing intraamniotic pressure, and thus, placental intravascular pressure, allowing redistribution of placental blood flow and normalization of amniotic fluid volumes in each sac. More aggressive therapies include abolishing the placental anastomoses by endoscopic laser coagulation or selective feticide by umbilical cord occlusion. Death of one fetus has been reported to result in the sudden transfusion of blood from the viable fetus to the low pressure system of the dead fetus, resulting in exsanguinations of the viable twin. If the gestational age is such that survival is likely, immediate delivery should be considered, recognizing that damage to the remaining viable fetus may already have occurred.

Twin Reversed Arterial Perfusion Syndrome/Sequence

Twin reversed arterial perfusion syndrome/sequence, also called an acardiac or acephalus twin, is a monozygotic fetus without a normally developed heart or brain, respectively, as the result of abnormal division of the zygote at the time of twinning. These fetuses are nonviable and survive antenatally only because they receive blood flow from their monochorionic co-twin. Because the "pump" twin is supplying blood flow to both its own body and that of its abnormal twin, death from heart failure is a common complication. Such pregnancies require close monitoring, with consideration of early delivery or selective feticide of the abnormal co-twin by umbilical cord occlusion if heart failure develops.

Multifetal Reduction and Selective Fetal Termination

Fetal reduction to triplet or twin gestations is associated with a significant risk of losing either another fetus or the whole pregnancy. Incidence of IUGR may be increased in surviving fetuses. Monochorionicity can complicate the reduction procedure; if one fetus of a monochorionic twin pair is inadvertently reduced, sudden hypotension and thrombotic phenomena could result in death or damage of the remaining twin fetus.

Risks of selective fetal termination of an anomalous or aneuploid fetus are higher than those associated with multifetal reduction. The pregnancy usually is more advanced by the time the anomaly is diagnosed (i.e., 18–22 weeks of gestation compared with 10–12 weeks of gestation), and location of anomalous fetus may be associated with increased risk. The risk of losing the whole pregnancy, having a preterm birth, or having an infant with a birth weight less than 2,500 g is highest when the reduced fetus overlies the cervix and when the pregnancy is at or beyond 20 weeks of gestation.

Intracardiac injection of potassium chloride has gained widespread acceptance for both selective termination and multifetal reduction because of proven safety and efficacy.

MANAGEMENT OF MULTIPLE PREGNANCIES

Clinical practice guidelines from Ireland have highlighted certain important points in care of these patients, listed below:[8]

- Where multiple gestations are identified on ultrasound examination, chorionicity should be assigned at the earliest opportunity. This is best achieved before 14 weeks gestation
- A record should be retained of the ultrasound image that supports assignment of chorionicity and a second opinion should be sought if there is uncertainty
- If chorionicity cannot be determined, monochorionicity should be assumed until proven otherwise, and a strategy of prenatal surveillance that includes screening for TTTS should be adopted accordingly
- Pre- and perinatal cares should be hospital-based for all multiple gestations, coordinated by an obstetrician experienced in the management of multiple gestations
- Indications for referral to a tertiary level fetal medicine unit:
  - Suspected monoamnionicity
  - Suspected TTTS
  - Fetal structural abnormality
  - Suspected intertwine growth: discordance more than 18%
  - Higher-order multiple gestations
  - Single fetal demise in a monochorionic twin gestation
- Monochorionic twin gestation should be regarded as "high-risk" and merits ultrasound examination every 2–3 weeks from 16 weeks' gestation as a means of screening for TTTS and fetal growth restriction
- Pregnancies complicated by TTTS prior to 26 weeks' gestation should be considered for laser ablation of communicating placental vessels as such therapy yields better perinatal outcomes than management by serial amnioreduction
- In the case of uncomplicated dichorionic twin gestation, serial growth evaluation should be performed at least every 4 weeks from 24 weeks' gestation
- Although mid-trimester determination of cervical length may predict preterm birth in twins, such evaluation is not recommended, on the basis that there is no preventative intervention that has been shown to reduce the risk of spontaneous preterm twin birth. Specifically, there is no evidence to support bed rest, elective placement of cervical cerclage, ultrasound-indicated cerclage, prophylactic tocolytic therapy, or progesterone for the purpose of prevention of preterm twin birth
- A course of antenatal corticosteroid therapy should be prescribed in the event of anticipated preterm delivery prior to 34 weeks' gestation, accepting that the benefit of antenatal corticosteroids in the prevention of respiratory morbidity may be less than that observed in singleton pregnancies. Corticosteroid therapy should be administered in a "timed" rather than in an untargeted (routine) manner
- Applying a strategy of close fetal surveillance, perinatal morbidity can be minimized by allowing uncomplicated monochorionic twin pregnancies continue to 37 weeks' gestation and dichorionic twins to 38 weeks. Among monochorionic twins, it must be acknowledged that this approach is balanced against a 1.5% risk of late *in utero* death
- Mode of twin delivery should be considered on the basis of individual case characteristics to include comorbidity, gestational age, availability of expertise in the management of vaginal twin birth and patient's preference
- Where no contraindications exist, mono- or dichorionic twins may be considered for vaginal birth. Women should be informed that where the first twin delivers by the vaginal route, the prospect of requiring a cesarean section for delivery of the second twin is approximately 4%
- An obstetrician experienced in vaginal twin birth should be immediately available in the event of twin labor.

CONCLUSION

Although the frequency of multiple gestations is lower than singleton gestations, multiple gestations account for a disproportionate share of neonatal morbidity and mortality. Much of this can be attributed to a higher rate of preterm delivery for multiple gestations. Neurologic outcomes also appear to be worse in multiple births. When matched for gestational age at delivery, infants born from multifetal pregnancies have an approximately 3-fold increase in cerebral palsy.

Maternal morbidity is also increased in a multifetal gestation. Women with multiples are more likely to be hospitalized with complications including preterm labor, preterm premature rupture of membranes, preeclampsia, placental abruption, pulmonary embolism, and postpartum hemorrhage. As a result, hospital costs are higher in these pregnancies. Information about multiple births and their consequences should be provided for couples considering treatment for infertility. For parents with multiple gestations, detailed information should be available throughout the pregnancy, birth and prenatal period and further into early childhood.

REFERENCES

1. Martin JA, Hamilton BE, Sutton PD, Ventura SJ, Menacker F, Kirmeyer S. Births: final data for 2004. Natl Vital Stat Rep. 2006;55(1):1-101.
2. National Institute for Health and Care Excellence (NICE). (2011). NICE guidelines [CG129]: Multiple pregnancy: The management of twin and triplet pregnancies in the antenatal period. [online]. Available from: www.ncbi.nlm.nih.gov/pubmed/22855972. [Accessed October, 2015].

3. Wani RJ. Twins, multiple gestations. In: Essential Obstetrics, 2nd edition. Mumbai, India: Bhalani Book Depot; 2010. pp. 394-405.
4. American College of Obstetricians and Gynecologists Committee on Practice Bulletins-Obstetrics; Society for Maternal-Fetal Medicine; ACOG Joint Editorial Committee. ACOG Practice Bulletin #56: Multiple gestation: complicated twin, triplet, and high-order multifetal pregnancy. Obstet Gynecol. 2004;104(4):869-83.
5. Barrett J, Bocking A. The SOGC Consensus Statement: management of twin pregnancies. J SOGC. 2000;91:5-15.
6. Crowther CA. Caesarean delivery for the second twin. Cochrane Database Syst Rev. 2000;(2):CD000047.
7. Christopher D, Robinson BK, Peaceman AM. An evidence-based approach to determining route of delivery for twin gestations. Rev Obstet Gynecol. 2011;4(3-4):109-16.
8. Institute of Obstetricians and Gynaecologists, Royal College of Physicians of Ireland and Directorate of Strategy and Clinical Care, Health Service Executive. (2012). Clinical Practice Guideline: Management of Multiple Pregnancy. [online]. Available from: www.hse.ie/eng/about/Who/clinical/natclinprog/obsandgynaeprogramme/pregmulti.pdf. [Accessed October, 2015].
9. American Congress of Obstetricians and Gynecologists (ACOG). Special problems of multiple gestations. Educational Bulletin No. 253. Washington DC, USA: ACOG; 1998.
10. Dickey RP, Taylor SN, Lu PY, Sartor BM, Storment JM, Rye PH, et al. Spontaneous reduction of multiple pregnancy: incidence and effect on outcome. Am J Obstet Gynecol. 2002;186(1):77-83.
11. Misra DP, Ananth CV. Infant mortality among singletons and twins in the United States during 2 decades: effects of maternal age. Pediatrics. 2002;110(6):1163-8.
12. Bejar R, Vigliocco G, Gramajo H, Solana C, Benirschke K, Berry C, et al. Antenatal origin of neurologic damage in newborn infants. II. Multiple gestations. Am J Obstet Gynecol. 1990;162(5):1230-6.
13. Pharoah PO, Adi Y. Consequences of in-utero death in a twin pregnancy. Lancet. 2000;355(9215):1597-602.
14. Cleary-Goldman J, D'Alton M. Management of single fetal demise in a multiple gestation. Obstet Gynecol Surv. 2004;59(4):285-98.
15. American Congress of Obstetricians and Gynecologists (ACOG). Intrauterine growth restriction. Practice Pattern No. 12. Washington DC, USA: ACOG; 2000.
16. Demissie K, Ananth C, Martin J, Hanley ML, MacDorman MF, Rhoads GG. Fetal and neonatal mortality among twin gestations in the United States: the role of intrapair birth weight discordance. Obstet Gynecol. 2002;100(3):474-80.
17. Goldenberg RL, Iams JD, Miodovnik M, Van Dorsten JP, Thurnau G, Bottoms S, et al. The preterm prediction study: risk factors in twin gestations. National Institute of Child Health and Human Development Maternal-Fetal Medicine Units Network. Am J Obstet Gynecol. 1996;175(4 Pt 1):1047-53.
18. American Congress of Obstetricians and Gynecologists (ACOG). Assessment of risk factors for preterm birth. ACOG Practice Bulletin No. 31. Washington DC, USA: ACOG; 2001.
19. Effect of corticosteroids for fetal maturation on perinatal outcomes. NIH Consens Statement 1994;12(2):1-24.
20. Quintero RA, Morales WJ, Allen MH, Bornick PW, Johnson PK, Kruger M. Staging of twin-twin transfusion syndrome. J Perinatol. 1999;19(8 Pt 1):550-5.

CHAPTER 40

Malpositions

Monica Chauhan

INTRODUCTION

Fetal malpositions and malpresentations are important as they are associated with an increased maternal and fetal morbidity and mortality.[1] In 96% of the deliveries near term, the fetus presents by vertex with the occiput lying anteriorly in 90% of them.[2,3] But if the fetus is in an occipitoposterior (OP) or occipitotransverse positions, a malposition is said to be present. If the fetal head is deflexed, brow or face can be the presenting parts. If the presentation of the fetus is nonvertex, a malpresentation is said to exist which may be breech or transverse. When malpositions and malpresentations present in labor, the birth can proceed normally; however, malpositions significantly prolong the second stage of labor and increase the incidence of operative delivery, postpartum hemorrhage and puerperal infection, with risks to both the mother and the baby. During labor and delivery, the OP position was associated with prolonged first and second stages of labor; oxytocin augmentation; use of epidural analgesia; chorioamnionitis; assisted vaginal delivery; third- and fourth-degree perineal lacerations; cesarean delivery; excessive blood loss; and postpartum infection. Newborns had lower 1-minute Apgar scores.[4]

DEFINITIONS

Presentation: fetal presentation refers to the part of the fetuses' body that is presenting at the pelvic outlet.

Normal presentation is cephalic with vertex as the presenting part.

Malpresentation (Figs 1A to D): it is said to occur when there exists any presentation other than a vertex, such as:
- Brow
- Face
- Breech
- Transverse or shoulder
- Compound.

Position: it is the location of the presenting part of the fetus in relation to the maternal pelvis.[5]

Normal position in a vertex presentation is occipito-anterior.

Malpositions: it refers to the relationship between the denominator and the pelvis that make spontaneous delivery unfavorable, e.g.:
- occipitoposterior or occipitotransverse in vertex presentation
- Sacroposterior in breech presentation
- Mentoposterior with face presentation.

PATHOPHYSIOLOGY

Incidence[6] (Table 1)

TABLE 1: Incidence of fetal presentation

Presentation	Percentage	Incidence
Cephalic	96.8	—
Breech	2.7	1: 36
Transverse lie	0.3	1: 335
Compound	0.1	1: 1,000
Face	0.5	1: 2,000
Brow	0.01	1:10,000
Occiput posterior	15% (early labor) 5% (at delivery)	—

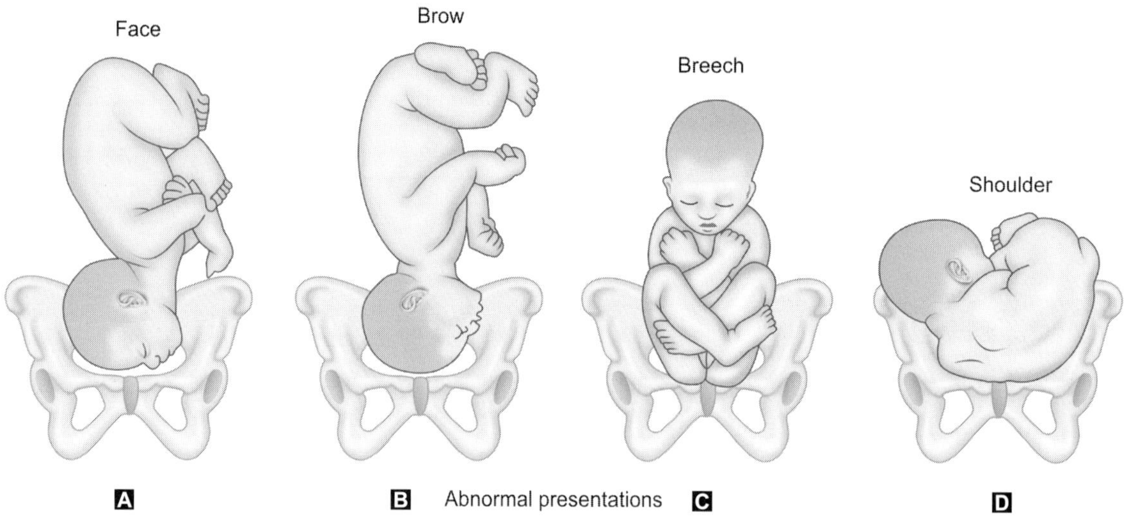

FIGS 1: Fetal malpresentations (abnormal presentations): **A,** Face; **B,** brow; **C,** breech and **D,** Shoulder (transverse lie).

Risk Factors for Malposition/Presentation

The risk factors responsible for malpositions and malpresentations can be classified as fetal and maternal.[6,7] They are as follows:

- Fetal factors:
  - Prematurity
  - Macrosomia
  - Fetal congenital anomalies: Anencephaly, hydrocephalous, muscle dystrophy, neurologic impairment, neck mass, or multiple nuchal cord loops (prevent flexion of the head)
  - Short umbilical cord
  - Intrauterine fetal death (IUFD)
- Maternal and uterine factors:
  - Contracted pelvis: prevents fetal descent into the pelvis
  - Multiparity resulting in lax abdominal wall
  - Multiple pregnancy
  - Uterine abnormalities (bicornuate, septate uterus)
  - Space occupying pelvic lesions (uterine fibroids/ ovarian tumors)
  - Placenta previa
  - Oligohydramnios/polyhydramnios.

Morbidity/Mortality

Malpositions and malpresentations are associated with possibility of adverse fetal and maternal outcomes, like:

- Preterm labor
- Increased incidence of premature rupture of membranes (PROM) which causes an increased risk of sepsis and cord prolapse
- Increased chances of operative vaginal deliveries by forceps/vacuum extraction or cesarean section
- Usually they result in unrecognized labor dystocia, uncoordinated painful uterine contractions, with slow or nonprogress of labor
- Obstructed labor, pathologic contraction rings, and possibility of rupture of lower uterine segment is also significant
- Increased chances of trauma to the genital tract
- Postpartum hemorrhage and sepsis
- Fetal and maternal distress which may lead to the death of the baby and/or the mother.

OCCIPITOPOSTERIOR POSITIONS (FIG. 2A AND B)

Occipitoposterior position is the most common type of malposition of the occiput.[8] The vertex is presenting, but the occiput lies in the posterior rather than the anterior part of the pelvis. As per Cochrane Database of Systematic Reviews 2011, approximately 15–32% of deliveries start with the head in an OP position, but the majority correct in labor.[8-11] The prevalence of persistent occiput-posterior position at delivery was 5–8%.[4] A persistent OP position results from a failure of internal rotation. Risk factors for OP positions include anthropoid and android pelvis [the anteroposterior (AP) diameter ≥ the transverse position]. There is a degree of partial deflexion which leads to this position. Persistence of the OP position is important because it can be associated with labor abnormalities and maternal and neonatal complications.[12] Labor is prolonged and operative interventions may be indicated.

Diagnosis

On Inspection

There is a saucer-shaped depression below the umbilicus (Figs 3A and B). This dip corresponds to the fetal neck. The abdomen looks flattened below the umbilicus due to absence of round contour of the fetal back. The outline created by the high, unengaged head can look like a full bladder.

On Palpation

- Fundal grip: the breech is easily palpable at the fundus
- Umbilical grip: the back is felt with difficulty in the flank, away from the midline. The anterior shoulder is about 3-inches from the midline. The limbs are easily felt near, or on both sides, of the middle line
- First and second pelvic grips: the head is usually not engaged, due to the deflexion. It is felt smaller as the bitemporal diameter palpated instead of the biparietal diameter in occipitoanterior.

On Auscultation

The fetal heart can be heard in the midline as the fetal back is not well flexed, so the chest is thrust forward.

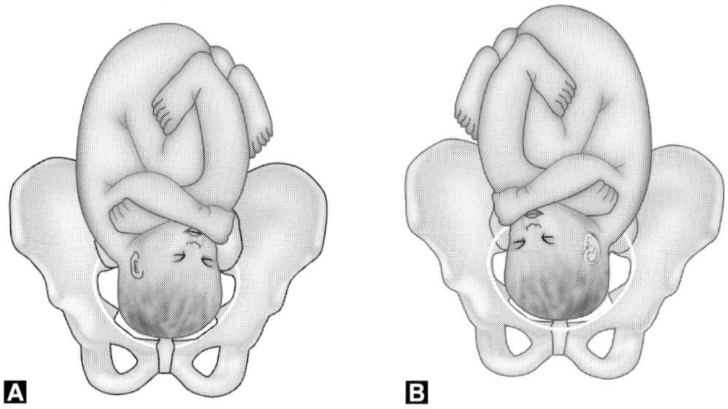

FIGS 2A AND B: Occipitoposterior (OP) positions: **A,** Right OP and **B,** Left OP positions.

Diagnosis During Labor

The uterine contractions may be incoordinate. The large and irregular presenting circumference does not fit well onto the cervix. Therefore, the membranes have a tendency to rupture spontaneously early in labor. Descent of the head can be slow even with good contractions. The woman may have a strong desire to push early in labor because the occiput is pressing on the rectum.

Vaginal examination: locating the anterior fontanel in the anterior part of the pelvis is diagnostic, but this may be difficult if caput succedaneum is present. The direction of the sagittal suture and location of the posterior fontanel (three radiating sutures) will confirm the diagnosis (Figs 4A to C).

Mechanism of Labor (Figures 5A and B)

Engagement occurs in oblique diameter with the occiput in the right OP position which is 5-times more common than left OP.[14] Engaging diameter is the suboccipitofrontal diameter of 10.5 cm, if the head is well flexed or the occipitofrontal of 11.5 cm, if the head is deflexed. Both are larger than the suboccipitobregmatic of 9.5 cm, in case of occipitoanterior position. These diameters give an oval-shaped presenting part which does not fit well on the cervix.

Normal Mechanism (90%)

Deflexion is corrected and complete flexion occurs. The occiput meets the pelvic floor first, and long anterior rotation through 3/8th of a circle occurs bringing the occiput anteriorly behind the symphysis pubis. The mechanism of labor will be the same as in occipitoanterior position and the fetus is delivered normally.

Abnormal Mechanism (10%)

- Direct OP (face to pubis) (6%): in 6% of cases, the sinciput touches the pelvic floor first and it will rotate anteriorly which means the occiput will rotate posteriorly by

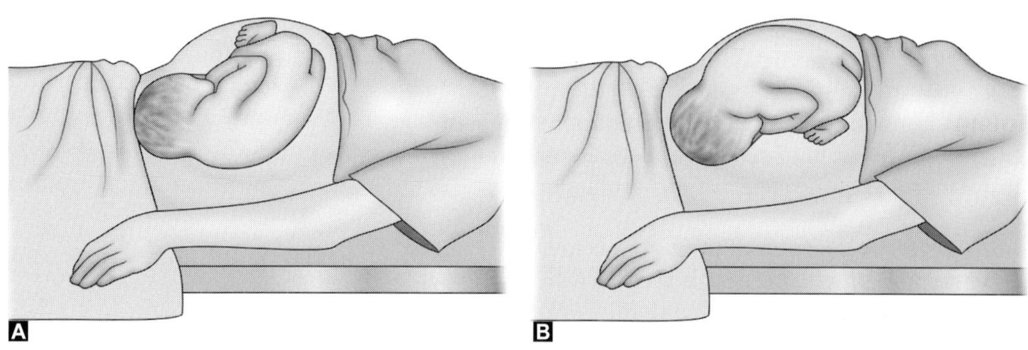

FIGS 3A AND B: Abdominal examination: **A,** Occipitoposterior (OP) position: note the suprapubic bulge formed by unengaged head and saucer shaped depression and **B,** Rounded abdominal contour in occipitoanterior position.

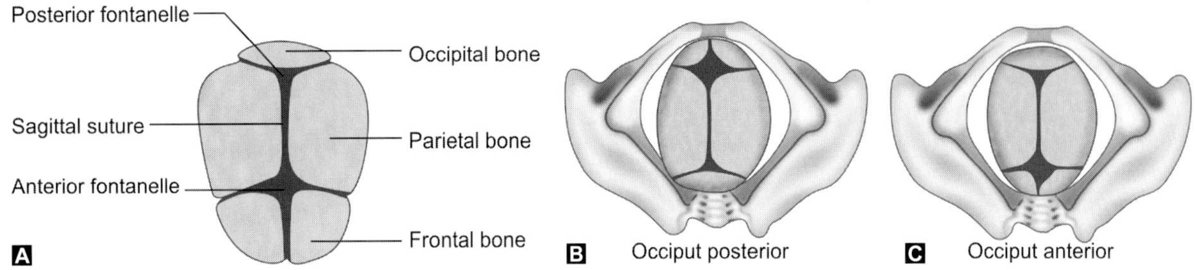

FIGS 4A TO C: **A,** Landmarks of the fetal skull; **B,** Occipitoposterior versus; **C,** Occipitoanterior positions.[13]

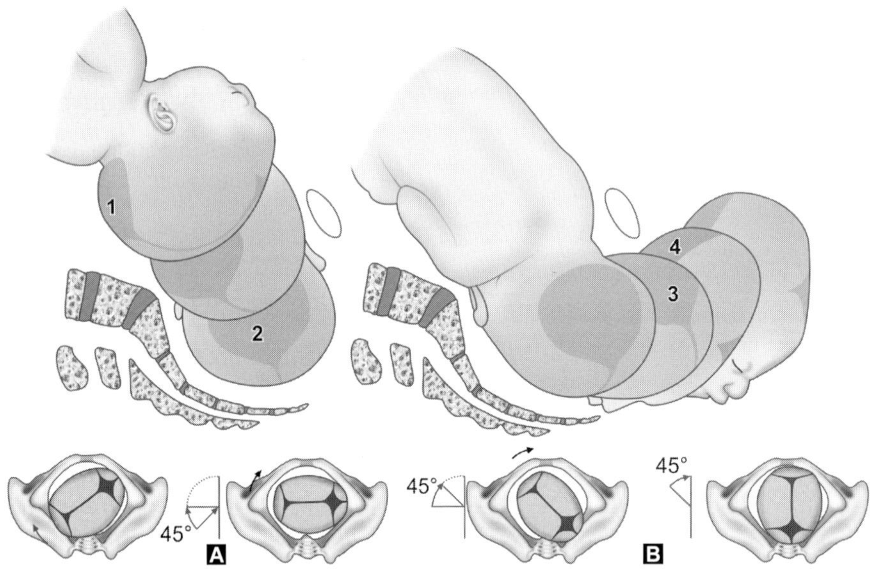

FIG. 5: Mechanisms of labor in occipitoposterior position.

1/8th of a circle (45° short rotation) to give a direct OP position. With further descent, the head will deliver by a combination of flexion and then extension at the outlet, provided that the uterine contractions are strong and there is no contracted pelvis. The emerging diameter is the large occipitofrontal diameter of 11.5 cm, which causes distention of the vulva causing perineal tears. If however, the labor fails to progress it is then called occipitosacral arrest

- Persistent OP (3%): in moderate deflexion, the occiput and sinciput meet the pelvic floor simultaneously. There is no internal rotation and the head persists in the oblique diameter (Fig. 6A)
- Deep transverse arrest (1%): in mild deflexion, the occiput rotates 1/8th circle anteriorly and the head is arrested with the sagittal suture in the transverse diameter (Fig. 6B). In deep transverse arrest and persistent OP, no further progress occurs and labor is obstructed as the head cannot be delivered spontaneously.

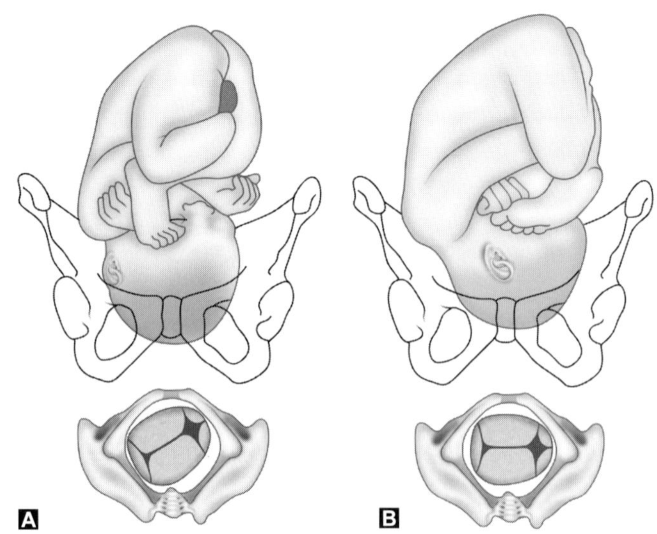

FIGS 6A AND B: **A,** Persistent occipitoposterior position and **B,** Persistent occiput-transverse position.

FACTORS FAVORING LONG ANTERIOR ROTATION

- Well-flexed head
- Good uterine contractions
- Roomy pelvis
- No PROM.

Causes of Failure of Long Anterior Rotation

- Deflexed head
- Uterine inertia
- Contracted pelvis: Rotation of the head cannot easily occur in android pelvis due to projection of the ischial spines and convergence of the side walls
- Lax or rigid pelvic floor
- Premature rupture of membranes early in labor.

Management of Labor

First Stage

Exclude contracted pelvis, cord presentation or prolapse.

Uterine inertia and prolonged labor are expected, so oxytocin should be used judiciously. Contractions are sustained, irregular, and accompanied by marked backache which needs analgesia. Premature rupture of membranes is prevented by providing adequate rest in bed, avoiding straining, avoiding high enema, and minimizing vaginal examinations.

The management remains same as in normal labor.

Second Stage

The mother and fetus are monitored carefully. Any evidence of uterine inertia is combated by using oxytocin, unless it is contraindicated. One of the following events is expected to occur:

- Long internal rotation 3/8th circle: delivery is completed as in normal labor in 45%[15]
- Direct OP (face to pubis): the head can be delivered spontaneously or by aid of outlet forceps. Liberal episiotomy is given to avoid perineal lacerations
- Deep transverse arrest (1%) and persistent OP (3%): the labor is obstructed and requires[15,16] (Fig. 7):
    - Vacuum extraction
    - Manual rotation to anterior position and forceps extraction
    - Forceps rotation and extraction
    - Cesarean section
    - Craniotomy.

Vacuum extraction (ventouse): proper application as near as possible to the occiput will promote flexion of the head.

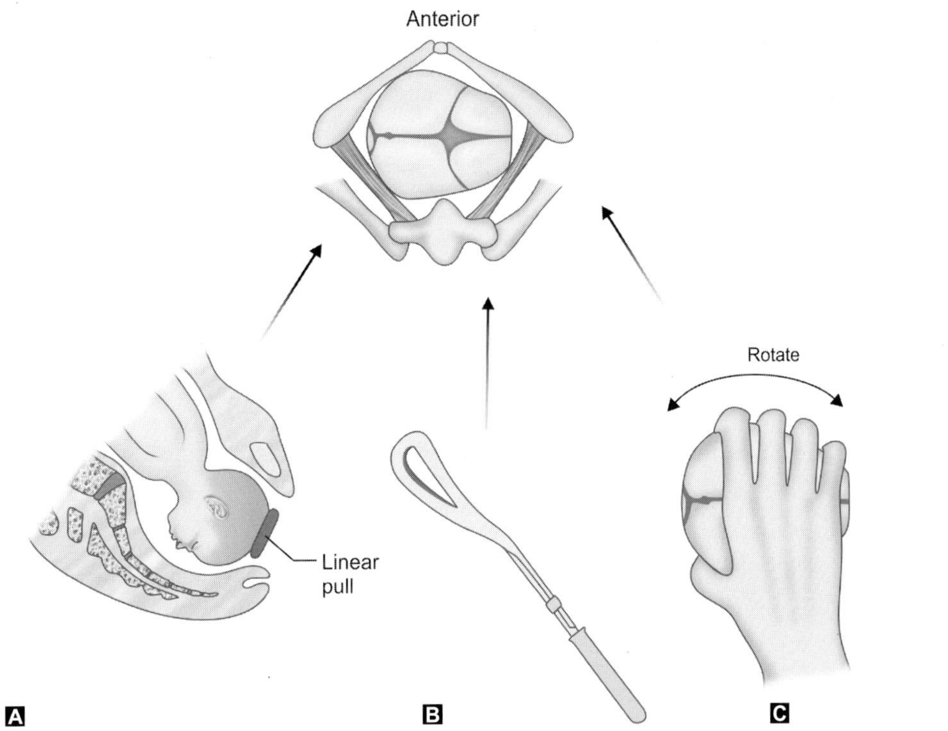

FIGS 7A TO C: Methods of delivering a baby in occipitotransverse position in the second stage of labor: **A,** Vacuum extraction; **B,** Rotation and extraction with Kielland's forceps; or **C,** Manual rotation of head and then forceps applied immediately, once occipitoanterior position is achieved.[8]

Traction will guide the head into the pelvis till it meets the pelvic floor where it will rotate.

Manual rotation and extraction by forceps: under general anesthesia the head is grasped bitemporally, and pushed slightly upwards and disimpacted. The head flexed. The occiput is rotated to anterior position is by the right hand introduced vaginally. This is aided by rotation of the anterior shoulder abdominally towards the midline by the left hand or by an assistant. The head is fixed abdominally by an assistant. This is followed by the application of forceps and extraction.

Rotation and extraction by a forceps: kielland's forceps have a minimal pelvic curve, thus it has the advantage of single application for rotation and extraction of the head. There are two methods of application: the wandering (or gliding method) and the direct application also known as the classical application.

Barton's forceps: it was originally designed for deep transverse arrest. It has a hinge in one blade between the blade proper and shank to facilitate application. The axis of the handle to that of the blades is 55°, i.e. the angle of the pelvic inlet to the outlet. It is used for rotation only, then conventional forceps is applied for extraction unless it has an axis traction piece so it can be used for rotation and extraction.

Scanzoni double application: the conventional forceps is applied to rotate the occiput anteriorly. Then the forceps is removed and reapplied so that the pelvic curve of the forceps is directed anteriorly and the head is extracted. This method is obsolete, as it is hazardous to the mother and fetus.

Cesarean section: it is indicated in the event of failure of the above methods or when there are other indications as in case of contracted pelvis, prolapsed cord before full cervical dilatation, etc.

Craniotomy: if the fetus is dead.

PERSISTENT OCCIPITOTRANSVERSE POSITION

It occurs when the fetal occiput is transverse to the maternal pelvis. The head engages in the left or right occipitotransverse position, the rotation to occipitoanterior takes place. If this fails to occur, the head remains in the transverse position in the second stage causing deep-transverse arrest. The occiput-transverse position is most likely transitory, because the occiput tends to rotate to the anterior position. In the absence of hypotonic uterine contractions, spontaneous anterior rotation usually occurs, allowing vaginal delivery.[5]

Management of Labor

Spontaneous rotation to the anterior position occurs in 90% of cases. Arrested labor may occur when the head does not rotate and/or descend. Delivery may be complicated by perineal tears or extension of an episiotomy. If there are signs of obstruction or the fetal heart rate is abnormal at any stage cesarean section has to be performed. If the membranes are intact, artificial rupture of the membranes has to be done. In case the cervix is not fully dilated and there are no signs of obstruction, labor should be augmented with oxytocin. But if the cervix is fully dilated but there is no descent in the expulsive phase, assess for signs of obstruction:[13]

- If there are no signs of obstruction, augment labor with oxytocin
- If the fetal head is more than 3/5th palpable above the symphysis pubis or the leading bony edge of the head is above –2 stations, perform cesarean section
- If the fetal head is between 1/5th and 3/5th above the symphysis pubis or the leading bony edge of the head is between zero station and –2 stations, perform delivery by vacuum extraction. But if the operator is not proficient in symphysiotomy, perform cesarean section
- If the head is not more than 1/5th above the symphysis pubis or the leading bony edge of the fetal head is at or below zero station, deliver by vacuum extraction or forceps.

The occiput may be manually rotated (anteriorly or posteriorly) and forceps delivery performed. Kielland's forceps may also be applied to the fetal head in the occipitotransverse position to rotate the occiput anteriorly and then deliver the head either with the same forceps or with Simpson or Tucker-McLane forceps.

In the platypelloid and the android pelvis, there is not adequate space to rotate the occiput to anterior or posterior position. In the android pelvis, the head may not be engaged, yet the scalp may be visible at the introitus due to supermolding and caput formation.

FACE PRESENTATION (FIGURE 8)

Face presentation is said to occur when the fetal head is hyperextended,[17] with the occiput resting against the upper back. The denominator is the chin (mentum) in face presentation.

Causes

- Anencephaly, as there is no bony skull
- Thyroid tumor/congenital tumor of the neck
- Umbilical cord coils around neck
- Polyhydramnios
- Contracted pelvis/cephalopelvic disproportion
- Multiparity and a lax abdominal wall.

Diagnosis

- On abdominal examination: longitudinal lie, cephalic presentation, groove can be felt between the head and the back. Cephalic prominence is on the same side as the fetal back

- On vaginal examination: the chin, mouth, nose, cheek bones, eyes, and supraorbital ridges are palpable (Fig. 9). The face might be mistaken with breech presentation since mouth may be mistaken for anus, facial bony prominence for buttocks and nose for genitalia
- Ultrasonogram or X-ray: it will confirm the diagnosis.

Mechanism of Labor (Figs 10A and B)

Labor begins in the brow position. But as the labor progresses, the fetus is pushed into the pelvis against the maternal tissues, the brow is either converted to vertex upon flexion, or becomes extended and turns into a face. The mentoposterior position has no mechanism of labor because the engaging diameter is the sternobregmatic of 16–18 cm, as the chest and the head try to pass the brim at the same time, requiring a cesarean section.

In mentoanterior position, engagement occurs in the transverse or oblique diameter of the inlet. All the cardinal movements of labor remain the same: engagement, descent , flexion, internal rotation, extension, and external rotation and expulsion. The exceptions being that there occurs extension instead of flexion and the head is delivered by flexion and not extension. Engagement, however, occurs late in the second stage at +3 station (compared to zero station in vertex presentation). Internal rotation will bring the chin anterior,

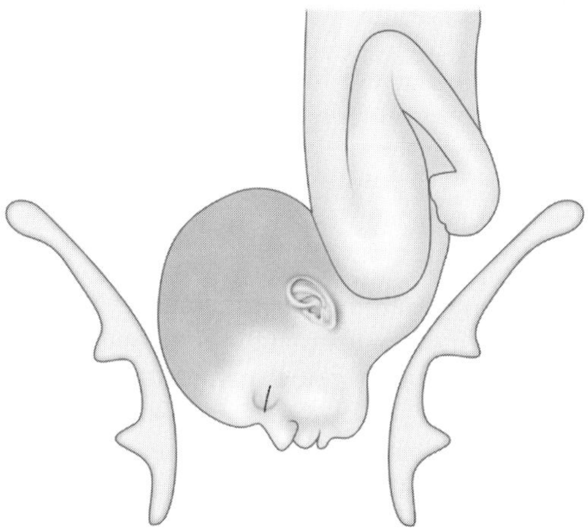

FIG. 8: Face presentation.[13]

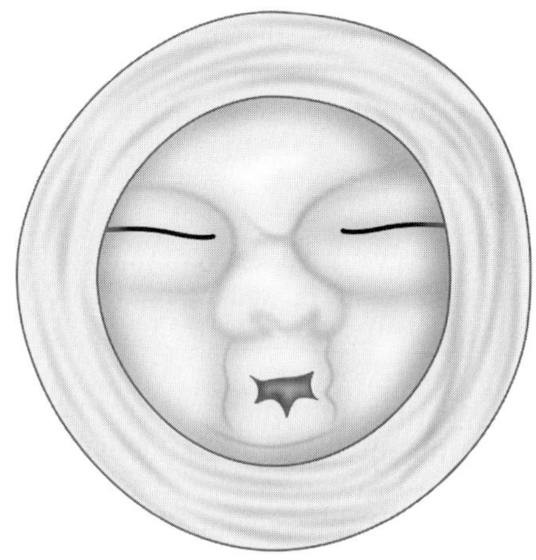

FIG. 9: Vaginal touch picture in face presentation.

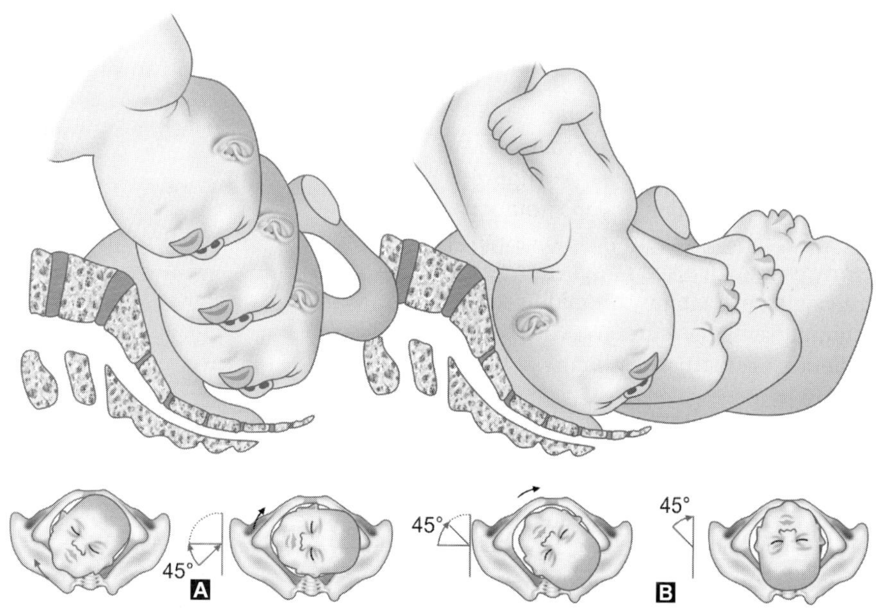

FIG. 10: Mechanism of labor in right mentoposterior position.

and the face delivers by flexion. The chin, nose, eyes, brow, vertex, and occiput appear successively. The second stage of labor is more prolonged due to the oblique line of thrust. The emerging diameter is the submentovertical of 11 cm, causing considerable stretching of the vulva and perineum. The chin rotates externally to the side it originally faced. The rest of the body delivers by the usual mechanism.

Management

Mentoanterior Position

- If the cervix is fully dilated, allow to proceed with normal childbirth
- If descent is unsatisfactory, deliver by forceps
- If the cervix is not fully dilated and there are no signs of obstruction, augment labor with oxytocin. Review progress as with vertex presentation.

Mentoposterior Position

- If the cervix is fully dilated, deliver by cesarean section
- If the cervix is not fully dilated, monitor descent, rotation and progress. If the features of obstruction appear, a cesarean section is indicated
- If the fetus is dead, deliver by craniotomy. But if the operator is not proficient in craniotomy, delivery by cesarean section is required.

If risks factors, like congenital malformation, contracted pelvis, and pre-eclampsia, have been excluded, normal vaginal delivery can be attempted. The first stage of labor has to be managed as in case of any other high-risk pregnancy. In the presence of risk factors and if the estimated fetal weight is more than 3.5 kg, then cesarean section should be considered. Attempts to manually convert the face to vertex (Thom maneuver) or to rotate a mentoposterior to mentoanterior positions are rarely successful. These maneuvers are associated with high perinatal mortality and maternal morbidity, including cord prolapse, uterine rupture and fetal cervical spine injury. Internal podalic rotation maneuvers are not justified, unless cesarean section cannot be performed. Rarely forceps may be used to deliver a face presentation. The use of vacuum extractor is contraindicated. Craniotomy may be required in neglected cases, where the baby is dead and the patient is in obstructed labor.

Outcomes

The perinatal morbidity, mortality, and maternal morbidity has decreased due to the increased use of cesarean section for malpresentations. Neonates delivered in the face presentation have facial and scalp edema, which usually resolves within 24–48 hours. Trauma during labor may cause tracheal and laryngeal edema immediately after delivery, with resultant neonatal respiratory distress. Fetal anomalies or tumors, such as fetal goiter that may have led to fetal malpresentation, may contribute to increased perinatal morbidity and mortality.

BROW PRESENTATION (FIGURE 11)

Brow presentation is the rarest of all the presentations and is also known as the military position. It is a variant of the face presentation. It occurs when there is incomplete extension of the head, i.e. in between a well flexed and hyperextended head.[13,17] It is usually transient and changes to face presentation if extension becomes complete, or changes to vertex if flexion occurs.

Causes

Causes of brow presentation are same as the causes for face presentation.

Diagnosis

- On abdominal examination, the findings are same as in face presentation except that the groove at the neck is less prominent and we are able to palpate the occiput and the chin
- On vaginal examination, the examiner can feel the nose on one side and supraorbital ridges, brow, and anterior fontanel on the other side. But the chin and mouth cannot be felt. The presence of a large caput may make it impossible for the examiner to make the diagnosis with confidence.

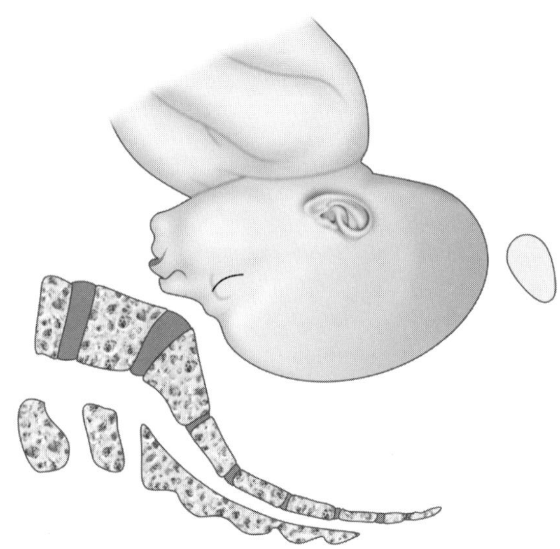

FIG. 11: Brow presentation.[13]

Mechanism of Labor

Engaging diameter is the mentovertical diameter of 14 cm; hence there is no mechanism of labor in a normal-sized fetus with an average-sized pelvis. Vaginal delivery can be possible only if the fetal head is small or the pelvis is very roomy (Fig. 12).

Management

Spontaneous correction usually occurs in labor and it converts to face or vertex, depending on whether extension or flexion occurs and then management can be tailored accordingly. Cesarean section is indicated if brow persists for more than 2 hours, hyperextension takes place or the head remains high up. Destructive procedures, such as craniotomy, are performed in cases presenting with IUFD, when the cervix is fully dilated, provided that rupture of uterus has been ruled out. If the operator is not proficient in craniotomy, or if the cervix is not fully dilated, deliver by cesarean section. The brow presentation should not be delivered by vacuum extraction, outlet forceps or symphysiotomy.

Prognosis

The complications of brow presentation are much the same as for other malpresentations:
- Obstructed labor and ruptured uterus
- Cord prolapse
- Facial bruising
- Cerebral hemorrhage.

COMPOUND PRESENTATION (FIGURE 13)

This type of presentation involves the prolapse of an extremity—a hand or arm—along with the presenting part, the fetal vertex/breech. Rarely a foot can present with the vertex if the knee is extended and the hip flexed, or a hand or arm may present along the side of the breech. Compound presentations are observed more commonly with preterm labor, after PROM, when a pelvic mass displaces the presenting part, or after induction of labor in unengaged presenting parts.

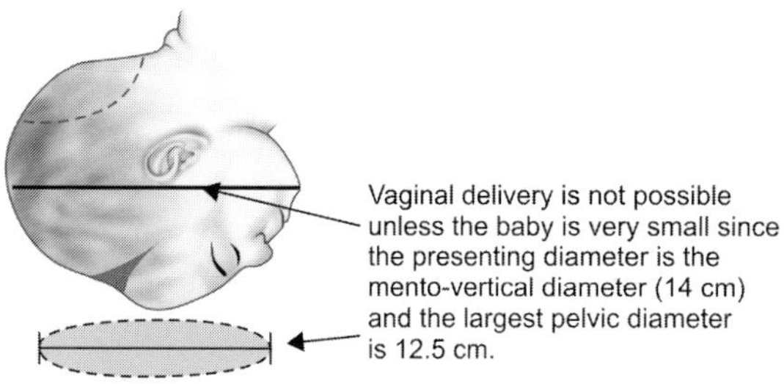

FIG. 12: Relationship of brow with respect to maternal pelvis.

On per vaginum examination, if the membranes are intact, with the process of labor this hand or leg is likely to regress spontaneously. If this does not happen then it can be reposited manually. If manual reposition does not succeed, then a cesarean section is required. If the hand or arm has prolapsed past the presenting part, vaginal delivery is abandoned and a cesarean section is performed.
Perinatal loss increased by:
- Prolapsed cord (as it can lead to death of the fetus)
- Traumatic obstetrical procedures.

TRANSVERSE LIE (FIGURES 14A AND B)

It occurs when the longitudinal axis of the fetus is perpendicular to that of the mother. Oblique lie is said if the fetal axis

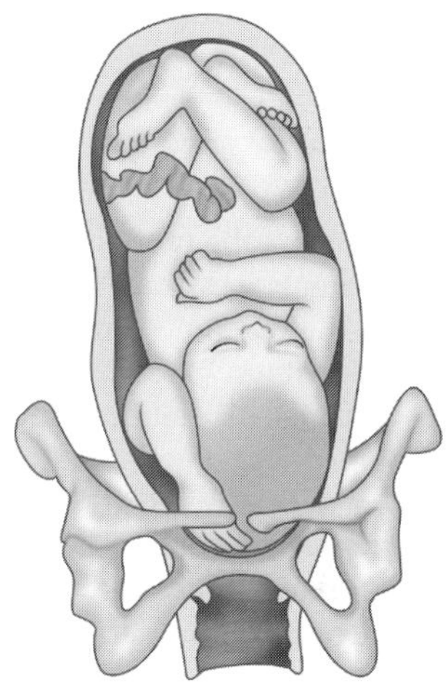

FIG. 13: Compound presentation: fetal hand alongside the fetal head.[13]

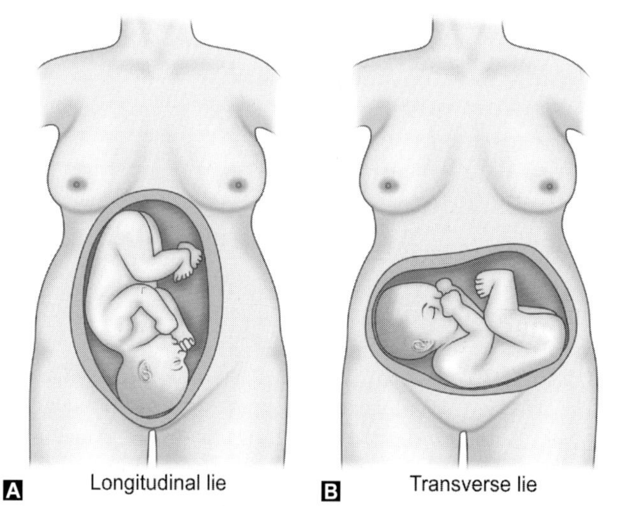

FIGS 14A AND B: Normal; **A,** longitudinal lie and **B,** transverse lie.

forms an acute angle (<90°) or if long axis of the fetus is not perpendicular. In both of these conditions, shoulder is the presenting part and acromion is the denominator.

Etiology

- Pendulous or flabby abdominal wall, particularly in multiparous patients
- Preterm fetus
- Placenta previa as the fetal head cannot be accommodated in the lower uterine segment because the placenta is occupying the lower segment
- Uterine malformation: Transverse lie usually occurs if uterus is "arcuate" shaped
- Excessive amniotic fluid (fetus is able to move around and assume different positions)
- Contracted pelvis/pelvic tumor
- Congenital fetal malformations/IUFD
- Multiple pregnancies.

Diagnosis

On abdominal examination, the uterus appears broader and the height of the fundus is less than that expected for the period of gestation as no fetal pole is occupying the fundus. Neither the head nor the buttocks can be felt at the symphysis pubis. The fetal head is usually felt in the flank on one side of the mother's abdomen and breech on the other (Figs 15A to D).

On vaginal examination, in early labor, the presenting part may not be felt. But when the labor is well progressed, examiner may feel the baby's shoulder. Shoulder is identified by the presence of acromion, scapula, clavicle, and axilla; "grid iron" of ribs and intercostal spaces may be felt. When the shoulder enters the pelvic brim, the baby's arm may prolapse and the elbow, arm, or hand may be felt in the vagina or become visible outside the introitus (Fig. 16).

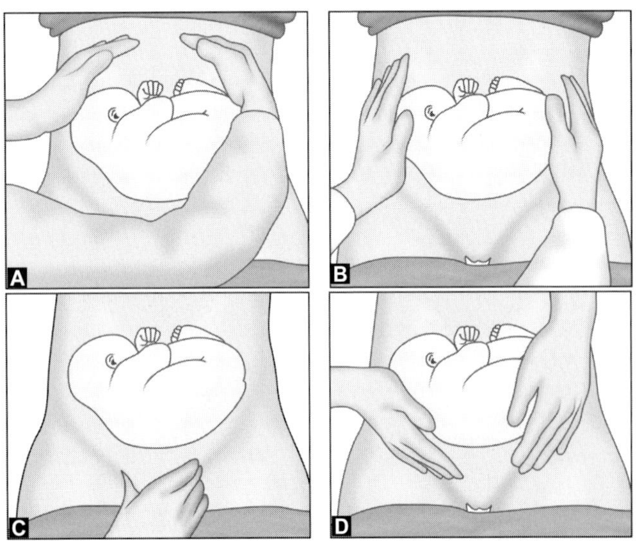

FIG. 15: Abdominal palpation (Leopold's maneuvers) in transverse lie.

Management

In a shoulder presentation, the baby cannot be delivered vaginally. It is possible only in very small fetuses (macerated stillborn and abortions with birth weight <800 g) and cannot occur in a full-term pregnancy. Fetus is delivered as conduplicato corpore, i.e., the head and thorax pass through the pelvic cavity at the same time.

The patient is admitted at around 36 weeks, as she may go into labor any time after 37–38 weeks and there is a high risk of PROM and cord prolapse. External cephalic version can be attempted after 39 weeks and if it is successful, stabilization and induction can be done. However, if even after 40 weeks the lie is unstable, an elective cesarean section is performed. If the woman is in early labor and the membranes are intact, external version can be attempted. If external version fails or is not advisable, the patient is delivered by cesarean section. If she presents late in labor, she should be taken up for a cesarean section. If she is left unattended, in a dorsoinferior transverse lie, further contractions will result in impacted shoulder in lower segment. But if it was dorsosuperior positio, the chances of cord prolapse are very high. Ruptured uterus may occur if the woman is left unattended. Destructive procedures are only performed in case of IUFD, by an experienced obstetrician after rupture of uterus has been ruled out. In modern practice, persistent transverse lie in labor is delivered by cesarean section whether the fetus is alive or dead.

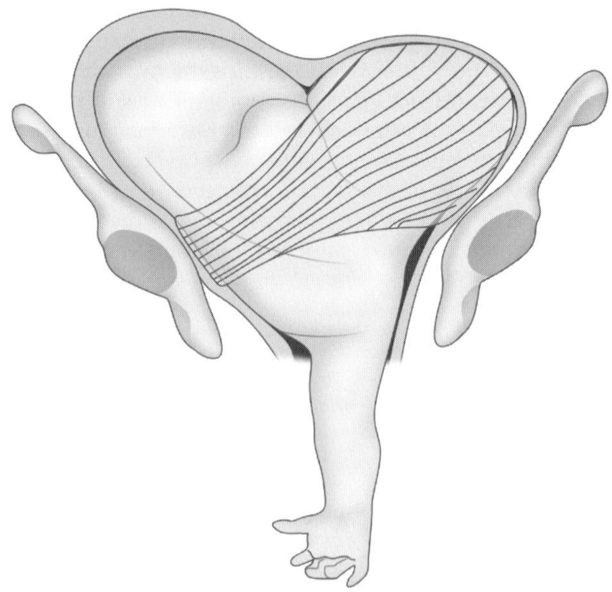

FIG. 16: Shoulder presentation with prolapsed arm in dorsoinferior position.

Complications

- Maternal risks:
  - Prolonged labor
  - Infection of the genital tract
  - Obstructed labor
  - Intrapartum hemorrhage
  - Postpartum hemorrhage
  - Lacerations of the genital tract and perineum
  - Risks of anesthesia
  - Deep vein thrombosis and pulmonary embolism
  - Vesicovaginal fistula
- Fetal risks:
  - Cord prolapse
  - Hypoxia
  - Infection
  - Traumatic injuries
  - Meconium aspiration.

REFERENCES

1. Edmonds DK, Whitfield CR (Eds). Dewhurst's Textbook of Obstetrics and Gynaecology for Postgraduates, 6th edition. Oxford, UK: Wiley-Blackwell Science; 1999.
2. Ratcliffe SD, Baxley EG, Cline MK, Sakornbut EL (Eds). Family Medicine Obstetrics, 3rd edition. Philadelphia, PA, USA: Elsevier Health Sciences; 2008.
3. Chakravarti S, Gupta K, Datta S. Malposition, malpresentation and cord prolapse. In: Arulkumaran S, Sivanesaratnam V, Chatterjee A, Kumar P (Eds). Essentials of Obstetrics, 2nd edition. New Delhi, India: Jaypee Brothers Medical Publishers; 2010.
4. Ponkey SE, Cohen AP, Heffner LJ, Lieberman E. Persistent fetal occiput posterior position: obstetric outcomes. Obstet Gynecol. 2003;101(5 Pt 1):915-20.
5. Wikipedia, The Free Encyclopedia. (2015). Shoulder dystocia. [online]. Available from: en.wikipedia.org/wiki/Shoulder_dystocia. [Accessed October, 2015].
6. Malpresentation and malposition. [online]. Available from www.pt.co.uk/reference/Malpresentation_and_Malposition.html. [Accessed October, 2015].
7. Cunningham FG, Leveno KJ, Bloom SL, Hauth JC, Rouse DJ, Spong CY, Williams JW (Eds). Williams Obstetrics, 23rd edition. New York, USA: McGraw-Hill Medical Publishing Division; 2010.
8. Chamberlain G, Steer P. ABC of labour care: unusual presentations and positions and multiple pregnancy. BMJ. 1999;318(7192):1192-4.
9. Gardberg M, Laakkonen E, Sälevaara M. Intrapartum sonography and persistent occiput posterior position: a study of 408 deliveries. Obstet Gynecol. 1998;91(5 Pt 1):746-9.
10. Peregrine E, O'Brien P, Jauniaux E. Impact on delivery outcome of ultrasonographic fetal head position prior to induction of labor. Obstet Gynecol. 2007;109(3):618-25.
11. Phipps H, de Vries B, Hyett J, Osborn DA. Prophylactic manual rotation for fetal malposition to reduce operative delivery. Cochrane Database Syst Rev. 2014;12:CD009298.
12. Cheng Y, Shaffer BL, Caughey A. The association between persistent occiput posterior position and neonatal outcomes. Obstet Gynecol. 2006;107(4):837-44.
13. World Health Organization (WHO). (2003). IRIS: Managing Complications in Pregnancy and Childbirth: A Guide for Midwives and Doctors. [online]. Available from hetv.org/resources/reproductive-health/impac/Symptoms/Malpositions__malpresetations_S69_S81.html. [Accessed October, 2015].
14. Dutta DC. Malposition, malpresentation and cord prolapse. In: Textbook of Obstetrics, 7th edition. New Delhi, India: Jaypee Brothers Medical Publishers; 2014. pp. 365-400.
15. Family Practice Notebook. (2015). Occipito posterior position. [online]. Available from www.fpnotebook.com/OB/LD/ocptPstr.htm. [Accessed October, 2015].
16. Family Practice Notebook. (2015). Manual rotation in occipitoposterior presentation. [online]. Available from www.fpnotebook.com/OB/procedure/MnlRtnlnOcptpstrPrsntn.htm. [Accessed October, 2015].
17. Gabbe SG, Niebyl JR, Galan HL, Jauniaux ER, Landon MB, Simpson JL, Driscoll DA (Eds). Obstetrics: Normal and Problem Pregnancies, 6th edition. Philadelphia, PA, USA: Saunder.

CHAPTER 41

Breech and Other Malpresentations

Smiti Nanda, Krishna Dahiya, Monika Dalal

INTRODUCTION

Breech is the most common abnormal presentation. When buttocks of the fetus lie over the maternal pelvis, it is called breech presentation. Breech presentation occurs in 25% of births before 28-weeks gestation, in 7% of births that occur at 32 weeks, and 1–3% of births that occur at term (Table 1). Perinatal mortality is increased 2-fold to 4-fold with breech presentation, regardless of the mode of delivery. Deaths most often are associated with malformations, prematurity, and intrauterine fetal demise.[1,2]

TYPES OF BREECH PRESENTATION

Breech can present in a variety of ways (Figs 1A to C).

- Frank breech (50–70%): buttocks are presenting part, hips flexed, knees extended
- Complete breech (5–10%): buttocks along with feet are presenting part, hips flexed, knees flexed
- Footling or incomplete breech (10–30%): one or both hips extended, either one or both feet are presenting part.

TABLE 1: Incidence of breech presentation according to gestational age

Gestation (weeks)	% Breech
21–24	33%
25–28	28%
29–32	14%
33–36	9%
37–40	3%

PREDISPOSING FACTORS FOR BREECH PRESENTATION[3]

- Prematurity is the most common predisposing factor. Smaller size of fetus and larger volume of amniotic fluid allow the fetus to undergo spontaneous version
- Maternal causes:
  - Contracted pelvis
  - Multiparae with lax abdominal wall (due to unstable lie)
  - Nullipara (uterine tone is greatest in nullipara, limiting the available space
  - Maternal anticonvulsant[4] and alcohol abuse[5] (influence on intrauterine fetal neurologic function)
- Uterine causes:
  - Mullerian duct abnormalities (septate and bicornuate uterus)
  - Fibriods
  - Uterine surgeries
- Abnormal placental location:
  - Cornufundal attachment of placenta, short cord
- Abnormality in liquor—oligohydraminos and polyhydrominos
- Fetal causes:
  - Twins
  - Fetus with extended legs
  - Hydrocephalus
  - Myelomeningocele (50% of all babies with hydrocephalus and myelomeningocele present by breech)
  - Intrauterine death (IUD) of fetus
  - Trisomy 13, 18, 21

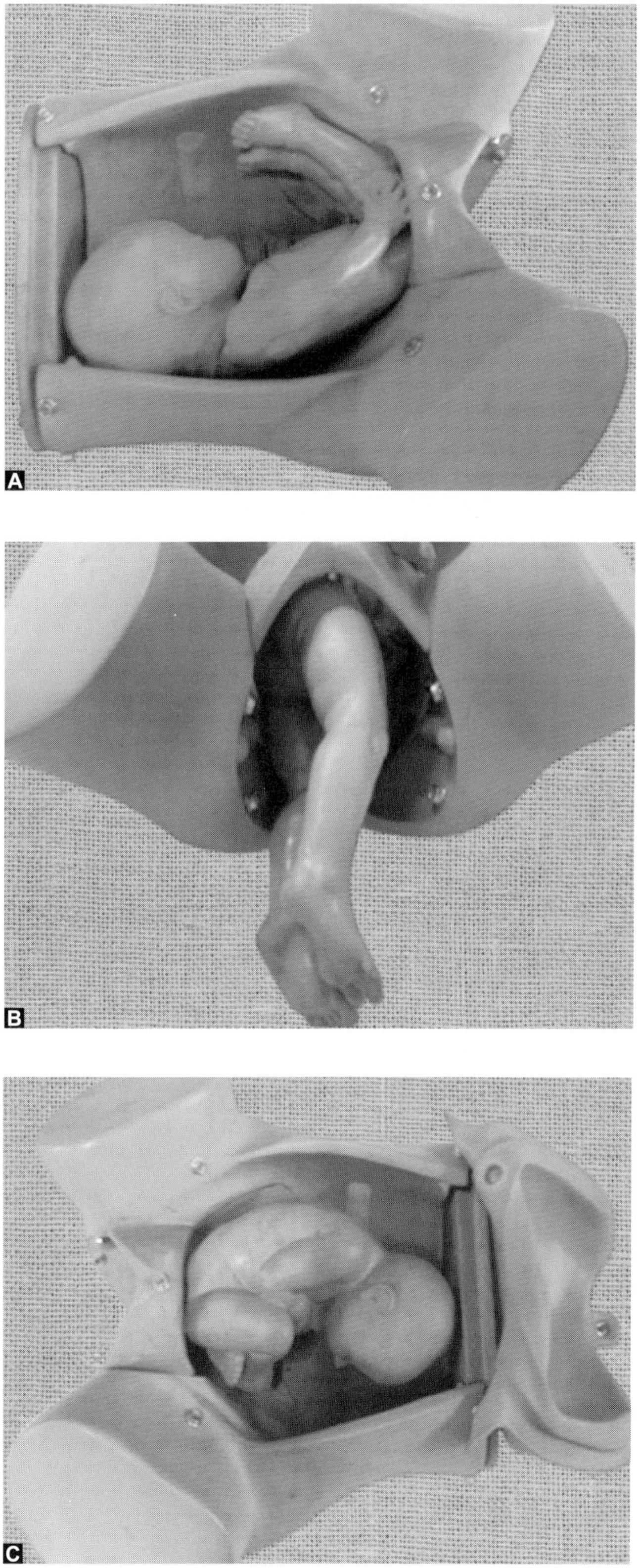

FIGS 1A TO C: Types of breech. **A,** Frank breech; **B,** Footling breech; **C,** Complete breech.

- Prader-Willi syndrome (50% present as breech)
- Anencephaly
- Myotonic dystrophy.

An active baby adapts position of best fit in normal intrauterine space.

Maternal or fetal mechanical risk factors are only found in between 7% and 15% of breech deliveries. Recurrence of breech delivery in successive siblings is high and there appears to be an increased risk of intergenerational recurrence, equally high transmitted via fathers or mothers.[6]

DIAGNOSIS

Prior to 32–35 weeks, the diagnosis is of no clinical significance.

Per-abdomen examination: Palpation only has a sensitivity of 28% and specificity of 94% in detection of breech presentation.[7]

- Fundal grip: ballottable head in the fundal area. Irregular small parts of feet may be felt by the side of head in frank breech
- Lateral grip: fetal back is felt on one side and limbs on the other side. Limbs are less felt in frank breech
- Pelvic grip: softer, irregular, broad mass felt in the pelvis. Breech is usually not engaged in complete breech and commonly engaged in frank breech
- Fetal heart sound (FHS): fetal heartbeat heard above the umbilicus.

Per-vaginal examination: The sacrum, ischial tuberosity, anus or foot can be palpated through the fornix. Foot can be identified by prominence of heel and lesser mobility of great toe.

Use of ultrasonography in breech is to confirm diagnosis, measurement of biparietal diameter, gestational age, estimated baby weight, localization of the placenta, assessment of liquor volume, fetal malformation, nuchal cord around the neck, congenital anomalies of the uterus. Fetal weight by ultrasound is measured less accurately in breech than cephalic. Fetal malformation (incidence of congenital malformations is 6%) and uterine malformation are more commonly associated with breech than cephalic presentation.

X-ray pelvimetry is increasingly abandoned because of possible long-term incidence of myelodysplasia.[8] Magnetic resonance imaging (MRI) has been used to assess the pelvic capacity in addition to all the above mentioned information. However, routine use of X-ray, computed tomography (CT), and MRI is not advisable.

Breech positions: the sacrum is the denominator of breech and there are four positions. In anterior position, the sacrum is directed towards the iliopubic eminence and in posterior positions, the sacrum is directed to the sacroiliac joints. The positions are: (1) first position—left sacroanterior (LSA) being the most common (2) second position—right sacroanterior (RSA) (3) third position—right sacroposterior (RSP), and (4) fourth position—left sacroposterior (LSP).

MECHANISM OF LABOR IN BREECH PRESENTATION

Sacroanterior Position

In the mechanism of breech delivery, the principal movements occur at three places; buttocks, shoulders, and the head. Buttocks and shoulders are bigger but more compressible while the head because of nonmoulding (due to rapid descent), present difficulties.

Delivery of Lower Limbs and Buttocks

Engagement: bitrochanteric diameter (10 cm) engages in right or left oblique diameter of inlet. Sacrum is directed towards one of the iliopubic eminence. Continuous descent occurs until anterior buttock touches the pelvic floor. Internal rotation of anterior buttock occurs after rotating one-eighth of circle and it comes behind the symphysis pubis, further descent occurs with lateral flexion and birth of buttocks and lower limbs occurs.

Delivery of Shoulders and Arms

Engagement: bisacromial diameter (12 cm, engaging diameter) engages in oblique diameter of inlet (same as that occupied by bitrochantric diameter). Engagement of shoulder occurs soon after delivery of breech. Descent is continuous. Internal rotation of shoulder brings the shoulders, in anteroposterior diameter of pelvic outlet. Simultaneously, there is external rotation of trunk by one-eighth of circle. First there is delivery of posterior shoulder followed by delivery of anterior shoulder by anterior flexion. Restitution is due to untwisting of trunk. After this, anterior shoulder comes towards the right thigh in left sacroanterior and towards left thigh in right sacroanterior. External rotation occurs in the same direction as of restitution. This is due to the internal rotation of occiput by one-eighth of circle anteriorly.

Birth of After-coming Head

- Engagement: engaging diameter is suboccipitofrontal (10 cm) enters into pelvis through opposite oblique diameter as that of buttocks. Flexion occurs along with descent. Internal rotation of occiput occurs by one-eighth of circle and occiput comes behind the symphysis pubis. Birth of the head with descent, subocciput hinges under the symphysis pubis. Head delivers by flexion; chin, mouth, nose, forehead, vertex, and occiput appear successively.

Sacroposterior Position

Only difference in mechanism is that head has to rotate by three-eighth of circle to bring the occiput behind the symphysis pubis.

Management

It includes reducing the incidence of breech presentation at term.

External Cephalic Version

It is the abdominal maneuver to bring the cephalic pole into lower pole of the uterus to convert a breech or transverse lie to a cephalic presentation.

The Royal College of Obstetricians and Gynecologists (RCOG)[8] currently recommends that all women with an uncomplicated breech pregnancy at term (37 weeks) should be offered external cephalic version (ECV), provided there are no contraindications. External cephalic version can be attempted in postdate women and can even be performed in early labor provided membranes are intact. External cephalic version is a safe procedure that has been shown not to increase the risk of IUD within and after 24 hours of the procedure, irrespective of the outcome of ECV.[9]

- Attempting ECV at term reduces the risk of a non-cephalic birth and cesarean section (CS)[9]
- Labor after a successful ECV has a higher rate of obstetric intervention than labor with a spontaneous cephalic presentation
- Success rates of ECV range between 30% and 80%. Factors contributing to successful ECV include: multiparity, non-white race, relaxed uterine tone, adequate liquor volume, and a station above the pelvic brim.
- Factors associated with failure:[10]
  - Nulliparity
  - Anterior or cornual placentation
  - Difficulty in palpating head
  - Oligohydramnios/polyhydraminos
  - Increased uterine tone
  - Descent of breech into pelvis
  - Maternal obesity
  - Frank breech
  - Short umbilical cord
  - Posteriorly located spine
  - Gestation >38 weeks.

External cephalic version at less than 36 weeks

- Iatrogenic preterm delivery can occur
- More likely to be associated with spontaneous reversion to breech.

External cephalic version after 36 week

- Fewer reversion
- Fewer spontaneous version
- Prompt management of complication
- No risk of prematurity.

Contraindications for External Cephalic Version

Absolute contraindication:
- If cesarean delivery is indicated irrespective of fetal position (contracted pelvis, placenta previa)
- Rupture of membranes
- Multiple gestation
- Uterine anomaly
- Nonreassuring fetal status
- Antepartum hemorrhage (placenta previa, abruption placentae)
- Fetal anomaly
- Fetal death.

Relative contraindication:
- Previous cesarean delivery
- Pre-eclampsia or hypertensive disorder
- Maternal cardiac disease
- Intrauterine growth restriction (IUGR)
- Oligohydraminos
- Bad obstetric history
- Elderly primigravida.

Spontaneous reversion to breech presentation can occur in less than 5% cases.

It should only be carried out by appropriately trained practitioners, where facilities for continuous fetal monitoring, ultrasound and emergency cesarean delivery are available. Patient should be fasting.

Preprocedure preparation

- Informed consent
- Bladder should be empty
- Ultrasonography (USG) to assess fetal position, amount of liquor, placental localization, rule-out congenital malformation
- Reactive nonstress test (NST) prior to procedure.

Procedure

Patient is asked to keep her abdominal muscles relaxed. Uterus may be relaxed using a tocolytic. Powder is sprinkled over the abdomen. Breech is disengaged from pelvis (scoop the breech out of pelvis). Basic principle in rotating the fetus is to keep the baby's back flexed and follow the shortest path to a cephalic position. (backwards flip or forwards somersault are two methods). Forward somersault is preferred. Slow and steady pressure should be used. Continuous cardiotocography (CTG) monitoring during the procedure is recommended. Maternal pulse and blood pressure should be taken every 5 minutes.[11] After successful version, the position of the fetus should be maintained manually for a few minutes.

Postprocedure care

- Nonstress test, fetal heart rate (FHR) tracing should be obtained
- In Rh -ve patients, anti-D immunoglobulin should be given
- Vaginal bleeding should be looked for.

Women should be advised that ECV can be painful (high pain levels reported in 5%) and the procedure will be stopped, if they wish. Beta-stimulants (when used to facilitate ECV) increase cephalic presentation in labor and birth, and reduce the CS rate in both nulliparous and multiparous women, but there are insufficient data on adverse effects.[9]

Complications[12]

- Discomfort to mother
- Need for emergency cesarean delivery
- Negative psychological effect in the event of failure
- Nonreassuring FHR
- Placental abruption
- Preterm labor pains
- Premature rupture of membrane (PROM)
- Uterine rupture
- Amniotic fluid embolism
- Pulsatility index is reduced in middle cerebral artery. This is merely a physiological response to manipulation to fetal head.[12]

Use of tocolysis in external cephalic version

Success rate increases with tocolysis. Use of tocolysis should be considered only when an initial attempt at ECV without tocolysis has failed.

Drugs: ritodrine, salbutamol, and terbutaline have been tried in different dosed by different routes. No effect has been observed with nifedipine and glyceryl trinitrate.

Insufficient evidence exists to support the use of postural techniques[13] (such as knee to chest), or moxibustion[14] (the burning of Chinese herbal medicine on acupuncture points) as alternatives to ECV.

MODE OF DELIVERY

The Royal College of Obstetricians and Gynecologists (2006)[8] has concluded that except in cases of advanced labor and imminent delivery, which are not otherwise defined, women with persistent singleton breech presentation at term should undergo a planned cesarean delivery. Cesarean section has been adopted as the "normal" mode of delivery for term breech presentations in Europe and the United State of America (USA), as the consensus is that this reduces the risk of birth-related complications. Cesarean delivery is associated with reduction in mortality from 13/1000 to 3/1000 and reduction in serious neonatal morbidity from 3% to 1.4%.

In the USA, over 85% of all breech births are now by CS (up from 14% in 1970). Intrapartum and neonatal deaths associated with breech presentation appear to have been declining. One study based on Scottish births between 1985 and 2004 showed a 75% decrease in deaths but the increased use of planned CS only partially explained the decrease.

Cochrane data base of systematic review concludes that policy of planned lower (uterine)-segment cesarean section (LSCS) is associated with a large decrease in perinatal and neonatal mortality and morbidity.[15]

Planned vaginal birth of term singleton breech may be reasonable under hospital-specific protocol guidelines for both eligibility and labor management.

Evidence has accumulated since term breech trial between 2000 and 2006, it supports offering an attempt at vaginal breech delivery in carefully selected and consenting woman.[16]

As per American Congress of Obstetricians and Gynecologists (ACOG) (2006), the decision regarding mode of delivery should depend on the experience of healthcare professional.

In developing countries like India, uniformly high rate of CS for breech must be brought down, because: (1) 50–60% pregnant woman are unbooked; (2) 64% deliveries are unsupervised; (3) postcesarean pregnancies are unattended; (4) median family size of 3.2; and (5) high infant and preschool mortality.[17]

Various scoring system have been proposed to help in selecting the mode of delivery. Two popular ones are the Zatuchni-Andros scoring system (Table 2) and Westin scoring system.

With scores of 0–4, CS is recommended.

Recommendation for Cesarean Delivery

- A large fetus (>3.5 kg)
- Any degree of contraction or unfavorable shape of pelvis

TABLE 2: Zatuchni-Andros Breech Scoring[18]

Parameters	0 Points	1 Points	2 Points
Parity	0	1	2
Gestational age (weeks)	39+	38	<37
EFW (lb)	8	7–8	<7
Previous breech	0	1	2
Dilatation	2	3	4
Station	–3	–2	–1

EFW, estimated fetal weight.

- A hyperextended head
- Incomplete or footling presentation
- Associated obstetric indication (instead of induction of labor)
- Uterine dysfunction (some use oxytocin augmentation)
- Viable preterm fetus in either active labor or in whom delivery is indicated
- Severe fetal growth restriction
- Previous perinatal death or children suffering from birth trauma
- Whenever there is a request for sterilization
- Lack of an experienced operator.

If delivery is required before the onset of spontaneous labor, elective cesarean section is preferable to induction of labor.

Criteria for Selection for Vaginal Breech Delivery

- Fetus neither too small nor too big (estimated fetal weight is 1500–3500 g)
- Well-flexed head
- Mother should have good capacity pelvis
- Fetus; either frank or complete breech.

Fetal Risk of Vaginal Breech Delivery

- Intracranial hemorrhage
- Medullary coning
- Severance of spinal cord
- Brachial plexus injury
- Occipital diastasis[19] (this is due to impact of occiput on maternal pubis during descent of fetal head into the pelvis during 2nd stage. Due to this injury, there can be separation of squamous part of occipital bone from lateral part. This produces a ridge in posterior fossa and hence bruising or laceration of cerebellum)
- Cerebellar bruising (can be present in the absence of occipital diastasis): damage to brain may not be apparent until 2 years of age, when child will manifest signs of clumsiness and poor co-ordination consequent upon its cerebellar damage
- Epiphyseal separation
- Genital damage in male
- Long-term neurologic damage
- Hypopituitarism
- Damage to mouth and pharynx
- Fracture of long bones
- Umbilical cord prolapse: incidence of cord prolapse in cephalic presentation, frank breech, complete breech and footling breech are 0.4%, 0.5%, 5%, and 15% respectively.
- Cerebral palsy.[20]

MANAGEMENT OF FIRST STAGE OF LABOR

- Informed consent explaining risk of head arrest and increased fetal and neonatal morbidity and mortality should be taken
- Part preparation and enema (routine enemas are not recommended)
- Vaginal examination is done at onset of labor for pelvis assessment, and after rupture of membranes to exclude cord prolapsed; repeated only when indicated to assess cervical dilatation, station, and descent
- Maintain maternal hydration and allow clear fluids only
- Epidural anesthesia is preferable but not routinely recommended
  - Advantage:
    - This will make any manipulation in the second stage more comfortable
    - Make any urge to push prior to full dilatation easier to resist
  - Disadvantage:[21]
    - Longer duration of second stage
    - Increased need for augmentation of labor with oxytocin infusion
    - Significantly higher CS rate in second stage of labor
- Maintain partogram.
  - Use of partogram in breech
    - Reduces the incidence of prolonged labor
    - Reduces the incidence of CS
    - Improves the condition of neonate at birth
- Monitoring of FHS and progress of labor to be done
- No premature bearing-down efforts
- Oxytocin infusion may be used for augmentation of labor. Oxytocin is particularly appropriate if there is primary dysfunctional labor (slow progress in the active phase, <1 cm cervical dilatation every 2 h).

Fetal Monitoring during Labor

- Fetal heart rate every 15 minutes
- After membrane rupture, per-vagiam examination to detect cord prolapse, FHR for first 5–10 minutes to detect occult cord prolapse.

Indication of Cesarean Section during Labor

- Arrest in progress of labor
- Nonreassuring fetal status
- Cord presentation or cord prolapse.

Meconium-Stained Liquor (MSL) in breech: in breech, predictive value of MSL for asphyxia is poor. When breech is still high in first stage, it may indicate fetal distress. Passage of meconium in second stage is almost universal.

MANAGEMENT OF SECOND STAGE OF LABOR

There are three methods of breech vaginal delivery.

1. Spontaneous breech delivery: usually occurs in a multigravida with a small baby. When the mother pushes the baby out with the normal bearing-down efforts and the baby is simply supported until delivered
2. Assisted breech delivery should be encouraged: baby is delivered with the assistance of obstetrician
3. Breech extraction: when the entire body of the fetus is extracted by the obstetrician with minimal aid from the mother. Indication includes fetal distress, and cord prolapse, after internal podalic version. It is carried out under anesthesia in cases of fully dilated cervix. It is done infrequently in a live baby.

Assisted Breech Delivery

Assisted breech delivery should always be conducted by a skilled obstetrician. The following are to be kept ready beforehand, in addition to those required for conduction of normal labor:

- Anesthetist and operation theatre; to administer anesthesia as and when required
- An assistant
- Availability of cross-matched blood
- Pudendal block and infiltration of perineum
- Instruments and suture materials for episiotomy
- Breech towel
- A pair of Piper's or long forceps for the after-coming head, if required
- Appliances for resuscitation of the baby, if asphyxiated
- Neonatologist.

Principles in Assisted Breech Delivery

- Never pull from below but push from above
- Always keep the fetus with the back anteriorly.

Disadvantages of Aggressive Traction

- Entrapment of the after coming fetal head can occur through the incompletely dilated cervix
- Slightest traction on the body may cause extension of head which increases the diameter of the head (longer occipitofrontal diameter, 11.5 cm) that must pass through the pelvic inlet.

Steps

- Time of shifting to delivery table: When the anterior buttock and fetal anus are visible and perineum start distending, she is placed in lithotomy position
- Parts are cleaned and draped
- Bladder should be empty

- To avoid aortocaval compression, the woman is tilted laterally (15 degree) using a wedge under the back
- If epidural has not been used earlier, pudendal block is given along with perineal infiltration
- A wide generous episiotomy will always be required. Advantages of episiotomy are:
  - To straighten the birth canal which specially facilitates the delivery of breech with extended legs where lateral flexion is inadequate
  - To facilitate intravaginal manipulation and for forceps delivery
  - To minimize compression of the after-coming head.

The best time for episiotomy is when the perineum is distended and thinned by the breech.

- The patient is encouraged to bear down
- Delivery is allowed by maternal efforts alone up to the umbilicus. Time must be noted
- In case of frank breech, the Pinard maneuver may be needed with a frank breech to facilitate delivery of the legs, only after the fetal umbilicus has been reached. Pressure is exerted against the inner aspect of the knee. Flexion of the knee follows, and the lower leg is swept medially and out of the vagina
- The umbilical cord is to be loosened and mobilized to one side of the sacral bay (away from pressure by presenting part) to minimize compression. There may be transient abnormality in cord pulsation at this stage, which has got no prognostic significance. Umbilical cord can be cut, if it is short
- The baby is wrapped with a sterile towel when held by the hands. Use of towel to cover the baby: (1) to prevent friction injury; (2) to improve the grip without the need for too much squeezing; (3) to keep the baby warm; (4) to prevent slipping; and (5) to prevent stimulus for respiration
- Fetal bony pelvis is grasped with both hands (Figs 2 and 3). Fingers should rest on anterior superior iliac crest and thumbs on sacrum, minimizing the chances of fetal abdominal soft tissue injury. If baby is grasped any higher than that, there is some risk of injury to the fetal kidneys and abdominal organs
- If the back remains posteriorly, gently rotate the torso so that the back comes anteriorly (sacroanterior)
- Assistant should apply suprapubic pressure to keep the fetal head flexed.

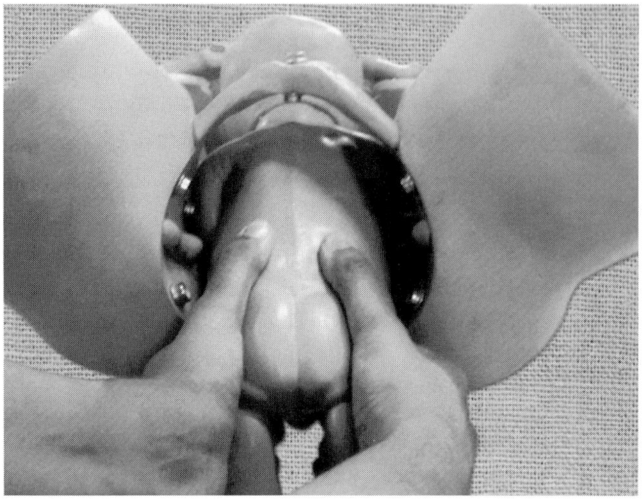

FIG. 2: Grasp the hips.

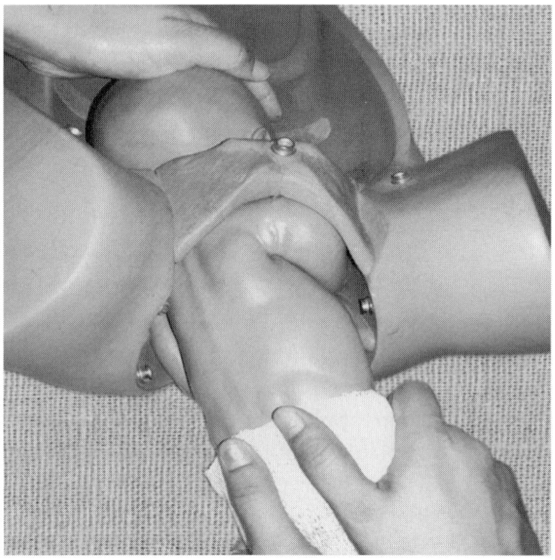

FIG. 3: Towel wrap and apply suprapubic pressure.

Delivery of the Arms

- Employ steady, gentle, downward traction until the lower angle of scapula is visible, note the position of the arms. If the vertebral border of the scapula remains parallel to vertebral column then the arms are flexed. If this is not parallel (winging of scapula), then the arms are extended (Figs 4 and 5)
- Make no attempts at delivery of shoulders and arms until one axilla becomes visible. When one axilla is visible, deliver the arms by simply hooking down each elbow with a finger one after the other. Lovset's maneuver should be used as first-line method for delivery of arms
- Keep the baby's body at or below the horizontal plane or axis of the birth canal. If the body is above the horizontal axis, there is risk of injury to the baby's spine through hyperextension.

Delivery of the After-coming Head

This is the most important stage of the breech delivery. There should be a time limit of around 5–10 minutes between delivery of umbilicus to delivery of mouth. There are three main methods for delivery of head; one of these can be used.

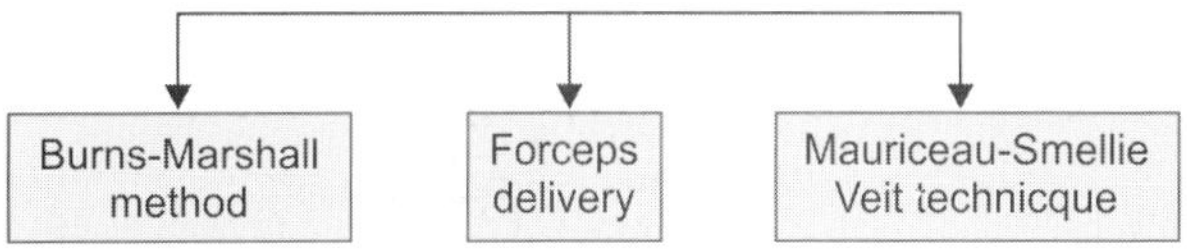

Burns-Marshall Method (Fig. 6)

The baby is allowed to hang till the nape of the neck is visible under the public arch. Suprapubic pressure by assistant is helpful to promote flexion of the head. The baby is grasped by the ankles with a finger in between the two maintaining a steady traction and forming a wide arc of circle, the truck is swing upward and forward direction. The left hand is used to guard the perineum, slipping the perineum off successfully the face and brow. Then trunk is depressed to complete the delivery of rest of the head.

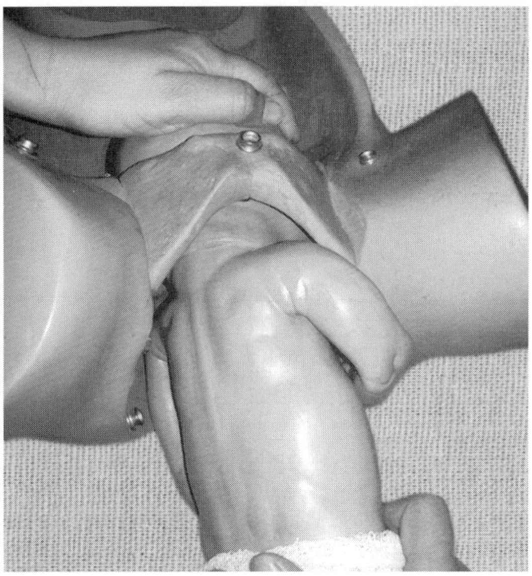

FIG. 4: Exert gentle outward traction, rotating the torso a small amount each way to free the scapulas.

Forceps Delivery

Two types of forceps can be used: Piper forceps (shanks of this are long and have a perineal curve with absent pelvic curve) and Laufe forceps. Forceps can be applied only in engaged head. The advantage of it is that delivery can be controlled by giving pull directly on the head and the force is not transmitted through the neck and flexion is better maintained. The head should be brought as low down as possible by allowing the baby to hang, aided by suprapubic pressure (Fig. 7). When the occiput lies under the back of the symphysis pubis, an assistant raises the legs of the child upwards to help in application of the blades from below. Extension of the head can be caused by extra elevation. The forces pull maintain an arc which follows the axis of the birth canal. The head should be delivered slowly (over 1 min).

Malar Flexion and Shoulder Traction (Modified Mauriceaue Smellie-Veit Technique)

These three great obstetricians described the use of the technique independently. Fetal body placed on the palm of the left hand and forearm. The middle and the index fingers of the left hand are placed over the malar bones on either sides (In the original method, index finger was introduced inside the mouth). Flexion is maintained by this. The ring and little fingers of the pronated right hand are placed on the

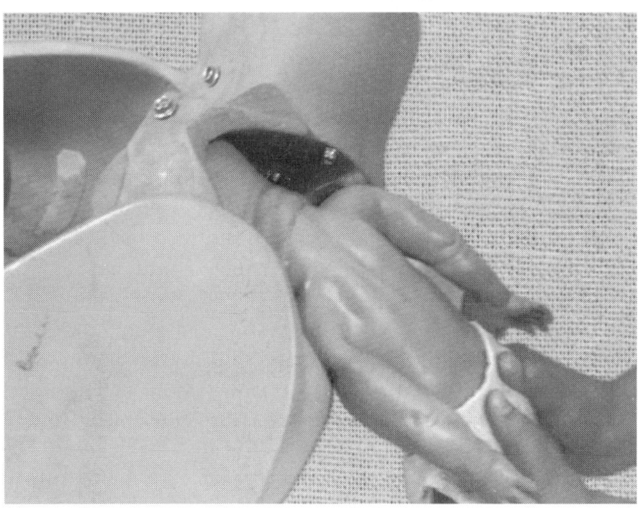

FIG. 5: Do not elevate the body, keep the body low.

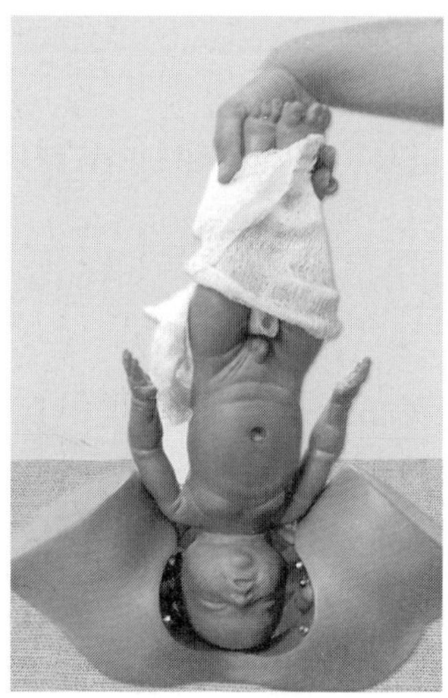

FIG. 6: Delivery of head.

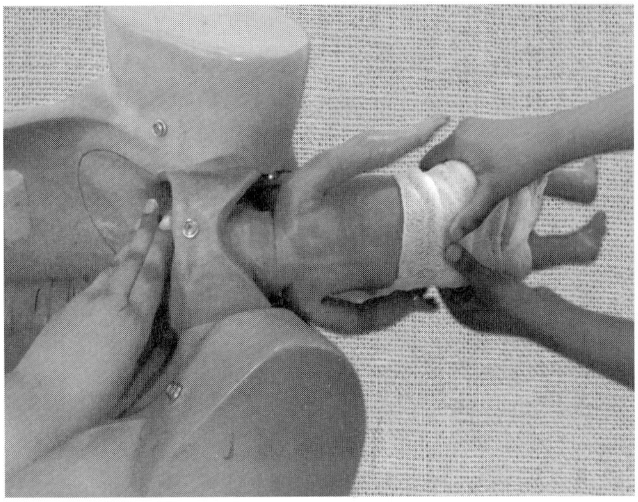

FIG. 7: Continue to exert suprapubic pressure as the head delivers.

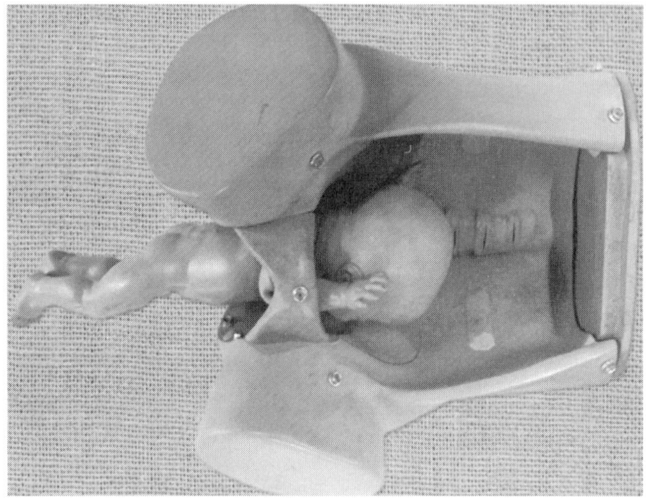

FIG. 8: Nuchal arm.

baby's right shoulder, the index finger is placed on the left shoulder, and the middle finger is placed on the suboccipital region. Now traction is given in downward and backward direction till the nape of the neck is visible under the pubic arch. The assistant helps by applying suprapubic pressure during this period to keep the head flexed. Thereafter, the body is elevated in upward and forward direction towards the mother's abdomen releasing the face, brow and lastly the trunk is depressed to release the occiput and vertex.

Third stage: Active management of third stage to be done.

Preterm breech: external cephalic version with preterm breech presentation is not recommended. Cesarean section (CS) is commonly done when fetal weight is less than 1500 g. However, it is not known whether the better perinatal outcome is due to the CS or the greater use of antenatal use of antenatal steroids and better neonatal care.

MANAGEMENT OF COMPLICATED BREECH DELIVERY

Arrest of breech (Tables 3 and 4) can be at level of outlet, ischial spines or above ischial spines.

Management of breech arrest at outlet is important to rule out outlet contraction of pelvis.

MANAGEMENT OF EXTENDED ARMS

One or both the arms may be extended and lies on the side of head or it lies behind the neck (nuchal displacement) (Fig. 8). Extended arms are diagnosed by noting the winging of scapula and absence of flexed limbs in front of chest.

TABLE 3: Management of breech arrest at outlet

Causes of arrest at outlet	Management
Outlet contraction	LSCS
Rigid perineum	Liberal episiotomy
Weak uterine contraction	Oxytocin augmentation
Big-size baby with extended legs	Groin traction (rule-out fetopelvic disproportion)

LSCS, lower (uterine) segment cesarean section.

TABLE 4: Management of breech arrest at or above the level of the ischial spines

Causes	Management
Contracted pelvis	LSCS
Weak uterine contractions	Oxytocin/LSCS
Fetopelvic disproportion	LSCS
With legs extended	Pinard's maneuver

LSCS, lower (uterine) segment cesarean section.

- Lovset's maneuver: this is the first line method to deliver the extended arms. General anesthesia is not required; no intrauterine manipulation is required
  - Principle: there is more space available in the posterior and lateral segments of the normal pelvis than anywhere. Due to curved birth canal, anterior shoulder remains above symphysis pubis and posterior shoulder will be below sacral promontory. When fetal trunk is rotated, posterior shoulder will appear below the symphysis pubis
  - Procedure: with the scapula visible, the trunk is rotated through 180°. Always keep the back anterior and maintain a downward traction. Posterior arm

will appear under the pubic arch and can be easily released and delivered first. The body of the fetus is then rotated in reverse direction to deliver the other shoulder and arm
- Classical method: patient is put under general anesthesia in lithotomy position. It needs intrauterine manipulation. Fetus is grasped by ankles and is slightly pulled upwards and to the side towards the ventral aspect of the fetus. Left hand is introduced along the curve of the sacrum until the band of elbow is reached. First the posterior arm is delivered. With firm pressure on the humerus, the arm is swept down over the child's face. The extended anterior arm is delivered in the same manner, while the trunk being depressed towards the perineum.

Nuchal Arm Reduction (Figs 9 and 10)

When arm is flexed at elbow and extended at shoulder and lies behind the fetal head.
- By rotating the fetus through half circle in such a direction that friction exerted by birth canal will serve to draw the elbow towards face
- Push the fetus upwards in an attempt to release the nuchal arm
- If rotation is still unsuccessful, nuchal arm is extracted by hooking a finger over it and forcing the arm over the shoulder and down the ventral surface of delivery of arm. In this case, fracture of humerus or clavicle is very common.

Occipitoposterior Position of Head

This situation arises when back of fetus fails to rotate to anterior. If this happens, rotation of back to anterior may be achieved by using stronger traction on fetal legs or bony pelvis. If back is still posterior, extraction by Mauriceau maneuver and deliver the fetus back down.

If this does not work, modified Prague maneuver can be used. Two fingers of one hand grasping the shoulders of the fetus from below. With the other hand, pull feet up over the maternal abdomen.

Entrapment of After-coming Head (Tables 5–7)

In this case, first rule-out contracted pelvis, incompletely dilated cervix and hydrocephalus.

A McRoberts maneuver can be used to facilitate delivery of the head, if it is arrested at the inlet and suprapubic pressure and the Mauriceau-Smellie- Veit maneuver have failed. This involves a sharp flexion of the maternal thighs towards the maternal abdomen and abduction of legs, in a way directly analogues to the management of shoulder dystocia in the vertex delivery.[22]

Delivery of Head through Incompletely Dilated Cervix

This can be in cases of preterm delivery, macerated baby, footling presentation, and breech extraction.

Management

Live baby: push cervix upwards, gentle traction on fetal body and delivery by malar flexion and shoulder traction.

Duhrssen's incision can be made at 2 and 10 o'clock position on cervix.

Dead baby: perforation of head is better than watchful expectancy.

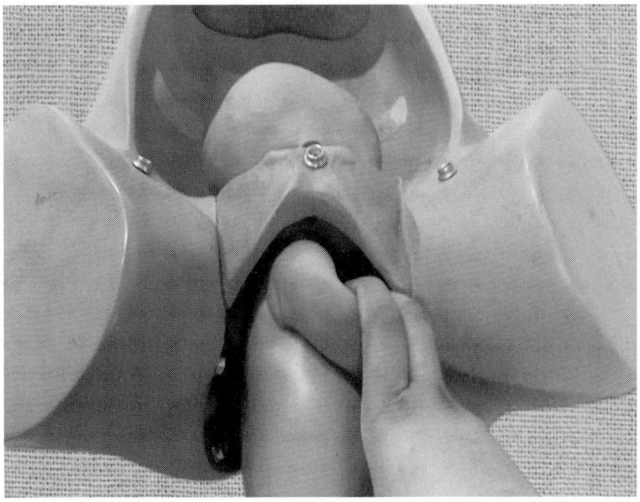

FIG. 9: Reach the humerus and sweep it over the chest toward you.

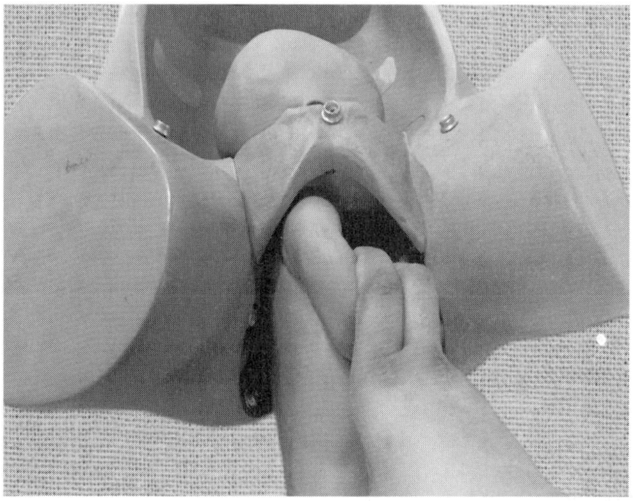

FIG. 10: Continue to bring the arm down and out.

TABLE 5: Entrapment of after-coming head at outlet

Cause	Management
Rigid perineum	Episiotomy
Deflexed head	Jaw flexion and shoulder traction or forceps

TABLE 6: Entrapment of after-coming head at mid-pelvis

Cause	Management
Deflexed head	Jaw flexion and shoulder traction
Contracted pelvis	Baby may be lost and craniotomy may be required

TABLE 7: Entrapment of after-coming head at brim

Cause	Management
Extended head	Jaw flexion and shoulder traction, GA is required for manipulation. Head is negotiated by keeping the sagittal suture in the transverse diameter of the inlet.
Contracted pelvis	Craniotomy through occipital bone/ hard palate.
Hydrocephalus	Decompression using an epidural needle through abdominal or vaginal route (ultrasound guided). Cerebrospinal fluid is drained through epidural needle.

GA, general anesthesia.

Difficulties during Cesarean Section in Breech

- In elective CS, lower-uterine segment may not be well formed and difficulty in delivery of head can occur
- Head can be trapped by well, contracted lower uterine segment. Incision should be enlarged in a J-shaped manner to increase the access
- Forceps may be applied for the delivery of head
- Cesarean section, at full dilatation and absent liquor may be difficult, because an arm may prolapse through the uterine incision. This arm should be immediately pushed back and a leg should be grasped and brought through incision
- Uterine malformation can be associated with breech. A rudimentary horn may be excised. In case of uterine malformation, also look for renal malformation (absent or pelvic kidney). Any uterine malformation should be noted down in operative notes.

Vaginal breech delivery will continue to occur and obstetricians need to preserve and acquire necessary skills to conduct assisted breech delivery without jeopardizing mother or baby. Continuing to train the next generation of obstetricians in principles and conduct of vaginal breech delivery is imperative.

TRANSVERSE LIE

The fetus is in a transverse lie when its longitudinal axis is perpendicular to the long axis of the maternal spine or uterine axis. When the fetal axis is placed oblique to maternal spine, this is oblique lie (Figs 11A to C). Both are collectively known as shoulder presentation. Mostly, the shoulder presents over the pelvic inlet in a transverse lie, but alternative presentations are hand and arm (may be prolapsed into the vagina), cord, or nil (fetal back is presenting). The fetal position is described with the fetal acromion as a denominator and is termed left or right acromion, according to which side of the mother the fetal shoulder is directed. The position may be dorsoanterior [more common (60%)], dorsoposterior, dorsosuperior or dorsoinferior.

Shoulder presentations are classified into four types, based on the location of the scapula:

- Left scapulaanterior (LSA)
- Right scapulaanterior (RSA)
- Left scapulaposterior (LSP)
- Right scapulaposterior (RSP).

Incidence

The incidence of transverse lie is 2% in early third trimester but only one in 300 deliveries (0.3%) at term.[23] The transverse lie diagnosed early in pregnancy, usually converts to a cephalic (or breech) presentation by term. The later in pregnancy the transverse lie is diagnosed, the more likely it is to persist.[24]

Causes of Shoulder Presentation

Maternal Causes:

- Multiparity (80% of cases occur in women who are para three or more); Lax abdominal and uterine muscles; imperfect uterine tone; and extreme uterine obliquity
- Uterine abnormality (arcuate or subseptate)
- Contracted pelvis
- Pelvic tumors (fibroid, ovarian cyst)
- Placenta previa
- Bony abnormalities of pelvis
- Distended urinary bladder (causes temporary change in lie, resolution occurs after emptying of the bladder).

Fetal causes:

- Preterm labor
- Multiple pregnancy (40%, more common for second baby than first)
- Polyhydramnios
- Intrauterine damage (due to loss of tone)
- Oligohydraminos (by restricting fetal movements)
- Fetal macrosomia (produces same effect as pelvic contracture)
- Fetal abnormality (hydrocephalus, tumor of fetal neck, sacral tumor, fetal ascites, and fetal neuromuscular dysfunction).

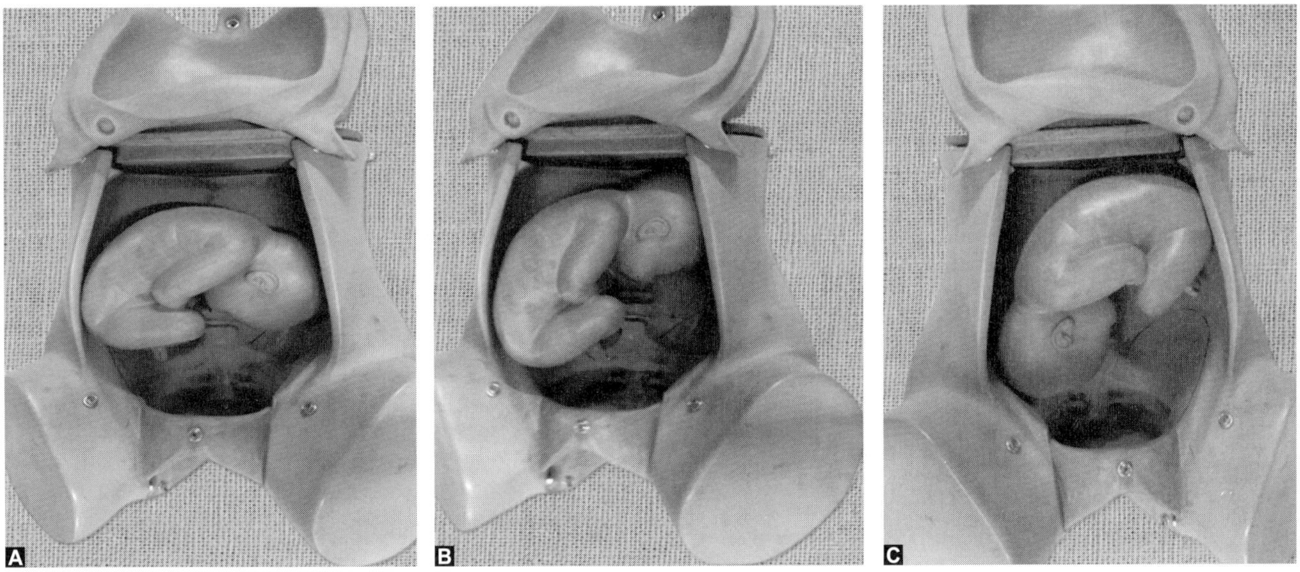

FIGS 11A TO C: Types of shoulder presentation: **A,** Transverse lie; **B,** oblique lie; and **C,** oblique lie

Diagnosis

- Inspection: the uterus appears broader and asymmetrical
- On abdominal palpation: the height of the fundus is less than expected for the period of gestation
- Fundal grip: the fundal grip is empty (not occupied by either the baby's head or buttocks)
- Lateral grip: soft, broad, and irregular breech felt on one side of the midline and smooth, hard, and irregular head is felt on other side

  When the back is anterior, hard resistance is felt across the abdomen and irregular nodules are felt, when back is posterior.
- Auscultation: FHS is heard at higher level and more distinct in dorso-anterior position
- Pelvic examination: in early labor, the presenting part may not be felt, but when the labor is well progressed, may feel the baby's ribs. When the shoulder enters the pelvic brim, the baby's hand, may prolapse and become visible outside the vagina.

Per-vaginam Examination

- During pregnancy: high presenting part
- During labor: in early labor, cervix is generally hanging lose. Presenting part is high. Long conical bag of membranes is present which may occasionally contain either a small loop of cord or a limb.

Later in labor, shoulder is identified by palpating the following parts: acromion process, scapula, clavicle, and axilla. On further palpation, chest of fetus can be felt by noting the ribs and have typical grid iron feel.

After rupture of membrane, hand may be prolapsed and the side to which it belongs can be determined by shaking hand with it.[7] There is very high chance of cord prolapse after rupture of membranes.

Ultrasonography should be done to ascertain fetal maturity, placental localization, position of back, liquor, fetal anomalies, and uterine anomalies.

Mechanism of Labor

There is no mechanism of labor in shoulder presentation. Spontaneous delivery of term-size fetus is impossible with persistent transverse lie. Usually, when the women go in labor, membrane rupture prematurely and hand prolapses. The hand becomes swollen, edematous and cyanosed. After some descent, shoulder is arrested by margins of pelvic inlet. As labor proceeds, the shoulder is impacted firmly in upper part of pelvis. The mother gets exhausted and features of dehydration and ketoacidosis develop; evidence of sepsis usually become apparent .The uterine contractions increase and there is retraction of upper segment, with thinning of lower segment, leading to formation of Bandl's ring which gradually rises higher and higher. Gradually, features of obstructed labor supervene in neglected shoulder presentation and eventually uterus ruptures.[8]

If the fetus is premature, small or macerated and pelvis is large, following favorable outcome can happen:

- Spontaneous rectification or correction of lie
- Spontaneous version into breech
- Spontaneous evolution—during labor, the shoulder comes under symphysis pubis, the trunk and breech deliver first followed by shoulder and head
- Spontaneous expulsion is possible by mechanism known as conduplicatio corporis where the fetal head and thorax and body of fetus doubled upon itself and expelled.

Management

Obstetric Management

Whenever a fetal transverse lie is encountered near term or in labor, the woman needs to be evaluated carefully with history, examination, and ultrasound, to determine if there are any predisposing factors, such as a placenta previa, uterine anomalies, or pelvic kidney that could modify management of the patient.

Antenatal Management

External cephalic version if not contraindicated, should be done at 36 weeks. If it fails repeat after 1 week. Admit the patient to hospital if the lie is persistently changing after 37 weeks. Rule-out wrong dates, multiple pregnancy, placenta previa, and pelvic tumors by history, examination, and ultrasound.[25] If unstable lie persists do ECV at 38–39 weeks and stabilizing induction can be planned.

Labor Management

External version may also be attempted in early labor; provided the membranes are intact and no fetal part has entered the pelvis.[26,27]

There is no mechanism of labor in transverse lie and an average-size baby fails to pass through an average-size pelvis. The route of choice of delivery is CS except in grossly premature less than 0.5 kg or a dead macerated up to 1 kg. If period of gestation is considered viable, not congenitally malformed, FHS positive, CS is done. Because of exceedingly high morbidity and mortality for both mother and fetus, there is no role for internal version and extraction in the management of transverse lie in a live singleton gestation.

Difficulties during Cesarean Section

- Lower-uterine segment not well formed, give liberal incision; J-shaped incision may be required
- Difficulty in extraction of baby especially when fetal back is over the pelvic inlet, inverted T- or U-shaped incision is often required to deliver the baby
- Difficulty in extraction due to liquor drained out, chances of extension.

Surgeon needs to look for uterine anomalies. If there is extension during CS, or malformation of uterus is detected, patient should be advised to have CS during next pregnancy.

If the Baby is Dead

Internal podalic version (IPV) with breech extraction may be attempted after ruling out contraindications. Destructive operations like decapitation (neck accessible) or evisceration are other options. After destructive operation, the uterine cavity must be explored to rule out rupture uterus.

Internal Podalic Version

Internal podalic version involves an intrauterine manipulate of the fetus to convert a transverse lie to a breech presentation, by grasping the foot and bringing it down and to facilitate delivery by breech extraction. There is no role for internal version and extraction in the management of transverse lie in singleton gestation.[28]

Delivery of the Second Twin

The delivery of the second twin in a transverse lie with a shoulder presentation represents a special situation that may be amenable to a vaginal delivery. As the first twin has just been delivered and the cervix is fully dilated, the obstetrician may perform an internal version, that is inserting one hand into the uterus, find the baby's feet, and then bring the baby into a breech position and deliver the baby as such.

Contraindications of Internal Podalic Version

- Big baby
- Contracted pelvis
- Obstructed labor with impending rupture
- Scanty liquor
- Uterine anomaly.

Timing and Prerequisites

- Cervix must be fully dilated
- Membranes recently ruptured, ensuring adequate liquor
- Baby of average size
- No contraindications to vaginal delivery.

Preprocedure Preparation

- Informed consent is mandatory; explaining the nature, risks, and success of the procedure
- Bladder should be empty
- Good uterine relaxation is necessary
- The procedure should be performed by an experienced operator
- Pediatrician should be available
- Per-abdominal examination should be done to assess fetal position, amount of liquor, and FHSs
- Per-vaginam examination should confirm that cervix is fully dilated and pelvis is adequate.

Procedure

- It is performed under deep anesthesia, preferably general anesthesia
- Place the woman in lithotomy position and continuously monitor fetal heart rate
- Under all aseptic precaution, one hand is introduced into the uterine cavity and taken along the thigh of the baby

- The foot is identified by the prominence of heel and one or both feet brought down gently
- The abdominal hand/assistant aids in pushing the head up towards the fundus to facilitate rotation
- The baby is delivered by breech extraction.

Postprocedure Care

- Uterine rupture should be ruled out
- Lacerations to the genital tract must be looked for
- Oxytocics should be given to avoid postpartum hemorrhage.

Complications of Internal Podalic Version

- Maternal injuries in the form of uterine rupture and tears of the cervix, vaginal, and perineal lacerations can occur, resulting in postpartum hemorrhage[29]
- Fetal birth asphyxia, intracranial injuries, and still birth may occur.

Complications of Transverse Lie

Maternal complications of transverse lie are prolonged labor, obstructed labor, rupture uterus, hemorrhage, shock, and even maternal death.

Fetal complications are cord prolapse, hand prolapse, fetal distress, and IUD.

COMPOUND PRESENTATION

Compound presentation (Fig. 12) means when more than one part presents at the brim at a time or, when a fetal extremity prolapses alongside the presenting part, and both enter the maternal pelvis at the same time. The most common associated combination is cord prolapse which may occur in 20% of cases.

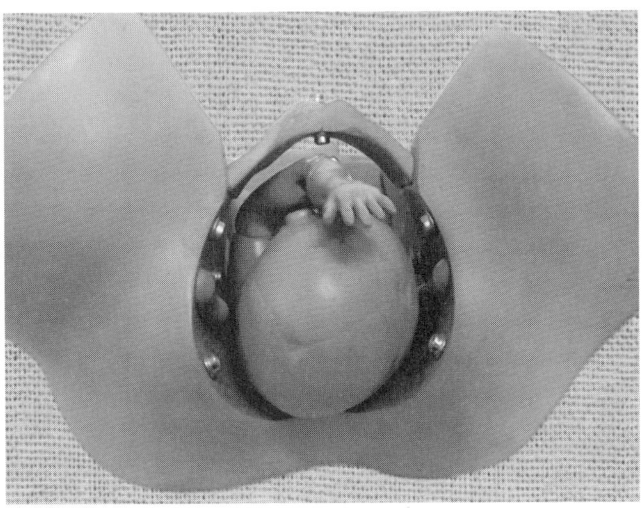

FIG. 12: Compound presentation.

- Head-hand or cord
- Breech-hand or cord
- Hand and foot
- Head-arm-foot (rarest)
- Incidence: 0.1%.

Causes

- Fetal: multiple pregnancy, prematurity
- Maternal: multiparity, polyhydramnios, contracted pelvis.

Diagnosis

Impossible to diagnose by abdominal palpation. May be suspected when arrest of labor occurs in active phase or there is failure of engagement of presenting part. Vaginal examination is the only method of diagnosis.[30]

Cord prolapse occurs in up to 20% of cases.

Management

In the majority of cases, the prolapsed extremity is gently pushed upwards with the normal course of labor and vaginal delivery. If the fetus and arm are relatively large in comparison to the maternal pelvis, obstructed labor will occur and a cesarean will be needed. There is increased risk of mechanical injury to the arm and shoulder, including fractures, nerve injuries, and soft tissue injury.

Indication of CS in compound presentation is cord prolapse, nonreassuring fetal heart, arrest of labor, and nonvertex compound presentation.

FACE PRESENTATION

The presentation is face when the head is fully extended and occiput is in contact with the back, and the chin (mentum) is presenting. Chin is the denominator in face presentation.[31] Incidence is 1:500 deliveries.

Etiology[32]

- Maternal: multiparity, lateral obliquity of uterus, contracted pelvis (40%), and pelvic tumors
- Fetal: congenital malformations 15% (most common anencephaly), congenital goiter, tumors of neck, big baby, dolichocephalic head, loops of cord around neck, and spasm of extensor group of muscles.

Diagnosis

The characteristic feature is the palpation of cephalic prominence on the same side as the back. The back is distinctly felt only near the breech. In a thin woman, a deep groove may be palpable between the occiput and the back. The fetal heart is best heard below umbilicus and distinctly heard when back is posterior. The presenting part is high, soft, and irregular. Face presentation is confirmed on vaginal examination by palpation of facial features-the supraorbital ridges, eyes, nose, mouth and chin. It may be difficult to define in the presence of facial edema in labor. There may be confusion with a breech. Differentiating features are: anus has sphincter tone, whereas mouth does not have. Also, the ischial tuberosities are always in line with the anus whereas mouth and malar eminencies form a triangle.[33]

Ultrasound or X-ray helps to confirm the diagnosis and may identify associated fetal anomalies as anencephaly and estimated baby weight.

Mechanism of Labor

Four positions are described with the chin as denominator: left mentoanterior, right mentoanterior, left mentoposterior, and right mentoposterior (Figs 13A to C). Mentoanterior positions are more common (Fig. 13B). Mechanism of labor has some similarity to that of the vertex. There is descent with increasing extension, internal rotation of the chin, flexion, restitution, and external rotation. The transverse submentobregmatic diameter enters the pelvis. The presenting lateral (biparietal—9.5 cm) and anteroposterior (submentobregmatic—9.5 cm) diameters are conducive for vaginal delivery. Descent is by same factors as in cephalic presentations. In the mentoanterior position, it rotates through one eighth of circle forwards to be with the chin behind the symphysis pubis. The head is born with the chin emerging under the pubic arch followed by the forehead and sinciput.[34]

In mentoposterior position (Fig. 13A), anterior rotation of the mentum occurs in only 20–30% cases. In the rest (70–80%), incomplete anterior rotation, nonrotation, or short posterior rotation of the mentum occurs. Labor gets arrested. There is no possibility of spontaneous delivery in mentoposterior position because; the relatively short neck cannot clear off the total length of the sacrum, which measures about 12 cm in length. Fetal brow is pressed against maternal symphysis pubis. This position hinders flexion necessary to negotiate birth canal. Hence, birth of head is impossible from a mentoposterior position; CS is advisable.

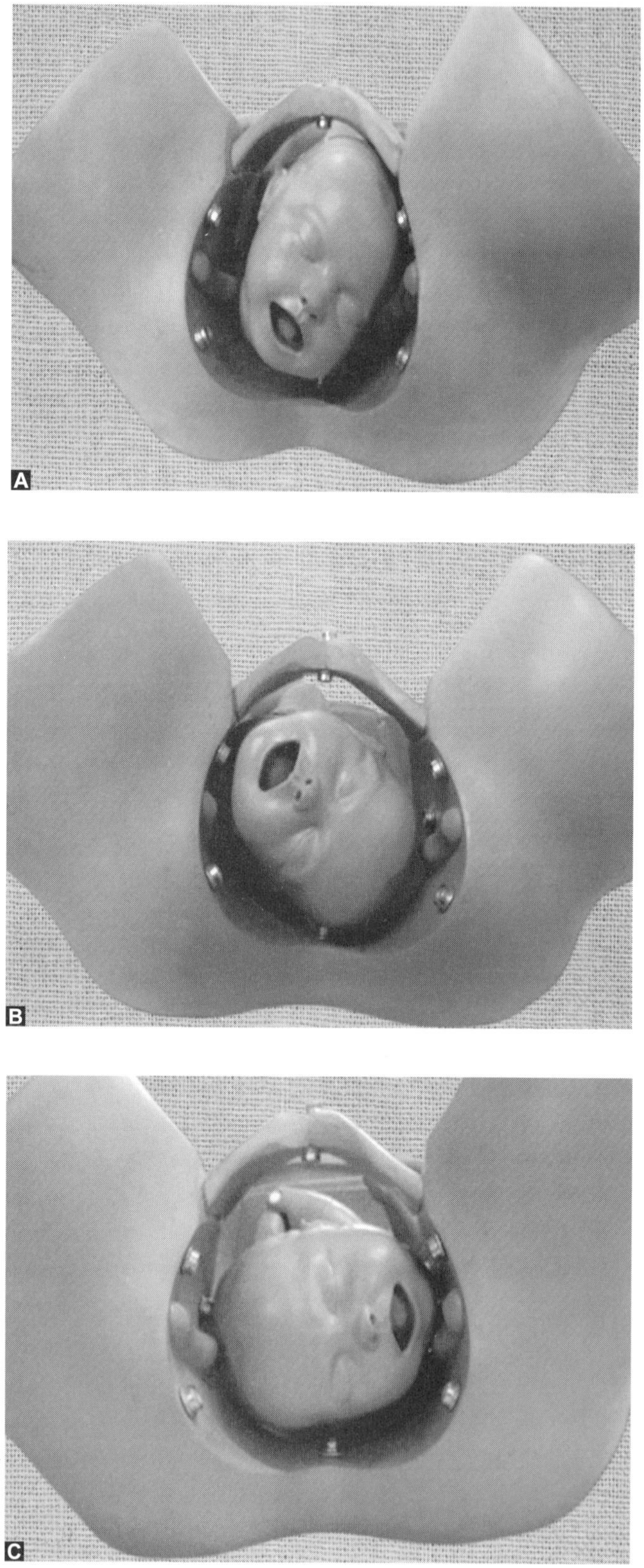

FIGS 13A TO C: Types of face presentation: **A,** Mentoanterior position; **B,** mentoanterior position; and **C,** mentotransverse position.

Management

Spontaneous vaginal delivery of mentoanterior should be expected in 60–80% of the cases. There is greater tendency of premature rupture of membranes and delayed engagement of presenting part. The partogram should be maintained. Any delay at the outlet should be dealt with forceps. Cesarean section is advisable for mentoposterior position.[35,36]

Complications include obstructed labor, rupture uterus, cord prolapse, facial bruising and cerebral hemorrhage.

BROW POSITION

Brow (Fig. 14) is the attitude adopted by the head between a face (complete extension) and a vertex (complete flexion). It is most unfavorable of all the cephalic presentations because its presenting diameter is the metovertical, i.e., 13.5 cm. The position is defined using anterior fontanella as the reference point. The lowermost part of head that is palpable on vaginal examination is the forehead which is termed brow because the orbital ridges and the bridge of the nose are the most definable part of the presentation.

Etiology

The causes of persistent brow presentation are the same as those for face presentation. A brow presentation is commonly unstable and often converts to a face or an occiput presentation.

Diagnosis

The brow presentation may be recognized through abdominal palpation, when both occiput and chin can be palpated easily. The cephalic prominence is felt at higher level and is on same side of back, and on opposite side chin may be felt at lower level. On vaginal examination, anterior fontanel is felt on one end and the orbital ridges, eyes, and root of nose are felt on the other end of the transverse diameter. But neither the mouth nor the chin is palpable.

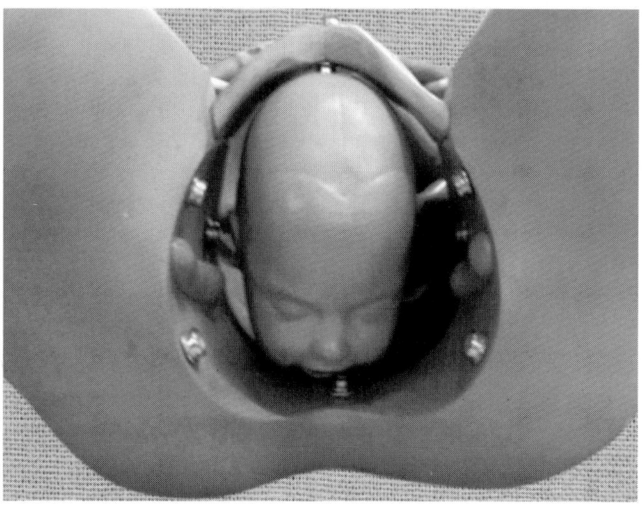

FIG. 14: Brow presentation.

Mechanism of Labor

Spontaneous conversion to face or vertex occurs in approximately 50% of cases, with 30% converting to face and 20% to vertex. The presentation may correct itself in labor by flexion and present as a vertex or undergo further extension and present as a face and may result in vaginal delivery. Persistence of brow presentation in labor at term is not compatible with vaginal delivery and necessitates a CS.

Complications[36]

Obstructed labor, rupture uterus, cord prolapse, facial bruising, cerebral hemorrhage, and intrapartam death.

CONCLUSION

Fetal malpresentations include breech, transverse lie, compound presentation, and face and brow presentations. At term 3-4% of all fetuses are in breech presentation, making this the commonest malpresentation. It can be diagnosed clinically by transabdominal examination during an antenatal checkup or by pervaginum examination during labour; however the diagnosis by ultrasonography is the most reliable modality. The strategies to deliver a patient with breech are external cephalic version with trail of labour, assisted breech vaginal delivery and elective caesarean section. Route of delivery is to be decided on presence of fully equipped set up and after taking informed consent and patient preference. Elective caesarean section has negligible maternal and neonatal mortality and morbidity but choice of vaginal delivery can be offered to patient in certain favourable conditions. The route of choice of delivery in transverse lie is CS, except in grossly premature less than 0.5 kg or a dead macerated up to 1 kg. Spontaneous vaginal delivery of mentoanterior should be expected in 60–80% of the cases. Caesarean section is advisable for mentoposterior and persistent brow presentation at term.

REFERENCES

1. Haughey F. Breech presentation: Is it a bad omen? Br J Obstet Gynaecol. 1982;60:417-20.
2. Coltart T, Edmonds DK, Al-Mufti R. External cephalic version at term: A survey of consultant obstetric practice in the United Kingdom and Republic of Ireland. Br J Obstet Gynecol. 1997;104:544-7.
3. Fruscalzo A, Londero AP, Salvador S, Bertozzi S, Biasioli A, Della Martina M, et al. New and old predictive factors for breech presentation: our experience in 14433 singleton pregnancies and a literature review. J Matern Fetal Neonatal Med. 2014;27:167-72.

4. Robertson IS. Breech presentation associated with anticonvulsant drugs. J Obstet Gynecol. 1984;4:174-7.
5. Manzke H. Morbidity among infants born in breech presentation. J Perinat Med. 1987;6:127-38.
6. Ford JB, Roberts CL, Nassar N, Giles W, Morris JM. Recurrence of breech presentation in consecutive pregnancies. BJOG. 2010;117:830-6.
7. Nassar N, Roberts CL, Cameron CA, Olive EC. Diagnostic accuracy of clinical examination for detection of non-cephalic presentation in late pregnancy: Cross-sectional study. Br Med J. 2006;333:578-80.
8. Royal College of Obstetricians and Gynecologists: The management of breech presentations at term. London, RCOG, 2006, Guideline No 20b.
9. Hofmeyr, GJ, Kulier, R. External cephalic version for breech presentation at term. Cochrane Database Syst Rev. 2012;10:CD000083.
10. Aisenbrey GA, Catanzarite VA, Nelson C. External cephalic version: Predictors of success. Obstet Gynecol. 1999;94:783-6.
11. Hofmeyr GJ. External cephalic version for breech presentation before term. Cochrane Database of Syst Rev. 2000;2:CD000084.
12. Lau TK, Leung TY, Lo KW, Fok WY, Rogers MS. Effect of external cephalic version at term on fetal circulation. Am J Obstet Gynecol. 2000;182:1239-42.
13. Hofmeyr GJ, Kulier R. Cephalic version by postural management for breech presentation. Cochrane Database of Systematic Reviews. 2012;1:CD000051.
14. Coyle ME, Smith CA, Peat B. Cephalic version by moxibustion for breech presentation. Cochrane Database of Systematic Reviews. 2012;5:CD003928.
15. Hofmeyr GJ, Hannah M, Lawrie TA. Planned caesarean section for term breech delivery Cochrane Database of Syst Rev. 2001;1:CD000166.
16. Edward R, Yeoman, Larry C, Gilstap. Breech Delivery–An evidence based approach Management of high risk pregnancy; 5th edition. Blackwell publishing; pp. 397-400.
17. Parikh MN, et al. External cephalic version. J Obstet Gynecol India. 2005;55:407-9.
18. Zatuchni GI, Andros GJ. Prognostic index for vaginal delivery in breech presentation at term–Prospective study. Am J Obstet Gynecol. 1967;98:854.
19. Wigglesworth JS, Husesmeyer RP. Intracranial birth trauma in vaginal breech delivery. Br J Obstet Gynecol. 1977;84:684-91.
20. Thorngren-Jerneck K, Herbst A. Perinatal factors associated with cerebral palsy in children born in Sweden. Obstet Gynecol. 2006;108:1499.
21. Chadha YC, Mahmood TA, Dick MJ, Smith NC, Campbell DM, Templeton A. Breech delivery and epidural analgesia. Br J Obstet Gynaecol. 1992;99:96-100.
22. Sushan A, Younis JS. McRoberts maneuver for the management of the after coming head in breech delivery. Gynecol Obstet Invest. 1992;32:188-9.
23. Depp R. Cesarean delivery. In: Obstetrics. Normal and Problem Pregnancies, Gabbe SG, Niebyl JR, Simpson JL (Eds). New York: Churchill Livingstone Elsevier; 2002. p. 551.
24. Cunningham FG, Gant NF, Leveno KJ, et al. Abnormal Labor. In: Williams Obstetrics. 23rd. 452-4.
25. Royal College of Obstetricians and Gynaecologists (RCOG). Umbilical cord prolapse. Green-top Guideline No. 50. 2014.
26. Collaris RJ, Oei SG. External cephalic version: a safe procedure? A systematic review of version-related risks. Acta Obstetrics and Gynecology Scandanavia. 2004;83:511-8.
27. Phelan JP, StineLE, Edwards NB. The role of external cephalic version in the intrapatum management of transverse lie presentation. Am J Obstet Gynecol. 1985;151:724-26.
28. Okonofua FE. Management of neglected shoulder presentation. BJOG. 2009;116:1695.
29. Chauhan AR, Singhal TT, Raut VS. Is internal podalic version a lost art? Optimum mode of delivery in transverse lie. J Postgrad Med. 2001;47:15.
30. Gardberg M, Leonova Y, Laakkonen E. Malpresentations-impact on mode of delivery. Acta Obstet Gynecol Scand. 2011;90:540-2.
31. MacKenzie IZ. Unstable lie, malpresentations, and malpositions. In: James DK, Weiner CP, Steer PJ, Gonik B, Crowther CA, Robson SC, (Eds). High risk pregnancy. Fourth edition. Philadelphia: Elsevier; 2011. pp. 1123-37.
32. Shaffer BL, Cheng YW, Vargas JE, Laros RK, Caughey AB. Face presentation: predictors and delivery route. Am J Obstet Gynecol. 2006;194:e10-2.
33. Royal College of Obstetricians and Gynaecologists (RCOG). Umbilical cord prolapse. Green-top Guideline No. 50. April 2008.
34. Borell U, Fernstrom I. The mechanism of labour in face and brow presentation: a radiographic study. Acta Obstet Gynecol Scand. 1960;39:626-44.
35. Duff P. Diagnosis and management of face presentation. Obstet Gynecol. 1981;57:105-12.
36. Coates T. Malpositions of the occiput and malpresentations. In: Fraser DM, Cooper MA, (Eds). Myles Textbook for Midwives. 15th edition. Sydney: Churchill Livingstone; 2009. pp. 573-605.

CHAPTER 42

Hypertensive Disorders in Third Trimester of Pregnancy and Puerperium

Joshi Suyajna D

INTRODUCTION

Hypertension is the most common medical problem encountered during pregnancy, complicating 10% of all pregnancies. Eclampsia and pre-eclampsia account for about half of these cases worldwide. Hypertensive disorders account for 5–10% of maternal deaths in the developed world.

Rates of perinatal mortality are also increased 2–3-fold in hypertensive mothers, and women with early-onset pre-eclampsia have a 4-fold increased risk of stillbirth.[1,4]

DIAGNOSIS AND CLASSIFICATION OF HYPERTENSIVE DISORDERS OF PREGNANCY

Diagnosis of Hypertensive Disorders of Pregnancy

Measurement of Blood Pressure

There is consensus across hypertensive disorders of pregnancy (HDP) guidelines that blood pressure (BP) should be measured with women seated and upright with the arm at the level of the heart, when possible. If upright posture is not possible, BP should be measured in the left lateral recumbent position, though it should be recognized that modestly lower BP readings can result in this position, because the right arm is usually elevated above heart level. Standard technique requires that the patient rest undisturbed, not talking, for 5–10 minutes with feet on the floor and back supported. Caffeine and tobacco should be avoided for at least 30 minutes prior to BP measurement. An appropriately sized cuff (i.e., length of 1.5-times the circumference of the arm) should be used. Korotkoff phase V should be used to designate diastolic BP (DBP).

Definition of Hypertension

Hypertension in pregnancy is defined as a sustained systolic BP (SBP) of 140 mmHg or more and/or a DBP of 90 mmHg or more. This is best confirmed on two occasions at least 6 hours apart but within 7 days using the same arm.

Severe hypertension should be defined as a SBP of 160 mmHg or a DBP of 110 mmHg. For severe hypertension, a repeat measurement should be taken for confirmation after 15 minutes using the same arm. The inclusion of SBP elevation in the definition of hypertension in pregnancy reflects evidence that both diastolic and systolic elevated readings have been associated with adverse outcomes such as perinatal morbidity.

Although the National High Blood Pressure Education Program (NHBPEP) report and American Congress of Obstetricians and Gynecologists (ACOG) practice bulletin for pre-eclampsia caution that a relative rise in SBP of 30 mmHg or diastolic relative rise of 15 mmHg warrants close observation, there is no systematic evidence that this relative rise in BP is predictive of pregnancy outcomes. Therefore, defining hypertension in pregnancy by a relative rise is no longer endorsed in published guidelines. In addition, relative BP rise as a criterion for defining hypertension has a high false-positive rate, especially because of the variability of BP across trimesters of pregnancy.

Previous terminology, such as "pregnancy-induced hypertension (PIH)", has been abandoned.

Measurement of Proteinuria

Proteinuria is defined as the excretion of more than 300 mg of protein in a 24-hour urine collection. Alternatively, a timed excretion that is extrapolated to this 24-hour urine value, or a protein-to-creatinine ratio of at least 0.3 (each measured as mg/dL). The dipstick method is discouraged for diagnostic use unless other approaches are not readily available. Cutoff for the diagnosis of proteinuria is considered as 1 +. A dipstick value of 1+ proteinuria has low sensitivity (55%; 95% confidence interval (CI) = 37–72%); a negative or "trace" result should not exclude further investigation if pre-eclampsia is suspected. Urinary dipstick testing has reasonable specificity (84%; 95% CI = 57–95%) for significant proteinuria.

Classification of Hypertensive Disorders of Pregnancy

The terminology and classification recommended by National Institute of Health (NHBPEP Working Group) is preferred over the older, but widely used term PIH because it is more precise. Hypertensive disorders of pregnancy have been classified into four categories:

1. Pre-eclampsia-eclampsia (BP elevation after 20 weeks of gestation with proteinuria or any of the severe features of pre-eclampsia listed below)
2. Chronic hypertension (of any cause that predates pregnancy or first diagnosed before 20 weeks of gestation)
3. Chronic hypertension with superimposed pre-eclampsia (chronic hypertension in association with pre-eclampsia)
4. Gestational hypertension (BP elevation after 20 weeks of gestation in the absence of proteinuria or any of the severe features of pre-eclampsia listed below).

PRE-ECLAMPSIA

Pre-eclampsia occurs in approximately 5% of all pregnancies, 10% of first pregnancies and 20–25% of women with a history of chronic hypertension. It is apparent from clinical practice and epidemiologic studies that pre-eclampsia represents gestational hypertension with end-organ manifestations, most commonly renal with proteinuria, but may also manifest as liver dysfunction, renal insufficiency, cerebral manifestations, or pulmonary involvement such as pulmonary edema (PE). The ACOG task force (2013), therefore, revised the definition of pre-eclampsia to include these alternate end-organ indications in an effort to be more inclusive of patients with atypical presentations. The task force also made two recommendations concerning proteinuria, once pre-eclampsia is diagnosed. These are:

1. No further quantitation of proteinuria is necessary following the diagnosis of pre-eclampsia
2. Delivery decisions should not be based upon the amount of proteinuria nor change in the amount of proteinuria.

The Task Force suggests that the diagnostic criteria for pre-eclampsia be changed to include the usual hypertensive thresholds (i.e., SBP ≥140 mmHg and DBP ≥90 mmHg, respectively, occurring twice, 4 hours apart, after 20 weeks) with either proteinuria (i.e., ≥300 mg per 24 hours, protein-to-creatinine ratio ≥0.3 day or 1+ urinary protein dipstick reading) or, in the absence of proteinuria, new onset of any of the following systemic findings:

- Thrombocytopenia (platelet counts <100,000 μL)
- Renal insufficiency (i.e., creatinine >1.1 mg/dL or 2-fold increase in creatinine in the absence of underlying renal disease)
- Abnormal liver function (i.e., hepatic transaminase levels twice normal)
- Pulmonary edema
- Cerebral or visual symptoms.

One key conclusion was to abandon the requirement that proteinuria be present to confirm the diagnosis. This decision reflects our growing understanding that the disease affects multiple organ systems and that renal involvement is not required for attendant maternal and perinatal morbidity and mortality.

Similarly, eliminated from measures of severe pre-eclampsia are massive proteinuria (i.e., >5 g/day) and fetal growth restriction because the extent of proteinuria does not predict morbidity, and fetal growth restriction occurs commonly in the absence of associated pre-eclampsia.

The new definition of severe pre-eclampsia includes any of the following:

- Systolic BP more than or equal to 160 mmHg or DBP more than or equal to 110 mmHg, respectively, occurring twice, 4-hours apart at bed rest
- Thrombocytopenia (platelet counts <100,000 μL)
- Impaired liver function defined as either otherwise unexplained right-upper-quadrant (RUQ)-epigastric pain unresponsive to medications, or hepatic transaminase levels twice normal
- Progressive renal insufficiency as defined above
- Pulmonary edema
- New-onset cerebral or visual disturbances.

One assumes that last four finding (mentioned above), if isolated, must occur in the setting of hypertension because other disorders [such as gestational thrombocytopenia, hepatitis, acute tubular necrosis (ATN), peripartum cardiomyopathy, and new-onset migraine] can present with these isolated "severe features". Obviously the combination of hepatic dysfunction and thrombocytopenia with hemolysis still constitutes hemolysis, elevated liver enzyme levels and low-platelet levels (HELLP) syndrome.

Etiopathogenesis of Pre-eclampsia

The etiology of pre-eclampsia remains unknown. For more than 100 years, there has been a plaque at the University of Chicago's Lying-in Hospital reserved for the individual who discovers the cause of pre-eclampsia.

This plaque may remain empty forever as the etiology of eclampsia may run the gamut of immunology, embryology, perinatology, chemistry, biochemistry, genetics, and a host of other biological and physical sciences.

There may be thousands of names needing a very large plaque.

Risk Factors

Maternal Personal Risk Factors for Pre-eclampsia

The following are maternal personal risk factors for pre-eclampsia:
- First pregnancy
- New partner/paternity
- Age younger than 18 years or older than 35 years
- History of pre-eclampsia
- Family history of pre-eclampsia in a first-degree relative
- Black race
- Obesity [body mass index (BMI) ≥30]
- Interpregnancy interval less than 2 years or longer than 10 years.

Maternal Medical Risk Factors for Pre-eclampsia

The following are maternal medical risk factors for pre-eclampsia:
- Chronic hypertension, especially when secondary to such disorders as hypercortisolism, hyperaldosteronism, pheochromocytoma, or renal artery stenosis
- Pre-existing diabetes (type 1 or type 2), especially with microvascular disease
- Renal disease
- Systemic lupus erythematosus (SLE)
- Obesity
- Thrombophilia
- History of migraine
- Use of selective serotonin uptake inhibitor antidepressants (SSRIs) beyond the first trimester.

Placental/Fetal Risk Factors for Pre-eclampsia

The following are placental/fetal risk factors for pre-eclampsia:
- Multiple gestations
- Hydrops fetalis
- Gestational trophoblastic disease
- Triploidy.

Pathophysiology

Although the exact pathophysiologic mechanism (Fig. 1) is not clearly understood, pre-eclampsia is primarily a disorder of placental dysfunction leading to a syndrome of endothelial dysfunction with associated vasospasm. In most cases, pathology evaluation demonstrates evidence of placental insufficiency with associated abnormalities such as diffuse placental thrombosis, an inflammatory placental decidual vasculopathy, and/or abnormal trophoblastic invasion of the endometrium.

Theories Associated with the Etiology of Pre-Eclampsia

Placental Implantation with Abnormal Trophoblastic Invasion

In a normal pregnancy, trophoblast-induced vascular changes extend from the intervillous space to the origin of spiral arterioles from radial arteries in the inner-third of the myometrium. These vascular changes are affected in two stages: (1) the conversion of decidual segments of the spiral arterioles by a wave of endovascular trophoblast migration in the first trimester and (2) the myometrial segments by a subsequent wave in the second trimester. This results in the conversion of 100–150 spiral arterioles into distended, tortuous and funnel-shaped vessels that communicate through multiple openings into the intervillous space.

In pre-eclampsia, above vascular changes are usually found in the decidual segments and the myometrial segments are left with their musculo-elastic architecture, leaving them responsive to hormonal influences.

Pre-eclampsia thus is characterized by inadequate trophoblastic invasion with loss of vascular refractoriness (Figs 2A and B).

Vasospasm

While failure of trophoblastic invasion of the spiral vessels seems to be the fundamental defect, the altered prostacyclin (PGI2)-to-thromboxane A2 (TXA2) ratio favoring TXA2 seems to be a major player in causing pre-eclampsia. Vasoconstrictor prostanoid profile and the lack of non-prostanoid vasodilators play a major role in generalized vascular constrictor activity resulting in a failure of necessary expansion of the blood volume. As a result, there is poor perfusion of peripheral organs and tissues including the placenta. The renin angiotensin system now functions as in a nonpregnant individual leading to worsening vasoconstriction, hypertension and fluid retention. Gant and coworkers (1973) demonstrated that increased vascular sensitivity to angiotensin II clearly preceded the onset of hypertension.

Endothelial Dysfunction

Endothelial dysfunction is accepted to be a central pathophysiological event in pre-eclampsia, leading to altered vascular reactivity and loss of vascular integrity. Soluble fms-like tyrosine kinase-1 (sFlt-1), a protein produced by

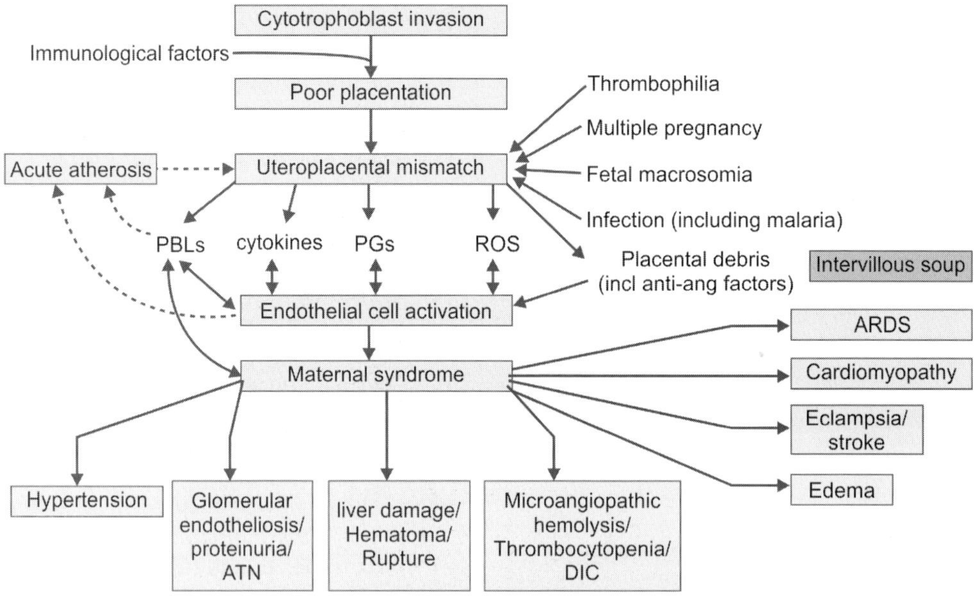

ARDS, acute respiratory distress syndrome; ATN, acute tubular necrosis; DIC, disseminated intravascular coagulopathy; PBLs, peripheral blood leukocytes; PGs, prostaglandins; ROS, reactive oxygen species.

FIG. 1: The pathogenesis of pre-eclampsia. In this model of pre-eclampsia, the maternal syndrome develops from a number of alternative pathways, leading to uteroplacental mismatch, whereby the fetoplacental demands outstrip the maternal circulatory supply. In response to the mismatch, and probably caused, in part, by recurrent ischemia-reperfusion injury within the intervillous (maternal blood) space of the placenta and accelerated placental apoptosis, a soup of endothelium-damaging substrates is released, with resulting endothelial cell activation and consequent development of the maternal syndrome of pre-eclampsia. Some elements of the soup—namely, activated peripheral blood leukocytes (PBLs)—can cause direct end-organ damage. There is cross talk between elements of the soup (not illustrated). Activated protein C could modify both the inflammatory and coagulation consequences of the endothelial cell activation.

placenta, acts by binding to the receptor-binding domains of vascular endothelial growth factor (VEGF) and placental-like growth factor (PLGF). Increased levels of this protein in maternal circulation result in reduced levels of free-VEGF and free-PLGF, with resultant endothelial cell dysfunction.

Cellular fibronectin, an isoform of fibronectin synthesized locally by endothelial cells in response to tissue injury, is elevated in pre-eclampsia. Other cellular markers of endothelial dysfunction like soluble intercellular adhesion molecule 1 (sICAM 1), soluble vascular cell adhesion molecule 1 (sVCAM 1), E-selectin, and plasma fibronectin are also elevated in patients with pre-eclampsia (Fig. 3).

Immunological Factors

The immunological reactions could result in the abnormalities of implantation and invasion. The risk of hypertension in pregnancy is appreciably enhanced in circumstances, where the formation of blocking antibodies to antigenic site on the placenta might be impaired. This may arise where the number of antigenic sites provided by the placenta is unusually, great compared with the amount of antibody as with multiple fetuses. Immunization concept is supported by the observation that pre-eclampsia develops more frequently in multiparous women impregnated by a new consort. Hoff and associates found a maternal-fetal human leukocyte antigen (HLA)-DR relation with pre-eclampsia.

Genetic Predisposition

Cooper and Chesley (1986) concluded that the single-gene hypothesis fits well in the etiology but multifactorial inheritance cannot be excluded. Women carrying the angiotensinogen gene variant T235 had a higher incidence of pre-eclampsia. Some found high incidence of Factor V Lei den mutation in preeclamptic women. The high expression of tumor necrosis factor-α (TNF-α) gene may have a major role in mediating endothelial disturbances predisposing women for hypertension. The role of endothelial NO synthase (eNOS) gene in the development of familial pre-eclampsia was evaluated by analysis among affected sister pairs. Chromosome 7q36 encoding the eNOS gene has been localized.

Management of Pre-eclampsia

Management of pre-eclampsia poses a stiff challenge as it is an unpredictable disorder whose only definitive cure is termination of pregnancy. Hence, management is directed

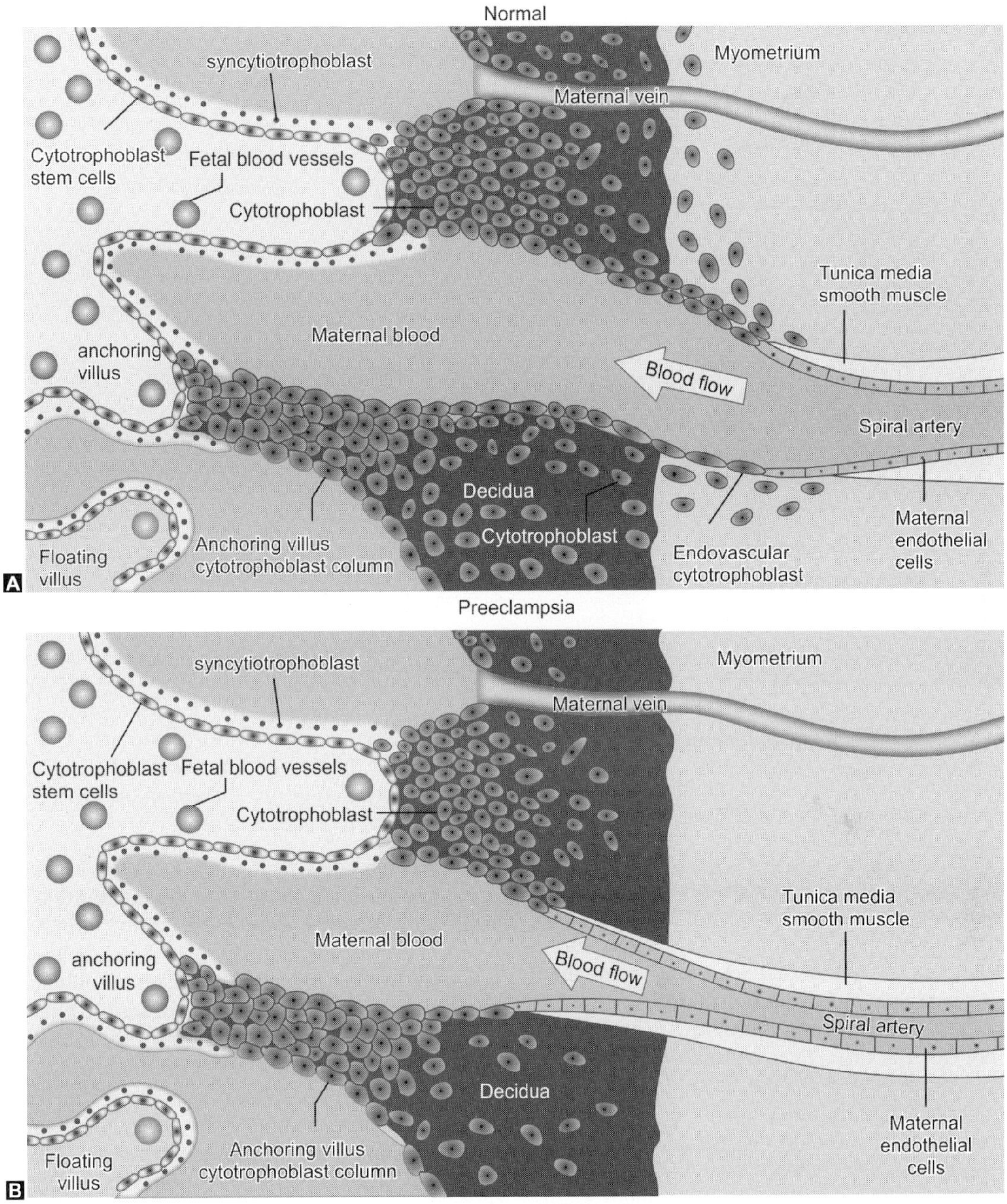

FIGS 2A AND B: Abnormal placentation in pre-eclampsia. In normal placental development, invasive cytotrophoblasts of fetal origin invade the maternal spiral arteries, transforming them from small-caliber resistance vessels to high-caliber capacitance vessels capable of providing placental perfusion adequate to sustain the growing fetus. During the process of vascular invasion, the cytotrophoblasts differentiate from an epithelial phenotype to an endothelial phenotype, a process referred to as "pseudo-vasculogenesis" or "vascular mimicry" (upper panel). In pre-eclampsia, cytotrophoblasts fail to adopt an invasive endothelial phenotype. Instead, invasion of the spiral arteries is shallow, and they remain small-caliber, resistance vessels (lower panel).

towards early detection and amelioration of its progression, the objective being to continue the pregnancy to achieve fetal maturity and prevent maternal complications, especially in mild hypertension. In order to prolong the pregnancy, day-to-day assessment of maternal and fetal condition is of vital importance. Management is determined by the following factors:

- Gestational age
- Severity of the disease
- Bishop score

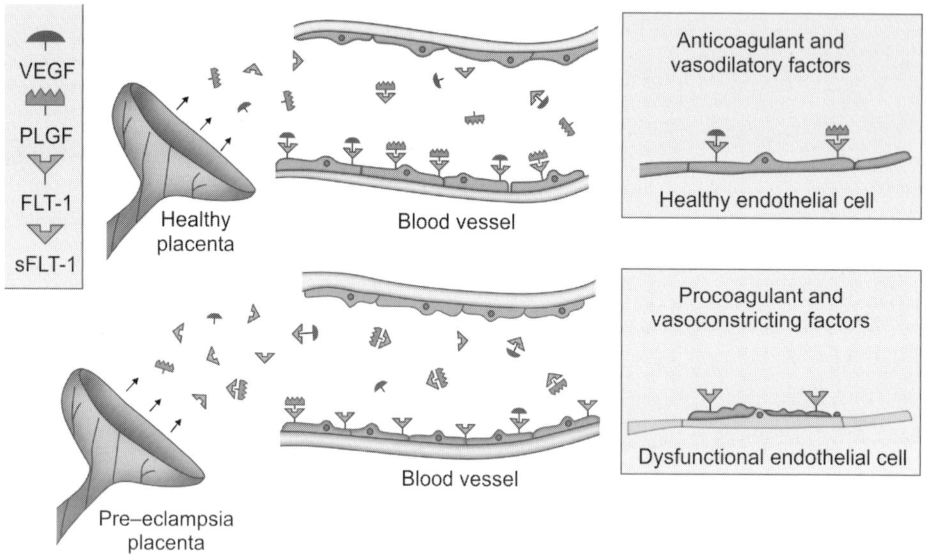

VEGF, vascular endothelial growth factor; PLGF, placental-like growth factor; sFlt-1, soluble fms-like tyrosine kinase-1.

FIG. 3: Schematic representation of endothelial dysfunction.

- Maternal condition
- Fetal condition.

Laboratory Abnormalities in Pre-eclampsia

The tests are usually normal in case of mild pre-eclampsia. The laboratory tests reflect the effect of disease on the various systems.

Complete blood count: hemoglobin levels greater than 13 g/dL suggest the presence of hemoconcentration. Low levels may be due to microangiopathic hemolysis or iron deficiency. In cases in which an incidental platelet count is less than 150,000/μL, 75% are secondary to dilution thrombocytopenia of pregnancy, 24% are due to pre-eclampsia, and about 1% of cases are due to other platelet disorders not related to pregnancy. Counts less than 100,000/μL suggest pre-eclampsia or idiopathic thrombocytopenic purpura (ITP). This may occur in 7% of the mild disease and 50% of the severe patients. Thrombocytopenia is characteristic of pre-eclampsia since it does not occur in essential hypertension. Examination of the peripheral blood smear for evidence of microangiopathic hemolysis and thrombocytopenia may reveal the presence of red blood cell (RBC) fragments. In this setting, the diagnoses of hemolytic-uremic syndrome (HUS), thrombotic thrombocytopenic purpura (TTP), and HELLP syndrome is a form of severe pre-eclampsia.

Liver function tests: hepatic dysfunction is observed in 10% cases of severe pre-eclampsia and is indicated by elevated levels of gamma glutamase, serum glutamic-oxalocetic transaminase (SGOT) [asparate aminotransferase (AST)], serum glutamic-pyruvic transaminase (SGPT) [alanine transaminase (ALT)], lactate dehydrogenase (LDH), and alkaline phosphatase. It should be noted that even placenta contributes to the concentration of alkaline phosphatase. Elevated hepatic transaminases may occur in the absence of epigastric/right upper quadrant (RUQ) pain. Bilirubin is rarely increased in pre-eclampsia but when elevated, the indirect fraction predominates.

Renal function tests: decreased clearance of uric acid usually precedes the changes of glomerular filtration rate (GFR). Tubular dysfunction occurs earlier to glomerular dysfunction. A serum uric acid level greater than 5 mg/dL is abnormal and is a sensitive but nonspecific, marker of tubular dysfunction in pre-eclampsia. A rising level of serum uric acid in pre-eclampsia during the last trimester may indicate poor fetal prognosis. However, it is a poor predictor of the disease as it rises along with the clinical appearance of the disease. Blood urea and serum creatinine are lower in pregnant women than in nonpregnant state due to increased GFR and the rise in plasma volume. Serum creatinine more than 0.8 mg/dL during pregnancy suggests intravascular volume contraction or renal involvement in pre-eclampsia.

Coagulation studies: prothrombin time (PT) and/or international normalized ratio (INR) and/or activated partial PT (aPTT) results may be abnormal in consumptive coagulopathy and disseminated intravascular coagulopathy (DIC) complicating severe pre-eclampsia. Checking the PT/INR/aPTT is not necessary in the absence of abnormal liver transaminases or thrombocytopenia.

Serum electrolytes: serum sodium and potassium levels are low during normal pregnancy due to hemodilution.

Persistent low levels of potassium in a hypertensive woman may indicate accelerated hypertension or an underlying mineralocorticoid producing tumor of the adrenal gland (Conn syndrome).

Management of Gestational Hypertension and Pre-eclampsia without Severe Features

In cases of mild hypertension, the pregnancy is continued up to 37 weeks if possible with close maternal and fetal surveillance to ensure adequate growth and maturity of the child (Flowchart 1). In such cases, pregnancy outcome is similar to that found in normotensive pregnancy. Maternal evaluation includes measurements of BP, weight, urine protein and questioning about symptoms of head ache, upper abdominal pain and visual disturbances. The BP should be checked every 15 minutes until the woman is stabilized and every 30 minutes in the initial phase of assessment. Blood pressure should be checked every 4 hours if the patient is stable and asymptomatic. Laboratory evaluation should be done weekly for mild hypertension and twice weekly for severe hypertension.

Fetal evaluation includes ultrasonography (USG), daily fetal movement count, and nonstress testing. In the acute setting, an initial assessment with cardiotocography should be undertaken. This gives information about fetal wellbeing at that time, but does not give any predictive information.

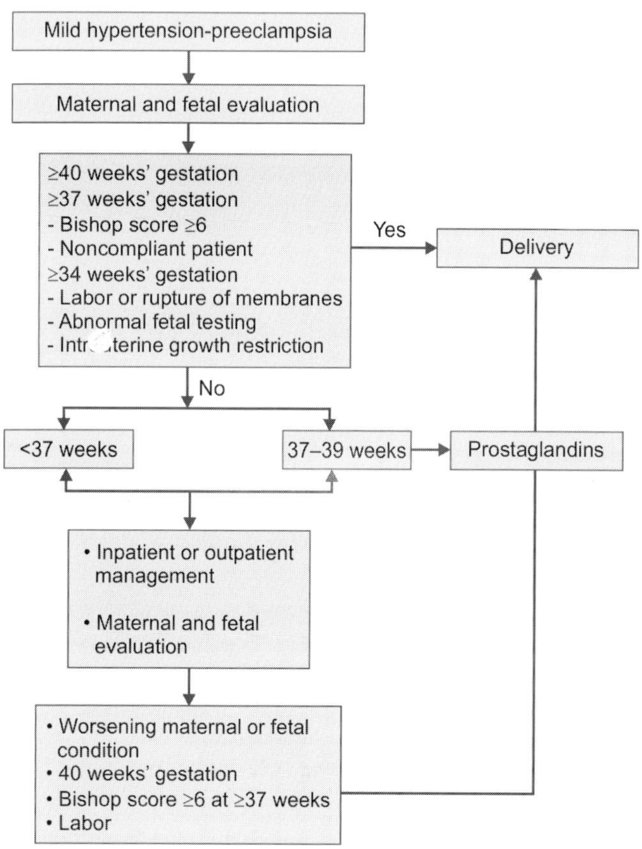

FLOWCHART 1: Management of mild hypertension: pre-eclampsia.

If conservative management is planned, then further assessment of the fetus with ultrasound measurements of fetal size, umbilical artery Doppler and liquor volume should be undertaken. Serial assessment will allow timing of delivery to be optimized. The value of Doppler in other fetal vessels has yet to be clarified.

The main pathology affecting the fetus, apart from prematurity, is placental insufficiency leading to intrauterine growth restriction/retardation (IUGR) that occurs in around 30% of preeclamptic pregnancies. Ultrasound assessment of fetal size, at the time of the initial presentation with hypertension, is a valuable one-off measurement to assess fetal growth.

Growth restriction is usually asymmetrical so measurement of the abdominal circumference is the best method of assessment. Reduced liquor volume is also associated with placental insufficiency and fetal growth restriction. Serial estimations of liquor volume can detect fetal compromise. Randomized trials have shown that investigation with umbilical artery Doppler assessment, using absent or reversed end-diastolic flow, improves neonatal outcome and serial investigations of this and other fetal vessels can be used to follow pregnancies under treatment and optimize delivery.

Management of Pre-eclampsia with Severe Features

It is mandatory to admit a woman with a diagnosis of severe pre-eclampsia (Flowchart 2). The management of severe pre-eclampsia is based on careful assessment, stabilization, continued monitoring and delivery at the optimal time for the mother and her baby. This means controlling BP; and if necessary preventing the convulsions. Senior obstetric and anesthetic staff and experienced midwives should be involved. Women in labor should have continuous electronic fetal monitoring. There is general consensus that severe hypertension should be considered as urgency and treated in pregnancy to decrease maternal morbidity and mortality even in the absence of symptoms.

Antihypertensive treatment should be started in women with a SBP over 160 mmHg or a DBP over 110 mmHg (Table 1). In women with other markers of potentially severe disease, treatment can be considered at lower degrees of hypertension. Labetalol, given orally or intravenously, nifedipine given orally or intravenous (IV) hydralazine can be used for the acute management of severe hypertension.

Atenolol, angiotensin-converting enzyme (ACE) inhibitors, angiotensin receptor-blocking drugs (ARB), and diuretics should be avoided. Nifedipine should be given orally not sublingually. Doctors should use the drug with which they are familiar.

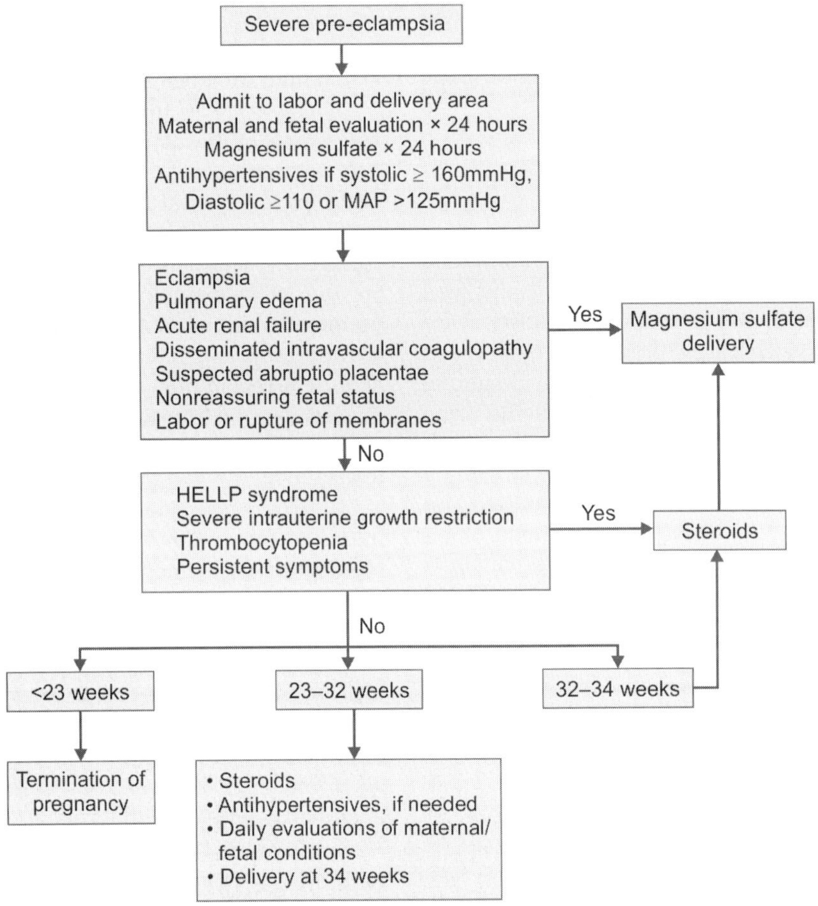

MAP, mean arterial pressure; HELLP syndrome, hemolysis elevated liver enzymes levels and low platelet levels.

FLOWCHART 2: Management of severe pre-eclampsia.

TABLE 1: Antihypertensive agents in acute hypertension

Drug	Mechanism of action	Dosage	Comment
Hydralazine hydrochloride	Arterial vasodilator	5 mg intravenous (IV), then 5–10 mg IV/20 minutes	Must wait 20 minutes for response between IV doses; possible maternal hypotension
Labetalol	Selective α- and nonselective β-antagonist	20 mg IV, then 40–80 mg IV/10 minutes (300 mg total dose); IV infusion 1–2 mg/min, titrated	Less reflex tachycardia and hypotension than with hydralazine
Nifedipine	Calcium-channel blocker	10 mg by mouth, may repeat after 30 minutes	Oral route only; possible exaggerated effect if used with magnesium sulfate ($MgSO_4$)
Nitroglycerin	Relaxation of venous (and arterial) vascular smooth muscle	5 µg/min infusion, double every 5 minutes	Requires arterial line for continuous blood pressure (BP) monitoring; potential methemoglobinemia
Sodium nitroprusside	Vasodilator	0.25 µg/kg/min infusion; increase 0.25 µg/kg/min/every 5 minutes	Requires arterial line for continuous BP monitoring; potential cyanide toxicity
Diazoxide	Peripheral arteriolar vasodilator	30–60 mg IV/5 minutes; IV infusion 10 mg/min, titrated	Possible rapid hypotension, hyperglycemia, decreased uterine contractility
Captopril, enalapril	Angiotensin-converting enzyme (ACE) inhibitor	Oral route only	Contraindicated during pregnancy due to potential fetal side-effects (anuria or renal failure)
Methyldopa	Dopa decarboxylase inhibitor	1 g loading dose; then 250–500 mg IV/6 hour	Slow onset of action (4–6 hour) after IV injection; not ideal for hypertensive crises

TABLE 2: Doses of most commonly used agents used for treatment of a blood pressure of 140–159 mmHg or 90–105 mmHg

Agent	Dosage	Comments
Methyldopa	250–500 mg PO BID-QID (maximum 2 g/day)	There is no evidence to support a loading dose of methyldopa.
Labetalol	100–400 mg PO BID-QID (maximum 1,200 mg/day)	Some experts recommend a starting dose of 200 mg PO BID.
Nifedipine	PA tablets (10–20 mg PO BID-QID, maximum 180 mg/day) or XL preparation (20–60 mg PO OD, maximum 120 mg/day)	Caution should be exercised in ensuring that the correct form of nifedipine has been prescribed.

PO, per oral; QID, four times a day; BID, twice a day; OD, once a day.

There is continuing debate concerning women with a DBP between 100 mmHg and 110 mmHg. Maternal treatment is associated with a reduction of severe hypertensive crises and a reduction in the need for further antihypertensive therapy; however, there appears to be a small reduction in infant birth weight. With treatment, a prolongation of pregnancy of an average of 15 days is possible as long as there is no other reason to deliver (Table 2).

Prophylactic Anticonvulsant Therapy

Magnesium sulfate ($MgSO_4$) should be considered for women with pre-eclampsia for whom there is concern about the risk of eclampsia. This is usually in the context of severe pre-eclampsia once a delivery decision has been made and in the immediate postpartum period. In women with less severe disease the decision is less clear and will depend on individual case assessment.

The magnesium sulpate for the prevention of eclampsia (MAGPIE) study has demonstrated that administration of $MgSO_4$ to women with pre-eclampsia reduces the risk of an eclamptic seizure. Women allocated $MgSO_4$ had a 58% lower risk of an eclamptic seizure, (95% CI = 40 - 71%). The relative risk reduction was similar regardless of the severity of pre-eclampsia.

Fluid Management

Fluid management in severe PIH consists of crystalloid infusions of normal saline or lactated Ringer's solution, at a rate of 80–100 mL/hour or 1-2 mL/kg/hour. Additional fluid volumes, in the order of 1,000 mL, may be required prior to use of epidural anesthesia or vasodilator therapy to prevent maternal hypotension and fetal distress. Fluid restriction is advisable to reduce the risk of fluid overload in the intrapartum and postpartum.

Intravenous fluids are known to cause a decrease in colloid oncotic pressure (COP) in laboring patients. In addition, baseline COP is decreased in patients with pre-eclampsia and may decrease further in postpartum period as a result of mobilization of interstitial fluids. This may be clinically relevant with respect to the development of PE in patients who are receiving beta mimetic. Therefore, close monitoring of fluid intake and output, hemodynamic parameters and clinical signs must be undertaken to prevent an imbalance of hydrostatic and oncotic forces that potentiate the occurrence of PE. Over the last 20 years, PE has been a significant cause of maternal death. Fluid administration should not be routinely administered to treat oliguria (<15 mL/hour). For persistent oliguria, neither dopamine nor furosemide is recommended. Central venous access is not routinely recommended, and if a central venous catheter is inserted, it should be used to monitor trends and not absolute values.

The regime of fluid restriction should be maintained until there is a postpartum diuresis, as oliguria is common with severe pre-eclampsia. If there is associated maternal hemorrhage, fluid balance is more difficult and fluid restriction is inappropriate.

Delivery

For women with any hypertension in pregnancy, vaginal delivery should be considered unless a cesarean section is required for the usual obstetric indications. If vaginal delivery is planned and the cervix is unfavorable, then cervical ripening agents should be used to increase the chance of a successful vaginal delivery. The delivery should be well planned, done on the best day, performed at the best place, by the best route, and with the best support team. A few hours' delay in delivery may be helpful if it allows the neonatal unit to be more organized or to transfer a mother to a place where a cot is available. This assumes the mother is stable before delivery and prior to transfer.

If the gestation is greater than 34 weeks, delivery after stabilization is recommended. Vaginal delivery is generally preferable but consultant obstetrician should discuss the mode of delivery with the mother. Vaginal prostaglandins (PGs) will increase the chance of success. Antihypertensive treatment should be continued throughout assessment and labor. Continuous fetal monitoring is performed as these fetuses are most often growth restricted with oligoamnios, and are vulnerable for fetal distress. Adequate pain relief is necessary to decrease the hypertensive response to labor pain. Epidural analgesia is highly effective helps to easily control BP and improves the perinatal and maternal outcome.

Regional analgesia and/or anesthesia are appropriate in a woman with a platelet count more than 75,000/µL unless there is coagulopathy; falling platelet concentration; or coadministration of an antiplatelet agent (e.g., ASA) or anticoagulant (e.g., heparin).

The third stage should be managed with 5 units intramuscular (IM) syntocinon or 5 units IV syntocinon given slowly. Ergometrine or syntometrine should not be given for prevention of postpartum hemorrhage, as this can further increase the BP.

Clinicians should be aware of the risk of late seizures and ensure that women have a careful review before discharge from hospital. Antihypertensive medication should be continued after delivery as dictated by the BP. It may be necessary to maintain treatment for up to 3 months, although most women can have treatment stopped before this. Clinicians should be aware that up to 44% of eclampsia occurs postpartum, especially at term, so women with signs or symptoms compatible with pre-eclampsia should be carefully assessed.

Complications of Severe Pre-eclampsia

Hemolysis, Elevated Liver Enzymes Levels, and Low Platelet Level Syndrome

The HELLP syndrome is a variant of severe pre-eclampsia, affecting up to 12% of patients with pre-eclampsia-eclampsia. As mentioned earlier, HELLP syndrome is characterized by Hemolysis, Elevated Liver enzymes and Low Platelets (Weinstein, 1982). The acronym, HELLP syndrome, was coined by Louis Weinstein in 1982, but the hematological changes were described by Pritchard et al. in 1954. Pritchard et al. credited association of thrombocytopenia with severe pre-eclampsia to Stahnke in 1922, and hepatic changes to Sheehan in 1950. Unlike most forms of pre-eclampsia, HELLP syndrome is not primarily a disease of primigravidas. Several studies have found that nearly half of HELLP syndrome patients were multigravidas, the incidence being almost twice that seen in primigravid patients (Table 3).

Subtypes of HELLP syndrome

- Mississippi classification:
  - Class 1 (most severe): platelets <50,000/mm^3
  - Class 2: platelets 50,000–100,000/mm^3
  - Class 3 (least severe): platelets 100,000–150,000/mm^3
- Tennessee classification:
  - True or complete: platelets <100,000/mm^3, AST >70 IU/L, LDH >600 IU/L
  - Partial or incomplete: severe pre-eclampsia with any one of the following: Absence of hemolysis (ELLP), absence of low platelets (HEL), elevated liver function (EL) and low platelets (LP).

TABLE 3: Recommended criteria for HELLP syndrome

Hemolysis (at least 2 of these):	• Peripheral smear (schistocytes, burr cells) • Serum bilirubin (>1.2 mg/dL) • Low serum haptoglobin • Severe anemia unrelated to blood loss
Elevated liver enzymes	• ALT or AST ≥twice upper level of normal
Low platelets	• <100,000/mm^3

ALT, alanine transaminase; AST, asparate aminotransferase.

Clinical findings: the clinical signs and symptoms of patients with HELLP syndrome are classically related to the impact of vasospasm on the maternal liver. Thus, the majority of patients present with signs or symptoms of liver compromise. These include malaise, nausea (with or without vomiting) and epigastric pain. In most series, hepatic or RUQ tenderness to palpation is seen consistently in HELLP syndrome patients.

Clinically, many HELLP syndrome patients do not meet the standard BP criteria for severe pre-eclampsia. In one series of 112 women with severe pre-eclampsia-eclampsia complicated by HELLP syndrome, admission of DBP was less than 110 mmHg in 31% of cases and less than 90 mmHg in 15% (Sibai, 1986). Some patients may first be seen because of jaundice, gastrointestinal (GI) bleeding, hematuria, or pain abdomen. They may be misdiagnosed as having other diseases (Box 1). Numerous misdiagnoses are associated with this syndrome, and a delay in diagnosis may be life-threatening, a pregnant woman with thrombocytopenia, elevated serum transaminase levels, or epigastric pain should be considered to have HELLP syndrome until proven otherwise. A rare but interesting complication of HELLP syndrome is transient nephrogenic diabetes insipidus.

Management: as with other severe pre-eclampsia variants, delivery is ultimately the treatment of choice (Flowchart 3). The timing of delivery, however, remains controversial.

Box 1: Medical and surgical disorders confused with the HELLP syndrome

- Acute fatty liver of pregnancy
- Appendicitis
- Diabetes mellitus
- Gallbladder disease
- Gastroenteritis
- Glomerulonephritis
- Hemolytic uremic syndrome
- Hepatic encephalopathy
- Hyperemesis gravidarum
- Idiopathic thrombocytopenia
- Kidney stones
- Peptic ulcer
- Pyelonephritis
- Systemic lupus erythematosus (SLE)
- Thrombotic thrombocytopenic purpura (TTP)
- Viral hepatitis

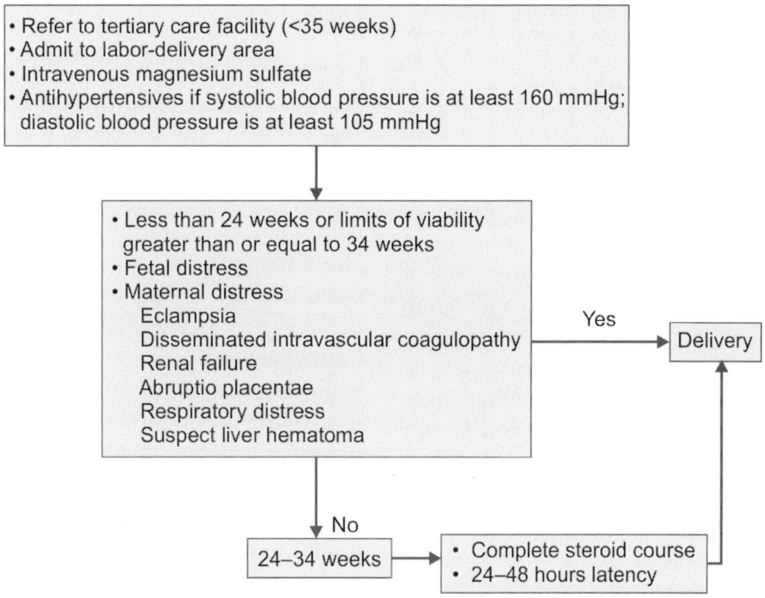

FLOWCHART 3: Management of HELLP syndrome.

Several investigators recommend immediate delivery, while others reasonably suggest that under certain conditions with marked fetal immaturity, delivery may safely be delayed for a short time.

Clark and associates have demonstrated transient improvement in patients with HELLP syndrome following bed rest and/or corticosteroid administration (Clark, 1986). Following an initial improvement, however, each patient's clinical condition worsened. Thus in a mother with a very premature fetus and borderline disturbances in platelet count or serum transaminase values, and in the absence of other absolute indications for delivery, careful hospital observation may at times be appropriate. Certainly, uncontrollable BP, significantly rising liver enzymes or a serum creatinine would mandate immediate delivery irrespective of gestational age.

The mode of delivery should depend on the state of the cervix and other obstetric indications for cesarean birth. HELLP syndrome, by itself, is not an indication for cesarean delivery. A high percentage of patients with HELLP syndrome, however, will undergo operative delivery. A commonly encountered situation involves a mother with a premature fetus, an unfavorable cervix, and a platelet count less than 100,000/μL. In such patients, cesarean delivery is often preferred to avoid the necessity of later operative delivery for failed induction in the face of more significant thrombocytopenia. Maintain platelet counts more than 20,000/μL for vaginal delivery, 40,000/μL for cesarean delivery. Platelet transfusion may 6–10 units of be necessary before cesarean section in cases below 40,000/μL. Laboratory abnormalities usually return to normal within a short time after delivery; it is not unusual, however, to see transient worsening of both thrombocytopenia and hepatic function in the first 24–48 hours postpartum. An upward trend in platelet count and a downward trend in lactate dehydrogenase concentration should occur in patients without complications by the 4th postpartum day. The treatment of patients with postpartum HELLP syndrome is same as that of antepartum period including the use of $MgSO_4$.

In a study of postpartum HELLP syndrome (Martin et al. 1997), dexamethasone 10 mg intravenously at 12-hour intervals was given until disease remission was noted in treated patients, at which time up to two additional 5 mg IV doses were given at 12-hour intervals. Most impressive was a clinically significant reduction of indicated transfusion and respiratory therapy, invasive hemodynamic monitoring, infectious or bleeding-related morbidity and length of postpartum hospital course. Cochrane data-base review (2004) concludes that there is insufficient evidence to determine whether adjunctive steroid use in HELLP syndrome decreases maternal and perinatal mortality, major maternal and perinatal morbidity. However, in this review, patients treated with dexamethasone had faster resolution of laboratory parameters.

Maternal and perinatal outcome: the presence of HELLP syndrome is associated with an increased risk of maternal death (0–24%) and increased rate of maternal morbidities, such as PE (8%), acute renal failure (ARF) (3%), DIC (15%), abruptio placentae (9%), acute respiratory distress syndrome (ARDS), sepsis, and stroke. There is an also increased rate of wound hematoma and increased need for blood and blood products. Development of HELLP syndrome in the postpartum period increases the chance of ARF and PE. The chances of placental abruption in HELLP syndrome patients are 20-times higher than that seen in the general obstetric population. The reported perinatal death is 7–20%.

Pulmonary Edema

Sibai and colleagues reported a 2.9% incidence of PE in severe pre-eclampsia-eclampsia. Seventy percent of these cases developed postpartum. A higher incidence of PEs was noted in older patients, multigravidas, and patients with underlying chronic hypertension. The etiology of PE in preeclamptic patients appears to be multifactorial.

Chest X-ray and arterial blood gases confirm the diagnosis. Other life-threatening conditions, such as thromboembolism, should be considered and ruled out as quickly as possible. Initial management of PE includes oxygen administration and fluid restriction. A pulse oximeter should be placed so that oxygen saturation may be monitored continuously. A pulmonary artery catheter may be considered for severe pre-eclamptic patients who develop PE antepartum, in order to distinguish between fluid overload, left ventricular dysfunction, and nonhydrostatic PE, each of which may require different approaches to therapy.

Furosemide (Lasix) administered in a 10–40 mg dose IV over 1–2 minutes represents the first line of conventional therapy for patients with PE associated with fluid overload. If adequate diuresis does not commence within 1 hour, an 80 mg dose may be slowly administered to achieve diuresis. In severe cases of PE, a diuresis of 2–3 L needs to be achieved. Prior to diuresis appropriate fluid management for these hemodynamically complex patients may be clarified by complete hemodynamic evaluation, using parameters derived by a pulmonary artery catheter.

When hypoxemia persists despite initial treatment, mechanical ventilation may be required for respiratory support, pending correction of the underlying problem. In all cases, close monitoring of the patient's respiratory status with frequent arterial blood gases should be performed. Fluid balance is maintained by careful monitoring of intake and output.

Renal Complications of Pre-eclampsia

Renal plasma flow and GFR are diminished significantly in pre-eclamptic patients. Renal biopsy of pre-eclamptic patients often demonstrates a distinctive glomerular capillary endothelial cell change, termed glomerular endotheliosis.

Acute renal failure in pre-eclamptic pregnancies is uncommon. Precipitating factors include abruption, coagulopathy, hemorrhage, and severe hypotension. If ARF occurs, hemodialysis or peritoneal dialysis may be required.

Liver Rupture

Hepatic infarction may lead to intrahepatic hemorrhage and development of a subcapsular hematoma, which may rupture into the peritoneal space and result in shock and death. The diagnosis of a liver hematoma may be aided by use of ultrasonography, radionuclide scanning, computed tomography (CT), and selective angiography. The maternal and fetal prognosis of liver rupture are poor. When the diagnosis of liver hematoma is suspected in severe pre-eclampsia prior to delivery of the fetus, immediate exploratory laparotomy and cesarean section should be considered in order to prevent rupture of the hematoma secondary to increased abdominal pressure in the second stage of labor, in vomiting, or during eclamptic convulsions. Prompt delivery is also mandatory. When the diagnosis of liver hematoma is made in the postpartum period, conservative management with blood transfusion and serial ultrasonography may be reasonable. Liver rupture with intraperitoneal hemorrhage, when suspected, requires laparotomy. Hemostasis may be achieved by compression, simple suture, topical coagulant agents, arterial embolization, omental pedicles, ligation of the hepatic artery, or lobectomy, depending on the extent of the hepatic damage.

Cerebral Edema

Cerebral hemorrhage and cerebral edema are two major causes of maternal mortality in pre-eclampsia. The three most important etiologic factors include: (1) increased intravascular pressure, (2) damage to vascular endothelium, and (3) reduced plasma COP. In pre-eclampsia, cerebral edema is thought to occur secondary to anoxia associated with eclamptic seizures or secondary to loss of cerebral autoregulation as a result of severe hypertension. General therapeutic principles in the treatment of cerebral edema include correction of hypoxemia and hypercarbia, avoidance of volatile anesthetic agents, control of body temperature and control of BP. Assisted hyperventilation reduces intracranial hypertension and the formation of cerebral edema. The administration of hypertonic solutions such as mannitol increases serum osmolality and draws water from the brain into the vascular compartment, thus reducing brain tissue water and volume. A 20% solution of mannitol is given as a 0.5–1.0 g/kg dose over 10 minutes or as a continuous infusion of 5 g/hour. Steroid therapy (dexamethasone, betamethasone, or methylprednisolone) is thought to be most effective in the treatment of focal chronic cerebral edema, which may occur in association with a tumor or abscess. Steroid therapy is less beneficial in cases of diffuse or acute cerebral edema.

Temporary Blindness (Amaurosis)

Temporary blindness may complicate 1–3% of cases of pre-eclampsia-eclampsia. The injury is usually the result of severe damage to the retinal vasculature or occipital lobe ischemia. Cunningham and colleagues evaluated over a 14-year period the clinical courses of 15 women with severe pre-eclampsia or eclampsia who developed cortical blindness (Cunningham, 1995). Blindness persisted from 4 hours to 8 days but resolved completely in all cases. Based on data from CT imaging and magnetic resonance imaging (MRI), cortical blindness results from petechial hemorrhage and focal edema in the occipital cortex.

Transient blindness usually resolves spontaneously after delivery of the fetus. Focal neurological deficits such as this require ophthalmologic and neurological consultation and CT/MRI of the brain. Paralysis of the sixth cranial nerve has been reported as a complication of eclampsia.

ECLAMPSIA

Eclampsia is the inevitable consequence of the disease progression in pre-eclampsia characterized by grand mal tonic-clonic seizures occurring in a patient with pre-eclampsia with other neurological and medical disorders ruled out.

Physicians of ancient civilizations of Egypt, Greece, India, and China possibly knew of the syndrome. Mention about eclampsia can be found in records of 2200 BC. Kahun Papyrus which mentions "to prevent women from biting her tongue, avite means a small wooden stick pound upon her jaws". The term eclampsia (to flash out suddenly, to come on suddenly, flash of lightning, to shine forth) was coined by Verandeus in 1668.

Mauriceaus recognized that the disease could be treated by prompt delivery. The incidence of eclampsia varies from 1 in 100 to 1 in 1,700 in developing countries and 1 in 2,000 in developed countries. Incidence in India varies from 1 in 30 to 1 in 500. In 80–85% cases, it is preceded by a stage of imminent eclampsia characterized by warning signs and symptoms that include headache, giddiness, and visual disturbances (flashes of light, dimmed vision, photophobia, and complete blindness). It arises without any obvious symptoms in 15–20% of the cases. Eclampsia unheralded by hypertension and proteinuria occurred in 38% of cases reported in the United Kingdom (Douglas, 1994). Douglass and Redman conclude that "the term pre-eclampsia is misleading because eclampsia can precede pre-eclampsia". Eclamptic seizures occur prior to the delivery in roughly 80% of patients. In the remainder, convulsions occur postpartum usually within 48 hours and they have been reported up to 23 days following delivery. An awareness of the diverse presentations is important to allow prompt and adequate treatment. The differential diagnosis includes epilepsy, coincidental cerebrovascular accident (CVA) and space-occupying lesions, infections (meningitis, encephalitis) metabolic disturbances and hysteria.

The precise cause of seizures in pre-eclampsia remains unknown. Hypertensive encephalopathy, as well as vasospasm, hemorrhage, ischemia, and edema of the cerebral hemispheres, have been proposed as etiologic factors. Thrombotic and hemorrhagic lesions have been identified on autopsy of pre-eclamptic women.

Risk Factors for Eclampsia

The following are considered risk factors for eclampsia:
- Nulliparity
- Family history of pre-eclampsia, previous pre-eclampsia and eclampsia
- Poor outcome of previous pregnancy, including IUGR, abruptio placentae, or fetal death
- Multifetal gestations, hydatid mole, fetal hydrops, primigravida
- Teen pregnancy
- Primigravida
- Patient older than 35 years
- Lower socioeconomic status.

The following preexisting medical conditions are also considered risk factors:
- Obesity
- Chronic hypertension
- Renal disease
- Thrombophilias-antiphospholipid antibody syndrome
- Protein C deficiency and protein S deficiency
- Antithrombin deficiency
- Vascular and connective tissue disorders
- Gestational diabetes
- SLE.

Stages of Convulsive Attack

The convulsive attack consists of four stages:
1. Stage 1 (premonitory stage): lasting for a few seconds to half a minute: patient becomes unconscious, pupils dilate, eyes roll from side to side, turned to one side and fix, twitching of the face and the hands
2. Stage 2 (tonic stage): lasts for a few seconds: the body becomes rigid with distorted features, hands are clenched, arms flexed
3. Stage 3 (the clonic stage): lasts for half a minute to 2 minute, alternative contraction and relaxation of the muscles, clenching of the jaw, tongue bites, twitching in the face starting around the angle of the mouth extending to the arm and leg of one side of the body. The face becomes cyanosed, tongue protrudes out with frothing in the mouth, and breathing becomes steratorius

4. Stage 4 (stage of coma): the movements cease, the patient lies quiet, coma supervenes, and respiration gradually quietens down. The patient wakes up after a short time with amnesia of the events, sometimes patient may go into deep coma from which she may not recover. Fits may occur in quick succession leading to a condition called "status eclampticus". During convulsions the temperature rises (rise of >39° is a grave sign suggestive of cerebral hemorrhage), the pulse rate and BP rises.

The first convulsions is usually the forerunner for others with the number of convulsions varying from 1 or 2 in mild cases to even 100 or more in untreated severe cases. As a rule, death does not occur until after frequent repetitive convulsions occur. During convulsions the placental blood flow decreases and this combined with maternal hypoxemia and lactic acidosis causes fetal bradycardia. However this usually recovers in 3–5 minutes, persistence of bradycardia for more than 10 minutes needs other causes like placental abruption to be ruled out. It is at times difficult to distinguish between postpartum eclampsia and postpartum cerebral vein thrombosis.

Clinical Features

Eclampsia always should be considered in a pregnant patient with a seizure episode. A pregnant patient who has been involved in an unexplained trauma (such as a single vehicle auto accident) and has exhibited seizure activity should be evaluated for eclampsia. Eclampsia can occur during the ante-, intra- and postpartum periods. 90% of eclampsia cases occur after 28 weeks' gestation.

Features of eclampsia include the following:
- Seizure or postictal state (100%)
- Headache (80%), usually frontal
- Generalized edema (50%)
- Vision disturbance (40%), such as blurred vision and photophobia
- Right upper quadrant abdominal pain with nausea (20%)
- Amnesia and other mental status changes

The incidences of signs or symptoms before seizure include the following:
- Headache (83%)
- Hyperactive reflexes (80%)
- Marked proteinuria (52%)
- Generalized edema (49%)
- Visual disturbances (44%)
- Right upper quadrant pain or epigastric pain (19%).

The absence of signs or symptoms before seizure includes the following:
- Lack of edema (39%)
- Absence of proteinuria (21%)
- Normal reflexes (20%).

The relation of seizure to delivery is as follows:
- Before delivery (>70%)
- Before labor (antepartum) (25%)
- During labor (intrapartum) (50%)
- After delivery (postpartum) (25%).

Although, patients with severe pre-eclampsia are at greater risk for seizures, 25% of patients have symptoms consistent with mild pre-eclampsia before the seizures.

A study by Cooray et al. found that the most common symptoms that immediately precede eclamptic seizures are neurologic symptoms (i.e., headache, with or without visual disturbance), regardless of degree of hypertension. This suggests that closely monitoring patients with these symptoms may provide an early warning for eclampsia.

Physical Findings

Most patients with eclampsia present with hypertension and seizures, along with some combination of proteinuria and edema. Findings at physical examination may include the following:
- Sustained SBP greater than 160 mmHg or DBP greater than 110 mmHg
- Tachycardia
- Tachypnea
- Rales
- Mental status changes
- Hyperreflexia
- Clonus
- Papilledema
- Oliguria or anuria
- Localizing neurologic deficits
- Right upper quadrant or epigastric abdominal tenderness
- Generalized edema
- Small fundal height for the estimated gestational age
- Apprehension.

Cervical examination of the patient with eclampsia should not be overlooked, because the delivery mode may largely depend upon the patient's cervical status.

Computed Tomography and Magnetic Resonance Imaging of the Head

Computed tomography scanning of the head, with or without contrast, can exclude cerebral venous thrombosis, intracranial hemorrhage, and central nervous system lesions, all of which can occur in pregnancy and present with seizures.

Although obtaining a CT scan in eclampsia is not routine, abnormalities have been observed in up to 50% of women imaged. Characteristic CT scan findings include cortical hypodense areas, particularly in the occipital lobes, and diffuse cerebral edema, which is believed to correspond to petechial hemorrhages and diffuse edema noted in postmortem studies.

Computed tomography scan findings may include the following:

- Cerebral edema
- Diffuse white matter low-density areas
- Patchy area of low density
- Occipital white matter edema
- Loss of normal cortical sulci
- Reduced ventricular size
- Cerebral hemorrhage
- Intraventricular hemorrhage
- Parenchymal hemorrhage (high density)
- Cerebral infarction
- Low-attenuation areas
- Basal ganglia infarctions.

Abnormal MRI findings of the head have been reported in up to 90% of women imaged. These include an increased signal at the gray-white matter junction on T_2-weighted images, as well as cortical edema and hemorrhage. The syndrome of posterior reversible encephalopathy (PRES), indicative of central vasogenic edema, has been increasingly recognized as a component of eclampsia.

Consider CT/MRI scanning in patients who have been involved in trauma, are refractory to $MgSO_4$ therapy, or have atypical presentations (e.g., seizures >24 hour after delivery, absence of severe hypertension).

Management: Basic Approach

The basic approach revolves around the following principles:

- General management
- Anticonvulsant management
- Antihypertensive management
- Obstetric management.

General Management

Patients with eclampsia require nursing in specialized intensive care units with all necessary equipment. All external provoking stimuli are reduced to the minimum. They are nursed on railed cots in quiet dark rooms with minimum handling and examinations.

Anticonvulsants are given as per the hospital protocol, suction apparatus is used to keep the throat clear. The head end may be lowered to facilitate postural drainage. Sometimes a left lateral position may be needed. Oxygen is given by mask at 8–10 L/minute to correct maternal and fetal hypoxia. During a convulsion soft, firm mouthgag is used to prevent injury to the tongue. If asphyxia sets in patients are intubated and positive pressure ventilation given, tracheostomy may be needed. One of the most important aspects of management is the maintenance of fluid balance. Fluid replacement should be with Ringer's lactate/normal saline at the rate of 60 mL/hour up to a maximum of 125 mL/hour. Once the patient is little stable and not restless, she is catheterized with an indwelling Foley's catheter and vaginal examination performed to assess the cervical status. Care is taken to prevent bedsores/pneumonia.

Anticonvulsant Treatment

Parenteral $MgSO_4$ has emerged as the drug of choice for treating and preventing eclampsia with its major advantages of efficacy and relative safety to the mother/baby. Eclampsia Collaborative Trial Group concluded that "there is now compelling evidence in favor of $MgSO_4$ for the treatment of eclampsia". In 2002 the results of the "MAGPIE trial" another large Multicentric Trial was published which showed beyond any reasonable doubt the efficacy of $MgSO_4$ in reducing the risk of eclampsia.

Pritchard gets the credit for popularizing $MgSO_4$ for pre-eclampsia and eclampsia in modern obstetrics by his famous Parkland Hospital regimen popularly known as the "Pritchard's regimen". Others who made significant contribution to establish $MgSO_4$ as the first-line anticonvulsant in eclampsia were Zuspan, Sibai, Duley, Flowers, Chesley and Pepper, Eastman, and Cruik Shant.

Convulsion-treatment interval: in our resource-restricted settings patient must be given $MgSO_4$ and antihypertensive at the site of convulsions with maximum importance to keep the airway patent. After stabilizing, the patient has to be transferred to tertiary-care center for definitive, disciplined management of these cases. Thus, crucial time is not wasted and almost seizure-free transportation can be ensured. Convulsion to medication interval is brought to minimum with optimum fetomaternal outcome.

Continuing the administration of $MgSO_4$ for 24 hours after the last fit in patients with eclampsia is at best empirical. The challenge of such a regimen giving $MgSO_4$ maintenance dose is enormous and unsatisfactory in poor-resource countries.

The anticonvulsant regimen alone cannot change maternal and fetal outcomes. The other principles of eclampsia management should be simultaneously and effectively instituted.

Sibai BM recommends that the patient should be stabilized regarding BP and control of convulsion before transport and the patient should be sent in an ambulance with medical personnel in attendance. In tertiary-care centers other causes of maternal mortality like hypertensive crises, left ventricular diastolic dysfunction, ARF, coagulatory disorders, etc. can be closely monitored and treated to reduce maternal mortality and morbidity.

Three-stage management protocol of eclampsia: the need of the hour is to arrest seizures at the earliest especially in Primary Health Care (PHC) settings so that convulsion to treatment interval is brought to minimum. "Three-stage

management strategy" for management of eclampsia include the following:
1. Primary management, at or near the place of convulsion
2. "Seizure-free transportation" of the patient
3. Tertiary-level management in high-dependency unit (HDU) or higher center.

Primary treatment should be basically very practical to be instituted anywhere, e.g., at the site of convulsion, house of the patient, family physician, primary health unit, etc. This strategy will help in improving the maternal and fetal outcomes. 10% of these patients may convulse again after receiving loading dose. This recurrence may be acceptable considering the potential benefits of seizure control during transportation to higher centers. According to Sibai most of eclamptic women will become seizure free after an additional dose 2 g $MgSO_4$. Administration and clinical monitoring of $MgSO_4$ can be done by medical, midwifery, or nursing staff, provided that they are appropriately trained. This achievement has obvious implications for care, particularly in low- and middle-income countries.

Mechanism of action: the precise mechanism of action of $MgSO_4$ in eclampsia is not clear with a great deal of controversies still existing. The postulated mechanisms include:

- Central action: blockade of N-methyl-D-aspartate (NMDA) subtype of glutamate-channel receptor in a voltage-dependent manner. Preferential uptake by the hippocampus and cerebral cortex rich in NMDA receptors with potent cerebral vasodilatation is demonstrated by Doppler studies. Increased $MgSO_4$ concentration was demonstrated in cerebrospinal fluid (CSF) after infusion
- Peripheral action: at the neuromuscular junction, causing blockage of calcium entering the cell and blocking calcium at the intracellular sites/membranes, reducing the presynaptic acetylcholine release at the endplate, reducing the motor endplate sensitivity to acetylcholine (reducing neuromuscular irritability). Direct action of a neuromuscular block though suggested seems unlikely, as the serum concentration for its anticonvulsive action is well below that needed for neuromuscular block.

Magnesium sulfate is also known as the Epsom salt. It is $MgSO_4.7H_2O$.USP. It has a molecular weight of 246 and 1 g of the salt contains 98 mg of elemental magnesium. The normal serum levels vary from 1.6 mEq/L to 2.1 mEq/L. Magnesium is not absorbed orally, it attracts water in the colon (basis for its use as a laxative). By about 90 minutes 50% of the infused magnesium move intracellular and by 4 hours about 50% are excreted in urine. Tubular reabsorption of magnesium depends on parathyroid hormone level.

Magnesium administered parenterally promptly crosses the placenta and achieves equilibrium in the fetal serum and less in the amniotic fluid (Table 4). The kidneys excrete magnesium. Calcium is the physiological antidote for magnesium.

TABLE 4: Serum levels of magnesium toxicity

Normal therapeutic level	4–6 mEq/L
Loss of patellar reflex	8–12 mEq/L
Feelings of warmth, flushing	9–12 mEq/L
Somnolence	10–12 mEq/L
Slurred speech	10–12 mEq/L
Muscular paralysis	15–17 mEq/L
Respiratory difficulty	15–17 mEq/L
Cardiac arrest	30–35 mEq/L

Magnesium sulfate is commercially available as 25% or 50% w/v, with 1 g of $MgSO_4$ containing 98 mg of elemental ion. Sibai, in 1984 found no therapeutic advantages of IV over IM administration except for avoidance of muscle pain.

Intravenous dose is always diluted because bolus may cause cardiac arrhythmia/arrest. Magnesium sulfate is not an innocuous drug, so strict monitoring of patients on $MgSO_4$ is needed to prevent serious side-effects to mother/fetus.

Fetal effects may include:
- Neurological, neuromuscular depression
- Protective effect against cerebral palsy
- Hyporeflexia
- Decreases fetal heart rate (FHR) variability.

Management of $MgSO_4$ toxicity is by calcium. Calcium is the logical antidote for magnesium. Intravenous calcium as 10 mL of 10% calcium gluconate infusion is given slowly over 3 minutes. It increases the acetylcholine liberated at the neuromuscular junction by the action potential. If respiratory arrest ensues, prompt endotracheal intubation and ventilation are lifesaving.

Magnesium Sulfate Regimens

- Joshi's classification of $MgSO_4$ regimens:
  - High-dose regimens, e.g., Pritchard's, Lucas, loading dose >10 g
  - Low-dose regimens, e.g., Zuspan, Suman Sardesai loading dose <10 g
  - Single-dose regimen, e.g., Joshi's single-dose regimen: VIMS
- Pritchard's protocol:
  - Loading dose: 4 g (20 mL of 20%) IV over not less than 3 minutes immediately to be followed by 10 g (20 mL of 50%) IM, 5 g in each buttock
  - If convulsions persist, after 15 minutes 2 g (10 mL of 20%) is given over 2 minutes. If women is large, 4 g is given
  - Maintenance dose: 5 g (10 mL of 50%) is given every 4 hours at alternate sites after assuring presence of knee reflex ultra and respiratory rate more than 14 breaths/min; urine output more than 100 mL

- Baha M Sibai regimen:
  - 6 g IV (30 mL of 20%) in 100 mL of 5% dextrose over 10–15 minutes 20 g of 50%; added to 1,000 mL of 5% dextrose given as IV infusion at 100 mL/hour (2 g/hour)
  - Adjust to get a serum magnesium level of 4.8–9.6 g/dL.

Modifications of standard regimens: in the last decade, researchers in the developing countries are constantly striving to steadily decrease the dosage of both loading and maintenance doses of $MgSO_4$ regimens to suit the local conditions. Disciplined use of standard Western regimens is hard to achieve in developing countries. There is definitely a transnational difference in response to $MgSO_4$ in the Third World with racial characteristics being important in determining the response; there is danger in applying the results of the trials as such in different countries. As discussed in the MAGPIE Trial report 2002, the most important question would be "what is the minimal effective dose?" If a woman is known to be or appear to be small, the dose should probably be limited (Pritchard). In recent years, Andrea Witlin in her review article on eclampsia, comments "one may also speculate that $MgSO_4$ dosing should vary according to the patients' weights or BMI. However, this has never adequately been evaluated".

Sardesai S et al. considering the small weights of Indian women tried low-dose $MgSO_4$ therapy in eclamptic women for control of convulsion and in imminent eclampsia as seizure prophylaxis. In a study of 570 eclamptic women, they gave 4 g of $MgSO_4$ as loading-dose intravenously and subsequently 2 g of $MgSO_4$ was given every 3 hours IV/IM with a recurrence rate of 7.89%. Begum et al. used low-dose "Dhaka regimen" comprising 10 g of loading dose, following this 2.5 g was given intramuscularly 4 hour in 65 patients. Only one (1.53%) developed recurrence. She concluded that half of the standard dose appeared to be sufficient to control convulsions.

Mahajan et al. in a study of 95 women used 6 g loading dose and 4 g maintenance dose reports recurrence rate of 1.05%. In Chowdhury et al. study of 630 women, 480 women received IM $MgSO_4$ as maintenance dose according to the Pritchard's regimen and 150 women were subjected to a low-dose IV regimen of $MgSO_4$ (0.6 g/hour). There was no significant difference in recurrence of convulsion (3.3% in IM and 2% in IV Groups).

The results of the MAGPIE trial suggest that a shorter course of treatment may be adequate. In this study, most of the women probably received only the loading-dose injection before being referred on to the recruiting hospital. For these women, there was no difference in outcome between those given further $MgSO_4$ or placebo (relative risk = 1–24; 95% CI = 0.49–3.11). The argument for a short course is further supported by the trial data, which suggest that the drug may continue to be beneficial long after the treatment has been given. Since eclamptic fits can occur at any time up to 7 days after delivery, for most of the time at which the women were at risk, they would have had subtherapeutic serum concentrations of $MgSO_4$. Despite this situation, prophylaxis seems to have been successful. To make $MgSO_4$ available to women at risk from eclampsia, a short regimen is suitable for use in underdeveloped countries, ideally this would include a single $MgSO_4$ injection (Andrew D Weeks, Lancet 2002).

Newer initiative in safe motherhood: however, it should be noted that most of these regimens are used at medical colleges and many eclampsia cases occur in rural places where immediate treatment to arrest the seizures is not readily available. Despite the compelling evidence in favor of $MgSO_4$, health personnel at primary-care level do not administer $MgSO_4$. Most of these women receive either no immediate treatment or receive some anticonvulsants like diazepam and sent to tertiary-care centers for further management. Transportation of these highly irritable eclamptic women is far from ideal in most of the Third World countries including India.

In the year 1998, Joshi SD started "single-dose $MgSO_4$ regimen" for eclampsia. Joshi et al. studied the effect of single-dose $MgSO_4$ "VIMS regimen" (4 g diluted IV plus 4 g IM) on 513 patients with a recurrence rate of 9.1% and 3.3% maternal mortality. The results of the study are comparable to other standard regimens. The need of the hour is to arrest seizures at the earliest, especially in PHC settings so that convulsion to treatment interval is brought to minimum. This strategy will help in improving the maternal and fetal outcomes. 10% of these patients may convulse again after receiving loading dose. This recurrence may be acceptable considering the potential benefits of seizure control during transportation to higher centers. According to Sibai most of these women will become seizure free after an additional dose 2-g $MgSO_4$. Administration and clinical monitoring of $MgSO_4$ can be done by medical, midwifery, or nursing staff, provided that they are appropriately trained. This achievement has obvious implications for care, particularly in low- and middle-income countries. Single-dose $MgSO_4$ VIMS regimen is simple and efficient. Single-dose regimen can be safely used outside the established obstetric centers (at PHC level itself where maximum cases of eclampsia occur) and transferred to tertiary care center for definitive, disciplined management of these cases. Thus, crucial time is not wasted and almost seizure-free transportation can be ensured. Convulsion to medication interval is brought to minimum. Thus many more lives of mothers can be saved.

Seizures refractory to standard $MgSO_4$ regimens may be treated with a slow 100 mg IV dose of thiopental sodium (pentothal) or 1–10 mg of diazepam. Alternatively, sodium amobarbital (up to 250 mg) may be administered IV. Alternatively, as advocated by Lucas, 1,000 mg of phenytoin is infused over a period of 1 hour and 500 mg of oral dose is given 10 hours later.

Antihypertensive Management

Magnesium sulfate alone cannot improve maternal outcome. The other principles of eclampsia management should be effectively instituted. Persistent and severe elevations of BP must be treated to prevent CVAs, PE, and ARF. The management has already been discussed in severe pre-eclampsia section.

Obstetric Management

Eclamptic patients require delivery without respect to gestational age (Cunningham, 1994). Cesarean delivery should be reserved for obstetric indications or deteriorating maternal condition. The gestational age, cervical status, fetal condition and position need to be considered before determining the most appropriate route of delivery. Cervical ripening agents can be used for induction of labor. However, prolonged induction should be avoided.

Maternal mortality rates are increased in patients with eclampsia, but the rates have declined dramatically in recent years. Contemporary maternal mortality rates range from 0% to 14%. Mortality rates are more in developing countries as most of these women are admitted to tertiary hospitals in moribund state. Mortality depends on the early referral, immediate anticonvulsant treatment, experience of the physicians and associated adverse pregnancy conditions. PE and intracerebral hemorrhage are the leading causes of death in eclampsia. Eclampsia still remains an important cause of maternal mortality in India. Along with sepsis and hemorrhage the other leading causes; it is called as "lethal triad" of maternal mortality. Overall, the contemporary perinatal mortality rate among eclamptics ranges from 7% to 30% and is most commonly secondary to placental abruption, prematurity and perinatal asphyxia. Antenatal deaths account for a significant proportion of the overall perinatal mortality. Depending on the gestational age and the clinical circumstances, it is advisable to have neonatologist available at delivery.

Complications of Eclampsia

As many as 56% of patients with eclampsia may have transient deficits, including cortical blindness. However, studies have failed to demonstrate evidence of persisting neurologic deficits after uncomplicated eclamptic seizures during the follow-up period. Studies suggest that there is an increased risk for CVAs and coronary artery disease (CAD) in eclamptic mothers later in life.

Other potential complications of eclampsia include the following:

- Permanent neurologic damage from recurrent seizures or intracranial bleeding
- Renal insufficiency and ARF
- Fetal changes: IUGR, abruptio placentae, oligohydramnios
- Hepatic damage and rarely hepatic rupture
- Hematologic compromise and DIC
- Increased risk of recurrent pre-eclampsia/eclampsia with subsequent pregnancy
- Maternal or fetal death.

Outcome

Although the incidence of eclampsia has declined in recent years, mainly due to the improvement of healthcare, serious adverse outcomes still exist. About 5% of patients with hypertension develop severe pre-eclampsia, and about 25% of women with eclampsia have hypertension in subsequent pregnancies. About 2% of women with eclampsia develop eclampsia with future pregnancies.

Multiparous women with eclampsia have a higher risk for the development of essential hypertension; they also have a higher mortality rate in subsequent pregnancies than do primiparous women.

Hypertensive Disorders in the Postpartum

Hypertensive disorders can develop during pregnancy, labor, and the puerperium. Postpartum period continues to pose a risk of pre-eclampsia, with up to 40% of eclamptic convulsions occurring in this period. Most will occur within 48 hours after delivery, with only 26% of seizures developing more than 48 hours after delivery.

The incidence of pre-eclampsia first appearing during the postpartum period is around 5–7%. HELLP syndrome can also occur during the postpartum period, up to 30% of cases presenting after delivery.

Blood Pressure Changes in the Postpartum

It has been suggested that increased resistance in the uteroplacental circulation resulting in an impaired blood flow and subsequent poor placental perfusion. If this is correct there should not be threat of pre-eclampsia and eclampsia during postpartum. After a normal delivery arterial BP rises progressively during the first 5 days.

This is due to the profound fluid shifts that occur in the postpartum. There is mobilization of extravascular fluid is observed, which results in a rise in the intravascular volume, and consequently an increase in the BP.

In a pregnancy complicated by pre-eclampsia, these changes will be occurring on a background of an already compromised vascular system of diffuse vasospasm secondary to endothelial cell damage. This shift of fluid from the extravascular to the intravascular space may also increase the risk of pulmonary edema, cerebral edema and eclampsia.

Pre-eclamptic women show persistently elevated central retinal artery systolic velocity in the postpartum period, because of distal vasoconstriction. These changes appear to resolve spontaneously before 6 weeks' postpartum.

Management of Postpartum Hypertension

The principles of management of postpartum hypertension are the same as for antepartum hypertension, the aim being to prevent severe hypertension (DBP >120 mmHg on any one occasion or DBP >110 mmHg on two consecutive occasions >4 hours apart). Extreme hypertension (mean arterial pressure >140 mmHg) causes direct arterial injury, which predisposes to cerebral hemorrhage. The aim of emergency antihypertensive treatment is to maintain BP less than 160/110 mmHg, thereby preventing cerebral injury from occurring.

Non-steroidal anti-inflammatory agents may contribute to increased BP and should be replaced by other analgesics in women with hypertension that persists for more than 1 day postpartum.

Acute Treatment of Postpartum Hypertension

The principle treatment of acute severe hypertension is same as in the antenatal period. There is no evidence to support the superiority of intravenous labetalol in comparison to intravenous hydralazine. The evidence for the use of short-acting antihypertensives for the treatment of severe hypertension is not robust enough to guide clinical practice, and as a result the decision regarding which agent to use remains in the hands of the treating clinician.

Nifedipine: it is a calcium-channel blocker, which inhibits the entrance of calcium into cardiac and smooth muscle cells of the coronary and systemic arterial beds, decreasing muscle tone and vascular resistance. It functions mainly as an arteriolar vasodilator and thus has minimal effects on cardiac conduction and heart rate, making it one of the most useful therapies available in the treatment of hypertension.

Nifedipine acts rapidly when given orally, which is its main route of administration. It can cause dangerously abrupt falls in BP within 10–15 minutes, which could lead to myocardial or cerebrovascular ischemia. The advent of slow-release nifedipine capsules has alleviated this problem, allowing an onset of action of 60 minutes and a more prolonged effect. Adverse effects are given in Table 5.

Chronic Treatment of Postpartum Hypertension

In the immediate postpartum period, women should be closely monitored for signs and symptoms of pre-eclampsia, including strict BP measurement and changing trends in their renal function, platelet count, liver enzymes, and coagulation profile. After a 48 hour inpatient stay, women can be reasonably discharged from hospital if their BP remains stable (<150/100 mmHg) on their postpartum antihypertensive medication and their blood tests do not

TABLE 5: Drugs used in the acute management of postpartum hypertension

	Labetalol	Hydralazine	Nifedipine
Indication	First- or second-line	First- or second-line	First- or second-line
Route of administration	Oral, IV	IV, IM, SC	Oral
Dose	100 mg BD orally; 20 mg/hour IV doubled every 30 min; maximum 2.4 g daily orally or IV infusion 160 mg/hour IV infusion	200–300 µg/min IV infusion; maintenance dose 50–150 µg/min	10 mg BD orally, adjusted infusion, according to response to a maximum dose of 60 mg daily in divided doses
Side-effects	Postural hypotension, dizziness, tiredness, headache, rashes, scalp tingling, difficulty in micturition, gastrointestinal symptoms (epigastric pain, nausea, or vomiting), liver damage, lichenoid rash	Headaches, nausea, sweating, arrhythmias, precipitation of angina, anxiety, restlessness, hyperreflexia	Tachycardia, palpitations, dizziness, flushing, headache, rash, pruritus, urticaria, nausea, diarrhea, constipation, increased frequency of micturition, eye pain, visual disturbances, myalgia, tremor, cholestasis, depression
Contraindications	Asthma, uncontrolled heart failure, Prinzmetal's angina, marked bradycardia, hypotension, sick sinus syndrome, second- or third-degree atrioventricular block, cardiogenic shock, metabolic acidosis, severe peripheral arterial disease, pheochromocytoma	Idiopathic systemic lupus erythematosus, severe tachycardia, high-output heart failure, myocardial insufficiency due to mechanical obstruction, pulmonale, dissecting aortic cor aneurysm, porphyria	Cardiogenic shock, advanced aortic stenosis, within 1 month of myocardial infarction, unstable or acute attacks of angina, porphyria
Safe in breast-feeding	Yes	Yes (but monitor infant)	Yes

IV, intravenous; IM, intramuscular; SC, subcutaneous; BD, twice a day.

show any worrying trends. They should be reviewed in the community by the midwife on the tenth postpartum day or by the General Practioner after 2 weeks.

Long-term Treatment of Postpartum Hypertension

In order to achieve BP control, drugs such as β-blockers, calcium-channel blockers and ACE inhibitors can be used in a stepwise manner. Maintenance therapy for postpartum hypertension should be managed in the same way as in the antepartum period, with the exception of the use of methyldopa, which should be avoided because it causes depression and psychosis in the postnatal period. If a woman is on methyldopa for PIH or pre-eclampsia, this can be changed to a β-blocker such as labetalol 200–800 mg/day in divided doses. If this is contraindicated, i.e., in asthma and heart failure, the woman can be started on second-line therapy, nifedipine 20–60 mg/day in divided doses. If she needs further antihypertensive medication, enalapril 2.5–10 mg daily can be added in Table 6.

Labetalol and nifedipine: they are the most common agents used for the chronic management of postpartum hypertension. Nifedipine has a more rapid clearance and lower peak serum concentration in postpartum patients with pre-eclampsia than when used in women in their third trimester taking nifedipine for PIH. As a result, dosage and dosing intervals need to be altered accordingly. Although labetalol is widely used in the puerperium, atenolol, acebutolol, nadolol, and sotalol are not recommended because they are excreted in the breast milk. Most other β-blockers are excreted in amounts too small to harm the infant.

Enalapril: ACE inhibitors are contraindicated during pregnancy. Women who have been on these drugs prior to pregnancy should discontinue them preconception because of their proven fetal toxicity. However, some can be used safely during the puerperium. Enalapril is excreted in very small amounts in breast milk and is not thought to be harmful. It is inadvisable to use newer drugs, such as captopril and lisinopril. Angiotensin converting enzymes inhibitors prevent the conversion of angiotensin I to angiotensin II. They are effective antihypertensives and generally well tolerated, although they can cause profound hypotension and renal impairment. Other side-effects are listed in Table 6.

Long-term Effects

The pre-eclamptic group had a higher incidence of pre-eclampsia in their second pregnancies (46.8% vs. 7.6%) and in subsequent pregnancies (20.7% vs. 7.7%) when compared with the normotensive group (Sibai 1986). According to Chesley, the recurrence of pre-eclampsia depends on:

- Time required becoming normotensive in the postpartum period; longer the time required higher the chance of recurrence

TABLE 6: Drugs used in the chronic management of postpartum hypertension

Type of drug	Labetalol	Nifedipine	Enalapril
	Beta-blocker	Calcium-channel antagonist	Angiotensin converting enzymes (ACE) inhibitor
Indication	First-line	Second-line	Third-line
Route of administration	Oral	Oral	Oral
Dose	200 mg/day in divided doses, up to a maximum of 800 mg/day in divided doses	20 mg/day in divided doses, up to a maximum of 60 mg/day in divided doses	2.5 mg daily, up to a maximum of 10 mg daily
Side-effects	As for acute management (see Table 5)	As for acute management (see Table 5)	Profound hypotension, renal impairment, persistent dry cough, angioedema, rash, pancreatitis, upper respiratory tract symptoms, gastrointestinal effects, altered liver function tests, cholestatic jaundice, hepatitis, blood disorders, palpitations, arrhythmias, angina, chest pain, Raynaud's syncope, cerebrovascular accident, myocardial ischemia, dermatological side-effects including Stevens-Johnson syndrome, toxic epidermal necrolysis, exfoliative dermatitis and pemphigus
Contraindications	As for acute management (see Table 5)	As for acute management (see Table 5)	Hypersensitivity to ACE inhibitors (including angioedema), known or suspected renovascular disease, pregnancy
Safe in breast-feeding	Yes	Yes	Yes

- Body mass index: larger the BMI, higher the chance of recurrence in subsequent pregnancies
- Time of onset of eclampsia: there is inverse relation between the gestational age and the chance of recurrence in subsequent pregnancy, later the onset lesser the incidence in next pregnancy
- Average SBP during pregnancy: higher the BP, higher the chance of recurrence.

Multiparous women with eclampsia will have higher incidence of chronic hypertension than do normal control groups or nulliparous eclamptic women. The overall incidence of chronic hypertension was significantly higher in the pre-eclamptic eclamptic group (14.8% vs. 5.6% Sibai). Patients remaining normotensive in subsequent pregnancies had the lowest incidence of chronic hypertension. Mann et al. reports a greater incidence of myocardial infarction in women with a history of pre-eclampsia (3-fold). According to Royal College of General Practitioners, women who were recruited for oral contraception study showed that women with a history of hypertension in pregnancy had a significantly increased risk of hypertension, myocardial infarction, and ischemic heart disease later in life. Pre-eclampsia Doubles the Risk for Premature Maternal Death; Katrina 2005.

CONCLUSION

Hypertension is the most common medical problem encountered during pregnancy, complicating 2–3% of pregnancies. The use of the term PIH should be abandoned as its meaning in clinical practice is unclear and often confusing. Pre-eclampsia is characterized by inadequate trophoblastic invasion with resultant placental ischemia and predominance of vasoconstrictor profile. The diagnosis of severe pre-eclampsia is no longer dependent on the presence of proteinuria. Primarily the management of pre-eclampsia is determined by the gestational age and the severity of the disease. Labetalol, nifedipine, and methyldopa are the preferred antihypertensive agents. Fluid restriction is advisable to reduce the risk of fluid overload in the intrapartum and postpartum. The presence of pre-eclampsia does not guarantee accelerated lung maturation and antenatal corticosteroid therapy should be considered for all women who present with pre-eclampsia before 34 weeks' gestation. The clinical signs and symptoms of patients with HELLP syndrome are classically related to the impact of vasospasm on the maternal liver. Eclampsia Collaborative Trial Group concluded that "there is now compelling evidence in favor of $MgSO_4$ for the treatment of eclampsia". Magnesium sulfate acts both centrally and peripherally. Magnesium toxicity is treated by 10% calcium gluconate. There are several modifications of standard $MgSO_4$ regimens in the developing countries. Joshi's single dose $MgSO_4$ (VIMS regimen) can be administered by health personnel at first referral unit (FRU) levels and then patient is transferred to tertiary centers for definitive management. This would ensure almost seizure-free transport. Eclamptic patients require delivery without respect to gestational age (Cunningham, 1994). Cesarean delivery should be reserved for obstetric indications or deteriorating maternal condition. Non hydrostatic factors (pulmonary capillary leak and deceased COP) may cause or contribute to PE in patients with pre-eclampsia. ARF in preeclamptic pregnancies is uncommon. Cerebral hemorrhage and cerebral edema are two major causes of maternal mortality in pre-eclampsia. Temporary blindness may complicate 1–3% of cases of pre-eclampsia-eclampsia due to occipital lobe ischemia. The patients with gestational hypertension have increased incidence of preterm delivery and small-for-gestational-age (SGA) babies. Unfortunately currently there is no clinically useful screening test to predict PE [World Health Organization (WHO), 2004]. The only group where low-dose aspirin may be justified is in women at risk of developing early-onset pre-eclampsia. Prevalence of remote hypertension is increased in multiparous who develop pre-eclampsia, and women with severe early-onset disease of any parity (Working Group Report on High Blood Pressure in Pregnancy 2001).

REFERENCES

1. Seneviratne HR, Wijeyaratne CN. Pregnancy-induced Hypertension, 1st edition. Hyderabad, India: Orient Longman; 1998.
2. John S, Seang LT, Chervenak F (Eds). Progress in Obstetrics and Gynecology, 17th edition. UK: Churchill Livingstone; 2007.
3. Leveno KJ, Bloom S, Cunningham FG, Spong CY, Rouse D, Hauth J. Williams Obstetrics, 23rd edition. Philadelphia, PA, USA: Tata McGraw Hill Medical Publishers; 2009.
4. Royal College of Obstetricians and Gynaecologists (RCOG). (2006). Severe pre-eclampsia/eclampsia, management (Green-top Guideline No. 10A). [online] Available from www.rcog.org.uk/en/guidelines-research-services/guidelines/gtg10a/. [Accessed February, 2016].
5. Clarke SL, Dildy GA, Belfort MA, Saade GR, Phelan JP, Hankins GD (Eds). Critical Care Obstetrics, 4th edition. Oxford, UK: Blackwell Science; 2004.
6. Landon MB, Gabbe SG, Bruner JP, Ludmir J. Doppler umbilical artery velocimetry in pregnancy complicated by insulin-dependent diabetes mellitus. Obstet Gynecol. 1989;73(6):961-5.
7. Queenan JT, Spong CY, Lockwood CJ (Eds). Queenan's Management of High-Risk Pregnancy: An Evidence-Based Approach, 6th edition. Oxford, UK: Wiley-Blackwell Science; 2012.
8. Misra R. Ian Donald's Practical Obstetrics Problems, 6th edition. New Delhi, India: BI Publications; 2007.
9. American Congress of Obstetricians and Gynecologists (ACOG). (2013). Hypertension in Pregnancy (Report of the ACOG Task Force on Hypertension in Pregnancy). [online] Available from www.acog.org/~/media/Districts/District%20VIII/HypertensionPregnancy.pdf?dmc=1&ts=20140527T0350044350. [Accessed February, 2016].
10. Woznicki K. (2005). Preeclampsia doubles the risk for premature maternal death. [online] Available from www.medpagetoday.com/OBGYN/Pregnancy/886. [Accessed February, 2016].

CHAPTER 43

Disorders of Fetal Growth

Pratap Kumar, Alok Sharma, Geetika G Syal

INTRODUCTION

Fetal growth is important because weight at delivery defines the perinatal outcome. Abnormal fetal growth includes intrauterine growth restriction (IUGR) or small for gestational age (SGA) fetuses and large for gestational age (LGA) or macrosomic neonates. The perinatal mortality and morbidity of the two extreme ends of fetal growth is increased from that of a normally grown population. However, the etiopathogenesis and management of the two remain different. This chapter has concentrated on fetal growth restriction (FGR) or also called as IUGR and LGA or macrosomia.

INTRAUTERINE GROWTH RESTRICTION

The most common sonography-based definition of FGR is a weight below the tenth percentile for gestational age, although other definitions employing a variety of criteria have been advocated. Some authors take third percentile as the cutoff, as 70% of infants with weight below tenth percentile are constitutionally small and hence not at increased risk.[1,2]

Normal Growth

There are three phases in the process of fetal growth, and this is somewhat overlapping on each of the phases. The first phase is the phase of cellular hyperplasia and encompasses the first 16 weeks of gestation. The second phase, known as the phase of concomitant hyperplasia and hypertrophy, occurs between 16 and 32 weeks and involves increase in cell size and number. The third and final phase, called the phase of cellular hypertrophy, occurs between the 32 week and term and is characterized by a rapid increase in cell size. Any insult to any of the phases leads to FGR (Fig. 1).

SYMMETRIC AND ASYMMETRIC GROWTH RESTRICTION

The pattern of normal growth described above forms the basis for the clinical classification of FGR. There are two kinds of FGR:

1. Symmetric FGR: comprises 20–30% of growth-restricted fetuses, refers to a growth pattern in which all fetal organs are decreased proportionally due to global impairment of early fetal cellular hyperplasia. The cause of this group of IUGR is ascribed to the fetus and includes genetic disorder or infection
2. Asymmetric FGR: characterized by a relatively greater decrease in abdominal size (e.g., liver volume and subcutaneous fat tissue) than head circumference and is found in the remaining 70–80% of the FGR population. Asymmetric fetal growth is thought to result from the capacity of the fetus to adapt to a hostile environment

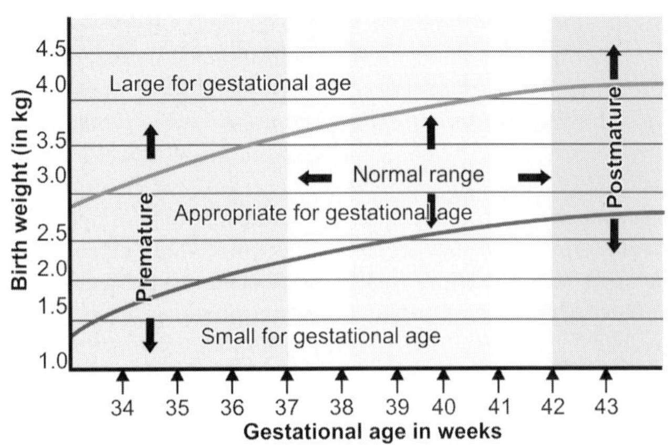

FIG. 1: Birth weight according to gestational age.

by redistributing blood flow in favor of vital organs (e.g., brain, heart, and placenta) at the expense of nonvital fetal organs (e.g., abdominal viscera, lungs, skin, kidneys). Here the cause is decreased uteroplacental blood flow thus having the maternal origin. This type happens in the later half of the pregnancy.[3]

Etiopathogenesis

Fetoplacental Causes

Congenital infections

Intrauterine infections account for 5–10% cases of IUGR; the common infectious agents implicated are TORCH group of infections. The various infections may cause cytolysis (e.g., cytomegalovirus), microvascular endothelial damage (e.g., syphilis), resulting in defect at the stage of cellular hyperplasia and thus disrupting fetal growth in early stage. Other infectious agents responsible for causing FGR include influenza virus, herpes zoster virus, poliovirus, malaria parasite, and *Listeria monocytogenes*.[4]

Chromosomal abnormalities, genetic syndromes, congenital malformations

These account for less than 10% of IUGR infants. Trisomies (13, 18, and 21) are common. About 53% cases of trisomy 13, and 64% cases of trisomy 18 are IUGR. Turner's syndrome is also associated with IUGR.

Genetic syndromes associated with FGR include Lowe's syndrome, Meckel's syndrome, Robert's syndrome, progeria. These are rare conditions.

Congenital malformations like neural tube defects, achondroplasia, osteogenesis imperfecta, and renal anomalies are responsible for increased incidence of IUGR fetuses.[5]

Placental perfusion defects

Factors, which lead to decrease in placental perfusion, result in FGR fetuses. Placenta previa is one of the causes as it is not favorable for nutrient exchange. Also a decrease in exchange area of placenta as in cases of abruption and infarction result in growth restriction. Other placental causes include circumvallate placenta, velamentous cord insertion, placenta accreta, hemangioma, and single umbilical artery.

Multiple pregnancy

It is associated with 30–40% risk of IUGR. The mechanisms consist of decreased space for growth, anomalies, twin-to-twin transfusion.

Maternal Causes

There are various maternal factors operating for the cause of IUGR.

Constitutionally small

Women who are constitutionally small, may give birth to SGA fetus that are otherwise normal and not at increased risk. It has been observed that women with prepregnancy body mass index (BMI) less than 19 have a 19% chance of having growth-restricted fetus, compared to 8% of normal BMI patients.

Poor maternal weight gain

The other factor responsible for growth restriction is poor maternal weight gain. Women with undernutrition, those with malabsorption like inflammatory bowel disease, enterocolitis and mothers who have had gastric bypass operation are at increased risk of giving birth to IUGR infants.

Poor uteroplacental blood flow

Various maternal diseases associated with poor uteroplacental blood flow are other important reasons for poor fetal growth. Hypertensive diseases of pregnancy, diabetes with vasculopathy, antiphospholipid antibody (APLA), hyperviscosity syndromes and collagen vascular diseases are important causes.

Decreased oxygenation

Maternal pathologies, which decrease maternal as well as fetal oxygenation, namely anemias, cyanotic heart diseases, parenchymal lung diseases are also responsible for limited growth of the fetus. Same reason can be attributed to IUGR observed in females living at high altitudes.

Medications and intoxicants

Medications like warfarin, folic acid antagonists, and immunosuppressive drugs are associated with increased risk of FGR. Cigarette smoking during pregnancy decreases intervillous blood flow and causes decrease in prostaglandin I2 production, in turn causing IUGR. Alcohol consumption, and use of heroin and cocaine have been associated with IUGR infants.

Idiopathic

Forty percent cases of IUGR are however idiopathic.[5]

Antenatal Diagnosis

The prerequisite for detection of IUGR remains accurate estimation of gestational age, which requires early baseline measurements.

Clinical Assessment

Clinical assessment is a reasonable screening tool for FGR in low-risk pregnancies.

Symphysis-fundal height measurement

This totally inexpensive technique is the measurement of the distance between the upper edge of the pubic symphysis and the top of the uterine fundus using a tape, to detect fetuses that are poorly grown. The first suspicion of FGR often arises when this length is noted to be discordant with the expected size for dates. Discordancy has been defined in various ways, the most common criteria is a fundal height in centimeters that is at least 4 cm below the gestational age in weeks (e.g., fundal height 32 cm at 36 weeks of gestation).

There is a controversy in the accuracy of fundal height measurements for screening and diagnosis of FGR. A systematic review concluded that there was not enough evidence (one trial) to recommend the use of this technique versus abdominal palpation for detecting abnormal fetal growth.[6] The method performs best when all of the measurements are done by the same clinician using the unmarked side of the tape (to reduce bias)[7] and are plotted to reflect fetal growth for the individual patient ("customized"), rather than against a standardized norm. There are other factors which may affect sensitivity which includes maternal BMI, bladder volume, parity, lie of the fetus and ethnic group.

Sonographic screening

Although early identification of growth-restricted fetuses allows for closer surveillance and earlier intervention in case of decompensation, the use of ultrasound in the third trimester to screen for fetal growth disturbance in low-risk women is practiced but is not effective for reliably detecting these fetuses or improving outcome. In a 2008 cochrane review of eight studies including 27,024 unselected or low-risk women, there was no difference in antenatal or neonatal interventions between women undergoing routine late ultrasound examination (after 24 weeks) and those who did not.[8]

Sonographic diagnosis

Ultrasound is useful, and there is a general consensus that once the suspicion of FGR has arisen same should be used to try to confirm or exclude the diagnosis. Clinical assessment alone is not adequate in pregnancies at high risk for FGR, given the low sensitivity and specificity. Risk factors that should prompt an ultrasound examination include significant lag of the fundal height on physical examination; suboptimal growth on a prior ultrasound; history of a prior birth of a SGA infant; poor maternal weight gain; or maternal conditions (e.g., pre-eclampsia and lupus erythematosus) associated with suboptimal fetal growth.

The simplest sonographic criteria to screen and diagnose fetal growth restriction is estimation of fetal weight.

The other morphometric tests discussed below are more likely to overlook fetuses with symmetric FGR, but can be used as confirmatory tests of suspected asymmetric FGR.

Abdominal circumference

During the phase of fetal hypoxia, due to the consumption of glycogen, fetal liver shrinks. Since fetal liver occupies major portion of fetal abdomen, the abdominal circumference (AC) becomes less.

Most studies report that reduced AC is the most sensitive single morphometric indicator of FGR, which is further increased by having serial measurements at least 14 days apart.[9,10] Measurement of AC was more predictive of FGR than measurement of either head circumference (HC) or biparietal diameter (BPD) or the combination of AC with either one of these two variables.[11] The optimal time to screen for FGR was at approximately 34 weeks of gestation. Biparietal diameter is the least sensitive and specific parameter to detect IUGR because firstly head is one of the last organs to be affected, and secondly late in pregnancy the fetal head on entering into the pelvis undergoes molding which makes the assessment difficult and erroneous.

Estimated fetal weight

Abdominal circumference alone can be used for predicting weight in normally growing fetuses at term and in low-risk populations; however, this method has limitations when used in preterm or growth-restricted fetuses. Therefore, additional sonographic variables have been incorporated into models for predicting fetal growth abnormalities. Formulas which include femur length (FL) have been shown to increase the accuracy of estimation of fetal weight. Fetal weight estimation has become one of the most common methods of identifying the growth-restricted fetus, since pediatricians use birth weight as their primary variable for defining growth restriction in the infant.

Growth velocity

Gestational age assessment is absolutely essential. Since, the use of any parameter (e.g., AC, estimated fetal weight) in the prediction of FGR is based upon accurate assessment of gestational age, if dates are unknown, serial sonographic examinations at two-week intervals should be performed to evaluate the rate of interval growth (i.e., growth velocity). Fetuses with normal growth velocity, amniotic fluid volume, and, Doppler velocimetry are at low risk of complications associated with FGR.

Body Proportions

The HC/AC ratio, FL/AC ratio, and ponderal index have also been used to identify the growth-restricted fetus, particularly in the setting of asymmetric FGR.[12,13]

HC/AC ratio: the HC/AC ratio has been proposed for evaluating fetuses with asymmetric FGR. In these infants, the size of the liver tends to be disproportionately small compared to the circumference of the head or length of the femur, which are initially spared from the effects of nutritional deficiency. Hence, HC/AC ratio remains larger for asymmetric IUGR infants and is normal in symmetric growth-restricted fetuses.

FL/AC ratio: the FL/AC ratio uses sonographic elements that relate to both weight and length in the prediction of FGR. An FL/AC ratio greater than 23.5% has a sensitivity of around 56% and specificity of about 74% for identification of asymmetric FGR.[14]

This ratio is independent of gestational age in normally grown fetuses in the last half of pregnancy. However, an abnormal FL/AC ratio does not accurately diagnose symmetric FGR.

Transverse cerebellar diameter

In a fetus with FGR, growth of the transverse cerebellar diameter (TCD) is not affected, thus TCD may serve as an independent indicator of gestational age against which other potential deviations of growth may be compared. Transverse cerebellar diameter/abdominal circumference ratio exceeding 2 SD above the mean is predictive of asymmetrical growth restriction.[15]

Amniotic fluid volume

Oligohydramnios refers to amniotic fluid-volume that is less than expected for gestational age. The decrease in amniotic fluid volume may be the first ultrasonographic sign of IUGR, and it occurs due to shift of blood flow from kidney to brain.[16] This is further supported by the findings of decreased renal perfusion and urine output in infants with IUGR.[17] It is typically diagnosed by ultrasound examination and may be described qualitatively or quantitatively by various methods. It is diagnosed, when the single maximum vertical pocket of amniotic fluid is less than 2 cm or amniotic fluid index (AFI) is less than 8 cm. Oligohydramnios is one of the sequelae of FGR. The proposed mechanism is diminished fetal urine production due to hypoxia-induced redistribution of blood flow to vital organs at the expense of less vital organs, such as the kidney. Fetal compromise is more, when there is presence of oligohydramnios. This is a diagnostic tool to predict both the presence of FGR and the level of associated fetal compromise, i.e., the pregnancies associated with oligohydramnios are at increased risk of perinatal mortality.

Biophysical Profile

It is a relatively easy and reliable sonographic tool for evaluating the fetal well-being. Modified biophysical profile (BPP) which incorporates nonstress test (NST) and AFI is also used nowadays.

Doppler velocimetry

To assess fetal perfusion, Doppler ultrasound is a noninvasive technique commonly used. FGR is associated with diminished flow and abnormal Doppler waveforms in both maternal and fetal vessels. Thus it reliably differentiates the fetus with pathological growth restriction from a constitutionally small but healthy fetus. Assessment of Doppler flow with appropriate intervention can reduce perinatal morbidity and mortality in pregnancies complicated by FGR.

Uterine artery

Uterine artery Doppler flow velocimetry has limited diagnostic accuracy for prediction of FGR and is not useful as a screening tool.

Umbilical artery

Doppler velocimetry in umbilical artery should be performed using mid-level free-floating loop of the cord and during fetal apnea. Doppler velocimetry in umbilical artery measures peak-systolic and end-diastolic blood flow through the umbilical artery. In normal pregnancy, as the diastolic blood flow through the umbilical artery increases with the gestational age, the systolic/diastolic (S/D) ratio falls. Hence, when there is increase resistance to blood flow in the placenta, as observed in IUGR fetuses, S/D ratio increases. An average S/D ratio greater than 3 after 30 weeks or more predicts IUGR with a sensitivity of 78% and specificity of 85%.[18]

Normal umbilical artery Doppler indicates that the fetus is not compromised and can be safely managed on outdoor basis with repeat tests fortnightly. However, increased S/D ratio in the presence of end-diastolic flow requires intensive fetal monitoring in the form of weekly Doppler and twice weekly NST, BPP or modified BPP (Fig. 2).

In case of absent end-diastolic flow (AEDF), daily fetal surveillance with umbilical artery Doppler, NST, BPP is required because of association of fetal hypoxia in 65–80% of cases. But if the gestational age is above 32 weeks, delivery must be considered (Fig. 3).

Reversal of end-diastolic flow (REDF) is indicative of immediate termination of pregnancy (Fig. 4).

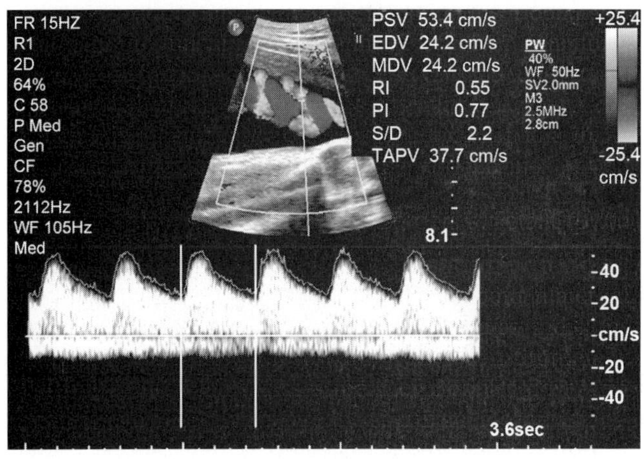

FIG. 2: Normal umbilical artery Doppler *(For color version, see Plate 5).*

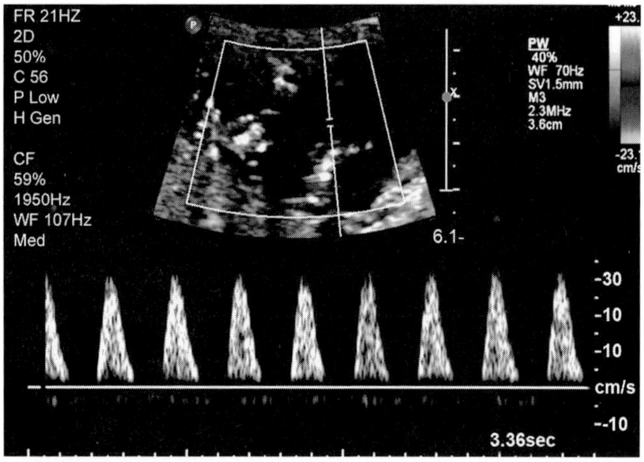

FIG. 3: Absent end-diastolic flow (umbilical artery Doppler) *(For color version, see Plate 5).*

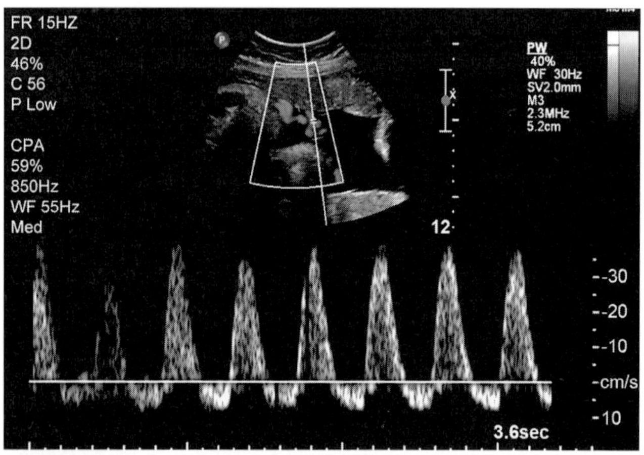

FIG. 4: Reversal of end-diastolic flow (umbilical artery Doppler) *(For color version, see Plate 5).*

Middle cerebral artery

Initially, there is normal or increased middle cerebral artery (MCA) blood flow to supply this vital organ at the expense of other organs and is due to the dilatation of fetal intracranial vessels. Decreased MCA flow has been associated with significant increase in perinatal mortality. Doppler cerebroplacental ratio (MCA pulsatility index/Umbilical artery pulsatility index) indicates severe fetal compromise and impending fetal death.

Fetal descending aorta

As with other Doppler tests, the pulsatility index (i.e., peak systolic minus minimal diastolic velocity divided by the mean velocity or systolic–diastolic/mean) of the fetal descending aorta is not useful for screening and diagnosis of FGR in the general obstetric population. It performs best for predicting the FGR in fetus who is beginning to decompensate from chronic hypoxia and malnutrition.

Normal blood flow in the fetal descending aorta is highly pulsatile, with a minimal end-diastolic component. This part of the aorta provides perfusion to the fetal abdominal organs, umbilical-placental circulation, and lower limbs. Increased placental impedance combined with redistribution of blood flow from nonvital to vital organs may result in changes in the aortic velocity waveforms. Assessment of these waveforms is limited to the pulsatility index because of the lack of diastolic flow.

Ductus venosus flow

If the flow in ductus venosus is absent or is of pulsatile nature, it calls for immediate delivery irrespective of period of gestation.

Biochemical Markers

These include fetal erythropoietin and amino acid concentrations. There are increased fetal erythropoietin concentrations in response to hypoxia and/or anemia. Glycine-to-valine ratio is increased. There is hypertriglyceridemia due to adipose tissue mobilization by the IUGR fetus.

Management

The goal of management of IUGR fetuses involves the management of the underlying cause of IUGR if present and to monitor fetal growth and well-being. Apart from this, selection of appropriate timing and mode of delivery can help in the reduction of perinatal morbidity and mortality. Involvement of a neonatologist forms an important part in the management of such cases.

The general measures include resting in lateral position, increasing the calorie intake in those with poor weight gain. Treating the contributing factor may be helpful. Low-dose aspirin has been found effective in cases of APLA and hypertensive diseases. Avoidance of smoking and alcohol are beneficial. Plasma volume expansion; maternal hyperoxygenation; amino acid infusions have been tried, but are of limited benefit.

Fetal Evaluation

This includes monitoring of fetal growth and fetal well-being. The two should be done clinically and sonographically.

Fetal growth

The clinical evaluation consists of maintaining a weekly gravidogram in which serial measurements of fundal height, symphysis-fundal height, and maternal weight are recorded.

The sonography should be done 2–3 weekly and should include measurements of BPD; AC; FL; HC/AC and FL/AC ratios; estimated fetal weight; and amniotic fluid volume.

Fetal well-being

Clinically the mother should be told about daily fetal movement count and asked about the same.

Since the growth-restricted fetuses have a high incidence of intrauterine death, intensive monitoring with NST, BPP, modified BPP, and Doppler studies are required for fetal well-being.

The indicators for fetal compromise on BPP include nonreactive NST, persistent late decelerations, poor baseline variability, oligohydramnios or if the total BPP score is less than 4. These parameters are further evaluated and supplemented by Doppler studies.

Timing of delivery

Timing of delivery is crucial as growth-restricted fetuses are at risk of IUD. The timing should be based on the tests which suggest that the risk of fetal death exceeds neonatal death.

Indications for delivery

Indications for delivery include: gestational age 38 weeks, low BPP score, oligohydramnios at or above 34 weeks and absent or reversed end-diastolic flow. In no case, the EDD be crossed.

In cases of prematurity, consideration should be given to the assessment of lung maturity, which can be done by measuring amniotic fluid lecithin-sphingomyelin ratio. In patients who are likely to deliver before 34 weeks, glucocorticoids should be administered.

Mode of delivery

When mild IUGR is present and the antenatal surveillance is normal, vaginal delivery is a reasonable approach. However, growth-restricted fetuses are prone for intrapartum hypoxia, and hence continuous and careful fetal heart monitoring is required. If there is any evidence of fetal compromise during labor, immediate intervention should be done.

In cases of unfavorable cervix prostaglandin E2 may be considered, though some authors consider IUGR as a relative contraindication for the use of prostaglandins.

In most cases of AEDF, cesarean delivery is a reasonable choice.

In cases of REDF or severe growth restriction or ominous fetal surveillance results, cesarean delivery is indicated.

The IUGR neonate is prone for many complications in the intranatal (Box 1), postnatal, and later in life.

The appearance of IUGR neonate is typically described as "old man-like", with little subcutaneous fat and having dry peeling skin. The head is relatively large (specially in asymmetric IUGR) with scaphoid abdomen. Fingernails are large along with hands and feet, which appear disproportionately larger than rest of the body. Yellow staining of fingernails, etc. denotes in utero meconium whereas petechiae, rashes, hepatosplenomegaly, etc. lead us to infectious causes of IUGR. The neonate might be hypertonic and appear more restless than usual other than in severe IUGR where the neonate is apathetic and sleepy (Fig. 5).

In the intranatal period, fetal distress due to hypoxia and cord compression can occur. Hence, a neonatologist must be present at the time of delivery and all equipment for resuscitation of the newborn should be available at hand.

Immediately after birth, the complications seen are: birth asphyxia and acidosis which require resuscitation. It may further lead to meconium aspiration, encephalopathy, and even persistent fetal circulation.

Metabolic alterations are also frequently seen. There may be hypoglycemia due to less glycogen reserves in the liver and less subcutaneous fat in growth-restricted infants.

- Hypocalcemia: because of relative hypoparathyroidism due to chronic hypoxia and increased tissue catabolism
- Hypothermia: less subcutaneous fat

Box 1: Problems in intrauterine growth restriction

- Intrauterine fetal demise
- Perinatal asphyxia
- Meconium-aspiration syndrome
- Persistent pulmonary hypertension of the newborn
- Pulmonary hemorrhage
- Hypoglycemia
- Hyperglycemia
- Polycythemia/hyperviscosity
- Temperature instability

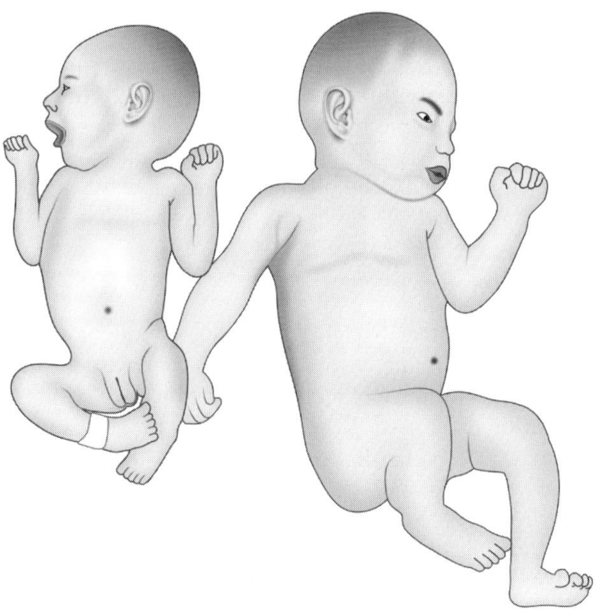

FIG. 5: Neonatal outcome.

- Hyperviscosity syndrome and polycythemia: again due to hypoxia there is increase in the levels of erythropoietin
- Hyperbilirubinemia: due to polycythemia and hemolysis because of asphyxia.

Disseminated intravascular coagulation, necrotizing enterocolitis, and intraventricular hemorrhage are other complications which are attributable to hypoxia.

In later period of life, the asymmetric infants catch up with growth in first 6 months of life. Growth-restricted infants are prone for neurological as well as intellectual deficits. The IUGR infants are likely to develop cardiovascular diseases, diabetes, and hypercholesterolemia in the adult life.

CONCLUSION

The optimal management of IUGR fetus is right antenatal surveillance and timed delivery.

LARGE FOR GESTATIONAL AGE

Large for gestational age refers to birth weight more than 90th percentile for that gestational age. Macrosomia refers to neonates weighing greater than 4,000 g or 4,500 g, regardless of the fetal gestational age. Majority of the studies support the use of 4,500 g as the weight at which a fetus should be considered macrosomic. Macrosomia poses increased risk to the mother as well as the fetus.

Etiopathogenesis

Diabetes

Poorly-controlled diabetes is the most important risk factor for developing fetal macrosomia. This can be explained by Pedersen's hypothesis, which states that maternal hyperglycemia leads to fetal hyperglycemia which stimulates increased production of insulin in the fetus. This hyperinsulinemia in the fetus results in excessive fetal growth. The increase in insulin-like growth factors is also responsible for increased glycogen synthesis, increased fat deposition and hence increased fetal growth.

Maternal Obesity

Large prepregnancy weight or excessive weight gain in pregnancy contribute to macrosomia. The reason can be attributed to presence of glucose intolerance which may or may not be diagnosed. However, the exact reason remains unclear.

Parity

It is well known that the average birth weight increases by 80–120 g with each successive pregnancy. Hence, multiparity becomes a contributory factor for LGA fetus.

- Postdatism: it has been estimated that 3–10% of postdated pregnancies are associated with macrosomia compared to only 1% of term deliveries. The proposed mechanism is the continued delivery of nutrients and also oxygen supply to the fetus[19]
- Genetic factors: beckwith-Wiedemann syndrome, Sotos' syndrome, Weaver's syndrome, and Nevo's syndrome are genetic disorders of overgrowth which are associated with LGA fetuses
- Congenital anomalies: hydrops fetalis, transposition of great vessels are the conditions associated with LGA
- Constitutional factors: taller and or heavier parents are likely to have LGA fetuses. Also if it is a male baby, chances of being LGA is more because male fetuses weigh 150 g on an average more than their matched female counterparts.

Diagnosis

Diagnosis of LGA depends on the clinical findings and sonography.

- Excessive maternal weight gain: the recommended weight gain in pregnancy is 11.2–15.9 kg for females with normal BMI, and 6.8 kg for obese women. If there is excessive weight gain in an already obese female, chances of macrosomia is increased
- Measurement of fundal height: fundal height that is 3–4 cm larger than the gestational age can be due to LGA fetus. The other causes which must be ruled out in this situation are wrong dates, full bladder, polyhydramnios, hydatidiform mole, fibroid uterus, and any pelvic mass
- Leopold maneuvers: they help in the estimation of fetal size with sensitivity and specificity of 10–43% and 99–99.8% respectively[20,21]
- Ultrasonography: the most important parameter for calculation of fetal weight remains AC. The AC greater than 35 cm or more in the third trimester identifies more than 90% of macrosomic infants, and the obstetrician must anticipate the same and be prepared for the management.

Glucose screening according to the guidelines must be done in every patient to rule out diabetes.

Complications

Maternal Complications

Cesarean section: elective cesarean section rate is increased in cases of suspected fetal macrosomia. Also, the incidence of emergency cesarean section is increased specially in primigravida for indications like prolonged labor, non-progress of labor, and fetal distress.

Traumatic and or operative vaginal delivery: the risk of third or fourth degree perineal trauma is increased fivefold in case of vaginal delivery of a macrosomic infant. There are increased chances of vaginal and cervical lacerations and tears.

Postpartum hemorrhage may be atonic and or traumatic in the form of vaginal and cervical lacerations or uterine rupture in neglected cases.

Fetal Complications

Shoulder dystocia and birth injuries: the incidence in macrosomic infants is 5–24%. The risk is increased around fourfold in diabetic mother and history of previous shoulder dystocia. One-fourth of these infants have brachial plexus injury (Erb–Duchenne palsy), facial nerve injury, or even fracture of the clavicle.

These injuries may also occur in macrosomic infants without shoulder dystocia. Injury to abdominal organs leading to hepatic and adrenal hemorrhage has also been reported.

Birth asphyxia: the cause remains uncertain. Stillbirths are also increased due to association with diabetes and postdatism.

Management of shoulder dystocia

Shoulder dystocia cannot be anticipated and is diagnosed when the fetal shoulders fail to deliver shortly after the delivery of fetal head. It is an emergency situation and requires an extra help. Involvement of a pediatrician and an anesthesiologist will be helpful. Another important step would be to give a wide episiotomy, if not made earlier or widen the existing one.

The first step should be McRoberts' maneuver. In this the maternal thighs are hyperflexed over her abdomen, which causes rotation of symphysis pubis upwards and flattening of the sacrum which in turn decreases the angle of pelvic inclination. At the same time, the assistant must give suprapubic pressure which helps in dislodging the anterior shoulder, while the head and neck are given downward traction.

Rubin or Wood's maneuver are the next steps in which the posterior shoulders are pushed towards the fetal chest or towards the fetal back in a corkscrew fashion respectively. These should be done under general anesthesia.

If the above maneuvers fail, the next step is Barnum maneuver. In this, delivery of posterior arm is done. By inserting his hand posteriorly into the hollow of sacrum, the operator identifies the posterior arm of the fetus and by giving gentle pressure on antecubital fossa flexes the fetal arm across its chest. At this point, the forearm is grasped and delivered.

Cleidotomy is the next step which helps in reducing the bisacromial diameter and facilitates the delivery.

Zavanelli maneuver is the final step in which after flexing the fetal head, it is replaced in the uterus followed by emergency cesarean section. Subcutaneous symphysiotomy is the other option which allows the disimpaction of fetal shoulders.

Neonatal complications

Hypoglycemia, hypocalcemia, polycythemia, and electrolyte disturbances are associated with a macrosomic infant.

Treatment

Treatment of diabetes to achieve euglycemia with diet control with or without insulin can help in treating early macrosomia. To prevent macrosomia in obese women, the role of dietary restriction is controversial.

According to recommendations by the American College of Obstetricians and Gynecologists, prophylactic cesarean may be considered for estimated fetal weight of more than 5,000 g in nondiabetic and more than 4,500 g in a diabetic pregnant woman. Maternal age and maternal preferences must also be borne in mind while deciding on the mode of delivery. However, in Indian scenario a baby more than 4 kg should be managed with guarded prognosis for vaginal delivery.

When the estimated fetal weight is more than 4.5 kg, and there is either a prolonged second stage or arrest of descent in the second stage, immediate cesarean must be done. Vacuum should not be used in such cases because of the risk of shoulder dystocia.

Induction of labor: elective induction has been widely recommended to prevent macrosomia and its complications, but many studies suggest that this increases the chances of cesarean section without altering the perinatal outcomes.

In summary, delivery of a suspected macrosomic baby must occur in a tertiary care center where facilities for cesarean section, blood and blood products, anesthesia, and neonatologists are available.

REFERENCES

1. American College of Obstetricians and Gynaecologists. Intrauterine growth restriction. Washington, DC: American College of Obstetricians and Gynaecologists; 2000.
2. Unterscheider J, Daly S, Geary MP, Kennelly MM, McAuliffe FM, O'Donoghue K, et al. Optimizing the definition of intrauterine growth restriction: results of the multicenter prospective PORTO study. Am J Obstet Gynecol. 2013;208(290):e1-6.
3. Wollmann HA. Intrauterine growth restriction: definition and etiology. Horm Res. 1998;49(Suppl 2):1-6.
4. Bernstein PS, Divon MY. Etiologies of fetal growth restriction. Clin Obstet Gynecol. 1997;40:723-9.
5. Baschat AA, Galan HL, Ross MG, Gabbe SG. Intrauterine growth restriction. In: Gabbe SG, Niebyl JR, Simpson JL, (Eds). Obstetrics: Normal and Problem Pregnancies. 6th edition. Philadelphia, PA: Elsevier Saunders; 2012.

6. Robert Peter J, Ho JJ, Valliapan J, Sivasangari S. Symphysial fundal height (SFH) measurement in pregnancy for detecting abnormal fetal growth. Cochrane Database Syst Rev. 2012;7:CD008136.
7. Jelks A, Cifuentes R, Ross MG. Clinician bias in fundal height measurement. Obstet Gynecol. 2007;110:892-9.
8. Bricker L, Neilson JP, Dowswell T. Routine ultrasound in late pregnancy (after 24 weeks' gestation). Cochrane Database Syst Rev. 2008;4:CD001451.
9. Sabbagha RE, Minogue J, Tamura RK, Hungerford SA. Estimation of birth weight by use of ultrasonographic formulas targeted to large-, appropriate-, and small-for-gestational age fetuses. Am J Obstet Gynecol. 1989;160:854-60.
10. Divon MY, Chamberlain PF, Sipos L, Manning FA, Platt LD. Identification of the small for gestational age fetus with the use of gestational age-independent indices of fetal growth. Am J Obstet Gynecol. 1986;155:1197-201.
11. Tamura RK, Sabbagha RE, Pan WH, Vaisrub N. Ultrasonic fetal abdominal circumference: Comparison of direct versus calculated measurement. Obstet Gynecol. 1986;67:833-5.
12. Crane JP, Kopta MM. Prediction of intrauterine growth retardation via ultrasonically measured head/abdominal circumference ratios. Obstet Gynecol. 1979;54:597-601.
13. Seeds JW. Impaired fetal growth: ultrasonic evaluation and clinical management. Obstet Gynecol. 1984;64:577-88.
14. Benson CB, Doubilet PM, Saltzman DH, Jones TB. FL/AC ratio: poor predictor of intrauterine growth retardation. Invest Radiol. 1985;20(7):727-30.
15. Malik A, Pandya VK, Shrivastava P. Gestational age estimation using transcerebellar diameter with grading of fetal cerebellum and evaluation of TCD/AC (Transcerebellar diameter/abdominal circumference) ratio as a gestational age independent parameter. Obstetrics. 2003;13(1):95-7.
16. Queenan JT. Management of High-Risk Pregnancy. 3rd edition. Boston: Blackwell Scientific; 1994. pp 402-12.
17. Veille JC, Kanaan C. Duplex Doppler ultrasonographic evaluation of the fetal renal artery on normal and abnormal fetuses. Am J Obstet Gynecol. 1989;161(6 Pt 1):1502-7.
18. Fleischer A, Schulman H, Farmakides G, Bracero L, Blattner P, Randolph G. Umbilical artery velocity waveforms and intrauterine growth retardation. Am J Obstet Gynecol. 1985;151:502-5.
19. Spellacy WN, Miller S, Winegar A, Peterson PQ. Macrosomia--maternal characteristics and infant complications. Obstet Gynecol. 1985;66(2):158-61.
20. Smith GC, Smith MF, McNay MB, Fleming JE. The relation between fetal abdominal circumference and birth weight: findings in 3512 pregnancies. Br J Obstet Gynaecol. 1997;104(2):186-90.
21. Chauhan SP, Hendrix NW, Magann EF, Morrison JC, Kenney SP, Devoe LD. Limitations of clinical and sonographic estimates of birth weight: experience with 1034 parturients. Obstet Gynecol. 1998;91(1):72-7.

CHAPTER 44

Disorders of Amniotic Fluid

Poonam V Shivkumar, Manisha Rewatkar

INTRODUCTION

The amniotic fluid in the womb of the pregnant women is actually a necessary requirement for the fetus as it is an essential component for its proper growth and development. It cushions the fetus from physical trauma, permits fetal lung growth, and provides a barrier against infection. Normal amniotic fluid volume (AFV) varies with gestational age and with every individual. Normally the volume of amniotic fluid increases with gestational age, peaking at 800–1,000 mL, which coincides with 36–37 weeks of gestation, remains stable for a while and then starts reducing as the gestational age crosses 40 weeks. An abnormally high level of amniotic fluid is called *polyhydramnios,* and it alarms the obstetrician for possibilities of fetal anomalies or medical disorder like diabetes. In pregnancies affected by polyhydramnios, approximately 20% of neonates are born with a congenital anomaly. Inadequate volume of amniotic fluid is termed as *oligohydramnios* which results in poor development of the lung tissue and can lead to fetal death. This article presents the causes, outcomes, and treatments of polyhydramnios and oligohydramnios, as well as their effects on the developing fetus and neonate.

AMNIOTIC FLUID AND ITS CONTENTS

Amniotic fluid is a clear, slightly yellowish liquid that surrounds the fetus during pregnancy. It encircles the fetus and is contained in the amniotic sac.

At first, it is mainly water with electrolytes, but by about the 12–14 week, the liquid also contains proteins, carbohydrates, lipids and phospholipids, and urea, all of which aid in the growth of the fetus.

In an Iranian study in 2007, the biochemical composition of amniotic fluid was assessed (Table 1). The pregnancies were divided into five stages as: stage I (0–30 days), stage II (31–60 days), stage III (61–90 days), stage IV (91–120 days), and stage V (121 days to term).

TABLE 1: Means ± SD of the analyzed variables of amniotic fluid at different stages of gestation and stages of pregnancy

Contents	Stage I	Stage II	Stage III	Stage IV	Stage V
Sodium (mmol/L)	123.3±10.9	125.0±8.3	115.9±14.6	122.0±12.1	120.8±17.8
Potassium (mmol/L)	6.2 ± 1.6	5.2 ± 1.3	5.8 ± 0.9	4.9 ± 0.9	5.6 ± 0.09
Chloride (mmol/L)	101.4 ± 31	115.1 ± 15	117.3 ± 17.8	106.6 ± 2	94.9 ± 18.5
Glucose (mg/dL)	7.1 ± 4.5	1.5 ± 5.7	8.8 ± 3.6	4.9 ± 3.2	3.6 ± 3.3
Urea (mg/dL)	43.7 ± 30.3	69.3 ± 25.6	84.8 ± 24.2	117 ± 68.5	91.7 ± 101.3
Uric acid (mg/dL)	0.4 ± 0.6	0.1 ± 0.1	0.1 ± 0.06	0.3 ± 0.1	0.7 ± 0.3
Creatinine (mg/dL)	1.5 ± 1.9	0.6 ± 0.8	0.6 ± 0.2	5 ± 3.2	5.9 ± 4.6
Total protein (mg/dL)	54.2 ± 79.9	26.6 ± 14.1	37.6 ± 6.9	44.4 ± 20	29.3 ± 15.7

Source: Derakhshanfar A, Bidadkosh A, Kazeminia S. Vitamin E protection against gentamicin-induced nephrotoxicity in rats: a biochemical and histopathologic study. Iranian J Vet. 2007;8:231-8.

DEVELOPMENT OF AMNIOTIC FLUID

Early Gestation

There are two fluid sacs that surround the embryo during early pregnancy: the amniotic sac containing amniotic fluid (AF) and the exocoelomic cavity containing coelomic fluid (i.e., extraembryonic coelomic fluid). These sacs contain large amounts of liquid relative to the size of the embryo/fetus.

Celomic Fluid

Celomic fluid is present between the developing chorionic and amniotic membranes beginning at about the 7th week of gestation, reaching a maximal volume around the 10th week, and subsequently decreasing in amount until it completely disappears at 12–14 weeks of gestation with subsequent fusion of the amniotic and chorionic membranes. It is likely that solutes and fluid from the excoelomic cavity cross the amniotic membrane into the AF and that celomic fluid is an early source of AF.

Mid Gestation

Fetal urine begins to enter the amniotic sac and the fetus begins to swallow AF in conjunction with the transition from embryo to fetus, although the daily volume flows are quite small at mid gestation.[1,2] The fetal lungs also begin to secrete liquid into the AF at this time.

Late Gestation

There appear to be two major sources for both AF production and clearance near term:

- Production—fetal urine and fetal lung liquid.
- Clearance—fetal swallowing and intramembranous pathway.

The intramembranous pathway refers to water and solute exchange that occurs directly between AF and fetal blood.[3-5] This occurs primarily across microscopic fetal vessels present on the fetal surface of the placenta. Smaller contributions may occur across the umbilical cord and fetal skin, however, transcutaneous flow ceases with skin keratinization at 22–24 weeks of gestation. Aquaporins (cell membrane water channel proteins) in the chorioamniotic membrane and placenta may play a role in intramembranous fluid resorption.[6]

The minor sources of AF production and clearance include:

- Production—secretions from the fetal oral-nasal cavities
- Clearance—transmembranous pathway.

The transmembranous pathway refers to water and solute exchange between AF and maternal blood across the decidua and myometrium. In contrast to intramembranous flow, which occurs from one fetal compartment to another, transmembranous flow takes place between maternal and fetal compartments. Transmembranous water and solute fluxes are immeasurably small, although these exchanges were once considered major contributors to AFV and composition.[3]

Both the transmembranous and intramembranous pathways permit flow of water and solutes in opposite directions (i.e., osmotic flow of water and diffusion of solutes), while the other pathways only allow flow of water and solutes in the same direction (i.e., bulk flow).[3]

Aside from transmembranous flow, all AFV ultimately derives from water flow across the placenta from mother to fetus. Alterations in maternal hydration can result in changes in AFV, presumably due to changes in transplacental water flow.[7,8]

Daily fetal urine excretion and fetal swallowing are the best-described processes for AF production and clearance. However, there remain major differences in the magnitude of current estimates of human fetal urine production.[9-11] We feel the best estimates of daily amniotic volume flows in the near-term fetus are:[12]

- Fetal urine production: 800 –1,200 mL/day
- Fetal lung liquid secretion: 170 mL/day
- Fetal swallowing: 500–1,000 mL/day
- Intramembranous flow: 200–400 mL/day
- Oral-nasal secretions: 25 mL/day
- Transmembranous flow: 10 mL/day.

These values are experimentally derived, in many cases using animal models.

Fetal Urination

The daily volume of fetal urine excreted is approximately 30% of fetal body weight.[3] Hourly flow rates progressively increase from 2 to 5 mL at 22 weeks of gestation to 30–50 mL at 40 weeks.[13,14] The reduction in maternal plasma sodium concentration (about 5 meq/L) during pregnancy may increase the fetal urine output and contribute to AF formation by enhancing osmotic flow of water across the placenta.[15] Fetal urinary flow rates decrease with conditions associated with placental insufficiency (e.g., pre-eclampsia, fetal growth restriction) and increase with conditions associated with cardiac failure (e.g., fetal anemia, supraventricular tachycardia, twin-twin transfusion syndrome). Fetal urination (and therefore AFV) is also adversely affected by obstructions in the fetal urinary tract.

Fetal Lung Secretions

The fetal lung secretes 100-times as much fluid as is needed to expand the developing lungs to facilitate their growth. The excess fluid exits the trachea, primarily during episodes of fetal breathing.[16] Approximately 50% of this fluid (170 mL/day) is swallowed and the remainder enters the AF compartment, which is the basis for fetal lung maturity testing.[17,18]

Fetal Swallowing

Fetal swallowing increases throughout gestation. Although swallowing-type movements can be noted by ultrasound late in the first trimester, these movements do not become well-coordinated until the third trimester.[19,20] Direct and indirect measurements of ovine fetal swallowing suggest that the fetus swallows AF equivalent to 20–25% of body.

Fetal swallowing is decreased with a consequent increase in AFV in some fetuses with neurologic abnormalities, such as anencephaly. Fetal swallowing may be also be impaired by obstruction in the fetal esophagus or duodenum.

Intramembranous Flow

Intramembranous flow is thought to be largely driven by the large osmotic gradient between fetal plasma and AF.

Oral-nasal Secretions and Transmembranous Flow

These pathways account for small volumes of fluid exchange. They are difficult to measure and have not been studied.[3,5] This firstly water-like fluid originates from the maternal plasma, and passes through the fetal membranes by osmotic and hydrostatic forces. As the placental and fetal vessels develop, the fluid passes through the fetal tissue, as the exsudativum of the skin. After 20–25 weeks of pregnancy, when the keratinization of skin occurs, the quantity of amniotic fluid begins to depend on the factors that comprise the circulation of AF.

The volume of AF is positively correlated with the growth of fetus. From 10–20 weeks, it increases from 25–400 mL approximately. From the 8th week, when the fetal kidneys begin to function, fetal urine is also present in the AF. Approximately in the 10th week, the breathing and swallowing of the fetus slightly decrease the amount of AF, but neither urination nor swallowing contributes significantly to AF quantity changes, until the 25th week, when keratinization of skin is complete. Then the relationship between AF and fetal growth stops. It reaches the plateau of 800 mL at the 28 week of gestational age. The amount of fluid declines to roughly 400 mL at 42 weeks of gestational age.

FUNCTIONS OF AMNIOTIC FLUID

The AF constantly moves (circulates) as the baby swallows and "inhales" the fluid, and then releases it.

- It helps to protect the fetus from trauma to the maternal abdomen and protect the baby from outside injury by cushioning sudden blows or movements
- It cushions the umbilical cord from compression between the fetus and uterus
- It has antibacterial properties that provide some protection from infection
- It serves as a reservoir of fluid and nutrients for the fetus
- It provides the necessary fluid, space, and growth factors to permit normal development of the fetal lungs and musculoskeletal and gastrointestinal systems
- The developing baby to move in the womb, which allows for proper bone growth
- The lungs to develop properly
- Keep a relatively constant temperature around the baby, protecting from heat loss.

ABNORMALITIES OF AMNIOTIC FLUID VOLUME IN PREGNANCY

The two major abnormalities of AF are:
1. Oligohydramnios: reduced amount of AF expected for that gestational age
2. Polyhydramnios: increased amount of AF expected for that gestational age.

Oligohydramnios

Multiple definitions of oligohydramnios are used, because no ideal cutoff level for intervention exists.
Oligohydramnios is characterized by the following features:
- Diminished AFV
- Amniotic fluid volume (AFV) of less than 500 mL at 32–36 weeks of gestation—Amniotic fluid volume depends on the gestational age; therefore, the best definition may be amniotic fluid index (AFI) less than the fifth percentile
- Single deepest pocket (SDP) of less than 2 cm
- Amniotic fluid volume of less than 5 cm or less than the fifth percentile.

An adequate volume of AF is critical to allow normal fetal movement and growth, and to cushion the fetus and umbilical cord. Oligohydramnios may inhibit these processes and can lead to fetal deformation, umbilical cord compression, and death.

Incidence

Oligohydramnios occurs in 4% of pregnancies.

A study of 3,050 uncomplicated pregnancies with singleton nonanomalous fetuses between 40 and 41.6 weeks of gestation noted oligohydramnios (defined as AFI less than 5) in 11%.[3] The incidence is high in laboring women, largely due to rupture of fetal membranes during or just before labor.[21-23]

Pathophysiology

The volume of AF is ultimately determined by the volume of fluid flowing into and out of the amniotic sac. Fetal urination, lung fluid, and swallowing all make important contributions to fluid movement in late gestation, with minimal contributions from other sources. Fetal disorders that affect any of these processes will affect the AFV.

Homeostatic mechanisms, such as intramembranous absorption (transfer of amniotic fluid across the amnion into the fetal circulation), also exist and work to maintain AFV. These mechanisms appear to be more successful in limiting excess fluid volume than in preventing reduced fluid volume.

Etiology

Conditions commonly associated with oligohydramnios are listed in the Table 2. The most likely etiologies vary according to severity and the trimester in which they are diagnosed. The majority of borderline/low normal AFV have no identifiable cause.

First trimester: the etiology is often unclear. Reduced AF prior to 10 weeks of gestation is rare because gestational sac fluid is primarily derived from the fetal surface of the placenta, transamniotic flow from the maternal compartment, and secretions from the surface of the body of the embryo.

Criteria for determining reduced AF at this gestational age included a difference between mean gestational sac size and crown-rump length of less than 5 mm or a mean gestational sac diameter/crown-rump length ratio outside the normal range for gestational age.[1,2,4,24,25]

TABLE 2: Causes of oligohydramnios

Maternal
• Medical or obstetrical conditions associated with uteroplacental insufficiency (e.g., pre-eclampsia, chronic hypertension, collagen vascular disease, nephropathy, thrombophilia) • Medications (e.g., angiotensin converting enzyme inhibitors, prostaglandin synthetase inhibitors, trastuzumab)
Placental
• Abruption • Twin-to-twin transfusion (i.e., twin polyhydramnios-oligohydramnios sequence) • Placental thrombosis or infarction
Fetal
• Chromosomal abnormalities
• Congenital abnormalities, especially those associated with impaired urine production
• Growth restriction
• Demise
• Post-term pregnancy
• Ruptured fetal membranes
Idiopathic

Second trimester: by the beginning of the second trimester, fetal urine begins to enter the amniotic sac and the fetus begins to swallow AF. Therefore, disorders related to the fetal renal/urinary system begin to play a prominent role in the etiology of oligohydramnios. Maternal and placental factors, as well as rupture of the fetal membranes, are also common causes of oligohydramnios in the second trimester.

The etiologies and relative frequencies of mid-trimester oligohydramnios were illustrated in a series of 128 fetuses first noted to have oligohydramnios at 13–24 weeks of gestation.[5] The following etiologies were observed:

- Fetal anomaly (51%)
- Preterm premature rupture of membranes (PPROM) (34%)
- Placental abruption (7%)
- Fetal growth restriction (FGR) (5%)
- Unknown (4%)[5]
- Six of the 65 anomalous fetuses were aneuploid.

Second trimester oligohydramnios related to amniocentesis appears to have a better prognosis. The membranes often "reseal" with re-accumulation of AF and normal pregnancy outcome. There are a few reports of the occurrence and outcome of oligohydramnios after chorionic villus sampling.[6,7]

Third trimester: oligohydramnios first diagnosed in the third trimester is often associated with PPROM or with uteroplacental insufficiency due to conditions such as preeclampsia or other maternal vascular diseases. Oligohydramnios frequently accompanies fetal growth restriction related to uteroplacental insufficiency. Fetal anomalies and abruptio placentae also play a role at this gestational age. Amniotic fluid volume normally decreases post-term and oligohydramnios can develop in these pregnancies. In addition, many cases of third trimester oligohydramnios are idiopathic.

There may also be an association between pregnancy during the summer season and oligohydramnios, likely related to suboptimal maternal hydration in hot weather.[8] Mechanisms of isolated oligohydramnios also may include alterations in the expression of water pores (aquaporin 1, aquaporin 3) in fetal membranes and placenta.[9]

Clinical Manifestations and Diagnosis

Oligohydramnios may be first suspected because the uterine size is less than expected for gestational age. Clinical diagnosis is based on the finding of decreased AF on ultrasound examination.

We use the AFI for diagnosing oligohydramnios. The AFI provides a means of quantifying normal and abnormal fluid volumes and comparing assessments of AFVs across gestation. As the fifth percentile for AFI averages approximately 7 cm throughout gestation, an AFI less than 5 cm is greater than two standard deviations below the mean value.[10] Most studies that found significant morbidity associated with oligohydramnios used an AFI less than 5 cm as the cutoff, rather than the percentile for gestational age.[11]

Evaluation of Pregnancies with Oligohydramnios

- A thorough maternal history and targeted physical examination is performed to look for maternal conditions that may be associated with oligohydramnios. The effect of maternal medications (e.g., prostaglandin synthase inhibitors) may be limited to oligohydramnios, whereas maternal medical disorders often cause a combination of fetal growth restriction and oligohydramnios
- A comprehensive sonographic evaluation with fetal biometry is performed, as well as a search for fetal anomalies, markers suggestive of aneuploidy (e.g., increased nuchal translucency), fetal growth restriction, or placental abnormalities (e.g., abruption) that may account for decreased AFV
- If PROM (premature rupture of membranes) is suspected but the diagnosis is uncertain after noninvasive assessments (e.g., examination for vaginal pooling, nitrazine and fern tests, Amnisure), indigo-carmine dye can be injected into the AF. Fetal membrane rupture is confirmed if dye is observed on a tampon placed in the vagina at the time of the procedure
- If there are fetal anomalies, amniocentesis may reveal an abnormal karyotype. Trisomy 13 and triploidy are the most common chromosomal abnormalities associated with early oligohydramnios.

Maternal serum a-fetoprotein screening, if elevated, also has prognostic significance and can be helpful in counseling.[6-9]

Methods of Increasing Amniotic Fluid Volume

There is no treatment of oligohydramnios that has been proven to be effective long-term. However, short-term improvement of AFV is possible and may be considered under certain circumstances, such as when a fetal anatomic survey is needed.

Amnioinfusion

Amnioinfusion temporarily increases AFV. It has been used in the following settings:

- To improve detection of fetal anomalies: during the second trimester, oligohydramnios may limit optimal ultrasound assessment of the fetus. In such cases, transabdominal amnioinfusion of approximately 200 milliliters of saline under ultrasound guidance can provide better visualization of fetal anatomy and thus improve diagnostic precision. It is a reasonable option when the information obtained is likely to affect pregnancy management

  Fetal magnetic resonance imaging, alone or in combination with amnioinfusion, has been used as a complementary imaging method for detecting fetal anomalies in second-trimester oligohydramnios.
- To facilitate cephalic version: decreased AF is considered a relative contraindication to version and increases the failure rate
- To prevent fetal sequelae of oligohydramnios: although investigational, serial transabdominal amnioinfusions have been used to improve fetal outcome in pregnancies with idiopathic oligohydramnios[12] or early oligohydramnios due to PROM.[13] A comparative study using an ovine model with complete obstructive uropathy found that serial amnioinfusions through an intra-amniotic port-a-cath prevented pulmonary hypoplasia compared to controls who did not undergo serial amnioinfusion.[14]

Maternal Hydration

Oral hydration is a means of transiently increasing AFV, and is less invasive than amnioinfusion. Hydration with oral water reduces maternal plasma osmolality and sodium concentration, resulting in an osmotically driven maternal to fetal water flux. Increased placental blood flow volume, fetal urine output, and possibly decreased reabsorption of amniotic fluid via swallowing or intramembranous flow increases the AFV.[15]

Three randomized trials of hydration in patients with oligohydramnios have been performed:

1. In the first trial, patients with oligohydramnios were randomly assigned to one of four groups: (1) intravenous hypotonic fluid for 2 hours, (2) intravenous isotonic fluid for 2 hours, (3) oral water for 2 hours, or (4) no therapy.[26] Only the groups who received intravenous hypotonic fluid or oral water, had an increase in AFI compared with the controls (2.8 cm and 3.8 cm, respectively, versus 0.5 cm in controls), emphasizing that maternal plasma osmolality reduction rather than maternal plasma-volume expansion is etiologic in increasing the AFI
2. The second randomized trial of hydration therapy of women with oligohydramnios compared the AFI effect of maternal intravenous hydration with 0.45% normal saline versus placebo therapy.[27] There were no significant differences in AFI between groups, but a slight increase in AFI in both groups
3. The third randomized trial of pregnancies complicated by third trimester idiopathic oligohydramnios found that long-term hydration (6 days) of intravenous isotonic infusion (1,500 mL/day) increased the mean AFI from

39.68 ± 11.11 to 77.70 ± 15.03 mm.[28] Patients were then randomized to home oral-hydration therapy of 1,500 mL/day or 2,500 mL/day and the higher volume group demonstrated significantly increased AF at delivery compared to the lower volume group (112.45 ± 14.92 mm versus 86.21 ± 16.89 mm, respectively P <0.001).

In cases of oligohydramnios in which delivery is not indicated, we feel that oral hydration may have some benefit, particularly in patients with evidence of maternal dehydration.

The combined use of oral water ingestion and desmopressin (DDAVP) markedly and transiently increases AFV.[16,17] This effect is attributed to both of maternal hydration and antidiuresis, and thus maternal plasma hypo-osmolality. Use of DDAVP for this indication should be considered experimental, and used only under approved research protocols.

Fetal membrane sealants: a variety of tissue sealants (e.g., fibrin glue, gelatin sponge, amniopatch) have shown some success in stopping leakage from ruptured membranes in case reports. Neither the safety nor the efficacy of these sealants has been established.

Prognosis and Management

The fetal/neonatal prognosis depends on the cause, severity, gestational age at onset, and duration of oligohydramnios. In fetuses with renal anomalies, the type of extra-renal anomalies, if present, also affects prognosis. In all cases, the clinician must consider the complete clinical picture and the risks of intervention prior to clinical management decisions.

First trimester

Reduced AF at this time is an ominous finding; the pregnancy usually aborts. In one series, 15 of 16 patients (94%) with a normal fetal heart rate and small sac noted on first trimester sonogram went on to spontaneously abort compared with only 4 of 52 control patients (8%) with normal sac size.[24]

These patients should be counseled, regarding the poor prognosis and inform them of the signs of miscarriage. Serial sonographic examinations are helpful for following the natural history of the process [e.g., worsening oligohydramnios, embryonic/fetal demise, or (rarely) resolution].

Second trimester

In the second trimester, prognosis and management depend upon the underlying etiology and the severity of oligohydramnios.

- Borderline/low normal amniotic fluid volume: pregnancies with borderline/low normal AFV generally have a good prognosis.[18,19] Serial sonographic examinations are helpful for following the natural history of the process, which may remain stable, resolve, or progress to development of oligohydramnios and/or fetal growth restriction
- Oligohydramnios: in the second trimester, oligohydramnios often ends in fetal or neonatal death. In the large series described above (128 fetuses first noted to have oligohydramnios at 13–24 weeks of gestation), survival occurred in 9/43 (21%) fetuses with PPROM, 2/9 (22%) fetuses with abruption, 1/5 (20%) idiopathic cases, 1/65 (1.5%) fetuses with congenital anomalies, and 0/6 fetuses with fetal growth restriction. Many of these women chose pregnancy termination because of the poor prognosis.

Preterm delivery, either spontaneous or indicated by maternal or fetal complications, occurs in more than 50% of cases.[20,29,30] Infants may have anatomical and functional abnormalities, such as skeletal deformations, contractures, and pulmonary hypoplasia. We initially perform a fetal anatomic survey to look for fetal malformation, which may influence future management. We administer oral maternal hydration or perform amnioinfusion in pregnancies in which the fetus cannot be visualized adequately. If rupture of membranes is uncertain, amnioinfusion with instillation of indigo-carmine dye facilitates both diagnosis of PPROM and visualization of fetal anomalies. Serial sonographic examinations are obtained to monitor AFV, fetal growth, and fetal well-being. Specific pregnancy complications associated with oligohydramnios are managed as appropriate for the condition. (See individual topic reviews on specific chromosomal and congenital anomalies, mid-trimester PPROM, maternal medical disorders, pre-eclampsia, abruptio placenta, etc.).

Third trimester

Some,[21,31] but not all,[32] studies have shown an inverse relationship between AFV in the third trimester and the incidence of adverse pregnancy outcome. Small sample size likely affected the results of negative studies. Adverse outcomes are related to umbilical cord compression, uteroplacental insufficiency, and meconium aspiration. In particular, uteroplacental insufficiency and cord compression are associated with fetal heart rate abnormalities that result in cesarean delivery and low Apgar scores.[5,33-36]

A study on 28,555 pregnancies to estimate pregnancy and neonatal outcomes in women with decreased AFI between 24 weeks and 34 weeks of gestation found that major malformations were more common in pregnancies with oligohydramnios (AFI <5 cm) and borderline AFI (5–8 cm) than in those with normal fluid: major malformations were present in 25%, 10%, and 2% of fetuses, respectively (P <0.001).[19]

The duration of oligohydramnios is also a prognostic factor. Patients who present with idiopathic oligohydramnios at an earlier gestational age are at risk for adverse perinatal outcomes compared with those presenting later in gestation.[5,37]

Given the potential high risk of adverse outcome, these pregnancies should undergo assessment of the acute and chronic fetal condition at each prenatal visit and fetal heart rate monitoring during labor. A nonstress test (NST) and AFI [or biophysical profile (BPP)] once or twice weekly until delivery should be performed, depending upon the maternal and fetal condition. Combined use of the NST and AFI is associated with a low rate of unexpected fetal death.[38-40]

Doppler velocimetry may have a role in identifying patients with idiopathic oligohydramnios who are at higher risk of adverse outcome.[41] In one retrospective series of 76 patients with oligohydramnios unrelated to PROM or congenital anomalies, the 46 patients with normal systolic/diastolic ratios demonstrated markedly reduced perinatal morbidity compared with the 30 patients with abnormal systolic/diastolic ratios (11% versus 80%).[42] These findings, and observations from other studies,[43] suggest that avoiding intervention in pregnancies with oligohydramnios and normal Doppler velocimetry may decrease iatrogenic morbidity related to prematurity. Although the role of Doppler velocimetry in managing fetal growth restriction is well established, its use in other circumstances remains to be validated.

Timing of Delivery

Timing of delivery in pregnancies complicated by idiopathic oligohydramnios is controversial.[44] Only one small, randomized trial has evaluated outcomes with intervention versus expectant management. In this trial, 54 pregnancies beyond 40 weeks of gestation with isolated oligohydramnios were randomly assigned to either induction of labor or expectant management.[45] No differences were found for any important maternal or neonatal outcome.

Observational studies have reported conflicting results. In one retrospective series, the corrected perinatal mortality rate in structurally normal fetuses with oligohydramnios was significantly lower when delivery was initiated upon diagnosis (in gestations of at least 28 weeks) than with conservative management (18 versus 90 per 1,000 births);[46] this suggests that intervention is indicated. However, the groups came from different institutions and time periods, so they may not have been comparable.

Our indications for delivery in patients with idiopathic oligohydramnios include, but are not limited to, nonreassuring fetal testing or reaching 37–38 completed weeks of gestation, regardless of the cervical Bishop score. Delivery as early as 36–37 weeks has been suggested.[47,48] Although induction increases the risk of cesarean delivery,[49,50] there is insufficient evidence to assure us that perinatal outcome with continued conservative management of oligohydramnios at term is comparable to that with delivery, even in the presence of an appropriately grown, noncompromised fetus, and absence of maternal disease.

We do not typically confirm pulmonary maturity prior to delivery in well-dated pregnancies beyond 36 weeks. Amniocentesis can be challenging in the presence of oligohydramnios due to the lack of a fetus- or placenta-free site for needle insertion.

Alternatively, the patient can be followed with serial NST and BPPs until term gestation is reached; the risks and benefits of various management plans should be discussed with the patient.

Labor

Neither AFI nor SDP performed on admission to the labor unit accurately predicts the risk of peripartum complications.[51-53] We recommend obtaining a short electronic fetal heart rate recording upon admission of patients in labor to help determine whether the fetal heart rate should be monitored continuously or whether intermittent monitoring is likely to be sufficient. If the fetal heart rate is not reactive or fetal heart rate decelerations are present, then we recommend continuous electronic fetal heart rate monitoring during labor. We also consider transcervical amnioinfusion for patients with oligohydramnios and variable fetal heart rate decelerations in labor.

Polyhydramnios

Polyhydramnios (also known as hydramnios) is an excessive volume of AF. It has been associated with an increased risk of various adverse pregnancy outcomes, including preterm birth, placental abruption, and fetal anomalies.[54-56] The diagnosis is made prenatally by ultrasound examination using a noninvasive qualitative or quantitative approach.

Incidence

The incidence of polyhydramnios in a general obstetric population generally ranges from 1 to 2%.[57-61]

Pathophysiology

The volume of AF reflects the balance between fluid production and movement of fluid out of the amniotic sac; the regulation of this process is incompletely understood. In late gestation, the primary sources of AF production are fetal urination and secretion of lung fluid; oral and nasal secretions make minimal contributions. The main routes of AF removal are fetal swallowing and absorption via the intramembranous pathway. Even a relatively minor increase in daily fetal urine production or decrease in fetal swallowing can result in a marked increase in AFV.[62-64]

Etiology

The most common cause of severe polyhydramnios are:

- Fetal anomalies (often associated with an underlying genetic diagnosis)
- Maternal diabetes
- Multiple gestation
- Idiopathic factors are more often associated with milder cases.

Polyhydramnios has been associated with fetal anomalies in most organ systems. The most common structural anomalies associated with polyhydramnios are those that interfere with fetal swallowing and/or absorption of fluid.[65,66] Decreased swallowing may be due to a primary gastrointestinal obstruction (e.g., duodenal, esophageal, or intestinal atresia), neuromuscular disorders (e.g., anencephaly), or to secondary obstruction of the gastrointestinal tract (e.g., massive unilateral dysplastic kidneys).

The combination of intrauterine growth restriction and polyhydramnios is suggestive of trisomy 18; other sonographic markers of trisomy 18 are typically present. Excess AF in this syndrome may be related to difficulty swallowing or to intestinal abnormalities. Other aneuploidies have also been associated with polyhydramnios, most commonly trisomy 21.

Increased urine production may occur in high-fetal cardiac-output states (e.g., fetal anemia due to alloimmunization, parvovirus infection, fetomaternal hemorrhage, α-thalassemia, and glucose-6-phosphatase deficiency) or, rarely, from entities such as fetal Bartter syndrome.[67] The antenatal form of Bartter syndrome is an autosomal recessive disorder associated with intrauterine presentation of renal tubular hypokalemic alkalosis. As a result, the fetus develops polyuria and subsequent polyhydramnios between 24 and 30 weeks of gestation. Prenatal diagnosis can be made by AF and maternal urine electrolyte testing. In monochorionic multiple gestation, polyhydramnios/oligohydramnios sequence is diagnostic of twin-twin transfusion syndrome.

The mechanism for polyhydramnios in pregnancies complicated by maternal diabetes is unclear. Fetal hyperglycemia leading to polyuria is one likely etiology, and is supported by the observation that polyhydramnios is often associated with high maternal glycated hemoglobin (A1C) levels and fetal macrosomia.[68,69] Decreased fetal swallowing or an imbalance in water movement between the maternal and fetal compartments in diabetic pregnancies are other possible mechanisms.

A simple rule of thumb is that in the first trimester, the fluid is more than the embryo/fetus; in the second trimester, the fluid is equal to the fetus; and in the third trimester, the fluid is less than the fetus.

Clinical Manifestations

Physical examination

- Polyhydramnios should be suspected by uterine size large for gestational age
- The increase in AFV is usually asymptomatic
- However, persistent shortness of breath, uterine irritability and contractions, and abdominal discomfort when uterine distention is severe are the other clinical features.

Clinical Significance

Many idiopathic cases resolve spontaneously.[1] However, polyhydramnios has been associated with an increased risk of several adverse outcomes in addition to the poor outcomes related to the associated morphologic abnormalities:[69]

- Maternal respiratory compromise
- Preterm labor, PROM, preterm delivery
- Fetal malposition
- Macrosomia
- Umbilical cord prolapse
- Abruption upon rupture of membranes
- Postpartum uterine atony.

These complications increase the risk of cesarean delivery and neonatal intensive care admission.

Maternal respiratory compromise, fetal malposition, cord prolapse, and postpartum uterine atony are related to uterine over-distention from excessive AFV. Although preterm labor and PROM may lead to spontaneous preterm delivery, preterm birth in affected pregnancies is also caused by iatrogenic intervention for management of pregnancy complications.

Overall perinatal mortality in polyhydramnios is increased two-fold to five-fold compared to pregnancies without polyhydramnios.[70] The combination of a small for gestational age fetus and polyhydramnios has a particularly poor prognosis (including perinatal death) due to the high prevalence of fetal chromosomal and structural abnormalities in this setting.[71-72]

Diagnosis

The diagnosis of polyhydramnios is based upon sonographic visualization of increased AFV. This may be qualitative or quantitative, but generally has a strong subjective component. Commonly used quantitative thresholds for polyhydramnios are:

- Single deepest pocket >8 cm
- Amniotic fluid index >25 cm
- Two diameter pocket >50 cm^2.

Postdiagnosis Evaluation

- Fetal chromosomal analysis should be offered when congenital anomalies are detected and this information will affect management, given the high risk of aneuploidy. In one large series, the prevalence of aneuploidy in anomalous fetuses with polyhydramnios was 10%.[58] Whether chromosomal analysis should be offered in the absence of anomalies or growth restriction is controversial, as the likelihood of aneuploidy is much lower in the setting of a normal sonogram (1%)[58]
- A monochorionic multiple gestations with polyhydramnios/oligohydramnios sequence are suggestive of twin-twin transfusion syndrome
- Screening for diabetes is appropriate if not previously performed
- If fetal hydrops is identified, the next step is evaluation for an immune or nonimmune etiology. In cases of fetal hydrops associated with polyhydramnios, evaluation of potential fetal anemia includes assessment of peak systolic velocity of the middle cerebral artery with a value >1.5 multiples of the median, suggesting moderate or severe anemia, irrespective of the cause. Workup for fetal anemia also includes testing for fetomaternal hemorrhage, acute parvovirus infection, and hemoglobinopathy
- Congenital infection may be associated with maternal signs or symptoms of infection and/or fetal abnormalities (e.g., hydrops, growth restriction, hepatosplenomegaly, cerebral ventriculomegaly, intracranial and intra-abdominal calcifications, and hyperechogenic fetal bowel, ascites). In the absence of maternal signs and symptoms or fetal findings (other than polyhydramnios), congenital infection (rubella, cytomegalovirus, and toxoplasmosis, syphilis) is an unlikely cause of isolated polyhydramnios[73]
- A detailed medical history should be obtained to evaluate for heritable diseases associated with polyhydramnios. These conditions often present with multiple congenital contractures (arthrogryposis), which should be identified by ultrasound. Most cases are recessive inheritance or new mutations. If suspected, the patient should be referred to a genetics specialist for three-generation pedigree and parental examination.

Management of Polyhydramnios

Management of idiopathic polyhydramnios depends on:

- Gestational age
- Severity
- Presence of symptoms
- Cause.

Antepartum fetal monitoring: no randomized trials have evaluated whether pregnancies complicated by idiopathic polyhydramnios benefit from any method of antenatal surveillance. Given the increase in risk of adverse pregnancy outcomes and the two-fold to five-fold increase in risk of perinatal mortality in these cases, antenatal fetal monitoring should be done in all high risk women.

Mild to moderate polyhydramnios: a NST and BPP should be performed upon diagnosis and then every 1–2 weeks until 37 weeks, and then weekly from 37 weeks to delivery. The BPP includes assessments of AFI so that the trajectory of amniotic volume change can be tracked. In severe polyhydramnios, a NST and BPP should be performed every week until delivery. In interpreting the BPP score, clinicians should be cautious about conclusions of fetal well-being with a borderline score (6/8), since the two points for AFV in these cases is not reassuring.

Indications for intervention: no randomized trials have directly compared expectant management and amnioreduction for management of polyhydramnios. In women with preterm singleton pregnancies, amnioreduction can be offered only if polyhydramnios is both severe and symptomatic (associated with significant maternal discomfort or preterm labor). The goal of amnioreduction is to relieve maternal discomfort and prolong pregnancy.[74] Two methods are available: decompression amniocentesis (i.e., removal of a large volume of AF via amniocentesis) and maternal administration of a prostaglandin synthetase inhibitor.[75-77]

Gestational age based approach

Pregnancies under 32 weeks

For severe symptomatic polyhydramnios, decompression amniocentesis (to normalize fluid volume) followed by treatment with indomethacin to maintain normal AFV without exposing the fetus to the risks of serial invasive procedures is suggested. A prophylactic maternal steroid is appropriate prior to the decompression amniocentesis in those pregnancies, because of the increased risk of preterm birth.

During indomethacin therapy, AFV at least weekly while titrating the indomethacin dose to AFV changes, is monitored. If there is no reduction in AFV, then the dose is gradually increased to a maximum of 2–3 mg/kg per day.[75] The drug is tapered when a reduction in AFV is observed. It may be possible to discontinue indomethacin if severe polyhydramnios does not recur as the indomethacin is tapered.[78] Indomethacin is discontinued no later than 32–34 weeks because of the risk of premature fetal ductal constriction.

During indomethacin therapy, serial fetal echocardiographic evaluations are obtained if the duration of therapy exceeds 48 hours and the pregnancy is over 24 weeks of gestation. Doppler velocimetry is performed at intervals of two days to one week.

Following the discontinuation of indomethacin, the AFV is assessed weekly, and continue NSTs/BPPs even if the AFV returns to normal, since polyhydramnios may recur.

Amniocentesis and/or indomethacin treatment can be reinitiated if severe polyhydramnios recurs.

Pregnancies over 32 weeks

For severe symptomatic polyhydramnios between 32 and 34 weeks of gestation, decompression amniocentesis is suggested. After 34 weeks, amniocentesis is offered for fetal lung maturity and delivers if maturity is confirmed.

Indomethacin is rarely utilized at ≥32 weeks, and only if the potential benefits (avoidance of serial decompression amniocentesis procedures) is likely to exceed the risks of premature ductal closure and maternal side effects.

Interventions

Decompression amniocentesis: there is no consensus about how much fluid to remove, how rapidly to remove the fluid, use of tocolytic medications, or use of antibiotics.

Technique

- Cleanse the site with a surgical scrub and then administer local anesthesia into the skin and subcuticular tissues[74]
- An 18-gauge spinal needle is inserted with the tip directed in a caudal direction, and the hub of the needle positioned cranially so as to prevent the needle tip from touching the uterine wall as the uterus becomes smaller with decompression
- Hard-walled arterial line tubing with a three-way stopcock is attached to the needle and connected to a vacuum-suction bottle
- The fluid may be suctioned directly into the container or, alternatively, removed with a 50 mL syringe under controlled suction
- A reasonable guideline is to remove the fluid no faster than 1,000 mL over 20 minutes and not to remove more than 5 L at one time
- The procedure is terminated when the AFI is normalized (generally 15–20 cm) or when intra-amniotic pressure is less than 20 mmHg[79]
- Sometimes the procedure will need to be terminated early because of patient discomfort, a clogged needle, or membrane separation. Use of antibiotic prophylaxis not needed, and initiate tocolytic drugs only if increased contractions occur.

On average, two procedures are needed to reduce AFV chronically, although some patients require many more procedures.[74,80]

Following decompression amniocentesis, AFV is monitored every one to three weeks, as indicated by the progression and severity of the process. Decompression amniocentesis is repeated if severe polyhydramnios recurs and the patient again becomes symptomatic.

Complications occur in 1–3% of procedures and include preterm labor, abruptio placentae, PROM, intra-amniotic infection, and hypoproteinemia.[74,80] In cases presenting with uterine contractions, decompression has reduced symptoms within a few hours of the procedure.[81]

Prostaglandin synthetase inhibitors

Maternal administration of prostaglandin synthetase inhibitors reduces AFV in pregnancies with normal or abnormal AFV at baseline. These drugs may stimulate fetal secretion of arginine vasopressin and facilitate vasopressin-induced renal antidiuretic responses and reduced renal blood flow, thereby reducing fetal urine flow. They also may impair production or enhance reabsorption of lung liquid.[82]

Indomethacin

Various regimens have been used, but a common approach is an initial dose of 25 mg orally four times daily. If there is no reduction in AFV after two or three days, then the dose is gradually increased up to 2–3 mg/kg per day.[75] Drug is tapered when there is a reduction in AFV, and discontinue it when polyhydramnios is no longer severe. A literature review found this therapy to be effective in 48 of 52 patients studied.[83]

Maternal side effects, such as nausea, esophageal reflux, gastritis, and emesis, have been studied primarily in women receiving the drug for inhibition of preterm labor; the prevalence of side effects in this population is 4%. Platelet dysfunction may occur. Alterations in maternal cardiovascular physiology are minimal.

The primary fetal concern with use of indomethacin is constriction of the ductus arteriosus. If the duration of therapy exceeds 48 hours and the pregnancy is over 24 weeks of gestation, we suggest serial fetal echocardiographic evaluation with Doppler velocimetry at intervals of two days to one week. Sonographic signs of ductal narrowing include tricuspid regurgitation and right ventricular dysfunction. The risk of ductal constriction increases with advancing gestational age and is almost 50% at 32 weeks of gestation. Constriction generally resolves within 24 hours after discontinuing the drug.

Sulindac

Sulindac is a nonsteroidal anti-inflammatory drug that also results in reduction of AFV, but appears to have less of a constrictive effect on the fetal ductus than indomethacin.[84-87] However, there are no clinical studies evaluating this agent for treatment of polyhydramnios. We do not use it for this indication.

Investigational approaches

- Investigational therapeutic approaches for polyhydramnios include the use of intra-amniotic pharmacologic agents to reduce fetal-fluid production. In bovine pregnancy, intra-amniotic administration of either arginine vasopressin (AVP) or desmopressin (DDAVP) results in rapid fetal plasma absorption and a marked decrease in fetal urine flow,[88] although there is no effect on fetal swallowing[89]
- Modulation of the amniotic membrane aquaporin water channels, which have been reported to be altered in the amnion and chorion of patients with unexplained polyhydramnios, may represent a potential future therapeutic opportunity to normalize AFV.[90,91]

Management of labor

During labor, fetal position is checked frequently to confirm maintenance of vertex presentation. The excess AF allows greater fetal mobility, so conversion to a breech, compound, or transverse presentation may occur.

Spontaneous rupture of membranes can cause sudden severe uterine decompression with risk of cord prolapse or abruption.

Prophylactic gradual abdominal or transcervical amnioreduction with a needle may prevent these complications during labor.

Controlled amniotomy is performed by using a small gauge needle to puncture the fetal membranes in one or more places in the operating room.

Induction

Although, there is no absolute contraindication to use of oxytocin or prostaglandins in cases of polyhydramnios, these agents should be used with caution. There is a marked increase in the incidence of postpartum hemorrhage related to atony in patients with polyhydramnios; use of uterine stimulants may increase this risk and that of AF embolism.[92,93] However, prostaglandins for cervical ripening and oxytocin for induction are used, as clinically indicated.

Timing of delivery

Mild to moderate polyhydramnios with normal NST and BPP: labor is induced at 39–40 weeks of gestation.

Severe cases: labor is induced at 37 weeks to minimize the risk of umbilical cord prolapse and/or abruption upon rupture of membranes. With intolerant maternal symptoms before 37 weeks, amniocentesis is performed as early as 34 weeks and delivers if the fetal lungs are mature.

REFERENCES

1. Nazari A, Check JH, Epstein RH, et al. Relationship of small-for-dates sac size to crown-rump length and spontaneous abortion in patients with a known date of ovulation. Obstet Gynecol. 1991;78:369-73.
2. Dickey RP, Olar TT, Taylor SN, et al. Relationship of small gestational sac-crown-rump length differences to abortion and abortus karyotypes. Obstet Gynecol. 1992;79:554-7.
3. Locatelli A, Zagarella A, Toso L, et al. Serial assessment of amniotic fluid index in uncomplicated term pregnancies: prognostic value of amniotic fluid reduction. J Matern Fetal Neonatal Med. 2004;15:233-6.
4. Rowling SE, Coleman BG, Langer JE, et al. First-trimester US parameters of failed pregnancy. Radiology. 1997;203:211-7.
5. Shipp TD, Bromley B, Pauker S, et al. Outcome of singleton pregnancies with severe oligohydramnios in the second and third trimesters. Ultrasound Obstet Gynecol. 1996;7:108-13.
6. Dyer SN, Burton BK, Nelson LH. Elevated maternal serum alpha-fetoprotein levels and oligohydramnios: poor prognosis for pregnancy outcome. Am J Obstet Gynecol. 1987;157:336-9.
7. Richards DS, Seeds JW, Katz VL, et al. Elevated maternal serum alpha-fetoprotein with oligohydramnios: ultrasound evaluation and outcome. Obstet Gynecol. 1988;72:337-41.
8. Koontz WL, Seeds JW, Adams NJ, et al. Elevated maternal serum alpha-fetoprotein, second-trimester oligohydramnios, and pregnancy outcome. Obstet Gynecol. 1983;62:301-4.
9. Los FJ, Hagenaars AM, Cohen-Overbeek TE, Quartero HW. Maternal serum markers in second-trimester oligohydramnios. Prenat Diagn. 1994;14:565-8.
10. Bronshtein M, Blumenfeld Z. First- and early second-trimester oligohydramnios-a predictor of poor fetal outcome except in iatrogenic oligohydramnios post chorionic villus biopsy. Ultrasound Obstet Gynecol. 1991;1:245-9.
11. Cheng EY, Luthy DA, Hickok DE, et al. Transcervical chorionic villus sampling and midtrimester oligohydramnios. Am J Obstet Gynecol. 1991;165:1063-8.
12. Feldman I, Friger M, Wiznitzer A, et al. Is oligohydramnios more common during the summer season? Arch Gynecol Obstet. 2009;280:3-6.
13. Zhu XQ, Jiang SS, Zhu XJ, et al. Expression of aquaporin 1 and aquaporin 3 in fetal membranes and placenta in human term pregnancies with oligohydramnios. Placenta. 2009;30:670-6.
14. Moore TR, Cayle JE. The amniotic fluid index in normal human pregnancy. Am J Obstet Gynecol. 1990;162:1168-73.
15. Mabie WC, Gonzalez AR, Sibai BM, Amon E. A comparative trial of labetalol and hydralazine in the acute management of severe hypertension complicating pregnancy. Obstet Gynecol. 1987;70:328-33.
16. Hofmeyr GJ, Gülmezoglu AM. Maternal hydration for increasing amniotic fluid volume in oligohydramnios and normal amniotic fluid volume. Cochrane Database Syst Rev. 2000;CD000134.
17. Doi S, Osada H, Seki K, Sekiya S. Effect of maternal hydration on oligohydramnios: a comparison of three volume expansion methods. Obstet Gynecol. 1998;92:525-9.
18. Yan-Rosenberg L, Burt B, Bombard AT, et al. A randomized clinical trial comparing the effect of maternal intravenous hydration and placebo on the amniotic fluid index in oligohydramnios. J Matern Fetal Neonatal Med. 2007;20:715-8.
19. Patrelli TS, Gizzo S, Cosmi E, et al. Maternal hydration therapy improves the quantity of amniotic fluid and the pregnancy outcome in third-trimester isolated oligohydramnios: a controlled randomized institutional trial. J Ultrasound Med. 2012;31:239-44.
20. Ross MG, Nijland MJ, Kullama LK. 1-Deamino-[8-D-arginine] vasopressin-induced maternal plasma hypoosmolality increases ovine amniotic fluid volume. Am J Obstet Gynecol. 1996;174:1118-25.

21. Rutherford SE, Phelan JP, Smith CV, Jacobs N. The four-quadrant assessment of amniotic fluid volume: an adjunct to antepartum fetal heart rate testing. Obstet Gynecol. 1987;70:353-6.
22. Sarno AP Jr, Ahn MO, Brar HS, et al. Intrapartum Doppler velocimetry, amniotic fluid volume, and fetal heart rate as predictors of subsequent fetal distress. I. An initial report. Am J Obstet Gynecol. 1989;161:1508-14.
23. Mercer LJ, Brown LG, Petres RE, Messer RH. A survey of pregnancies complicated by decreased amniotic fluid. Am J Obstet Gynecol. 1984;149:355-61.
24. Bromley B, Harlow BL, Laboda LA, Benacerraf BR. Small sac size in the first trimester: a predictor of poor fetal outcome. Radiology. 1991;178:375-7.
25. Tadmor OP, Achiron R, Rabinowiz R, et al. Predicting first-trimester spontaneous abortion. Ratio of mean sac diameter to crown-rump length compared to embryonic heart rate. J Reprod Med. 1994;39:459.
26. Turhan NO, Atacan N. Antepartum prophylactic transabdominal amnioinfusion in preterm pregnancies complicated by oligohydramnios. Int J Gynaecol Obstet. 2002;76:15-21.
27. Locatelli A, Ghidini A, Verderio M, et al. Predictors of perinatal survival in a cohort of pregnancies with severe oligohydramnios due to premature rupture of membranes at <26 weeks managed with serial amnioinfusions. Eur J Obstet Gynecol Reprod Biol. 2006;128:97-102.
28. Nicksa GA, Yu DC, Kalish BT, et al. Serial amnioinfusions prevent fetal pulmonary hypoplasia in a large animal model of oligohydramnios. J Pediatr Surg. 2011;46:67-71.
29. Nijland MJ, Ross MG, Kullama LK, et al. DDAVP-induced maternal hyposmolality increases ovine fetal urine flow. Am J Physiol. 1995;268:R358-65.
30. Fisk NM, Ronderos-Dumit D, Soliani A, et al. Diagnostic and therapeutic transabdominal amnioinfusion in oligohydramnios. Obstet Gynecol. 1991;78:270-8.
31. Chamberlain PF, Manning FA, Morrison I, et al. Ultrasound evaluation of amniotic fluid volume. I. The relationship of marginal and decreased amniotic fluid volumes to perinatal outcome. Am J Obstet Gynecol. 1984;150:245-9.
32. Petrozella LN, Dashe JS, McIntire DD, Leveno KJ. Clinical significance of borderline amniotic fluid index and oligohydramnios in preterm pregnancy. Obstet Gynecol. 2011;117:338-42.
33. Moore TR. Superiority of the four-quadrant sum over the single-deepest-pocket technique in ultrasonographic identification of abnormal amniotic fluid volumes. Am J Obstet Gynecol. 1990;163:762-7.
34. Mercer LJ, Brown LG. Fetal outcome with oligohydramnios in the second trimester. Obstet Gynecol. 1986;67:840-2.
35. Morris JM, Thompson K, Smithey J, et al. The usefulness of ultrasound assessment of amniotic fluid in predicting adverse outcome in prolonged pregnancy: a prospective blinded observational study. BJOG. 2003;110:989-94.
36. Magann EF, Doherty DA, Chauhan SP, et al. Dye-determined amniotic fluid volume and intrapartum/neonatal outcome. J Perinatol. 2004;24:423-28.
37. Sarno AP Jr, Ahn MO, Phelan JP. Intrapartum amniotic fluid volume at term. Association of ruptured membranes, oligohydramnios and increased fetal risk. J Reprod Med. 1990;35:719-23.
38. Chauhan SP, Sanderson M, Hendrix NW, et al. Perinatal outcome and amniotic fluid index in the antepartum and intrapartum periods: A meta-analysis. Am J Obstet Gynecol. 1999;181:1473-8.
39. Phelan JP. The postdate pregnancy: an overview. Clin Obstet Gynecol. 1989;32:221-7.
40. Alchalabi HA, Obeidat BR, Jallad MF, Khader YS. Induction of labor and perinatal outcome: the impact of the amniotic fluid index. Eur J Obstet Gynecol Reprod Biol. 2006;129:124-7.
41. Vink J, Hickey K, Ghidini A, et al. Earlier gestational age at ultrasound evaluation predicts adverse neonatal outcomes in the preterm appropriate-for-gestational-age fetus with idiopathic oligohydramnios. Am J Perinatol. 2009;26:21-5.
42. Clark SL, Sabey P, Jolley K. Nonstress testing with acoustic stimulation and amniotic fluid volume assessment: 5973 tests without unexpected fetal death. Am J Obstet Gynecol. 1989;160:694-7.
43. Nageotte MP, Towers CV, Asrat T, Freeman RK. Perinatal outcome with the modified biophysical profile. Am J Obstet Gynecol. 1994;170:1672-6.
44. Miller DA, Rabello YA, Paul RH. The modified biophysical profile: antepartum testing in the 1990s. Am J Obstet Gynecol. 1996;174:812-7.
45. Carroll BC, Bruner JP. Umbilical artery Doppler velocimetry in pregnancies complicated by oligohydramnios. J Reprod Med. 2000;45:562-6.
46. Skotnicki MZ, Rybaczuk M, Urban J. [Doppler examination of fetal cerebral circulation in pregnancies complicated with idiopathic oligohydramnios]. Ginekol Pol. 2004;75:128-32.
47. Bastide A, Manning F, Harman C, et al. Ultrasound evaluation of amniotic fluid: outcome of pregnancies with severe oligohydramnios. Am J Obstet Gynecol. 1986;154:895.
48. Danon D, Ben-Haroush A, Yogev Y, et al. Prostaglandin E2 induction of labor for isolated oligohydramnios in women with unfavorable cervix at term. Fetal Diagn Ther. 2007;22:75.
49. Bannerman CG, Chauhan SP. Oligohydramnios at 34-36 weeks: observe or deliver. Am J Obstet Gynecol. 2011;205:163.
50. Ek S, Andersson A, Johansson A, Kublicas M. Oligohydramnios in uncomplicated pregnancies beyond 40 completed weeks. A prospective, randomised, pilot study on maternal and neonatal outcomes. Fetal Diagn Ther. 2005;20:182-5.
51. Manzanares S, Carrillo MP, González-Perán E, et al. Isolated oligohydramnios in term pregnancy as an indication for induction of labor. J Matern Fetal Neonatal Med. 2007;20:221-4.
52. Magann EF, Chauhan SP, Kinsella MJ, et al. Antenatal testing among 1001 patients at high risk: the role of ultrasonographic estimate of amniotic fluid volume. Am J Obstet Gynecol. 1999;180:1330-6.
53. Spong CY, Mercer BM, D'alton M, et al. Timing of indicated late-preterm and early-term birth. Obstet Gynecol. 2011;118:323-33.
54. Golan A, Wolman I, Sagi J, et al. Persistence of polyhydramnios during pregnancy--its significance and correlation with maternal and fetal complications. Gynecol Obstet Invest. 1994;37:18-20.
55. Many A, Hill LM, Lazebnik N, Martin JG. The association between polyhydramnios and preterm delivery. Obstet Gynecol. 1995;86:389-91.
56. Smith CV, Plambeck RD, Rayburn WF, Albaugh KJ. Relation of mild idiopathic polyhydramnios to perinatal outcome. Obstet Gynecol. 1992;79:387-9.
57. Hill LM, Breckle R, Thomas ML, Fries JK. Polyhydramnios: ultrasonically detected prevalence and neonatal outcome. Obstet Gynecol. 1987;69:21-5.
58. Dashe JS, McIntire DD, Ramus RM, et al. Hydramnios: anomaly prevalence and sonographic detection. Obstet Gynecol. 2002;100:134-9.
59. Thompson O, Brown R, Gunnarson G, Harrington K. Prevalence of polyhydramnios in the third trimester in a population screened by first and second trimester ultrasonography. J Perinat Med. 1998;26:371-7.
60. Biggio JR Jr, Wenstrom KD, Dubard MB, Cliver SP. Hydramnios prediction of adverse perinatal outcome. Obstet Gynecol. 1999;94:773-7.
61. Pri-Paz S, Khalek N, Fuchs KM, Simpson LL. Maximal amniotic fluid index as a prognostic factor in pregnancies complicated by polyhydramnios. Ultrasound Obstet Gynecol. 2012;39:648-53.
62. Harding R, Bocking AD, Sigger JN, Wickham PJ. Composition and volume of fluid swallowed by fetal sheep. Q J Exp Physiol. 1984;69:487-95.

63. Pritchard JA. Deglutition by normal and anencephalic fetuses. Obstet Gynecol. 1965;25:289-97.
64. Pritchard JA. Fetal swallowing and amniotic fluid volume. Obstet Gynecol. 1966;28:606-10.
65. Ben-Chetrit A, Hochner-Celnikier D, Ron M, Yagel S. Hydramnios in the third trimester of pregnancy: a change in the distribution of accompanying fetal anomalies as a result of early ultrasonographic prenatal diagnosis. Am J Obstet Gynecol. 1990;162:1344.
66. Stoll CG, Alembik Y, Dott B. Study of 156 cases of polyhydramnios and congenital malformations in a series of 118,265 consecutive births. Am J Obstet Gynecol. 1991;165:586-90.
67. Sieck UV, Ohlsson A. Fetal polyuria and hydramnios associated with Bartter's syndrome. Obstet Gynecol. 1984;63:22S-24S.
68. Vink JY, Poggi SH, Ghidini A, Spong CY. Amniotic fluid index and birth weight: is there a relationship in diabetics with poor glycemic control? Am J Obstet Gynecol. 2006;195:848-50.
69. Idris N, Wong SF, Thomae M, et al. Influence of polyhydramnios on perinatal outcome in pregestational diabetic pregnancies. Ultrasound Obstet Gynecol. 2010;36:338-43.
70. Ross MG, Brace RA, National Institute of Child Health and Development Workshop Participants. National Institute of Child Health and Development Conference summary: amniotic fluid biology--basic and clinical aspects. J Matern Fetal Med. 2001;10:2-19.
71. Magann EF, Chauhan SP, Doherty DA, et al. A review of idiopathic hydramnios and pregnancy outcomes. Obstet Gynecol Surv. 2007;62:795-802.
72. Erez O, Shoham-Vardi I, Sheiner E, et al. Hydramnios and small for gestational age are independent risk factors for neonatal mortality and maternal morbidity. Arch Gynecol Obstet. 2005;271:296.
73. Sickler GK, Nyberg DA, Sohaey R, Luthy DA. Polyhydramnios and fetal intrauterine growth restriction: ominous combination. J Ultrasound Med. 1997;16:609-14.
74. Fayyaz H, Rafi J. TORCH screening in polyhydramnios: an observational study. J Matern Fetal Neonatal Med. 2012;25:1069-72.
75. Elliott JP, Sawyer AT, Radin TG, Strong RE. Large-volume therapeutic amniocentesis in the treatment of hydramnios. Obstet Gynecol. 1994;84:1025-7.
76. Cabrol D, Landesman R, Muller J, et al. Treatment of polyhydramnios with prostaglandin synthetase inhibitor (indomethacin). Am J Obstet Gynecol. 1987;157:422-6.
77. Hickok DE, Hollenbach KA, Reilley SF, Nyberg DA. The association between decreased amniotic fluid volume and treatment with nonsteroidal anti-inflammatory agents for preterm labor. Am J Obstet Gynecol. 1989;160:1525-30.
78. Kirshon B, Mari G, Moise KJ Jr. Indomethacin therapy in the treatment of symptomatic polyhydramnios. Obstet Gynecol. 1990;75:202-5.
79. Rode L, Bundgaard A, Skibsted L, et al. Acute recurrent polyhydramnios: a combination of amniocenteses and NSAID may be curative rather than palliative. Fetal Diagn Ther. 2007;22:186-9.
80. Fisk NM, Tannirandorn Y, Nicolini U, et al. Amniotic pressure in disorders of amniotic fluid volume. Obstet Gynecol. 1990;76:210.
81. Leung WC, Jouannic JM, Hyett J, et al. Procedure-related complications of rapid amniodrainage in the treatment of polyhydramnios. Ultrasound Obstet Gynecol. 2004;23:154-8.
82. Jauniaux E, Holmes A, Hyett J, et al. Rapid and radical amniodrainage in the treatment of severe twin-twin transfusion syndrome. Prenat Diagn. 2001;21:471-6.
83. Kramer WB, Van den Veyver IB, Kirshon B. Treatment of polyhydramnios with indomethacin. Clin Perinatol. 1994;21:615-30.
84. Moise KJ Jr. Polyhydramnios. Clin Obstet Gynecol. 1997;40:266.
85. Bartfield M, Carlan SJ. The safety and efficacy of prolonged outpatient sulindac to prevent the recurrence of preterm labor: a prospective double-blind study. Prim Care Update Ob Gyns. 1998;5:178.
86. Kramer WB, Saade GR, Belfort M, et al. A randomized double-blind study comparing the fetal effects of sulindac to terbutaline during the management of preterm labor. Am J Obstet Gynecol. 1999;180:396-401..
87. Peek MJ, McCarthy A, Kyle P, et al. Medical amnioreduction with sulindac to reduce cord complications in monoamniotic twins. Am J Obstet Gynecol. 1997;176:334-6.
88. Gilbert WM, Cheung CY, Brace RA. Rapid intramembranous absorption into the fetal circulation of arginine vasopressin injected intraamniotically. Am J Obstet Gynecol. 1991;164:1013-20.
89. Kullama LK, Nijland MJ, Ervin MG, Ross MG. Intraamniotic deamino(D-Arg8)-vasopressin: prolonged effects on ovine fetal urine flow and swallowing. Am J Obstet Gynecol. 1996;174:78.
90. Mann SE, Dvorak N, Gilbert H, Taylor RN. Steady-state levels of aquaporin 1 mRNA expression are increased in idiopathic polyhydramnios. Am J Obstet Gynecol. 2006;194:884-7.
91. Zhu X, Jiang S, Hu Y, et al. The expression of aquaporin 8 and aquaporin 9 in fetal membranes and placenta in term pregnancies complicated by idiopathic polyhydramnios. Early Hum Dev. 2010;86:65763.
92. Kramer MS, Rouleau J, Baskett TF, et al. Amniotic-fluid embolism and medical induction of labour: a retrospective, population-based cohort study. Lancet. 2006;368:1444-8.
93. Harman CR. Amniotic fluid abnormalities. Semin Perinatol. 2008;32:288-94.

CHAPTER 45

Third Trimester Bleeding

Uma Pandey, Stephen W Lindow

ANTEPARTUM HEMORRHAGE

Bleeding into or from the genital tract after the period of viability (from 24 weeks gestation in high-resource countries and from 28 weeks in resource-poor settings) but before the baby is born is termed antepartum hemorrhage (APH). The term APH includes hemorrhage that occurs in the first and second stage of labor. Despite the above definition, women with similar bleeding between 20 weeks and 28 weeks gestation are managed as an APH.[1,2]

Incidence: APH occurs in 3–5% of all pregnancies.

Causes of APH in general:[1,2]

- Maternal bleeding:
  - Placental bleeding:
    - Abruptio placentae ~35% of cases
    - Placenta previa ~35% of cases
  - Nonplacental causes:
    - Bloody show
    - Cervical ectopy
    - Cervicitis (Chlamydia)
    - Cervical polyp
    - Cervical intraepithelial neoplasia (CIN) and cancer cervix
    - Vaginal varicosities
    - Trauma.
- Fetal bleeding:
  - Vasa previa (accounts for <%)
  - Other placental and umbilical cord anomalies:
    - Velamentous insertion of the umbilical cord
    - Circumvallate placenta
    - Succenturiate lobe
    - Congenital arteriovenous malformations
    - Aberrant blood vessel.

PLACENTA PREVIA

Definition: placenta previa is when the placenta abnormally implants in the lower segment of uterus near or over the cervical os instead of attaching to the corpus or fundus (this definition is more appropriate as the lower segment forms later in the pregnancy). Previa is a Latin word that means the placenta is present before the presenting part of the fetus.[3]

Incidence: it varies from one study to another but estimates vary from 1.2/1,000 to 2.8/1,000 pregnancies.[4]

Etiology and Risk Factors[5]

No specific etiology has been found for placenta previa but associations exist.

- Previous placenta previa (12 times the risk)
- Uterine scarring (previous lower segment cesarean section, previous dilatation and curettage): This is possibly due to damage to endometrium and/or myometrium that leads to abnormal placental implantation
- Age more than 35 years
- Multiple gestations, multiparity
- Reduced interpregnancy interval
- Tumors (commonly fibroids) distorting the uterine cavity.

Classification

Before ultrasound (especially transvaginal) became a routine practice traditionally it was classified in to four types of placenta previa.[6] The grading system does not accuratly identify women at risk of major hemorrhage.

1. Total placenta previa: the internal cervical os is covered completely covered by the placenta (grade 4)

2. Partial placenta previa: the internal cervical os is covered partially by placenta (grade 3)
3. Marginal placenta previa: the edge of the placenta is at the margin of the internal os (grade 2)
4. Low-lying placenta: placental edge is not near the internal cervical os but is in the lower segment (grade 1).

Cause of Bleeding

This is due to relative growth of the lower uterine segment due to which the placenta shears off from its attachment. As a result, maternal uteroplacental vessels open and lead to an episode of bleeding. The most important fact is that bleeding is "maternal" unlike in vasa previa. The bleeding stops by various mechanisms: thrombosis of open sinuses, placental infarction and mechanical pressure by the presenting part.

Clinical Presentation[6]

- Sudden onset, painless and profuse, bright red vaginal bleeding: ususally there are warning hemorrhages but not always. These warning hemorrhages are small bouts of bleeeding which ususally brings patients to the hospital. Bleeding can become profuse and lead to fetal distress, preterm labor or fetal death. The maternal condition can also be jeopardized due to hemorrhagic shock and it extreme cases can lead to maternal death
- The uterus usually is soft and nontender (unlike cases of placental abruption)
- Fetal malpresentation is common (placenta previa does not allow engagement of fetal head)
- Fetal bradycardia, repeated decelerations or fetal distress could be present along with bleeding.

Diagnosis

Placenta previa should always be suspected in a women who presents with bleeding in the second half of pregnancy. Table 1 describes differentating features of placenta previa and abruptio placentae. Ultrasonography is a necessity for the diagnosis.[7]

The ultrasonographic picture showing placenta previa is given in Figure 1.

The diagnosis can rarely be established by clinical examination. Digital cervical examination is never allowed unless the woman is in the operating theater with all the preparations for immediate delivery—even the most gentle finger examination can result in torrential blood loss. Although digital vaginal examination is contraindicated in a woman who presents with undiagnosed vaginal bleeding during pregnancy a gentle speculum is allowed and may yield useful information.

TABLE 1: Differentiating features of placenta previa and abruptio placentae

Characteristics of	Placenta previa	Abruptio placentae
Amount of blood loss	Variable	Variable, may be concealed
Duration	Usually 2–3 hours	Continues for longer
Abdominal pain	None unless in labor	Dominant feature
FHR pattern	Usually normal	Usually abnormal
Coagulation defect	Normal	DIC is a feature
Associated risk factors	None	Often present

FHR, fetal heart rate; DIC, disseminated intravascular coagulation.

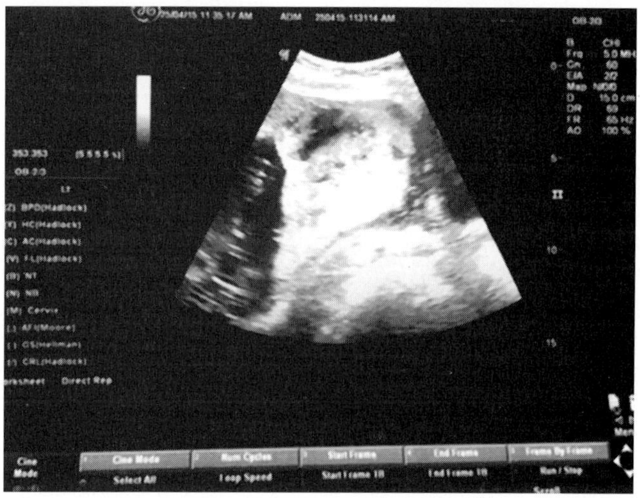

FIG. 1: Ultrasonogrphic picture of placenta previa.

Society of Obstetricians and Gynaecologists of Canada Clinical Practice Guidelines, 2007[8]

The modern recommedation is:

- Sonographers are encouraged to report the actual distance from the placental edge to the internal cervical os at transvaginal scan, using standard terminology of millimeters away from the os or millimeters of overlap. A placental edge that exactly reaching the internal os is described as 0 mm. When the placental edge reaches or overlaps the internal cervical os between 18 weeks' and 24 weeks' gestation (incidence 2–4%), a follow-up examination for placental location in the third trimester is recommended. Overlap of more than 15 mm is associated with an incresed likelihood of placenta previa at term
- When the placental edge lies between 20 mm away from the internal os and 20 mm overlap after 26 weeks' gestation, ultrasound should be repeated at regular

intervals depending on the gestational age, distance from the internal os, and bleeding, because continued change in placental location is likely. Overlap of 20 mm or more at any time in the third trimester is highly predictive of placenta previa.

Endovaginal ultrasound has a positive predictive value of 93.3% and a negative predictive value of 97.6% for the diagnosis of of placenta previa.[9] With transperineal sonography positive predictive value was 98% and negative predictive value was 100%.[10]

Explanation of Placental Migration

Placental migration is clearly a misnomer. At 20 weeks of gestation the length of the lower uterine segment is less than 1 cm. With progressive enlargement of the uterus the lower uterine segment enlarges and extends to more than 5 cm in size towards term. This is the explanation for "placental migration" i.e., a placenta which covers the internal os in the first trimester appears to move up and lies in the upper segment of the uterus in the end of pregnancy.

A placenta which is found in the lower uterine segement in the first trimester has a 90% chance it will migrate as pregnancy progresses towards term. Patients should be counseled regarding this in the first trimester (to avoid unneccesary anxiety). Transvaginal sonography is safe and more accurate than transabdominal ultrasound because the placental edge and the internal os are often obscured by the symphysis pubis or the fetus.[11]

Maternal Complications

- Per vaginal bleeding and resulting anemia.
- Malpresentation
- Long hospital stay
- Hypotension
- Acute respiratory distress syndrome (ARDS)
- Acute renal failure
- Morbid adherent placenta and recurrence
- Increased operative intervention
- Increased incidence of postpartum hemorrhage (PPH)
- Maternal death
- Venous thomboembolism (VTE)
- Anesthetic and surgical complications
- Air embolism.

Fetal Complications

- Increased perinatal mortality ranges from 7% to 25% (due to prematurity, asphyxia or congenital malformations)
- Increased preterm deliveries and low birth weight
- Fetal asphyxia
- Increased risk of congeintal malformation (2–4 times)
- Fetal malpresentaion
- Fetal exsanguination
- Intrauterine growth restriction
- Unexpected fetal death.

Management

Thorough preoperative evaluation allows better planning. Factors to be considered are adequate blood bank facilites, competent surgical and possibly gynecology oncosurgical team and urology team. Patient should ideally be mananged in a tertiary referral center.

Management depends upon the maternal and fetal condition and facilites available for resuscitation. Cases of morbidly adherent placenta (accreta, increta and percreta) should be transferred to higher units which have facilitites available for management of PPH (including vascular radiology for uterine artery embolization).

The definitive treatment is delivery of the placenta (and fetus) but the timing of this depends on:
- Amount of uterine bleeding
- Gestational age and viability of the fetus.

Expectant therapy (if preterm fetus and no severe bleeding):
- Hospitalization until bleeding settles
- Tocolysis (although controversial)
- Maternal corticosteroids for fetal lung maturation
- Some patients with a non-bleeding placenta previa can be managed on an outpatient basis.

Delivery: it is needed when:
- Mother is bleeding to an extent that affects or will affect her health
- Gestation is greater than 36 weeks
- Fetal distress in a viable fetus.

Patients who suffer massive blood loss will need adequate resuscitation along with packed cell transfusion, intensive unit care. It is important to deliver (by cesarean) before resuscitation is complete when there is a massive blood loss as the rate of loss is too fast to allow adequate blood replacement. The most important aspect is to remove the bleeding part (the placenta) to terminate the bleeding.

Patients with mild bleeding can be managed conservatively:
- With steroid cover (from 25 weeks to 35 weeks gestation)
- McAfee and Johnson regime (Fig. 2)
- Until the baby is mature
- Adequate blood is arranged for any eventuality
- Mother counseled
- Adequate neonatal facilities available
- Patient is in a unit in which she can be operated on round the clock if she starts to bleed
- Cervical cerclage has a controversial role as the data is insufficient.

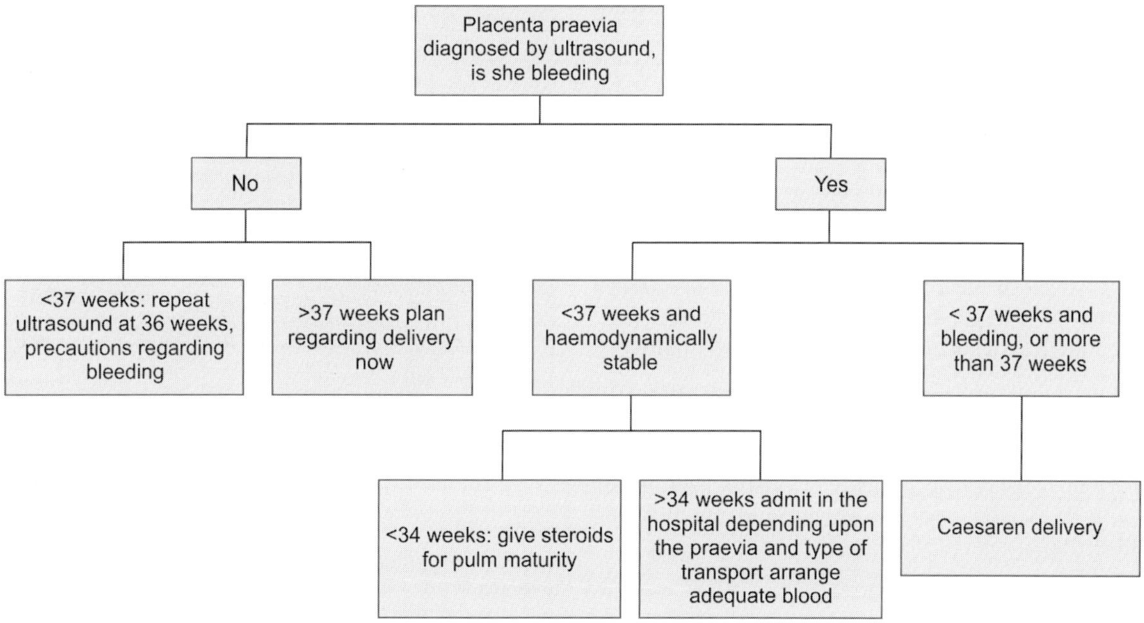

FIG. 2: Management of placenta previa.

*McAfee and Johnson regimen (McAfee UK and Johnson USA 1945): Expectant Management

Aim: to continue pregnancy for fetal maturity without compromising maternal safety in a center where there is a facility for cesarean delivery and blood bank. It can only be allowed to a mother whose Hb is more than 10 g%, gestation less than 37 weeks, normal fetal heart rate (FHR) and no vaginal bleeding.

Cesarean Section

Cesarean section should be performed by an experienced obstetrician. Regional blockade by an expert anesthetist can be used. Cesarean can be done by lower segment method or by classical route, the operating surgeon should decide the approach. Classical cesarean has the advantage that the operation can be done quickly, baby can be delivered without cutting through placenta, so there is no question of fetal exsanguination. But the disadvantage of classical is that many obstetricians of modern days might not be familiar with the procedure. When the lower segment approach is performed the placenta should preferably be separated manually to get the lower margin and the membranes are ruptured or if not possible the placenta can be divided promptly to enter into the amniotic sac to deliver the baby. In either case the cord is clamped quickly to prevent further fetal exsanguination.

Once the placenta has been delivered, uterotonic agents are adminstered. There are number of medications available which can be used. Oxytocin IM or IV, methyl ergometrine, prostaglandin $F_{2\alpha}$, and misoprostol as a part of medical management of PPH. The surgical management of PPH involves:

- Bimanual uterine compression
- Call for help: senior obstetricians, senior anesthetist, hematologists
- Continue maternal resuscitation
- Start blood transfusion
- If oozing from the placental bed continues then hemostatic sutures may be used, i.e., oversewing the implantation site
- If the placental bed continues to bleed, then selective devascularization can be attempted (bilateral ligation of the uterine and ovarian vessels)
- If this does not control the blood loss, bilateral internal iliac artery ligation is performed
- Failing these attempts to achieve hemostasis, hysterectomy is the last option to save the life of the mother
- Where facilities and expertise exist, selective uterine artery embolization can be done under radiological guidance either preoperatively or more commonly, postoperatively.

Evidence Regarding Cervical Cerclage (The Cochrane Collaboration)

Intervention for suspected placenta previa (review): three trials were included, involving a total of 114 women. Both tested interventions (home versus hospitalization and cervical cerclage versus no cerclage) were associated with reduced lengths of stay in hospital antenatally: weighted mean difference (WMD) respectively -18.50 days (95% confidence interval (CI) -26.83 to -10.17), -4.80 days (95% CI -6.37 to -3.23). Otherwise, there was little evidence of any clear advantage or disadvantage to a policy of home versus hospital care. The one woman who had hemorrhage severe enough to require immediate transfusion and delivery was in the home care group. Cervical cerclage may reduce the risk of delivery before 34 weeks: relative risk (RR) 0.45 (95% CI 0.23–0.87), or the birth of a baby weighing less than 2 Kg RR 0.34 (0.14–0.83) or having a low five minute Apgar score RR 0.19 (0.04–1.00). In general, these possible benefits were more evident in the trial of lower methodological quality.

Conclusions*:* there are insufficient data from trials to recommend any change in clinical practice. Available data should, however, encourage further work to address the safety of more conservative policies of hospitalization for women with suspected placenta previa, and the possible value of insertion of a cervical suture.[12]

PLACENTAL ABRUPTION

Placental abruption is defined as the separation of a normally implanted placenta from the uterine site before the delivery of the fetus (Figs 3 and 4). Placental abruption occurs in 0.5–1.8% of all pregnancies. Abruptio placentae are an important cause of maternal and fetal mortality and morbidity.[13]

Note that the classifications of abruptio placenta and placenta previa are mutually exclusive therefore "a previa that abrupts" cannot occur.

Abruption is called "revealed" when blood tracks between the membranes and the decidua, trickles through the cervix and comes out of vagina. Less frequently encountered one is the "concealed" abruption in which blood accumulates behind the placenta and there is no external bleeding. The process of abruption may involve the whole of placenta or part of it. The "Rule of 50%" is about 50% of cases occur before the onset of labor and abruption involving more than 50% of the placenta is frequently associated with fetal death.

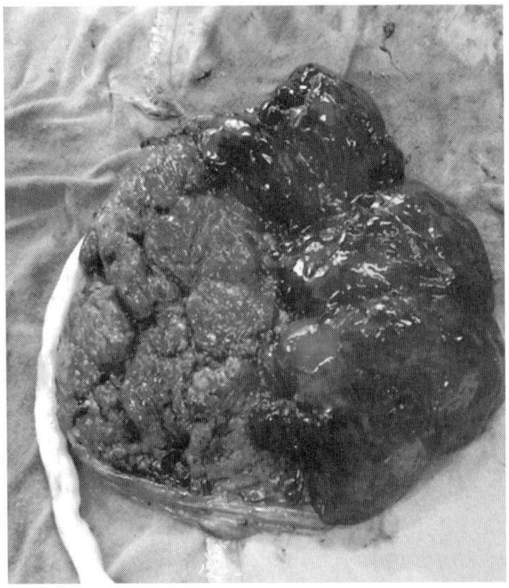

FIG. 3: Placental abruption *(For color version, see Plate 5).*

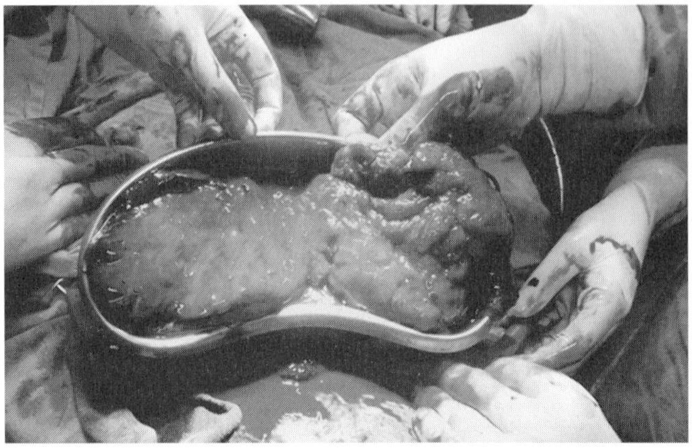

FIG. 4: Placental abruption after cesarean section *(For color version, see Plate 6).*

There is significant discrepancy between the rates of diagnosis of abruption between clinicians, ultrasonographers and pathologists. Therefore it is frequent clinical practice to diagnose cases of abruption clinically and not rely on ultrasound finding or histopathological examination.

Predisposing Factors[14]

- Previous placental abruption (15–20 fold increase)
- Chronic hypertension or pregnancy induced hypertension, pre-eclampsia
- Thrombophilia
- Cigarette smoking
- Cocaine use
- Multiparity and advanced maternal age
- Multifetal gestation
- Vascular deficiency or deterioration (e.g., diabetes mellitus, collagen diseases)
- Pprom
- Sudden reduction in uterine volume (e.g., sudden amniotic fluid loss, delivery of a first twin)
- Short umbilical cord (<20 cm)
- Hydramnios
- Trauma (car accident, maternal abdominal trauma), external or internal fetal version
- Intrauterine infection
- Mean levels of homocysteine are higher among patients with abruption than controls
- Elevated second-trimester maternal serum α-fetoprotein is associated with 10 fold increased risk. Notching in the uterine artery Doppler in the second trimester is also associated with an increased risk.

Pathophysiology

Abruption results from hemorrhage at the decidual-placental interface. The process involves vasospasm and thrombosis of the decidual vessels with necrosis and hemorrhage.

An abruption can be acute or chronic. An acute process is seen in cases of trauma, sudden decompression of uterus in cases of hydramnios or after delivery of first twin.

In the majority of cases an abruption is long standing process which may start in the first trimester. Pre-eclampsia, intrauterine growth restriction and aburption have possibly a common causative factor "uteroplacental insufficiency", as in each case the placenta shows evidence of thrombosis, fibrinoid necrosis, hemosiderinladen macrophages and evidence of villous hemorrhage.[15,16]

Thrombin is a potent uterotonic agent and presence of old placental blood during the histological examination of abruptio placentae support the concept that thrombin production is implicated in preterm birth.[17]

Classification

Grade I (mild): the diagnosis of abruptio placentae is made retrospectively on postpartum detection of a small retroplacental clot.
Grade II (intermediate): this diagnosis is based on the classic features of abruptio placentae with uterine hypertonicity, but the fetus is still alive.
Grade III (severe): the fetus is dead (separation of 50% or more of the placental area usually is incompatible with fetal life)
Grade IIIA: overt coagulopathy is not present.
Grade IIIB: together with overt coagulopathy.

Normal values of blood coagulation profile are given in Table 2. It is imperative that regular investigations to be performed in case of abruption for maternal condition in regular interval as shown in (Table 3).

Diagnosis

Diagnosis is a clinical one, and ultrasonography and the Kleihauer-Betke test are of limited diagnostic value.

Signs and Symptoms

- Blood loss, external (revealed in about 80% of patients) or concealed hemorrhage
- Sudden severe abdominal (uterine) or back pain
- Uterine tenderness
- Persistent uterine hypertonus
- Evidence of fetal distress
- Maternal hypovolemic shock

TABLE 2: Reference range of blood coagulation profile

Test	Value
Bleeding time	1–3 minute (Duke's method)
Coagulation time	3–7 minute (Wright's tube method)
Clot observation test (Weiner's)	6–12 minutes
Clot retraction time	30 minutes
Prothrombin time	11–17 sec
Thrombin time	11–15 sec
Platelet count	1.5–4 Lakh/mm^3
Fibrinogen degradation products	0–5/μg/mL
Fibrinogen	300–600 mg%
D-Dimer	0–200 mg/mL

TABLE 3: Frequency of coagulation tests in abruptio

Clotting time	2 hourly
Coagulation profile	4 hourly
Fibrinogen	4 hourly
FDPs	4 hourly
FBC	4 hourly

FDPs, fibrinogen degradation products; FBC, full blood count.

- Coagulation defects/disseminated intravasular coagulopathy.

May present with no symptoms and can also present as idiopathic preterm labour.

Patients with a mild placental abruption may be asymptomatic. The amount of vaginal bleeding correlates poorly with the degree of placental separation.

Complications

- Renal: acute tubular necrosis can present due to acute hypovolemia which is a reversible process in most of the cases. But acute cortical necrosis can also lead to oliguria and renal failure and it is due to cortical damage from the products which are released from the coagulations cascade. Renal cortical necrosis may result in chronic renal failure[18]
- Hemorrhage (intraperitoneal/couvelaire uterus/broad ligament hematoma)
- Shock
- Postpartum hemorrhage and sepsis
- Blood coagulation abnormalities
- Fetal: prematurity, asphyxia, fetal death.

Differential Diagnosis

The differential diagnosis of an abruptio placenta varies according to the presentation, e.g. the presentation may be one of APH or one of lower abdominal pain with a concealed abruption.

Placenta previa, appendicitis, urinary tract infection, preterm labor, fibroid degeneration, ovarian pathology, other causes of APH mentioned in the begining of the chapter and muscular pain.

Management

Cases of placental abruption cannot be predicted or prevented. It can only be optimsed through attention to the risks and benefits of conservative management, monitoring of maternal and fetal well-being and timely delivery once indicated.

Urgent Hospitalization

- Maternal vital signs should be monitored
- Electronic fetal heart rate monitoring
- Ultrasonography may useful to exclude placenta previa
- Blood test for hemoglobin, hematocrit, platelet count, coagulation profile
- 2–6 units of typed and cross-matched blood and 2–6 units of fresh frozen plasma must be prepared initially.

Fetal complications:
- Preterm Birth 10%
- Increased perinatal mortality rate (25–30%, due to prematurity, asphyxia, SGA, congenital anomalies)
- Increased rate of fetal intraventricular hemorrhage
- Increased rate neonatal cystic periventricular leukomalacia
- Fetal growth restriction
- Congenital malformations 4.4%.

Maternal complications:
- Hemorrhagic shock
- Disseminated intravascular coagulopathy
- Renal failure
- Postpartum hemorrhage
- Need for blood and blood product transfusion
- Hysterectomy
- Maternal death
- Puerperal sepsis
- Sheehan's syndrome
- Fetomaternal hemorrhage.

Delivery

Cesarean section is indicated for the majority of abruptio placentae cases with a viable fetus even if there is no evidence of fetal distress. It is difficult to predict the extension of the abruption which can occur quickly.

Vaginal delivery is indicated:
- If no fetal distress is evident and the diagnosis of an abruptio placenta is not secure
- When the fetus is dead and absence of life-threatening bleeding.

Fluid and blood replacement therapy: for adequate resuscitation of mother.

Correction of the Coagulopathy

Check if disseminated intravascular coagulation (DIC) has developed, replace adequate amount of coagulations factors, fresh frozen plasma and platlets.

Amniotomy

Should be performed as early as possible in labor. The rationale behind this is the as the amount of amniotic fluid is reduced or drained it may allow better spiral artery compression and serve to decrease bleeding from the implantaion site and also reduce the entry of thromboplastin in the maternal circulation.

Expectant Therapy

If the fetus is immature, bleeding is small, no fetal distress, and uterine irritability is absent:
- Tocolytics (controversial opinion because side-effect of tachycardia can mask the clincal sign of blood loss. So if used at all should be with very cautious approach)
- Steroids for fetal lung maturation.

Future Pregnancies[19]

- Adequate counselling regarding recurrence rate (10%)
- Control hypertension
- Serial growth scans with umbilical artery Doppler
- Folic acid prophylaxis periconceptionally
- Patients with a thrombophillia may need heparin and aspirin.

VASA PREVIA

Definition

It is the presence of fetal blood vessels crossing the amniotic membranes over the cervical os, due to velamentous isertion of umbilical cord into the membranes in the lower uterine segment. This is due to the absence of protective Wharton's gelatin the vessels may be easily lacerated at the time of membrane rupture. There is increased perinatal mortality with this condition. It is very uncommon, incidence being only 1:2,500 births.[20] The condition is associated with fetal hemorrhage and a 33–100% rate of perinatal mortality.

Hemorrhage occurs as the cervix dilates or membranes rupture either spontaneoulsy or by artificial techniques.

Risk Factors[21,22]

- *In vitro* fertilization
- Low-lying and second trimester placenta previa
- Marginal cord insertion
- Mutiple gestation
- Succenturiate—lobed and bilobed placentae.

Ultrasound scan remains the mainstay of antenatal diagnosis of vasa previa. Determing placental cord insertion during the anomaly scan can be done and which may prove useful.

Presentation

The mother starts to have painless heavy bleeding upon rupture of the membranes. The condition is rare, but the fetus can exsanguinates witihin minutes as the total blood volume is only 250 mL at term. Emergency delivery of fetus is the management of choice.[23]

An apt test can confirm that the blood is fetal but delivery should not deferred for confirmation of blood in women with hemorrhage and fetal heart rate abnormalities.[24]

Cervical Bleeding

- Cytologic sampling is mandatory
- Bleeding can be controlled with cauterization or packing
- Bacterial and viral cultures can be diagnostic.

Cervical Polyps

- Bleeding is usually self-limited
- Trauma should be avoided
- Cytologic sampling is mandatory
- Polypectomy may control bleeding and yield a histologic diagnosis.

Bloody Show

Bloody show is characteristically associated with cervical changes and blood-tinged mucus.

Vulvovaginal Trauma

- Patient history frequently elucidates the cause
- Adequate pelvic examination should be performed, including an examination under anesthesia, if necessary
- Penetration of the cul-de-sac necessitates exploretory laparotomy
- Foreign bodies must be removed
- Wounds should be debrided and closed, of clean
- Hematomaqs should be evacuated. Hemostasis should be obtained. Drains as needed should be placed
- Tetanus prophylaxis is indicated.

Hematuria

Hematuria as a souce of vaginal bleeding can be diagnosed by urinalysis.

REFERENCES

1. James DK, Steer PJ, Weiner CP, Gonik B. High Risk Pregnancy, 4th edition. Philadelphia: Elsevier Saunders; 2011.
2. Sharma JB. Textbook of Obstetrics, 1st edition. New Delhi: Avichal Publishing Company; 2012.
3. Queenan JT, Hobbins JC, Spoong CY. Protocols for high risk pregnancies, 4th Edition. Massachusetts: Blackwell; 2005.
4. Crane JM, Van Den Hof MC, Dods L, Armson BA, Liston R. Neonatal outcomes with placenta previa. Obstet Gynecol. 1997;177:210-4.
5. Konar H. DC Dutta's Textbook of Obstetrics, 7th edition. New Delhi: Jaypee Brother Medical Publishers (P) Ltd.; 2013.
6. Cunningham FG, Macdonald PC, Grant NF, Leveno KJ. Obstetrical Haemorrhage. In: Willliams' Obstetrics, 20th edition. Norwalk, Connecticut: Appleton & Lang; 1997.pp.745-82.
7. Mustafa SA, Brizot ML, Carvalho MH. Transvaginal ultrasonography in predicting placenta previa at delivery: a longitudinal study. Ultrasound Obstet Gynecol. 2002;20:356-9.
8. Oppenheimer L. SOGC Clinical Practice Guideline, Diagnosis and Management of Placenta Previa. JOGC. 2007:189.
9. Leerentveld RA, Gilberts ECAM, Arnold KJCW, Wladimiroff JW. Accuracy and safety of transvaginal sonographic placental localisation. Obstet Gynecol. 1990;76:759-62.
10. Rani PR, Harith PH, Gowri R. Comparative study of transperineal and tranabdominal sonography in the diagnosis of placenta previa. J Obstet Gynaecol. 2007;33(2):134-7.
11. Timor-Tritsch IE, Yunis RA. Confirming the safety of transvaginal sonography in patients suspected of placenta previa. Obstet Gynecol. 1993;81(5 pt 1):742-4.
12. The Cochrane Collaboration. Interventions for suspected placenta previa. Neilson JP. Evidence regarding Cervical Cerclage. 2007;4.
13. Ananth CV, Berkowitz GS, Savitz DA, Lapinski RH. Placental abruption and adverse perinatal outcome. J Am Med Assoc. 1999;282:1646-51.
14. Sheiner E, Shoham-Vardi I, Hallak M, Hadar A. Placental abruption in term pregnancies: clinical significance and obstetric risk factors. J Matern Fetal Neonatal Med. 2003;13:45-9.
15. Bernischke K, Kaufmann P. Pathology of the human placenta, 4th edition. New York: Springer; 2000.
16. ACOG Educational Bulletin. Obstetric aspects of human trauma management. Number 251, September 1998. American College of Obstetricians and Gynaecologists. Int J Gynaecol Obstet. 1999;64:87-94.
17. Rana A, Sawhney H, Gopalan S, Panigrahi D, Nijhawan R. Abruptio placentae and chorioamnionitis-microbiological and histologic correlation. Acta Obstet Gynecol Scand. 1999;78:363-6.
18. Sakornbutt E, Leeman L, Fontaine P. Late pregnancy bleeding. Am Fam Physician. 2007;75:1199-1206.

19. Towers CV, Pircon RA, Heppard M. Is tocolysis safe in the management of third trimester bleeding? Am J Obstet Gynecol. 1999;180(6 pt 1):1572-8.
20. Rasmussen S, Irgens LM, Dalaker K. Outcome of pregnancies subsequent to placental abruption: a risk assessment. Acta Obstet Gynecol Scand. 2000;79:496-501.
21. Oyalese KO, Tuner M, Lees C, Campbell S. Vasa Previa: an avoidable obstetric tragedy. Obstet Gynecol Surv. 1999;54:138-45.
22. Faiz AS, Ananth CV. Etiology and risk factors for placenta previa: an overview and metaanalysis of observational studies. J Matern Fetal Neonatal Med. 2003;13:175-90.
23. Hladky K, Yankowitz J, Hansen WF. Placental abruption. Obstet Gynecol Surv. 2002;57:299-305.
24. Nelle M, Zilow EP, Kraus M, Bastert G, Linderkamp O. The effect of Leboyer delivery on blood viscosity and other hemorheologic parameters in term neonate. Am J Obstet Gynecol. 1993;169:189-93.

CHAPTER 46

Isoimmunization

Ajay S Dhawle

INTRODUCTION

Isoimmunization or alloimmunization is the production of antibodies by an individual against constituents of the tissues of another individual of the same species. In obstetrics, when any fetal blood group factor inherited from the father is not possessed by the mother, antepartum or intrapartum fetal-maternal bleeding may stimulate an immune reaction in the mother. The antibodies thus produced can travel transplacentally, leading to destruction of the fetal red blood cell (RBC). In severe cases the anemic fetus develops ascites, subcutaneous edema, and pleural and pericardial effusions (hydrops fetalis) and dies in the womb. Many different antibodies (anti-D, anti-Kell, anti-c, anti-E, etc.) can cause hemolytic disease of the fetus and newborn. Sometimes the sensitization results even prior to pregnancy as a result of a mismatched blood transfusion.

INCIDENCE

The incidence of Rh incompatibility varies by race and ethnicity. Approximately 15% of whites are Rh-negative, compared with only 5–8% of African Americans and 1–2% of Asians and Native Americans.

There are limited data available on immunization rates in pregnant women from India or on the antigens responsible for any immunization. In a study from Delhi[1] that included parous women, the overall prevalence of alloantibodies was 1.25%. There was a statistically significant difference between alloimmunization rates in the Rh antigen D-negative and D antigen-positive groups (10.7% vs. 0.12%, respectively). Anti-D antibody contributed to 78.4% of total alloimmunizations.[1] The high incidence of isoimmunization amongst the parous Rh-negative women in India might be because of the lack of implementation of standardized and universal anti-D immunoprophylaxis. The rest of minor antigens that may result in isoimmunization are discussed in Table 1. Many western countries follow the universal screening for all antibodies at the first trimester checkup.

TABLE 1: Minor red blood cell antigens associated with hemolytic disease of the newborn (HDN)

Blood System	Specific Antigens	Severity of hemolytic diseasesof the newborn
Kell	• K • K • Kp(a) Mild • Kp(b) • Js(a) • Js(b)	• Mild to severe • Mild • Mild • Mild • Mild • Mild
Duffy	• Fy(a) • Fy(3)	• Mild to severe • Mild
Kidd	• Jk(a) • Jk(b) • Jk(3)	• Mild to severe • Mild to severe • Mild
Lewis	• Y • Fy(b) • P1	• Not a cause of HDN • Not a cause of HDN • Not a cause of HDN
MNSs	• M • N • S • S • U • Mi(a) • Mf(a) • Vw	• Mild to severe • Mild • Mild to severe • Mild to severe • Mild to severe • Moderate • Moderate • Mild

Continued

Continued

Blood System	Specific Antigens	Severity of hemolytic diseasesof the newborn
	• Mur • Hil • Hut	• Mild • Mild • Mild
Lutheran	• Lut(a) • Lut(b)	• Mild • Mild
Diego	• Di(a) • Di(b)	• Mild to severe • Mild to severe
Xg	• Xg(a)	• Mild
P	• PP1(k) • P1	• Mild to severe • Not a cause of HDN

Source: Adapted from Weinstein, L. Clin Obstet Gynecol 1982;25:327 and Reid, ME, Toy, PTCY. in Hematology and Infancy and Children, 5th ed, Nathan, DG, Drkin, SH (Eds)m WBH Saunders, Philadelphia, 1998, p. 1768.

ETIOLOGY

Blood group isoimmunization generally arises from one of pathogenic incidents:

- Incompatible blood transfusion
- Fetomaternal hemorrhage (FMH).

Incompatible Blood Transfusion

Transfusion isoimmunization, although uncommon, is generally related to development of atypical antibodies and are of little clinical consequence; however, severe hemolytic disease of the fetus and newborn can be related to a few atypical antibodies.

Fetomaternal Hemorrhage

Fetomaternal bleeding is a much more common cause of RhD isoimmunization than incompatible blood transfusion, and it is a significant cause of atypical antibody development as well.

Antepartum hemorrhage, pregnancy-induced hypertension, manual removal of the placenta, cesarean delivery and external version are all associated with larger volumes of blood less than transplacental hemorrhage. Amniocentesis, for genetic or other indications, has also been associated with increased risk of maternal sensitization, particularly if the placenta is traversed during amniocentesis. A 5–7% incidence of FMH has been identified after abortion, both spontaneous and therapeutic. Maternal response to the introduction of Rh-positive fetal cells into maternal circulation is a two-step phenomenon. The first, primary Rh immune response is frequently slow and weak in the development. This may be related to the relatively compromised immune response seen in the pregnant patient. Immunoglobulin M (lgM) anti-D is often not identified before 8–9 weeks after exposure, and as many as 6 months may elapse before this primary response is seen.

The pregnant patient then frequently switches rapidly to the production of IgG anti-D, which does cross the placenta.

After the establishment of the primary response, a second exposure with a very small inoculum generally produces a rapid and profound increase in IgG anti-D.

ABO INCOMPATIBILITY

It appears that the risk of Rh immunization is approximately 16% when an Rh-negative woman has her first pregnancy with an ABO-compatible Rh-positive fetus. If the mother is not immunized by the first pregnancy, the risk appears approximately the same for the second pregnancy. Although subsequent pregnancy risks for nonresponding patients decreases, a patient undergoing five Rh-positive ABO-compatible pregnancies has a 50% likelihood of becoming Rh immunized. As ancillary consideration is the impact of fetal ABO incompatibility, which confers partial protections, thereby decreasing immunization risks markedly. Woodrow calculated that the risk of Rh immunization after an ABO-incompatible Rh-positive pregnancy is approximately 2%. Although, FMH sufficient to cause immunization can occur throughout the pregnancy and delivery process, as many as 2% of Rh-negative women become Rh immunized during otherwise uncomplicated pregnancies between 28 weeks of gestation and delivery. This represents 12% of all Rh-negative women who would become Rh immunized as a result of Rh-positive pregnancies. This has led to the recommendation for the administration of Rh immunoglobulin to all unsensitized Rh-negative pregnant women at 28 weeks of gestation.

PATHOPHYSIOLOGY

When a RhD-negative woman is pregnant with a RhD-positive fetus (having inherited the RhD antigen from its father), isoimmunization can occur. Any FMH can potentially lead to maternal exposure to fetal RBCs, which can trigger a maternal immune response. This FMH can result from antenatal or peripartum sensitizing events, which includes threatened miscarriage, ectopic pregnancy, any invasive prenatal procedure (chorionic villous sampling, amniocentesis, etc.), antepartum hemorrhage, external cephalic version, manual removal of placenta and closed abdominal injury. Only approximately 1–2% of Rh alloimmunization is caused by antenatal FMH.[2] An amount as little as 0.1 mL of RhD-positive blood is sufficient to cause isoimmunization.[3] Without immune prophylaxis, there is a 16% risk that an Rh-negative woman bearing a Rh-positive child will become Rh-isoimmunized.[4]

The initial response of the maternal immune system against the Rh factor is production of IgM antibodies, which typically cannot cross the placenta. This is why the chance of significant fetal or neonatal compromise is unlikely in the first pregnancy and the baby escapes insult. However, in the next pregnancy, exposure of maternal immune system to Rh-positive fetal RBCs (that escape into maternal circulation through the placenta) elicits an anamnestic response leading to rapid and robust production of antibodies. This secondary response is characterized by production of IgG antibodies that cross the placenta freely into the fetal circulation and bind to the antigenic sites on fetal RBCs. These cells are then hemolyzed via complement mediated pathways, releasing bilirubin. Inability of the fetus to replenish the RBCs and to keep pace with ongoing hemolysis due to huge influx of maternal antibodies results into anemia. Severe fetal anemia can lead to a high output cardiac failure resulting in fluid accumulation in body cavities. This combination of fluid accumulation in at least two extravascular compartments (pericardial effusion, pleural effusion, ascites, or subcutaneous edema) is referred to as hydrops fetalis. The excess bilirubin from the hemolyzed RBCs can accumulate in the fetal basal ganglia resulting in neurological damage and even death (kernicterus).

Once alloimmunization has occurred, irrespective of the type of antibody involved, the principles of management remain essentially similar. The only exception may be Kell alloimmunization as here the antibody levels do not always correlate with disease severity and there is much greater suppression of erythropoiesis rather than intravascular hemolysis.

RISK FACTORS

Although the numbers are equivocal, it appears that approximately 2% of women having spontaneous or therapeutic abortion are at risk of becoming Rh immunized. It is suggested that early abortion (6–8 weeks) carries a much lower risk than later abortion. The risk increases to 5% after 20 weeks of gestation.

The diagnosis and management of the Rh immunized pregnancy depends on the early initial evaluation and identification patients at risk. A blood sample should be taken from every woman at her first antenatal visit for blood type, Rh blood grouping and antibody screening. This test should be universal and carried out independent of reported results of prior screening tests.

EVALUATION

All patients should be evaluated for prior sensitization. It is incumbent on the practitioner to follow sensitized pregnancies closely with both maternal and fetal surveillance.

Antibody Titers

Serial antibody titers are the mainstay of maternal assessment. After it is determined that there is maternal sensitization and the possibility of fetal antigen positivity, additional antibody titer determinations should be performed at the pregnancy progress. A second maternal antibody titer is performed at 18–20 weeks of gestation and then repeated monthly for the rest of the pregnancy. Rarely does significant hemolytic disease in the fetus occur before 20 weeks of gestation.

Fetal Assessment

Fetal antigen status can be inferred from information gained from antigen testing of the father. When necessary, fetal antigen status can be determined directly by cord-blood sampling or from fetal cells obtained by amniocentesis. Fetal anemia can be diagnosed from fetal blood obtained from cord-blood sampling. Ultrasound is the primary tool for fetal surveillance throughout the pregnancy. It can provide several types of information, all of which are critical to successful management:

- Fetal growth
- Fetal well-being by biophysical profile scoring
- Presence of ascites or hydrops as indicators of fetal anemia
- Assessment of middle cerebral artery (MCA) blood flow by Doppler technology as a direct assessment of fetal anemia and risk of intrauterine death.

Antepartum fetal testing is used to monitor the development of fetal hypoxia due to fetal anemia.

PREVENTION OF ISOIMMUNIZATION

Anti-D Ig is indicated only in nonsensitized Rh-negative women for prevention of isoimmunization. Following administration of anti-D, a positive antibody screen will be found in the woman.[5] This response is typically of low titer and weakly reactive (not exceeding 1:8). Anti-D crosses the placenta and binds to fetal RBCs, without causing hemolysis, anemia or jaundice.[6] Postnatal anti-D to Rh-negative women reduces the risk of sensitization from around 16% to approximately 2%. The residual 2% risk is believed to result from sensitization occurring during the course of pregnancy, especially during the third trimester. This is the reason why routine antenatal prophylaxis at the beginning of the third trimester is advocated.

Antenatal

Anti-D Ig 300 μg (1,500 IU) should be given routinely to all Rh-negative nonsensitized women at 28 weeks' of gestation when fetal blood type is unknown or known to be Rh-positive.[7] Without antenatal anti-D prophylaxis, 1.6–1.9%

of Rh-negative women risk becoming sensitized.[8] The Royal College of Obstetricians and Gynaecologists (RCOG) alternatively advises two doses of 100 µg (500 IU) at 28 weeks and 34 weeks of gestation.[9]

The RCOG recommends anti-D for miscarriage (threatened or spontaneous), only if:
- The gestational age is beyond 12 weeks
- There is no medical or surgical intervention needed for completion of miscarriage.[9]

An intramuscular dose of 500 IU of anti-D will neutralize a FMH of up to 4 mL of fetal RBCs. For each milliliter in excess of 4 mL, a further 125 µg of anti-D is necessary. Minimum recommended doses of anti-D at less than 20 weeks of gestation and at 20 + 0 weeks of gestation and above are 250 IU and 500 IU respectively.[9]

Postnatal

The postnatal dose varies in different countries 1,500 IU (300 µg) is the standard dose in the USA and India, 500–600 IU (100–120 µg) in Canada and 1,000–1,250 IU in many European countries. It is important to note that the countries using a smaller dose use a routine Kleihauer-Betke test for estimation of FMH and need for additional anti-D. For successful immunoprophylaxis, anti-D should be given as soon as possible after the potential sensitizing event, but always within 72 hours. If it is not given before 72 hours, every effort should still be made to administer the anti-D, as a dose given within 10 days may provide some protection. Ideally, anti-D should be administered intramuscularly into the deltoid muscle.[9]

Who Needs Extra Dose?

Certain circumstances may be associated with heavier FMH[10] and may need additional dose of anti-D. These include:
- Traumatic deliveries including cesarean section
- Manual removal of the placenta
- Stillbirths and fetal deaths
- Abdominal trauma during the third trimester
- Twin pregnancies (at delivery)
- Unexplained hydrops fetalis.

Here it is important to quantify the FMH using the Kleihauer acid elution test and calculate the dose of anti-D accordingly. Patients who are weak-D positive (D^u) are not at risk for isoimmunization and should not receive anti-D immunoprophylaxis.

ANTENATAL MANAGEMENT OF AN ISOIMMUNIZED MOTHER

Screening

All pregnant women should be tested at the time of the first prenatal visit for ABO blood group and RhD type. Some countries universally screen for the presence of erythrocyte antibodies. If the woman is positive for certain antibodies, the severity of immune response is determined by titers using the indirect Coombs test. Critical titer is the titer at which the fetus is at a significant risk of developing severe hemolysis, anemia and hydrops. This is generally different for different labs and can range between 1:8 and 1:32. Hence, it is important to perform testing in the same laboratory, maintaining uniformity. Also, the antibody titers only represent maternal antibody response severity and not the fetal status. If the initial antibody titer is 1: 8 or less, the patient may be monitored with titer assessment every 4 weeks. For patients with alloimmunization involving antigens other than D, similar titer levels should be used to guide care except in Kell-sensitized patients because Kell antibodies do not correlate with fetal status.[11]

Maternal titers are not useful in predicting the onset of fetal anemia after the first affected gestation. In a woman who has already had a sensitized pregnancy, the titers become less reliable, and fetal surveillance should be initiated at the earliest gestational age at which fetal transfusion is an option, usually 18 weeks.[12,13]

Husband's Blood Group/Rh Type and Fetal Status

Once a woman is found to be isoimmunized to a particular antigen, it is important to know the status of her partner for that particular erythrocyte antigen. Further testing is unnecessary, if the partner is negative for the given antigen. With regards to the RhD antigen, if the father is homozygous for the D antigen, all his children will be Rh-positive and the fetus will need surveillance; if he is heterozygous, there is a 50% likelihood that each pregnancy will have an Rh-negative fetus that is not at risk of anemia.

The fetal antigen type should be assessed when the paternal genotype is thought to be heterozygous or is unknown. This can be accomplished by subjecting an amniocentesis sample to a polymerase chain reaction (PCR). Alternatively, detection of fetal DNA in maternal plasma for RhD antigen status is a newer technique that uses molecular analysis with greater than 99% accuracy in the second trimester.[14,15] However, if access to either of these techniques is a problem or if invasive testing is not desired, these isoimmunized pregnancies can be managed with noninvasive ultrasound assessment of the fetal MCA using Doppler.

Paternal antigen testing should be performed, and if the father is antigen negative, there is no risk of fetal hemolytic disease, no matter what the maternal antibody titer.

As extramarital pregnancies do occur, patients should be made aware of the potential for catastrophic complications should be wrong male be tested as the father of the baby. If there is any uncertainty about paternity, the pregnancy should be treated as having unknown paternal antigen status with presumption of risk for Rh immunization or fetal disease to occur.

Traditionally, the management of isoimmunized pregnancies used amniocentesis to determine the optical density of the amniotic fluid at 450 nm using spectrophotometry. Bilirubin in the amniotic fluid results in a deviation of the optical density at this wavelength. This difference [optical density difference (Δ OD_{450})] is then plotted on the Liley chart or the Queenan curve (for earlier gestations) to assess the degree of severity of hemolysis or fetal anemia and the need for intrauterine transfusion (IUT). Fetuses affected by hemolytic disease secrete abnormally high levels of bilirubin into the amniotic fluid. The amount of bilirubin can be quantitated by spectrophotometrically measuring absorbance at the 450 nm wavelength in a specimen of amniotic fluid that has been shielded from light. Alternatively, percutaneous umbilical blood sampling (PUBS) may be used to determine all blood parameters directly.

If amniocentesis is used to monitor the fetus, the results (Δ 450) are plotted on a 'Liley' curve (Fig. 1).

The Liley curve is divided into three zones:

- A result in zone I indicates mild or no disease. Fetuses in zone I are usually followed with amniocentesis every 3 weeks
- A result in zone II indicates intermediate disease. Fetuses in low zone II are usually followed by amniocentesis every 1–2 weeks
- A result above the middle of zone II may require transfusion or delivery.

Patients with results in zone I or low zone II can be allowed to proceed to term, at which point labor should be induced. In most cases, patients in the middle of zone II can progress to 36–38 weeks of gestation. Depending on gestational age, patients in zone III should either be delivered or should receive intrauterine fetal transfusion.

Although serial determinations of delta optical density at 450 nm and PUBS are the most common methods for the evaluation of fetal status, Doppler ultrasonography of the MCA has also been used to identify fetuses at risk for moderate to severe hemolytic disease.

Lastly, in women with extremely high titers (>256), at less than 28 weeks, where the fetus does not demonstrate hydrops, and there is a documented history of fetal death due to hydrops intravenous immunoglobulin (IVIg) might be offered. The dose is 400 mg/kg/day for 5 days, with repeat infusions every 15–21 days. Specific contraindications to IVIg use include a previous episode of intravenous immunoglobulin-induced anaphylaxis (rare) and selective IgA deficiency.

MIDDLE CEREBRAL ARTERY: PEAK SYSTOLIC VELOCITY

The current management uses the MCA peak systolic velocity (PSV) to diagnose fetuses with severe anemia. Fetal anemia results in a hyperdynamic circulation which increases the PSV of the MCA. MCA-PSV is more than 1.5 times the median for a given gestational age, predicts moderate-to-severe anemia with a sensitivity of 100% and a false-positive rate of 12%.[16]

Of course, the MCA Doppler has certain pitfalls. Firstly, the angle of insonation to the MCA should be as close to zero

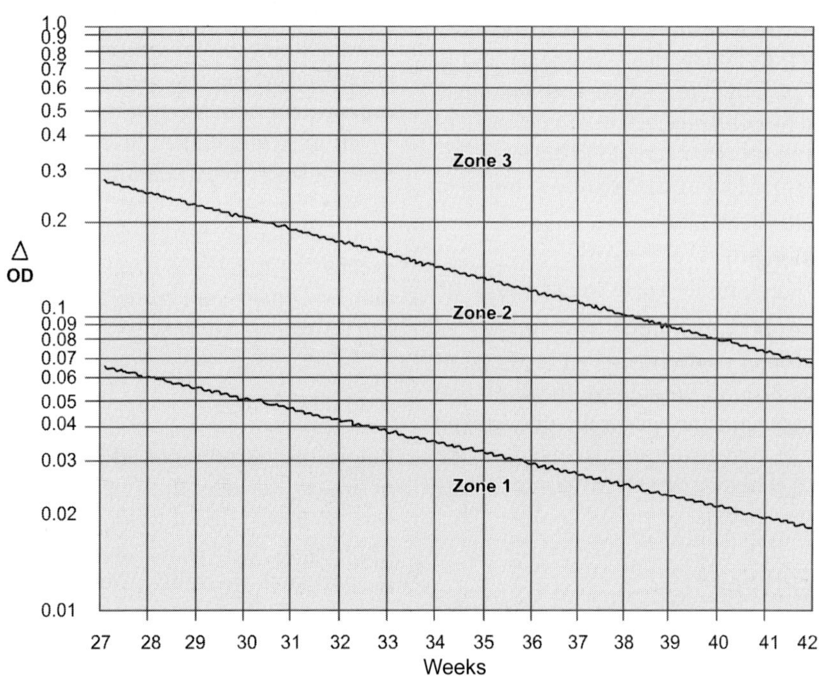

FIG. 1: Liley graph.

as possible. Any angulation of the probe induces an error in the PSV reading. Thus, this should be undertaken only by experienced sonographers. Secondly, sampling should be done as close to the origin of MCA as possible and whole length of the MCA should be visualized. The baby should be resting; not moving or breathing. Thirdly, there is a higher false-positive rate with this technique after 34–35 weeks of gestation.[17]

CORDOCENTESIS AND INTRAUTERINE BLOOD TRANSFUSION

Once the MCA-PSV reaches 1.50 MoM, cordocentesis is recommended and is the gold standard for detection of fetal anemia. In general, the average fetal hematocrit is 36–44% and with severe anemia, it is less than 30%.[18] The patient should be counseled that there is a fetal loss rate related to the procedure and that it depends on the gestation, site of sampling and underlying pathology. The risk of an uncomplicated fetal blood sampling (FBS) is 1–3%, but if the fetus is hydropic it may be as high as 20%. Fetal blood can be taken either from the placental cord insertion site or from the intrahepatic vein. Complications of FBS include fetal bradycardia, hemorrhage, cord hematoma and tamponade, and fetal death. The procedure is done under continuous ultrasound guidance, and facilities for immediate analysis of the fetal blood should be available.

The common sites for IUT are the cord insertion and the intraperitoneal. These transfusions can also be in the intrahepatic umbilical vein or even intracardiac. A combined technique of intravascular and intraperitoneal allows for longer intervals between transfusions. The ideal red cells used for IUT are: type O, RhD-negative, cytomegalovirus-negative, hemoglobin S-negative, irradiated and leukocyte poor. The red cells should be tightly packed to a hematocrit of 75–90% in an effort to avoid volume overload in the fetus.[13,17] There are many formulae to calculate the volume of blood to be transfused. A commonly used one is:

Volume of blood transfusion [mL] = [Gestational age in weeks - 20] × 10.

An intravenous dose of vecuronium (0.1 mg/kg of ultrasonogram-estimated fetal weight) is given at the start of the intravascular transfusion to immobilize the baby and prevent fetal injury. Transfusions are generally undertaken at 2-week intervals for the first two transfusions, then the interval is lengthened to 3–4 weeks. Weekly MCA monitoring is essential in between transfusions.

DELIVERY AND POSTPARTUM

Timing of delivery: there is no consensus as to the best timing of delivery. The pregnancy should be prolonged until the fetus reaches a gestational age necessary for survival. In mild hemolysis, it would be reasonable to wait until 37–38 weeks of gestation. With severely sensitized pregnancies requiring multiple invasive procedures, however, the risks of continued cord blood sampling and transfusions must be considered and compared with those neonatal risks associated with early delivery. Given that the overall neonatal survival rate after 32 weeks of gestation in most neonatal intensive care nurseries is greater than 95%, it is prudent to time procedures so that the last transfusion is performed at 30–32 weeks of gestation, with delivery at 32–34 weeks of gestation after maternal steroid administration to enhance fetal pulmonary maturity.[19] Some other authors recommend IUT up to 36 weeks of gestation, when intravascular transfusion is feasible in order to limit neonatal morbidity.[20] Delivery can then be accomplished between 37 weeks and 38 weeks of gestation. At delivery, cord blood should be collected for analyses of hemoglobin, packed cell volume and bilirubin, and for a direct antiglobulin test (DAT). The mode of delivery is dependent on standard obstetric grounds. Prior intrauterine therapy is not an indication for an elective cesarean section.

PROGNOSIS

Fifty percent of all isoimmunized fetuses are mildly affected. The fetal anemia is mild at birth, and bilirubin levels do not rise to dangerous levels.

Twenty-five to thirty percent of isoimmunized fetuses have moderate disease. In these cases, hematopoiesis is sufficient to keep up with the rate of hemolysis. Hepatic function is not compromised. *In utero*, the placenta is able to clear the breakdown products of hemolysis. After delivery, neonatal bilirubin levels rise rapidly. Exchange transfusion is needed to prevent neonatal death or severe neurologic impairment from kernicterus.

In the remaining 20–25% of affected fetuses, severe anemia leads to extramedullary hematopoiesis, particularly in the liver. Liver obstruction and decreased hepatic synthetic-activity lead to portal and umbilical hypertension, ascites, hydrops and fetal death. Without either IUT or delivery, only a small proportion of severely affected fetuses can be expected to survive.

OUTCOMES

Before the introduction of fetal or neonatal treatment, the perinatal mortality from hemolytic disease of the newborn was 40–50%.[21] The development of the neonatal exchange transfusion in 1945 was accompanied by a 50% reduction in perinatal mortality. Despite this innovative neonatal therapy, hydropic fetuses continued to die *in utero*. With IUT, the overall survival was noted to be 84% with nonhydropic fetuses having better outcomes (92%) than hydropic fetuses (70%).[22] The neonate may face early anemia due to ongoing hemolysis from the passively transferred maternal antibodies or sometimes late anemia as a result of suppressed erythropoiesis secondary to transfusions. Normal neurodevelopmental outcome can be expected in more than 90% of cases. The incidence of sensorineural hearing loss is increased in babies because of the toxic effect of prolonged exposure of bilirubin on the developing eighth cranial nerve.[23]

NEWER TREATMENT MODALITIES

Extensive plasmapheresis with partial replacement using 5% albumin and IVIg or the administration of IVIg at 1 g/kg body weight weekly has been shown to be moderately effective in early-onset severe disease. The mechanism of action appears to be blockage of Fc receptors in the placenta, reducing antibody transport across to the fetus, Fc receptors on the phagocytes in the fetal reticuloendothelial system and feedback inhibition of maternal antibody synthesis. However, these techniques only postpone the need for cordocentesis and transfusion until 20–22 weeks' gestation, when these procedures can be performed at a more acceptable risk. A review of IVIg use found that it is useful in preventing the onset of fetal hydrops and in delaying the need for IUT.[24]

REFERENCES

1. Pahuja S, Gupta SK, Pujani M, et al. The prevalence of irregular erythrocyte antibodies among antenatal women in Delhi. Blood Transfus. 2011;9:388-93.
2. Davey M. The prevention of rhesus-isoimmunization. Clin Obstet Gynaecol. 1979;6:509-30.
3. Zipursky A, Pollack J, Neelands P, et al. The transplacental passage of foetal red blood-cells and the pathogenesis of Rh immunization during pregnancy. Lancet-1963;2:489-93.
4. Bowman JM. Controversies in Rh prophylaxis: who needs Rh immune globulin and when should it be given? Am J Obstet Gynecol. 1985;151:289-94.
5. Hartwell EA. Use of Rh immune globulin. ASCP practice parameter. American Society of Clinical Pathologists. Am J Clin Pathol. 1998;110:281-92.
6. Trolle B. Prenatal Rh-immune prophylaxis with 300 µg immune globulin anti-D in the 28th week of pregnancy. Acta Obstet Gynecol Scand. 1989;68:45-7.
7. Fung Kee Fung K, Eason E, Crane J, Armson A, De La Ronde S, et al. Prevention of Rh Alloimmunization. SOGC clinical practice guideline. J Obstet Gynaecol Can. 2003;25(9):765-73.
8. Hadley A, Kumpel B. The role of Rh antibodies in haemolytic disease of the newborn. Baillieres Clin Haematol. 1993;6:423-44.
9. The Royal College of Obstetricians and Gynaecologists (RCOG). (2011). The use of Anti-D immunoglobulin for rhesus D prophylaxis: Green top Guideline no 22. [online] Available from www.rcog.org.uk/en/guidelines-research-services/guidelines/gtg22/. [Accessed December, 2015].
10. The American College of Obstetricians and Gynecologists (ACOG). Prevention of Rh D Alloimmunization. ACOG Practice Bulletin 4. Obstet Gynecol. 1999;93(5).
11. Hackney DN, Knudtson EJ, Rossi KQ, et al. Management of pregnancies complicated by anti-c isoimmunization. Obstet Gynecol. 2004;103:24-30.
12. Spinnato JA. Hemolytic disease of the fetus: a plea for restraint. Obstet Gynecol. 1992;80:873-7.
13. Bowman JM. Hemolytic disease (erythroblastosis fetalis). In: Creasy RK, Resnik R, (Eds). Maternal-fetal medicine. 4th edition. Philadelphia, PA, USA: WB Saunders; 1999. pp. 736-67.
14. Lo YM, Hjelm NM, Fidler C, Sargent IL, Murphy MF, Chamberlain PF, et al. Prenatal diagnosis of fetal RhD status by molecular analysis of maternal plasma. N Engl J Med. 1998;339:1734-8.
15. Gautier E, Benachi A, Giovangrandi Y, Ernault P, Olivi M, Gaillon T, et al. Fetal RhD genotyping by maternal serum analysis: a two-year experience. Am J Obstet Gynecol. 2005;192:666-9.
16. Mari G, Deter RL, Carpenter RL, Rahman F, Zimmerman R, Moise KJ, et al. Noninvasive diagnosis by Doppler ultrasonography of fetal anemia due to maternal red-cell alloimmunization. Collaborative Group for Doppler Assessment of the Blood Velocity of Anemic Fetuses. N Engl J Med. 2000;342:9-14.
17. Moise KJ. Management of rhesus alloimmunization in pregnancy. Obstet Gynecol. 2002;100:600-11.
18. Maxwell DJ, Johnson P, Hurley P, Neales K, Allan L, Knott P. Fetal blood sampling and pregnancy loss in relation to indication. Br J Obstet Gynaecol. 1991;98(9):892-7.
19. Bowman JM. Maternal alloimmunization and fetal hemolytic disease. In: Reece EA, Hobbins JC (Eds). Medicine of the fetus and mother, 2nd edition. Philadelphia: Lippincott-Raven; 1999. pp. 1241-69.
20. Boggs TR. Survival rates in Rh sensitizations: 140 interrupted versus 141 uninterrupted pregnancies. Pediatrics 1964;33:758-62.
21. Bowman JM. The management of Rh-isoimmunization. Obstet Gynecol. 1978;52:1-16.
22. Schumacher B, Moise KJ. Fetal transfusion for red blood cell alloimmunization in pregnancy. Obstet Gynecol. 1996;88:137-50.
23. Hudon L, Moise KJ, Hegemier SE, Hill RM, Moise AA, Smith EO, et al. Long-term neurodevelopmental outcome after intrauterine transfusion for the treatment of fetal hemolytic disease. Am J Obstet Gynecol. 1998;179:858-63.
24. Voto LS, Mathet ER, Zapaterio JL, Orti J, Lede RL, Margulies M. High-dose gamma globulin (IVIg) followed by intrauterine transfusions (IUTs): a new alternative for the treatment of severe fetal hemolytic disease. J Perinat Med. 1997;25(1):85-8.

Section 7

Medical and Surgical Complications

CHAPTER 47

Cardiovascular Diseases and Chronic Hypertension

Suman Puri, Sandeep Puri, Kanupriya Jain, Arshdeep Singh, Gurleen Wander

INTRODUCTION

The cardiovascular system is the most severely affected by the physiological changes of pregnancy. The cardiac disease is identified particularly in the third trimester when the cardiac output doubles. Usually pregnancy comes as a temporary complication in the disease process of the patient's cardiac lesion, a process which in any case is likely to shorten life. Under good supervision, provided that the extra demands of pregnancy are met, it should be possible for a cardiac patient to emerge from the experience of childbirth without any degradation in her underlying condition.

INCIDENCE OF HEART DISEASES IN PREGNANCY

Although the reported incidence of heart disease in pregnancy varies between 0.1% and 4%,[1] cardiac disease remains a significant cause of maternal death worldwide.[2] In west, the traditional preponderance of rheumatic heart disease (RHD) is becoming progressively less. In contrast, mitral stenosis is a common condition in pregnant women with heart disease in developing countries. Rheumatic mitral stenosis forms 88% of the heart diseases complicating pregnancy in the tertiary referral center in India.[3] Congenital heart diseases (CHD) are the most common birth defects in humans, affecting approximately 0.8% of all live births.[4] With the advances in medical and surgical care, many women with CHD are now reaching reproductive age. Although rare, the incidence of acute myocardial infarction is estimated at 0.6–1 per 10,000 pregnancies.[5] Myocardial infarction occurs more commonly in the third trimester and most commonly involves the anterior wall.[6] With the increasing age and fertility of mothers the incidence of coronary artery disease in pregnancy is likely to increase. The incidence of peripartum cardiomyopathy is estimated at between 1 in 1,500 and 1 in 4,000 deliveries in United States.[7]

PREPREGNANCY EVALUATION

Ideally, patients with known cardiac disease should be properly assessed before pregnancy. Prepregnancy evaluation should focus on identifying and quantifying risks for both mother and offspring. Assessment should include a full history and examination, and an echocardiogram. If patients are already symptomatic, serious consideration should be given to interventional therapy or surgery prior to pregnancy to avoid life-threatening complications. It is important to assess the functional capacity of the heart. This is done according to the New York Heart Association (NYHA) Classification for symptoms, like angina, dyspnea, palpitations and fatigue as shown in table 1.

TABLE 1: New York Heart Association Classification

Class I	Patient with cardiac disease, but without limitation of the physical activity
Class II	Patient with cardiac disease resulting in slight limitation of the physical activity
Class III	Patient with cardiac disease resulting in marked limitation of the physical activity
Class IV	Patient with cardiac disease resulting in inability to carry out any physical activity without discomfort

COMPLICATIONS OF PREGNANCY WITH CARDIAC DISEASE

The type of complication depends on the specific cardiac pathology. Arrhythmias and cardiac failure are the two most common complications encountered.

Atrial fibrillation complicating pregnancy has a high mortality. Szekely and Snaith[8] demonstrated that in cases fibrillating before pregnancy, the incidence of frank heart failure developing during pregnancy or in puerperium was 25% as compared to 70% in patients who developed fibrillation during pregnancy. Atrial fibrillation is a medical emergency. Pharmacological therapy includes digoxin and β-blockers. Electric cardioversion is performed, if the pharmacological therapy fails. It is safe for the fetus.

In patients with atrial fibrillation, anticoagulant therapy is mandatory irrespective of the severity of the cardiac lesion. During the first trimester, there is significant risk of embryopathy and fetal hemorrhage with vitamin K antagonists.[9] However, these can be used safely during the second and third trimester, provided that heparin is substituted at week 36[10] or a cesarean section is planned. Therapy with low molecular weight heparin (2,500 IU S/C once daily) instead of conventional heparin is gaining popularity due to less stringent monitoring of the coagulogram. The effects of heparin can be immediately corrected by protamine whereas those of warfarin and similar anticoagulants take many hours to reverse. Postpartum, when the immediate risk of hemorrhage has passed, warfarin cover is resumed.

Valvular heart diseases, like mitral stenosis produce pulmonary hypertension and subsequent pulmonary edema. All patients with heart failure during pregnancy should be admitted for bed rest. Medical treatment includes salt and fluid restriction, diuretics and antihypertensive therapy. Angiotensin converting enzyme (ACE) inhibitors are generally contraindicated in pregnancy due to their poor safety profile.

Infective endocarditis is a potentially fatal complication during pregnancy. Antibiotic prophylaxis is required to prevent this at the time of delivery. It should be administered, if patient is suspected for bacteremia and if cardiac lesion is a high-risk lesion like prosthetic cardiac valves, history of prior endocarditis, complex cyanotic congenital cardiac malformation or there is presence of surgical shunt. Prophylaxis includes ampicillin (2 g) plus gentamicin (1.5 mg/kg) followed by 1 g ampicillin 6 hours later.

DIAGNOSIS DURING PREGNANCY

Identifying deterioration of an existing cardiac condition is a diagnostic challenge as normal physiological changes also produce similar signs and symptoms which mimic cardiac diseases. A thorough physical examination is of prime importance. Appearance of a diastolic murmur merits further investigations. Some symptoms of cardiac disease in pregnancy are progressive dyspnea, nocturnal cough, hemoptysis, syncope and chest pain. Some of the important signs are cyanosis, clubbing of fingers, persistent neck vein distension, systolic murmur grade III or more, diastolic murmur, cardiomegaly, persistent arrhythmia, split second heart sound and any evidence of pulmonary hypertension. Electrocardiography, echocardiography, magnetic resonance imaging and cardiac biomarkers [CPK-MB, troponin I, brain natriuretic peptide (BNP), pregnancy associated plasma protein A (PAPP-A)] can be useful adjuncts. Most relevant investigation is the echocardiography which allows noninvasive evaluation of cardiac structure and function. Moreover, it does not involve X-ray exposure.

GENERAL MANAGEMENT DURING PREGNANCY

Patient with heart disease should be supervised in a tertiary care center. Initial assessment should be made in consultation with the cardiologist. The patient's NYHA class should be decided in first few months of pregnancy. Table 2 mentions the safety profile of the cardiovascular drugs to be used during pregnancy.

Adequate rest should be ensured and physical activity permitted only to a degree which falls short of producing discomfort. Pregnant ladies with lower NYHA class need monthly antenatal visits, but those in NYHA class III and IV need to be assessed every week. These patients need to be informed about the inherent risks of pregnancy continuation. If seen early enough consideration should be given to termination of pregnancy. If pregnancy is continued planned care should be stressed upon. Weight gain should be

TABLE 2: Safety profile of commonly used cardiovascular drugs in pregnancy[12]

Drug	FDA category
Atenolol	D
Other β-blockers	C
ACE inhibitors/ARBs	D
Amiodarone	D
Aspirin/clopidogrel	B
Calcium channel antagonists	C
Digoxin	C
Loop diuretics	C
Thiazide diuretics	B
Low molecular weight heparin	C
Spironolactone	D
Statins	X

ACE, angiotensin converting enzyme; ARB, angiotensin receptor blocker.

restricted as far as possible by diet and reducing salt intake. Anemia needs vigorous management. Women should avoid contact with people who have respiratory infections to protect against endocarditis. Pneumococcal and influenza vaccines are recommended. Cigarette smoking should be stopped. The condition of teeth should be attended thoroughly. The onset of pre-eclamptic toxaemia should be taken even more seriously than usual as there is increased fluid retention.[11]

Reassessment of the patient's functional class should be done between 28 and 32 week. Any deterioration in functional class should be reversed by bed rest and medical therapy before labor.

A need for interventional therapy may arise when cardiac functions deteriorate during pregnancy. Such procedures are performed in second trimester (13–28 weeks). Radiation of the fetus and its teratogenic effect are an important consideration. first trimester irradiation will be associated with higher incidence of fetal malformation.

Cardiac surgery should be done only if all other treatment modalities have failed. Due to increased risk of malformations, surgery is best avoided in first trimester. Second trimester is favored period for any invasive procedure. However, intraoperative complications, embolic phenomenon, placental hypoperfusion and risk of preterm labor can cause increased fetal mortality and morbidity. In third trimester, the risk of prematurity should be weighed against the risk of surgery.

Management During Labor

Most of the patients with cardiac disease can be delivered vaginally unless there is an obstetric indication for cesarean delivery. Delivery should be conducted in a tertiary health institution where a cardiologist and anesthesiologist are available round the clock.

Induction of Labor

This is seldom necessary in patients with heart disease. But it may be done for obstetric reasons keeping a watch on development of cardiac failure and pulmonary edema. It is usually safe to induce labor.

First Stage of Labor

Patients who are NYHA class III or IV may require invasive monitoring during labor. The role of encouragement and assurance to the patient to keep up the morale is not to be undermined.

- Pelvic assessment: trial of labor in a contracted pelvis is absolutely contraindicated
- Position: the patient should be confined to bed and propped up with a lateral tilt. Oxygen can be given by mask, if required. Patient can be given digoxin, if the pulse rate exceeds 110/minute or respiratory rate increases to 24/minute. Vitals should be monitored frequently
- Fluids: restrict fluid infusion to less than 75 mL/hour to prevent pulmonary edema
- Antibiotics: prophylactic antibiotics during labor are considered appropriate to prevent endocarditis. Dose, number and duration of antibiotics required are decided according to the cardiac lesion
- Analgesia: epidural (bupivacaine/fentanyl). It has long been recognized that potentially dangerous intrapartum fluctuations in cardiac output can be minimized by using epidural anesthesia.[13] Tachycardia secondary to labor pains is averted by epidural analgesia. Hypotension should be avoided
- Assessment of progress of labor: uterine contractions, fetal heart rate, cervical dilatation and descent of head and color of the liquor should be assessed.

The average duration of labor is usually shortened in the cardiac case and 8 hours in the first stage would be an average figure.

Second Stage of Labor

Constant supervision is mandatory. Fetal heart rate is recorded at every 5 minutes. A Swan-Ganz catheter is a useful adjunct as it helps to determine the fluid status and the pressure in the left heart. Some schools of thought recommend cardiac catheterization in all the patients with moderate to severe mitral stenosis during labor.[14]

In general, a term vaginal delivery in a well-managed cardiac patient is the best solution to various problems presented by maternal heart disease and pregnancy.

Second stage is the stage of effort and effort on the part of the patient has to be avoided or curtailed by instrumentation. A golden practice is to prepare the instrument trolley as soon as the patient is fully dilated. As soon as the head is at the perineum, episiotomy is worthwhile as it facilitates effortless delivery. The forceps should not be used unless the patient is unlikely to deliver herself within the next 20 minutes. Ventouse is preferable to forceps as it can be applied without putting the patient in lithotomy position. This is a huge advantage as raising legs increases the venous return and puts strain on the already burdened heart.

In cases of severe disease, pelvic disproportion, prolonged labor, pre-eclampsia and in coarctation of aorta, cesarean section has been advocated as the preferred mode of delivery.

Third Stage of Labor

It is the most crucial stage of labor. Placental separation and its descent into vagina are allowed to occur spontaneously. Constant watch is mandatory. Active management of third stage is done. Oxytocin infusion is preferred over ergometrine. Ergometrine will increase the heart's load by causing additional blood to be squeezed into circulation and also it shuts down the uterine arteriovenous shunt. Injection furosemide can be given intravenously usually in a dose of 40 mg to decrease the cardiac load.

As soon as the delivery is completed, the patient should be propped up. Early ambulation is recommended as these patients are at an increased risk of thromboembolic phenomenon. In order to increase the venous return, the use of elastic stockings is encouraged.

Puerperium

The most hazardous time for these women appears to be the immediate postpartum period. Such patients often enter the postpartum period already operating at maximum cardiac output and cannot accommodate the volume shifts that follow delivery. Signs of pulmonary congestion must be carefully watched for. Patient is not allowed out of bed, until all signs of cardiac failure, if present have disappeared. Any infection in puerperium is taken seriously. Visitors are to be restricted to minimum.

Patient should be kept under observation in the hospital for a minimum of 5 days. Discharge from hospital should be more delayed in case any complications arise. A good follow-up system is essential. It is a part of the responsibility of the obstetrician and cardiologist to prepare pregnant women with heart disease for responsible motherhood. During pregnancy a flexible plan of continuing care should be developed, and its importance emphasized during the postpartum period.

Contraception

These patients need contraception counseling. Steroidal contraception is contraindicated. Intrauterine devices are capable of inducing infection. Barrier methods of contraception are advocated. Sterilization should be considered at the end of first week of puerperium under local anesthesia. If heart is not well compensated, husband is advised for vasectomy.

RHEUMATIC HEART DISEASE

Of all forms of RHD, mitral stenosis is the most common and accounts for around 75% of all the cases. Sometimes it is first diagnosed during pregnancy. The symptoms may peak at around 20–24 weeks gestation as cardiac output and intravascular volume peaks, and then stabilize. Patients with severe mitral stenosis remain at risk of heart failure and pulmonary edema throughout the third trimester and into the puerperium as well.

Pregnant women with RHD of moderate-severe mitral stenosis, severe pulmonary hypertension and atrial fibrillation are at high-risk of heart failure. Fetal outcome is also poor in cases of NYHA class III and IV. An acute attack of rheumatism, superimposed on a damaged heart, can be precipitated during pregnancy.[15] It poses a very serious threat and death may rapidly follow delivery in cases of active rheumatic carditis. All patients with RHD or a past history of rheumatic fever should be placed on antibiotic prophylaxis against recurrent rheumatic fever as soon as possible. Infective endocarditis is a real risk and should be suspected when patient shows tachycardia at rest, dyspnea, fever, edema, anemia and occasionally proteinuria. Splenic enlargement and embolic phenomenon may be demonstrated.[15]

Women with valvular replacement surgery can undertake a pregnancy only after serious consideration. Before pregnancy anticoagulation with warfarin is appropriate. During early pregnancy warfarin is not advisable as spontaneous abortions, malformed fetuses are more common. This drug also has a long half-life so is inappropriate at the time of labor. Recommendations are to switch to unfractionated heparin between 6 weeks and 12 weeks and after 36 weeks. Regular monitoring of coagulation parameters is done. Heparin is stopped just before delivery and then restarted 6 hours after vaginal delivery or 24 hours after cesarean section.

CONGENITAL HEART DISEASE

A patient management plan should already be drawn up before the onset of pregnancy by a pediatric cardiologist. Patients with CHD are at a greater risk of pulmonary thromboembolism. Every decision regarding anticoagulation during pregnancy must take account of the risks for the mother and child. The administration of low dose acetylsalicylic acid is useful in these patient populations.

Background

- There has been a marked increase in the incidence of pregnancies complicated by CHD because patients who would have died in childhood before modern medical and surgical techniques are surviving to reproductive age
- Fetal risks include:
    - Growth restriction due to maternal cyanosis (i.e. tetralogy of Fallot and Eisenmenger syndrome) or decreased uterine blood flow (i.e. coarctation of the aorta and aortic stenosis)
    - Inheritance of CHD (between 5% and 20% risk for most lesions).

ATRIAL SEPTAL DEFECT

If the diagnosis of a large atrial septal defect (ASD) associated with hemodynamically significant shunt is known before pregnancy, the patient should have ASD closed prior to planned pregnancy. In general, uncomplicated ASD need not be treated during pregnancy. However, in the presence of risk factors, ASD may need to be closed (transcatheter/surgical) during pregnancy.

Background

- Atrial septal defect is the most common heart lesion complicating pregnancy
- Hemodynamic effects
  - Most patients are asymptomatic, and the lesion is discovered by auscultation of a murmur
  - The left-to-right shunting will cause an increase in pulmonary blood flow, but pulmonary hypertension is a relatively late finding.

Effect of Pregnancy

- In the absence of pulmonary hypertension, this lesion is well tolerated in pregnancy and should not threaten maternal health. In fact, peripheral vasodilation may reduce left-to-right shunting during pregnancy
- If the patient has experienced pulmonary hypertension, then she is at risk for Eisenmenger syndrome (discussed below), a diagnosis that carries a maternal mortality of 50%
- When counseling the patient with an ASD, it is critical to evaluate her for pulmonary hypertension either by noninvasive testing such as an echocardiogram or by right-sided heart catheterization.

Treatment

- Management during pregnancy
  - In the absence of pulmonary hypertension, there are no special requirements during pregnancy
  - With pulmonary hypertension, the management should be as for any patient at risk for Eisenmenger syndrome
  - A small percentage of patients with ASD have atrial fibrillation or flutter, which may be managed conservatively with antiarrhythmic agents such as digoxin.

VENTRICULAR SEPTAL DEFECT

The size of the septal defect is the most important clinical predictor of the prognosis during pregnancy. Large defects are frequently associated with congestive cardiac failure, arrhythmias or pulmonary hypertension. Shunt reversal (Eisenmenger syndrome) in ventricular septal defect (VSD) is associated with maternal mortality. Isolated small to moderate VSD imposes a low-risk for cardiac complications during pregnancy and labor and delivery are well tolerated by these patients.

Background

Hemodynamic Effects

- The size of the defect determines the degree of disability
- A small lesion is hemodynamically insignificant and is well tolerated.

With a large defect with significant left-to-right shunting, the initial abnormality would be left ventricular hypertrophy to compensate for the decrease in forward flow, followed by the development of pulmonary hypertension caused by the increased pressures delivered to the pulmonary vasculature and, finally, biventricular hypertrophy with the side pumping against a significant afterload.

Effect of Pregnancy

- The impact of pregnancy will depend on the hemodynamic abnormalities of the individual patient
- Without pulmonary hypertension, the decrease in systematic vascular resistance caused by pregnancy may be beneficial, causing an increase in forward flow. However, the increase in blood volume may lead to congestive heart failure in the patient with long-standing left ventricular hypertrophy
- When there is pre-existing pulmonary hypertension, Eisenmenger syndrome may develop, a diagnosis that carries a risk of maternal morbidity of 50% (discussed below)
- The patient with an uncomplicated, repaired VSD is not at risk during pregnancy.

Treatment

- Management during pregnancy
  - In the absence of pulmonary hypertension, there are no special requirements during pregnancy except for bacterial endocarditis prophylaxis
  - With pulmonary hypertension, the management should be as for any patient at risk for Eisenmerger syndrome.

PATENT DUCTUS ARTERIOSUS

Patent ductus arteriosus (PDA) is uncommon during pregnancy as it is detected and corrected in neonatal period. Still if present, it is well tolerated. During delivery, epidural anesthesia is avoided as systemic hypotension can lead to shunt reversal and subsequent development of Eisenmenger syndrome.

Background

- Historically, PDA was one of the more common congenital cardiac lesions complicating pregnancy. It is rare today as a result of early surgical repair.
- Hemodynamic effects and consequences are similar to those described for VSD.

Effect of Pregnancy

- With a small lesion, pregnancy is well tolerated
- With pulmonary hypertension, there is significant risk for Eisenmenger syndrome, with its attendant risks (see below)
- With a corrected PDA, there is no additional risk as a result of pregnancy.

Treatment

- Management during pregnancy
  - In the absence of pulmonary hypertension, there are no special requirements during pregnancy except for bacterial endocarditis prophylaxis
  - With pulmonary hypertension, the management should be as for any patient at risk for Eisenmenger syndrome.

EISENMENGER SYNDROME

In the presence of left-to-right shunt, progressive increase in the pulmonary blood flow and pulmonary vascular resistance results in pulmonary hypertension. Ultimately a state is reached when the pressure in the pulmonary circulation exceeds the pressure in the systemic circulation. This leads to shunt reversal called Eisenmenger syndrome. Once the Eisenmenger pathophysiology is established, pulmonary hypertension is irreversible and any surgical intervention is a waste.

Maternal mortality in the presence of Eisenmenger syndrome varies between 30% and 60%.[16] Because of the high mortality associated with continuing pregnancy, pregnancy termination in first (dilatation and curettage) or second trimester (dilatation and evacuation) is preferred.[17] However, if pregnancy is continued, all attempts are made, to avoid increase in pulmonary vascular resistance, by using pulmonary vasodilators (inhaled nitric oxide, prostacyclin analogs), avoidance of hypotension and anemia and continuous oxygen administration.

Background

- This is a syndrome describing reversal of flow when there is an anatomic defect, allowing communication between the right circulation and left circulation
- This syndrome is associated, in descending order of frequency, with a large VSD, a large PDA, ASD, tetralogy of Fallot and other complex cyanotic CHD.

Hemodynamic Effects

- The underlying anatomic defect initially creates a left-to-right shunt secondary to higher pressures in the left side of the heart
- Prolonged exposure of the pulmonary circulation to increased pressures from the left ventricle results in pulmonary hypertension
- When pulmonary pressures equal systemic pressures, the shunt will become bidirectional
- When pulmonary pressures exceed systemic pressures, the shunt will become predominately right to left with delivery of desaturated blood to the systemic circulation
- Compensatory polycythemia then develops, increasing the risk for thromboembolic phenomenon.

Effect of Pregnancy

- Pregnancy is hazardous in patients with pre-existing Eisenmenger syndrome, as well as in patients with pulmonary hypertension and an anatomic shunt because of their risk for Eisenmenger syndrome
- Several cardiovascular changes predispose to shunt reversal or increasing a pre-existing right-to-left shunt. These include the normal decrease in systemic vascular resistance, the hypercoagulable state with risk for thromboembolic phenomena and consequent increased pulmonary vascular resistance, and hypovolemia (from obstetric causes such as bleeding) resulting in an acute decrease in systemic vascular resistance
- Maternal mortality is estimated to be 50% in patients with Eisenmenger syndrome as a result of intractable hypoxia
  - The time of greatest risk is during the intrapartum and immediate postpartum periods, as a result of the major fluid shifts occurring at these times
  - The woman at greatest risk for death is the one with advanced, fixed pulmonary hypertension unresponsive to oxygen therapy.

Treatment

Management during pregnancy

- Termination of pregnancy should be strongly encouraged
  - Patients who choose not to terminate must be carefully monitored throughout pregnancy
  - Prolonged bet rest is advised with an existing right-to-left shunt to limit the need for increased oxygen consumption
  - Prevention of hypovolemia is essential to avoid either the development of right-to-left shunting in those at risk or increasing a pre-existing right-to-left shunt
  - It is also important to avoid conditions such as hypoxia, acidosis and hypercarbia, which will increase pulmonary vascular resistance
  - Some have recommended prophylactic heparin to decrease the risk of thromboembolic phenomenon, which would acutely increase with pulmonary pressures. However, the few studies addressing the use of prophylactic heparin in this setting have not shown an improvement in maternal mortality
  - Vaginal delivery is preferred to cesarean section because the risk for maternal mortality has been

reported to be as high as 75% with cesarean delivery. The validity of this statistic has been questioned because confounding factors leading to a decision for a rapid delivery may be responsible for a significant portion of the risk
    - It is crucial to watch for signs of shunt reversal or a worsening right-to-left shunt and to treat this development aggressively.

The intrapartum period confers the greatest risk. Recommendations are for:
- Invasive monitoring with arterial and pulmonary artery catheters
- Oxygen therapy
- Strict attention to preload and systemic vascular resistance
- Vasoconstrictor agents as needed to maintain systemic pressures
- A shortened second stage labor.

COARCTATION OF AORTA

Hemodynamically significant coarctation should be repaired before pregnancy is contemplated. Aneurysms may also develop below the coarctation or in the cerebral circulation, and may lead to rupture. In the presence of aneurysms termination of pregnancy should be strictly considered.[18]

When the gestation is continued, elective cesarean section should be considered in patients with an unrepaired coarctation and enlargement of the proximal aorta. In addition to the dangers of aortic rupture, there is increased risk of cerebral hemorrhage, subacute bacterial endocarditis, hypertensive encephalopathy and acute circulatory failure following delivery.

Background

Coarctation is frequently associated with other cardiovascular abnormalities such as bicuspid aortic valve and congenital berry aneurysm of the circle of Willis.

Hemodynamic Effects

- Upper extremity hypertension is common secondary to the obstruction to outflow, and there is compensatory left ventricular hypertrophy
- Visible and palpable collateral arteries in the scapular region and lower extremity hypotension are found commonly.

Effect of Pregnancy

- With uncomplicated coarctation of the aorta, pregnancy is usually well tolerated
- A minority of cases will be complicated by congestive heart failure secondary to the effect of maternal hormones on the blood vessel wall architecture.

Treatment

Management during pregnancy
- Hypertension should be controlled to decrease the risk for aortic dissection and rupture
- Bacterial endocarditis prophylaxis is recommended.

TETRALOGY OF FALLOT

Background

- This is the most common cyanotic lesion complicating pregnancy
- It is a syndrome of pulmonary stenosis, right ventricular hypertrophy, large VSD and dextroposition of the aorta that overrides the right ventricle
- The vast majority of pregnant women will already have full or partial surgical repair because the disease is otherwise usually fatal in childhood or early adulthood.

Hemodynamic Effects

- There is right outflow obstruction with resultant right-to-left shunting. This delivers blood with decreased oxygen saturation to the systematic circulation
- Right ventricular hypertrophy will develop as a result of the right outflow obstruction.

Effect of Pregnancy

- Patients with a full surgical repair before pregnancy are not at increased risk during pregnancy
- Pregnancy is poorly tolerated in patients who have not had surgical repair, because the decrease in systemic vascular resistance will cause an increase in right-to-left shunting with further desaturation of blood flowing to the systemic circulation. Patients believed to have an especially poor prognosis in pregnancy are those with:
    - A baseline hematocrit greater than 60%
    - Arterial oxygen saturation less than 80%
    - A history of syncopal episodes, and
    - Significant right ventricular hypertension.
- Patients with palliative (partial) repairs such as the Blalock-Taussig (anastomosis of the subclavian artery to the right pulmonary artery), Potts (anastomosis of the descending aorta to the left pulmonary artery) or Waterston-Cooley (anastomosis of the ascending aorta to the right pulmonary artery) may be minimally symptomatic before pregnancy and yet may be at risk for decompensation during pregnancy.

Therefore, it is important to evaluate functional status by the parameters just mentioned.

Treatment

Management during pregnancy

- It is essential to avoid hypovolemia and decreased venous return so as not to increase right-to-left shunting
  - Pressure-graded elastic support hose are recommended
  - Supplemental oxygen should be used as necessary.

AORTIC STENOSIS

Background

It may result from congenital or acquired heart disease.

The most common congenital lesion is a bicuspid valve, and there frequently are other associated cardiovascular anomalies. The lesion may not be stenotic at birth, but will become progressively stenotic with aging.

Hemodynamic Effects

- When the valve reaches a critical narrowing in an area of less than 1 cm^2, there is obstruction to left ventricular outflow with development of left ventricular hypertrophy. This, in turn, may result in a fixed stroke volume and ischemia as a result of poor perfusion of the coronary blood vessels
- Decompensation may occur with additional stress, progressing to left ventricular dilation and failure.

Effect of Pregnancy

Pregnancy is poorly tolerated in the patient with critical aortic stenosis.

The patient has a fixed stroke volume and is able to increase cardiac output to meet the increased demands of pregnancy only by increasing heart rate. An increase in heart rate will decrease relatively the diastolic portion of the cardiac cycle, and this will result in decreased time for coronary perfusion and ventricular filling. In addition, the decreased systemic vascular resistance is also detrimental because the heart may be unable to fill a dilated vascular bed. This may result in syncope and hypertension.

The risk of maternal mortality with critical aortic stenosis is approximately with severe aortic stenosis.

Treatment

Management during pregnancy

- In a patient with critical aortic stenosis, strict limitation of activity is essential to minimize the need for cardiac output augmentation during pregnancy
- Avoid situations that will further impede venous return such as hypovolemia
- Use of support hose may help to maintain venous return
- Left-sided heart failure should be treated as in the nonpregnant patient
- Bacterial endocarditis prophylaxis is recommended.

PULMONARY STENOSIS

Background

Unlike aortic stenosis, this lesion is not usually progressive.

Hemodynamic Effects

- Mild degree of pulmonary stenosis usually cause no symptoms or hemodynamic compromise
- With severe stenosis there will be obstruction to right ventricular outflow, causing the development of right ventricular hypertrophy. The patient with severe stenosis may be unable to argument cardiac output, leading to symptoms of exertional dyspnea and fatigue.

Effect of Pregnancy

- Most patients with pulmonary stenosis tolerate pregnancy well.
- The patient with severe stenosis may be unable to meet the demands for augmented cardiac and may not tolerate the volume expansion of pregnancy, leading to right-sided heart failure.

Treatment

Management during pregnancy

- Hypervolemia and hypovolemia should be avoided
- Right-sided heart failure should be treated as in the nonpregnant patient

If medical therapy fails, a transvenous balloon valvuloplasty may be performed safely during pregnancy

Bacterial endocarditis prophylaxis is recommended.

ISCHEMIC HEART DISEASE

The management of ischemic heart disease in pregnancy should be a multidisciplinary team approach. In early pregnancy, pregnancy termination may be an option. Survival is the primary concern and revascularization should not be withheld because the patient is pregnant. Coronary reperfusion by means of percutaneous transluminal coronary angioplasty or coronary artery bypass graft surgery has been reported to be successful during pregnancy although experience is still limited.

In the case of acute myocardial infarction, delivery should be postponed, if possible, for at least 2 weeks from the time of infarction.[19] Maternal mortality is significantly higher during this time, possibly due to the increased hemodynamic requirements during labor that increase myocardial demand and the risk of myocardial ischemia. The patient in labor with acute myocardial infarction should be managed in the coronary intensive care unit. Preload reduction is a recognized potential disadvantage of epidural anesthesia. This complication can be prevented by ensuring that the patient is adequately hydrated at the time of induction of the epidural. If desired, cardiac output can be increased by placing the patient in the left lateral decubitus position. Because of the risk of coronary artery spasm, ergot alkaloids should be avoided immediately after delivery. Patient should be monitored for 48 hours postpartum in an intensive care unit due to the significant hemodynamic changes that occur during this time.

Previous myocardial infarction is not an absolute contraindication to pregnancy. But subsequent pregnancy in a patient with myocardial infarction is associated with a small, but definitely increased risk of perinatal loss.

PERIPARTUM CARDIOMYOPATHY

It is a dilated cardiomyopathy that occurs in the peripartum period. It is defined as cardiac failure developing in the last month of pregnancy or within 6 months of delivery in women without previous cardiac disease, and there is no other detectable cause of cardiac failure. When peripartum cardiomyopathy occurs in the last trimester of pregnancy, delivery is indicated. The cardinal requirement for defining peripartum cardiomyopathy is echocardiographical findings of left ventricular dysfunction, i.e., ejection fraction is less than 45%, fractional shortening is less than 30% and end diastolic dimension is more than 2.7 cm/m^2.[20]

Myocardial biopsy shows myocarditis in majority of the cases. Infections (viral), autoimmune processes, unique hormonal environment and possible maladaptive responses to the hemodynamic changes of the pregnancy are the contributory causes. Early endomyocardial biopsy has been suggested to identify a subgroup of patients who have a histologic picture of inflammatory myocarditis and who may be responsive to immunosuppressive therapy.[21] Intravenous immunoglobulins have also shown improvement in ejection fraction.

Cardiac transplant is always the last resort in this condition with left ventricular assist device needed to bridge recovery or time to transplant as it buys time.

It has been observed in United States that the peak incidence of peripartum cardiomyopathy occurs in first postpartum month and is more frequent amongst older, multiparous, black females. Other risk factors include twin pregnancy, pregnancy-induced hypertension, infections, selenium deficiency,[22] tocolytic therapy, surgical delivery or history of previous peripartum cardiomyopathy. It may be wise to continue ACE inhibitor and β-blocker till 1 year after recovery of ventricular function. Annual two-dimensional echocardiography is advised to monitor left ventricular ejection fraction (LVEF). Future pregnancy is contraindicated in all patients with persistent cardiomegaly accompanying left ventricular dysfunction. Patients who have recovered normal left ventricular function, seem to have good prognosis. Such patients, if wish to have further pregnancy, should undergo dobutamine stress echocardiography.[23] If this is normal, a normal pregnancy can be expected, though the experience and information is sparse.

CHRONIC HYPERTENSION IN PREGNANCY

Hypertension in pregnancy is defined as a systolic of 140 mmHg or greater or a diastolic of 90 mmHg or greater. The National High Blood Pressure Education Program classifies hypertensive disorders of pregnancy into following categories: gestational hypertension, chronic hypertension, pre-eclampsia and pre-eclampsia superimposed on pre-existing hypertension.

Chronic hypertension complicates between 1% and 5% of pregnancies. Chronic hypertension in pregnancy may be an increasing clinical problem. This has been attributed to increasing maternal age, obesity and the pandemic of metabolic syndrome.

Chronic hypertension is associated with increased maternal and fetal risks, such as perinatal mortality superimposed preeclampsia, placental abruption and progression to severe hypertension. The presence of hypertension itself, irrespective of blood pressure medication use, has been shown to result in lower birth weights. Increasing evidence supports the association between hypertensive pregnancy disorders and increased risks for cardiovascular disease (CVD) later in life.[24]

Management

The 2007 European Society of Hypertension/European Society of Cardiology guidelines, recommend treatment for a blood pressure is more than or equal to 140/90 mmHg[25] in women with gestational hypertension, pre-existing hypertension with superimposed gestational hypertension, or hypertension with subclinical organ damage or symptoms at any time during pregnancy. In the presence of renal disease, proteinuria, left ventricular hypertrophy, hypertensive retinopathy, microvascular disease, stroke and age greater than 40, therapy should be initiated for a diastolic blood pressure more than or equal to 90 mmHg.

Current guidelines for the prevention of CVD in women recommend referral of patients with a history of hypertensive pregnancy to primary care or cardiology, in order to facilitate monitoring and control of risk factors, and though there are currently no guidelines, routine screening for renal disease with blood urea nitrogen, serum creatinine and urinalysis may be indicated in affected women. The goals of treating hypertension during pregnancy are prevention of cardiovascular complications and other target organ disease.

Nonpharmacological Therapeutic Approach

Lifestyle interventions, such as weight loss and a reduction in salt intake, are of proven benefit in nonpregnant hypertensive patients. There is currently no evidence from prospective, randomized trials that instituting such programs during pregnancy is effective in preventing pre-eclampsia in at risk individuals.[26]

In 2009, the Institute of Medicine revised their guidelines for gestational weight gain and recommended that women who are overweight prior to pregnancy [body mass index (BMI) 25–29.9] gain only 15–25 lbs during pregnancy, as opposed those with normal weight (BMI 18.5–24.9) prior to pregnancy, who should gain 25–35 lbs. Obese women with a BMI more than 30 should gain only 11–20 lbs, according to the new recommendations.[27]

Pharmacological Approach

Patients with chronic hypertension which is adequately controlled on medications that are safe for pregnancy should continue this regimen throughout pregnancy. In fact, during the first trimester, these women may require a decrease in the dose of antihypertensive medications as their blood pressure gradually decreases.

According to the Working Group Report of the National High Blood Pressure Education Program (NHBPEP), methyldopa and hydralazine, respectively, are recommended as initial oral or intravenous therapy. Methyldopa acts centrally by decreasing sympathetic tone, and therefore can have many side effects, including sedation and impaired sleep patterns. One potential side effect is that it may cause mild elevations of liver enzymes, which can lead to diagnostic confusion with HELLP syndrome. Hydralazine is a direct vasodilator that can be administered orally or intravenously, and is often used in the setting of hypertensive urgency, given its fast onset of action. However, hydralazine has been associated with hypotension, oliguria and fetal distress.[28] It is also associated with a lupus-like syndrome and peripheral neuropathy. Hydralazine remains, however, commonly used when other treatment regimens have failed to achieve adequate blood pressure control, as most obstetricians are quite familiar with its pharmacological actions and find its side effect profile acceptable. Although, the use of methyldopa and hydralazine results in vasodilatation, blood pressure is often not lowered sufficiently with these agents, as therapeutic doses may lead to intolerable side effects (methyldopa) and significant fluctuations in blood pressure (hydralazine), which may necessitate their discontinuation during pregnancy.

In current practice, antihypertensive medications other than methyldopa and hydralazine are being used more often in pregnancy, and particularly in patients for whom blood pressure control either cannot be achieved with these agents or because of intolerable side effects.

Diuretics, β-blockers and calcium channel blockers (CCBs) are acceptable medications that can be continued in patients with pre-pregnancy hypertension.

Diuretics are the most commonly used medication among women of child-bearing age with chronic hypertension. The use of diuretic therapy during pregnancy remains controversial, primarily due to theoretical concerns. A possible side effect of any diuretic is vascular volume contraction, which may paradoxically cause further elevations of blood pressure in pre-eclamptic women. In a randomized trial of women with chronic hypertension in pregnancy, the use of diuretics reduced plasma volume, but was not associated with adverse pregnancy outcomes. Therefore, if a woman is on a diuretic prior to pregnancy, this can be continued during pregnancy, with the exception of spironolactone, which may have fetal antiandrogen effects.

Beta-blockers appear to be more effective than methyldopa in avoiding episodes of severe hypertension in women with preconception hypertension. Fetal growth restriction and low placental weight in patients have been associated with the use of atenolol during the second trimester,[29] but not with other β-blocking agents, such as labetalol. Labetalol is becoming one of the favored therapies for hypertension in pregnancy. It is a nonselective β-blocker that antagonizes both β and α-1 receptors. Its side effects include fatigue, decreased exercise tolerance, as well as bronchospasm in individuals with reactive airway disease. Labetalol has been compared to methyldopa in prospective trials and neither medication was associated with adverse maternal or fetal outcomes.

Although only limited trials exist, nifedipine has been shown to decrease blood pressure without affecting the blood flow in the umbilical artery.

The effects of clonidine on fetal growth have been shown to be mediated through the maternal hemodynamic response to medication. Clonidine may impair fetal growth, especially if the mother has a reduction in heart rate after therapy is initiated.[30] It can cause significant rebound hypertension and does not have as strong a record of safety as methyldopa. It should be considered in cases of intolerance to methyldopa.

Concern regarding the potential adverse effects relates to certain classes of antihypertensive medications, such as ACE inhibitors and angiotensin receptor blockers (ARBs), due to their mechanisms of action that exert adverse effects on a growing fetus.[31] A study published in 2006 by Cooper and colleagues demonstrated that exposure to ACE inhibitors in the first trimester can be associated with significant congenital malformations affecting both the cardiovascular and central nervous systems. If a woman becomes pregnant while on one of these agents, she should be switched immediately to an alternative therapy and offered an ultrasound and fetal echocardiography at 18 weeks gestation, and providers should discuss the possible risks for congenital malformations with the patient. There is little data regarding direct renin inhibitor Aliskiren in pregnancy, but it is also considered category D by the US Federal Drug Administration.

Secondary hypertension should be considered in women with difficult to control blood pressure requiring three or more antihypertensive agents, including a diuretic, and/or indicative laboratory and clinical findings and should be evaluated for the same. The detailed discussion on secondary hypertension is beyond the scope of this chapter.

REFERENCES

1. Klein LL, Galan HL. Cardiac disease in pregnancy. Obstet Gynecol Clin N Am. 2004;31:429-59.
2. Saving Mothers. A report of the National Committee on Confidential Enquiries into maternal deaths in South Africa (1999–2001) DOH. Pretoria: 162–174.
3. Kannan M, Vijayanand G. Mitral stenosis and pregnancy: Current concepts in anaesthetic practice. Indian J Anaesth. 2010;54:439-44.
4. Harris IS. Management of Pregnancy in Patients with Congenital Heart Disease. Prog Cardiovasc Dis. 2011;53(4):305-11.
5. James AH, Jamison MG, Biswas MS, Brancazio LR, Swamy GK, Myers ER. Acute myocardial infarction in pregnancy: A United States population-based study. Circulation. 2006;113:1564-71.
6. Roth A, Elkayam U. Acute myocardial infarction associated with pregnancy. Ann Intern Med. 1996;125:751-62.
7. Demakis JG, Rahimtoola SH, Sutton GC, Meadws WR, Szanto PB, Tobin JR, et al. Natural course of peripartum cardiomyopathy. Circulation. 1971;44:1053-61.
8. Szekely P, Snaith L. Atrial fibrillation and pregnancy. Br Med J. 1961;1(5237):1407-10.
9. Montavon C, Hoesli I, Holzgreve W, Tsakiris DA. Thrombophilia and anticoagulation in pregnancy: indications, risks and management. J Matern Fetal Neonatal Med. 2008;21(10):685-96.
10. Salazar E, Izaguirre R, Verdejo J, Mutchinick O. Failure of adjusted doses of subcutaneous heparin to prevent thromboembolic phenomena in pregnant patients with mechanical cardiac valve prostheses. J Am Coll Cardiol. 1996;27(7):1698-1703.
11. Donald I. Practical obstetric problems. 5th edition. London: Lloyd Luke (Medical books) Ltd; 1979. pp.164-6.
12. Ruys TP, Cornette J, Roos-Hesselink JW. Pregnancy and delivery in cardiac disease. J Cardiol. 2013;61(2):107-12.
13. Ueland K, Akamatsu TH, Eng M Bonica JJ, Hansen JM. Maternal cardiovascular dynamics. VI. Cesarean section under epidural anesthesia with epinephrine. Am J Obstet Gynecol. 1972;114:775.
14. Brady K, Duff P. Rheumatic heart disease in pregnancy. Clin Obstet Gynaecol. 1989;32(1):21-40.
15. Donald I. Practical obstetric problems, 5th edition. London: Lloyd Luke (Medical books) Ltd; 1979. pp. 155.
16. Avila WS, Grinberg M, Snitcowsky R, Faccioli R, Da Luz PL, Bellotti G, et al. Maternal and fetal outcome in pregnant women with Eisenmenger syndrome. Eur Heart J. 1995;16:460-4.
17. Elkayam V, Gleicher N. Cardiac problems in pregnancy. I. Maternal aspects: the approach to the pregnant patient with heart disease. JAMA. 1984;251:2838.
18. Clark SL. Structural cardiac disease in pregnancy. In: Clark SL, Cotton DB, Phelan JP (Eds). Critical Care Obstetrics, 3rd edition. Boston: Blackwell Scientific; 1997.
19. Hankins GD, Wendel GD, Leveno KJ, Stoneham J. Myocardial infarction during pregnancy: A review. Obstet Gynecol. 1985;65:139-46.
20. Pearson GD, Veille JC, Rahimtoola SH, Hsia J, Oakley CM, Hosenpud JD, et al. Peripartum cardiomyopathy: National Heart, Lung and Blood Institute and Office of Rare Diseases (National Institutes of Health) workshop recommendations and review. JAMA. 2000;283:1183-8.
21. Mason JW, O'Connell JB, Herskowitz A, Rose NR, McManus BM, Billingham ME, et al. A clinical trial of immunosuppressive therapy for myocarditis. N Engl J Med. 1995;333:269-75.
22. Fett JD, Ansari AA, Sundstrom JB, Coombs GF. Peripartum cardiomyopathy; a selenium disconnection and an autoimmune connection. Int J Cardiol. 2002;86:311-16.
23. Lampert MB, Lang RM. Peripartum cardiomyopathy. Am Heart J. 1995;130:860-70.
24. Report of the National High Blood Pressure Education Program Working Group on High Blood Pressure in Pregnancy. Am J Obstet Gynecol. 2000;183(1):S1-22.
25. Mancia G, De Backer G, Dominiczak A, Cifkova R, Fagard R, Germano G, et al. 2007. Guidelines for the management of arterial hypertension: The Task Force for the Management of Arterial Hypertension of the European Society of Hypertension (ESH) and of the European Society of Cardiology (ESC). J Hypertens. 2007;25(6):1105-87.
26. Artal R, O'Toole M. Guidelines of the American College of Obstetricians and Gynecologists for exercise during pregnancy and the postpartum period. Br J Sports Med. 2003 37(1):6-12.
27. Siega-Riz AM, Viswanathan M, Moos MK, Deierlein A, Mumford S, Knaack J, et al. A systematic review of outcomes of maternal weight gain according to the Institute of Medicine recommendations: birthweight, fetal growth, and postpartum weight retention. Am J Obstet Gynecol. 2009;201(4):339 e1-14.
28. Magee LA, Cham C, Waterman EJ, Ohlsson A, von Dadelszen P. Hydralazine for treatment of severe hypertension in pregnancy: meta-analysis. BMJ. 2003 327(7421):955-60.
29. Butters L, Kennedy S, Rubin PC. Atenolol in essential hypertension during pregnancy. BMJ. 1990;301(6752):587-9.
30. Rothberger S, Carr D, Brateng D, Hebert M, Easterling TR. Pharmacodynamics of clonidine therapy in pregnancy: a heterogeneous maternal response impacts fetal growth. Am J Hypertens. 2010;23(11):1234-40.
31. Cooper WO, Hernandez-Diaz S, Arbogast PG, Dudley JA, Dyer S, Gideon PS, et al. Major congenital malformations after first trimester exposure to ACE inhibitors. N Engl J Med. 2006;354(23):2443-51.

CHAPTER 48

Respiratory Diseases

Geetha D Balsarkar, Alok Sharma

INTRODUCTION

Like any other system, the respiratory system undergoes various changes that are beneficial to the mother and the fetus during the course of a normal pregnancy. However, these may predispose the patient to developing certain acute pulmonary disorders, such as aspiration, thromboembolic diseases, pulmonary edema and amniotic fluid embolism. These conditions can be very challenging to the clinician. Pregnancy can also alter the course of some chronic pulmonary diseases, most notably, asthma and sarcoidosis. Conversely, these chronic pulmonary conditions, if poorly controlled, can affect pregnancy and delivery.

RESPIRATORY PHYSIOLOGY

Anatomical Changes

Due to hormonal changes in pregnancy, there is increased blood flow in the upper respiratory tract and airway mucosa, producing hyperemia, mucosal edema, hypersecretion and increased mucosal friability. Estrogen is probably responsible for tissue edema, capillary congestion and hyperplasia of mucous glands. These changes may be more pronounced in patients with preexisting atopic disease, chronic sinusitis, or pre-eclampsia and these patients are more prone during the third trimester to have epistaxis.

The enlarging uterus changes the anatomy of the thoracic cage. As the uterus enlarges; the diaphragm is displaced upward by as much as 4 cm; the anteroposterior and transverse diameter of the thorax increases effectively increasing the chest wall circumference. However, diaphragm function remains normal, and diaphragmatic excursion is maintained.

Pulmonary Function

The various anatomical changes of the thorax produce a progressive decrease in functional residual capacity, which is reduced 10–20% by term. Majority of the patients complain of having to take deep breaths in the third trimester. Because the diaphragm is displaced upward, there is a decrease in residual volume and expiratory reserve volume, resulting in a decreased functional residual capacity. Conversely, inspiratory capacity and tidal volume increases, so that vital capacity and total lung capacity remains the same. This increase is thought to be caused by increased progesterone levels. Hormonal changes do not significantly affect airway function. Pregnancy does not appear to affect lung compliance, but chest wall and total respiratory compliance are reduced towards term.[1]

Ventilation

The minute ventilation increases significantly, reaching 20–40% above baseline at term for adequate oxygenation. Alveolar ventilation increases by 50–70% at term. The increase in ventilation occurs because of increased metabolic carbon dioxide production and because of increased respiratory drive due to the high serum progesterone level. The tidal volume increases by 30–35%. The respiratory rate remains relatively constant or increases slightly.

Arterial Blood Gases

Dyspnea is a usual symptom during pregnancy, affecting 60–70% of women with no previous history of cardiac or pulmonary disease. Although the etiology is unknown, it is thought to be related to physiologic hyperventilation

Physiological hyperventilation causes respiratory alkalosis with compensatory renal excretion of bicarbonate, maintaining an arterial pH in the range of 7.40–7.47. Oxygen consumption by the mother increases by 20–33% by term because of fetal demands and increased maternal metabolic processes.

In active labor, hyperventilation further increases and tachypnea caused by labor pains result in marked hypocapnia and respiratory alkalosis, adversely affecting fetal oxygenation. In some patients, severe pain and anxiety can lead to rapid shallow breathing with alveolar hypoventilation and mild hypoxemia.

Fetal Oxygenation

Oxygen released to the placenta and fetus is dependent on maternal arterial oxygen content and uterine blood flow. Small changes in maternal (partial oxygen) PaO_2 can cause large changes in fetal oxygen saturation because the fetus is operating on the steep portion of the oxygen dissociation curve.

Pulmonary Pharmacology[2]

- Xanthine derivatives: both theophylline and aminophylline are often used in pregnancy, crosse the placenta, but no fetal adverse effects or malformations have been reported. Theophylline absorption and excretion are unaffected by pregnancy, and this drug also appears in breast milk
- Beta-agonists: these have little systemic absorption and a more potent bronchodilatory effect when used via inhalation. Hence, they can be used both orally or through inhalation. There is no difference in perinatal mortality, congenital malformations, birth weight, or Apgar scores[3]
- Corticosteroids: the use of corticosteroids during pregnancy continues to be controversial, although numerous reports confirm their use without adverse fetal effects. Both inhaled as well as oral corticosteroids can be used
- Antihistamines and decongestants: these medications are routinely prescribed for nasal symptoms, mucosal edema and hyperemia that accompany normal pregnancy. Brompheniramine when used for prolonged period has been associated with congenital malformations
- Antibiotics used for respiratory infections: the antibiotics considered safe during pregnancy are penicillin, cephalosporins and azithromycin. Although penicillin and ampicillin readily cross the placenta, no adverse effects to the fetus are reported. Cephalosporins also traverse the placenta to a moderate degree, but no adverse fetal effects occur. Antibiotics that have relative contraindications during pregnancy and puerperium include sulfonamides, trimethoprim, aminoglycosides, nitrofurantoin, antituberculosis drugs, tetracyclines and quinolones
- Teratogens used in pulmonary disease: these drugs mainly include iodine-containing compounds. Brompheniramine, antihistamine, coumarin and anticoagulants cause various teratogenic effects. Ciprofloxacin, sulfonamides, tetracyclines, chloramphenicol, streptomycin and rifampicin have been associated with various effects, like deafness. Ionizing radiation exposure to the fetus is associated with growth retardation, central nervous system (CNS) effects on the fetus, microcephaly and eye malformations. Maternal radiation exposure of less than 0.05 Gy is associated with no adverse effects, a dose of 0.05–0.1 Gy is considered the gray zone, and exposure to more than 0.1 Gy is associated with significant fetal effects. Fetal ionizing radiation might cause increases in childhood leukemia.[2]

PREGNANCY-SPECIFIC DISORDERS

Amniotic Fluid Embolism

Amniotic fluid embolism is an extremely rare (1 case per 8,000–80,000 births), but potentially catastrophic complication, with a mortality rate of 10–80%. As long as the fetal membranes remain intact, fluid cannot enter the maternal circulation. In addition, there must also be disruption of the uterine veins and a pressure gradient favoring fluid entry. This is precipitated with labor and delivery and is seen with uterine manipulation like rupture of membranes, uterine trauma like delivery, and the early postpartum period. Two possible sites of entry are the uterine veins at the site of placental separation and small tears in the lower uterus and endocervix. Amniotic fluid containing particulate fetal debris, like desquamated squamous cells, meconium, lanugo hair and mucin enters the vascular circulation through open blood vessels of endocervical veins or uterine tears, obstructs the pulmonary vessels, and causes vascular spasms, resulting in pulmonary hypertension. Acute left ventricular failure might occur with embolism probably due to humoral events mediated by cytokines.

Clinical Features

Clinical presentation usually involves a sudden onset of severe dyspnea, hypoxemia and cardiovascular collapse in a delivered patient. Less common presentations are hemorrhage caused by disseminated intravascular coagulation and fetal distress. The predisposing factors are polyhydramnios, multiple gestation, traumatic delivery, meconium staining of amniotic fluid, advanced age, and the use of uterine stimulants during labor and delivery.

Diagnosis

The diagnosis of amniotic fluid embolism is usually based on suspicion and is often a diagnosis of exclusion. Fetal squamous cells in a wedged pulmonary capillary aspirate have been used to confirm the diagnosis postmortem, but are not specific. Other conditions including septic shock, pulmonary thromboembolism, ruptured placentae, tension pneumothorax and myocardial ischemia have to be ruled out first.

Treatment and Clinical Course

Treatment involves ABC, maintenance of airway, breathing and cardiopulmonary resuscitative and supportive measures with prompt attention to inotropic support. No single therapy has been shown to be effective in treatment, although corticosteroids have been suggested. The survivors develop complications of disseminated intravascular coagulation or adult respiratory distress syndrome.

Tocolytic Pulmonary Edema

Beta-adrenergic agents, like isoxsuprine, ritodrine and terbutaline, are used widely and indiscriminately to inhibit preterm labor. They predispose to pulmonary edema during pregnancy. Conditions like multiple gestation, prolonged exposure to catecholamines (which cause myocardial dysfunction), increased capillary permeability like in sepsis, malarial infestation, administration of general anesthesia, and a concomitant use of large volume of intravenous fluid that may have been administered in response to maternal tachycardia. Glucocorticoids administered in preterm labor can also contribute to fluid retention.

Clinical Features

Symptoms include chest pain, dyspnea, tachypnea, tachycardia and cough. On auscultation, whistling or bubbling sound is heard and chest X-ray suggests pulmonary edema. It can happen during administration of beta-adrenergic agents or even 24–48 hours after discontinuation of the drug.

Diagnosis

The diagnosis is mainly clinical, in an acute condition, but suspicion is very important. The other conditions which have the same symptoms are cardiogenic pulmonary edema, amniotic fluid embolisms and aspiration pneumonia.

Treatment and Clinical Course

Beta-adrenergic agent must be immediately stopped; pulmonary edema usually resolves rapidly. The additional treatment is supportive and includes adequate oxygenation, diuresis and improving cardiac function. The response is usually rapid. If there is no improvement within 24 hours, an alternative cause for pulmonary edema should be considered.

Pre-eclampsia and Pulmonary Edema

Pulmonary edema rarely occurs along with pre-eclampsia due to increased capillary permeability. Approximately 3% of all patients with pre-eclampsia have pulmonary complications. Patients with pre-eclampsia are usually volume depleted and pulmonary edema most commonly occurs in the early postpartum period and is often associated with aggressive fluid replacement. Reduced albumin concentration, loss of fluid in third space and myocardial dysfunction contribute to edema formation.

Clinical Features and Diagnosis

The symptom is of acute breathlessness in a patient with pre-eclampsia. On auscultation rales and rhonchi could be present.

Management

The most important approach is to restrict fluid and administer supplemental oxygen and cause diuresis. Invasive monitoring with central catheter, might be useful, if inotropic vasodilator therapy becomes necessary.

Peripartum Cardiomyopathy

Cardiogenic cause of pulmonary edema is important in the differential diagnosis of acute respiratory failure in pregnancy. Cardiac failure due to overload or loss of contractility of the cardiac muscle can occur in the absence of preexisting heart disease as a result of severe hypertensive disease of pregnancy and peripartum cardiomyopathy. This idiopathic condition can present during the last month of pregnancy or during the postpartum period and is associated with significant mortality. During labor and early postpartum, tachycardia and increased cardiac output can precipitate acute pulmonary edema.

ASTHMA

Asthma is one of the most common comorbid medical conditions affecting pregnant women and the outcome of pregnancy. The course of asthma during pregnancy is very variable; one-third of patients improve, one-third remains stable and one-third worsen. In patients with symptomatic asthma, gestational weeks 24–36 tend to be the most difficult. Only 10% of women experience asthma exacerbation during labor and delivery, and the severity tends to revert to that of pregnancy by 3 months' postpartum. Asthma is generally expected to follow a similar course during successive pregnancies.

A summary of observations during the 20th century suggests that infant outcome might be worse as asthma severity increases and that outcome with aggressive asthma management is usually good.[4]

Asthma exacerbations during pregnancy that require medical intervention occur in about 20% of women, with approximately 6% of women being admitted to the hospital. These exacerbations occur primarily in the late 2nd trimester and are either triggered by viral infection or nonadherence to inhaled corticosteroid medication. Severe exacerbations during pregnancy are a significant risk factor for a low-birth weight baby and inhaled corticosteroid use may reduce the risk.

Objective assessment with pulmonary function tests is essential to assess the presence of airflow obstruction.[5]

Inadequate asthma control or factors that are associated with increased asthma severity during pregnancy lead to lower pulmonary function, which is associated with increased gestational hypertension and premature delivery.

Therapy

Avoidance and Control of Asthma Triggers

Asthma is usually triggered by known factors, including allergy, upper respiratory tract infection, sinusitis, exercise, aspirin, nonsteroidal anti-inflammatory agents, and irritants like tobacco smoke, chemical fumes, humidity, emotional upset and stress. Avoiding these triggers can help the pregnant patient by reducing her medications required for control. Smoking is emerging as a strong trigger in urban population. Gastroesophageal reflux is also known to trigger asthma, and approximately one-third of pregnant woman have symptomatic reflux. This needs to be dealt with small meals and raising the head of the bed or patient sleeping in semi-reclining positions. Some patients might require antacids or H2-receptor blocking medications to prevent cough and asthma.[6]

Medications during Pregnancy

Clinicians have to weigh the drugs used in asthma for their side effects on the mother and the fetus with the control the asthmatic patient has during pregnancy. When required, the drugs are added in a step-wise fashion at regular intervals.[7]

Office Management of Asthma

In outpatient asthma management, β-2 agonists are used for symptomatic benefit. Inhaled corticosteroids remain the mainstay of therapy for asthma control. Initiate treatment with the lowest possible dose of inhaled steroids; the dose can be increased further as required by symptomatic and objective asthma assessment.[8]

Long-acting adrenergic agonists might be used in symptomatic patients on adequate corticosteroid therapy. The leukotriene antagonists are the newest agents available for asthma management. Their exact role in the treatment of asthma during pregnancy is unclear. No widespread experience has been gained with the use of these agents in pregnant patients. Theophylline might be used as a third-line agent after beta-agonist therapy and inhaled steroids. Extensive experience has been gained with the use of theophylline during pregnancy, and it does not appear to cause developmental risk.[2]

Fetal Outcome

Asthma can have a number of morbid effects on pregnancy outcome. An increased incidence of preterm births, low-birth weight and increased prenatal mortality largely related to poor asthma control, has been reported. Physicians and patients should not inappropriately avoid the use of effective pharmacologic therapy because of concerns for fetal effects of drugs.[3]

Acute Asthma Exacerbation

Acute exacerbations that necessitate emergency department visits typically require a course of systemic corticosteroids. Oxygen should be used liberally, and the oxygen saturation should be maintained at or above 95% to ensure fetal well-being. A beta-agonist with or without ipratropium should be given via a metered-dose inhaler with a spacer or in nebulized form. Theophylline has limited use in acute exacerbations. Aggressive management of asthma exacerbation is recommended because of greater risk to the fetus from untreated asthma.[9]

VENOUS THROMBOEMBOLISM

Venous thromboembolism (VTE) is the leading cause of morbidity during pregnancy and the puerperium and is increasingly the leading cause of nonobstetric maternal mortality. In 2011, the American College of Obstetricians and Gynecologists (ACOG) issued an updated practice bulletin for thromboembolism in pregnancy, emphasizing recommendations for diagnosing, preventing, and managing VTE.[10]

Pregnant patients are at increased risk for thromboembolic disease for the following reasons: (1) reduced venous tone and blood flow in the lower limbs, causing venous stasis; (2) pressure on the inferior vena cava and left iliac vein by the uterus, leading to venous outflow obstruction and stasis and (3) an increase in several clotting factors and a decrease in fibrinolytic activity, leading to a hypercoagulable state.

Pathophysiology

Venous thromboembolism is approximately 5 times more common in pregnant women compared with nonpregnant women of the same age. The most constant predisposing factor is increased venous stasis. The physiologic changes of pregnancy due to progesterone effect result in increased venous distensibility and capacitance, which are seen from the 1st trimester. Other factors that contribute to VTE are pregnancy-induced hypertension (PIH), cesarean delivery, advanced maternal age, prolonged bed rest, hemorrhage, sepsis, multiparity and obesity. The entire coagulation cascade is altered toward coagulation in pregnancy. Coagulation factors II, VII and X increase significantly by mid-pregnancy. Fibrin production increases as protein S levels decrease. Protein C levels remain unchanged; the fibrinolytic system is inhibited, particularly, in the third trimester. Activated protein C resistance increases the risk of VTE many folds. Other inherited and acquired factors such as systemic lupus erythematosus (SLE) and autoimmune disorders also increase the risk of VTE.[11]

Diagnosis

Three-fourths of cases of venous thrombosis occur during antepartum period, with approximately 50% occurring by week 15 of gestation. Deep venous thrombosis (DVT) begins in veins of the calf and thigh in pregnancy, similar to nonpregnant women, but involvement of the left lower extremity is seen commonly. The clinical diagnosis of DVT is more difficult in pregnant women than in nonpregnant women because swelling and leg discomfort are common symptoms in pregnancy compared with antepartum periods and postpartum periods, death from VTE in pregnancy most often known to occur during the peripartum period.

Diagnostic Testing

Venography is considered the gold standard for diagnosis, but is difficult to perform and interpret and might cause appreciable pain in the foot and calf or hypersensitivity reactions. Increasingly, noninvasive studies like venous Doppler have replaced venography.[12]

Doppler Ultrasonography

Doppler ultrasonography is the mainstay of testing. The most reliable ultrasound criterion for thrombosis is a failure to collapse the vascular lumen completely with gentle probe pressure. The sensitivity and specificity for Doppler ultrasound for proximal thrombi is very high. False-positive test results can occur during pregnancy.

PULMONARY EMBOLISM

Suspicion is most important in pulmonary embolism. Commonly seen in obese, hypertensive patients with prolonged immobilization and major pelvic surgery. Signs and symptoms of pulmonary embolism are more evading the diagnosis because dyspnea and tachypnea are common in pregnancy compared to nonpregnant patients, where tachypnea, dyspnea, chest pain (pleuritic), apprehension, and rales and rhonchi are present in at least 50% of patients.

Diagnosis

Pulmonary embolism requires diagnostic testing to confidently confirm or exclude the diagnosis. This is particularly true in pregnancies because the diagnosis of DVT or pulmonary embolism requires management as in (1) prolonged therapy, entire nine months with heparin, which is costly, (2) prophylaxis during all future pregnancies, and (3) avoidance of oral contraceptive pills and hormone replacement therapy

The first diagnostic test offered should be Doppler ultrasonography. If the Doppler leg study fails to get any positive findings, then ventilation-perfusion lung scanning is advised. Perfusion scanning alone is done primarily, and the ventilation scan is added, if perfusion defects are noted. Pulmonary angiography might also be necessary, if lung scan findings are not conclusive and clinical suspicion is very high.[12]

Management

Patients, irrespective of gestational age with strong suspicion of pulmonary embolism, should be treated immediately with heparin. Heparin is the safest anticoagulant to use during pregnancy because it does not cross the placenta and hence no effect on the fetus. The initial loading should be 5,000–10,000 units and then, an infusion should be started. The patient's activated partial thromboplastin time should be sent and repeated at regular intervals and kept in the therapeutic range, which is 1.5–2 times the baseline value. Nowadays low molecular weight heparin (LMWH) can be given once a day and this does not require monitoring. LMWH does not increase the risk of bleeding with delivery or cesarean section.

Warfarin should be avoided throughout pregnancy as it results in embryopathy characterized by mental retardation, optic atrophy, cleft lip, cleft palate and cataracts in addition to hemorrhage. The teratogenic effects are seen when accidentally taken during the 1st trimester. Warfarin during any gestation of pregnancy crosses the placenta and it can cause fetal and neonatal hemorrhage with placental abruption.

Duration of Anticoagulation

Patients who sustain a DVT or pulmonary embolism in the antepartum period and started on anticoagulation therapy with heparin should continue throughout the pregnancy. After delivery, warfarin can be started and the heparin can be tapered off. Warfarin should be continued for at least 6 weeks postpartum or until at least 3 months of anticoagulant therapy have been completed.

Side Effects of Treatment

Osteopenia is seen with unfractionated heparin administered for more than 6 months. The problem of osteopenia and osteoporosis might be reduced with use of LMWH. It is not definite whether administration of calcium and vitamin D supplementation really helps the patient on heparin, but all pregnant patients are given this supplementation.

Prophylaxis

In pregnant patient with VTE during pregnancy, the recurrence rate in a subsequent pregnancy has been estimated to be 4–15%. Women with any known hypercoagulable state are also at increased risk of VTE during pregnancy and should receive prophylaxis. LMWH is most appropriate for prophylaxis as it requires a single daily dose, does not require frequent laboratory monitoring, and may be associated with a lower risk of osteoporosis and bleeding.[11]

PNEUMONIA

Pneumonia is relatively infrequent, but serious complication of pregnancy is the most frequent cause of nonobstetric infection. It is the third most frequent cause of indirect maternal mortality. Although, pneumonia can occur during any time of pregnancy, the presence of pneumonia in the third trimester can lead to preterm labor. When associated with other medical conditions, such as HIV infection, diabetes mellitus or chronic respiratory disease, it causes poor outcome both in the mother and the fetus.

Bacteriology

Streptococcus pneumonia is the most common pathogen implicated. Others are *Mycoplasma pneumoniae, Haemophilus influenzae* and *Legionella* species, influenza and other viruses, but virtually any infectious agent can cause pneumonia in a pregnant patient.

Clinical Features

A history of upper respiratory tract infection, cough with sputum, fever, dyspnea and chills should raise suspicion of pneumonia which could be unilobar or multilobar. A delay in diagnosis might lead to the development of complications of pneumonia, such as respiratory failure or empyema.

Therapy for Bacterial Pneumonia

The antibiotics that are safe in the pregnant patient are penicillins, cephalosporins, and macrolides and clindamycin. Viral pneumonia and fungal pneumonia are also common in pregnant patients, usually with secondary bacterial infections. Influenza has an acute onset after an incubation of 1–4 days and presents as high fever, headache, malaise and cough. Varicella pneumonia is a serious respiratory tract infection leading to high maternal mortality. This might need acyclovir for better control.[13]

Pneumonia with HIV infection in pregnancy is due to *Pneumocystis carinii.* Patients with *P. carinii* pneumonia require treatment with trimethoprim-sulfamethoxazole with folate supplementation and the use of new proteinase inhibitors.

TUBERCULOSIS

Child-bearing women are at significant risk for both tuberculosis infection and its progression to disease. With prompt diagnosis and early institution of proper therapy, a good outcome is seen for the mother and child. All pregnant patients are candidates for screening for tuberculosis infection as they present to the doctor, and if found to have the disease, should receive therapy during pregnancy.

HIV infection and drug-resistant tuberculosis present special challenges in the pregnant patient. Knowledge of drugs used to treat these with their interactions and teratogenic effects of antiretrovirals and second-line antituberculosis agents, is needed to treat these patients properly. Tuberculosis in pregnancy is usually treated with isoniazid and rifampin. Ethambutol may be added initially until sensitivities are available. These drugs cross the placental barrier, but they are associated with a low-risk of adverse fetal effects. Streptomycin and other injectable antituberculous drugs are contraindicated because of fetal toxicity, deafness and potential teratogenic effects during pregnancy.

OTHER PULMONARY DISORDERS

Acute Respiratory Distress Syndrome

Pregnant patients are at very high-risk of increased membrane permeability. The reduced albumin level due to hemodilution and resultant reduced plasma oncotic pressure of pregnancy, lowers the critical pulmonary capillary pressure at which pulmonary edema develops.

The pregnant patient develops acute respiratory distress syndrome (ARDS) from obstetric complications as well as from medical conditions. Obstetric complications, such as amniotic fluid embolism, chorioamnionitis and placental abruption, can produce acute toxic lung injury. Pregnancy also predisposes the patient to other pulmonary insults that can cause ARDS, such as gastric aspiration, pneumonia, air embolism and massive hemorrhage. Repeated renal tract infection causing pyelonephritis also causes ARDS during pregnancy. Iatrogenic factors, like excessive fluid administration and tocolytic therapy have been implicated.[14]

Adequate maternal oxygen saturation is essential for fetal wellbeing. Prompt and aggressive management improves prognosis. Hit hard, hit fast should be the dictum in these critical patients. Excessive alkalosis can have adverse effects on placental perfusion, while maternal acidosis appears to be reasonably well-tolerated by the fetus.

Pleural Diseases

Pleural effusions can accompany obstetric complications such as pre-eclampsia. Asymptomatic pleural effusion in the postpartum period is also known in hypoproteinemic patients. The increased blood volume and reduced colloid osmotic pressure that occur in pregnancy and the impaired lymphatic drainage due to Valsalva maneuvers during pregnancy cause pleural effusion. Moderately sized effusions or the presence of symptoms need a full clinical evaluation.[15]

Obstructive Sleep Apnea

With polycystic ovarian syndrome (PCOS) and obesity on the rise, snoring and sleep apneas are very common among pregnant women. However, few come forward with the history. Limited polysomnographic recordings are available that systematically investigate the causes of these complaints.

In pregnancy, respiratory physiology is temporarily altered by physical and hormonal changes that can profoundly change breathing during sleep. This is countered by the high circulating level of progesterone which increases the ventilatory drive, and is a protective effect. Obesity predisposes individuals to sleep-related breathing disorders and weight gain and increased nasal obstruction during pregnancy are considered contributory to sleep breathing disorders. The enlarging uterus alters diaphragmatic function, thus resulting in reduced functional residual capacity and potentially causing shunting and hypoxemia leading to hypoxemia during hypoventilation in sleep.[16,17]

Pregnancy may precipitate or worsen sleep apnea. Nasal continuous positive airway pressure (CPAP) is a safe and effective treatment of sleep disordered breathing during pregnancy.

Diagnostic Modalities

Spirometry

Forced vital capacity (FVC) and forced expiratory volume in 1 second (FEV1) are unchanged during pregnancy.

Radiologic Imaging

The chest X-ray (2 views) and chest computed tomography are acceptable for use in pregnancy with proper shielding of the maternal abdomen as they expose the fetus to 0.02–0.07 mrad and less than 1 rad respectively.[18]

Risks of fetal anomalies, growth restriction, or abortions are not increased with radiation exposure of less than 5 rad. Cumulative dosimetry should be calculated, if multiple X-rays are anticipated.

One to two rad of fetal radiation exposure may increase the risk of leukemia from the background rate of 1 in 3,000–1 in 2,000 children.

SWINE FLU (H1N1)

Background

Novel influenza A H1N1 (hemagglutinin 1 and neuraminidase 1) virus, a new strain of influenza A virus, that originated in swine and initially popularly termed "Swine flu", had spread from an initial outbreak in Mexico and southern US in April 2009, to many countries of Europe and Asia. In June 2009, the WHO raised the level of alert for an influenza pandemic to 6 – the highest possible level and the first such declaration in the past 41 years.[19]

Etiology

Influenza viruses are a group of RNA viruses belonging to the family Orthomyxoviridae. They are classified into three distinct genera: influenza A, B and C. Influenza A can be further divided into a number of subtypes according to the expression pattern of two viral antigens: hemagglutinin (which mediates viral attachment) and neuraminidase which mediates viral release). There are 16 hemagglutinin and 9 neuraminidase variants. Thus, H1N1 designates a specific subtype of influenza A. Influenza B and C are not divided into subtypes. Both influenza A and B strains cause seasonal infections of viral influenza (flu). Influenza C typically causes a mild respiratory illness.[20,21]

Pathogenesis

This type of influenza (H1N1) virus had never been previously recognized in either pigs or humans. The term "Novel" reflects the unique genetic makeup of the virus: a reassortment of several swine strains, a human strain and an avian strain. In contrast to genetic drift, reassortment (genetic shift) creates completely new antigens, thereby limiting the ability of the immune system to recognize and destroy the new virus.

Transmission

- Direct transmission from pigs to humans and vice versa.
- Human-human transmission mainly occurs through droplet infection
- Disease spreads very quickly in crowded places and in cold, dry weather
- People may become infected by touching or handling something contaminated with flu viruses on it and then touching their mouth or nose.

Clinical presentation

Manifestations of H1N1 influenza (swine flu) are similar to those of seasonal influenza. Patients present with symptoms of acute respiratory illness, including at least 2 of the following:

- Fever
- Cough
- Sore throat
- Body aches
- Headache
- Chills and fatigue
- Diarrhea and vomiting (possible)

Risk factors

Pregnancy itself is a risk factor for severe disease. Others include:

- Pregnant woman in late gestation
- Women with any other underlying medical disease

Symptoms commonly develop within 1 week of exposure and patients are contagious for = 8 days thereafter. In pregnant women novel H1N1 viral infection may present with any of the following:

- Uncomplicated influenza
  - Typical acute respiratory illness (fever/feverishness), cough, sore throat, nasal congestion or rhinorrhea, fatigue, headache, muscle pain, malaise but not shortness of breath or dyspnea
  - Diarrhea and/or vomiting may be found, not accompanied with dehydration
- Complicated or severe influenza
  - For some women, illness might progress rapidly resulting in dyspnea, tachypnea or hypoxia
  - Other complications may include pneumonia. CNS involvement (encephalopathy, encephalitis) and severe dehydration
  - There can be exacerbation of any underlying medical illness
  - Hospital admission is mandatory
- Signs and symptoms of progressive disease

  Patients who are present initially with uncomplicated influenza may progress to more severe disease. Progression can be rapid (within 24 hours). Indicators of progression are:
  - Shortness of breath (with activity or at rest), difficulty in breathing, tachypnea, presence of cyanosis, bloody or colored sputum, chest pain and low blood pressure
  - Altered mental status, unconsciousness, drowsiness, or difficult to awaken and recurring or persistent convulsions, confusion, severe weakness, or paralysis
  - Severe dehydration, manifested as decreased activity, dizziness, decreased urine output and lethargy.

Clinical guidelines on specimen collection and testing for H1N1 influenza A virus.[22]

Obtain an upper respiratory specimen, preferably a nasopharyngeal swab. Where appropriate, bronchoalveolar lavage (BAL) may also be submitted for severe causes.

A rapid influenza antigen test is commonly used in suspected cases. Centres of disease control and prevention (CDC) defines a confirmed case of novel H1N1 influenza A as an individual with an influenza-lime illness and detection by real-time reverse transcriptase-polymerase chain reaction (RT-PCR), culture or 4-fold rise in specific antibody titer based on acute compared to convalescent sera. A probable case is defined as an individual with an influenza A by RT-PCR, but in whom the strain of infection has not been determined. Current guidelines suggest that viral shedding is 2 days prior to the illness and until 7 days from illness onset or until fever has resolved, which ever happens last.

Specimen Collection

- Wear gloves, gown, eye protection for personal protection (a N95 respirator with eye protection is only recommended while performing an aerosol-generating medical procedure)
- Patients with copious discharge should be requested to gently clean their nose by washing or with tissue
- Incline the patient's head as required and insert the cotton swab perpendicular to the face to the depth of 2–3 cm into the nostril
- Swab around the inside of the nostril and along the floor of the nasal cavity by rotating the swab shaft between the fingers
- Break or cut off the swab shaft and place into the accompanying vial of transport media and tighten the lid securely
- Label the container with patient's full name and date of birth.

Pregnancy-related Complications

- There can be spontaneous abortions and premature rupture of membranes leading to preterm labor
- Nonreassuring fetal nonstress test (NST) (most commonly fetal tachycardia), fetal distress, may at times leading to intrauterine death
- Increase in number of emergency cesarean section
- There is not much information on whether this virus is transmitted to the fetus via the placenta, although this class of viruses is not considered teratogenic in humans. But it can indirectly affect the fetus possibly from high fever. Hyperthermia in early pregnancy has been associated with neural tube defects and other congenital anomalies and fever during labor and birth is the risk factor for neonatal seizures, newborn encephalopathy, cerebral palsy and death
- Increase in number of hospital and intensive care unit (ICU) admissions
- Mortality occurs to be higher in pregnant women especially if infection occurs in the third trimester.

Management[23,24]

Early treatment is recommended for women especially in the third trimester and those presenting with fever since they are at the highest risk of serious outcomes.

The CDC currently recommends antiviral treatment and chemoprophylaxis with oseltamivir and zanamivir, neuraminidase inhibitor antiviral medications, which target the early phase of the infection. Their mechanism of action involves a crucial step in the life cycle of influenza A and B. A viral surface glycoprotein (hemagglutin) binds to sialic acid residues on respiratory epithelial surface glycoproteins, which is necessary for the initiation of infection. After the virus replicates, it is also attached to the host cell the same way until neuraminidase cleaves this link and frees the new virions. However, novel H1N1 strain is resistant to adamantanes, such as amantadine and rimantadine.

Oseltamivir

It is a prodrug that is hydrolyzed by the liver to its active metabolite, oseltamivir carboxylate, with an elimination half-life of 6–10 hours.

Therapeutic dose: 75 mg BD for 5 days. Therapy should be initiated within 48 hours of the initial symptoms to capture the early phase of viral replication

Prophylactic dose: 75 mg OD for 10 days after exposure.

Drug safety in pregnancy and lactation:[23]

- Studies have shown that the drug is extensively metabolized by the human placenta and that trans-placental transfer of the metabolite was incomplete with minimal accumulation on the fetal side
- Therapeutic dosages taken during the 1st trimester may be associated with increased risk of abortions, trisomy 21 and anencephaly, though further research is required in the field
- It is C category drug
- The maximum milk concentrations of the drug and its active metabolite are reported to be 38.2 ng/mL and 39.5 ng/mL. (equivalent to 43.4 ng/mL of oseltamivir), respectively when mother is on therapeutic dosage of the drug. This shows that the infant is exposed to milk containing a maximum of 81.6 ng/mL of the drug, which corresponds to 0.012 mg/kg/day, which is much smaller to the pediatric dosage of 2–4 mg/kg/day
- Side effects—nausea and vomiting.

Zanamivir

- Administered by inhalation with a dry powder inhaler
- Bioavailability of the drug: 10–20% by inhalation and 21% by oral administration
- Approximately 90% of the absorbed dose is excreted unchanged in the urine
- Elimination half-life in serum is between 2.5 hours and 5.1 hours.

Therapeutic dose: 10 mg inhaled once daily for 10 days after exposure.

Drug safety in pregnancy and lactation:

- Data is very insufficient for its use during pregnancy. Clinical trials have reported one case of spontaneous miscarriage, I case of pregnancy termination and another case reporting a healthy term baby
- It is a category C drug
- Peak concentration after a single dose ranges from 34 ng/mL to 96 ng/mL
- Assuming a maternal serum concentration of 100 ng/mL, a milk to plasma ratio of 1.0 and an intake of milk of 150 mL/kg/day, the maximum amount of drug that a 5 kg infant would ingest would be 0.075 mg/day, which is much lower than the recommended prophylactic dosage for children of 10 mg/day inhalation.

Side effects: nausea and vomiting. There can be respiratory distress, especially in asthmatic patients.

BREASTFEEDING[24]

If pregnant patient delivers child infected with H1N1, she should avoid close contact with her infant until she has been on antiviral medications for at least 48 hours, her fevers have resolved and she can control her coughing and secretions. During this time, healthy adults should provide bottle feedings of the expressed breast milk. After this initial period of isolation, the mother should continue to practice good hand hygiene and cough etiquette and wear a facemask for the next 7 days.

Breastfeeding is advised to be continued after this even if mother is receiving remaining treatment or post-exposure prophylaxis for novel H1N1 influenza virus. Breastfeeding is known to strengthen the neonatal immense response, and infants who are not breastfed, may actually be more vulnerable to viral infection.

INFLUENZA VACCINE

The WHO strongly recommends vaccination of high-risk individuals including pregnant women against influenza infection.

In general, there are two types of influenza vaccines. One is the inactivated influenza vaccine ("flu-shot") that is given with a needle, usually in the art. This is the type of vaccine that Advisory Committee on Immunization Practices (ACIP) recommends pregnant women should receive.

The influenza A (H1N1) 2009 inactivated (flu-shot) vaccines that have been licensed are available in both single dose and multidose preparations. Multidose preparations are formulated with thimerosal, a mercury-containing preservative used to ensure that the vaccine does not become contaminated after the vial has been opened. Single dose preparations contain no thimerosal, or only trace amounts. Studies have shown that there is no known harm from thimerosal preservative-containing vaccine. Thus, pregnant women may receive either preservative-free or thimerosal preservative-containing influenza vaccine.

The other type of influenza vaccine, "nasal-spray" influenza vaccine (sometimes called LAIV for "live attenuated influenza vaccine") is made with live weakened influenza virus. The LAIV is not recommended by the ACIP for use in pregnancy.

The CDC and FDA recommend that pregnant women receive both the inactivated influenza A H1N1 (2009) monovalent vaccines can be soreness at the injection site, mild fever, body aches, and fatigue for a few days after the inoculation.

All influenza vaccines continue to be produced using eggs. For this reason, a previous history of severe, life-threatening allergies to eggs are a contraindication to the use of influenza vaccine.

REFERENCES

1. Leighton B, Fish J. Pulmonary Disease in Pregnancy. Glob Libr Women's Med. 2008;1756-2228.
2. National Asthma Education and Prevention Program. Managing asthma during pregnancy: recommendations for pharmacologic treatment. National Guideline Clearinghouse. Jan 2005.
3. Bakhireva LN, Jones KL, Schatz M, Johnson D, Chambers CD. Asthma medication use in pregnancy and fetal growth. J Allergy Clin Immunol. 2005;116(3):503-9.
4. Murphy VE, Clifton VL, Gibson PG. Asthma exacerbations during pregnancy: incidence and association with adverse pregnancy outcomes. Thorax. 2006;61(2):169-76.
5. Schatz M, Dombrowski MP, Wise R, Momirova V, Landon M, Mabie W. Spirometry is related to perinatal outcomes in pregnant women with asthma. Am J Obstet Gynecol. 2006;194(1):120-6.
6. Carroll KN, Griffin MR, Gebretsadik T, Shintani A, Mitchel E, Hartert TV. Racial differences in asthma morbidity during pregnancy. Obstet Gynecol. 2005;106(1):66-72.
7. Cockcroft DW. Treatment of asthma during pregnancy. Ann Allergy Asthma Immunol. 2005;95(3):213-4.
8. Liccardi G, Cazzola M, Canonica GW, D'Amato M, D'Amato G, Passalacqua G. General strategy for the management of bronchial asthma in pregnancy. Respir Med. 2003;97(7):778-89.
9. Murphy VE, Gibson P, Talbot PI, Clifton VL. Severe asthma exacerbations during pregnancy. Obstet Gynecol. 2005;106(5 Pt 1):1046-54.
10. James A. Committee on Practice Bulletins—Obstetrics. Practice bulletin no. 123: thromboembolism in pregnancy. Obstet Gynecol. 2011;118(3):718-29.
11. Liu S, Rouleau J, Joseph KS, Sauve R, Liston RM, Young D, et al. Epidemiology of pregnancy-associated venous thromboembolism: a population-based study in Canada. J Obstet Gynaecol Can. 2009;31(7):611-20.
12. Heit JA, Kobbervig CE, James AH, Petterson TM, Bailey KR, Melton LJ. Trends in the incidence of venous thromboembolism during pregnancy or postpartum: a 30-year population-based study. Ann Intern Med. 2005;143(10):697-706.
13. Chen YH, Keller J, Wang IT, Lin CC, Lin HC. Pneumonia and Pregnancy Outcomes: A Nationwide Population-based Study. Amer J Obstet Gynecol. 2012;207(4):288.e1-7.
14. Paternoster DM, Pascoli I, Parotto M, Cester M, Nanhornguè K, Merati E, et al. Pulmonary hypertension during pregnancy: management of two cases. Arch Gynecol Obstet. 2010;281(3):431-4.
15. Streit M, Speich R, Fischler M, Ulrich S. Successful pregnancy in pulmonary arterial hypertension associated with systemic lupus erythematosus: a case report. J Med Case Reports. 2009;3:7255.
16. Pien GW, Schwab RJ. Sleep disorders during pregnancy. Sleep. 2004;27(7):1405-17.
17. Guilleminault C, Kreutzer M, Chang JL. Pregnancy, sleep disordered breathing and treatment with nasal continuous positive airway pressure. Sleep Med. 2004;5(1):43-51.
18. Cunningham FG, Gant NF, Leveno KJ, Gilstrap LC, Hauth JC, Wenstrom KD. General considerations and maternal evaluation. Williams Obstetrics, 21st edition. New York: McGraw-Hill; 2001. pp. 1143-58.
19. World Health Organization (2010). WHO guidelines for pharmacological management of pandemic influenza A (H1N1) 2009 and other influenza viruses. [online]. Available from http://www.who.int/csr/resources/publications/swineflu/h1n1_guidelines_pharmaceutical_mngt.pdf. [Accessed December, 2015].
20. Management guidelines for pregnant women and neonates born to women with suspected or confirmed pandemic H1N1 influenza (Swine origin A/H1N1 influenza), Perinatal services BC, May 2011.
21. Mirdamadi K, Einarson A. H1N1 and influenza viruses. Canadian Family Physician. 2011;57:1003-4.
22. Carlson A, Thung SF, Norwitz ER. H1N1 influenza in pregnancy: what all obstetric care providers ought to know. Rev Obstet Gynecol. 2009;2(3):139-45.
23. Bozzo P, Djokanovic N, Koren G. H1N1 influenza in pregnancy; risks, vaccines and antivirals. J Obstet Gynaecol Can. 2009;31(12):1171-75.
24. Tanaka T1, Nakajima K, Murashima A, Garcia-Bournissen F, Koren G, Ito S. Safety of neuraminidase inhibitors against novel influenza A (H1N1) in pregnant and breastfeeding women. CMAQJ. 2009;181(1-2):55-8.

CHAPTER 49

Gastrointestinal Disorders

Ramaraju H Ediger

INTRODUCTION

Gastrointestinal physiology is poorly studied during pregnancy even though gastrointestinal symptoms are the cause of a significant number of queries and concerns. Nonspecific symptoms of vomiting, epigastric pain, abdominal cramps and diarrhea can occur frequently in pregnancy. Motor dysfunction of the gastrointestinal system and increasing uterine size are believed to be contributing factors. These gastrointestinal problems are self-limiting and most do not affect maternal and fetal outcome. Their importance in obstetric practice is to differentiate them from diseases with similar presentation requiring diagnosis and management.

During normal pregnancy, the gastrointestinal tract and its appendages undergo remarkable anatomical, physiological and functional changes. These changes can appreciably alter clinical findings normally relied on for diagnosis and treatment of gastrointestinal disorders. Nausea and vomiting, which is frequent early in normal pregnancy is one among them. If these symptoms persist beyond early pregnancy or develop later, they may be erroneously attributed to normal physiological changes and a serious pregnancy complications or nonobstetrical problems may be overlooked. In another instance, most obstetricians, but not most internists or gastroenterologists, are aware that epigastric or right upper quadrant pain can be an ominous sign of severe pre-eclampsia. Finally, as pregnancy progresses, gastrointestinal symptoms become more difficult to assess and physical findings are often obscured by the large gravid uterus; which displaces abdominal organs and can alter the location and intensity of pain and tenderness.

GENERAL CONSIDERATIONS

Diagnostic Techniques

In general, today's technological advances have made gastrointestinal tract evaluation completed without having to depend on conventional radiological techniques.

Endoscopy

Fiberoptic endoscopic instruments which have revolutionized diagnosis and management of most gastrointestinal are well-suited for use during pregnancy. Cappell[1] estimated 20,000 pregnant women annually needed endoscopy to evaluate the esophagus, stomach, duodenum and colon. The proximal jejunum can also be studied and the ampulla of Vater cannulated to perform endoscopic retrograde cholangiopancreatography [(ERCP) (Alhashem and colleagues)]. In most endoscopies, sedation is required and special considerations are given to complications unique to pregnancy.

Upper gastrointestinal endoscopy is used for management as well as diagnosis of a number of problems. Common bile duct exploration and drainage are used for choledocholithiasis. It is also used for sclerotherapy as well as placement of percutaneous endoscopic gastrostomy (PEG) tubes.

Flexible sigmoidoscopy can be used safely in pregnant women (Siddiqui and Denise-Proctor). Colonoscopy is used to view the entire colon and distal ileum for diagnosis and management of inflammatory bowel disease. Bowel preparation is completed using polyethylene glycol (PEG) electrolyte or sodium phosphate solutions with care to avoid serious maternal dehydration. Reports of colonoscopy during pregnancy are limited, but preliminary results are encouraging and it should be performed, if indicated.

Noninvasive Imaging Techniques

The most common technique for gastrointestinal evaluation is abdominal sonography. Because computed tomography (CT) use is limited in pregnancy due to radiation exposure, magnetic resonance imaging (MRI) is now commonly used for evaluating the abdomen and retroperitoneal space.

Laparotomy and Laparoscopy

Surgery is life-saving for certain gastrointestinal conditions, perforated appendicitis being the most common example. In the first study using the Swedish Registry database through 1981, Mazze and Kallen[2] reported that abdominal exploration by laparotomy or laparoscopy was performed in 1,331 of 720,000 pregnancies—approximately 1 in every 500. Kort and associates reported a similar incidence of 1 in 635 in nearly 50,000 pregnancies. In both the studies, the most common indications for surgery were appendicitis, an adnexal mass and cholecystitis.

Laparoscopic procedures have replaced traditional surgical techniques for many abdominal disorders during pregnancy.[3] Reports from the Swedish registry database, Reedy[4] and associates described 2,181 pregnant women underwent laparoscopy and 1,522 had gone through laparotomy for nonobstetrical indications. The incidence for all procedures was approximately 1 in every 800 pregnancies. Both were mostly performed before 20 weeks and they were found to be safe. Finally, long-term surveillance studies suggest no deleterious effects for either mother or child (Rizzo).

The most common nongynecological procedures performed during pregnancy are cholecystectomy and appendectomy.[5] Guidelines for diagnosis, treatment and use of laparoscopy for surgical problems during pregnancy have been provided by the Society of American Gastrointestinal and Endoscopic Surgeons.

Nutritional Support

Specialized nutritional support can be delivered enterally, usually via nasogastric tube feedings, or intravenously with peripheral or central venous access. When possible, enteral alimentation is preferable because it has fewer serious complications.[6] In obstetrical patients, very few conditions prohibit enteral nutrition as a first effort to prevent catabolism.

The purpose of parenteral feeding or hyperalimentation is to provide nutrition when the intestinal tract must be kept quiescent. Peripheral venous access may be adequate for short-term supplemental nutrition, which derives calories from isotonic fat solutions. Central venous access is necessary for total parenteral nutrition because its hyperosmolarity requires rapid dilution in a high flow vascular system. These solutions provide 24–40 kcal/kg/day principally as a hypertonic glucose solution. Heyland[7] and colleagues reviewed 26 randomized controlled trials (RCTs) involving more than 2,200 critically ill nonpregnant patients and reported that overall mortality rates were not influenced by parenteral nutrition.

Parenteral Nutrition during Pregnancy

There have been a variety of conditions for which total parenteral nutrition was employed during pregnancy (Box 1). Gastrointestinal disorders are the most common indication and in the many studies cited, duration of feeding averaged 33 days. It is imperative to emphasize that complications of parenteral nutrition are frequent and they may be severe. The myriad gastrointestinal complications were recently reviewed by Guglielmi[8] and colleagues. Russo-Stieglitz and associates described 26 pregnancies with a 50% rate of complications, which includes pneumothorax, hemothorax and brachial plexus injury. The most frequent serious complication is catheter sepsis and Folk and coworkers described 25% incidence in 27 women with hyperemesis gravidarum (HG). Although bacterial sepsis is most common, *Candida* septicemia has been described (Paranyuk and associates). The Centers for Disease Control and Prevention (CDC) has published detailed guidelines for management to

Box 1: Indications for parenteral nutrition during pregnancy[9]

- Anorexia nervosa
- Appendiceal rupture
- Bowel obstruction
- Burns
- Cholecystitis
- Crohn disease
- Diabetic gastropathy
- Esophageal injury
- Hyperemesis gravidarum
- Jejunoileal bypass
- Malignancies
- Pancreatitis
- Pre-eclampsia syndrome
- Preterm labor/ruptured membranes
- Short bowel syndrome
- Small bowel obstruction
- Stroke

Source: From Kirby (1988) and Russo-Stieglitz (1999), and all their colleagues.

prevent catheter-related sepsis. Perinatal complications are uncommon however; fetal subdural hematoma caused by maternal vitamin K deficiency was described by Sakai and colleagues.

There is also appreciable morbidity from a peripherally inserted central catheter (PICC). Ogura[9] and colleagues reported infection with long-term access in 31 of 52 pregnant women. Holmgren and coworkers reported complications in 21 of 33 women in whom a PICC line was placed for hyperemesis. Infections were the most common and half of infected women also had bacteremia. One review of 48 reports of nonpregnant adults, Turcotte and associates concluded that there were no advantages to peripherally placed catheters compared with centrally placed ones.

DISORDERS OF THE UPPER GASTROINTESTINAL TRACT

Hyperemesis Gravidarum

Many women commonly experience mild to moderate nausea and vomiting especially until approximately 16 weeks. Few women experience it in a severe and unresponsive form not responding to simple dietary modification and antiemetics. To quantify the severity of nausea and vomiting, Lacasse[10] and colleagues have proposed a pregnancy-unique quantification of emesis and nausea (PUQE) scoring index. Hyperemesis gravidarum (HG) is defined variably as vomiting sufficiently severe to produce weight loss, dehydration, alkalosis from loss of hydrochloric acid and hypokalemia. Acidosis develops from partial starvation (Chihara and coworkers). In some women, transient hepatic dysfunction develops. In population-based studies from California and Nova Scotia, the hospitalization rate for hyperemesis was 0.5–0.8%.[11] Hospitalization is less common in obese women (Cedergren and associates). There is recurrence rate of 20% in women hospitalized in a previous pregnancy for hyperemesis.[12] Hyperemesis appears to be related to high or rapidly rising serum levels of pregnancy-related hormones. With limited external stimulus, putative culprits include human chorionic gonadotropin (hCG), estrogens, progesterone, leptin, placental growth hormone, prolactin, thyroxine and adrenocortical hormones.[13] Studies by Goodwin and coworkers implicate the vestibular system. There seems to be no doubt that in some but not nearly all acute cases, there are interrelated psychological components (Buckwalter and Simpson). In some, hyperemesis is given a reason for elective termination (Poursharif and colleagues). Other factors that increase the risk for admission include hyperthyroidism, previous molar pregnancy, diabetes, gastrointestinal illnesses and asthma (Fell and coworkers). And for some unknown reasons, a female fetus increases the risk by 1.5 times (Schiff and colleagues, Tan and coworkers).

Helicobacter pylori Infection

Association of *H. pylori* infection with hyperemesis has been proposed, but evidences are not conclusive. Goldberg[14] and colleagues performed scholarly systematic review of 14 case control studies. At this time, it is not recommended to do test for or treat for gastric infection in women with hyperemesis. Because the "cocktail(s)" required for eradication of *H. pylori* would most likely cause vomiting in most pregnant women. Ponzetto[15] and colleagues reported that *H. pylori* seropositivity was linked to an increased risk for pre-eclampsia. In the population-based California study by Dodds and associates, however, the incidence of gestational hypertension was not different from that in control women. *H. pylori* infection has also been linked to iron deficiency in pregnancy (Weyermann and associates).

Complications

Vomiting may be prolonged, frequent and severe. Plasma zinc levels are increased, copper levels decreased and magnesium levels unchanged (Dokmeci and associates). Preliminary findings are that a third of women with hyperemesis have an abnormal electroencephalogram (EEG) [(Vaknin and colleagues)]. A list of potentially fatal complications is given in Box 2.

Various degrees of acute renal failure from dehydration are encountered in some women. The extreme example which was described by Hill and colleagues is a woman who required 5 days of dialysis when her serum creatinine level rose to 10.7 mg/dL. Life-threatening complications of continuous retching include Mallory-Weiss tears. Others are esophageal rupture, pneumothorax, and pneumomediastinum (Yamamoto and colleagues).[16]

At least two serious vitamin deficiencies have been reported with hyperemesis in pregnancy. Wernicke encephalopathy from thiamine deficiency is not uncommon. Chiossi[17] and colleagues reviewed 49 cases and reported that only half had the triad of confusion, ocular findings, and ataxia. Usually, there are MRI findings. At least three maternal deaths have been described and long-term sequel is common and includes blindness, convulsions

Box 2: Some life-threatening complications of recalcitrant hyperemesis gravidarum

- Depression: cause versus effect
- Esophageal rupture: Boerhaave syndrome
- Hypoprothrombinemia: vitamin K
- Hyperalimentation complications
- Mallory-Weiss tears: bleeding, pneumothorax, pneumomediastinum, pneumopericardium
- Renal failure: may require dialysis
- Wernicke encephalopathy: thiamine deficiency

and coma (Selitsky and coworkers). Vitamin K deficiency has been reported causing maternal coagulopathy and fetal intracranial hemorrhage (Kawamura, Robinson).

Management

A Cochrane Database review by Jewell and Young[18] confirmed a salutary effect from a number of antiemetic given orally or by rectal suppository as first-line agents. When simple measures fail, intravenous crystalloid solutions are given to correct dehydration, ketonemia, electrolyte deficits and acid-base imbalances.

Thiamine, 100 mg is given to prevent Wernicke encephalopathy previously discussed. If vomiting persists after rehydration and failed outpatient management, hospitalization is recommended [American Congress of Obstetricians and Gynecologists (ACOG), 2004]. Antiemetics such as promethazine, prochlorperazine, chlorpromazine or metoclopramide are given parenterally. There is little evidence that treatment with glucocorticosteroid is effective. Two small trials found no benefits of methylprednisolone compared with placebo but the steroid treated group had significantly fewer readmissions.[19] In a study of 110 women at Parkland Hospital, Yost and colleagues compared placebo with intravenous methylprednisolone plus tapered oral steroids. A third in each group required readmission. In a study by Bondok[20] and coworkers, pulsed hydrocortisone therapy was superior to metoclopramide to reduce vomiting and readmissions. Serotonin antagonists are the most effective agents for controlling chemotherapy-induced nausea and vomiting (Hesketh). When used in one trial for HG, however, ondansetron was not superior to promethazine (Sullivan and associates). Reports of serotonin antagonist use in pregnancy are limited, but there is no evidence of teratogenicity (Briggs and associates).[21] With persistent vomiting after hospitalization, appropriate steps should be taken to exclude possible underlying diseases as a cause of hyperemesis. Endoscopy did not change management in 49 women reported by Debby and coworkers. Examples include gastroenteritis, cholecystitis, pancreatitis, hepatitis, peptic ulcer and pyelonephritis. In addition, severe pre-eclampsia and fatty liver are considerations after mid-pregnancy. Although clinical thyrotoxicosis has been implicated as a cause of hyperemesis, it is more likely that abnormally elevated serum thyroxine levels are surrogate for higher than average serum hCG levels. Tan[22] and colleagues have described this as "chemical hyperthyroidism". Of interest, Panesar[23] and associates showed that a cohort of women with hyperemesis had lower serum thyrotropin levels. In few clinical experiences, serum free thyroxine levels normalize quickly with hydration. Following treatment, most women have had a salutary response and may be sent home with antiemetic therapy. Their readmission rate is 25–35% in most prospective studies. If associated, psychiatric and social factors contribute to the illness, the woman usually improves remarkably while hospitalized, but may relapse after discharge. In these women, assistance with psychosocial problems is beneficial.[24]

Nutritional Support

Vaisman[25] and coworkers described successful use of nasojejunal feeding for up to 21 days in 11 such women. Percutaneous endoscopic gastrostomy with a jejunal port PEG (J) tube was described by Schrag and coworkers.

In their study of 166 women, Folk and colleagues reported that in 16%, central venous access was established for nutrition. The list of complications included line sepsis in 25% and thrombosis and infective endocarditis in one woman each.

Reflux Esophagitis

Heartburn or pyrosis is common in late pregnancy. The retrosternal burning sensation is caused by esophagitis from gastro-esophageal reflex related to relaxation of the lower esophageal sphincter.[26] Common folklore has held that women with excessive heartburn give birth to infants with more hair. And although this may seem strange, Costigan and associates recently confirmed this. They proposed a shared biological mechanism. Pregnancy hormones caused both relaxation of the esophageal sphincter—thus more reflux, more heartburn and they also modulated hair growth.

Symptoms usually respond to raising the head of the bed and treatment with oral antacids. If severe symptoms persist, H2-receptor antagonists such as cimetidine or ranitidine are prescribed. These are considered safe but misoprostol is contraindicated because it may stimulate labor. The commonly used proton-pump inhibitor, omeprazole is also safe for use in pregnancy.[27,21] If there still is no relief, then endoscopy should be considered. Biertho[28] and associates described 25 women who had undergone laparoscopic Nissen fundoplication for reflux prior to pregnancy. Only 20% had reflux symptoms requiring antacids during pregnancy.

Hiatal Hernia

Rigler and Eneboe performed upper gastrointestinal radiographs in 195 women in late pregnancy (Fig. 1). Almost 20% of 116 multiparas and 5% of 79 nulliparas had a hiatal hernia. Notably, in only 3 of 10 women, a hernia persisted for 1-18 months postpartum.

The relationship of hiatal hernia with reflux esophagitis and thus symptoms are not clear. Cohen and Harris[29] demonstrated no relationship between reflux and hernia and showed that the lower esophageal sphincter functioned effectively even when displaced intrathoracically. Nevertheless, during pregnancy, these hiatal hernias

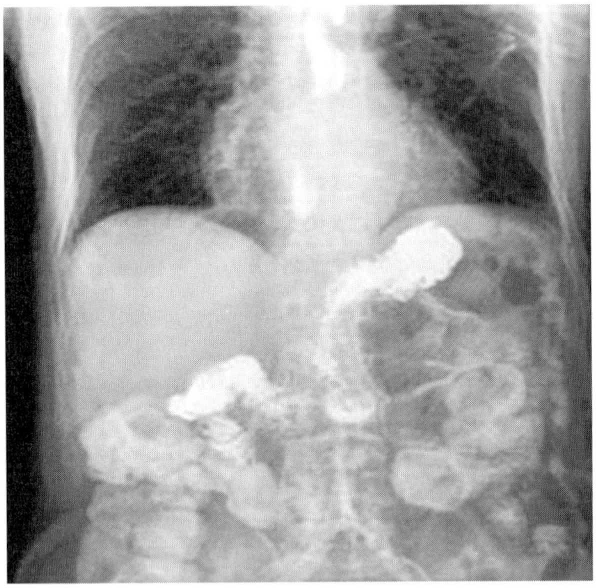

FIG. 1: Picture of hiatal hernia.

may cause vomiting, epigastric pain and bleeding from ulceration. Curran and colleagues described a 30-week pregnancy complicated by gastric outlet obstruction from a paraesophageal hernia, which they subsequently successfully repaired. Biertho and associates reported a woman with a prior Nissen fundoplication whose pregnancy was complicated by gastric herniation into the thoracic cavity. Emergency surgical intervention was followed by spontaneous abortion.

Diaphragmatic Hernia

These are caused by herniation of abdominal contents through either the foramen of Bochdalek or foramen of Morgagni. Fortunately, they rarely complicate pregnancy. Kurzel[30] and associates reviewed the outcomes of 18 pregnant women with such a hernia and who developed acute obstruction. Because the maternal mortality rate was 45%, they recommend repair during pregnancy even if a woman is asymptomatic. Flick and coworkers reported a 23-week pregnancy complicated by maternal intrathoracic bowel herniation through an old traumatic diaphragmatic defect. Finally, several case reports describe spontaneous diaphragmatic rupture from increased intra-abdominal pressure during delivery (Ortega-Carnicer)

Achalasia

The word literally means "failure to relax". Achalasia is a motility disorder in which the lower esophageal sphincter fails to relax properly with swallowing and there are nonperistaltic contractions of the esophageal muscularis (Khudyak and colleagues). The defect is caused by inflammatory destruction of the myenteric, i.e., Auerbach's plexus of smooth muscle of the lower esophagus and its sphincter. Postganglionic cholinergic neurons are unaffected thus there is unopposed sphincter stimulation. Symptoms are dysphagia, chest pain and regurgitation. Barium swallow radiography demonstrates "bird beak" or "ace of spades" narrowing at the distal esophagus. Endoscopy is performed to exclude gastric carcinoma, and manometry is confirmatory. If dilatation of the esophagus and medical therapy does not provide relief, myotomy is considered. [31]

Pregnancy

Normal relaxation of the lower esophageal sphincter during pregnancy theoretically should not occur with achalasia. Even so, in most women pregnancy does not seem to worsen achalasia. Mayberry and Atkinson interviewed 20 affected women who reported no excessive reflux esophagitis. In their review of 35 pregnancies, Khudyak[32] and colleagues described most as symptom free, although esophageal dilatation was needed in a few. A maternal death at 24 weeks associated with a 14 cm diameter mega esophagus was described by Fassina and Osculati.

Management includes soft diet and anticholinergic drugs. With persistent symptoms, other options include nitrates, calcium channel antagonists, and botulinum toxin injection (Khudyak and coworkers). Balloon dilatation of the sphincter may be necessary and 85% of nonpregnant patients respond to this. Satin and colleagues and Fiest and associates reported successful use of pneumatic dilatation in pregnancy. It is important to remember that esophageal perforation is a serious complication of dilatation.

Peptic Ulcer

Erosive ulcer disease more often involves the duodenum rather than the stomach in young women. Gastroduodenal ulcers in nonpregnant women may be caused by chronic gastritis from *H. pylori* or they develop from use of aspirin or other nonsteroidal anti-inflammatory drugs. Acid secretion is also important and thus the efficacy of antisecretory agents (Suerbaum and Michetti). Gastro-protection during pregnancy is probably due to reduced gastric acid secretion, decreased motility and considerably increased mucus secretion (Hytten). Despite this, Cappell and Garcia theorize that ulcer disease may be under-diagnosed because of frequent treatment for reflux esophagitis. In the past 40 years at Parkland Hospital, whom they cared for more than 400,000 pregnant women, they have encountered very few symptomatic ulcer disease cases. Before appropriate therapy was commonplace, Clark[33] studied 313 pregnancies in 118 women with proven ulcer disease and reported a clear remission during pregnancy in almost 90%. Benefits were short lived however and symptoms recurred in over half by 3 months postpartum and in almost all by 2 years.

Management

Antacids are first-line therapy and H2 receptor blockers are reserved for those who do not respond. Proton pump inhibitors are effective and at least two studies have shown no apparent teratogenic effects.[21,27] Sucralfate is the aluminum salt of sulfated sucrose that provides a protective coating at the ulcer base. Only approximately 10% of the aluminum salt is absorbed and it is considered safe for pregnant women.

With active ulcers, a search for *H. pylori* is undertaken. Diagnostic aids include the urea breath test, serological testing or endoscopic biopsy. If any of these are positive, antimicrobial therapy is indicated. There are a number of effective oral treatment regimens that do not include tetracycline and that can be used during pregnancy. These include amoxicillin, 1000 mg twice daily; clarithromycin, 500 mg twice daily or metronidazole, 500 mg twice daily, used in paired combination for 7 days.[34]

Upper Gastrointestinal Bleeding

Occasionally, persistent vomiting is accompanied by worrisome upper gastrointestinal bleeding. Occasionally, there is a bleeding peptic ulceration. However, most of these women have small linear mucosal tears near the gastro-esophageal junction (Mallory-Weiss tears). Bleeding usually responds promptly to conservative measures, including iced saline irrigations, topical antacids and intravenously administered H2-blockers. Transfusions may be needed and if there is persistent bleeding, then endoscopy is indicated.[35] With persistent retching, the less common, but more serious, esophageal rupture Boerhaave syndrome may develop from greatly increased esophageal pressure.

DISORDERS OF THE SMALL BOWEL AND COLON

The small bowel has diminished motility during pregnancy. Using a nonabsorbable carbohydrate, Lawson[36] and colleagues showed that small bowel mean transit times were 99, 125 and 137 minutes in each trimester, compared with 75 minutes when nonpregnant. One study by Everson, mean transit time for a mercury-filled balloon from the stomach to the cecum was 58 hours in term pregnant women compared to 52 hours in nonpregnant women.

Muscular relaxation of the colon is accompanied by increased absorption of water and sodium that predisposes to constipation, which is reported by almost 40% of women at some time during pregnancy.[37] These symptoms are usually only mildly bothersome and preventive measures include a high fiber diet and bulk-forming laxatives. Treatment option has been reviewed by Wald.[38] Some have encountered several pregnant women who developed mega-colon from impacted stool. These women almost invariably had chronically abused stimulatory laxatives.

Infectious Diarrhea

The large variety of viruses, bacteria, helminthes and protozoa that cause diarrhea in adults inevitably afflict pregnant women. For example, the incidence of *Clostridium difficile*, pseudomembranous colitis has tripled in the past decade.[39] Traveler's diarrhea is usually mild and responds to loperamide (Medical Letter).

Inflammatory Bowel Disease

The two presumably noninfectious forms of intestinal inflammation are ulcerative colitis and Crohn's disease. The latter also is known as regional enteritis, Crohn ileitis and granulomatous colitis. Differentiation between the two is important because treatment differs for either of them. Though, they both share common factors and sometimes it is impossible to distinguish them if Crohn disease involves the colon. The salient clinical and laboratory features shown in table 1 permit a reasonably confident diagnostic differentiation in most cases. The etiopathogenesis of both disorders is enigmatic, but there is genetic predisposition towards either. Inflammation is thought to result from inappropriate response of the mucosal immune system to normal bacterial flora with or without an autoimmune component.[40]

Diagnostic Criteria for Inflammatory Bowel Syndrome (Rome III Criteria for the Diagnosis of IBS 2006)

Recurrent abdominal pain or discomfort at least 3 days per month in the last 3 months with symptom onset at least 6 months prior to diagnosis, associated with two or more of the following:
- Relieved with defecation
- Onset associated with change in frequency of stool
- Onset associated with change in form (appearance) of stool

Supportive symptoms that are not part of Rome III criteria include:
- Abnormal stool frequency (three bowel movements per week or more than three bowel movements per day) abnormal stool form (lumpy/hard or loose/watery)
- Defecation straining, urgency or a feeling of incomplete bowel movement
- Passing of mucus and bloating

TABLE 1: Some differentiating characteristics of ulcerative colitis and Crohn disease[43, 40]

Characteristics	Ulcerative colitis	Crohn disease
Genetics and heredity	Polygenic, 6–20% monozygous twin concordance, HLA Bw35, B27, DR2, chromosomes[3,5,7,12,16]	Polygenic, 50–58% monozygous twins, HLA A2, B27, DR5, DQ1; chromosome 16 (IBD1–IBD9)
Natural History		
Bowel involvement	Large bowel mucosa and submucosa, continuous involvement beginning at rectum (40% proctitis only)	Small and large bowel mucosa and deeper layers, transmural involvement common; may affect small or large bowel only, or both, discontinuous and segmental involvement, strictures or fistulas common
Colonoscopy	Mucosal erythema with granularity and friability with superficial ulceration, rectal involvement almost always	Patchy involvement, rectum usually spared, perianal involvement common
Symptoms	Diarrhea with blood or mucus, tenesmus	Cramping abdominal pain and
		watery diarrhea, vomiting; malnutrition, low-grade fever; weight loss
Clinical course	Exacerbations and remission, acute and intermittent common, may be chronic and unremitting	Exacerbations and remission; surgery commonly required
Extraintestinal manifestations	Arthritis, erythema nodosum, pyoderma gangrenosum, uveitis	Arthritis, erythema nodosum, uveitis, anemia, carcinoma
Serum antibodies	Anti-neutrophil cytoplasmic-antibody (pANCA) approximately 70%	Anti-saccharomyces cerevisiae ~50%
Complications	Toxic mega-colon (5%), strictures; reactive arthritis, sclerosing cholangitis, cancer (3–5%)	Fistulas; reactive arthritis; toxic mega-colon
Management	Medical, proctocolectomy curative	Medical, segmental resection if indicated

HLA, human leukocyte antigen; IBD, inflammatory bowel disease.
Source: Farrell and Peppercorn, Friedman and Blumberg, Lichtenstein and colleagues; and Podolsky.

Ulcerative Colitis

Inflammation is confined to the superficial luminal layers of the colon typically beginning at the rectum and extending proximally for a variable distance. Half of afflicted patients have disease confined to the rectum and rectosigmoid. Endoscopic findings include mucosal granularity and friability interspersed with mucosal ulcerations and a mucopurulent exudate. The extent of inflammation is proportional to symptoms, and bloody diarrhea is the cardinal presenting finding. The disease is characterized by exacerbations and remissions. For unknown reasons, prior appendectomy protects against development of ulcerative colitis.[41] Toxic mega-colons are particularly dangerous complication that frequently necessitates colectomy. Extraintestinal manifestations include arthritis, and erythema nodosum. Another serious problem is that the risk of cancer approaches 1% per year.

Management

Ulcerative colitis is treated medically. Drugs that deliver 5 aminosalicyclic acid (5-ASA) or mesalamine are used for active colitis as well as maintenance therapy. Sulfasalazine is the prototype, and its 5-ASA moiety inhibits prostaglandin synthase in the colon. Glucocorticoids are given orally, parenterally or by enema for more severe disease that does not respond to 5-ASA. Immunomodulating drugs include azathioprine, 6-mercaptopurine, cyclosporine and methotrexate used in conjunction with prednisone in nonpregnant in patient for maintenance. High-dose intravenous cyclosporine may be beneficial for severely ill patients and used in lieu of colectomy. For recalcitrant disease, proctocolectomy is performed and a permanent ileostomy or an ileoanal anastomosis with a continent ileal pouch is created. Within the past few years, the anti-tumor necrosis factor (TNF) antibody infliximab has been reported to be modestly effective for treatment and maintenance of moderate to severe active disease.[42]

Crohn Disease

This disorder has more protean manifestations than ulcerative colitis. It involves not only the bowel mucosa but also the deeper layers and sometimes there is transmural involvement. The disease is typically segmental. Approximately 30% of patients have small bowel involvement, 25% have isolated colon involvement and 40% have both usually, with the terminal ileum and colon involved. Symptoms depend on which bowel segment(s) is involved. Thus, complaints may include cramping, abdominal pain, diarrhea, weight loss, low-grade fever, and obstructive symptoms. The disease is chronic with exacerbations and remissions and importantly, it cannot be cured medically or surgically.[43] Almost 30% of patients requires surgery during the first year after diagnosis and thereafter, 5% per year require surgery. Reactive arthritis is common, and the risk of cancer although not as great as with ulcerative colitis, is increased substantively.

Management

There is no regimen that is universally effective for maintenance during asymptomatic periods. Sulfasalazine is effective for some, but the newer 5-ASA formulations are better tolerated. As a class, they appear to be safe in pregnancy.[44] Prednisone therapy may control moderate to severe flares, but is less effective for small-bowel involvement. Immunomodulators such as azathioprine, 6-mercaptopurine, methotrexate and cyclosporine are used for active disease and for maintenance.[45] With the exception of methotrexate, most of these drugs appear relatively safe during pregnancy (Briggs and coworkers, Moskovitz and associates). Methotrexate is categorized as Class X drug. In the past few years, anti-TNF-α antibodies like infliximab, adalimumab, and certolizumab, have been found effective for active Crohn's disease and maintenance (Sandborn Sands). This class of immunomodulators are considered category B, but data supporting safety in pregnancy are limited (Roux and colleagues).

Conservative surgery is indicated for complications. Patients with small-bowel involvement more likely will require surgery for complications that include fistulas, strictures, abscesses and intractable disease. Some develop perineal communications that interfere with vaginal delivery (Forsnes and coworkers).

Inflammatory Bowel Disease and Fertility

Subfertility is commonly linked to any chronic medical disease (Bradley and Rosen). Despite this, Mahadevan cited a normal fertility rate unless surgery is performed for bowel disease. It may also be partially due to sulfasalazine which causes reversible sperm abnormalities (Feagins and Kane). Alstead[46] and Nelson-Piercy reported that decreased female fertility from active Crohn disease returned to normal with remission. After ileal pouch anal anastomosis, however, up to half of women with ulcerative colitis are infertile (Waljee and associates). Thus, subfertility may be associated with active or severe disease.

Inflammatory Bowel Disease and Pregnancy

Both disorders are relatively common in young women and thus are encountered during pregnancy. The consensus is that pregnancy does not increase the likelihood of an inflammatory bowel disease flare. Pertinent to this, Riis and colleagues performed a 10-year surveillance of women in the European Collaborative on inflammatory bowel disease. The likelihood of a flare during pregnancy was decreased compared with their preconceptional course. This diminished rate persisted for years after pregnancy and was attributed to close attention and monitoring of enrolled patients. Although most women with quiescent disease in early pregnancy uncommonly have relapses when a flare develops, it may be severe. Conversely, active disease in early pregnancy increases the likelihood of poor pregnancy outcome. In general, most usual treatment regimens may be continued during pregnancy. If needed to direct management, diagnostic evaluations should be undertaken and if indicated, surgery should be performed.

Regarding effects on pregnancy, it is likely that overall adverse perinatal outcomes are increased. Kornfeld[47] and coworkers described outcomes in a population based cohort study of 756 Swedish women with pre-existing ulcerative colitis or Crohn disease. Rates of preterm birth, low birth weight, fetal growth restriction and cesarean delivery were all increased 1.5–2-fold. According to Reddy and associates, these are more likely in women with multiple recurrences. Importantly, despite these results, perinatal mortality rates were not increased in either study. Also, it is evident that much of this excessive morbidity is attributable to Crohn disease.[48]

Ulcerative Colitis and Pregnancy

There is no evidence to suggest that pregnancy has any significant effects on ulcerative colitis. In a meta-analysis of 755 pregnancies, Fonager[49] and colleagues reported that ulcerative colitis quiescent at conception worsened in approximately a third of pregnancies. In women with active disease at the time of conception, approximately 45% worsened, 25% remained unchanged and only 25% unproved. These observations were similar to those previously described in an extensive review by Miller.

Management for colitis for the most part is the same as for nonpregnancy. Flares may be caused by psychogenic stress and reassurance is important. Calcium supplementation is provided because osteoporosis is common. Maintenance of colitis is continued with 5-ASA derivatives and flares are treated with corticosteroids. Recalcitrant disease is treated with immune modulators. Okada and associates described a dramatic response in a 13-week pregnant woman treated with leukocyte apheresis. Parenteral nutrition may be necessary for women with prolonged exacerbations.

Colorectal endoscopy is performed as indicated (Katz). Colectomy for fulminant colitis may be lifesaving and it has been performed during each trimester. Dozois and colleagues reviewed 42 such cases and found that, in general, outcomes have been good in reports published after 1980. Most women underwent partial or complete colectomy, but decompression colostomy with ileostomy was described by Ooi and coworkers in a 10- and a 16-week pregnancy.

Proctocolectomy improves sexual function and fertility (Cornish and coworkers). Women who have had a colectomy and ileal pouch anal anastomosis can safely deliver vaginally. Hahnloser and colleagues reviewed routes of delivery in women with 235 pregnancies before and 232 pregnancies after continent pouch surgery. Functional outcomes were similar and these researchers concluded that cesarean delivery should be for obstetrical indications. In at least one case, however, adhesions to the growing uterus led to pouch perforation (Aouthmany and Horattas). Pouchitis is an inflammatory condition of the ileoanal pouch, probably due to bacterial proliferation, stasis and endotoxin release. It usually responds to cephalosporins or metronidazole.

By most accounts, ulcerative colitis has minimal adverse effects on pregnancy outcome. Modigliani reviewed outcomes in 2,398 pregnancies in women with colitis. Perinatal outcomes were not substantively different from those in the general obstetrical population. Specifically, the incidences of spontaneous abortion, preterm delivery and stillbirths were remarkably low. In a population based cohort study from Washington state, Dominitz and coworkers described pregnancy outcomes in 107 women with ulcerative colitis. With two exceptions, perinatal outcomes were similar to those of 1,308 normal pregnancies. One exception was an inexplicably increased incidence of congenital malformations, and the other was the cesarean delivery rate that was increased from 20 to 29% compared with controls.

Crohn Disease and Pregnancy

There is no evidence that pregnancy affects Crohn disease. One report suggested that disease activity might even be decreased (Agret and colleagues). In general, disease activity is related to its status around the time of conception. In their cohort study, Fonager and associates analyzed outcomes in 279 pregnancies based on disease activity at conception. For 186 women whose disease was inactive at conception, only a fourth relapsed during pregnancy. In contrast, of the 93 with active disease at conception; two-thirds either worsened or had no change.

Maintenance therapy is similar to that for nonpregnant women. Oral or topical 5-ASA derivatives, usually with azathioprine, 6-mercaptopurine or cyclosporine are continued as they appear to be safe during pregnancy (Briggs and colleagues). Methotrexate is contraindicated and recently mycophenolate mofetil and mycophenolic acid have been reported to cause serious congenital anomalies (FDA). Katz and coworkers described treatment with the monoclonal antibody infliximab in 96 pregnancies.

In 31 of these, treatment was given in the first trimester with no adverse sequelae. Calcium supplementation is given to combat osteoporosis. Parenteral hyperalimentation has been used successfully during severe recurrences (Russo-Stieglitz and colleagues). Endoscopy or surgery is performed as indicated. An abdominal surgical procedure was required during 5% of pregnancies described by Woolfson and colleagues. In one instance, a woman with known Crohn disease at 32 weeks underwent emergent cesarean delivery for a presumed abruption. Instead, an abscess was found around the hepatic flexure (Panayotidis and Triantafyllidis).

As discussed previously, Crohn disease is associated with increased adverse perinatal outcomes usually related to disease activity. Based on a 20-year review, Korelitz[50] concluded that perinatal outcomes were generally good with quiescent disease. In one case control Danish study, Norgard[51] and colleagues reported a 2-fold risk of preterm neonates. Dominitz and coworkers reported 2–3 fold increase in preterm delivery, low birth weight, and fetal growth restriction in fetuses of 149 women with Crohn disease. The rate of cesarean delivery in this study was also increased compared with normal controls 28 versus 20%. As discuss consequently, women with an ileal loop colostomy may have significant problems. Women with perianal fistula unless these are rectovaginal, usually can undergo vaginal delivery without complications (Takahashi and colleagues).

Colostomy/Ileostomy and Pregnancy

Colostomy or an ileostomy can be problematic during pregnancy because of its location. Gopal and colleagues described 82 pregnancies in 66 women with an ileostomy. Although normal dysfunction was common, it responded to conservative management in all cases. But surgical intervention was necessary in three of six women who developed bowel obstruction and in another four with ileostomy prolapse—almost 10% over. Although only a third of 82 women underwent cesarean delivery. Takahashi and associates described six of seven cesarean deliveries in women with enterostoma created for Crohn disease.

Colectomy with mucosal proctectomy and ileal pouch, anal anastomosis is the preferred surgical procedure for ulcerative colitis and familial colonic polyposis. Disadvantages include frequent bowel movements, fecal incontinence including nocturnal soilage in almost half of patients and pouchitis. Although these disadvantages temporarily worsened during pregnancy, they abated postpartum. Importantly, Farouk and associates reported that pregnancy did not worsen long term colostomy function. Most have concluded that vaginal delivery is acceptable in these women.

Intestinal Obstruction

The incidence of bowel obstruction is not increased during pregnancy although it generally is more difficult to diagnose. Meyer and colleagues reported a 20-year incidence of 1 in 17,000 deliveries at two Detroit hospitals. As shown in Table 2, approximately 50% cases are due to adhesions from previous pelvic surgery that includes cesarean delivery. When women of all ages are considered, small-bowel obstruction eventually develops in only 1 per 1000 cesarean deliveries performed (Al-Sunaidi and Tulandi). Another 25% of bowel obstruction is caused by volvulus-sigmoid, cecal, or small bowel (Fig. 2). These have been reported in late pregnancy or early puerperium (Biswas, Lal).[52] Intussusception is occasionally encountered (Gould and coworkers). A degenerating uterine leiomyoma causing small bowel obstruction was described by MacDonald and associates.

TABLE 2: Causes of intestinal obstruction during pregnancy and the puerperium

Causes of obstruction	Percent
• Adhesions: ○ First and second trimester: 10–15% ○ Third trimester: 2% ○ Postpartum: 10%	60
• Volvulus: ○ Midgut: 2% ○ Cecal: 5% ○ Sigmoid: 10%	25
• Intussusception	5
• Hernia, carcinoma, other	5

Courtesy: Connolly (1995) and Redlich (2007) and all their colleagues.

Etiopathogenesis

Most cases of intestinal obstruction during pregnancy result from pressure of the growing uterus on intestinal adhesions. According to Davis and Bohon[53], this more likely occurs—(A) around mid-pregnancy, when the uterus becomes an abdominal organ; (B) in the third trimester, when the fetal head descends; or (C) immediately postpartum, when there is an acute change in uterine size. Perdue and colleagues reported that 80% of pregnant women had nausea and vomiting. Importantly, 98% of all women had either continuous or colicky abdominal pain. Abdominal tenderness was found in 70% and abnormal bowel sounds in only 55%. Plain abdominal radiographs following soluble contrast showed evidence of obstruction in 90 % of women. Plain radiographs are less accurate for diagnosing small-bowel obstruction and CT and MRI are useful (McKenna).[54]

Pregnancy Outcomes

Mortality rates with obstruction during pregnancy can be excessive because of difficult and thus delayed diagnosis, reluctance to operate during pregnancy and the need for emergency surgery (Firstenberg and Malangoni).

Of 66 pregnancies, Perdue and associates described 6% maternal mortality rate and 26% fetal mortality rate. Perforation from massively dilated bowel may cause sepsis. Two of the four women who died had sigmoid or cecal volvulus caused by adhesions late in pregnancy.

Colonic Pseudo-obstruction

Also called as Ogilvie syndrome, pseudo-obstruction is caused by adynamic colonic ileus (Fig. 3). Approximately 10% of all cases are associated with pregnancy. The

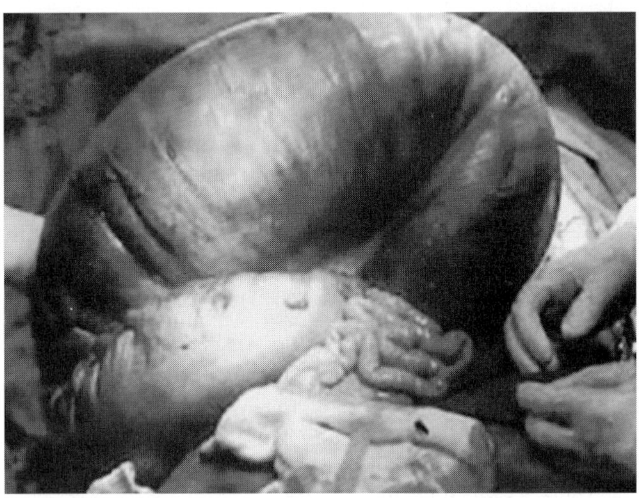

FIG. 2: Massively dilated colon in volvulus ***(For color version, see Plate 6).***

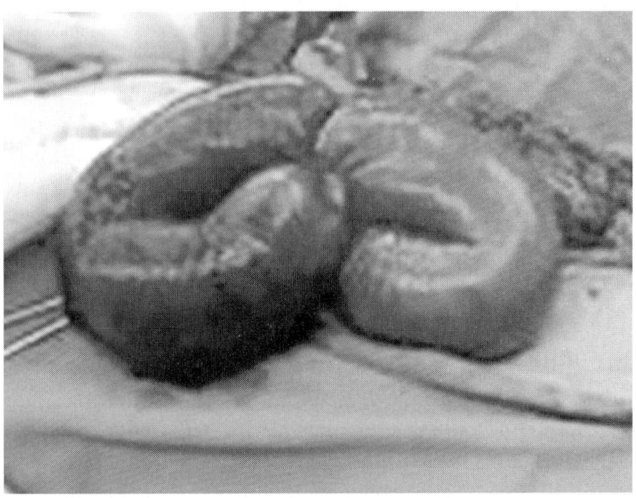

FIG. 3: Picture of colonic pseudo-obstruction ***(For color version, see Plate 6).***

syndrome usually develops postpartum but it has been reported occasionally antepartum (Tung and associates). It is characterized by massive abdominal distension with cecal dilatation. Although unusual, the large bowel may rupture (Singh and colleagues). In most cases, intravenous infusion of neostigmine, 2 mg, results in prompt decompression.[55] In some cases, colonoscopic decompression is performed, but laparotomy is done for perforation.[56]

Appendicitis

Suspected appendicitis is one of the most common indications for abdominal exploration during pregnancy. Mazze and Kallen reported this in approximately 1 in 1,000 pregnant women in the Swedish registry of 720,000 pregnancies. Appendicitis was confirmed in 65% for an incidence of approximately 1 in 1,500 pregnancies. It is interesting and inexplicable that the incidence was much lower in the Danish registry of more than 320,000 pregnancies. Hee and Viktrup[57] reported the confirmed appendicitis rate of only 1 per 5,500 pregnancies. There is some evidence that appendicitis is less common during pregnancy compared with its incidence in age-matched nonpregnant controls.[58]

It is repeatedly and appropriately emphasized that pregnancy makes diagnosis of appendicitis more difficult. This is partly because nausea and vomiting accompany normal pregnancy. In addition, as the uterus enlarges, the appendix commonly moves upward and outward so that pain and tenderness are "displaced" (Baer and colleagues). Another often stated reason is that some degree of leukocytosis accompanies normal pregnancy.

For all of these reasons, pregnant women and especially those late in gestation frequently do not have clinical findings "typical" for appendicitis. It commonly is confused with cholecystitis, preterm labor, pyelonephritis, renal colic, placental abruption or degeneration of a uterine leiomyoma.

Most reports indicate increasing morbidity and mortality rates with increasing gestational age. And as the appendix is progressively deflected upward by the growing uterus, omental containment of infection becomes increasingly unlikely. It is indisputable that appendiceal perforation is more common during later pregnancy. In the studies by Andersson and Lambe and Ueberrueck and associates, the incidence of perforation averaged approximately 8, 12 and 20% in successive trimesters.

Diagnosis

Persistent abdominal pain and tenderness are the most reproducible findings. As discussed, although most have reported that pain migrates upward with appendiceal displacement, this has been disputed.

Graded compression sonography during pregnancy is difficult because of cecal displacement and uterine imposition (Pedrosa). Appendiceal CT is more sensitive and accurate than ultrasound (USG) to confirm suspected appendicitis (Paulson, Raman) [59] (Fig. 4). Specific views can be designed to decrease fetal radiation exposure. In one study, Wallace and coworkers reported that the negative appendectomy rate was 54% with clinical diagnosis alone, but only 8% if sonography and CT scanning were used. MRI may be preferable; few have had good results with its use (Israel and associates). Although not as accurate as preliminary findings suggested, Pedrosa and associates reported no false-negative diagnoses with MRI, but a 30% false positive rate in 140 pregnant women with suspected appendicitis. Finally, appendiceal scanning following administration of native leukocytes tagged with technetium 99 was not successful in 13 pregnant women reported by Stewart and associates.

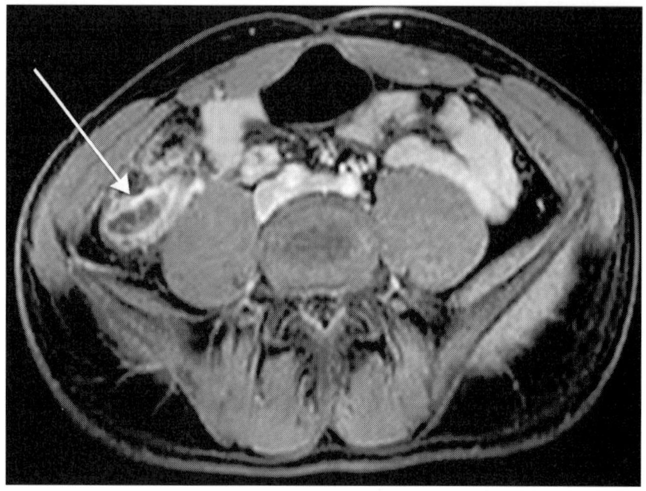

FIG. 4: CT Scan picture of nonperforative appendicitis.

Management

When appendicitis is suspected, treatment is prompt surgical exploration. Although diagnostic errors sometimes lead to removal of a normal appendix, surgical evaluation is superior to postponed intervention and generalized peritonitis. In most reports the diagnosis is verified in 60–70% of pregnant women who undergo surgical exploration. Related to the successive perforation rate by trimester discussed above, the accuracy of diagnosis is inversely proportional to gestational age. Mazze and Kallen reported that 77 % of first-trimester diagnoses were correct. In the next two trimesters, however, only 57% were found to be correct.

During the first half of pregnancy, laparoscopy for suspected appendicitis has become the norm. From the Swedish database, Reedy[60] and colleagues reported similar perinatal outcomes in nearly 2,000 laparoscopic appendectomies compared with those of more than 1,500 laparotomies done before 20 weeks. In many centers, laparoscopic appendectomy is performed in the third trimester (Barnes and colleagues; Rollins and associates). Parangi and coworkers are less enthusiastic about this approach, it is recommended that laparoscopic surgery in pregnancy past 26–28 weeks should be performed only by the most experienced surgeons. For laparotomy, most surgeons prefer a McBurney incision.

Before exploration, intravenous antimicrobial therapy is begun, usually with a second-generation cephalosporin or third-generation penicillin. Unless there is gangrene, perforation, or a periappendiceal phlegmon, antimicrobial therapy can usually be discontinued after surgery. Without generalized peritonitis, the prognosis is excellent. Seldom is cesarean delivery indicated at the time of appendectomy. Uterine contractions are common and although some clinicians recommend tocolytic agents. De Veciana and colleagues reported that tocolytic use increased the risk for maternal pulmonary permeability edema with sepsis syndrome .If appendicitis is undiagnosed before delivery, often when the large uterus rapidly empties, walled-off infection is disrupted, causing an acute surgical abdomen. New onset appendicitis during the immediate puerperium is uncommon. However, it is important to remember that puerperal pelvic infections typically do not cause peritonitis.

Effects on Pregnancy

Appendicitis increases the likelihood of abortion or preterm labor, especially if there is peritonitis. Mazze and Kallen and Cohen Kerem[61] and associates reported that spontaneous labor ensued with greater frequency following surgery for appendicitis compared with other indications after 23 weeks. In the former study, fetal loss was 22% if surgery was performed after 23 weeks. McGory and colleagues surveyed the California inpatient file of 3,133 pregnant women undergoing surgery for suspected appendicitis. Overall, the fetal loss rate was 23%. The rate was doubled -6 versus 11% with simple versus complicated disease. Interestingly, it was higher in those with negative appendiceal pathology compared with those with simple appendicitis 4 versus 10%.

Mays and colleagues have suggested a link between sepsis and neonatal neurological injury. Viktrup and Hee found that appendicitis during pregnancy was not associated with subsequent infertility.

SPECIAL CONSIDERATIONS

Medications

Physician's inexperience and the lack of prospective trials in pregnancy make medication choice during pregnancy an anxiety-provoking task. If possible, all medications should be avoided, especially during the first trimester. During organogenesis (first 16 weeks), medications are potentially more harmful to the fetus than in the second and third trimester. The risks and benefits must be weighed and it is not uncommon to postpone treatment and carefully observe the patient until the pregnancy is further along or finished.

Medications commonly used in gastrointestinal diseases (Table 3) and their classification according to current pregnancy categories (Table 4) are mentioned here.

TABLE 3: Medications used in gastrointestinal diseases according to pregnancy categories

Medications	Pregnancy category*	Special consideration
Antiulcer		
Antacids	B	Drug of choice for dyspepsia
Cimetidine	B	Crosses the placenta and excreted in maternal milk but toxicity has not been observed
Ranitidine	B	4–13 times more potent than cimetidine. Excreted in breast milk.
Famotidine	B	3 times more potent than ranitidine
Nizatidine	B	Not recommended in pregnancy. Spontaneous abortion, low birth weight and congenital malformations in animals. Little data in humans
Sucralfate	B	Animal studies negative, no human studies
Misoprostol	X	Contraindicated (In one study complete or incomplete abortion induced in 7%)
Lansoprazole	B	Safer than omeprazole
Omeprazole	C	Little available from either animal or human studies, questionable teratogenicity
Pantoprazole	B	No fetal teratogenicity. Limited data in human pregnancy
Rabeprazole	B	No fetal teratogenicity. Limited data in human pregnancy
Esomeprazole	B	No fetal teratogenicity. Limited data in human pregnancy
Simethicone	C	No data
Pepto-Bismol	C	No data
Inflammatory bowel		
Corticosteroids	C	Low risk, possible increased risk of cleft palate, adrenal insufficiency in neonate
Sulfasalazine	B	Patients with IBD on sulfasalazine fare better than those with untreated disease

Continued

Continued

Medications	Pregnancy category*	Special consideration
Mesalamine (oral and topical)	B	Similar to sulfasalazine
Balsalazide	B	Similar to mesalamine
Olsalazine	C	Low risk, similar to mesalamine
Azathioprine/6-MP	D	Safety during pregnancy has been shown in the renal transplant and IBD population
Cyclosporine	C	May be used in severe Crohn's disease to avoid surgery
Methotrexate	X	Should not be used during pregnancy
Infliximab	B	Limited data on safety in human pregnancy
Adalimumab	B	Limited data on safety in human pregnancy
Tacrolimus	C	Limited data, use if mother's health mandates
Antiemetics:		
Pyridoxine (B6)	A	Safe and effective in humans. (dose of 25 mg orally every 8 hr)
Doxylamine	B	Available over-the-counter
Meclizine	B	Questionable safety and efficacy
Diphenhydramine	B	Questionable safety and efficacy
Metoclopramide	B	Safe and effective in humans
Promethazine	C	Effective but safety is questioned
Prochlorperazine	C	Effective but safety is questioned
Droperidol	C	Limited data
Ondansetron	C	Limited data
Granisetron	B	No human studies
Antidiarrheals:		
Loperamide Hydrochloride	B	Opioid. May be used for symptomatic treatment in mild Crohn's disease.
Diphenoxylate/ atropine	C	Opioid plus anticholinergic, teratogenic in animals
Pepto-Bismol	C	Not safe during pregnancy
Kaopectate		Not safe in pregnancy, now contains bismuth

Continued

Continued

Medications	Pregnancy category*	Special consideration
Laxatives:		
Metamucil	A	Safe during pregnancy
Docusate sodium	C	Safe during pregnancy
Lactulose/sorbitol	B	Poorly absorbed sugars, act as osmotic laxatives
Polyethylene glycol	C	Probably first choice in pregnancy
Bisacodyl	C	Low risk short term
Senna	C	Probably safe in pregnancy
Sodium phosphate oral/enema	C	Avoid long-term use, hypermagnesemia, hyperphosphatemia, dehydration

IBD, inflammatory bowel disease; MP, mercaptopurine.

TABLE 4: Definition of Food and Drug Administration classification

FDA classification	Definition
Category A	Wellcontrolled studies in human show no fetal risk
Category B	Animals studies show no risk, but human studies inadequate Or Animal studies show some risk, but not supported by human studies
Category C	Animal studies show risk, but human studies are inadequate or lacking Or No studies in humans or animals
Category D	Definite fetal abnormalities in human studies, but potential benefits may outweigh the risks
Category X	Contraindicated in pregnancy, fetal abnormalities in animals or humans, risks outweigh benefits.

FDA, Food and Drug Administration

CONCLUSION

Variety of gastrointestinal conditions may occur during pregnancy ranging from hyperemesis to hiatal hernia, infectious diarrhea, and IBD. Inflammatory bowel is a chronic, idiopathic disorder of the gastrointestinal tract. The two main types of IBD are Crohns disease and ulcerative colitis. These two entities share clinical and epidemiologic characteristics and are managed similarly. Inflammatory bowel disease is associated with the patterns of relapse and remission. The peak age of onset occurs in adolescence and early adulthood, so most women with IBD are of child bearing age. The course of these IBDs during pregnancy largely depends on disease activity at conception, and they can be associated with pregnancy complications. Management requires continuation of appropriate medications and close surveillance, with aggressive treatment of any flare. Several commonly used medications for IBDs have been shown to be safe in pregnancy. With current management, most women with IBD will have normal pregnancy outcomes.

REFERENCES

1. Cappell MS. The fetal safety and clinical efficacy of gastrointestinal endoscopy during pregnancy. Gastroenterol Clin North Am. 2003;32(1): 123-79.
2. Mazze RI, Källén B. Appendectomy during pregnancy—a Swedish registry study of 778 cases. Obstet Gynecol. 1991;77(6):835-40.
3. Carter JF, Soper DE. Operative laparoscopy in pregnancy. JSLS. 2004; 8(1):57-60.
4. Reedy MB, Kallen B, Kuehl TJ. Laparoscopy during pregnancy—a study of five fetal outcome parameters with the use of the Swedish Health Registry. Am J Obstet Gynecol. 1997;177(3): 673-9.
5. Fatum M , Rojansky N. Laparoscopic surgery during pregnancy. Obstet Gynecol Surv. 2001;56(1):50-9.
6. Hamaoui E, Hamaoui M. Nutritional assessment and support during pregnancy, Gastroenterol Clin North Am. 2003;32(1):59-121.
7. Heyland DK, MacDonald S, Keefe L, Drover JW. Total parenteral nutrition in the critically ill patient. Journal of the American Medical Association.1998; 280(23):2013-9.
8. Guglielmi FW, Baggio–Bertinet D, Federico A, Forte GB, Guglielmi A, Loguercio C. Total parenteral nutrition related gastrointestinal complications. Dig Liv Dis. 2006;38(9):623-42.
9. OguraJM, Francois KE, Perlow JH, Elliott JP. Complications associated with peripherally inserted central catheter use during pregnancy. Am J Obstet Gynecol. 2008;188(5):1223-5.
10. Lacasse A, Rey E, Ferreira E, Morin C. Bérard A. Validity of a modified pregnancy-unique quantification of emesis and nausea PUQE scoring index-to assess severity of nausea and vomiting in pregnancy. Am J Obstet Gynecol. 2008;198(1):71-7.
11. Bailit JL: Hyperemesis gravidarum—epidemilogical findings from a large cohort. Am J Obstet Gynecol. 2005;193(3Pt 1):811-4.
12. Dodds L, Fell DB, Joseph KS, Allen VM, Butler B. Outcome of pregnancies complicated by hyperemesis gravidarum. Obstet Gynecol. 2006;107(2 Pt 1):285-92.
13. Verberg MF, Gillot JD,Fardan NA, et al. Hyperemesis gravidarum—a literature review. Hum Reprod Update. 2005;11(5):527-39.
14. Goldberg D, Szilyagi A, Graves L. Hyperemesis gravidarum and *Helicobactor pylori* infection—a systematic review. Obstet Gynecol. 2007;110(3):695-703.
15. Ponzetto A, Cardaropoli S, Piccoli E, Rolfo A,Gennero L, Kanduc D, et al. Preeclampsia associated with *Helicobacter pylori* seropositivity in Italy. J Hypertens. 2006;24(12):2445-9.
16. Schwartz M, Rossoff L. Pneumomediastinum and bilateral pneumothoraces in a patient with hyperemesis gravidarum. Chest. 1994;106(6):1904-6.
17. Chiossi G, Nerri I, Cavazzuti M, Basso G, Facchinetti F. Hyperemesis gravidarum complicated by Wernicke encephalopathy—background, case report and review of the literature. Obstet Gynecol Surv. 2006: 61(4):255-68.
18. Jewell D, Young G. Interventions for nausea and vomiting in early pregnancy. Cochrane Database Syst Rev. 2000; 2:1-47.
19. Safari HR, Fassett MJ, Souter IC, Alsulyman OM, Goodwin TM. The efficacy of methylprednisolone in the treatment of hyperemesis gravidarum—a randomized double-blind controlled study. Am J Obstet Gynecol. 1998; 179(4):921-4.
20. Bondok RS, Sharnouby NM, Eid HE, Abd Elmaksoud AM. Pulsed steroid therapy is an effective treatment for intractable hyperemesis gravidarum. Crit Care Med. 2006;34(11):2781-3.
21. Mahadevan U, Kane S: American gastroenterological association institute technical review on the use of gastrointestinal medications in pregnancy. Gastroenterology. 2006;131(1):283-311.
22. Tan JY, Loh KC, Yeo GS, Chee YC: Transient hyperthyroidism of hyperemesis gravidarum. Br J Obstet Gynaecol. 2002;109(6):683-8.
23. Panesar NS, Chan KW, Li CY, Rogers MS. Status of anti-thyroid peroxidase during normal pregnancy and in patients with hyperemesis gravidarum. Thyroid. 2006;16(5):481-4.
24. Swallow BL, Lindow SW, Masson EA, Hay DM. Psychological health in early pregnancy—relationship with nausea and vomiting. J Obstet Gynaecol. 2004;24(1):28-32.
25. Vaisman N, Kaidar R, Levin I, Lessing JB. Nasojejunal feeding in hyperemesis gravidarum—a preliminary study. Clin Nutr. 2004;23(1):53-7.
26. Hytten FE. The alimentary system. In: Hytten F, Chamberlain G (Eds). Clinical Physiology in Obstetrics. London:Blackwell; 1991.p.137.
27. Diav-Citrin O, Arnon J, Shechtman S, Schaefer C,van Tonningen MR, Clementi M, et al. The safety of proton pump inhibitors in pregnancy—a multicentre prospective controlled study. Aliment Pharmacol Ther. 2005; 21(3):269-75.
28. Biertho L, Sebajang H, Bamehriz F, Head K, Allen C, Anvari M. Effect of pregnancy on effectiveness of laparoscopic Nissen fundoplication. Surg Endosc. 2006; 20(3): 385-8.
29. Cohen S, Harris LD. Does hiatus hernia affect competence of the gastroesophageal sphincter? N Engl J Med. 1971;284(19):1053-6.
30. Kurzel RB, Naunheim KS, Schwartz RA. Repair of symptomatic diaphragmatic hernia during pregnancy. Obstet Gynecol. 1988;71(6 Pt 1): 869-71.
31. Torquati A, Lutfi R, Khaitan L, Sharp KW, Richards WO. Heller myotomy vs Heller myotomy plus Dor fundoplication—cost-utility analysis of a randomized trial. Surg Endosc. 2006;20(3):389-93.
32. Khudyak V, Lysy J, Mankuta D. Achalasia in pregnancy. Obstet Gynecol Surv. 2006;61(3):207-11.
33. Clark DH. Peptic ulcer in women. Br Med J.1953;1(4822):1254-7.
34. Dzieniszewski J, Jarosz M. Guidelines in the medical treatment of *Helicobacter pylori* infection. J Physiol Pharmacol. 2006;57(3):143-54.
35. O'Mahony S. Endoscopy in pregnancy. Best Pract Res Clin Gastroenterol. 2007;21(5):893-9.
36. Lawson M, Kern F, Everson GT. Gastrointestinal transit time in human pregnancy—prolongation in the second and third trimesters followed by postpartum normalization. Gastroenterology.1985;89(5):996-9.
37. Everson GT. Gastrointestinal motility in pregnancy. Gastroenterol Clin North Am.1992;21(4):751-76.
38. Wald A. Constipation, diarrhea, and symptomatic hemorrhoids during pregnancy. Gastroenterol Clin North Am. 2003;32(1):309-22.
39. Kelly CP, LaMont JT. *Clostridium difficile*—more difficult than ever. N Engl J Med. 2008;359(18):1932-40.
40. Friedman S, Blumberg RS. Inflammatory bowel disease. In: Fauci AS, Braunwald E, Kasper DL, Stephen L. Hauser, Dan L, J. Larry Jameson, Joseph Loscalzo (Eds). Harrison's Principles of Internal Medicine, 17th edition. New York: McGraw-Hill; 2008. pp.1886-98.
41. Selby WS, Griffin S, Abraham N, Solomon MJ. Appendectomy protects against the development of ulcerative colitis but does not affect its course. Am J Gastroenterol. 2002;97(11):2834-8.

42. Rutgeerts P, Sandborn WJ, Feagan BG, Reinisch W, Olson A, Johanns J, et al. Infliximab for induction and maintenance therapy for ulcerative colitis. N Engl J Med. 2006;353(23):2462-76.
43. Lichtenstein GC, Hanauer SB, Sandbord WJ. Management of Crohn's disease in adults. Am J Gastroenterol. 2009;104(2): 465-83.
44. Rahimi R, Nikfar S, Rezaie A, Abdollahi M. Pregnancy outcome in women with inflammatory bowel disease following exposure to 5-aminosalicylic acid drugs—a meta-analysis. Reprod Toxicol. 2008;25(2):271-5.
45. Prefontaine E, Sutherland LR, Macdonald JK. Azathioprine or 6-mercaptopurine for maintenance of remission in Crohn's disease. Cochrane Database Syst Rev. 2010;6:1-25.
46. Alstead EM, Nelson-Piercy C. Inflammatory bowel disease in pregnancy. Gut. 2003;52(2):159-61.
47. Kornfeld D, Cnattingius S, Ekbom A. Pregnancy outcomes in women with inflammatory bowel disease—a population based cohort study. Am J Obstet Gynecol. 1997;177(4):942-6.
48. Dominitz JA, Young JC, Boyko EJ. Outcomes of infants born to mothers with inflammatory bowel disease—a population based cohort study. Am J Gastroenterol. 2002;97(3):641-8.
49. Fonager K, Sorensen HT, Olsen J, Dahlerup JF, Rasmussen SN. Pregnancy outcome for women with Crohn's disease—a follow-up study based on linkage between national registries. Am J Gastroenterol. 1998;93(12):2426-3.
50. Korelitz BI. Inflammatory bowel disease and pregnancy. Gastroenterol Clin North Am. 1998;27(1):213-24.
51. Norgård B, Hundborg HH, Jacobsen BA, Nielsen GL, Fonager K. Disease activity in pregnant women with Crohn's disease and birth outcomes—a regional Danish cohort study. Am J Gastroenterol. 2007;102(9):1947-54.
52. Alshawi JS. Recurrent sigmoid volvulus in pregnancy—report of a case and review of the literature. Dis Colon Rectum. 2005;48(9):1811-3.
53. Davis MR, Bohon CJ. Intestinal obstruction in pregnancy. Clin Obstet Gynecol. 1983;26(4):832-42.
54. Essilfie P, Hussain M, Stokes IM. Small bowel infarction secondary to volvulus during pregnancy—a case report. J Reprod Med. 2007;52(6):553-4.
55. Ponec RJ, Saunders MD, Kimmey MB. Neostigmine for the treatment of acute colonic pseudo-obstruction. N Engl J Med. 1999;341(3):137-41.
56. DeGiorgio R, Knowles CH. Acute colonic pseudo-obstruction. Br J Surg. 2009;96(3):229-39.
57. Hée P, Viktrup L. The diagnosis of appendicitis during pregnancy and maternal and fetal outcome after appendectomy. Int J Gynaecol Obstet. 1999;65(2):129-35.
58. Andersson RE, Lambe M. Incidence of appendicitis during pregnancy. Int J Epidemiol. 2001;30(6):1281-5.
59. Gearhart SL, Silen W. Acute appendicitis and peritonitis. In: Fauci AS, Braunwald E, Kasper DL, Stephen L. Hauser, Dan L, J. Larry Jameson, Joseph Loscalzo (Eds). Harrison's Principles of Internal Medicine, 17th edition. New York: McGraw-Hill; 2008. pp.1914-17.
60. Reedy MB, Källén B, Kuehl TJ. Laparoscopy during pregnancy—a study of five fetal outcome parameters with use of the Swedish Health Registry. Am J Obstet Gynecol. 1997;177(3):673-9.
61. Cohen-Kerem R, Railton C, Oren D, Lishner M, Koren G. Pregnancy outcome following non-obstetric surgical intervention. Am J Surg. 2005;190(3):467-73.

CHAPTER 50

Liver Diseases

Shashank Shekhar

PHYSIOLOGICAL CHANGES DURING PREGNANCY

Blood supply to liver during pregnancy remains unchanged despite an increase in cardiac output and so does the liver size. Telangiectasia and palmar erythema which are otherwise clinical markers of liver disease, are seen commonly during pregnancy (due to hyperestrogenic state). Decreased gall-bladder motility with increased secretion of cholesterol in second and third trimesters increases the lithogenicity of bile.

LIVER FUNCTION TESTS

Alanine transaminase, aspartate transaminase, γ-glutamyl transpeptidase (GGT) and bilirubin values remain unchanged during pregnancy; however, their range is changed with reduction in the upper end. This is a consequence of hemodilution of pregnancy. Alkaline phosphatase is elevated up to 300% but is placental in origin. There is increase in the hepatic synthesis of coagulation factors VII, VIII, X and fibrinogen, yet the range for prothrombin time (PT) and activated partial thromboplastin time (APTT) remain unchanged. It is believed that prolonged PT is a good early marker of hepatic synthetic dysfunction. Serum albumin concentrations fall due to hemodilution.

LIVER DISEASES RELATED TO PREGNANCY

Liver diseases unique to pregnancy fall into two main categories depending upon their association with or without pre-eclampsia (Box 1). The pre-eclampsia associated liver diseases are pre-eclampsia itself, the hemolysis, elevated liver enzymes, low platelet count (HELLP) syndrome and acute fatty liver of pregnancy (AFLP). Hyperemesis gravidarum (HG) and intrahepatic cholestasis (ICP) have no relation to pre-eclampsia.

Box 1: Classifying liver diseases during pregnancy

- Liver disease related to pregnancy
  - Pre-eclampsia/hypertension-associated liver diseases
    - Pre-eclampsia
    - HELLP Syndrome
    - Acute fatty liver of pregnancy
  - Not associated with pre-eclampsia/hypertension
    - Hyperemesis gravidarum associated liver dysfunction
    - Intrahepatic cholestasis of pregnancy
- Liver diseases unrelated to pregnancy
  - Pre-existing
    - Cirrhosis and portal hypertension
    - Hepatitis B and C
    - Autoimmune liver disease
    - Wilson's disease
  - Liver diseases coincidental with pregnancy
    - Viral hepatitis
    - Gallbladder and biliary disease
    - Budd-Chiari syndrome
    - Drug-induced hepatotoxicity

HELLP, hemolysis, elevated liver enzymes, low platelet count.

Hyperemesis Gravidarum

Hyperemesis gravidarum (HG) complicates 0.3–2.0% of pregnancies.[1,2] It is characterized by intractable vomiting in the first trimester (typically, 4–10 weeks) leading to dehydration, ketosis and weight loss of 5% or more and necessity to hospitalize. HG is not a liver disease in strict sense but it leads to liver dysfunction in 50% of cases. The mechanism of liver involvement in HG is multifactorial and not well understood.

Transient hyperthyroidism is seen in 60% cases.[3] HG associated liver dysfunction should be a diagnosis of exclusion. A woman presenting with liver dysfunction with or without HG in first trimester must be carefully investigated to rule out other causes of liver dysfunction (viral hepatitis, drug-induced liver injury).

Liver Function Abnormalities

There is mild to up to 20-fold elevations in aspartate aminotransferase (AST) and alanine aminotransferase (ALT), [(ALT > AST)] and rarely mild jaundice. Liver function abnormalities and other biochemical abnormalities resolve on resolution of vomiting.

Management

Management of HG is supportive and includes intravenous rehydration with short period of fasting followed by reintroduction of diet rich in carbohydrates and low in fat. Antiemetics such as dopamine antagonists (metoclopramide, domperidone), phenothiazine (chlorpromazine, prochlorperazine) or antihistamine H1 receptor antagonists (cyclizine, promethazine) are used safely during pregnancy.[3] Thiamine supplementation is given with dextrose infusion particularly in women who give history of prolonged (over weeks) vomiting to prevent Wernicke's encephalopathy.

Intrahepatic Cholestasis of Pregnancy

Intrahepatic cholestasis of pregnancy is the most frequent cause of cholestasis during pregnancy. However, occurrence of cholestasis during pregnancy does not always imply the clinical diagnosis of ICP as pregnancy itself is a cholestatic condition and chronic liver diseases may be unmasked for the first time during pregnancy with clinical presentation of cholestasis. Differentiation of ICP from other chronic liver diseases is important as both maternal and fetal prognosis varies. ICP prevalence varies according to countries and 0.5–1.5% prevalence is seen in European countries. South Asia including India has higher incidence of ICP.

Clinical Presentation

Pruritus is the main symptom. Though it is generalized, it might be severe in palms and soles and shows worsening during night. Pruritus usually develops after 25 weeks with 80% cases occurring after 30 weeks. It usually disappears within first few days after delivery. Jaundice develops in 10% cases, 2–4 weeks after pruritus and is usually less than 5 mg/dL.

Liver Function Tests

Fasting serum bile acid levels of more than 10 μmol/L is the key diagnostic test, however, it is not available everywhere. ALT and AST are usually raised 2–10 times but may be elevated up to 20 times in few. Transaminases are elevated secondary to increased membrane permeability of hepatocytes. GGT levels are not raised. Infact raised GGT activity is considered a marker of chronic liver disease.

How to Make a Diagnosis of Intrahepatic Cholestasis?

The diagnosis of ICP should be made on the following grounds:

- Typical clinical presentation of pruritus occurs in second half of pregnancy. History of itching during previous pregnancy or on contraceptive pills adds weight
- Abnormal liver function tests as described above
- Exclusion of other liver diseases (viral hepatitis, autoimmune liver disease)
- A complete recovery of pruritus and liver function tests soon after delivery. Hence, ICP is a presumptive diagnosis until resolution of symptoms postpartum.

Pathogenesis: intrahepatic cholestasis is associated with abnormal biliary transport across the canalicular membrane, the etiology of which is complex and heterogeneous. Literature suggests that genetic, hormonal and exogenous factors all play a role in occurrence of ICP.[4]

- Genetic: clustering of ICP cases in families and high incidence in certain ethnic groups suggested a genetic predisposition. Identification of mutations and polymorphism of genes involved in hepatobiliary transport have provided the evidence to the theory.[5, 6]The discussion of these genes and their mutations is beyond the scope of this chapter
- Hormonal: role of estrogens is supported by the fact that ICP is more common in twin pregnancies (where estrogen levels are higher) and ICP symptoms are sometimes seen in women given exogenous estrogens in the form of contraceptive pill. Abnormalities of progesterone metabolism with accumulation of sulfate metabolites saturating the hepatobiliary transport system are also implicated in ICP. There are case reports of ICP triggered by prescription of natural progesterone for preventing preterm delivery in third trimester[7, 8]
- Exogenous: had the etiology of ICP been only genetic, then all the pregnancies of predisposed women should have been complicated by ICP. However, such is not the case as ICP recurs only in 60–70% of subsequent pregnancies. This suggests a role of extraneous factors influencing the occurrence of ICP in genetically predisposed women. Other facts which support the role of exogenous factors are geographical variation in occurrence, seasonal variability in several countries and decreasing prevalence of ICP in Chile.[9]

Prognosis for Mother and Fetus

ICP has a benign prognosis for mother. There is no serious short- or long-term maternal morbidity seen with ICP. However, a recent longitudinal retrospective population based cohort study has shown an association of ICP with several liver diseases.[10] ICP does carry a risk for fetus. Fetal complications of ICP are prematurity, chronic placental insufficiency, anoxia, meconium passage and sudden intrauterine fetal death (IUFD). The risk of sudden IUFD is currently 1% in developed countries and is rarely seen before the last month of pregnancy.

Medical and Obstetrical Management

Management of ICP is 2-fold, symptomatic therapy for mother with close surveillance and early delivery for fetus.

Symptomatic management of mother: ursodeoxycholic acid (UDCA) in the doses of 10–15 mg/kg per day is the treatment of choice for ICP at present. It provides relief against pruritus, improves liver function tests and appears to be safe during pregnancy. At molecular level, it offers cytoprotective against hepatotoxic effects of hydrophobic bile acids improve hepatobiliary bile acid transport and decreases plasma bile acid. Hydroxyzine (25 mg/day) or aqueous cream with 1% menthol may be used to alleviate pruritus. Other drugs such as cholestyramine are less effective and may lead to vitamin K deficiency. S-Adenosyl-L-methionine is less effective than UDCA but may have additive effect.

Management for fetus: close fetal monitoring and early delivery (preferably 37 weeks but no later than 38 weeks) remains the cornerstone of obstetric management, though the evidence is lacking. An even early delivery is advocated when cholestasis is severe. [11] However, sudden IUFD cannot be totally avoided even with this approach.

Pre-eclampsia/Hypertension Related Liver Diseases and Pregnancy

Preeclmapsia/Eclampsia

Pre-eclampsia is defined as hypertension and proteinuria after 20 weeks of pregnancy and within 48 hours of delivery. It complicates 10% of the pregnancies. It is a multisystem disorder and liver is involved in 20–30% cases of preeclampsia. It is the most common cause of liver dysfunction and hepatic tenderness in pregnancy [12]. Liver involvement is secondary to vasospasm of hepatic vascular bed. Aminotransferase levels are usually elevated mildly to up to 10 times, however they might occasionally be elevated up to 20 times normal values. Jaundice occurs only occasionally (5%) and is usually less than 5 mg/dL. The liver involvement in pre-eclampsia is an indicator of the severity of pre-eclampsia and no specific therapy for liver involvement is required.

Hemolysis, Elevated Liver Enzymes, Low Platelet Count Syndrome

It is a severe variant of pre-eclampsia and complicates around 2–12% of pre-eclampsia cases.[13]

It is defined by the presence of hemolysis, elevated liver enzymes and low platelet counts.

Etiology: there is andothelial injury and fibrin deposition in blood vessels which leads to microangiopathic hemolytic anemia (schistocytes and burr cells on smear) with platelet activation and consumption. Consequently, small to diffuse areas of hemorrhage and necrosis develop from zone 1 to involve the whole lobule. This may occasionally lead to large hematomas, capsular tears and intraperitoneal hemorrhage.

Clinical features: majority of patients present in third trimester (28–36 weeks of gestation) but 30% cases occur in postpartum period. There is no typical presenting sign or symptom which distinguishes HELLP from pre-eclampsia. Midepigastric or right upper quadrant abdominal pain is the most common feature. Other symptoms are nausea, vomiting, malaise, and headache. Jaundice is present in about 5% cases.[14]

Differential diagnosis: occasionally, HELLP syndrome must be distinguished from other conditions, especially AFLP (with which it has significant overlap) [15] or from the rare conditions of thrombotic thrombocytopenic purpura, hemolytic uremic syndrome or antiphospholipid syndrome (especially, in the presence of hepatic infarction).

Management: cornerstone of management in HELLP syndrome is prompt delivery.[16] Women must be hospitalized and managed in high dependency obstetric units. Along with all relevant hematological and biochemical investigations, liver imaging with CT scan (limited views) or magnetic resonance imaging (MRI) should be done to identify hepatic complications of infarction, liver parenchymal hemorrhage or subcapsular hematoma, as ultrasound is not a reliable tool to identify these complications. Hypertension must be aggressively controlled and blood or blood products should be used, if required to improve anemia or coagulation disorders. After initial optimization, delivery must be immediately affected in pregnancies at or beyond 34 weeks of gestation or with evidence of multiorgan dysfunction, disseminated intravascular coagulation (DIC), renal failure, abruption placenta or fetal distress.

Management of HELLP syndrome remote from term with fetal lung immaturity and stable maternal condition is controversial.[15,16] We believe that delivery must be immediately affected after temporizing management and corticosteroid therapy for 24–48 hours in such cases. A longer conservative therapy in such cases will lead to deterioration of maternal disease within 1–10 days with a high risk of fetal loss.

Hepatic complications of HELLP syndrome/pre-eclampsia: major hepatic complications of HELLP syndrome are rare and seen in 5% of cases and are following: [17]

- Intraparenchymal hemorrhage
- Liver infarction
- Subcapsular hematoma
- Hepatic rupture
- Hepatic failure.

Hepatic infarction: right upper quadrant pain and fever with marked elevation in serum aminotransferases is characteristic of liver infarction. It can be confirmed on CT scan. Patient may have an underlying procoagulant state such as antiphospholipid antibody syndrome. It is less frequent than subcapsular hematoma formation.

Hepatic parenchymal hemorrhage and subcapsular hematoma: This complication correlates with severity of thrombocytopenia. Presenting feature is severe upper abdominal pain with pyrexia and anemia. Serum aminotransferases values are in the range of thousands. Hepatic intraparenchymal hemorrhages with contained hematomas in hemodynamically stable patients are managed conservatively with aggressive correction of coagulopathy and anemia. However, there is a possibility of rapid expansion of hematoma and liver rupture hence intensive hemodynamic monitoring should be done. Moreover, there should be immediate availability of large volumes of blood/blood products for transfusion and surgical intervention, if the need arises. Exogenous trauma such as abdominal palpation, convulsions, emesis and unnecessary transportation must be avoided. Management of hemodynamically unstable patient is aggressive resuscitation with immediate laparotomy.

Liver rupture: it is a life-threatening complication and is usually preceded by intraparenchymal hemorrhage progressing to contained subcapsular hemorrhage in the right lobe in patients with severe thrombocytopenia. Maternal mortality is 50% and survivability depends on rapid aggressive supportive care and immediate laparotomy. Most effective surgical management is evacuation of hematoma with pressure packing and drainage along with hepatic artery ligation.

Acute Fatty Liver of Pregnancy

Acute fatty liver of pregnancy is a rare (1 in 20,000 deliveries) and catastrophic disease with a high maternal and fetal mortality. As a rule, AFLP is a disease of third trimester. Abnormalities in fatty acid oxidation lead to microvesicular fatty infiltration of hepatocytes resulting in widespread damage.

Etiology

Principal abnormality found so far in certain cases of AFLP is a defect in the mitochondrial fatty acid oxidation (FAO) in mother and her fetus. Two enzymes involved in mitochondrial FAO and whose mutations are closely linked with AFLP are mitochondrial trifunctional protein and it is α subunit long-chain 3-hydroxyacyl-CoA dehydrogenase (LCHAD). Our current understanding from a number of studies is that a mother is heterozygous for LCHAD deficiency and she carries a fetus who is homozygous or heterozygous for LCHAD mutation. The maternal reduced capacity to oxidize long-chain fatty acids coupled with placental and fetal deficiency to do so leads to abnormal accumulation of long chain fatty acid metabolites in maternal circulation. These metabolites then get deposited in hepatocytes (fatty infiltration) and cause hepatotoxicity. Apart from AFLP, FAO defects in mother and fetus have led to development of HELLP syndrome as well.

Clinical Features

Unlike HELLP, majority of women are nulliparous. Clinical presentation is variable however most frequent symptoms are anorexia for a couple of weeks, nausea, vomiting, right upper abdominal pain and headache. Woman is ill looking, jaundiced and may be hypertensive and edematous. Patient may have ascites (partly due to portal hypertension) and liver is small or normal. In severe forms, patient may demonstrate hepatic encephalopathy with or without coma. Up to half of the patients with AFLP will have hypertension and/or proteinuria (pre-eclampsia), and hence classified with pre-eclampsia/hypertension associated liver disease in pregnancy.[18] Polyuria and polydipsia are pathognomonic symptoms in the setting of liver disease in pregnancy, however, they are present only in 5% cases.

Laboratory Abnormalities

Liver function tests: AST and ALT are elevated up to 300–500 times usually but not as high as in viral hepatitis. Hyperbilirubinemia is common but usually is not higher than 5 mg/dL.

Coagulation profile: in severe cases, PT is raised and fibrinogen levels are decreased (due to hepatic synthetic defect and DIC). Thrombocytopenia is common. A clinical vignette is that low platelets in late pregnancy should prompt one to perform liver function tests to rule out AFLP.

Hematological abnormalities: typical abnormalities are normocytic normochromic anemia and leukocytocis.

Other biochemical abnormalities: hypoglycemia is characteristic and is a poor prognostic sign. Other biochemical abnormalities are metabolic acidosis, renal dysfunction, high ammonia and biochemical pancreatitis.

Diagnosis

Microvesicular steatosis on liver biopsy is diagnostic, but it is rarely necessary besides coagulopathy precluding it in most of the situations. So, in majority of the cases a presumptive diagnosis of AFLP is made based on clinical and laboratory findings. Swansea diagnostic criteria have been proposed as an alternative to liver biopsy (Box 2).[19]

Differential diagnosis: presence of hypertension, proteinuria and other clinical and laboratory features are seen overlapping between AFLP and HELLP syndrome. However, as compared to HELLP syndrome, patient with AFLP are more likely to have hepatic failure with coagulopathy, hypoglycemia, encephalopathy and renal failure (Table 1). Viral hepatitis must be ruled out by serological testing in every case.

Management

Prompt delivery is the primary therapy. There are no reports of recovery before delivery in literature. Management begins with hospitalization and initial stabilization (correction of coagulation and other abnormalities). Delivery should be effected promptly which is usually by cesarean section after correction of coagulation disorders. Though a vaginal delivery would reduce the chances of major peritoneal bleeding, it should be tried only if it seems possible in less than 24 hours in the presence of international normalized ratio of less than 1.5 and platelet counts of more than 50,000. A hepatologist should be involved early on. Prophylactic antibiotics are recommended to prevent uterine infections. Blood sugar levels must be closely monitored.

Most patients recover within 1–4 weeks (though a phase of cholestasis may persist longer). Recovery is complete with no signs of chronic liver disease. With early delivery and advances in supportive care, maternal mortality is now 7–18%. Infections and bleeding remain most life-threatening

Box 2: Swansea diagnostic criteria for diagnosis of acute fatty liver of pregnancy

Swansea diagnostic criteria for diagnosis of acute fatty liver of pregnancy

Six or more of the following feature required in the absence of another explanation:

- Vomiting
- Abdominal pain
- Polydipsia/polyuria
- Encephalopathy
- High bilirubin (>14 μmol/L)
- Hypoglycemia (<4 μmmol/L)
- High uric acid (>340 μmol/L)
- Leukocytosis (>11×109 cells/L)
- Ascites or bright liver on ultrasound
- High AST/ALT (>42 IU/L)
- High ammonia (>47 μmol /L)
- Renal impairment (creatinine>150 μmol/L)
- Coagulopathy (PT>14 seconds or APTT>34 seconds)
- Microvesicular steatosis on liver biopsy

PT, prothrombin time; APTT, activated partial thromboplastin time; AST, aspartate aminotransferase; ALT, alanine aminotransferase; IU, international unit.

TABLE 1: Distinguishing features of intrahepatic cholestasis of pregnancy, the HELLP syndrome and acute fatty liver of pregnancy

	Intrahepatic cholestasis of pregnancy	HELLP	Acute fatty liver of pregnancy
% Pregnancies	0.1(USA) Higher in India	0.2–0.5	0.5–0.01
Onset/Trimester	25–32 weeks	third or postpartum	third or postpartum
Family history	Often	No	Occasionally
Presence of pre-eclampsia	No	Yes	50%
Typical clinical features	Pruritus Mild jaundice	Hemolysis Thrombocytopenia	Liver failure with coagulopathy, encephalopathy, hypoglycemia, DIC
Aminotransferases	Mild to 10–20 fold	Mild to 10–20 fold	300–500 typical but may be high
Bilirubin	<5mg/ dL	<5 mg/dL unless massive necrosis	Often <5mg/dL but higher in severe disease
Hepatic Imaging	Normal	Hepatic infarcts, hematoma, rupture	Fatty infiltration
Histology	Normal—mild cholestasis. No necrosis	Patchy/extensive necrosis and hemorrhage	Microvesicular fatty infiltration of hepatocytes in zone 3
Maternal mortality	0%	1–25%	7–18%
Fetal/Perinatal mortality	0.4–1.4%	11%	9–23%
Recurrence in subsequent pregnancies	45–70%	4–19%	With LCHAD mutations —yes No mutation—may occur but rarely

DIC, disseminated intravascular coagulation; LCHAD, long-chain 3-hydroxyacyl-C coenzyme A dehydrogenase; USA, United States of America; HELLP, hemolysis, elevated liver enzymes, low platelet count.

complications. Liver transplantation has a limited role in those with fulminant hepatic encephalopathy and those who fail to recover after delivery.

Recurrence and Screening

Most women would not become pregnant again either by choice or due to necessity of hysterectomy to control postpartum hemorrhage (PPH). There is 20–70% chance of recurrence in case of repeat pregnancy. All women with AFLP and their offspring must be screened for abnormalities of FAO.

PRE-EXISTING LIVER DISEASES

Cirrhosis and Pregnancy

Most women with advanced cirrhosis will not conceive as they are amenorrheic and infertile due to hypothalamic dysfunction.[20,21] Nonetheless, pregnancy is achieved by many and even successfully completed in those with well compensated disease and mild portal hypertension. Fetal loss, maternal morbidity and mortality remain high in pregnant women with cirrhosis and hence such cases should be managed by high-risk obstetricians and hepatologists. Most common complication is variceal bleeding (25%) during second trimester and second stage of labor as portal hypertension worsens. [12] All women with cirrhosis and portal hypertension planning to conceive should undergo variceal screening and banding of varices before pregnancy. Additionally, those with no varices before pregnancy should undergo endoscopy during second trimester, and if found to have varices should be managed with β-blocker therapy. Acute variceal bleeding is managed endoscopically as in nonpregnant women though vasopressin is contraindicated during pregnancy. Other complications are hepatic decompensation with worsening synthetic liver functions, jaundice, thrombocytopenia, ascites and rarely rupture of splenic aneurysms. The best route of delivery is unknown. However, those with known large varices are best delivered by cesarean section. In the absence of large varices, assisted vaginal delivery with shortening of second stage can be accomplished.

Acute Viral Hepatitis

Viral hepatitis due to hepatitis A, B, C, D, and E, herpes simplex, cytomegalovirus and Epstein-Barr virus accounts for the 40% of cases of jaundice seen in pregnant women in the western world. [22]

Hepatitis A

The course of hepatitis A in pregnancy is similar to that seen in nonpregnant state. Hepatitis A in third trimester is associated with increased risk of prematurity. [23] Treatment remains supportive.

Hepatitis B and C

The incidence of hepatitis B and C in pregnancy is same as outside pregnancy. The clinical and serological course of hepatitis B and C during pregnancy does not differ from nonpregnant state nor does it have any adverse effect on pregnancy itself. Treatment is supportive. Vertical transmission and measure to reduce vertical transmission are discussed separately.

Hepatitis E

Hepatitis E is endemic in India and pregnant women are more vulnerable to hepatitis E than hepatitis A, B or C. Hepatitis E tends to run a severe course in pregnancy especially in our country with patients more likely to develop fulminant hepatic failure in third trimester. [24 25] Maternal and fetal mortality secondary to fulminant hepatic failure is very high (41–54% and 69% respectively).[26] Importantly, delivery does not change the outcome and management remains supportive with patient being ideally managed in intensive care unit.

Herpes Simplex Virus Hepatitis

Herpes simplex viral hepatitis is a rare entity, however, pregnant women are more susceptible than general population. The course during pregnancy is usually severe and fulminant with high maternal mortality. Herpes simplex viral hepatitis leads to "anicteric hepatitis" with normal levels of bilirubin in the presence of severe derangements in liver function tests. Mucocutaneous manifestation of herpes simplex infection occurs in only 50% cases [27]. A high degree of suspicion would be lifesaving as treatment with intravenous acyclovir is effective.

Viral Hepatitis and Vertical Transmission

Primary concern with chronic hepatitis B infection in pregnancy is possibility of vertical transmission. In fact, vertical transmission is the leading cause of most hepatitis B virus (HBV) infections worldwide. Foremost in the strategy to reduce vertical transmission of HBV infection is routine screening of pregnant women for hepatitis B virus at initial booking visit. Women who are without immune antibodies and display a high-risk behavior (intravenous drug abuse, multiple sex partners) are at increased risk of acquiring hepatitis B during pregnancy and can be given hepatitis vaccine with little risk to the fetus. The key factors in vertical transmission are presence of hepatitis B e-antigen (suggesting active viral replication), anti HB e-antibodies and the viral load. Vertical transmission is maximum with presence of hepatitis B e-antigen and viral load (50–80%), lower with anti-HBe (25%) and lowest in carriers (5%).[12] Vertical transmission can be significantly reduced (up to 95%) by passive-active immunoprophylaxis of the babies by hyperimmune B immunoglobulin within 12 hours of birth and hepatitis B vaccination within first 6 months. Cesarean section does not reduce the transmission rates.

Use of antiviral therapy during pregnancy to reduce the vertical transmission of hepatitis B is a controversial issue and no guidelines exist at present. Some people advocate use of lamivudine monotherapy after 32 weeks of pregnancy when viral load is in excess of 10^6 viral copies per milliliter.[28] This can be considered in women who have infected their child in previous pregnancy. However, there are concerns of viral resistance with lamivudine monotherapy.

Vertical transmission with maternal hepatitis C infection is very low. However, two factors which increase the transmission rates are maternal coinfection with HIV and fetal exposure to a large volume of maternal blood or secretion during delivery in the presence of high viral load.

Vertical transmission of hepatitis A and D is very rare and occurs only with high viral loads (acute phase) during delivery. Hence, newborns of mothers with hepatitis A in the third trimester should be administered immune globulin within 48 hours of birth.

Gallbladder Disease and Pregnancy

Pregnancy favors gallstone formation for the following reasons—cholesterol secretion increases in second and third trimester compared to other constituents of bile, and hence bile gets supersaturated with cholesterol. Secondly, gall-bladder volumes are higher during pregnancy due to decreased rate and volume of emptying. Thus, large residual volumes of supersaturate bile eventually leads to stone formation in up to 10% of pregnant women. Interestingly, despite high prevalence of gallstones formation during pregnancy women usually becomes symptomatic following the delivery. In fact symptomatic gallstone disease remains the number 1 nonobstetric reason for hospital admission in the year following delivery.

Principal clinical presentations of gallstone disease in order of frequency during pregnancy are—acute biliary colic, acute cholecystitis and gallstone pancreatitis (rare). Management of uncomplicated acute biliary colic and cholecystitis during pregnancy is supportive, with bed rest, intravenous hydration and antibiotics. However, cholecystectomy is indicated for intractable biliary colic, severe acute cholecystitis, not responding to conservative management and acute gallstone pancreatitis. Due to 50% recurrence of biliary colic before delivery, it is also recommended that those presenting with symptomatic gallstone disease in first and second trimester should undergo cholecystectomy during second trimester. Surgery is avoided in first trimester due to risk of abortion with anesthesia and in third trimester due to risk of preterm labor. Extrahepatic ductal stone are best managed by endoscopic retrograde cholangiopancreatography (ERCP), sphincterotomy and stone extraction under antibiotic coverage.

CONCLUSION

About 3% of the pregnancies are affected by liver diseases. Severe liver disease in pregnancy is rare. Liver diseases during pregnancy can be divided into those related to pregnancy and those just incidental to pregnancy and this distinction is important as cornerstone of management in most pregnancy related disease (except HG) is termination of pregnancy. Pregnancy related liver diseases are most frequent cause of liver dysfunction during pregnancy. Pregnancy related liver diseases has characteristic timing in relation to the trimesters of pregnancy. HG occurs in first trimester, intrahepatic cholestasis in late second and third trimester, HELLP, eclampsia and AFLP mainly occur in third trimester.

REFERENCES

1. Fairweather DV. Nausea and vomiting during pregnancy. Obstet Gynecol Annu. 1978; 7: 91-105.
2. Källén B. Hyperemesis during pregnancy and delivery outcome: a registry study. Eur J Obstet Gynecol Reprod Biol. 1987; 26(4): 291-302.
3. Bottomley C, Bourne T. Management strategies for hyperemesis. Best Pract Res Clin Obstet Gynaecol. 2009; 23(4):549-64.
4. Arrese M, Macias RIR, Briz O, Perez MJ, Marin JJG. Molecular pathogenesis of intrahepatic cholestasis of pregnancy. Expert Rev Mol Med. 2008;10: e9.
5. Oude Elferink RP, Paulusma CC. Function and pathophysiological importance of ABCB4 (MDR3 P-glycoprotein). Pflügers Arch. 2007; 453(5):601-10.
6. Jacquemin E, Cresteil D, Manouvrier S, Boute O, Hadchouel M. Heterozygous nonsense mutation of the MDR3 gene in familial intrahepatic cholestasis of pregnancy. Lancet. 1999; 353(9148):210-1.
7. Laatikainen T, Tulenheimo A. Maternal serum bile acid levels and fetal distress in cholestasis of pregnancy. Int J Gynaecol Obstet. 1984; 22(2):91-4.
8. Benifla JL, Dumont M, Levardon M, Foucher E, Cadiot G, Crenn-Hebert C, et al. Effects of micronized natural progesterone on the liver during the third trimester of pregnancy. Contracept Fertil Sex.1997; 25(2):165-9.
9. Reyes H, Báez ME, González MC, Hernández I, Palma J, Ribalta J, et al. Selenium, zinc and copper plasma levels in intrahepatic cholestasis of pregnancy, in normal pregnancies and in healthy individuals, in Chile. J Hepatol. 2000; 32(4): 542-9.
10. Ropponen A, Sund R, Riikonen S, Ylikorkala O, Aittomäki K. Intrahepatic cholestasis of pregnancy as an indicator of liver and biliary diseases: a population-based study. Hepatology. 2006; 43(4):723-8.
11. Saleh MM, Abdo KR. Consensus on the management of obstetric cholestasis: National UK survey. BJOG. 2007;114(1):99-103.
12. Hay JE. Liver disease in pregnancy. Hepatology. 2008; 47(3):1067–76.
13. Baxter JK, Weinstein L. HELLP syndrome: the state-of the-art. Obstet Gynecol Surv. 2004; 59(12): 838-45.
14. Sibai BM, Ramadan MK, Usta I, Salama M, Mercer BM, Friedman SA. Maternal morbidity and mortality in 442 pregnancies with hemolysis, elevated liver enzymes, and low platelets (HELLP syndrome). Am J Obstet Gynecol. 1993;169(4):1000-6.

15. Barton JR, Sibai BM. Diagnosis and management of hemolysis, elevated liver enzymes, and low platelets syndrome. Clin Perinatol. 2004;31(4):807-33.
16. Sibai BM. Diagnosis, controversies, and management of the syndrome of hemolysis, elevated liver enzymes, and low platelet count. Obstet Gynecol. 2004;103(5 Pt 1):981-91.
17. Zarrinpar A, Farmer DG, Ghobrial RM, Lipshutz GS, Gu Y, Hiatt JR, et al. Liver transplantation for HELLP syndrome. Am Surg. 2007; 73(10):1013-6.
18. Bacq Y, Constans T, Body G, Choutet P, Lamisse F. Acute fatty liver of pregnancy. J Gynecol Obstet Biol Reprod. 1986;15(7):851-61.
19. Ch'ng CL, Morgan M, Hainsworth I, Kingham JG. Prospective study of liver dysfunction in pregnancy in Southwest Wales. Gut. 2002;51(6):876-80.
20. Russell MA, Craigo SD. Cirrhosis and portal hypertension in pregnancy. Semin Perinatol. 1998;22(2):156-65.
21. Brunt PW, Kew MC, Scheuer PJ, Sherlock S. Studies in alcoholic liver disease in Britain. I. Clinical and pathological patterns related to natural history. Gut. 1974;15(1):52-8.
22. Elinav E, Ben-Dov IZ, Shapira Y, Daudi N, Adler R, Shouval D, et al. Acute hepatitis A infection in pregnancy is associated with high rates of gestational complications and preterm labor. Gastroenterology. 2006; 130(4):1129-34.
23. Willner IR, Uhl MD, Howard SC, Williams EQ, Riely CA, Waters B. Serious hepatitis A: an analysis of patients hospitalized during an urban epidemic in the United States. Ann Intern Med. 1998; 128(2):111-4.
24. Sreenivasan MA, Banerjee K, Pandya PG, Kotak RR, Pandya PM, Desai NJ, et al. Epidemiological investigations of an outbreak of infectious hepatitis in Ahmedabad city during 1975-76. Indian J Med Res. 1978; 67:197-206.
25. Khuroo MS, Teli MR, Skidmore S, Sofi MA, Khuroo MI. Incidence and severity of viral hepatitis in pregnancy. Am J Med. 1981; 70(2):252-5.
26. Banait VS, Sandur V, Parikh F, Murugesh M, Ranka P, Ramesh VS, et al. Outcome of acute liver failure due to acute hepatitis E in pregnant women. Indian J Gastroenterol. 2007; 26(1):6-10.
27. Klein NA, Mabie WC, Shaver DC, Latham PS, Adamec TA, Pinstein ML, et al. Herpes simplex virus hepatitis in pregnancy: two patients successfully treated with acyclovir. Gastroenterology.1991; 100(1): 239-44.
28. Joshi D, James A, Quaglia A, Westbrook RH, Heneghan MA. Liver disease in pregnancy. Lancent. 2010; 375(9714):594-605.

CHAPTER 51

Renal Diseases

Reeti Mehra, Sanjay D Cruz

INTRODUCTION

Whenever nephrologists are called upon to give their opinion in a given pregnant patient of chronic kidney disease (CKD) there are two questions that confront him. These two key questions are what will be the impact of the CKD on the fetus, and secondly what are the effects of pregnancy going to be on the kidneys of the pregnant mother. Keeping these two questions in view, decisions are taken on further course of management of the patient. Needless to say management of such a patient is dependant upon a multidisciplinary approach involving an obstetrician and a nephrologist. The diagnosis and management of renal disease in pregnancy begins by taking a careful history and performing a thorough physical examination. There are several clues in history and examination which will help guide any future course of action. Particular attention should be directed toward any history of kidney ailment, proteinuria, hypertension, collagen vascular diseases or diabetes affecting either the patient or close relatives.

RENAL CHANGES IN PREGNANCY

The body of the pregnant woman adapts to pregnancy in myriad ways. Kidneys are no exception. The kidney size increases by 1 cm along with a corresponding increase in volume. The changes involving the urinary tract begin in the first trimester of pregnancy and can persist up to 16 weeks postpartum. These anatomical changes include dilatation of the renal collecting system and the ureters along with smooth muscle hypertrophy and connective tissue hyperplasia of the ureters. The peristaltic activity is reduced in the ureters, which leads to stasis of urine compared to the nonpregnant state, thereby increasing the risk of infection. These changes can be ascribed to a combination of mechanical and hormonal factors.[1]

The cardiac output increases by about 40% by middle of second trimester. Despite the increase in cardiac output, the blood pressure falls because of decrease in vascular resistance. The blood volume increases by about 50% which is contributed by an increase in plasma volume as well as red blood cell (RBC) volume. Throughout pregnancy there is a cumulative retention of Na to the tune of 500–900 meq. Retention of salt and water leads to edema in 35–80% of healthy pregnant women. With advancing gestational age, edema may be contributed by pressure of the gravid uterus on the inferior vena cava (IVC). Edema of pregnancy is usually localized to the legs whereas edema of the face and hands points towards pre-eclampsia. Salt retention of normal pregnancy does not lead to hypertension. Presence of edema and hypertension should raise the possibility of pre-eclampsia.[2]

The hemodynamics in the kidneys undergoes changes as well. The effective renal plasma flow (ERPF) significantly increases during pregnancy reaching a peak of 50–85% over baseline in mid-trimester and then shows a small decline during the third trimester. The glomerular filtration rate (GFR) follows the same pattern as EPRF and increases by 40–65% and decreases to 15–20% over baseline late in the third trimester.[3] The filtration fraction which is the ratio of GFR to ERPF is decreased initially. Both the ERPF and GFR are affected by posture, being maximal in recumbent position. Factors contributing to increase in GFR, plasma volume and renal plasma flow include nitric oxide (NO), endothelin and relaxin. In addition, there is altered glomerular porosity leading to hyperfiltration of glucose, amino acids and other water soluble vitamins.

TESTS FOR RENAL FUNCTION IN PREGNANCY

Tests to evaluate renal function during pregnancy must be interpreted in relation to the changes in plasma volume, glomerular filtration and tubular reabsorption during gestation. Test reports that may be considered as normal in the nongravid woman may indicate renal dysfunction during pregnancy.

During pregnancy, fractional excretion of uric acid increases leading to a decrease of serum uric acid level by 25%. Upper normal limit of serum uric acid level in pregnant women is 5 mg/dL.[4] However, it may be higher in women with multiple gestations. The physiological increase in GFR during pregnancy normally results in a decrease in concentration of blood urea nitrogen (BUN) and serum creatinine. BUN normally decreases from nonpregnant levels of 12 to 9 mg/dL and plasma creatinine levels decline from a nonpregnant mean value of 0.7 to 0.5 mg/dL.[1] Serum creatinine level consistently over 0.80 mg/dL at any stage of gestation is distinctly abnormal.

Kidney disease is often subclinical. Measurement of renal function and quantification of proteinuria is of paramount importance in recognizing subclinical disease. With the dramatic hormonal and hemodynamic changes of pregnancy, renal function is altered and these changes must be considered when assessing renal function in pregnancy. The modification of diet in renal disease (MDRD) formula, which estimates GFR (eGFR) using a combination of serum creatinine, age, sex and race is routinely used to estimate renal function in patients with CKD. However, this formula has not been validated in pregnant women and is not recommended. Creatinine-based formulae like Cockcroft-Gault formula also is inaccurate in pregnant subjects. This is due to several factors like low creatinine values due to hemodilution, water retention and weight gain of approximately 10 kg during a pregnancy. Given these issues, 24 hour urine collection for creatinine clearance remains the gold standard for GFR estimation in pregnancy.[5]

In nonpregnant women, spot urine protein/creatinine ratio (PCR) is appropriate when screening for proteinuria. However, in the pregnant state this is slight discordance between urine production rate (UPR) and 24-hour protein estimation in a timed collection. This is especially true for borderline cases in which proteinuria ranges between 250 and 400 mg over 24 hours. The pooled sensitivity and specificity of protein/creatinine ratio (PCR) is 90% and 78% respectively.[6] It is reasonable to use PCR as a tool, when pre-eclampsia is suspected with the 24-hour method reserved for equivocal cases. Dipsticks have their own limitations. The urine must be at room temperature for them to be reliable. If they have been exposed to air, they will give false-positive results for glucose and false-negative results for blood. False-positive test for protein may be due to concentrated urine, exercise, fever from any cause, many white blood cells (WBCs) in the urine or vaginal secretions with epithelial cells. Women with +1 (or more) dipstick positive proteinuria in the absence of infection should have the level of proteinuria quantified.

When confronted with a pregnant patient with increasing proteinuria associated with advancing pregnancy in a known patient of kidney disease, does not necessarily indicate that the kidney disease is progressing.

Glycosuria should be checked for with the help of glucose oxidase-impregnated dipstick. Not uncommon to find glycosuria in pregnant women. It can normally be found due to increased porosity of the glomerular membrane or could be pathological. Presence of glycosuria should always be confirmed with fasting blood glucose levels to differentiate between physiological glycosuria and diabetes, gestational or otherwise.

Urinary sediment should be examined in a freshly voided specimen. The presence of cellular (RBCs/WBCs/Pus cells) cast indicates that the origin of cells is from upper tract proximal to the collecting tubules. This feature is helpful in differentiating glomerular hematuria from other causes, pyelonephritis from simple urinary tract infection and should be carefully looked for.

Renal biopsy in the first and second trimester is safe. The incidence of complications and rate of complications are similar to the nonpregnant population.[7] However, it should not be performed in patients with uncontrolled hypertension. A renal biopsy should be performed only if it is likely to alter the course of management in special situations like rapidly progressive glomerulonephritis, rapid decline of renal function in early pregnancy especially unexplained renal failure. Unless warranted, kidney biopsy should be postponed to postpartum period.

At times imaging studies may be required to delineate the anatomy. Renal sonogram may be ordered for if a tumor, obstructive uropathy or stone disease is suspected. Radiological procedure with or without contrast agents like X-ray, kidneys, ureters, and bladder (KUB), intravenous pyelography (IVP) and computed tomography (CT) scan should be avoided. If they are necessary, proper shielding of abdomen limiting the exposure to less than 5 Rads is recommended. Magnetic resonance imaging (MRI) may be done safely in pregnant individuals if indicated.

ACUTE KIDNEY INJURY

It is a syndrome characterized by rapid reversible decline in renal function leading to retention of nitrogenous waste products. Acute kidney injury (AKI) has been classically classified as prerenal, renal [acute tubular necrosis (ATN)] and postrenal causes. All the causes that can lead to AKI in nonpregnant population can cause renal failure in pregnancy. However, there are certain causes that are unique to pregnancy. With the advancement of medical prenatal and perinatal care, legalization of abortions and availability of better and more potent antibiotics, the incidence of AKI has dramatically reduced. In the western countries, the rate of acute renal failure (ARF) is less than 0.004%. Pre-eclampsia, hemorrhage due to placenta previa, abruption placenta, uterine atony/lacerations/rupture and abortions are the leading causes and account for 95% of the obstetric causes of ARF.[8] Other conditions which are unique to the gravid state include disseminated intravascular coagulation (DIC) due to intrauterine death, hyperemesis gravidarum (HG), obstruction due to gravid uterus due to polyhydramnios and multiple gestations, amniotic fluid embolism, eclampsia, acute fatty liver of pregnancy and hemolysis, elevated liver enzymes, low platelet count (HELLP) syndrome.

Mortality rate due to AKI can reach as high as 14%. Most of the deaths from ARF in pregnancy are due to the underlying disease rather than the renal failure itself.

Acute tubular necrosis can result from any of the prerenal causes if the insult is severe and prolonged. Classically the oliguric phase lasts for 2 weeks followed by diuretic phase and renal recovery.

The management of ATN includes correction of the underlying inciting event. Replenishment of intravascular volume should precede diuretic therapy. During the oliguric phase fluid restriction, management of electrolyte imbalance and avoidance of nephrotoxic medications is the mainstay of therapy. Special care must be taken regarding the potassium intake in these patients. In patients with advanced azotemia, dialysis may be required. High calorie, high protein diet must be prescribed in those patients requiring dialysis. In the diuretic phase, meticulous attention must be paid to maintenance of fluid and electrolyte status most notably hypokalemia.

Acute cortical necrosis is most severe end of the spectrum of AKI. It results from prolonged and severe ischemia of the cortical tissue mostly due to torrential hemorrhage and shock in the peripartum setting. It is more common in older women, multigravidas and multiple gestations following an obstetric catastrophe. It should be suspected if ARF develops before 30 weeks of gestation and is associated with prolonged anuria or oliguria (of more than 10 days duration). It is characterized by the death of renal cortical tissue with sparing of the medulla. Cortical necrosis can be patchy or diffuse, the latter having a worse prognosis. Contrast enhanced CT (CECT) of the kidneys can help in differentiation of these two conditions. In cortical necrosis there is a hypodense rim sandwiched between hyperdense viable cortical tissue on the outside and the medullary tissue on the inside. Renal biopsy can also differentiate between these two conditions. Unlike ATN, the recovery of renal function is incomplete and the patients may require lifelong renal replacement therapy. Recovery can be expected up to 3 years and a prolonged trial of dialysis should be given in patients of cortical necrosis.[9]

HYPERTENSIVE DISORDERS OF PREGNANCY

Hypertension is the most common medical complication seen in pregnancy. It occurs in approximately 10% of pregnancies. Owing to the decrease in blood pressure (BP) in normal pregnancies, the upper limit of normal BP 140/90 is of little consequence. BP greater than 125/75 mmHg and mean arterial pressure (MAP) of 82 before 32 week of gestation and BP more than 125/85 and MAP greater than 92, thereafter is associated with increased fetal and maternal risk. Patients having hypertension during pregnancy usually would fall into one of the four categories:[10] (1) pre-eclampsia; (2) pre-eclampsia superimposed on chronic hypertension; (3) chronic essential hypertension and (4) gestational hypertension. Serum uric acid may be useful in differentiating these conditions with serum urate levels over 5.5 mg/dL is a strong indicator of the presence of pre-eclampsia.[2]

1. Preeclampsia: preeclampsia is defined by the American college of obstetricians and gynaecologists (ACOG) as the new onset of hypertension (BP greater than 140/90) and proteinuria (more than 300 mg protein in a 24-hour urine collection) after 20 week of gestation.[11] Hypertension that develops in pre-eclampsia is due to increased peripheral vascular resistance (PVR). Increased PVR leads to reduction of renal blood flow. Therefore, GFR, ERPF and the filtration fraction decrease in pre-eclampsia. These processes start much before any clinical signs or symptoms appear.

    The exact etiology is unknown but is thought to be due to endothelial damage. Endothelial damage in pre-eclampsia is mediated at least in part by disruptions in balance between proangiogenic [vascular endothelial growth factor (VEGF), Placental growth factor (PGF) and transforming growth factor (TGF-β)] and antiangiogenic [soluble fms-like tyrosine kinase-1 (sFlt1) and, soluble endoglin (sEng)] circulating factors.[5]

    There is growing evidence supporting the central role of placental antiangiogenic factors, including sFlt1 in the pathogenesis of pre-eclampsia. sFlt1 is a circulating antagonist to both VEGF and PlGF and is overexpressed in the placenta of women with pre-eclampsia. VEGF is important in maintaining glomerular endothelial cell health and healing and its absence induces proteinuria and thrombotic microangiopathy resembling pathologic glomerular changes of pre-eclampsia. Another molecule sEng, a proteolytic cleavage product of the TGF-β receptor endoglin seems to act synergistically with sFlt1.

    Heme oxygenase (HO), an anti-inflammatory enzyme with antioxidant properties, attenuates VEGF-induced sFlt1 expression. Diminished HO activity has been observed in women with pre-eclampsia and mediates increased placental sFlt1 and sEng expression.

    A potential role for agonistic autoantibodies to the angiotensin AT1 receptor (AT1-AA) in the pathogenesis of pre-eclampsia has been proposed. Elevated levels of AT1-AA have been linked to increased vascular reactivity to angiotensin II. In addition, AT1-AA has been linked to oxidative stress and decreased trophoblast invasion, stimulates trophoblast sFlt1 production *in vitro* and therefore may mediate excess sFlt1 production by the placenta in pre-eclampsia. The endothelial protective effect of VEGF and PlGF in normal pregnancy is mediated by NO, and impaired NO synthesis may contribute to endothelial dysfunction in pre-eclampsia.

These are novel molecules that have been linked to the pathogenesis of pre-eclampsia, the challenge is to diagnose pre-eclampsia early and in this these new molecules will have an important role to play. It remains to be seen whether angiogenic biomarkers will be sensitive and specific enough for widespread clinical use.

The pathology in the kidneys is characterized by pronounced swelling of the glomerular endothelial cells and deposits of fibrin like material within and under the endothelial cell, a process termed as endotheliosis. The capillaries are bloodless with swollen endothelial and mesangial cells. The exact etiology for the decline in renal function is unknown. After delivery, the renal function usually reverts to normal quickly but can progress to ATN if treatment is not initiated at an appropriate time.

The usual presentation is sudden weight gain associated with proteinuria and hypertension. Other accompaniments may include headache, visual disturbance and epigastric pain. Pre-eclampsia usually does not occur before 32 weeks, however it can occur earlier. If it occurs in the first trimester, it is pathognomonic of a hydatidiform mole.[12] The disease has a bimodal presentation being more common in young primiparous and older multiparous women. Others who are at risk of developing pre-eclampsia include those with underlying hypertension, diabetes, renal disease, twin pregnancies.

Pregnancies complicated by pre-eclampsia and ARF are associated with high morbidity and mortality. There is an increased incidence of preterm delivery seen in up to half of patients. Patient's renal function returns to normal within 8 weeks of parturition.

HELLP complicated by AKI does not significantly increase maternal morbidity or mortality rates. Acute fatty liver of pregnancy is a rare disorder characterized by acute onset of upper quadrant pain, jaundice and renal insufficiency. Though most patients have concomitant renal insufficiency, only a few require dialysis. This usually occurs beyond the 34th week of gestation, and is characterized by hyperbilirubinemia and elevated liver enzymes. Occasional patient may develop hypoglycemia, coagulopathy and hepatic failure. Liver histology shows micro vesicular steatosis of hepatocytes. Treatment is inducing delivery or terminating the pregnancy along with supportive care.

2. Preeclampsia superimposed on chronic hypertension: it is more common in older women with underlying renal disease. Should be suspected if the woman had hypertension prior to 20 weeks of gestation with one of the features like new onset proteinuria, sudden rise in blood pressure, increase in the level of proteinuria suddenly and/or thrombocytopenia and liver function abnormalities. Hyperuricemia may also be a clue to suspect this condition.
3. Chronic hypertension: chronic hypertension is to be considered when prepregnancy blood pressures are in the hypertensive range (more than 140/90 mmHg) or in those patients in whom hypertension appears before 20 weeks of gestation. The incidence of pre-eclampsia, abruption placenta, IUGR is increased in such patients.
4. Gestational hypertension: it is defined as new onset hypertension in midterm not associated with proteinuria. The hypertension resolves after delivery. The risk factors include obesity, multiparity and family history of hypertension. These women are at increased risk of developing chronic hypertension at a later stage in their lives.

The goal of the nephrologist is to prevent pre-eclampsia and its complications. Bed rest and meticulous control of blood pressure are the corner stones of therapy. α-Methyldopa is the first-line agent due to its proven safety track record. Side effects include sedation, postural hypotension, hemolytic anemia and elevated liver enzymes. Other options include labetalol, hydralazine and calcium channel blockers. Diuretics are usually not recommended, however they can be continued if they were effective in controlling chronic hypertension.

Aspirin has been tried considering the prominent alterations in prostacyclin-thromboxane balance in pre-eclampsia. The use of aspirin in two meta-analysis has shown a small but significant overall benefit with a relative risk for pre-eclampsia of 0.81–0.90 for aspirin-treated patients. A small reduction in the risk for early preterm birth was also observed in both analyses. Low dosage aspirin is safe in pregnancy. Aspirin prophylaxis should be offered to women who are at an increased risk of developing pre-eclampsia.[12]

Antioxidants, folic acid, calcium supplements have all been tried in the past with no proven benefit. NO donors or precursors such as L-arginine might be effective for the prevention or treatment of pre-eclampsia. Novel therapies like recombinant VEGF, monoclonal antibodies (mAbs) to sFLT1 and sENG are being tried in animal models.

Postpartum AKI usually resembles the related syndromes of hemolytic uremic syndrome and thrombotic thrombocytopenic purpura together broadly grouped under the head thrombotic microangiopathies (TMA). Pregnancy may be a risk facture for TMA because of several factors inherent with pregnancy like increased concentration of procoagulant factors decreased fibrinolytic activity, loss of endothelial cell thrombomodulin and decreased activity of ADAMTS13 (a disintegrin and metalloproteinase with a thrombospondin type 1 motif, member 13), also known as von Willebrand factor-cleaving protease (VWFCP). It usually occurs days to weeks after a normal delivery. These disorders have thrombocytopenia, microangiopathic hemolytic anemia, hypertension and AKI in common. It may be confused with HELLP syndrome and at times renal biopsy may be required to differentiate these two conditions. Hemolytic uremia syndrome/thrombotic thrombocytopenic purpura (HUS/TTP) typically shows fibrin thrombi and fibrinoid necrosis on histology. The mainstay of therapy is plasmapheresis or plasma exchange. Steroids have no role.

URINARY TRACT INFECTION

Asymptomatic bacteriuria is found in 2% of sexually active women and is more common (up to 7%) during pregnancy. Because of the dilatation of the calyces and ureters that occurs in pregnancy, 25% will go on to develop pyelonephritis which can cause fetal growth restriction, fetal death and premature labor. Pyelonephritis is common at around 20 weeks and in the puerperium. Asymptomatic bacteriuria and urinary tract infections (UTIs) in pregnancy should be treated with antibiotics.[13] Antibiotic prophylaxis should be given to women with recurrent bacteriuria or UTIs and kidney disease. About 20% of women having pyelonephritis in pregnancy have underlying renal tract abnormalities and an intravenous urogram (IVU) or ultrasound at 12 weeks postpartum should be considered.

REFLUX NEPHROPATHY

Patients with reflux nephropathy are prone to recurrent UTI and should be given prophylactic antibiotics during pregnancy. In addition they should be encouraged to practice double voiding. The degree of reflux and the presence of secondary glomerulosclerosis determine the prognosis in these patients. Serum creatinine level greater than 1.25 mg/dL is associated with significantly higher rate of fetal loss and a greater chance of pre-eclampsia and a decline in renal function. Patients in whom the serum creatinine level greater than 2.3 mg/dL may experience a marked and rapid decline in renal function.[14] The degree of proteinuria is a good indicator of prognosis because it reflects underlying secondary glomerular lesion. Reflux nephropathy also has a potential for inheritance and the mother should be educated about this.

NONDIALYSIS CHRONIC KIDNEY DISEASE AND PREGNANCY

Chronic kidney disease is defined as kidney damage for more than 3 months associated with structural or functional abnormalities of the kidney that can lead to a decline in GFR. It has been further subdivided into five stages depending on the GFR. Stage 1: More than 90 mL/min; Stage 2: 60–89 mL/min; Stage 3: 30–59 mL/min; Stage 4: 15–29 mL/min and Stage 5: Less than 15 mL/min. Initially, surviving nephrons hypertrophy in number and function. This initial maladaptation predisposes the remaining nephrons to sclerosis and unrelenting destruction. Diabetes, hypertension and glomerular diseases are major causes of CKD. Fertility declines progressively with increasing severity of renal disease.

Both maternal and fetal outcomes can be affected by the presence or absence and the stage of CKD. The outcome is not related to the type of renal disease but the degree of renal insufficiency and degree of proteinuria. The preconception level of renal function is again a significant indicator of the long-term prognosis. During pregnancy most women with CKD experience worsening of hypertension (25%) and increase in proteinuria (50%). In pregnant women with CKD the target blood pressure should be 140/90 mmHg. Such women are at an increased risk of pre-eclampsia and should be offered aspirin as prophylaxis. Women with a variety of mild underlying primary renal diseases (serum creatinine less than 1.4 mg/dL) often show increases in GFR during pregnancy, although of smaller magnitude than seen in normal pregnant women. The gestational rise in GFR becomes compromised as the severity of the underlying disease worsens. Renal allograft recipients also show a substantial increase in GFR during pregnancy provided that there is no underlying graft rejection and graft function is normal. Increased proteinuria often occurs but comes down after parturition in most women with mild renal disease; indeed, a small increase in protein excretion is seen even in normal pregnancy.

Patients who are at increased risk include those with GFR, 40 mL/min and proteinuria exceeding 1g/day before pregnancy.[14] These are the patients who are at high risk, and pregnancy in such patients should preferable be avoided. There is plenty of data to suggest that women with mild renal impairment (serum creatinineless than 1.4 mg/dL), little or no proteinuria and normal blood pressures have near normal maternal and fetal outcomes. There is little or no risk of progression to end-stage renal disease (ESRD) or preterm delivery. Women with moderate to severe CKD (serum creatinine more than 2.5 mg/dL) who conceive are at an increased risk of both maternal and fetal complications including preterm delivery, pre-eclampsia and accelerated decline in maternal renal function.

The largest study comprised 82 pregnancies in 67 women with primary renal disease and a serum creatinine level of more than 1.4 mg/dL. The underlying disorder was glomerulonephritis in 51% of the women and chronic tubule-interstitial disease in the remaining.[15] Of these women, 72% had moderate renal insufficiency (serum creatinine level

1.4–2.4 mg/dL) and 18% had severe (2.5 mg/dL or more). Overall, the total rate of decline in renal function was 43%. At 6 month postpartum, 31% of the women experienced a pregnancy-related decline that persisted, 10% had a decline between 6 weeks postpartum and 6 months, 8% experienced a pregnancy-related decline but recovered and the remaining 51% continued to be stable. Overall, the fetal survival rate was 93% and 59% delivered prematurely. The rates of preterm delivery and intrauterine growth retardation (IUGR) for women with severe renal disease were 73% and 57%, respectively; the rates for women with moderate disease were 55% and 31%, respectively.[16]

DIALYSIS CHRONIC KIDNEY DISEASE AND PREGNANCY

Fertility rates among women on dialysis are very low due to infrequent and irregular menstrual cycles, anovulatory cycles and existing hormonal abnormalities. They seldom become pregnant. However, it is possible to conceive and to carry to term. The frequency of conception has been reported to range from 0.3% to 2.2% per year; and the fertility rate is twice in hemodialysis patients compared to peritoneal dialysis patients.[17] Since these patients may be having irregular periods, pregnancies may go unrecognized, early spontaneous abortion may be mistaken for heavy menses in women with ESRD with irregular menstruation.

The outcome in women who conceived before dialysis is better than in those who conceived after beginning dialysis.[17] The infant survival has been reported to be in the range of 30–50%. In a study of 320 pregnancies, there were 42% surviving neonates, 6% stillborn infants and 7.5% neonatal deaths. The authors also concluded that a lower frequency of prematurity and low birth weight was associated with conception before initiation of dialysis. The length of time, women are on dialysis prior to conception has a bearing on the outcome. The frequency of preterm labor, pre-eclampsia, IUGR is higher in these patients. In a review of six studies, authors concluded the spontaneous abortion rate ranges from 12% to 46%, polyhydramnios was present in 42–79% and cesarean delivery rate 46–53%.

Dialysis prescription in a pregnant lady differs from that in a nonpregnant state. The hours and frequency of dialysis are increased by 50% to maintain a BUN in the ideal range 50–60 mg/dL. 20 hours of hemodialysis per week is recommended.[18] Intradialytic hypotension and rapid fluctuations in intravascular volume should be avoided. Anemia is common in patients receiving dialysis and is exacerbated by pregnancy and should be managed with erythropoietic stimulating agents. Approximately one-third of patients need to be transfused before or at delivery. Hypertension should be aggressively controlled. Patients should be advised high-calorie, high-protein diet in addition to supplements of calcium, iron and dialyzable vitamins. Patients should be counseled that they will be at an increased risk of pregnancy-related complications.

PREGNANCY IN A RENAL ALLOGRAFT RECIPIENT

Fertility returns rapidly after kidney transplantation. The fertility rates are higher in younger transplant patients as compared to those who receive the graft later in life. The first reported successful pregnancy occurred in a recipient of a kidney transplant from an identical twin sister performed in 1958. During the past 3 decades, there has been a steady increase in the number of pregnancies after renal transplantation and the results are encouraging. However, the pregnancy rates in allograft recipients is less than age matched general population.[19] Davison and Milne reviewed pregnancies in transplant patients. Fewer than 40% of conceptions did not continue beyond the first trimester of the remainder, 94% were successful.[20] Remarkably, like in a nontransplant pregnancy, the GFR rises during pregnancy in pregnant transplant patients, despite the fact that the kidneys are denervated and lie in an ectopic location. In 15%, there could be deterioration of renal function that could persist after delivery. The incidence of graft rejection is similar to that in the nonpregnant population. Pre-eclampsia is the most common maternal complication affecting 30% of pregnancies.

Standard markers of pre-eclampsia like changes in urinary protein excretion, plasma uric acid, platelet count or liver function tests seem to be less useful in transplanted patients than in the normal population. A transplanted kidney rarely obstructs labor and delivery by cesarean section is required only for obstetric reasons.

Steroids and standard immunosuppressive agents like prednisone, cyclosporine A and azathioprine are well tolerated by the fetus. No increase in congenital malformations has been reported. More than 50% of live born infants had no neonatal problems. Davison and Milne reported a 45–60% preterm delivery rate and an incidence of small for gestational age infants of greater than 20%.[20]

Before any woman with a renal transplant embarks contemplates a pregnancy, she should be counseled by experts in the field. Certain factors like absence of hypertension, stable graft function, 2 years post-transplant near normal baseline renal function ensure a better outcome. In addition, she should be receiving maintenance doses of immunosuppressive therapy. Pregnancy generally has no effect on graft function or survival, however, an important concern is that the mothers may not survive long after the pregnancy and childbirth. Current data suggest that 10% of mothers die within 7 years of pregnancy.

PRIMARY GLOMERULAR DISEASE AND PREGNANCY

Nephritic Syndrome

It is not uncommon to come across a woman with glomerular disease who gets pregnant. Acute glomerulonephritis is a syndrome characterized by the abrupt appearance of RBCs and RBC casts in the urine along with impaired renal function with sodium and water retention leading to edema and hypertension. Diseases presenting as acute glomerulonephritis include poststreptococcal glomerulonephritis, membranoproliferative glomerulonephritis, immunoglobulin A (IgA) nephropathy, lupus nephritis, and Goodpasture's syndrome. Laboratory tests like antinuclear antibody (ANA), IgA levels, complement levels, antistreptococcal antibodies and antiglomerular basement membrane (GBM) antibodies are required to differentiate these conditions. Careful attention should be paid to control of hypertension, electrolyte balance, and edema.

Nephrotic Syndrome

The nephrotic syndrome is a syndrome characterized by proteinuria greater than 3.5 g per 24 hours leading to hypoalbuminuria, edema, hyperlipidemia and lipiduria. The onset is insidious and renal function is normal at presentation. Common histological entities include minimal-change nephrotic syndrome, focal segmental glomerulosclerosis, mesangiocapillary glomerulonephritis and membranous nephropathy.

Complications include protein malnutrition, hypercoagulability leading to thromboembolic complications and ARF. Renal vein thrombosis is associated with nephrotic syndrome in pregnancy and manifests with acute loin pain, hematuria and deterioration of renal function. Prophylactic anticoagulation is indicated if serum albumin is less than 2 g/dL.[2] Diuretics can be used for intractable edema but should be avoided in volume depleted patients. Steroids may be used in these patients to ameliorate proteinuria in consultation with nephrologist.

Prognosis for a successful pregnancy outcome without deterioration in renal function depends on the etiology of nephrotic syndrome, degree of proteinuria, renal dysfunction and severity of hypertension. Successful pregnancy is unlikely in azotemic patients.

SECONDARY GLOMERULAR DISEASES AND PREGNANCY

Systemic Lupus Erythematosus

Systemic lupus erythematosus (SLE) is the most common collagen vascular disease in pregnancy because this disease is seen most commonly during the child-0bearing years. SLE does not affect the fertility of the woman. It is a multisystem disease affecting all the major organs of the body. Renal involvement is the major cause of morbidity and mortality in such patients. Several autoantibodies including ANA, anti-double stranded (dsDNA), anti single stranded (ssDNA), anti-Ro, anti-La, anti-Sm are seen in these patients, which may damage tissue directly or indirectly by forming antigen-antibody immune complexes as in lupus glomerulonephritis. Lupus nephritis has been classified into five classes, class I being the most benign and class V being the worse.

B obrie and colleagues reviewed 213 pregnancies (73 women) associated with lupus nephritis. Renal biopsy was performed in 66 women proliferative glomerulonephritis was seen in 48. After exclusion of therapeutic abortions (24/213), the overall percentage of live births was 87%.[21] Fetal loss is higher if the onset of SLE occurred during pregnancy or in the immediate postpartum period. When pregnancy occurs after the onset of SLE fetal prognosis depends on the disease activity prior to conception, the degree of proteinuria, hypertension or derangement of renal function. The fetal mortality rate appears to be independant of the presence or absence of lupus anticoagulant.The latter is closely associated with anticardiolipin antibodies. A high anticardiolipin level is a sensitive predictor of IUGR and intrauterine device (IUD).[22] Most of the offspring of SLE patients are normal, but a neonatal lupus syndrome is characterized by skin rash, congenital heart block (CHB) and ANA positivity in maternal and fetal sera may be seen in a few newborns. CHB is permanent. There is a close correlation between isolated congenital heart block and the presence of maternal antibody to soluble tissue ribonucleoprotein antigens anti-Ro (SS-A). Close monitoring of heart rate of newborns is mandated and a cardiologist should be available for pacemaker placement if need be.

In pregnant women with SLE, proteinuria is expected to increase during pregnancy and the serum creatinine level may either rise or not fall normally. Lupus flares are usually moderate and can easily be controlled by steroid therapy. However, the course of maternal lupus nephritis is especially poor when SLE presents during pregnancy. SLE with superimposed pre-eclampsia may present with signs and symptoms indistinguishable from a flare up of lupus nephritis. In such situations rising titers of anti-DNA antibodies or falling levels of complement C3 or C4 are compatible with a flare. Hypertension should be managed aggressively.[23]

Lupus nephritis used to be one of the most common reasons for recommending therapeutic abortion in SLE. However, therapeutic abortion is now rarely indicated. A favorable fetal outcome may be anticipated if the disease is in remission for at least 6 months prior to conception with a stable renal function and controlled hypertension. There is no evidence to suggest that pregnancy has an adverse effect on SLE.

Diabetic Nephropathy and Pregnancy

Diabetic nephropathy (DN) complicates 4–10% of pregnancies in women with diabetes. The classical presentation is with proteinuria, hypertension and azotemia. Urine sediment is benign. DN should not be considered if there are RBCs/RBC casts in urine. Literature is divided on the issue whether diabetic nephropathy is accelerated by pregnancy. Most of the studies favor the notion that proteinuria and hypertension worsen during pregnancy in such patients. However, there are data to suggest in the absence of severe hypertension or severe renal insufficiency, pregnancy does not alter the natural course of diabetic nephropathy. After delivery, proteinuria declines spontaneously. The perinatal survival rate for diabetic women with nephropathy is close to 90%. About one-third of pregnancies are complicated by preterm labor and another third are complicated with IUGR. Hypertensive complications and pre-eclampsia complicate up to 15% and 50% pregnancies respectively. DN is associated with higher perinatal rates of mortality and morbidity than in pregnant diabetic women without nephropathy. Outcome is superior if maternal glucose levels and blood pressure are tightly controlled. Having said all this, a recent systematic review and meta-analysis concluded that the heterogeneous evidence from studies on DN in pregnancy emphasizes the need for further perspective studies on this issue.[24]

GENERAL MANAGEMENT OF RENAL DISEASE IN PREGNANCY

Women with known renal disease should be counseled before they embark on a pregnancy to discuss the effects of pregnancy on the renal disease and to assess the severity of the extent renal disease.

The outcome of pregnancy is generally good if renal function and blood pressure are normal at conception. Frequent antenatal visits are advised to assess blood pressure, weight gain and renal function. Renal function should be assessed monthly to 28 weeks and then every 2 weeks until term. Fetal well-being and growth must be carefully monitored. Nonstress testing is indicated weekly from 26 weeks and twice weekly from 32 weeks until delivery. Ultrasonographic measurements of fetal growth should be performed at 26, 32 and 36 weeks.

If maternal blood pressure is well controlled, renal function is not deteriorating and fetal growth and well-being are satisfactory then pregnancy can be safely prolonged until term. In the absence of premature delivery or evidence of fetal distress, vaginal delivery may be anticipated.

DRUGS IN PATIENTS WITH KIDNEY DISEASE AND PREGNANCY

Some general principles should be adhered to while prescribing drugs during pregnancy. They should be administered only if necessary, avoid prescribing drugs in first trimester, choose medicines that are safe (Category A and B), polypharmacy should be avoided. One should use the lowest possible dose that is effective. In CKD patients, the excretion of medications is altered and the drugs should be prescribed according to the GFR to avoid toxicity.

Teratogenic effects of angiotensin-converting enzyme inhibitors (ACEI) include fetal hypotension, anuria-oligohydramnios, growth retardation, pulmonary hypoplasia, renal tubular dysplasia, neonatal acute renal failure and hypocalvaria. These effects carry a neonatal mortality rate as high as 25%.[5] A similar pattern of fetal anomalies has been reported with exposure to angiotensin II receptor antagonists (ARBs). Current recommendations are ACEIs and ARBs be discontinued before conception and that patients be educated regarding the use of appropriate birth control while taking these agents.

Calcineurin inhibitors like cyclosporine and tacrolimus, steroids and azathioprine are the mainstays of safe immunosuppressive therapy in pregnant transplant recipients.[5] There is evidence to suggest teratogenic effects of mycophenolate mofetil (MMF) in human pregnancy like fetal bone marrow suppression and structural malformations including hypoplastic nails, shortened fingers, microtia (ear malformations) and cleft lip/palate. Women on MMF-based regimens and are contemplating pregnancy should discontinue the medication at least 6 weeks before contemplating pregnancy. There are few human data on the safety of sirolimus in pregnancy, however animal studies do suggest teratogenicity and hence this drug should be avoided.

Aminoglycosides and quinolones should be avoided in pregnancy. Oral anticoagulants are contraindicated. Antibiotics which are safe for both the maternal kidneys and the fetus include penicillin, aminopenicillin, cephalosporin, nitrofurantoin, macrolides, doxycycline and clindamycin.

CONCLUSION

Renal and urinary tract disorders are commonly encountered in pregnancy and some may precede pregnancy. The physiological changes of pregnancy may worsen the renal diseases and the reverse is true too i.e., renal disease does affect the pregnancy predisposing to growth restricted fetus, preterm, IUD, and increased incidence of preeclampsia. Good prenatal and antenatal care can lead to favorable outcomes and no long-term sequelae.

REFERENCES

1. Lindheimer MD, Conrad KP, Karumanchi SA. Renal physiology and disease in pregnancy. In: Alpern RJ, Caplan MJ, Moe OW (Eds). The Kidney: Physiology and Pathophysiology, 5th edition. USA: Academic Press; 2012 .pp. 2689-762.
2. Brenner BM. The Kidney. In: Kincaid-Smith P, Fairley KF (Eds). The Kidney and Hypertension in Pregnancy. New York: Churchill Livingstone; 1993. pp. 1731-63.
3. Sturgiss SN, Dunlop W, Davison JM. Renal haemodynamics and tubular function in human pregnancy. Baillieres Clin Obstet Gynaecol. 1994; 8(2):209-34.
4. Lim KH, Friedman SA, Ecker JK, Kao L, Kilpatrick SJ. The clinical utility of serum uric acid measurements in hypertensive diseases of pregnancy. Am J Obstet Gynecol.1998;178(5):1067-71.
5. Maynard SE, Thadhani R. Pregnancy and the Kidney. J Am Soc Nephrol. 2009;20(1):14-22.
6. Price CP, Newall RG, Boyd JC. Use of protein: creatinine ratio measurements on random urine samples for prediction of significant proteinuria—a systematic review. Clin Chem. 2005;51(9):1577-86.
7. Lindheimer MD, Davison JM. Renal biopsy during pregnancy—"To b or not to b". Br J Obstet Gynaecol. 1987;94(10):932-4.
8. Turney JH, Ellis CM, Parsons FM. Obstetric acute renal failure 1956-1987. Br J Obstet Gynaecol. 1989;96(6):679-87.
9. Kleinknecht D, Grünfeld JP, Gomez PC, Moreau JF, Garcia-Torres R. Diagnostic procedures and long-term prognosis in bilateral renal cortical necrosis. Kidney Int. 1973;4(6):390-400.
10. Lindheimer MD, Taler SJ, Cunningham FG. Hypertension in pregnancy. J Am Soc Hypertens. 2010;4(2):68-78.
11. The American Congress of Obstetricians and Gynecologists. Hypertension in Pregnancy, 2013 [online] AICOG website. Available from http://www.acog.org/~/media/Task%20Force%20and%20Work%20Group%20Reports/HypertensioninPregnancy.pdf [Accessed December 2015].
12. Duley L, Meher S, Jones L. Drugs for treatment of very high blood pressure during pregnancy. Cochrane Database Syst Rev. 2013;7:1-156.
13. Schnarr J, Smaill F. Asymptomatic bacteriuria and symptomatic urinary tract infections in pregnancy. Eur J Clin Invest. 2008;38 Suppl 2:50-7.
14. Kincaid-Smith P, Fairley KF. Renal disease in pregnancy—three controversial areas—mesangial IgA nephropathy, focal glomerular sclerosis (focal and segmental hyalinosis and sclerosis), and reflux nephropathy. Am J Kidney Dis. 1987;9(4):328-33.
15. Imbasciati E, Gregorini G, Cabiddu G, Gammaro L, Ambroso G, Del Giudice A, et al. Pregnancy in CKD stages 3 to 5—fetal and maternal outcomes. Am J Kidney Dis. 2007;49(6):753-62.
16. Jones DC, Hayslett JP: Outcome of pregnancy in women with moderate or severe renal insufficiency. N Engl J Med. 1996;335(4):226-32.
17. Okundaye I, Abrinko P, Hou S. Registry of pregnancy in dialysis patients. Am J Kidney Dis. 1998;31(5):766-53.
18. Jones DC. Pregnancy complicated by chronic renal disease. Clin Perinatol. 1997;24(2):483-96.
19. Kashanizadeh N, Nemati E, Sharifi-Bonab M, Moghani-Lankarani M, Ghazizadeh S, Einollahi B, et al. Impact of pregnancy on the outcome of kidney transplantation. Transplant Proc. 2007;39(4):1136-8.
20. Davison JM, Milne JEC. Pregnancy and renal transplantation. Br J Urol. 1997;80(Suppl 1):29-32.
21. Bobrie G, Liote F, Houillier P, Grünfeld JP, Jungers P. Pregnancy in lupus nephritis and related disorders: Am J Kidney Dis. 1987:9(4);339-43.
22. Cameron JS, Hicks J, Frampton G, et al. The outcome of pregnancy in patients with lupus nephritis—proceedings of the European dialysis transplant association and the European Renal Association.1985;22:487.
23. Lateef A, Petri M. Managing lupus patients during pregnancy. Best Pract Res Clin Rheumatol. 2013;27(3):435-47.
24. Piccoli GB,Clari R,Ghiotto S,Castelluccia N,Colombi N,Mauro G,Tavassoli E, et al. Type 1 diabetes, diabetic nephropathy and pregnancy—a systematic review and meta-study. Rev Diabet Stud. 2013;10(1):6-26.

CHAPTER 52

Endocrinal Disorders: Diabetes Mellitus

Reeti Mehra, Yashdeep Gupta

INTRODUCTION

Incidence of Diabetes is on an increase worldwide . Centre for Disease control and Prevention in 2013 have estimated that in USA, the number of diabetics will range about 1 in 3 to 1 in 5 by 2050 .Obesity , increasing life expectancy and changing lifestyles are some of the contributary factors. A change in uterine environment is also a preceding and predisposing factor that leads to Type 2 diabetes . An understanding of its pathophysiology and management during pregnancy is of paramount importance for all; the mother, the fetus and the society at large, if the increasing burden of the disease has to be curbed

DEFINITION

Diabetes mellitus (DM) refers to a group of metabolic diseases characterized by hyperglycemia resulting from defects in insulin secretion, insulin action, or both.

PREVALENCE

In India, 65 million people had diabetes by 2013. The number of people with diabetes in India has been projected to increase to 101.2 million by 2030.[1]

The prevalence of gestational diabetes mellitus (GDM) as per Carpenter and Coustan criteria as well as by Diabetes in Pregnancy Study Group India (DIPSI) criteria has been estimated to be around 15%.[2,3] As per the 2013 International Diabetes Federation (IDF) Diabetes Atlas, the estimated age-standardized prevalence (20–49 years) of hyperglycemia in pregnancy for India is 27.5% with 90% of women affected by GDM [The figures are based on new criteria for diagnosis of GDM, proposed by International Association of Diabetes and Pregnancy Study Group (IADPSG), and adopted by World Health Organization (WHO)]. The figures imply that there are nearly 5.4 million women in India annually, whose pregnancy gets complicated by GDM.[4] This represents a huge number at risk for future diabetes, which if not managed properly would add to already huge burden of diabetes.

CLASSIFICATION OF DIABETES (GENERAL)

Diabetes mellitus is classified on the basis of the pathogenic process that leads to hyperglycemia, as opposed to earlier criteria, such as age of onset or type of therapy.[5] Table 1 provides a current classification of DM. The two broad categories of DM are designated types 1 and 2. Other specific types of diabetes include genetic defects in insulin secretion

TABLE 1: Etiologic classification of diabetes mellitus

I.	Type 1 diabetes • Immune mediated • Idiopathic
II.	Type 2 diabetes
III.	Other specific types of diabetes
	• Genetic defects of β-cell function • Genetic defects in insulin action • Diseases of the exocrine pancreas • Endocrinopathies • Drug or chemical induced • Infections • Uncommon forms of immune-mediated diabetes • Other genetic syndromes sometimes associated with diabetes
IV.	Gestational diabetes mellitus

or action, mitochondrial abnormalities, and a host of conditions that impair glucose tolerance.

Gestational diabetes mellitus is a separate entity in this classification.

CLASSIFICATION OF DIABETES (PREGNANCY)

Recent recommendations for GDM screening attempt to distinguish between overt diabetes and GDM, i.e., glucose elevations that precede pregnancy and glucose elevations that occur during pregnancy (Fig. 1).[5-7]

The two broad categories are:

1. Overt diabetes of diagnosis.
2. Gestational diabetes mellitus.

Distinction between overt diabetes and gestational diabetes is important, as management of women with level of hyperglycemia consistent with overt diabetes requires assessment of chronic complications, comorbidities and is more likely to require pharmacological intervention.[6] The maternal and fetal complications are also more as compared to women with GDM or normoglycemia. Therefore, early detection would help in decreasing the risk of associated complications.

The recent American Diabetes Association (ADA), Endocrine Society and WHO guidelines recommends distinction between these two entities in pregnancy.[5-7] Two important points that should be kept in this context are:

1. This distinction should be made by testing at first antenatal visit, preferably in first trimester itself.[5-7] Certain women, for example, with history of GDM in previous pregnancy, polycystic ovary syndrome, could be evaluated early than 24 weeks with oral glucose tolerance test (OGTT).
2. As Indians are high risk ethnicity, having high prevalence of diabetes and pre-diabetes in reproductive age group, the screening should be universal, even in first trimester. The recommended investigations for this are mentioned in flowchart. 1.[7]

American Diabetes Association, Endocrine Society and WHO guidelines recommends 75 g 2 hours OGTT for diagnosis of GDM at 24–28 weeks, if initial investigations are normal.[5-7] American College of Obstetricians and Gynecologists (ACOG) prefers 100 g OGTT (Carpenter and Coustan) criteria, preceded by glucose challenge test. A women with value greater than 130 mg% or greater than 140 mg% as per discretion of the provider, after 50 g glucose challenge test, should undergo screening with 100 g OGTT.[8] DIPSI recommends single 2 hours value ≥140 mg% as diagnostic cut-off for diagnosis (Flowchart 1).[9] As per DIPSI guidelines, a pregnant woman found to have normal glucose tolerance in the first trimester, should be tested for GDM again around 24th–28th week and finally around 32nd–34th week.

PATHOPHYSIOLOGY OF DIABETES IN PREGNANCY

Pregnancy is a metabolic stressor. During a healthy pregnancy, increases in placental hormones, including progesterone, human placental lactogen, cortisol, growth hormone lead to a

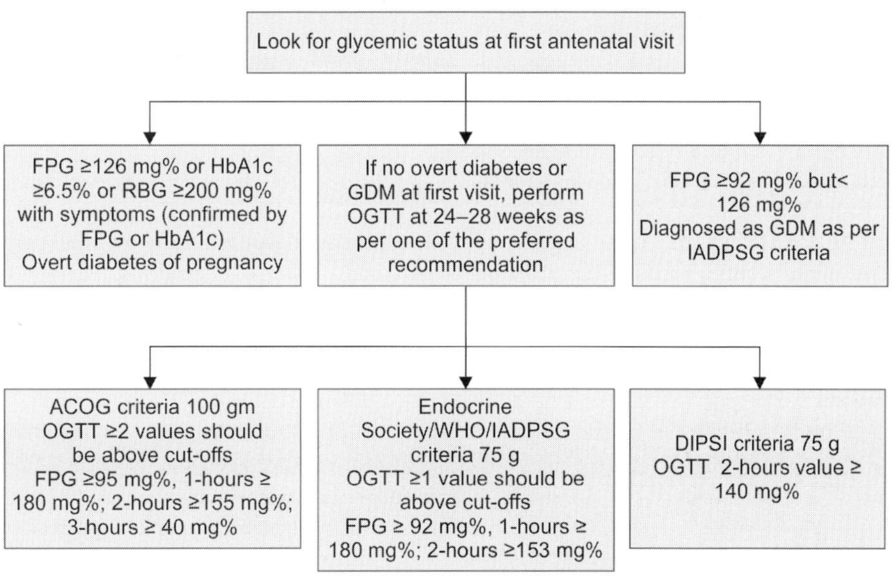

FPG, fasting plasma glucose; RBG, random blood glucose; GDM, gestational diabetes mellitus; OGTT, oral glucose tolerance test; DIPSI, Diabetes in Pregnancy Study Group of India; ACOG, American College of Obstetricians and Gynecologists; WHO, World Health Organization; IADPSG, International Association of Diabetes and Pregnancy Study Groups.

FLOWCHART. 1: Screening and diagnostic strategy for gestational diabetes mellitus with recommendations from various professional bodies.

progressive condition of insulin resistance, hyperinsulinemia and mild postprandial hyperglycemia. Maternal metabolic adaptations, particularly in the second half of pregnancy, direct glucose and amino acids to the growing fetus. Mild postprandial hyperglycemia serves to increase the amount of time that the maternal glucose levels are elevated above the basal after a meal, thereby increasing the flux of ingested nutrients from mother to the fetus.

During fasting, the fetal demand for glucose is met by 15–30% increase in maternal hepatic glucose output. This phenomenon is responsible for lower fasting values (55–65 mg/dL) which offset the postprandial elevations resulting in 24-hour mean glucose values similar to nonpregnant state.[10]

In diabetes in pregnancy, there is in addition a reduced insulin response because of β-cell dysfunction. At the same time, there is exaggerated resistance to the ability of insulin to stimulate glucose utilization and to suppress both glucose production and fatty acid levels resulting in worsening of hyperglycemia in case of overt diabetes or gestational diabetes (onset during pregnancy).[11]

IMPLICATIONS OF MANAGEMENT OF DIABETES DURING PREGNANCY

Fetal

Implications in First Trimester

The pregnant women with overt diabetes and insufficient blood glucose control in first trimester is at increased risk of having a fetus with congenital anomalies.[12] Endocardiac cushion defects are most common congenital malformations in overt diabetes during pregnancy. Sacral agenesis and caudal regression syndrome are most specific of diabetes but are very rare. The other congenital malformations seen are situs inversus, anencephaly, spina bifida, renal agenesis, cystic kidney, transposition of great vessels, and anal/rectal atresia.

The National Institute for Health and Care Excellence (NICE) guidelines recommend women with HbA1c >10% be advised against becoming pregnant, based on Danish data showing a 16% risk of serious adverse pregnancy outcome when HbA1c exceeds 10.4%.[12,13] It is important to know the association between glycemic control and congenital malformations, but the risk should not be exaggerated, since malformations occur only in a minority of diabetic pregnancies.[12]

Implications in Second Trimester

By the second trimester, maternal hyperglycemia stimulates fetal insulin secretion. Fetal hyperinsulinemia in turn results in accelerated fetal growth. Fetal insulin itself is an important growth factor. Other growth factors, including human placental growth hormone, fetal insulin-like growth factor (IGF), and tumor necrosis factor (TNFα) are also influenced by maternal hyperglycemia.[12] The macrosomia could predispose to further complications (Table 2). In addition, a detrimental lasting effect on fetal pancreatic islets and β-cell development from maternal hyperglycemia may potentially increase the long-term risk of diabetes in adult life.[12]

Implications in Third Trimester and in Perinatal Period

In later pregnancy, the metabolic environment resulting from fetal hyperinsulinemia predisposes to hypoxia, acidosis and stillbirth. At birth, fetal hyperinsulinemia is the cause of transient neonatal hypoglycemia.[12]

Impact on Long-term Offspring Health

Fetal exposure to a hyperglycemic environment increases the risk of developing obesity, metabolic syndrome and type 2 diabetes mellitus (T2DM) in future. In Growing Up Today Study, which included examination of offspring (aged 9–14 years) of mothers with GDM, it was found to be associated with an increased risk of adolescent overweight.[14]

Maternal

The pregnant women with overt diabetes are at increased personal risk of suffering from hypoglycemia and worsening of pre-existing microvascular and macrovascular complications, although these generally have no lasting

TABLE 2: Fetal complications

Intrauterine	During labor	Day 1	Day 2 and 3	Long term
• Increased spontaneous abortion rates • Still birth • Intrauterine growth retardation • Large for gestational age	• Birth trauma (shoulder dystocia, Erb's palsy, asphyxia, fractured bones) • Cesarean section	• Congenital malformations • Cardiomyopathy • Hypoglycemia • Respiratory distress syndrome	• Hypocalcemia • Hyperbilirubinemia • Polycythemia • Renal vein thrombosis	• Obesity • Visceral obesity • Insulin resistance • Hyperinsulinemia • T2DM • Cardiovascular disease • Metabolic syndrome

T2DM, type 2 diabetes mellitus.

Box 1: High risk diabetic complications in pregnancy

- Active proliferative retinopathy
- Severe diabetic nephropathy with GFR ≤30%
- Severe autonomic neuropathy
- Severe coronary heart disease

GFR, glomerular filtration rate.

detrimental effect.[12] In presence of high risk diabetic complications (Box 1), avoiding pregnancy should be recommended. If a patient is already pregnant, termination of pregnancy might occasionally be advisable to prevent severe fetal and maternal morbidity.[15]

Hypoglycemia

Women with type 1 diabetes mellitus (T1DM) are extremely susceptible to hypoglycemia, especially during the first 22 weeks of pregnancy when insulin sensitivity actually increases before decreasing in the second trimester. The rise in maternal insulin resistance after 22 weeks gestation lessens glucose variability and hypoglycemic risk.[15]

Diabetic Retinopathy

Diabetic retinopathy is more prevalent in women with T1DM of childbearing age compared to women with T2DM. Pregnancy may promote the onset of diabetic retinopathy in about 10% of cases, as well as contribute to its worsening when already present.[16] The short-term risk of progression of retinopathy during pregnancy is approximately double that during the nonpregnant state. However, long-term detrimental effects are rare. Although every structure of the eye can be affected by diabetes, retinal tissue, with all its vessels, is particularly susceptible.[16] Pregnancy can also cause macular edema; it spontaneously regresses during the postpartum and therefore does not require immediate treatment.[16] The evaluation and care of diabetic retinopathy from preconception to postpartum period is tabulated in Box 2.[7,13,15-17]

Box 2: Diabetic retinopathy: Evaluation and care from preconception to postpartum period

Risk factors that influence the development and progression of diabetic retinopathy during pregnancy

- Pregnant state itself
- Duration of diabetes and degree of metabolic control
- Degree of retinopathy at conception
- The presence of coexisting hypertension, pre-eclampsia
- Rapid glycemic improvements in pregnancy may cause progression of pre-existing retinopathy, particularly if previously moderate or severe

Preconception evaluation and care

- Detail ocular assessment by an ophthalmologist for all diabetic women
- Women with severe diabetic retinopathy should be advised to postpone conception until the condition is treated and is stable for at least 6 months
- Laser photocoagulation therapy is indicated to reduce the risk of vision loss in preconception patients with high risk proliferative diabetic retinopathy (PDR), clinically significant macular edema, and in some cases of severe nonproliferative diabetic retinopathy (NPDR). The same holds true during pregnancy also
- Glycemic and blood pressure control should be optimal

Evaluation and care during pregnancy

- Patients with no or minimal retinopathy should be evaluated in the first and third trimesters, mild retinopathy (every trimester), moderate to severe NPDR or PDR (monthly) at the discretion of eye care provider
- In rare cases of severe disease that may be refractory to laser coagulation, termination of pregnancy can be considered given the high risk of permanent blindness

Care during delivery

- In women with untreated PDR, vaginal delivery has been associated with retinal and vitreous hemorrhage. Assisted second-stage delivery or cesarean delivery should be considered
- Stable diabetic retinopathy is not considered a contraindication to vaginal delivery; however, elective cesarean delivery may be considered to avoid increased intraocular pressure in cases that necessitated, or were refractory to laser photocoagulation

Postpartum follow-up

- Establish retinopathy can rapidly progress even up to 1 year after delivery and can lead to sight-threatening deterioration. Woman with established retinopathy should be seen within 3 months of delivering and periodically thereafter till 1 year

Diabetic Nephropathy

Diabetic nephropathy complicates approximately 5% of insulin-dependent diabetic pregnancies.[18] Assessment for vasculopathy is important before pregnancy. The risk of potentially irreversible kidney damage during pregnancy is low in women with diabetic nephropathy who have normal or slightly elevated serum creatinine levels (<124 μmol/L).[15] The rate of decline in glomerular filtration rate (GFR) was comparable in a cohort of women with diabetic nephropathy who were pregnant or were not, during an observation period of up to 16 years.[19] However, in women with severely reduced kidney function, progression to end stage renal failure during or shortly after pregnancy has been observed.[15] The evaluation and care of diabetic nephropathy in preconception and pregnancy period is tabulated in Box 3.[7,12,13,15-19]

Cardiovascular Risk

There is 3- to 4-fold increased risk of myocardial infarction in pregnancy with greatest risk in the peripartum period.[20]

Box 3: Diabetic nephropathy: Evaluation and care from preconception to postpartum period

Diagnosis
- The diagnosis of microalbuminuria during pregnancy is based on repeated measures of urinary albumin excretion (UAE) 30–299 mg/day or albumin creatinine ratio (ACR) 30–299 mg/g in the absence of bacteriuria
- The diagnosis of overt diabetic nephropathy during pregnancy is presumed if there is persistent albuminuria (≥300 mg/day) or proteinuria (≥500 mg/day) before 20 weeks' gestation in the absence of bacteriuria or evidence of other renal or urinary tract disorders. Proteinuria in the second half of pregnancy may be due to pre-eclampsia

Maternal risks
- Deterioration of renal function
- Exacerbation of coexisting hypertension
- Development of pre-eclampsia
- Thrombosis if proteinuria exceeds 5 g/day

Fetal risks
- Intrauterine growth retardation
- Premature delivery
- Stillbirth

Preconception evaluation and care
- Renal function should be assessed before conception
- Glucose and blood pressure control should be optimal

Evaluation and care during pregnancy
- Assessment for diabetic nephropathy should be done during first antenatal visit, if previously not done
- In women with overt nephropathy, protein intake should be restricted to 1.1 g/kg body weight per day, but not to <60 g/day
- Patients with overt nephropathy can reach nephrotic levels of proteinuria in the third trimester (3–20 g/day), usually with regression of proteinuria postpartum
- Thromboprophylaxis should be considered if proteinuria exceeds 5 g/day

Nephrology referral should be made
- If the GFR (calculated by 24-hour CrCl) is <60 mL/min per 1.73 m^2 or
- Urinary protein excretion is >2 g/day or; serum creatinine is >120 µmol/L

GFR, glomerular filtration rate; CrCl, creatinine clearance.

Box 4: Cardiovascular assessment in women planning pregnancy and during pregnancy with diabetes

Who are at risk and should be evaluated
- Patients of age ≥35 years and duration of T1DM ≥15 years or T2DM ≥10 years
- Known case of coronary artery disease
- Presence of cardiac autonomic neuropathy, cardiomyopathy or heart failure
- Ischemic stroke or peripheral artery disease
- Presence of other cardiovascular disease (CVD) risk factors, such as hypertension

How to evaluate
- In a woman with diabetes having sufficient number of vascular risk factors (particularly the duration of the woman's diabetes and her age), screening studies for coronary artery disease should be undertaken before conception
- Screening should be done for presence of cardiovascular risk factors (hypertension, dyslipidemia, albuminuria, smoking, family history of premature CVD) in all diabetic women
- A resting ECG before or during pregnancy should be done in patients with diabetes of age ≥35 years
- Patients with symptoms or signs suggestive of CHD, or abnormal resting ECG, should have cardiology consultation

Action required
- Treat CVD risk factors, such as hyperglycemia, hypertension, dyslipidemia and smoking with interventions adapted for pregnancy
- Statins, fibrates and niacin should be stopped before pregnancy. Bile acid binding resins may be used to treat hypercholesterolemia, when required
- Women with diabetes should be treated to a SBP <130 mmHg and DBP <80 mmHg
- Angiotensin converting enzyme inhibitors and angiotensin receptor blockers are contraindicated. Blood pressure medications that are safe for pregnancy (methyldopa, long acting calcium channel blockers, selected β-adrenergic blockers) should be added sequentially until target blood pressure levels are achieved
- Excessive salt intake should be avoided, but women should not be severely salt restricted. Adequate potassium intake should be encouraged

ECG, electrocardiogram; CHD, coronary heart disease; SBP, systolic blood pressure; DBP, diastolic blood pressure.

Active or previously treated coronary heart disease is reported to occur in 1 of 10,000 pregnancies but in 1 of 350 diabetic pregnant women.[17] Women with a long duration of T1DM and older women with T2DM are potentially at risk, and those with previous or suspected cardiac history should be evaluated by cardiologist before pregnancy.[17] The assessment and optimization of cardiovascular risk and risk factors are tabulated in Box 4.[7,15,17,20]

Diabetic Ketoacidosis

Diabetic ketoacidosis (DKA) is a medical emergency that must be excluded in all pregnant women with T1DM who become unwell, even if blood glucose values are normal (euglycemic DKA can occur in pregnancy).[13,17] DKA is discussed ahead.

Others

Pre-eclampsia is a major cause of maternal morbidity and mortality. Women with diabetes are at increased risk of pre-eclampsia compared with the general population. Spontaneous preterm birth (<37 weeks) is 5-fold higher in diabetic pregnancies than for the general maternity population. This increases the risk of perinatal morbidity and mortality associated with prematurity.[12]

Long-term Implications in Case of Gestational Diabetes Mellitus

Gestational diabetes mellitus is associated with increased long-term risks of diabetes, metabolic syndrome and cardiovascular disorders. While most cases of GDM resolve with delivery, these individuals are at 7-fold increase risk of developing T2DM subsequently.[21]

The maternal complications are tabulated in Table 3.

SCREENING/INVESTIGATIONS NEEDED IN CASE OF DIABETES DURING PREGNANCY FOR FETAL WELL-BEING

A woman with diagnosis of diabetes and pregnancy should be assessed for glycemic control every 1–2 weeks. The fetal viability and gestational age should be confirmed with ultrasound at 6–8 weeks. Ultrasonographic examination of the fetal heart (four chambers and outflow tract) along with routine detailed anatomical ultrasound scan for congenital abnormalities should be done at 18–22 weeks. The ultrasound monitoring of fetal growth (using abdominal circumference measurements) and amniotic fluid volume should commence at 28 weeks, and then at 32 and 36 weeks. The monitoring of fetal well-being by regular non-stress test, biophysical profile should be individualized for women at risk of intrauterine growth restriction. For women without other complications and well-controlled glycemia, tests for fetal well-being can commence at 38 weeks.[12,13]

SCREENING/INVESTIGATIONS NEEDED IN CASE OF DIABETES DURING PREGNANCY FOR ASSOCIATED COMPLICATIONS FOR MOTHER

In view of increased risk of worsening of pre-existing complications, or risk of developing new complications, women with pre-existing diabetes should undergo thorough workup before conception as well as periodically through pregnancy. The recent recommendations by Endocrine Society on preconception evaluation and care apart from comorbidities and complications discussed above are tabulated in Box 5.[7] Women without preconception evaluation, and who present first time in pregnant state should undergo this evaluation and optimization at first antenatal visit.

TARGETS FOR GLYCEMIC CONTROL

Hyperglycemia and Adverse Pregnancy Outcome (HAPO) study showed that the association between maternal glycemia and poor outcomes was continuous, making it difficult to identify threshold criteria below which no risk was present.[22] During a healthy pregnancy, mean fasting blood glucose levels decline progressively to a remarkably low value of 75 ± 12 mg/dL. However, peak postprandial blood glucose values rarely exceed 126 mg/dL.[10] As per the latest recommendations by Endocrine Society, women with overt or gestational diabetes should strive to achieve a target preprandial blood glucose ≤95 mg/dL. Even lower fasting blood glucose ≤90 mg/dL, if can be safely achieved without undue hypoglycemia, should be targeted.[7] The target blood glucose levels 1 hour after the start of a meal should be ≤140 mg/dL and 2 hours after the start of a meal ≤120 mg/dL, when these targets can be safely achieved without undue hypoglycemia.[5,7] The pregnant women with overt diabetes should aim to achieve an HbA1c ≤7% (ideally ≤6.5%).[7]

Box 5: Preconception care of women with diabetes (recommendations by Endocrine Society)

- Preconception counseling: Aim to inform woman to have optimal glycemic control before pregnancy. Medications should be reviewed. Comorbidities and complications should be assessed and taken care of
- Optimization of insulin therapy preferably with multiple daily dose insulin or continuous subcutaneous insulin
- HbA1c levels should be as close to normal as possible without undue hypoglycemia
- Folic acid (5 mg) daily should be prescribed daily before conception to reduce the risk of neural tube defects
- For women with type 1 diabetes, measurement of serum TSH and thyroid peroxidase are recommended before conception

TABLE 3: Maternal complications

During pregnancy	During labor	During peurperium
• Spontaneous abortion • Infections especially urinary tract infections, vaginal candidiasis • Polyhydramnios • Pre-eclampsia • Ketoacidosis • Worsening of diabetic nephropathy, retinopathy • Preterm labor • Uncontrolled hyperglycemia • Hypoglycemia	• Ketoacidosis • Prolonged labor • Shoulder dystocia • Increased incidence of instrumental delivery • Increased incidence of operative delivery • Maternal soft tissue injuries, perineal tears, vaginal lacerations, cervical tears • Postpartum hemorrhage	• Subinvolution of uterus • Puerperal sepsis • Failed lactation

MONITORING OF BLOOD GLUCOSE LEVELS

Glycemic control can be achieved by frequent self-monitoring of blood glucose (SMBG). Experts recommend that finger-stick blood glucose measurement be performed 6-8 times/day.[23] Testing before and either 1 or 2 hours after the start of each meal, and, as indicated, at bedtime and during night are the recommended timings of monitoring.[5,7] 3.00 am blood glucose levels could help to differentiate between Dawn phenomenon or Somoygi phenomenon. Postprandial glucose values have the strongest correlation with fetal growth. In women managed with postprandial blood glucose levels, the mean (± SD) decrease in the glycated hemoglobin during treatment was greater (–3% ± 2.2% versus 0.6% ± 1.6%; P <0.001), birth weights were lower (3,469 ± 668 g versus 3,848 ± 434 g; P = 0.01), and the rates of neonatal hypoglycemia (3% versus 21%; P = 0.05) and macrosomia (12% versus 42%; P = 0.01) were lower.[24] There are no specific recommendations in favor of either 1 hour or 2 hours postprandial value by professional bodies.[5,7] Continuous glucose monitoring can be used during pregnancy in women with overt or gestational diabetes when self-monitored blood glucose levels are not sufficient to assess glycemic control (including both hyperglycemia and hypoglycemia).[7]

Box 6: Recommendations on medical nutrition therapy

- Women with overt or gestational diabetes should limit carbohydrate intake to 35–45% of total calories, distributed in 3 small- to moderate-sized meals and 2–4 snacks including an evening snack
- Diet should contain 175 g/day of digestible carbohydrate, 1.1 g/kg/day of protein and enough fiber intake (28 g/day), in form of vegetables, fruits, and whole grains
- Fat consumption should be limited to less than 30% of the total calories. Consumption of unsaturated fatty acids including the n-6 and n-3 fatty acids should be encouraged; saturated fat should be limited to more than 10% of energy intake and trans fats to the minimal amount possible
- The guidelines for the intake of minerals and vitamins are as for women without diabetes, with the exception of taking folic acid 5 mg daily beginning 3 months before withdrawing contraceptive measures or otherwise trying to conceive
- At 12 weeks gestation, the dose of folic acid can be reduced to 0.4–1.0 mg/day, which should be continued until the completion of breastfeeding

  Note: Folate supplementation may mask signs of B12 deficiency in women with type 1 diabetes who can have autoimmune gastritis. Therefore, consider obtaining baseline vitamin B12 levels in these patients.
- Women are encouraged to acquire micronutrients from natural food sources, but a prenatal supplement of vitamins and minerals should be considered in women with pre-existing diabetes
- Vegetarian pregnant women may need supplements of vitamin D and vitamin B12

TREATMENT

During Pregnancy Till Onset of Labor

Diet

Individualized medical nutrition therapy (MNT) is recommended for all pregnant women with overt or gestational diabetes to help achieve and maintain desired glycemic control while providing essential nutrient requirements.[5] Institute of medicine revised guidelines for weight gain during pregnancy should be followed.[10] Weight should be monitored at each visit. Obese women with overt or gestational diabetes should reduce their calorie intake by approximately one-third (compared with their usual intake before pregnancy) while maintaining a minimum intake of 1600-1800 kcal/day.[7] The recommendations as per ADA and Endocrine Society, on MNT are tabulated in Box 6.[4,7,17]

Goals for MNT in pregnancy include:

- Adequate nutrient intake to support a healthy pregnancy
- Excellent glucose control by balancing food/carbohydrate intake with physical activity and insulin treatment
- Adequate but not excessive weight gain
- Learning appropriate food and exercise behaviors that can contribute to long-term maternal health.

In women with pre-existing diabetes, MNT in conjunction with physical activity is advised in conjunction with drug therapy. Whereas, initial treatment of gestational diabetes should consist of MNT and daily moderate exercise for 30 minutes or more. Blood glucose-lowering pharmacological therapy is initiated if lifestyle therapy is insufficient to maintain normoglycemia in women with gestational diabetes.[7]

Physical Activity

Exercise facilitates the glucose uptake, improves glucose clearance sustains insulin sensitivity. Furthermore, exercise also regulates counter-regulatory hormones and decreases hepatic glucose output as evident in fasting blood glucose levels.[10] ADA recommends that pregnant women without medical and obstetric contraindications (Table 4) should be encouraged to use physical activity as part of their overall diabetes management, at least 30 min/day.[17,25]

The minimal target of 30 minute can be divided into three 10-minute sessions preferably after meals. Carbohydrate consumed before, during, and after physical activity will help avoid hypoglycemia, especially if glucose is <100 mg/dL.[17]

Insulin

Insulin has been the mainstay of therapy for glycemic control in pregnancy, because it does not cross the placenta into the fetus and has many decades of proven efficacy.[8] For women with pregestational diabetes, both the ADA and NICE advocate multiple daily injections combining a pre-meal insulin (short acting human insulin) or quick acting analogue with a bedtime (intermediate acting human insulin or long acting analogue).[5,13] Majority of women with GDM can be managed with diet and exercise. Insulin remains the first line drug if needed. Endocrine society suggests that women with a diagnosis of gestational diabetes before 25 weeks gestation and for those women with fasting plasma glucose levels >110 mg/dL should preferably put on insulin, as they are unlikely to respond to MNT even combined with glyburide/metformin.[7]

Insulin lispro and insulin aspart are safe in pregnancy and may improve postprandial glycemic control in women with T1DM.[7] However, a lack of data indicating improved fetal outcomes suggests that there is no imperative to switch to a short-acting analogue where the woman's diabetes is well controlled with human insulin.[26] There are no reports of the use of insulin glulisine in pregnancy and its use is not recommended.[26] A randomized controlled trial (RCT) comparing insulin detemir and neutral protamine hagedorn (NPH) insulin found no significant difference in fetal outcomes.[27] There was no significant difference in incidence of hypoglycemia. The greater evidence available for insulin detemir supports its use as the first line long-acting analogue in pregnancy but the lack of definitive fetal benefits means that there is no strong need to switch a woman who is well controlled on NPH insulin.[26] There seems little justification in using long acting insulin analogues in women with gestational diabetes or T2DM where the risk of hypoglycemia is low. There is lack of good evidence safety data for use of glargine in pregnancy.[26] The insulins available for use in pregnancy are summarized in Table 5.

TABLE 4: Contraindications to physical activity during pregnancy

Contraindications	Medical	Obstetric
Absolute	• Hemodynamically significant heart disease • Restrictive lung disease	• Incompetent cervix • Multiple gestation at risk for premature labor • Persistent second or third trimester bleeding • Placenta previa after 26 weeks gestation • Premature labor during the current pregnancy • Ruptured membranes • Pre-eclampsia, pregnancy induced hypertension
Relative	• Severe anemia • Unevaluated maternal cardiac arrhythmias • Chronic bronchitis • Uncontrolled type 1 diabetes • Extreme morbid obesity • Extreme underweight (body mass index <12 kg/m^2) • History of extremely sedentary lifestyle • Poorly controlled hypertension • Poorly controlled hyperthyroidism • Poorly controlled seizures • Orthopedic limitations • Heavy smoker	• Intrauterine growth restriction in the current pregnancy

TABLE 5: Insulin preparations that can be used in pregnancy

Preparation	Time of action		
	Onset, hour	Peak, hour	Effective duration, hour
Short/rapid acting			
Regular	0.5–1.0	2–3	4–6
Aspart	<0.25	0.5–1.5	3–4
Lispro	<0.25	0.5–1.5	3–4
Intermediate/long acting			
NPH	1–4	6–10	10–16
Detemir	1–4	Minimal peak activity	Up to 24
Glargine (less evidence based safety data)	1–4	Minimal peak activity	Up to 24

NPH, neutral protamine hagedorn.

Oral Antidiabetic Agents

Drug of choice for management of diabetes in pregnancy has always been insulin. But some of the drugs, metformin and glyburide, have now reasonable amount of data to support their use in pregnancy.[28]

The Endocrine Society guidelines suggest that glyburide is suitable alternative to insulin therapy for glycemic control in women with gestational diabetes who fail to achieve sufficient glycemic control after a 1-week trial of MNT and exercise, except for those women with a diagnosis of gestational diabetes before 25 weeks gestation and for those women with fasting plasma glucose >110 mg/dL, in which case insulin therapy is preferred. Regarding metformin, the suggestion for use is in those women with gestational diabetes, who do not have satisfactory glycemic control despite MNT, and who refuse or cannot use insulin or glyburide, and are not in the first trimester.[7]

ACOG and the UK NICE have recommended that either metformin or glibenclamide can be used to treat gestational diabetes.[8,13] By contrast, ADA recommends that both drugs should only be used during pregnancy in the context of clinical trials.[5] No oral hypoglycemic agent (OHA) has been approved by Food and Drug Administration (FDA) for use in pregnancy yet.[29] It should also be kept in mind that there is a paucity of long-term follow-up data on children exposed to oral agents *in utero*.

The treatment plan is summarized in flowchart. 2.

Glycemic Management after Antenatal Corticosteroid Therapy

Antenatal corticosteroids (ACS) are recommended for use in antenatal mothers at risk of preterm delivery before 34 weeks. One common side-effect of these drugs is their propensity to cause hyperglycemia. In women with diabetes, the need for

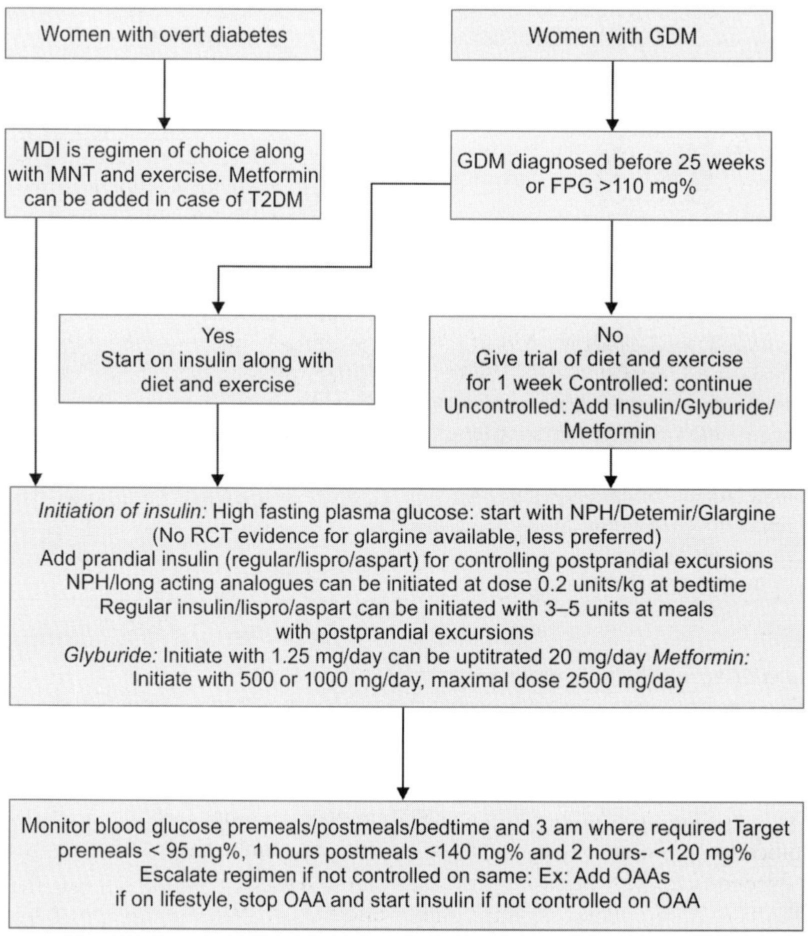

GDM, gestational diabetes mellitus; MDI, multiple dose insulin; MNT, medical nutrition therapy; T2DM, type 2 diabetes mellitus; FPG, fasting plasma glucose; NPH, neutral protamine hagedorn; RCT, randomized controlled trial; OAA, oral anti-diabetic agent.

FLOWCHART 2: Treatment plan for women with diabetes in pregnancy.

ACS is even more pronounced. Use of ACS may worsen the diabetic control, requiring initiation of insulin therapy or intensification of insulin regimen.[30] There are no suggestions from guidelines regarding glycemic management after ACS therapy. An increase in dose of 16–40% has been recommended by various authors.[30] However, an individualized approach is necessary because of the wider inter-individual and intra-individual variability noted in degree and duration of hyperglycemia after steroid injections.

Timing and Mode of Delivery

A woman with pregestational diabetes who is well controlled, delivery is recommended after 39 weeks of gestation and by the estimated date of delivery. Though there is no evidence based recommendation regarding timing of delivery in women with GDM that is controlled either with a diet and exercise regimen or with medication. Woman with good glycemic control can be managed expectantly. They usually do not require delivery before 39 weeks of gestation. The women with abnormal glucose profile may be delivered at 38 weeks of gestation. Pregnancy should not be allowed to go postdate. ACOG also recommends that women with GDM should be counseled regarding the option of scheduled cesarean delivery when the estimated fetal weight is 4500 g or more.

Management during Labor

Different forces are at play during labor: placental hormones giving insulin resistance, relaxin enhancing insulin sensitivity, uterine muscle using glucose, the woman frequently taking nothing by mouth, and there is the general stress, anxiety, and excitement associated with delivery. In the nondiabetic woman these stresses are well handled physiologically, but in the diabetic person controlling glucose in this environment is both crucial and challenging.[31]

Hyperglycemia in the mother gives rise to higher glucose levels in the baby with resultant fetal hyperinsulinemia and hence neonatal hypoglycemia.[12] Neonatal hypoglycemia occurs in 24–48% of offspring of women with pre-existing diabetes and 16–19% of offspring of women with GDM.[32-34] Poor glycemic control during pregnancy and fetal macrosomia are predisposing factors in addition to maternal hyperglycemia during labor. The fetus relies on the mother for its glucose supply but once the umbilical cord is clamped the neonate has to fend for itself. Glycogenesis and gluconeogenesis provides the required glucose to the neonate after the delivery to prevent neonatal hypoglycemia, requiring increase in glucagon and fall in insulin levels. However, this glucagon response is blunted in infants of diabetic mothers. The adaptive mechanism takes 12–24 hours to mature so that the normal glucose in the neonate is typically much lower than adults. The cortisol and growth hormone responses are also blunted in hypoglycemic neonates. The neonate tolerates these lower glucose values remarkably well, but very low values may be associated with twitching and possible seizures. Neonatal hypoglycemia likely accentuates the risk of brain injury from other insults.[31]

ACOG and the American College of Endocrinology (ACE) recommends target glucose range of 70–110 mg/dL in labor for both gestational and pregestational diabetics.[35,36] There is a significant negative correlation between more severe maternal glycemia (glucose >144 mg/dL) during labor and neonatal hypoglycemia.[37] Some studies suggests that maternal glycemia 15–30 mg/dL above the consensus threshold of 110 mg/dL may be permissible without significantly increasing neonatal risk.[38,39] The management during labor involves insulin infusion with or without dextrose based intravenous fluids.

Women with T1DM should be managed with dextrose based intravenous fluid along with insulin infusion to reduce the risk of ketosis.[40] Some women with T2DM and most with GDM can be managed without insulin during labor, if their insulin requirements were not too high during pregnancy (<0.5 u/kg/day). Requirements >1 u/kg/day during pregnancy will usually require infusion.[31] Women with T2DM and GDM may have sufficient glycogen stores to prevent hypoglycemia in the latent phase of labor. But, in cases or at centers where oral intake is restricted due to maternal aspiration risk, dextrose solutions should be supplemented, as labor demands necessitates glucose as an energy source. The glucose requirement increases with prolonged labor induction, during the active phase of labor, and with maternal pushing aspects. Most of the protocols keep fluid replacement rates at 125 mL/hour. Blood glucose monitoring should be done 1–2 hourly to keep the glucose levels within targets.[40] The plan is summarized in flowchart. 3.

Cesarean Section

In case of elective cesarean section, it should be planned early during daytime in order to prevent prolonged fasting related hypoglycemia. Night time insulin dose should be reduced appropriately. Woman should be regularly tested for a capillary blood glucose hourly starting in morning before surgery. Monitor blood glucose every 30 minutes from induction of anesthesia until after the baby is born.[13,40] The woman should be hydrated with nondextrose containing solution if glucose is 70–110 mg/dL, dextrose only if <70 mg% and insulin/dextrose infusion if glucose >110 mg/dL twice in a row.[40] Patient should be closely monitored after deliver for hypoglycemia. In cases of T1DM, insulin infusion with dextrose containing fluid should be used to avoid ketoacidosis.

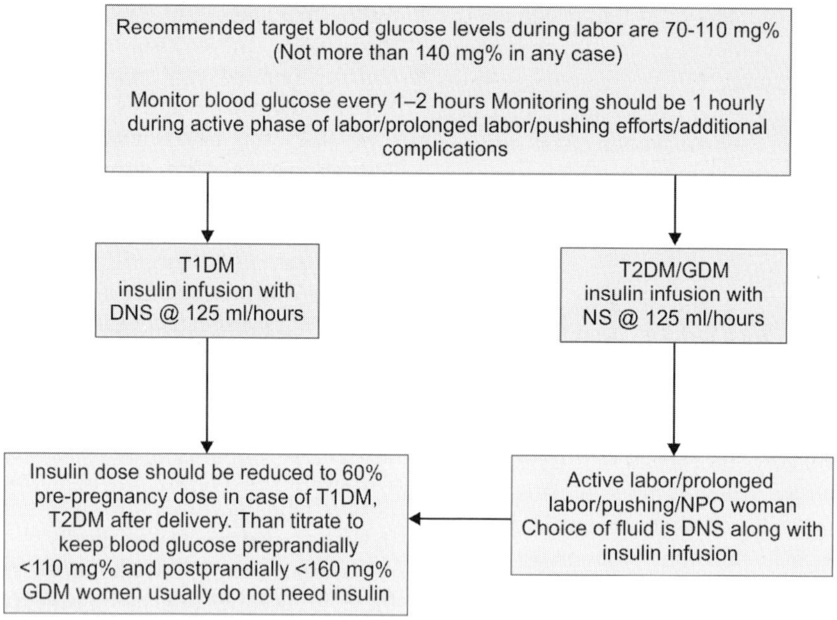

T1DM, type 1 diabetes mellitus; T2DM, type 2 diabetes mellitus; DNS, dextrose normal saline; NS, normal saline; GDM, gestational diabetes mellitus; NPO, normal pregnancy outcome.

FLOWCHART 3: Glycemic management during labor.

After Delivery in Postpartum Period

In the immediate postpartum period, there is rapid improvement in insulin sensitivity in the mother, making them particularly vulnerable to hypoglycemia. This enhanced insulin sensitivity is probably due the removal of insulin antagonistic placental hormones and blunted pituitary growth hormone reserve. Therefore, the rapid resolution of the insulin resistance gives IV insulin with its short half-life an additional theoretical advantage over subcutaneous insulin during labor.[31,40] After delivery, insulin dose should be reduced to 60% of the predelivery dose to prevent hypoglycemia.[15] This is the more important in women after a cesarean section who do not eat or are not allowed to eat for hours to days.[40] Hypoglycemic therapy should be discontinued immediately after the birth in women who were diagnosed with GDM. Breastfeeding which should be stimulated as much as possible, does lead to even lower insulin requirements and insulin dose should be decreased further if necessary to prevent hypoglycemia.[15] Monitor blood glucose levels carefully to establish the appropriate dose. The woman should be advised meal or snack before or during feed to avoid hypoglycemia.[17]

Any drugs that were discontinued for safety reasons in the preconception period should be avoided during breastfeeding also.[17] Women with T1DM should continue to use insulin. However, as per NICE guidelines, metformin and glibenclamide can be resumed or continued immediately after birth in women with pre-existing T2DM who are breast feeding.[13] The same is not universally agreed upon.[41] FDA has not approved any oral antidiabetic drug to be used during breastfeeding.[41] Blood glucose monitoring should be continued during hospital stay to exclude persisting hyperglycemia in woman with GDM.

The glucose targets are less stringent during postpartum period as compared to pregnancy. Fasting plasma glucose levels of <140 mg/dL and postprandial glucose levels of <180 mg/dL are acceptable. However, in woman who underwent cesarean section, the targets should be <110 mg/dL and 160 mg/dL respectively to facilitate wound healing. Even in others, more stringent glycemic control should be aimed, if safely achievable.[40]

Usually in women who undergo cesarean section, carbohydrate intake during first 24 hours may be difficult to anticipate. The administration of short acting insulin by sliding scale with meals can provide coverage until a solid diet can be tolerated. However, continuation of long acting basal insulin is extremely important (dose can be reduced as required) in women with T1DM, in order to prevent the risk of DKA.[40]

Women with GDM and normoglycemia postpartum should be advised 75 g OGTT (non-pregnant cut-offs) after 6 weeks of delivery and periodically thereafter.[5] Irrespective of type of diabetes, importance of lifestyle modification advice should be reinforced for each one of them.[5] Further follow-up of all women (with diabetes in pregnancy) with an endocrinologist or internist should be encouraged.

HYPOGLYCEMIA CARE

The postabsorptive plasma glucose declines by 10 mg/dL during early pregnancy. The threshold for secretion of counter-regulatory hormones is also lower (48-57 mg/dL) during gestation in diabetic women. Therefore, threshold of <60 mg/dL has been reasonably used to define hypoglycemia during pregnancy.[17] Hypoglycemia is more common with T1DM as compared to T2DM or GDM. Severe hypoglycemia occurs 3–5 times more frequently in early pregnancy than in the period prior to pregnancy, whereas in the third trimester the incidence of severe hypoglycemia is lower than in the year preceding pregnancy.[15] Risk factors for severe hypoglycemia during pregnancy include a history with severe hypoglycemia in the year preceding pregnancy, impaired hypoglycemia awareness, long duration of diabetes, low HbA1c in early pregnancy, fluctuating plasma glucose values and excessive use of supplementary insulin injections between meals. Pregnancy-induced nausea and vomiting have not been seen as contributing factors.[42]

All women should be educated and trained about the recognition and treatment of hypoglycemia, SMBG, and the need to carry glucose and a medical alert identification. Glucose (15–20 g) is the preferred treatment for the conscious woman with hypoglycemia, although any form of carbohydrate may be used. If SMBG 15 minutes after treatment shows continued hypoglycemia, the treatment should be repeated. Once SMBG glucose returns to normal, the woman should consume a meal or snack to prevent recurrence of hypoglycemia. Women should be advised to balance physical activity and the timing and amount of insulin doses and carbohydrate intake in meals and snacks to minimize iatrogenic hypoglycemia. The spouses, partners, and coworkers of women at risk for hypoglycemia should be instructed for the appropriate use of glucagon.[17]

MANAGEMENT OF DIABETES KETOACIDOSIS

Diabetic ketoacidosis is a serious complication of diabetes in pregnancy, occurring in approximately 1–3% of women with diabetes who become pregnant. It usually occurs in patients with T1DM especially with new-onset T1DM, but it may also affect women with T2DM or, more rarely, women with GDM. The marked increase in insulin resistance and enhanced lipolysis/ketosis associated with pregnancy account for the greater risk of DKA during gestation. DKA is rarely life threatening to the pregnant woman if it is recognized and treated promptly.[43] The risk of maternal mortality secondary to complications from DKA is not well established. However, fetal loss rates remain in the order of 10–25% for a single episode of DKA despite substantial improvements in perinatal and neonatal care. Prompt recognition and management of this medical emergency complicating pregnancy is essential in order to optimize perinatal outcome for both mother and fetus (Box 7).[43,44]

Box 7: Diabetic ketoacidosis in pregnancy

When to suspect DKA?

A high index of suspicion for DKA in diabetic pregnant women with nausea, vomiting, abdominal pain, fever, and poor oral intake, in addition to symptoms related to hyperglycemia.

Predisposing factors include

- Infection
- Omission of insulin doses
- Obstetrical use of β-sympathomimetic drugs and glucocorticoids
- Protracted vomiting, starvation and dehydration
- Undiagnosed diabetes
- Insulin pump failure
- Poor glycemic control

Risks to mother

- Acute renal failure
- Adult respiratory distress syndrome
- Myocardial infarction
- Cerebral edema
- Even death.

Risks to fetus

- Preterm delivery
- Acidosis and hypoxia could result in fetal demise
- Adverse neurobehavioral outcomes and lower IQ

Educate

- All women with pre-existing diabetes who are planning pregnancy or already pregnant should be educated about DKA; prevention with self-monitoring of blood glucose (SMBG), MNT, and appropriate insulin therapy; and sick day management
- The patient should be taught to perform urine ketone measurements at times of illness or when persistent glucose levels exceed 200 mg/dL and to promptly report positive values

Management of DKA during pregnancy include

- Correction of volume depletion
- Insulin infusion
- Monitoring and correcting electrolyte imbalances
- Identifying and treating precipitating factors

Fetal monitoring

- Continuous fetal heart rate monitoring and biophysical tests are used to assess fetal well-being in cases occurring after 24 weeks' gestation
- Immediate delivery may not be necessary for ominous patterns, since correction of DKA often reverts the patterns to normal (usually after 4–8 hours)
- If fetal status does not improve or if the maternal condition continues to deteriorate despite aggressive therapy, delivery is warranted

DKA, diabetic ketoacidosis; MNT, medical nutrition therapy.

PSYCHOSOCIAL MANAGEMENT OF WOMEN WITH DIABETES IN PREGNANCY

Emotional well-being is part of diabetes management. Psychological disorders, which can affect glycemic control, are detectable in up to one-third of diabetic patients, including women who are pregnant. Psychosocial therapies are of proven benefit in the management of diabetes.[17,45,46] Depression in diabetic women is strongly associated with poor self-care and glycemic control, micro- and macrovascular complications, and increased health care expenditures. The hormonal changes and other stresses of pregnancy are thought to increase vulnerability to the onset or return of depression, which is associated with poor perinatal outcome. Structured psychotherapy can be a useful first-line therapy for mild depression, but pharmacotherapy is needed for severe depression.[17]

CONCLUSION

Obstetric diabetology is a field of medicine marked by clinical equipoise and therapeutic ambiguity. The precious and fragile nature of the fetus or unborn child, the unique physiology of the gravid mother, and the temporary nature of pregnancy, combine to make obstetric diabetes practice different from routine diabetes care. GDM presents a window of opportunity to prevent diabetes and associated metabolic illness, not only in the mother, but also in the unborn generation. Active screening, diagnosis, lifestyle management, MNT, and drugs, if required, will help not only in improving short-term maternal and fetal outcomes, but will also bring down the long-term ill consequences.

REFERENCES

1. Ramachandran A, Snehalatha C, Ma RC. Diabetes in South-East Asia: an update. Diabetes Res Clin Pract. 2014;103(2):231-7.
2. Seshiah V, Balaji V, Balaji MS, et al. Gestational diabetes mellitus in India. J Assoc Physicians India. 2004;52:707-11.
3. Grewal E, Kansara S, Kachhawa G, Ammini AC, Kriplani A, Aggarwal N, et al. Prediction of gestational diabetes mellitus at 24 to 28 weeks of gestation by using first-trimester insulin sensitivity indices in Asian Indian subjects. Metabolism. 2012;61(5):715-20.
4. Guariguata L, Linnenkamp U, Beagley J, et al. Global estimates of the prevalence of hyperglycaemia in pregnancy. Diabetes Res Clin Pract. 2014:103(2);176-85.
5. American Diabetes Association. Standards of medical care in diabetes—2013. Diabetes Care. 2013;36(Suppl 1):S11-66.
6. World Health Organization, Geneva. (2013) WHO Guidelines Approved by the Guidelines Review Committee. Diagnostic Criteria and Classification of Hyperglycaemia First Detected in Pregnancy. [online] Available from http://www.ncbi.nlm.nih.gov/books/NBK169024/pdf/TOC.pdf [Accessed December 2015].
7. Blumer I, Hadar E, Hadden DR, Jovanovič L, Mestman JH, Murad MH, et al. Diabetes and pregnancy: an endocrine society clinical practice guideline. J Clin Endocrinol Metab. 2013;98(11):4227-49.
8. Committee on Practice Bulletins—Obstetrics. Practice Bulletin No. 137: Gestational diabetes mellitus. Obstet Gynecol. 2013;122(2 Pt 1):406-16.
9. Seshiah V, Das AK, Balaji V, Joshi SR, Parikh MN, Gupta S, et al. Gestational diabetes mellitus—guidelines. J Assoc Physicians India. 2006;54:622-8.
10. Inturrisi M, Lintner NC, Sorem KA. Diagnosis and treatment of hyperglycemia in pregnancy. Endocrinol Metab Clin North Am. 2011;40(4):703-26.
11. Tutino GE, Tam WH, Yang X, Chan JC, Lao TT, Ma RC. Diabetes and pregnancy: perspectives from Asia. Diabet Med. 2014;31(3):302-18.
12. Ali S, Dornhorst A. Diabetes in pregnancy: health risks and management. Postgrad Med J. 2011;87(1028):417-27.
13. Guideline Development Group. Management of diabetes from preconception to the postnatal period: summary of NICE guidance. BMJ. 2008;336(7646):714-7.
14. Gillman MW, Rifas-Shiman S, Berkey CS, et al. Maternal gestational diabetes, birth weight, and adolescent obesity. Pediatrics. 2003;111(3):e221-6.
15. Ringholm L, Mathiesen ER, Kelstrup L, et al. Managing type 1 diabetes mellitus in pregnancy—from planning to breastfeeding. Nat Rev Endocrinol. 2012;8(11):659-67.
16. Pescosolido N, Campagna O, Barbato A. Diabetic retinopathy and pregnancy. Int Ophthalmol. 2014;34(4)989-97.
17. Kitzmiller JL, Block JM, Brown FM, Catalano PM, Conway DL, Coustan DR, et al. Managing preexisting diabetes for pregnancy: summary of evidence and consensus recommendations for care. Diabetes Care. 2008;31(5):1060-79.
18. Landon MB. Diabetic nephropathy and pregnancy. Clin Obstet Gynecol. 2007;50(4):998-1006.
19. Rossing K, Jacobsen P, Hommel E, Mathiesen E, Svenningsen A, Rossing P, et al. Pregnancy and progression of diabetic nephropathy. Diabetologia. 2002;45(1):36-41.
20. El-Deeb M, El-Menyar A, Gehani A, et al. Acute coronary syndrome in pregnant women. Expert Rev Cardiovasc Ther. 2011;9(4):505-15.
21. Bellamy L, Casas JP, Hingorani AD, et al. Type 2 diabetes mellitus after gestational diabetes: a systematic review and meta-analysis. Lancet. 2009;373(9677):1773-9.
22. HAPO Study Cooperative Research Group, Metzger BE, Lowe LP, Dyer AR, Trimble ER, Chaovarindr U, et al. Hyperglycemia and adverse pregnancy outcomes. N Engl J Med. 2008;358(19):1991-2002.
23. Ballas J, Moore TR, Ramos GA. Management of diabetes in pregnancy. Curr Diab Rep. 2012;12(1):33-42.
24. De Veciana M, Trail PA, Evans AT, et al. A comparison of oral acarbose and insulin in women with gestational diabetes mellitus. Am J Obstet Gynecol. 2002;99(Suppl 4):S5.
25. ACOG Committee Obstetric Practice. ACOG Committee opinion. Number 267, January 2002: exercise during pregnancy and the postpartum period. Obstet Gynecol. 2002;99(1):171-3.
26. Lambert K, Holt RI. The use of insulin analogues in pregnancy. Diabetes Obes Metab. 2013;15(10):888-900.
27. Mathiesen ER, Hod M, Ivanisevic M, Duran Garcia S, Brøndsted L, Jovanovic L, et al. Maternal efficacy and safety outcomes in a randomized, controlled trial comparing insulin detemir with NPH insulin in 310 pregnant women with type 1 diabetes. Diabetes Care. 2012;35(10):2012-7.
28. Holt RI, Lambert KD. The use of oral hypoglycaemic agents in pregnancy. Diabet Med. 2014;31(3):282-91.
29. Berggren EK, Boggess KA. Oral agents for the management of gestational diabetes. Clin Obstet Gynecol. 2013;56(4):827-36.
30. Kalra S, Kalra B, Gupta Y. Glycemic management after antenatal corticosteroid therapy. N Am J Med Sci. 2014;6(2):71-6.
31. Ryan EA, Al-Agha R. Glucose control during labor and delivery. Curr Diab Rep. 2014;14(1):450.

32. Shand AW, Bell JC, McElduff A, Morris J, Roberts CL. Outcomes of pregnancies in women with pre-gestational diabetes mellitus and gestational diabetes mellitus; a population-based study in New South Wales, Australia, 1998-2002. Diabet Med. 2008;25(6):708-15.
33. Maayan-Metzger A, Lubin D, Kuint J. Hypoglycemia rates in the first days of life among term infants born to diabetic mothers. Neonatology. 2009;96(2):80-5.
34. Stenninger E, Schollin J, Aman J. Early postnatal hypoglycaemia in newborn infants of diabetic mothers. Acta Paediatr. 1997;86(12):1374-6.
35. ACOG Committee on Practice Bulletins. ACOG Practice Bulletin. Clinical Management Guidelines for Obstetrician-Gynecologists. Number 60, March 2005. Pregestational diabetes mellitus. Obstet Gynecol. 2005;105(3):675-85.
36. Garber AJ, Moghissi ES, Bransome ED Jr, Clark NG, Clement S, Cobin RH, et al. American College of Endocrinology position statement on inpatient diabetes and metabolic control. Endocr Pract. 2004;10(Suppl 2):4-9.
37. Taylor R, Lee C, Kyne-Grzebalski D, et al. Clinical outcomes of pregnancy in women with type 1 diabetes(1). Obstet Gynecol. 2002;99(4):537-41.
38. Barrett HL, Morris J, McElDuff A. Watchful waiting: a management protocol for maternal glycaemia in the peripartum period. Aust N Z Obstet Gynaecol. 2009;49(2):162-7.
39. Carron Brown S, Kyne-Grzebalski D, Mwangi B, et al. Effect of management policy upon 120 Type 1 diabetic pregnancies: policy decisions in practice. Diabet Med. 1999;16(7):573-8.
40. Garrison EA, Jagasia S. Inpatient management of women with gestational and pregestational diabetes in pregnancy. Curr Diab Rep. 2014;14(2):457.
41. Castorino K, Jovanovič L. Pregnancy and diabetes management: advances and controversies. Clin Chem. 2011;57(2):221-30.
42. Ringholm L, Pedersen-Bjergaard U, Thorsteinsson B, Damm P, et al. Hypoglycaemia during pregnancy in women with Type 1 diabetes. Diabet Med. 2012;29(5):558-66.
43. de Veciana M. Diabetes ketoacidosis in pregnancy. Semin Perinatol. 2013;37(4):267-73.
44. Sibai BM, Viteri OA. Diabetic ketoacidosis in pregnancy. Obstet Gynecol. 2014;123(1):167-78.
45. Kalra B, Sridhar GR, Madhu K, Balhara YP, Sahay RK, Kalra S. Psychosocial management of diabetes in pregnancy. Indian J Endocrinol Metab. 2013;17(5):815-8.
46. Kalra B, Kalra S, Balhara YP. Psychological assessment and management in diabetes. J Pak Med Assoc. 2013;63(12):1555-7.

CHAPTER 53

Endocrinal Disorders: Thyroid and Parathyroid

Saswati S Choudhury

INTRODUCTION

Thyroid gland is a highly vascular organ situated in lower part of the neck and consists of two lobes, connected across the median plane by isthmus. It gets enlarged during pregnancy. Two thyroid hormones are secreted by this gland out of which triiodothyronine is the chief agent and 3-5 times more potent than thyroxine which is responsible for cellular metabolism. Thyroxine mainly serves as pro-hormone for T3 or triiodothyronine. Plasma iodide enters thyroid under the influence of thyroid stimulating hormone (TSH) of anterior pituitary which also induces proteolytic process causing release of thyroid hormones from thyroglobulin, latter being the colloid serving as storage for them.[1]

The parathyroid glands are small ovoid or lentiform structures which usually lie between the posterior borders of the lobes of thyroid gland and capsule. There are usually four, two on each sides and known as superior and inferior parathyroid depending on their positions. The superior one is more consistent in position but the inferior ones may lie in various positions and at times numbers may vary as well. The hormone secreted by it is known as parathormone (PTH) which is concerned with the metabolism of calcium and phosphorus in the body both being vital for pregnant mother and fetus. Because ionic calcium is essential for life, PTH is necessary for life. Parathyroid are composed of chief cells which are source of PTH and the oxyphil cells of unknown function which appears around puberty and increase in number with age.[2]

Pregnancy needs intricate and well balanced functions of all the endocrine glands of the body which is also applicable to thyroid and parathyroid glands to have an optimum outcome. Thyroid disease is usually manifested in reproductive age group and therefore it is one of the most common endocrinopathy affecting pregnant women.[3]

THYROID PHYSIOLOGY IN THIRD TRIMESTER OF PREGNANCY, FETUS, AND NEONATE

Pregnancy produces an overall increase in thyroid activity which allows a healthy individual to remain in a net euthyroid state. Increased level of estrogens in pregnancy causes rise in thyroxine binding globulin (TBG) synthesized by liver. It reaches a plateau at 24 weeks and remains same till two weeks postpartum.[1]

Total T_3 and T_4 remains high throughout pregnancy but free T_3 and freeT_4 level are high in first trimester only due to TSH like activity of human chorionic gonadotropin (hCG) which is peaks around ten weeks. There is an inverse relationship of TSH and hCG level in pregnancy and so TSH is low at first trimester with relatively high free T_4. More the level of hCG less is the level of TSH with high T_4.

Fetal TSH increases and reaches a height at 28th week and remains high till term. At term fetal thyroxine level is higher than maternal level with fetal thyroid hyperactivity. Triiodothyronine level rise but concentration is relatively low, resembling hypothyroid adult. Reversed T3 level which is an inactive form of thyroid hormone is higher and remains high for 3-5 days after delivery and reached normal after two weeks.[1]

Thyroid Function Tests

Thyroid dysfunctions cause maternal and fetal complications. Objective of thyroid function tests is to treat disease before significant complication arises. Wide arrays of tests are available for determination of thyroid function out of which the most reliable markers are levels of TSH, T3 and T4. Immunometric methods of TSH assays can detect as low as 0.02 mIU/L and fourth generation of TSH assays have a sensitivity of 0.001–0.002 mIU/L and mostly used for research purpose. Nonpregnant level of TSH varies from 0.04-4.5 mIU/L and normal level of TSH excludes any thyroid dysfunction. The normal changes in thyroid activity and association of pregnancy with conditions that can cause hyperthyroidism needs careful interpretation of thyroid function tests in pregnancy.[4]

Pregnancy produces overall increase in thyroid activity which allows a healthy individual to remain in euthyroid state. Following changes occur in pregnancy:

- 2–3-fold increase of thyroid binding globulin (TBG) concentration
- 30–100% increase in total T3 and T4 concentration
- Increase in serum thyroglobulin
- Increased renal iodide clearance
- Human chorionic gonadotropin has mild thyroid stimulating activity

In first trimester T3 and T4 is high in response to thyroid stimulating activity of hCG and after that they fall.[3]

Level of Thyroid Hormones in Pregnancy

According to the guidelines of American Thyroid Association for the diagnosis and management of thyroid diseases in pregnancy and puerperium 2011 the upper level of TSH in nonpregnant state is taken as 4 mIU/L and the upper level in pregnancy is taken as 2.5–3 mIU/L. The guideline also recommended that the range of TSH in the laboratory who does not have their own reference range should use their range of TSH which is 0.1–2.5 mIU/L in first trimester, 0.2–3 mIU/L in second trimester and 0.3–3 mIU/L in third trimester. Normal nonpregnant level of free T4 is 0.7–2 ng/dL, total T4 5–12 µg/dL. Serum free T3 is lower in concentration and assay is problematic. Total T3 is 65–170 ng/dL and free T3 is 0.2–0.5 ng/dL.[5]

High doses of glucocorticoides and dopaminergic drugs inhibit TSH release. High doses of propranolol, β-adrenergic antagonists and glucocorticoids decrease T3 concentration. Drugs like phenytoin carbamazepine and phenobarbitone lower T3 and T4. High dose of frusemide, salicylate, some nonsteroidal anti-inflammatory drugs (NSAIDs) may transiently rise free T3 and T4 concentration. Box 1 shows causes of high TSH.

Thyroid Antibodies

The major thyroid antigens are thyroglobulin (Tg), thyroid peroxidase (TPO) and thyrotropin receptor (TSHR) Pregnant women who have high serum anti-Tg antibody concentrations are more likely to have postpartum thyroiditis. The presence of a high serum anti-TPO antibody concentration in during first trimester of pregnancy may predict the occurrence of postpartum thyroiditis. Anti-TPO antibody concentration is high in women with postpartum thyroiditis. Measurement of anti-TPO antibody is a more sensitive test of thyroid autoimmunity than anti-Tg antibody. It should be the main diagnostic tool for identification of autoimmune origin of thyroid disease.[3,4]

Box 1: Causes of high thyroid stimulating hormone

- Hypothyroidism
- Recovery from severe illness
- Pituitary excess due to pituitary tumors causing secondary hyperthyroidism (very rare)

Thyrotropin Receptor Antibodies

- TSH binding inhibitory immunoglobulin (TBII)
- TSHR-Stimulating Antibody—TSHR-SAb
- TSHR-blocking antibody—TSHR-BAb

In pregnant women transplacental passage of TSHR-SAb or TSHR-BAb can result in transient fetal and neonatal thyrotoxicosis or hypothyroidism. Measurement of maternal serum TBII is helpful in assessing fetal or neonatal thyrotoxicosis in pregnant women with Grave's thyrotoxicosis, neonatal hypothyroidism in pregnant women with hypothyroidism and chronic autoimmune thyroiditis. This test should be done in third trimester. If TBII is high, serum TSHR-SAb and TSHR-BAb can be measured. The risk of neonatal thyrotoxicosis is very low unless maternal serum TBII and TSHR-SAb activity is very high. Among postpartum women with thyrotoxicosis, measurement of serum TSHR antibodies may help to distinguish between Graves thyrotoxicosis and postpartum thyroiditis as the cause.[4]

Other Antibodies

- Tg-TPO antibody
- Antibody to second colloid antigen CA2
- Gp330
- Anti-NIS antibody

Measurement of anti-TPO antibodies is more helpful. Anti-Tg is done only when suspicion is high and anti-TPO antibody is normal. TBII measurement is done to identify or exclude Grave's disease as a cause of thyrotoxicosis.

Hypothyroidism in Pregnancy

In overt hypothyroidism cases pregnancy is not very common as hypothyroidism is also responsible for anovulation. But subclinical hypothyroidism is often encountered in pregnancy nowadays. Clinical diagnosis of hypothyroidism is difficult as one third cases of hypothyroid may not have any symptoms and another third will have moderate symptoms and only the rest will have the classic symptoms. Signs and symptoms of hypothyroidism are enumerated in Box 2.

Diagnosis is based on elevated serum TSH with low free T4 index value. But high TSH with normal T4 means subclinical hypothyroidism.

Box 2: Signs and symptoms of hypothyroidism

Symptoms of hypothyroidism
- Fatigue
- Sleeplessness
- Lethargy
- Mental slowing
- Depression
- Cold intolerance
- Decreased perspiration
- Hair loss
- Dry skin
- Deeper voice or hoarseness
- Weight gain
- Constipation
- Arthralgias
- Muscle aching
- Stiffness
- Paresthesias
- History of menstrual irregularity

Signs of hypothyroidism
- General slowing of speech
- Dry and pale skin
- Sparse thin hair
- Bradycardia
- Myxedema
- Hyporeflexia
- Carpal tunnel syndrome
- Diffuse or nodular goiter
- Anemia

Fetus is totally dependent on maternal source of thyroid hormone in early developmental state and deficiency in early pregnancy is related to delayed psychomotor development and low IQ in infants born to hypothyroid mothers.

Main maternal complication is high risk of pre-eclampsia. There is also increase incidence of premature delivery with its related mortality and morbidity. The women who are hypothyroid at conception but become euthyroid with treatment have 15–30% risk of pre-eclampsia. The hypertension tends to be milder and develops later than that of hypothyroid group. Patients who are still hypothyroid after second trimester have 22–44% chance of developing preeclampsia and preterm delivery. Cause of hypertension is poorly understood. Probabilities are reduced cardiac output and increased peripheral resistance in hypothyroid patients. Elevated TSH and low T4 is associated with endothelin which is a potent vasoconstrictor and may also be responsible.[6,7]

Hypothyroid mothers also have a higher incidence of abruptio placentae and postpartum hemorrhage. Inadequately treated cases are prone to intrauterine fetal death and low birth weight babies. Thyroid hormone is essential for central nervous system (CNS) development of fetus. Deficiency in later half of pregnancy may affect axon and dendrite migration, synapse formation, glial cell proliferation and myelination. Term deliveries are seen in almost 95% cases in patients with adequate replacement therapy of thyroid hormones but only 20% cases with inadequate T4 replacement.[8] Postpartum thyroid dysfunction is known late sequelae and may develop many months after childbirth.

Management of Hypothyroidism in Pregnancy

Ideally women should be euthyroid before planning of pregnancy and treatment needs readjustment in pregnancy. Levothyroxine is the drug of choice. If the patient is a known hypothyroid before pregnancy dose of levothyroxine should be increased by 50% as soon as pregnancy is diagnosed and dose to be titrated to a low normal TSH concentration prior to conception. Several studies have shown that 50–70% women need an increase of T4 dose, an average of 50 µg daily during pregnancy.[9,10] TSH should be measured after 4–6 weeks and dose to be increased if necessary till it is stabilized. After delivery, dosage should be reduced to pre-pregnancy level and repeat TSH estimation is done after 4–8 weeks to look for adequacy of treatment. For patients diagnosed in pregnancy dosage is usually 2 µg/kg actual body weight and then adjusted according to TSH level every 4–6 weeks.

Hyperthyroidism in Pregnancy and Puerperium

Grave's disease is the most common cause of hyperthyroidism which occurs due to stimulation of the thyroid by thyrotropin receptor stimulating antibodies (TRAb). Incidence is about one in 2000 pregnancy. Other causes of hyperthyroidism are toxic multinodular goiter and toxic nodule, Iodine induced hyperthyroidism, TSH-induced hyperthyroidism.

Signs and symptoms of hyperthyroidism are enumerated in Box 3.

Diagnosis is confirmed by low serum TSH and high T4 level. The TSHR-Ab test is done in extrathyroid manifestation like orbitopathy, large goiter and long-standing disease treated with ablation and come with unexplained fetal tachycardia.

Pre-eclampsia, heart failure due to cardiac muscle dysfunction, fetal loss, premature labor, LBW are more likely to occur in untreated or poorly controlled thyrotoxic women than in those receiving adequate treatment.[11] Preterm delivery, perinatal mortality and maternal heart failure are common in patients who remains thyrotoxic in spite of the treatment or patients diagnosed during pregnancy. Risk of spontaneous abortion is higher with thyroid autoimmunity.

Other causes of hyperthyroidism in third trimester of pregnancy are toxic multinodular goiter, single toxic adenoma, subacute thyroiditis, iodide induced hyperthyroidism, struma ovarii, and thyrotropin receptor activation. If the disease is properly treated and monitored, complications related to hyperthyroidism is much less.

Box 3: Signs and symptoms of hyperthyroidism

Symptoms
- Weight loss
- Tremor
- Palpitations
- Heat intolerance
- Increased appetite
- Tiredness
- Altered bowel functions
- Mood changes
- Poor concentration
- Insomnia
- Emotional lability
- Hyperactive tendon reflex

Signs
- Resting tachycardia
- Atrial fibrillation
- Bone loss
- Lid lag
- Grave's orbitopathy
- Infiltrative dermopathy

Clinical neonatal hyperthyroidism can occur in 1% of babies born to mothers with Grave's Disease. TRAb of Grave's disease can cross the placenta and may stimulate fetal thyroid causing hyperthyroidism in fetus with signs of fetal tachycardia, IUGR and cardiac failure as well as fetal goiter. In uncontrolled hyperthyroidism of mother in late pregnancy fetal pituitary thyroid axis is suppressed due to high fetal level of maternal thyroxine which crosses placenta and along with transplacental transfer of antithyroid drugs this rarely can cause hypothyroidism in infants born to hyperthyroid mothers.

According to guidelines of American thyroid Association for the diagnosis and management of thyroid disorders in pregnancy and postpartum 2011 TSH level can be as low as 0.03 mIU/L but one should take medical history in detail and measure free T_4 level if TSH level is less than 0.1 mIU/L to rule out the disease.

There is no adverse pregnancy outcome in subclinical hyperthyroidism reported till date.[12].Hyperthyroidism before pregnancy may remit during pregnancy due to Th2 immune response but may revert back in postpartum period when Th1 immune response predominates again.

Management of Hyperthyroidism

The dose of antithyroid drugs should be kept to the minimum consistent with euthyroidism. Propylthiouracil (PTU) and methimazole is the treatment of choice in pregnancy. Radioiodine is contraindicated. Revision of doses needed during pregnancy and free T4 level should be at upper end of reference range. The initial dose of PTU is 200–400 mg and can be increased to 600 mg if required, and that of methimazole is 20–40 mg daily in two divided doses. Some improvement of symptoms occurs after one week but 4–6 weeks needed for full effect. After hyperthyroidism is controlled the dose gradually needs to be reduced by 25% every third or fourth week to settle at 50–100 mg twice daily.[13] PTU is usually given in first trimester to avoid teratogenic effect of methimazole like aplasia cutis. From second trimester onwards methimazole is preferred to avoid long term deleterious hepatic effect of PTU.

Maternal thyroid status is a reliable marker for dose titration and level of TSH should be lowest normal and level of T4 should be higher normal to avoid neonatal hypothyroidism. Drug should be continued in maintenance doses till labor to avoid relapse especially during labor and delivery including operative delivery and to avoid thyroid crisis. Propranolol may be used in indicated cases but prolong use sometimes causes fetal growth restriction, impaired response to hypoxic stress, postnatal bradycardia and hypoglycemia.

Previous successful treatment of hyperthyroidism does not guarantee full cure as relapse may occur during pregnancy and after delivery.

Fetal Monitoring in Hyperthyroidism

Serial ultrasonography (USG) is to be done to rule out growth restriction, tachycardia, heart failure goiter, hydrops and advanced bone age. If fetal hyperthyroidism is suspected maternal antithyroid drug adjustment is done. Incidence of fetal hyperthyroidism is 1–5% of mothers with Grave's disease.[14,15] In fetal hypothyroidism intra-amniotic thyroxine may be considered.[16]

Thyroid Storm and its Management

Thyroid storm is a hypermetabolic state and associated with adverse outcome. This is characterized by fever, tachycardia out of proportion to fever, restlessness, confusion seizure, vomiting, profuse sweating, diarrhea and cardiac arrhythmia. Labor, operative delivery infection may precipitate the attack. In untreated case shock stupor and coma may occur. Management consists of oxygen, antipyretics, intensive monitoring and antithyroids like propylthiouracil and methimazole along with Lugol's iodine.

Hyperthyroidism in Postpartum Period

Breast-feeding is not contraindicated in mothers who are on antithyroids as there are no reports of any adverse outcome on neonate and only limited quantity of PTU and methimazole are found in breast milk but mothers are advised to take the medicine just after a feed.[17] Monitoring of neonatal thyroid function is needed periodically. Periodical monitoring of thyroid hormones of the infant should also be considered.

There is a significant risk of exacerbation of the disease in the postpartum mothers and thyroid function tests should be done at 6 weeks and 12 weeks after delivery. In mothers whose TRAb concentration was high at thirty weeks of gestation neonatal TSH and T4 is checked after 6 hours of delivery and treatment should be started accordingly.[18] Neonates whose mothers are on antithyroid drugs till delivery should be tested several days after delivery as baby may remain euthyroid at birth due to circulating antithyroid drug from maternal side. This neonatal hyperthyroid state is usually self-limiting till the circulating maternal TRAb disappears by three months.[14]

Neonatal Thyroid Physiology

Newborns respond to the stress of birth by a surge of TSH within 30 minutes and come to baseline by 48–72 hours, with consequent rise of T_3 and T_4. Level of both thyroid hormones reaches to peak at 24–48 hours in response to TSH rise and rise of T3 is more pronounced. High reverse T3 level in pregnancy is continued in first 3–5 days after birth and comes to normal by two weeks.[1] Test for thyroid function is done usually 2–4 days after birth or within 7 days. Preterm infants have attenuated TSH surge. Screening of all infants should be performed between two and four days of birth. False positive TSH elevation may be found if the test is done at 24–48 hours after birth. If hypothyroidism diagnosed treatment should be started as soon as possible with levothyroxine. Incidence of neonatal hypothyroidism is 1 in 4000 live births.[1]

Postpartum Thyroiditis

Postpartum thyroiditis occurs in 5% of population with iodine deficiency within 2–6 months after delivery or abortion. This is characterized by a phase of hyperthyroidism followed by hypothyroidism usually with spontaneous resolution. But sometimes thyroid function tests are necessary to differentiate from Grave's disease. Detection of anti-TPO antibody in antenatal period predicts 30–50% chance of development of postpartum thyroiditis developing. Initial thyrotoxic state does not need any medication but hypothyroid state should be treated with levothyroxine for at least six months in symptomatic patients and then discontinue and TSH should be checked to determine requirement of further treatment.

THYROID NODULES AND THYROID CANCER IN THIRD TRIMESTER

Thyroid nodules being a disease of reproductive age group may be encountered in pregnancy. As majority of thyroid cancer developed in solitary thyroid nodules so malignancy may also be present. Toxic adenomas are found in 2% of pregnant women and some studies also show an association with pregnancy but they are not confirmatory. Radioiodine is contraindicated for diagnostic purpose as well as treatment in pregnancy and USG remains as the mainstay for diagnosis and fine needle aspiration biopsy in rapidly enlarging nodules or solid and big size nodules for confirmation of malignancy. Management in third trimester comprises of confirmation by aspiration biopsy and immediate surgery in confirmed malignancy unless they are few weeks from delivery. In low grade malignancy surgery may be deferred till delivery. If patient is treated with radioactive iodine in pre-pregnancy period conception should be delayed for one year after treatment with high dose radioactive iodine.[19]

Parathyroid Hormone

Parathormone is a polypeptide hormone with 84 amino acids.[20] The release of parathyroid gland is controlled by circulating levels of calcium ion. Low calcium ion level increases release of parathormone and high level of ionic calcium decreases its release. The actions of parathormone are mostly in kidneys, gut and bones. It is responsible for bone mineral metabolism, renal reabsorption of calcium and excretion of phosphates. It also causes enhanced magnesium reabsorption and inhibition of exchange of hydrogen ions for sodium ions by the tubules. It enhances intestinal uptake of calcium indirectly through its effect on vitamin D_3 metabolism. Another major role of PTH is to stimulate biosynthesis of 1,25-dihydroxyvitamin D_3 from vitamin D precursor by the kidney. It possibly increases mitosis rate of red-cell progenitors and thymic lymphocytes.

For calcium homeostasis all the claciotropic hormones (PTH, Calcitonin and Vitamin D_3) are necessary for integrated action. Decreased or increased production of PTH leads to hypocalcemic or hypercalcemic states because of its important role in production of 1,25-dihydroxyvitamin D_3. Parathyroid hormone changes in pregnancy are not very clear. Some study has shown decrease of PTH in first and second trimester and some studies conclude that there is no change of this hormone.[21]

In normal pregnancy there is profound change in calcium homeostasis due increase requirement of the growing fetus more so in later half of pregnancy and lactation. Hypocalcemia and hypovitaminosis D_3 is been linked in some studies with pre-eclampsia.[21,22]

Hypoparathyroidism

Hypocalcemia occurs due to hypofunction of parathyroid. Low calcium ion results into hyperphosphatemia probably due to partial deficiency or suppression of

1,25-dihydroxyvitamin D_3 level. Tetany and convulsions are most serious complication of hypoparathyroid state which in late pregnancy may be confused with eclampsia. Latent tetany may be detected by Chvostek's sign (tapping over facial nerves causing facial muscle contraction) or Trousseau's sign [carpal spasm by occluding arterial blood supply with blood pressure (BP) cuff].[2]

Hyperparathyroidism

Primary hyperparathyroidism leads to hypercalcemia and elevated Vitamin D_3 level. It may occur due to adenomas or hyperplasia of parathyroids. Primary hyperthyroidism is a disease of elderly but in 25% cases it may occur in child bearing age.[23] Secondary hyperparathyroidism occurs due to chronic renal failure. Primary hyperparathyroidism is also been associated with endothelial damage insulin resistance and cardiovascular disorders and these are similar to pre-eclampsia. Hypovitaminosis D may be a predisposing factor for primary hyperparathyroidism.[24,25] Main cause of primary hyperparathyroidism is parathyroid adenoma. A study by Hella Hultin et al. in 2009[21] has shown a statistically significant relationship of parathyroid tumors with pre-eclampsia. This study concluded that a history of parathyroid adenoma should be taken as risk of pre-eclampsia. In classical hyperparathyroidism other than typical bone manifestation and nephrolithiasis, hypertension is present in half of the cases.

Neonatal hypocalcemia occur in mothers with hyperparathyroidism presumably due to maternal hypercalcemia which suppresses fetal parathyroid function.[20]

CONCLUSION

Thyroid and parathyroid are being vital for human life; minor alteration in their function can cause various implications in pregnant mother fetus and neonates. Profound physiological changes of immune function and different metabolism in pregnancy may result in dysfunctions of both thyroid and parathyroid hormones. Timely intervention will prevent all fetal and maternal complication and hence the importance of early diagnosis in pregnancy if not before. Newer studies showing relationship of parathyroid hormones and vitamin D_3 with pre-eclampsia which is a still a disease of theories may unfold the path of knowing the pathophysiology of this killer disease of pregnant mothers.

REFERENCES

1. Speroff L, Fritz MA. Reproduction and thyroid. In: Clinical Gynaecologic Endocrinology and Infertility, 7th edition. Pliladelphia: Lippincott Williams and Wilkins; 2005. pp.805-21.
2. Hadley ME. Endocrinology. 5th edition. Pearson Education; 2004. pp.191-219.
3. Glinoer D, de Nayer P, Bourdoux P, Lemone M, Robyn C, van Steirteghem A, et al. Regulation of maternal thyroid function during pregnancy. J Clin Endocrinol Metab. 1990;71:276-87.
4. Toft AD, Beckett G. Measuring serum thyrotropin and thyroid hormone and assessing thyroid hormone transport. In: Braverman LE, Utiger RD (Eds). Werner and Ingbar's The Thyroid-a fundamental and clinical text, 9th edition. Pliladelphia: Lippincott Williams and Wilkins; 2005. pp. 329-44.
5. Green AS, Abalovich M, Alexander E, Azizi F, Mestman J, Negro R, et al. Guidelines of American thyroid association for the diagnosis and management of thyroid disease during pregnancy and postpartum. Thyroid. 2011;21(10):1081-125.
6. Montoro MN. Hypothyroidism in pregnancy. In: Mishell DR, Goodwin TM, Brenner PF (Eds). Management of common problems in obstetrics & Gynaecology, 4th edition. Blackwell publishing; 2002. pp.12-4.
7. Abalovich M, Amino N, Barbour LA, Cobin RH, De Groot LJ, Glinoer D, et al. Management of thyroid dysfunction during pregnancy and postpartum: Endocrine Society clinical practice guideline. J Clin Endocrine Metab. 2007;92(8 Suppl):S1-47.
8. Chan S, Rovet J. Thyroid hormones in fetal central nervous system development. Fet Met Med Rev. 2003;14:1-32.
9. Mandel SJ, Larsen PR, Seely Ew, Brent GA. Increased need of thyroxine during pregnancy in women with primary hypothyroidism. N Eng J Med. 1990;323:91-6.
10. Kaplan MM. Monitoring thyroxine treatment during pregnancy. Thyroid. 1992;2:147-52.
11. Millar LK, Wing DA, Leung AS, Koonings PP, Montoro MM, Metsmen JH. Low birth weight and preeclampsia in pregnancies complicated by hyperthyroidism. Obstet Gynecol. 1994;84:946-9.
12. Casey BM, Dashe JS, Wells CE, McIntire DD, Leveno KJ, Cunninghum FG. Subclinical hyperthyroidism and pregnancy outcomes. Obstet Gynecol. 2006;107:337-41.
13. Goodwin TM, Mestman JH. Thyroid disease in pregnancy: hyperthyroidism. In: Mishell DR, Goodwin TM, Brenner PF Management of common problems in obstetrics & Gynaecology, 4th edition. Blackwell publishing; 2002. pp.15-7.
14. Polak M, Le Gac I, Vulliard E, Guibourdenche J, Leger J, Toubert ME, et al. Fetal and neonatal thyroid function in relation to maternal Grave's Disease. Best Pract Res Clin Endocrinol Metab. 2004;18:289-302.
15. Weetman AP. Graves' Disease. N Eng J Med. 2000;343:1236-48.
16. Luton D, Le Gac I, Vuillard E, Castanet M, Guibourdenche J, Noel M, et al. Management of Grave's disease during pregnancy: the key role of fetal thyroid gland monitoring. J Clin Endocrinol Metab. 2005;90:6093-8.
17. Abalovich M, Guitierrez S, Alcaraz G, Maccallini G, Garcia A, Levalle O. Overt and subclinical hypothyroidism complicating Pregnancy. Thyroid. 2002;12:63-8.
18. Laurberg P, Nygaard B, Glinoer D, Grussendorf M Orgiazzi J. Guidelines for TSH-receptor antibody measurement in pregnancy: results of an evidenced-based symposium organized by the Europian association. Eur J Endocrinol. 1998;139:584-6.
19. Kenyon AP, Nelson-Piercy C. Thyroid disease. In: James, Steer, Weiner, Gonik, Crowther, Robson (Eds). High risk pregnancy—management options, 4th edition. Elsevier Saunders publication; 2011. pp.813-25.

20. Bringhurst ER, Demay M, Kronenberg HM. Hormones and disorders of mineral metabolism. In: Melmed, Polonsky, Larsen, Kronenberg (Eds). Williams textbook of Endocrinology, 12th edition. Elsevier publication; 2011. pp.1260-78.
21. Hultin H, Hellman P, Lundgren E, Olovsson M, Ekbom A, Rastad J, et al. Association of parathyroid adenoma and pregnancy with preeclampsia. J clin Endocrinol Metab. 2009;94(9):3394-9.
22. Bodnar LM, Catov JM, Klebanoff MA, Ness RB, Roberts JM. Prepregnancy BMI and occurrence of severe hypertensive disorders of pregnancy. Epidemiology. 2007;18:234-9.
23. Schnatz PF, Curry SI. Primary hyperparathyroidism in pregnancy: evidence based management. Obstet Gynecol surv. 2002; 57:365-76.
24. Hagstrom E, Lundgren E, Rastad J Hellman P. Metabolic abnormalities in patient with normocalcemic hyperparathyroidism detected at population based screening. Eur J Endocrinol. 2006;155:33-9.
25. Nilsson IL, Aberg J, Rastad J, Lind L. Endothelial vasodilatory dysfunction in primary hypoparathyroidism is reversed after parathyroidectomy. Surgery. 1999;126:1049-55.

CHAPTER 54

Endocrinal Disorders: Pituitary and Adrenals

Suvarna S Khadilkar, Akanksha Sood

INTRODUCTION

Endocrinology disorders in pregnancy can have significant impact on pregnancy outcome, especially in third trimester. Diabetes is the most common endocrine disorder encountered during pregnancy followed by hypothyroidism and hyperthyroidism. Disorders of pituitary and adrenals, though rare, are important to be aware of due to potential for significant maternal and fetal morbidity or mortality, if not diagnosed and managed appropriately.[1]

PITUITARY

To optimize the pregnancy outcomes, it is essential for us to understand changes in the physiology of the gland with pregnancy. The anterior lobe of pituitary is almost doubled in size. The serum prolactin levels are increased to 10-fold with peak in late gestation and postpartum. Increase in estrogen and progesterone during pregnancy gives a negative feedback effect on anterior pituitary resulting in decreased levels of gonadotropins. Pituitary growth hormone is decreased and there is a progressive increase in the placental growth hormone. Adrenocorticotropic hormone (ACTH) levels increase throughout pregnancy, but absolute levels are less than nonpregnant. Thyrotropin levels are unaffected. Free T3 and T4 are unchanged, but due to increase in thyroxine-binding globulin (TBG), total T3 and T4 are increased.

Posterior pituitary hormone oxytocin is increased. Vasopressin levels remain unchanged, but plasma osmolarity is decreased so there is decreased threshold for secretion.

PITUITARY DISORDERS

Prolactinomas

Prolactins secreting pituitary tumors are a known cause of amenorrhea and an ovulation leading to infertility. With effective medical treatment with dopamine agonists and ovulation induction, we see many cases of pregnancy with prolactinomas. Rarely, they may be diagnosed first time in pregnancy.

During pregnancy due to increased estrogen there is hyperplasia of anterior pituitary lactotrophs, leading to enlargement of adenoma. Prolactinoma more than 10 mm in size is known as macroprolactinoma and less than 10 mm in size is known as microprolactinoma. Pregnant women with microprolactinomas usually tolerate pregnancy well. Those with macroprolactinomas more often have symptomatic enlargement, hence require vigilance.

Ideally the patient with prolactinoma should be thoroughly evaluated pre-pregnancy. This includes serum prolactin levels and radiology, magnetic resonance imaging (MRI) preferred. Pre-pregnancy, those with microadenoma should be started on dopamine agonist and macroadenoma should preferably be treated with surgery.

During pregnancy, patient should be under the care of a multidisciplinary team including obstetrician, endocrinologist and ophthalmologist.

For asymptomatic microadenoma, there is less than 5% chance of sudden symptomatic enlargement. Medication can be safely stopped for these patients. They should be educated for self-referral in case of any warning signs, like headache or visual disturbance. If any symptoms suggestive of enlargement are seen, it warrants urgent MRI. Headache is caused due to pressure over the dura and visual disturbance due to compression of optic nerve both as a consequence of tumor enlargement.

For asymptomatic macroadenomas, risk of symptomatic exacerbation is 30–35%. Regarding continuation of medical treatment with bromocriptine, the decision must be individualized. These patients must be evaluated every 3 months with visual testing.[2] Those with symptomatic macroadenoma should be evaluated monthly. Cabergoline is used in refractory cases. Bromocriptine or cabergoline have not been found to be teratogenic; however, long-term use of both has been associated with a small increased risk of mother developing heart valve fibrosis. Echocardiogram should be considered in women who have significant murmur.

Serum prolactin levels are not useful to monitor the disease activity, but if markedly increased outside the normal pregnancy range may suggest tumor enlargement. Ericsson et al. in 2013 suggested that screening or monitoring for exacerbation is best undertaken by vigilance of clinical features and prompt testing.[2,3]

Treatment of complications during pregnancy is influenced by gestational age and the severity of signs and symptoms. Medical treatment with bromocriptine or cabergoline is successful in most cases and is preferred.[4] Recent data indicate that cabergoline is safe for the developing fetus and for the mother.[4] Once the fetus is mature, induction of labor or cesarean section can be considered. Only in refractory cases, trans-sphenoid surgery is undertaken.[5] The complications of surgery include infection, hemorrhage, hypopituitarism leading to pituitary insufficiency and transient diabetes insipidus. After surgery the risk of preterm delivery is also increased.

Intrapartum care is essentially the same as other labouring women. Magnetic resonance imaging and serum prolactin should be done during the first postnatal visit though serum prolactin may be elevated, if the patient is lactating. These women, even if on treatment, should be encouraged to breastfeed. Although, lactation may be little suppressed. The patient must be referred to endocrinologist for discussion regarding further or definitive treatment, if required. She should still be asked to report, if headache or visual disturbance and asked to follow-up again after 6–8 weeks.

In a review of 73 patients with prolactinoma in pregnancy, Domingue ME et al. found that more than 40% of women with previous diagnosis of prolactinoma have normal prolactin level without medical treatment for a median follow-up of 22 months after pregnancy and lactation. The likelihood of remission is associated with a smaller initial adenoma size and normalization of pituitary MRI after pregnancy.[6]

Acromegaly

Acidophilic pituitary adenoma with increase in growth hormone (GH) production leads to acromegaly. Up to 40% also have hyperprolactinemia. These patients are mostly amenorrheic and pregnancy is occasional. During pregnancy there is increased risk of comorbidities, such as hypertension, insulin resistance and cardiomyopathy and also of tumor enlargement leading to visual field defects and hemorrhage. Medical treatment with somatostatin analog, octreotide has been successfully used in these patients during pregnancy. Ideally a definitive treatment in the form of radiotherapy or surgery should be done pre-pregnancy but if left untreated, 10% would require hypophysectomy during pregnancy. Overall, pregnancy in acromegaly is uneventful and newborns are unaffected. Dopamine agonists and somatostatin analogs have not been associated with major adverse effects to the fetus; however, more data are needed to validate their safety.[7]

Dias et al. (2013) in a prospective study of 10 pregnancies with acromegaly concluded that acromegaly control usually improved and tumor growth was not stimulated during pregnancy in spite of withdrawal of drug treatment. Drug treatment can be discontinued in most patients. Uncontrolled disease before pregnancy may pose a higher risk for diabetes and hypertension.[8]

Diabetes Insipidus

Diabetes insipidus is due to decreased vasopressin secretion from posterior pituitary. It usually follows pituitary surgery or autoimmune destruction. It is characterized by massive polyuria and with specific gravity of urine less than 1.005. Diagnosis is usually by water deprivation test, but this is not performed in pregnancy as dehydration is poorly tolerated by pregnant women. Most cases show deterioration in pregnancy due to increase in glomerular filtration rate (GFR) and vasopressinase enzyme secreted by placenta.

Due to vasopressinase, in some patients, transient diabetes insipidus of pregnancy can also occur. It is usually seen in the third trimester. It is also seen in association with HELLP syndrome, acute fatty liver of pregnancy and twin gestation. Postpartum, it can accompany Sheehan's syndrome.

Patients are managed with synthetic vasopressin 0.1–0.25 mg twice daily intranasal. Its use is safe in pregnancy and lactation. Although its structure is similar to oxytocin and it can potentially stimulate uterine contractions, there is no risk of increased preterm labor in those using intranasal DDAVP (desmopressin: 1-deamino-8-D-arginine vasopressin). DDAVP 4 µg/mL, it is a synthetic analog of the natural pituitary hormone 8-arginine vasopressin, an antidiuretic hormone (ADH) affecting renal water conservation. Intravenous doses of 0.1–0.4 µg/kg body weight, infused over a 10-minute period. One mL (4 µg) of DDAVP solution has an antidiuretic activity of about 16 IU; 1 μg of DDAVP is equivalent to 4 IU. When administered by injection, DDAVP has an antidiuretic effect about 10 times that of an equivalent dose administered intranasally. It is prudent to monitor plasma electrolytes, fluid status and specific gravity of urine to ensure optimal treatment.

Pituitary Insufficiency (Sheehan's Syndrome)

Pituitary insufficiency is usually seen in cases of autoimmune lymphocytic infiltration, pituitary apoplexy (Sheehan's syndrome), tumor and surgery. Massive postpartum hemorrhage (PPH) leading to hypoperfusion of hyperplastic pituitary and ischemic necrosis is the pathology behind Sheehan's syndrome. There is no correlation between the amount of PPH (blood lost) and the occurrence of Sheehan's syndrome.

It may present in postpartum period with failure to lactate, but in many cases it has insidious course over months to years. There is an average delay of 7 years from the onset to diagnosis. Most signs of Sheehan's syndrome are aspecific and classical signs, such as agalactia and amenorrhea are often difficult to detect, which can explain the long diagnostic delay.[9] Late onset disease may present with loss of pubic hair, oligomenorrhea, senile vaginal atrophy, hypothyroidism, etc. These women are usually infertile, but may conceive spontaneously.

For diagnosis during pregnancy, gonadotropin measurement has no value. Normal thyroid stimulating hormone (TSH) with low thyroxine suggests secondary hypothyroidism. Also, cortisol levels are low and do not increase in response to stress.

During pregnancy these patients require supplementation of thyroxine 100–200 μg/day and steroids; prednisolone 5 mg in the morning and 2.5 mg in the evening. Mineralocorticoid replacement is usually not required. Postpartum dosages need to be readjusted. Table 1 summarizes various disorders of pituitary in third trimester of pregnancy and puerperium.

TABLE 1: Summary of common disorders of pituitary in third trimester and puerperium

Hyperpituitarism	Hypopituitarism
• Prolactinoma m/c ○ Asymptomatic ○ Headache ○ Visual disturbances ○ Medical Rx may cause suppression of lactation	• Diabetes insipidus ○ Polyuria ○ Should be differentiated from psychogenic cause and GDM/DM
• Acromegaly ○ Hormonal–acromegaly phenotype ○ Enlargement: headache and visual disturbances	• Panhypopituitarism ○ Classical: agalactia, amenorrhea (postnatal) ○ Delayed: senile vaginal atrophy, loss of pubic hair, hypothyroidism, etc.

DM, diabetes mellitus; GDM, gestational diabetes mellitus.

ADRENAL

During pregnancy there is 2–3-fold increase in cortisol levels contributed by increase in free cortisol and also cortisol binding globulin due to hyperestrogenic state. ACTH levels are increased, but are less than nonpregnant state. During labor there is a surge of both ACTH and cortisol. ACTH does not cross placenta, it is produced by placenta as corticotropin-releasing hormone (CRH). Dehydroepiandrosterone (DHEA) production is increased in normal pregnancy which is aromatized to estradiol and estrone by the placenta.

Cushing's Syndrome

This is a state of adrenal excess and can be ACTH dependent or independent. In cases of primary pituitary disease (Cushing's disease) with adrenal hyperplasia there is increase in androgen production from adrenals which inhibit pituitary gonadotropin leading to amenorrhea and infertility. In adrenal adenomas there is overproduction of cortisol only and these are less likely to impair fertility. Therefore, primary adrenal disease, i.e., adrenal adenomas are more commonly encountered during pregnancy. Other causes of Cushing's syndrome can be neoplastic ectopic ACTH secretion or even excessive exogenous corticosteroids.

Clinically, many clinical features of Cushing's syndrome mimic signs and symptoms of normal pregnancy, like weakness, weight gain, edema, striae, hypertension and impaired glucose tolerance test (GTT).[10] The distinguishing features of Cushing's syndrome would be early onset hypertension, easy bruising and features of proximal myopathy. Clinical picture of Cushing's syndrome may be thus exacerbated by pregnancy and relieved postdelivery. Obstetric complications include increased rate of preterm birth (43%), increased stillbirth rate (6%), hypertension, pre-eclampsia and intrauterine growth restriction (IUGR). Many of these including unexplained stillbirth are attributable to hyperglycemia.

Preferred screening test in a suspected case is 24 hours urine free cortisol measurement. Serum cortisol levels are raised. Pregnancy specific range for plasma and urine cortisol should be used. Carr et al.[11] has given a reference range for pregnancy. 14.9 ± 4 mg/dL at 11 weeks' gestation and 35.2 ± 0 mg/dL at 26 weeks' gestation; the levels remained elevated until labor and delivery. Further diagnostic tests which may be useful include ACTH levels, high dose dexamethasone suppression test, ultrasonography (USG) and MRI of adrenals and MRI of pituitary.

Treatment significantly improves prognosis and live birth rate. First step is to identify the source of hormone and then institute proper therapy. Outside of pregnancy surgery is the treatment of choice. In pregnancy surgery is ideally performed in second trimester. Pricolo et al.[12] showed a comparison of the pregnancy outcome in patients with Cushing's syndrome based on the timing of surgical intervention in relation to pregnancy. In the study, a group of seven patients who were operated with unilateral adrenalectomy during pregnancy were compared with a group of 19 patients in whom adrenalectomy was done after delivery. Of the seven in the first group, one fetal death and no neonatal complications occurred, but fetal death and neonatal complications occurred in 12 of the 19 pregnancies in the second group. Bevan et al.[13] reported that surgical treatment during pregnancy is safe and significantly reduces fetal loss, premature labor and maternal morbidity. Before surgery a thorough evaluation should be done with MRI to rule out carcinoma. In third trimester, delivery should be expedited and definitive treatment given postpartum. Metyrapone (which blocks cortisol synthesis by blocking 11β-hydroxylase) is the most widely used medical therapy in pregnancy, although it can exacerbate hypertension and pre-eclampsia. Ketoconazole and mitotane are teratogenic and aminoglutethimide is associated with fetal masculinization, hence avoided in pregnancy.

Congenital Adrenal Hyperplasia

Congenital adrenal hyperplasias (CAH) are a group of heritable disorders associated with an inability or deficiency in the ability to produce cortisol. In affected individuals, the disease begins early in gestation and leads to disease that is manifested at birth. Without cortisol, there is a failure of negative feedback and excessive secretion of CRH from the hypothalamus and ACTH from the anterior pituitary. Continued secretion of ACTH causes stimulation of the adrenal cortex, leading to hyperplasia.

Although low fertility rates have traditionally been reported among women with classic CAH and especially among women with the salt-wasting variant, fertility rates are significantly improved. The various reasons are earlier treatment of CAH, improved results of medical and surgical therapy, more available choices for ovulation induction and assisted reproductive techniques. Once pregnant, these women have a high probability of successful outcome. Key issues should be emphasized in the management of CAH during gestation, including the need for assessing adrenal steroid replacement and adrenal androgen suppression, particularly in light of the interplay between maternal hyperandrogenism and the protective effect of placental aromatase activity, which provides a relatively large margin of safety for the female fetus. Maternal hormone levels should be evaluated in the context of laboratory-specific reference ranges for pregnancy. This disorder is seen as a simple autosomal recessive trait.

Prenatal treatment of the mother with glucocorticoids can prevent or reduce that the virilizing effects of fetal 21-hydroxylase deficiency.[14] This procedure has been used in cases where couples have previously had a child with virilizing CAH. In such cases, it is known that both parents are carriers, and since only female children require prenatal treatment, the probability that the current fetus is affected is 1 in 8. Treatment of the mother with glucocorticoids must begin at 6–7 weeks of gestation, at which time it is almost never known whether the fetus is affected. Hence, in seven of eight cases, the fetus does not actually require therapy. The long-term effect and safety of this procedure is poorly defined.

The baby should be examined for ambiguous genitalia and monitored for evidence of adrenal insufficiency. Although an affected female infant with classic CAH has not been reported as a pregnancy outcome of a mother with classic virilizing CAH, these concerns should be discussed during preconception counseling. Patients should also be aware of the importance of medication compliance and careful hormonal monitoring during the entire pregnancy. In most cases, successful gestational management requires the close coordination of care between the obstetrician and endocrinologist.

Conn's Syndrome

Primary aldosteronism is extremely rare in pregnancy presenting with hypertension and hypokalemia. Causes include adrenal aldosterone secreting adenoma, adrenal carcinoma or bilateral adrenal hyperplasia. Hypertension in presence of hypokalemia should warrant ultrasound imaging of adrenals. Due to hypertension there is increased risk of abruption, preterm delivery and stillbirth. Increased progesterone during pregnancy masks the action of aldosterone leading to amelioration of hypertension. So, in some cases, hypertension may only develop postpartum. Patient usually requires two or three antihypertensives for the control of blood pressure. Also, potassium sparing diuretics should be used to overcome hypokalemia. Spironolactone, however, should be avoided during pregnancy due to antiandrogenic effect leading to feminization of male fetus. Krysiak et al. described a case of primary aldosteronism secondary to bilateral adrenal hyperplasia in three subsequent pregnancies. They concluded that each case of treatment-resistant hypertension in pregnancy requires assessment for the presence of primary aldosteronism, and that amiloride seems to be a safe and effective agent in the nonsurgical treatment of this disorder in pregnant women with primary aldosteronism.[15] Open/laparoscopic adrenalectomy may be required in refractory cases.

Addison's Disease (Primary Adrenal Insufficiency)

Addison's disease is primarily caused by autoimmune destruction. It can also be secondary to granulomatous diseases as a sequelae of tuberculosis, fungal infection or AIDS and post-bilateral adrenalectomy. The symptoms of mineralocorticoid and glucocorticoid deficiency are mostly nonspecific including fatigue, weakness, anorexia, nausea, vomiting and nonspecific abdominal pain. These symptoms, if present with increased skin pigmentation (due to increased ACTH stimulation of melanocytes) should raise suspicion of Addison's disease. Investigations would reveal decreased cortisol levels coupled with increased ACTH levels. On ACTH stimulation there is no increase in cortisol levels.

Replacement therapy with prednisolone (5 mg in the morning and 2.5 mg in the evening) and fludrocortisone (0.05–0.1 mg daily) is necessary during pregnancy. Increased doses of corticosteroids should be considered in any stressful events like hyperemesis, infection and during labor. Vigilance should be kept for any signs of electrolyte imbalance and fluid overload like edema and excessive weight gain. It is crucial that a pregnant woman with primary adrenal insufficiency (PAI) and her partner are well educated regarding the adjustment of glucocorticoid dose in intercurrent illness and that both are trained in hydrocortisone emergency injection techniques.[14] Although, adrenal antibodies cross placenta, neonatal adrenal insufficiency is rarely encountered.

Acute adrenal crisis presents with nausea, vomiting and profound epigastric pain accompanied by hypothermia and hypoperfusion. In this emergent situation, patient must be given steroids and fluid replacement under critical care setting. Lebbe et al. (2013)[16] concluded that with the appropriate replacement therapy, these patients can expect to have an uneventful pregnancy and deliver a healthy infant.

Adrenal Medulla

Pheochromocytoma

Pheochromocytoma is a tumor of chromaffin cells of adrenal medulla and leads to excessive secretion of catecholamines. In a study by Harper et al. in 1980–87, 47 cases of pheochromocytoma with pregnancy were studied and reported that maternal and fetal mortality rate were 17% and 26%, respectively. Ahlawat et al.[17] in 1999, reported significant reduction in maternal and fetal mortalities rate 4% and 11%, respectively.

These are rare in pregnancy and diagnosis is often overlooked or confused with pre-eclampsia. Suspicion is raised in cases with postural hypotension with paroxysmal or labile hypertension associated with headache, perspiration, palpitation and tachycardia. Although hypertension is hallmark of pheochromocytoma, it may not be present in all the cases. Other typical presentations include arrhythmias, abdominal pain, visual disturbances, convulsions and sudden collapse.

Apart from clinical features, laboratory diagnosis with 24 hours urine collection for catecholamines and their metabolites is used for confirmation. MRI and sonography are the imaging modalities of choice for tumor localization in pregnancy, to avoid radiation exposure.

Phenoxybenzamine (α-adrenergic blocker) is safe in pregnancy and can be used in inoperable cases. It can also be given preoperatively and after surgical removal of the tumor. It should be initiated with relatively low doses 5–10 mg orally 3 times a day and increased every few weeks titrating with the symptoms. Propranolol (β-blocker) 10 mg 3–4 times a day can be added after starting α–blockers and can be increased, if tachycardia persists. Beta blockers induce a paradoxical increase in blood pressure in absence of α-blockade, so they should be administered only after effective α-blockage. Mode of delivery in these patients is a matter of debate. A study done by Schenker and Granat showed, higher maternal mortality rates with vaginal delivery (31%) than with cesarean delivery (19%). Kapoor et al. in 2013 concluded that selected multigravidae cases and those with previous history of short uncomplicated labor, may be considered for vaginal delivery under epidural analgesia and with backup facilities available to manage hypertensive crisis.[18]

Surgical removal of the tumor is the definitive management and should ideally be done prepregnancy and in pregnancy during the second trimester. Some studies have reported optimal fetal outcome, if surgery is deferred till fetal maturity. Higher maternal mortality rates have been associated with vaginal delivery as compared to cesarean section.

Table 2 summarizes common disorders of adrenal gland in third trimester and puerperium

TABLE 2: Summary of common disorders of adrenal gland in third trimester and puerperium

Hyperadrenalism	Hypoadrenalism

Adrenal cortex
• Adrenal adenoma
• Adrenal hyperplasia
• Adrenal carcinoma (only few cases reported in pregnancy)
  ○ Cushing's syndrome
    – Distinguishing from pregnancy: Early onset hypertension, easy bruising and features of proximal myopathy
    – Mimicking pregnancy: Weight gain, edema, striae, hypertension and impaired GTT
  ○ Adrenal hyperplasia
    – Congenital adrenal hyperplasia
  ○ Conn's syndrome
Adrenal medulla
• Pheochromocytoma
	Addison's disease
	• Fatigue
	• Weakness
	• Anorexia
	• Nausea and vomiting
	• Nonspecific abdominal pain
	• Increased skin pigmentation

REFERENCES

1. Laway BA, Mir SA. Pregnancy and pituitary disorders: challenges in diagnosis and management. Indian J Endocrinol Metab. 2013;17(6):996-1004.
2. Ericsson C, Lindblom B. [Risk of prolactinoma growth during pregnancy. Visual field tests required in macroadenoma, small risk in microadenomas]. Lakartidningen. 2012;109(25):1226-8.
3. Witek P, Zieli ski G. Management of prolactinomas during pregnancy. Minerva Endocrinol. 2013;38(4):351-63.
4. Bajwa SK, Bajwa SJ, Mohan P, Singh A. Management of prolactinoma with cabergoline treatment in a pregnant woman during her entire pregnancy. Indian J Endocrinol Metab. 2011;15(Suppl3):S267-70.
5. Maiter D, Primeau V. 2012 update in the treatment of prolactinomas. Ann Endocrinol (Paris). 2012;73(2):90-8.
6. Domingue ME, Devuyst F, Alexopoulou O, Corvilain B, Maiter D. Outcome of prolactinoma after pregnancy and lactation: a study on 73 patients. Clin Endocrinol (Oxf). 2014;80(5):642-8.
7. Cheng V, Faiman C, Kennedy L, Khoury F, Hatipoglu B, Weil R, et al. Pregnancy and acromegaly: a review. Pituitary. 2012;15(1):59-63.
8. Dias M, Boguszewski C, Gadelha M, Kasuki L, Musolino N, Vieira JG, et al. Acromegaly and pregnancy: a prospective study. Eur J Endocrinol. 2013;170(2):301-10.
9. Ramiandrasoa C, Castinetti F, Raingeard I, Fenichel P, Chabre O, Brue T, et al. Delayed diagnosis of Sheehan›s syndrome in a developed country: a retrospective cohort study. Eur J Endocrinol. 2013;169(4):431-8.
10. Garla V, Kheetan R, Saleem T. Cushing›s syndrome in pregnancy: a diagnostic conundrum. W V Med J. 2013;109(6):34-6.
11. Carr BR, Parker CR, Madden JD, MacDonald PC, Porter JC. Maternal plasma adrenocorticotropin and cortisol relationships throughout human pregnancy. Am J Obstet Gynecol. 1981;139(4):416-22.
12. Pricolo VE, Monchik JM, Prinz RA, DeJong S, Chadwick DA, Lamberton RP. Management of Cushing›s syndrome secondary to adrenal adenoma during pregnancy. Surgery. 1990;108(6):1072-78.
13. Bevan JS, Gough MH, Gillmer MD, Burke CW. Cushing›s syndrome in pregnancy: the timing of definitive treatment. Clin Endocrinol (Oxf). 1987;27(2):225-33.
14. Ritzen EM. Prenatal dexamethasone treatment of fetuses at risk for congenital adrenal hyperplasia: benefits and concerns. Seminars Neonatology. 2001;6:357-62.
15. Krysiak R, Samborek M, Stojko R. Primary aldosteronism in pregnancy. Acta Clin Belg. 2012;67(2):130-4.
16. Lebbe M, Arlt W. What is the best diagnostic and therapeutic management strategy for an Addison patient during pregnancy? Clin Endocrinol (Oxf). 2013;78(4):497-502.
17. Ahlawat SK, Jain S, Kumari S, Varma S, Sharma BK. Pheochromocytoma associated with pregnancy: case report and review of the literature. Obstet Gynecol Surv. 1999;54(11):728-37.
18. Kapoor G, Salhan S, Sarda N, Sarda AK, Aggarwal D. Phaeochromocytoma in pregnancy: safe vaginal delivery, is it possible? J Indian Med Assoc. 2013;111(4):266-7.

CHAPTER 55

Hematological Complications

Veerendrakumar CM, Joshi Suyajna D

INTRODUCTION

Normal pregnancy is characterized by significant changes in almost every organ and system to support the demands of fetus without compromising maternal well-being. In normal pregnancy, the physiological change in hemoglobin (Hb) concentration and platelet count during pregnancy are well known phenomena.[1] Significant changes in hematological and coagulation system will make the women more prone for certain complications during pregnancy, delivery and puerperium. During pregnancy the plasma volume increases by 50% and the red blood cell (RBC) volume increases only by 20–30%.[2] Increases in blood volume are mainly to cater to the demands of the fetoplacental circulation and to compensate for blood loss during parturition. Increase in blood volume is more pronounced in multifetal gestations and in iron deficient states. Leukocytosis, occurring during pregnancy is due to the physiologic stress induced by the pregnant state.[3] There is an absolute monocytosis during pregnancy, especially in the first trimester. Monocytes help in preventing fetal allograft rejection by infiltrating the decidual tissue.[4] Platelet counts decrease during pregnancy, particularly in the last trimester known as "gestational thrombocytopenia" which is due to hemodilution and may also be related to increased platelet activation and accelerated clearance. It is evident in 8% of the cases[5] and do not have significant effect on mother and fetus. It has hence been recommended that the lower limit of platelet count in late pregnancy should be considered as 1.15 lac/cumm.[6] Pregnancy-associated changes in the coagulation and fibrinolytic pathways favor thrombus formation. Fibrinogen and clotting factors VII, VIII, X, XII, von Willebrand factor (vWF) and ristocetin cofactor activity increase remarkably as gestation progresses. In pregnancy, partial thromboplastin time (aPTT) is usually shortened, by up to 4 seconds in the 3rd trimester, largely due to hormonally influenced increase in factor VIII. No marked changes in prothrombin time or thrombin time occured.[6] In contrast antithrombin III and protein C levels are either unchanged or increased and protein S levels are generally seen to decrease in pregnancy.[7] Acquired-activated protein C (APC) resistance has been found to occur in pregnancy, even when factor V Leiden and antiphospholipid antibodies are not present. This has been attributed to the high factor VIII and factor V activity and low free protein S levels. Hence, APC sensitivity ratio does not serve as a screening test for factor V Leiden during pregnancy.[8] Hypercoagulable state helps to decrease blood loss at delivery and at the same time puts the mother at risk of thromboembolic events during pregnancy and puerperium. This chapter gives overview about the hematological complications of pregnancy and puerperium and hence exhaustive coverage of all the complications is beyond its scope. Only important complications are considered.

ANEMIA IN PREGNANCY

Iron Deficiency Anemia

Iron deficiency anemia (IDA) remains the most common medical disorder in pregnancy in the developing world.[9] Fifty-one percent of the pregnant women are anemic and of all the anemias of the pregnancy 75% are due to iron deficiency.[10] Fall of Hb is a very late manifestation of iron deficiency and takes about 2.5 years to develop. Causes for depleted iron stores are poor nutritional status, recurrent infection, excessive menstrual loss and short birth interval. Anemia in pregnancy is a condition with effects that may be deleterious to mothers and fetus. Indeed, it is a known risk factor for many maternal and fetal complications.

Factors Responsible for High Prevalence of Anemia

Studies carried out in India have shown that iron deficiency is the major cause of anemia followed by folate deficiency.[11] In India, the prevalence of anemia is high because of:

- Low dietary intake, poor iron (<20 mg/day) and folic acid intake (<70 mg/day)
- Poor bioavailability of iron (3–4% only) in phytate and fiber-rich Indian diet
- Chronic blood loss due to infection such as malaria and hookworm infestations[12,13]
- Anemia gets aggravated by increased requirements during adolescence and during pregnancy.[14]

Maternal Consequences of Anemia

Mild Anemia

Women with mild anemia in pregnancy have decreased work capacity. Women with chronic mild anemia may go through pregnancy and labor without any adverse consequences, because they are well compensated.

Moderate Anemia

Women with moderate anemia have substantial reduction in work capacity. They are more susceptible to infections and recovery from infections may be prolonged. Premature births are more common in women with moderate anemia. Substantial proportion of maternal deaths due to antepartum and postpartum hemorrhage, pregnancy-induced hypertension and sepsis occur in women with moderate anemia.

Severe Anemia

Three distinct stages of severe anemia have been recognized: compensated, decompensated and that associated with circulatory failure. The cardiac output is raised even at rest, the stroke volume is larger and the heart rate is increased. Palpitation and breathlessness even at rest are symptoms of these changes. Maternal mortality rates show a steep increase when maternal Hb levels fall below 5.0 g/dL. Anemia directly causes 20% of maternal deaths in India and indirectly accounts for another 20% of maternal deaths.[15]

Fetal Consequences of Anemia

Most of the studies suggested that a fall in maternal Hb below 11.0 g/dL is associated with a significant rise in perinatal mortality rate.[16-18] There is usually a 2-3-fold increase in perinatal mortality rate when maternal Hb level fall below 8.0 g/dL and 8-10-fold increase when maternal Hb level fall below 5.0 g/dL.[19,20] A significant fall in birth weight due to increase in prematurity rate and intrauterine growth retardation has been reported when maternal Hb levels were below 8.0 g/dL.[19,20]

MANAGEMENT

A pregnant woman requires about 2–4.8 mg iron everyday. To have it from the dietary sources she must consume 20–48 mg of dietary iron. This is practically impossible in India because of average vegetarian diet does not contain more than 10–15 mg of iron and the phytate content in it further reduces iron absorption. Moreover, majority of Indian women enter pregnancy with iron depleted condition already. The iron store is markedly diminished when there is fall in Hb values. Therefore, in India there is a need for routine iron supplementation to all pregnant women.

The National Nutritional Anemia Control Programme (NNACP) was initiated in India in 1970 to provide free iron-folic acid (IFA) supplementation to all pregnant women commencing from the second trimester until 3 months of lactation. Nearly 40 years on, anemia still contributes 20% of the maternal mortality of 350–450/100,000 live births. Less readily measurable is the impact of IDA on childhood development and later adult disease.

ORAL IRON PREPARATIONS

Once women become iron deficient in pregnancy, it is not possible to ensure repletion through diet alone and oral supplementation is needed. Oral iron is an effective, cheap and safe way to replace iron. Oral iron supplementation should be taken on an empty stomach, as absorption is reduced or promoted by the same factors that affect absorption of dietary nonheme iron. The usual therapeutic dosage of oral iron is 60–120 mg/day.

Ferrous salts: table 1 shows ferrous salts and the amount of iron in various oral preparations.

Other oral iron preparations available are:

- Iron polysaccharide complex
- Carbonyl iron
- Sodium feredetate

PARENTERAL IRON THERAPY

Parenteral iron therapy is indicated when there is absolute noncompliance with, or intolerance to, oral iron therapy or

TABLE 1: Amount of iron in various oral preparations

Preparation	Molecular iron (mg/tab)	Elemental iron (mg/tab)
Ferrous sulfate	300	60
Ferrous fumarate	200	66
Ferrous gluconate	300	36

proven malabsorption [Royal College of Obstetricians and Gynecologists (RCOG), 2007]. It circumvents the natural gastrointestinal regulatory mechanisms to deliver nonprotein bound iron to the red cells.

Intravenous Iron Preparations

Iron Sucrose

Intravenous iron sucrose circumvents many of the obstacles that have contributed to the failure of the IFA program. Safe and efficacious in dialysis, nondialysis chronic kidney disease (CKD), inflammatory bowel disease (IBD), computed tomography-induced anemia, peripartum period, gastric bypass and heavy menstrual blood loss.

- There is irrefutable evidence that compared to oral iron, intravenously iron sucrose results in a much more rapid resolution of IDA and has minimal side effects
- As it is administered intravenously, it circumvents many of the problems that bedeviled the IFA program, including problems of compliance
- Unlike intravenous dextran iron, anaphylactic reactions are rare with iron sucrose. It cannot be administered as a total dose infusion and doses above 300 mg are not recommended.

Recommended dose: 200 mg infused over 20 minutes.

Test dose: Not indicated.

The most common adverse reactions more than 2 % following the administration of iron sucrose are diarrhea, nausea, vomiting, headache, dizziness, hypotension, pruritus, pain in extremity, arthralgia, back pain, muscle cramp, injection site reactions, chest pain and peripheral edema.

Iron III Carboxymaltose

It is a ferric hydroxide carbohydrate complex, which allows for controlled delivery of iron within the cells of the reticuloendothelial system (primarily bone marrow) and subsequent delivery to the iron binding proteins ferritin and transferrin.

- Molecular weight: 150,000 Daltons
- Concentration: 50 mg/mL
- Half-life: 16 hours
- It is administered intravenously, as a single dose of 1,000 mg over 15 minutes (maximum 15 mg/kg by injection or 20 mg/kg by infusion)
- Due to the stability of the complex, ferric carboxymaltose (FCM) does not release ionic iron under physiological conditions
- The iron hydroxide is tightly bound within a carbohydrate cage
- Once in the body, iron is released gradually, avoiding the acute toxicity.

Following a 1,000 mg iron dose, iron sucrose and gluconate cause oversaturation of transferrin, while with FCM a balance of apotransferrin, Fe-Tf and Fe2-Tf is observed. Randomized controlled trials (RCT) have shown noninferiority (Van Wyk et al. 2007; Breymann et al. 2007) and superiority (Seid et al. 2008) to oral ferrous sulfate in the treatment of iron deficiency anemia in the postpartum period, with rapid and sustained increases in Hb.

Iron III Isomaltoside (Monofer)

It is an intravenous preparation with strongly bound iron in spheroid iron-carbohydrate particles, providing slow release of bioavailable iron-to-iron binding proteins. Doses more than 1,000 mg iron can be administered in a single infusion (Gozzard, 2011), although there is little data on its use in the obstetrics setting.

Ferumoxytol

Super paramagnetic iron oxide nanoparticles coated with a low molecular weight semisynthetic carbohydrate.

Dose: Safe and efficacious as a 1,020 mg infusion over 15 seconds with no episodes of anaphylaxis. Currently, there are no published data on the safety and efficacy of ferumoxytol in pregnancy.

Ferric Gluconate Complex

- Composition: Sodium ferric gluconate complex in sucrose
- Molecular weight: 350,000 Daltons
- Approved for only intravenous use
- Dose: 125 mg of ferric gluconate, slow intravenous push at the rate of 12.5 mg/min
- Intravenous infusion: 125 mg in 100 mL over 30–60 minutes.

INTRAMUSCULAR PREPARATIONS

Iron Dextran

Compared with oral iron, intramuscular iron dextran has been shown in a RCT to reduce the proportion of women with anemia (Komolafe et al. 2003). However, injections tend to be painful and there is significant risk of permanent skin staining. The advantage of intramuscular iron dextran is that, following a test dose, it can be administered in primary care, although facilities for resuscitation should be available as there is a small risk of systemic reaction. Elemental iron 50 mg/mL can be given iv/im.

Test dose: Required 25 mg slow intravenous push over 5 minutes.

Adverse reaction less with low molecular weight preparations (<1:20,000) flushing, tingling of the hands, shivering, or dizziness may occur. The area around the injection site may be tender, irritated, or discolored (brown). Delayed reactions occur in 1–2 days after their treatment. These side effects usually lessen within 3–4 days, if the medication was injected into a vein or within 3–7 days, if the medication was injected into a muscle. Side effects persisting or worsen more than 4–7 days after treatment are: back/joint/muscle aches, chills, moderate to high fever, vomiting, backache and headache.

Iron Sorbitol

- Composition: iron sorbitol citric acid complex
- Molecular weight: 50,000 Daltons
- Route: intramuscular
- Concentration: 50 mg/mL
- Half-life: 30–60 days
- Test dose: Required
- Dosing: 100 mL

Iron sorbitol should not be administered concurrently with oral iron medication. Initial local discomfort, sometimes described as painful, may be experienced at the site of injection. Temporary skin discoloration at the injection site may occur. In a very small percentage of cases the injection may be followed by a localized or generalized urticaria.

A transient metallic taste is common, which may be accompanied by a temporary loss of taste. Nausea, vomiting, diarrhea, headache, dizziness, sweating and flushing of the face may occur. Hematuria has also been reported.

Severe systemic reactions with cardiac involvement are seen mostly in connection with overdose. Those reported include sensations of pressure in the chest, circulatory failure, hypertension, syncope, hypotension, arrhythmia, palpitation, atrioventricular block, bradycardia, atrial fibrillation and tachycardia. Adverse effects, like anaphylactic reactions, repeated multiple infusions, intramuscular injection site pain, staining and abscess formation make older preparations obsolete nowadays.

THALASSEMIAS

The thalassemias are a heterogeneous group of genetic disorders of Hb synthesis. Inheritance is in a Mendelian recessive manner. The mutation may result in a reduced rate of production of the affected gene or result in no chain synthesis at all.[21] Thalassemias are often classified by their clinical effects into thalassemia minor, thalassemia intermedia and thalassemia major. In general, thalassemia carriers are often symptomless and fall into the minor category. Intermediate levels are more severely affected and may often have anemia, although this does not require regular transfusion. In its major form, thalassemia presents with a lifelong transfusion dependency.

DIAGNOSIS OF THALASSEMIA

Thalassemia should be suspected in pregnant women, if:

- History of transfusion-dependant anemia in the patient herself or in the family
- Women with microcytic hypochromic blood picture, not responding to oral iron therapy.

INVESTIGATIONS

- Complete blood count and peripheral smear: showed low level of Hb and decreased mean corpuscular volume (MCV)
- Hemoglobin electrophoresis: the serum level of various types of Hb is assessed by electrophoresis. This helps in clinching the type of thalassemia and its severity
- Automated high performance liquid chromatography (HPLC): some variants of Hb unresolved by conventional electrophoresis can be diagnosed by HPLC
- Molecular genetic testing: this is indicated in pregnant women suffering from mild to moderate microcytic hypochromic anemia not responding to iron therapy with β-thalassemia excluded; it is done to detect α-chain deletions
- Genetic counseling and prenatal diagnosis: it is indicated in a thalassemic pregnant woman with a carrier spouse. The various methods are:
    - Chorionic villous sampling (CVS)
    - Amniocentesis
    - Cordocentesis
    - Ultrasonography (USG): useful for diagnosis of α-thalassemia.

Alpha Thalassemia

Women with one or two out of four alpha gene deletions are usually symptoms free and have a normal pregnancy outcome. When three of the four α-globin genes are absent, known as HbH disease, there are variable clinical features ranging from mild asymptomatic anemia to severe transfusion-dependant anemia, with jaundice, hepatosplenomegaly, growth restriction and bone abnormalities. Mild to moderate hemolysis is the predominant feature. This is worsened during pregnancy; prophylactic folic acid (5 mg/day) is recommended. A fetus affected by Hb Barts with no alpha chain production (both parents carrying two alpha deletions on the same chromosome) will develop hydrops, polyhydramnios and placentomegaly.[22] There is a high-risk of pre-eclampsia in the mother. The fetus is also at risk of congenital abnormalities. If iron deficiency is excluded, then carriage of thalassemia should be suspected and the diagnosis is confirmed with polymerase chain reaction (PCR) and globin gene analysis.

Beta Thalassemia

This condition is due to a defect in beta chain synthesis. It interferes with red cell maturation and increases red cell destruction within the marrow and spleen. Major forms have lifelong chronic dyserythropoietic anemia with splenomegaly and skeletal deformity. With inadequate transfusion profound anemia, marked skeletal deformity of the long bones and skull, recurrent infections and death occurs. With adequate transfusion anemia is controlled, but transfusion-related iron overload will result in endocrine abnormalities, pancreatic, hepatic and cardiac failure. This results in failure of pubertal growth, delayed sexual development and hypogonadotropic hypogonadism affecting fertility. Thus, only a small number of successful pregnancies are reported.[23-25] With β-thalassemia intermedia there is a reasonable pregnancy success rate with well-controlled disease. Transfusion requirements increase with increasing gestation with the aim to maintain Hb over 10 g/dL and thereby correct anemia, suppress hyperactive erythropoiesis and inhibit iron absorption. Most often, chelating agents are discontinued on diagnosis of pregnancy, and restarted after delivery. Folic acid supplements are required throughout pregnancy. β-thalassemia minor is usually symptom free, but anemia is common in pregnancy.[26]

POSTPARTUM CONSIDERATIONS

- Blood transfusion is continued as per requirement
- Iron chelation therapy can be restarted after 3 weeks
- Lactation is not contraindicated
- Oral contraceptive pills to be avoided in splenectomized patients due to the risk of thrombosis; no contraindication to other types of contraception.

MEGALOBLASTIC ANEMIA

This type of anemia is characterized by defective DNA synthesis caused by folic acid and/or vitamin B12 deficiency. Only 3–4% anemia have megaloblastic anemia and in many cases it is due to folic acid deficiency. Elevated homocysteine levels are important marker for folic acid and B12 deficiency. Elevated levels of homocysteine levels can also be due to environmental and genetic factors. Macrocytic anemia with hypersegmentation of neutrophils is consistently seen in true folic acid and B12 deficiency and is used for diagnosis in pregnant women. Associated neuropsychiatric symptoms suggest B12 deficiency. Neural tube defects are well related to folic acid deficiency. Neural tube defects (NTD) affected births were reduced by 72% with folic acid treatment.[27] Institute of medicine recommends 600 μg of folate daily and prior NTD affected pregnant women receive 4 mg of folate daily. Miscarriage occurs commonly in women with homocystinuria and there is a hope that vitamin treatment may allow these women to complete their pregnancies. Pre-eclampsia, intrauterine growth restriction (IUGR) are possibly related to hyperhomocysteinemia and theoretically folic acid and B12 can lower homocysteine levels. More clinical trials are needed in this area. Both folate and B12 deficiency can mask iron deficiency because of impaired hematopoiesis. Treatment of folic acid deficiency requires 1 mg/day of folate. Treatment of megaloblastic anemia due to B12 deficiency requires 1,000 μg parenteral cyanocobalamin every week for 6 weeks followed by 1,000 μg, intramuscular every month.

OTHER RARE ANEMIAS

Occasionally, obstetrician may encounter hemolytic anemias. The most common form of hemolytic anemia during pregnancy is microangiopathic anemia seen in H (hemolysis) EL (elevated liver enzymes) LP (low platelets) (HELLP) syndrome due to intravascular hemolysis. Sickle cell disease (SCD) anemia may also be seen infrequently. Rarely autoimmune hemolytic anemia and hemolytic anemia due to glucose-6-phosphate dehydrogenase deficiency may be seen. Very rarely microangiopathic hemolytic anemia may be encountered in clinical situations, like thrombotic thrombocytopenic purpura, hemolytic uremic syndrome (HUS) or in herpetic hepatitis. Hemoglobin electrophoresis is necessary in every pregnant patient with microcytic anemia who is refractory to oral iron therapy. In β-thalassemia minor patients characteristically show Hb A2 levels more than 3.5%. These patients have low Hb levels, but unlike IDA they have normal RBC counts. In patients from Southeast Asia, the Mediterranean, or of African descent, Hb electrophoresis to evaluate for sickle Hb and thalassemia is recommended. Prenatal diagnostic tests for SCD anemia and thalassemia comprise PCR of fetal DNA extracted from amniotic cells, of trophoblasts from chorionic villus sampling, and of erythroblasts obtained from cordocentesis. Magnetic cell sorting, pyrophosphorolysis-activated polymerizations (PAP) and digital PCR are being evaluated as noninvasive methods by testing the scanty fetal cells in the maternal circulation.[28,29]

PLATELET DISORDERS

Thrombocytopenia is a common hematological disease occurring in 10% of the patients.[30] Physiological drop in platelet count occurs in 5–7% of pregnancies, and accounts for 75% of all cases of thrombocytopenia in pregnancy.[31] If platelet count is less than 70,000/μL, a pathological cause must be found out.

Causes of Thrombocytopenia

Physiological: gestational thrombocytopenia.
Pathological:

- Diminished production, e.g., aplastic anemia and severe megaloblastic anemia

- Increased destruction, e.g., idiopathic thrombocytopenic purpura (ITP) and heparin-induced thrombocytopenia
- Increased consumption, e.g., HELLP syndrome, pre-eclampsia, thrombotic thrombocytopenic purpura (TTP), disseminated intravascular coagulation (DIC).

Idiopathic Thrombocytopenic Purpura

Idiopathic thrombocytopenic purpura is the most common of the pathological causes. Unlike gestational thrombocytopenia ITP starts in 1st trimester and platelet count worsens as the pregnancy advances. ITP affects the fetus as well due to transplacental passage of IgG antiplatelet antibodies. Severe thrombocytopenia (<20,000/μL) is seen in 5% of the neonates. Management is not different from nonpregnant patients. Corticosteroids are the main stay in most of the cases. Other therapies aimed at improving the maternal platelet count in anticipation of delivery include intravenous immunoglobulin (IVIg) and intravenous anti-D IgG. The patient may require platelet transfusion during delivery, if the platelet count drops below 20,000/μL. Splenectomy is reserved for severe cases only.

Management of Neonatal Thrombocytopenia

Evaluation of the fetal platelet count by percutaneous umbilical blood sampling (PUBS) or fetal scalp sampling is controversial as it causes bleeding and hence it is not recommended (risks >> benefits). Avoid scalp electrodes/forceps/ventouse during delivery. Measure cord blood platelet count immediately after birth and daily platelet count till day 4. If neonate's platelet count is less than 20,000/mm^3 administer IVIg 1 g/kg. If life-threatening hemorrhage is suspected give both IVIg and platelet transfusion.

PRE-ECLAMPSIA AND ECLAMPSIA, AND HEMOLYSIS, ELEVATED LIVER ENZYMES, LOW PLATELETS SYNDROME

In Pre-eclampsia-eclampsia the incidence of developing isolated thrombocytopenia is 18% and chances of developing HELLP syndrome is 15–20%. HELLP syndrome is seen in 0.5–0.9% of all pregnancies and rate of recurrence of HELLP syndrome in subsequent pregnancies is 3%. It usually develops in 3rd trimester of pregnancy. Pathophysiology of this condition is generalized damage/alteration in endothelium causing microthrombus. Clinical features include nausea, malaise, vomiting, epigastric pain or right upper quadrant pain, headache and visual disturbances.

Diagnostic criteria of HELLP syndrome includes:

1. Microangiopathic hemolytic anemia (MAHA) suggested by fragmented RBC's and increased lactate dehydrogenase (LDH)
2. Elevated liver enzymes: aspartate transaminase (AST), alanine transaminase (ALT) more than 70 U/L
3. Low platelet count: platelet count less than100,000/mm^3.

Complications of Hemolysis, Elevated Liver Enzymes, Low Platelets Syndrome

- Disseminated intravascular coagulation is seen in 20% of cases
- Abruption is seen in 16% of cases
- Maternal mortality is 1–4%
- Perinatal mortality: 10–40% which is mainly caused by placental ischemia, abruption and prematurity.

Management of Hemolysis, Elevated Liver Enzymes, Low Platelets Syndrome

Conduct delivery as early as possible. If there is evidence of DIC, platelet is transfused along with fresh frozen plasma (FFP) to correct clotting factor deficiency and cryoprecipitate is used to correct hypofibrinogenemia. HELLP syndrome usually resolves after delivery. If there is persistence or worsening of the condition even after 2–3 days of delivery plasma exchange for 2–4 days is considered where 1–1.5 volume of plasma of the patient is replaced with FFP of donors.

ACUTE FATTY LIVER OF PREGNANCY

Incidence is less than 0.0001%. It is seen in 3rd trimester. Etiology is believed to be due to fetal deficiency of long-chain 3-hydroxyacyl-CoA dehydrogenase or mitochondrial enzymes involved in fatty acid oxidation.

Clinical features include malaise, nausea, dyspepsia, epigastric or right upper quadrant pain. There is development of acute DIC because of consumption of fibrinogen and antithrombin.

Investigations show evidence of hypoglycemia, abnormal liver function tests, electrolyte imbalance and coagulopathy. Thrombocytopenia is seen, but there is no MAHA. Diagnosis of acute fatty liver of pregnancy (AFLP) is mainly clinical and it is confirmed by liver biopsy with oil o red stain, where it shows fat globules.

THROMBOTIC THROMBOCYTOPENIC PURPURA

It is a clinical trial of MAHA, thrombocytopenia and neurological symptoms, like headache, confusion, visual hallucination, paresis and coma which are seen in 75% cases. Along with these renal dysfunction and fever, i.e., clinical pentad is seen in only 40% of cases.

Diagnostic criteria:

- Indirect coomb's test is negative (r/o immune-mediated hemolytic anemia)

- Increased LDH
- Increased indirect bilirubin
- Decreased haptoglobin levels.

Salient investigation findings are as follows:

- Platelet count is low usually less than 1 lakh/mm^3
- Peripheral smear shows schistocytes
- Urine analysis normal [r/o systemic lupus erythematosus (SLE) which shows red cell casts]
- Serum creatinine more than 2 mg/dL
- Proteinuria - + or ++ on dip stick (rule out preeclampsia).

Treatment of Thrombotic Thrombocytopenic Purpura

Plasma exchange is the main stay of treatment option which should be initiated within 24 hours of presentation. Plasma exchange removes ADAMTS13 antibodies and replaces deficient enzyme from FFP used for it. Rituximab-monoclonal antibody against CD20 is under trial. In congenital TTP-FFP transfusion is done 3–4 weekly. TTP platelet transfusion is contraindicated because it causes appearance or worsening of symptoms by initiation of microthrombi which is composed of platelets. Maternal mortality in TTP without treatment is 90% with treatment mortality rate decreases to 20%.

Recommendations for Treatment of Thrombotic Thrombocytopenic Purpura

- The diagnosis of TTP should be treated as a medical emergency
- The initial diagnosis of TTP should be made on clinical history, examination and routine laboratory parameters of the patient including blood film review
- In view of the high-risk of preventable early deaths in TTP, treatment with plasma exchange should be initiated as soon as possible preferably within 4–8 hours regardless of the time of day at presentation, if a patient presents with a MAHA and thrombocytopenia in the absence of any other identifiable clinical cause
- Platelet transfusions is contraindicated in TTP unless there is life-threatening hemorrhage.

HEMOLYTIC UREMIC SYNDROME

It is a rare disorder characterized by MAHA, thrombocytopenia and renal involvement. Onset is usually in postpartum period. Mean time duration from delivery to onset is average 27 days. Childhood HUS is associated with *Escherichia coli* H7: O157 shiga like toxin. Other causes of HUS are cyclosporine and other cytotoxic drugs, oral contraceptive pill. Thrombocytopenia is of mild variety. Only 50% patients of HUS have platelet count less than 1 lakh/mm^3 at the time of diagnosis. But platelet count decreases as disease progresses. It finally progresses to DIC usually.

Treatment of Hemolytic Uremic Syndrome

Plasma exchange removes toxins responsible for the disorder. Maternal mortality is about 50%. Long-term prognosis is poor because of subsequent development of hypertension and chronic renal failure. About 15–25% patients will develop chronic kidney disease.

DIFFERENTIATING BETWEEN THROMBOTIC THROMBOCYTOPENIC PURPURA AND HEMOLYTIC UREMIC SYNDROME

Thrombotic thrombocytopenic purpura most commonly develops in antenatal period where as HUS onsets during postnatal period. In TTP thrombocytopenia and its manifestations are seen predominantly whereas renal involvement is predominant in HUS.

COAGULATION DISORDERS

von Willebrand's Disease

A good history and physical examination is essential for the evaluation of bleeding disorder in pregnancy. Mucocutaneous bleeding is generally due to primary hemostatic dysfunction [platelet/vWF deficiency] and deep bleeding is usually due to clotting factor deficiency. Congenital disorders are rare in pregnancy. The most common inherited disorder in pregnancy is von Willebrand's disease (vWD).[32] vWF is essential mediator of primary hemostasis as it acts as a bridging molecule for both platelet adhesion and aggregation. Estrogen and thyroid hormone have direct influence on vWF concentration. In 3rd trimester increased estrogen concentration can correct milder forms of vWF deficiency, while hypothyroidism can result in an acquired deficiency of vWF. vWD must be suspected in any pregnant woman with abnormal tendency for bleeding especially repeated postpartum bleeding. Such patients require platelet function assay (PFA-100), aPTT, prothrombin and platelet count. If platelet count is normal and PFA-100 and aPTT are abnormal chance of vWD is high. Definitive diagnosis requires determination of vWF and VIII levels.

Desmopressin (DDAVP) is the drug of choice given at a dose of 0.3 mg/kg for 15–30 minutes for type 1 vWD. Humate-P (factor VIII concentrate) and cryoprecipitate when Humate-P is not available can be used for type 2 and 3 vWD.

Thrombophilia

Pregnancy is hypercoagulable state. Pregnancy complications such as severe pre-eclampsia, intrauterine growth retardation, abruptio placentae and stillbirths have been shown to be associated with thrombophilia. Recurrent miscarriage has also been associated with thrombophilia. Thromboembolism in pregnancy as in the nonpregnant state is linked to thrombophilia.

Important hereditary thrombophilia are:

- Factor V Leiden (FVL) mutation
- Prothrombin promoter mutation
- Protein S deficiency
- Protein C deficiency
- Hyperhomocysteinemia
- Methylenetetrahydrofolate reductase (MTHFR) mutations.

Antiphospholipid antibody syndrome is the most important acquired thrombophilic condition. Placenta is the most preferred target organ for hereditary thrombophilias in view of low pressure system coupled with prothrombotic changes of pregnancy.

Factor V Leiden Mutation

Factor V Leiden mutation is responsible for 20–50% of the cases of deep vein thrombosis (DVT) during pregnancy.[33] Its presence is associated with early pregnancy losses, pre-eclampsia and IUGR. FVL mutation is significant risk factor for DVT, cerebral vein thrombosis, pulmonary embolization and placental thrombosis. Advanced maternal age, obesity, multiparity, smoking, prolonged bedrest, lower segment cesarean section (LSCS) increase the risk of DVT in women with FVL mutation. History of deep vein thrombosis in patient herself or in first-degree relative is the most important risk factor. Heterozygous carriers of FVL mutation require prophylactic anticoagulation either with regular heparin 5,000–10,000 units 12th hourly or low molecular weight heparin (LMWH) 40 mg once daily. However, following conditions require therapeutic anticoagulation:

- History of DVT and pulmonary embolism
- Double heterozygous with other thrombophilia
- History of stillbirth. Due to high thrombogenic potential of protein S and protein C deficiency, pregnant women with these affected conditions must be treated with therapeutic anticoagulation.

Deep Vein Thrombosis

Early studies have estimated the incidence of symptomatic venous thrombosis during pregnancy using radiographic investigations to be 0.5–3.0%. Antenatal DVT is at least as common as postpartum DVT and can occur at any time during pregnancy, although pulmonary emboli are more common postpartum.[34]

REFERENCES

1. Yip R. Significance of an abnormally low or high hemoglobin concentration during pregnancy: special consideration of iron nutrition. Am J Clin Nutri. 2000;72(1):272S-9S.
2. Guyton & Hall. Textbook of Medical Physiology, 11th edition. Philadelphia: Saunders; 2005. p. 103.
3. Fleming AF. Hematological changes in pregnancy. Clin Obstet Gynecol. 1975;2:269.
4. Kline AJ, Williams GW, Hernandez-Nino J. D-Dimer concentration in normal pregnancy: new diagnostic thresholds are needed. Clin Chem. 2005;51(5):825-9.
5. Burrows RF, Kelton JG. Thrombocytopenia at delivery: a prospective survey of 6715 deliveries. Am J Obstet Gynecol. 1990;162:731-4.
6. Ramsay Margaret Normal hematological changes during pregnancy and the puerperium. In: Pavord S, Hunt B (Eds). The Obstetric Hematology Manual. Cambridge University Press, Cambridge; 2010. pp. 1-11.
7. Davis GL Hemostatic changes associated with normal and abnormal pregnancies. Clin Lab Sci. 2000;13:223-8.
8. Clark P, Brennard J, Conkie JA, McCall F, Greer IA, Walker ID. Activated protein C sensitivity, protein C, protein S and coagulation in normal pregnancy. Thromb Hemost. 1998;79:1166-70.
9. Bernard BJ, Hakimi M, Palletier D. An analysis of anemia and pregnancy related maternal mortality. J Nutr. 2001;131:604S-15S.
10. Sifakis S and Pharmakides G. Anemia in pregnancy. Ann N Y Acad Sci. 2000;900:125-36.
11. Kalaivani K. Prevalence & consequences of anaemia in pregnancy. Indian J Med Res. 2009;130(5):627-33.
12. Toteja GS, Singh P. Micronutrient profile of Indian population. Indian Pediatr. 2003;40(5):477-9.
13. National Nutrition Monitoring Bureau (NNMB). (2003). Prevalence of Micronutrient Deficiencies. [online] Available from nnmbindia.org/NNMB%20MND%20REPORT%202004-Web.pdf. [Accessed December, 2015].
14. DLHS on RCH. Nutritional status of children and prevalence of anaemia among children, adolescent girls and pregnant women 2002-2004. [online] Available from www.rchindia.org/nr_india.htm 2006. [Accessed December, 2015].
15. Government of India. (2006). Maternal Mortality in India: 1997-2003. Registrar General of of Census Operation, New Delhi. 2006 India. [online] Available from www.censusindia.net/Maternal_Mortality_in_India_1997-2003.doc. [Accessed December, 2015].
16. Ramachandran P. Nutrition in pregnancy. In: Gopalan C, Kaur S (Eds). Women and Nutrition in India, Special Publication No. 5. New Delhi: Nutrition Foundation of India; 1989. pp. 153-93.
17. Ramachandran P. Anaemia in pregnancy. In: Ratnam SS, Bhasker Rao K, Arulkumaran S (Eds). Obstetrics and Gynaecology for postgraduates. Madras: Orient Longman; 1992. pp. 42-53.
18. Prema K, Ramalakshmi BA, Madhavapeddi R, Babu S. Effect of intramuscular iron therapy in anaemic pregnant women. Indian J Med Res. 1982;73:534-46.
19. Prema K, Neela Kumari S, Ramalakshmi BA. Anaemia and adverse obstetric outcome. Nutr Rep Int. 1981;23:637-43.
20. Lister VG, Rossiter CE, Chong M. Perinatal mortality. Br J Obstet Gyn. 1985;92 (Suppl 5):88-99.
21. Old J. Screening and genetic diagnosis of haemoglobin disorders. Blood Rev. 2003;17:43-53.
22. Chui D, Waye J. Hydrops fetalis caused by α-thalassaemia: an emerging health care problem. Blood. 1998;91:2213-22.
23. Aessopos A, Karabatsos F, Farmakis D, Katsantoni A, Hatziliami A, Youssef J, et al. Pregnancy in patients with well-treated β-thalassaemia: outcome for mothers and newborn infants. Am J Obstet Gynecol. 1999;180:360-5.

24. Mordel N, Birkenfeld A, Goldfarb AN, Rachmilewitz EA. Successful full-term pregnancy in homozygous β-thalassaemia major: case report and review of the literature. Obstet Gynecol. 1989;73:837-9.
25. Jensen CE, Tuck SM, Wonke B. Fertility in β-thalassaemia major: a report of 16 pregnancies, preconceptual evaluation and a review of the literature. Br J Obstet Gynaecol. 1995;102:625-9.
26. Sheiner E, Levy A, Yerushalmi R, Katz M. β-thalassemia minor during pregnancy. Obstet Gynecol. 2004;103:1273-7.
27. Kang SS, Wong PW, Zhou JM, Sora J, Lessick M, Ruggie N, et al. Thermolabile methylenetetrahydrofolate reductase in patients with coronary artery disease. Metabolism. 1988;37(7):611-3.
28. Phylipsen M, Yamsri S, Treffers EE, Jansen DT, Kanhai WA, Boon EM, et al. Non-invasive prenatal diagnosis of β-thalassemia and sickle-cell disease using pyrophosphorolysis-activated polymerization and melting curve analysis. Prenat Diagn. 2012;32(6):578-87.
29. Barrett AN, McDonnell TC, Chan KC, Chitty LS. Digital PCR analysis of maternal plasma for noninvasive detection of sickle cell anemia. Clin Chem. 2012;58(6):1026-32.
30. Mcrae KR, Samuels P, Scheiber AD. Pregnancy associated thrombocytopenia: pathogenesis and management. Blood.1992;80:2697-714.
31. Shehata N, Burrows R, Kelton JG. Gestational thrombocytopenia. Clin. Obstet.Gynecol. 1999;42:327-34.
32. Rodeghiero F, Castaman G, Dini E. Epidemiological investigation of the prevalence of von Willebrandt's disease.Blood. 1987;69(2):454-9.
33. Koster T, Rosendaal FR, Ronde H, Briet Ernest, Vandenbroucke JP, Bertina RM. Venous thrombosis due to poor anticoagulant response to activated protein C: Leiden Thrombophilia study. Lancet. 1993;342:1503.
34. Gates S. Thromboembolic disease in pregnancy. Curr Opin Obstet Gynecol. 2000;12:117.

CHAPTER 56

Immunological Complications

K Aparna Sharma, Alka Kriplani

INTRODUCTION

Autoimmunity is an aberration in the capacity to distinguish biologic "self" from "non-self". Persistent immunologic activation results in an autoimmune disease. These diseases are characterized by a typical pattern of clinical signs and symptoms and confirmed by the serologic presence of autoantibodies. Susceptibility to specific diseases depends on subset of human leukocyte antigen (HLA) alleles and the genes, mainly responsible for immunoglobulins, immune receptors on T-cells and major histocompatibility complex genes.

These disorders have a major predilection to the female gender, especially women of reproductive age, and these are frequently encountered during pregnancy. Estrogens accelerate disease while androgens are protective. Diseases with strong cellular pathophysiology undergo remission during pregnancy [rheumatoid arthritis (RA) and multiple sclerosis] while diseases with autoantibody production, tend to increase in severity during pregnancy [systemic lupus erythematosus (SLE) and Graves' disease].

The list of autoimmune disorders is quite exhaustive. The commonly encountered autoimmune disorders in pregnancy are the antiphospholipid antibody syndrome (APS), SLE, immune thrombocytopenic purpura (ITP), scleroderma and RA. These conditions would be discussed in detail.

ANTIPHOSPHOLIPID ANTIBODY SYNDROME

Antiphospholipid antibody syndrome is the most common cause of acquired thrombophilias. From the time that it was first coined in 1986 by Nigel Harris it became one of the few, if any treatable cause of fetal loss and pregnancy morbidity. Antiphospholipid antibody syndrome is characterized by the presence of antibodies against negatively charged phospholipids on the cell membrane. It is more commonly seen in females as compared to males in the ratio of 5:1. Antiphospholipid antibody syndrome can occur as primary APS or secondary APS in conjunction with the other connective tissue disorders.

The two main types of antiphospholipid antibodies (aPL) of concern to obstetricians are lupus anticoagulants (LAC) and anticardiolipin antibodies (aCL),[1] although the presence of anti-β_2-glycoprotein-I (anti-β_2-GPI) antibodies may be a risk factor for later miscarriages and/or thromboembolic complications.[2]

Antiphospholipid antibody syndrome in women is associated with: arterial or venous thrombosis or specific pregnancy complications, and laboratory evidence of antibodies to proteins bound to anionic phospholipids.

Pregnancy Morbidity

Because of a lot of controversy over the definition of pregnancy morbidity, a uniform criteria defining pregnancy morbidity was proposed by an International Committee in 2006.[2]

- More than or equal to one unexplained fetal deaths; more than or equal to 10 weeks of gestation with normal morphology by prenatal ultrasound examination or direct postnatal examination
- More than or equal to one preterm deliveries of a morphologically normal infant before 34 weeks of gestation due to severe preeclampsia, eclampsia, or

features consistent with placental insufficiency. Generally, accepted features of placental insufficiency include:
- Abnormal or nonreassuring fetal surveillance test (e.g., nonreactive nonstress test)
- Abnormal Doppler flow velocimetry waveform analysis (e.g., absent end-diastolic flow in the umbilical artery)
- Oligohydramnios, or
- Birth weight less than the 10th percentile for the gestational age

- More than or equal to three unexplained, consecutive, spontaneous pregnancy losses less than 10 weeks of gestation, after exclusion of maternal anatomic and hormonal abnormalities and paternal and maternal chromosomal abnormalities.

The majority of pregnancy losses are preclinical occurring in up to 40% of cases while early pregnancy losses occur in 13% of cases. Pregnancy losses after 12 weeks occur in up to 1% of cases. Preeclampsia (25%) and intrauterine growth retardation (IUGR; 15–30%) occur in significant proportion of cases.

Thromboembolic Disease

Pregnancy and the puerperium are associated with an increased risk of thromboembolic disease, and this risk is particularly high in pregnant women with APS. In prospective studies, the risk of thromboembolic disease during pregnancy or postpartum was 5–12% among women with known APS (compared with 0.025–0.10% in the general obstetrical population).[3,4]

Laboratory Criteria

- Anticardiolipin (aCL) antibodies of immunoglobulins G or M (IgG/IgM) type in medium or high titer (>40 GPL or >40 MPL) on two or more occasions, at least 12 weeks apart
- Anti-β_2-GPI in medium or high titer (99th percentile) on two or more occasions, at least 12 weeks apart
- LAC on two or more occasions at least 12 weeks apart.

These antibodies are seen in 1–4% of healthy individuals, in 30–50% of SLE patients and in 5–20% patients with recurrent pregnancy loss (RPL). The sensitivity and specificity of various laboratory parameters are mentioned in Table 1.

Antiphospholipid antibody syndrome is diagnosed, if one clinical and one laboratory criteria are met.

Potential Mechanisms for Morbidity

The pathogenesis of pregnancy morbidity in APS is incompletely understood, but is thought to involve platelet and endothelial cell activation, as well as procoagulant effects of aPL.[5]

TABLE 1: Laboratory diagnosis of antiphospholipid antibody syndrome

Antibodies	Test of detection	Sensitivity (%)	Specificity (%)
Lupus anticoagulant (LAC)	dRVVT	83	95
Anticardiolipin (IgG, IgM)	ELISA	95	75 (IgG more specific)
Anti-β2-glycoprotein I (Anti-β2-GPI)	ELISA	81	91

IgG, immunoglobulin G; IgM, immunoglobulin M; dRVVT, diluted Russell's viper venom test; ELISA, enzyme-linked immunoassay.

Although thrombosis may be one mechanism for adverse pregnancy outcome, not all affected placentas have signs of thrombosis or infarction. aPL also appears to have a direct effect on human placental trophoblast, inhibiting the expression of human chorionic gonadotropin, inducing apoptosis, decreasing trophoblast fusion, altering expression of adhesion molecules, limiting trophoblast invasiveness and inhibiting decidualization of cultured endometrial stromal cells.[6,7]

Management Algorithm

Heparin can be used to prevent venous thrombosis and low-dose aspirin [acetylsalicylic acid (ASA)] or a combination of low-dose ASA and heparin can be used to prevent arterial thrombosis and pregnancy-morbidity in pregnant women with APS. Low-molecular-weight heparin (LMWH) is preferred because of its potential greater safety and efficacy compared with unfractionated heparin, but unfractionated heparin is an acceptable alternative.

Pregnant Women with Antiphospholipid Antibody Syndrome with Previous Thrombotic Event

Antepartum: therapeutic anticoagulation with LMWH and aspirin is recommended.

Postpartum: in the postpartum period, there is a general consensus that long-term anticoagulation is required;[8] however, certain guidelines advocate only 6 weeks of prophylaxis upfront and a hematological review of the prevalent risk factors to decide on the long-term requirements.[9,10]

Pregnant Women with Antiphospholipid Antibody Syndrome with Pregnancy Morbidity (No History of Thrombosis)

Antepartum: aspirin along with LMWH in a prophylactic dose should be given throughout the antenatal period.

Aspirin can be started in the periconceptional period, while heparin should be started after the confirmation of intrauterine pregnancy even before the cardiac activity is confirmed. The gestation till which both need to be continues remains controversial. The Royal College of Obstetricians and Gynaecologists (RCOG, UK) recommends administration till 35 weeks[9] while the American College of Obstetricians and Gynecologist (ACOG)[8] and the American College of Chest Physicians (ACCP)[10] advocate its continuation till the time of labor and delivery.

Postpartum: presence of associated risk factors for thrombosis decides the duration of postpartum thromboprophylaxis. In the absence of any such risk factors an anticoagulation of 7 days appears to be enough[9] while it should be continued for 6 weeks in the presence of additional risk factors.[8-10]

Pregnant Women with Antiphospholipid Antibodies without Antiphospholipid Antibody Syndrome Diagnosis

Antepartum: it is unclear whether asymptomatic healthy women with aPL who do not meet criteria for APS are at increased risk of pregnancy morbidity. The bulk of evidence suggests little or no increase in risk in this group.[11,12] So it reasonable to follow these patients with antenatal clinical surveillance.[9]

Postpartum: as the postpartum period carries the highest risk of thrombosis, prophylactic anticoagulation can be advised for a period of 7 days.[9]

SYSTEMIC LUPUS ERYTHEMATOSUS

Systemic lupus erythematosus is a multisystem chronic inflammatory disease, characterized by periods of remission and relapse. Most commonly affected organs are joints, skin, kidneys, lung and nervous system, and the most common symptoms are extreme fatigue, fever, weight loss, myalgia and arthralgia. The prevalence of SLE is 3–5 per 100,000 individuals and is 5–10 times more common in females. As it frequently involves women in the reproductive age-group, their pregnancies may be associated with complications. The prognosis for both mother and child is best when SLE has been quiescent and when renal disease in remission for at least 6 months prior to the pregnancy.

THE EFFECT OF SYSTEMIC LUPUS ERYTHEMATOSUS ON PREGNANCY

Systemic lupus erythematosus can affect both the mother and the fetus. The mother is at risk of developing lupus flare (15–63%), pre-eclampsia (30%), lupus nephritis (40–50%) and lupus cerebritis (20%). Fetal complications include pregnancy early- or late-pregnancy losses (11–29%), intrauterine growth retardation (IUGR), preterm birth, neonatal lupus (rare) and congenital heart block (CHB; rare). For the optimal management of pregnancies with SLE, it is important to identify women who are at a higher risk of developing these complications. Also, these women should be managed by a multidisciplinary team in a tertiary center well equipped to handle these complications.[13]

Patients with SLE with one or more of the following features should be followed by an obstetrician experienced in management of high-risk pregnancies as the presence of these factors are predictors for development of complications:[14]

- Prior history of poor obstetric outcomes
- Cardiac involvement (heart failure)
- Pulmonary hypertension (mean pressure >50 mmHg)
- Interstitial lung disease
- Restrictive lung disease (forced vital capacity <1 L)
- Evidence of active lupus
- Chronic renal failure (creatinine >2.8 mg/dL)
- Active renal disease
- Stroke within the previous 6 months
- aPL/APS
- Antibodies to Ro/La (predisposing to neonatal lupus)
- High-dose glucocorticoid therapy
- Immunosuppressive therapy
- Multiple gestations.

The major issues unique to pregnant patients with SLE and their fetuses, especially later in pregnancy, are:

- Exacerbation of the disease
- Fetal loss, IUGR and preterm delivery (often in the setting of aPL)
- Neonatal lupus
- Breastfeeding.

Exacerbation of Systemic Lupus Erythematosus

Flares may occur during any trimester or postpartum. Remission for a period of 6–12 months before conception decreases the chances for SLE exacerbations during pregnancy and postpartum. The significant risk factors for lupus flares include:

- Active disease at the time of conception
- Active nephritis
- Abruptly stopping drug therapy
- Evidence of APS
- Hormone manipulation for in-vitro fertilization.

In the past, exacerbation of SLE occurred in over 50% of patients during pregnancy. However, the incidence of exacerbation during pregnancy and the postpartum period has been progressively diminishing in the past few decades.

The frequency of exacerbation (or persistently active disease) varies with the state of disease activity at conception, ranging from 7–33% in women who have been in remission for at least 6 months and from 61–67% in women who have active disease at the time of conception.[15,16]

The diagnosis of flare and management of SLE flare based on the disease activity index are mentioned in tables 2 and 3.

Renal Disease

Patients with organ damage at the time of pregnancy may have difficulty since pregnancy imposes an added burden on malfunctioning organs. This phenomenon is particularly important in patients with renal disease.

Lupus Nephritis

Pregnancy in women with lupus nephritis is associated with an increased risk of fetal loss (up to 75%) and with worsening of the renal and extrarenal manifestations in most,[15] but not all[16] studies. The main cause is immune complex deposition and complement activation leading to inflammatory renal damage. It occurs in about 50% of patients. The most common presentation proteinuria (75%) and 40% have hematuria or pyuria.

Glucocorticoids are the first-line of therapy in active lupus nephropathy, i.e., oral prednisone, 40–50 mg/day. Cytotoxic agents may be indicated for severe proliferative lesions, as in moderate-to-severe diffuse proliferative glomerulonephritis. Cyclophosphamide, in a divided monthly dose of 0.5–1.0 g/m^2, can be used.

TABLE 2: Systemic lupus erythematosus disease activity index: American College of Rheumatology 2011 Guidelines

Score	Present descriptor
8 (for each symptom)	• Neurological symptoms: seizure, psychosis, organic brain syndrome, visual disturbance, cranial nerve disorder, lupus headache, cerebrovascular accident
4 (for each symptom)	• Vasculitis • Arthritis or myositis • Renal: urinary casts, hematuria, proteinuria, pyuria
2 (for each symptom)	• Cutaneous: new rash, alopecia, mucosal ulcers • Pleurisy, pericarditis, low complement decrease in CH50, C3, or C4, increased DNA binding

TABLE 3: Treatment of systemic lupus erythematosus flair based on disease activity index

Mild or moderate flare	Severe flare
>3 points	>12 points
Treatment	
• Increase in prednisone, but not to >0.5 mg/kg/day • Add non-steroidal anti-inflammatory drug (NSAID) or chloroquine	• Prednisone >0.5 mg/kg/day • Add new drugs cytoxan, azathioprine, methotrexate • Hospitalization

Pre-eclampsia

It is a common complication of pregnancy with SLE occurring in about 13% of cases. The incidence is much higher in patients with renal disease, underlying hypertension, APS and those on high-dose steroids. It is often difficult to distinguish from lupus nephropathy. Laboratory testing may be, but is not always, useful in distinguishing pre-eclampsia from nephritis or a lupus flare:

- Proteinuria: lupus nephritis is often associated with proteinuria and/or an active urine sediment (red and white cells and cellular casts), whereas only proteinuria is seen in pre-eclampsia
- Hypocomplementemia and anti-DNA antibodies: SLE flare is likely to be associated with hypocomplementemia and increased titers of anti-DNA antibodies while in pre-eclampsia they are normal[17]
- Thrombocytopenia, elevated serum levels of liver enzymes and uric acid, and decreased urinary excretion of calcium: more prominent in pre-eclampsia than lupus nephritis.

Fetal Loss: Pregnancy Loss

Prospective studies have reported losses ranging from 11 to 29%. IUGR is a frequent complication because of underlying risk factors like renal disease, pre-eclampsia and APS. Preterm birth occurs in around 20% of cases. But with improved antenatal care the frequency of pregnancy losses are decreasing.[18]

Neonatal Lupus

It is a passively transferred autoimmune disease that occurs 1 in 20,000 livebirths. It is seen in babies born to mother with anti-Ro and/or anti-La/SSB antibodies, many of whom do not have lupus or other autoimmune disease. The common manifestations can be CHB, skin lesions, thrombocytopenia, anemia and hepatitis. CHB is the most serious manifestation seen in 2% of cases. It can develop before birth, after infancy, or in adults. For antenatal diagnosis, the finding of a structurally normal heart with atrioventricular (AV) dissociation is suggestive of the diagnosis. The presence of anti-Ro/La anti-idiotypic antibody is indicative of a better future outcome. Fetal hydrops due to CHB is another important predictor of fetal outcome. Steroids for prophylaxis of this condition are not recommended. If the diagnosis of anti-Ro/La associated heart block is made before 27 weeks, it is associated with a high mortality of 20%. The recurrence rate in future pregnancy is as high as 17%. Maternal use of hydroxychloroquine (HCQ) may be associated with reduced rates of the cardiac manifestations in the newborn, including CHB and isolated cardiomyopathy, and maternal HCQ use is also associated with a decreased risk of recurrence of cardiac neonatal lupus in subsequent pregnancies.[19,20] The antenatal management of CHB is summarized in Flowchart 1.

Vaginal delivery is possible in cases of CHB, if there is the availability of fetal pulse oximeter. Around 30–80% of neonates would need pacemakers. The indications for putting pacemakers are:

- Second/third-degree AV block associated with symptomatic bradycardia, congestive cardiac failure (CCF)
- Third-degree AV block in the infant with ventricular rate less than 50–55 beats/min or with congenital heart disease with ventricular rate less than 70 beats/min
- Third-degree AV block beyond first year with rate less than 50 beats/min or abrupt pauses in ventricular rate
- Complex CHD with rate less than 35 beats/min or pauses in ventricular rate more than 3 seconds
- Asymptomatic sinus bradycardia in the adolescent when the longest RR interval is less than 3 seconds and the minimum heart rate is more than 40 beats/min.

Breast-feeding

Breast-feeding is feasible for most women with SLE. However, some medications may enter breast milk.[21] Short-acting non-steroidal anti-inflammatory drugs (NSAIDs), anti-malarials, low-dose prednisone (<15–20 mg/day), warfarin and heparin are safe for the nursing infant, as little or no active drug is secreted in breast milk while the disease-modifying antirheumatic drugs (e.g., etanercept, infliximab, adalimumab, rituximab) have a doubtful safety profile.

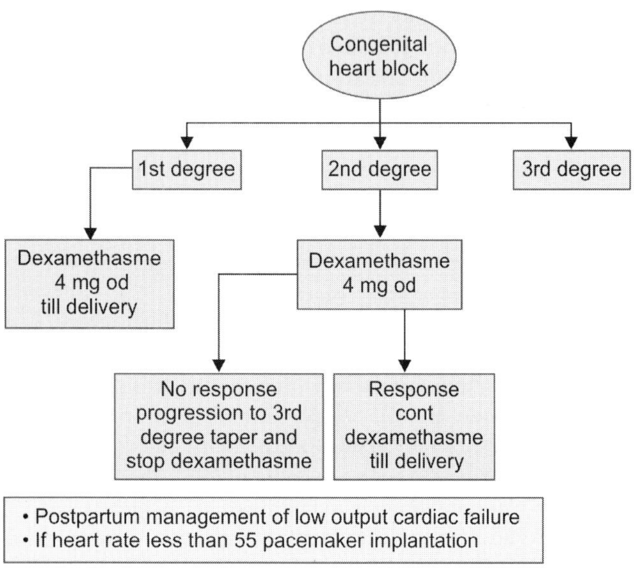

FLOWCHART 1: The antenatal management of congenital heart block.

MANAGEMENT

There are two issues related to therapy of women with lupus who become pregnant: monitoring of disease activity in both asymptomatic and symptomatic patients and treatment of active disease. The schedule for monitoring is shown in table 4.

RHEUMATOID ARTHRITIS

It is a chronic symmetrical inflammatory arthritis of the synovial joints occurring in about 2.5–7.0 people per 10,000 per year. Its prevalence is about 1% in the adult population and reduces to 0.5% in pregnancy. The peak age of occurrence is in the 40 and 50s with a greater female predominance of 2: 1 to 3:1. Rheumatoid factor (RF) is an autoantibody made by oligoclonal activated B cells when they react with antigens on the Fc (fragment crystallizable) portion of IgG.

Effect of Pregnancy on Rheumatoid Arthritis

Rheumatoid arthritis dramatically improves during pregnancy. Approximately, 50–80% of women with RA improve during pregnancy.[23] Improvement starts in the first trimester by a reduction in joint stiffness and pain. Peak improvement occurs in second or third trimester.

Postpartum Flare

Approximately, 90% of patients flare during the postpartum period, usually, within the first 3 months.[24] In addition, one study suggested an increased risk of developing RA in the first 3 months postpartum, particularly after a woman's first pregnancy.[25]

Effect of Rheumatoid Arthritis on Pregnancy

Pregnancy Outcome

There is no adverse effect of RA on pregnancy. Although one case-control study demonstrated a slight increase in spontaneous abortion in women with RA,[26] most reports have failed to show any increase in fetal morbidity or in fetal losses.[27] Atlanto axial subluxation can be a rare complication of general anesthesia (GA) for cesarean section. Very rarely limitation of hip abduction is severe enough to impend vaginal delivery.

Antenatal Management

Management of this condition requires a multidisciplinary management. The treatment plan should be made in conjunction with an obstetrician and a physician or a rheumatologist. Physiotherapy is an important aspect of therapy.

TABLE 4: Monitoring schedule for pregnant females with systemic lupus erythematosus

First visit[22]	At the end of each trimester	Monthly	Last trimester of pregnancy	Postpartum
Physical examination, including blood pressure	Glomerular filtration rate, urine protein/ urine creatinine ratio	A platelet count (or CBC)	Weekly biophysical profile score or nonstress test (if no heart block) with amniotic fluid assessment	Postpartum flare can occur. Tests recommended following an uncomplicated delivery:
Renal function (glomerular filtration rate, urinalysis, urine protein/urine creatinine ratio)	aCL		If intrauterine growth retardation (IUGR), then umbilical artery Doppler	Urinalysis, urine protein/ urine creatinine ratio
Complete blood count (CBC)	Complement (CH50 or C3 and C4)			Renal function, if the urinalysis is abnormal
Anti-Ro/SSA and anti-La/SSB antibodies	Anti-dsDNA			CBC
Lupus anticoagulant (LAC) and anticardiolipin antibody (aCL) assays				Anti-dsDNA
Anti-double stranded DNA antibodies (Anti-dsDNA)				Complement (CH50, or C3 and C4)
Complement (CH50, or C3 and C4)				
Uric acid level				
Women who have antibodies to Ro/ SSA and/or La/SSB should undergo fetal monitoring for heart block				

Drug Therapy in Pregnancy

In patients whose RA becomes active during pregnancy, NSAIDs can be used up to the beginning of the third trimester. In patients in whom high-dose, daily NSAIDs is required to control symptoms or in whom NSAID use is inadequate, a lowest dose of prednisone may be necessary for disease control. The dose of prednisone should be limited to not more than 10 mg/day. HCQ and sulfasalazine can be used in patients with an inadequate response to NSAIDs or prednisone.

Persistent or Flaring Disease Activity

Glucocorticoids in doses higher than 10 mg/day can be used to manage disease flares or persistent moderately to highly active disease that is not adequately controlled with other medications. Patients should be counseled that use of glucocorticoids before 14 weeks of gestation can increase the risk of cleft palate formation and can contribute to pregnancy-induced hypertension and to gestational diabetes later during pregnancy. In patients with disease refractory to routine management or with continued flares during pregnancy despite the use of glucocorticoids, the decision to initiate or resume therapy with a tumor-necrosis factor (TNF) inhibitor can be considered, although the patient needs to be aware of the balance of benefits and risks of this treatment.

Antenatal visits should be scheduled every 2–4 weeks throughout pregnancy.

Labor and Delivery

Mode of delivery can be decided according to the obstetrical indications. However, the physical abilities should be taken into consideration on an individual basis.

Postpartum

Patient should be monitored for RA exacerbations which should be managed in consultation with a rheumatology subspecialist.

Medication Use During Breast-feeding

Many of the same restrictions on medication use apply also to breast-feeding mothers:[28] NSAIDs can be used, but aspirin should be avoided. Prednisone can be taken in low doses. In patients taking 20 mg/day or more, it is recommended to wait 4 hours after the dose prior to nursing. Azathioprine, cyclosporine, cyclophosphamide, methotrexate and chlorambucil should be avoided in nursing.

IMMUNE THROMBOCYTOPENIC PURPURA

Immune thrombocytopenic purpura is a common autoimmune disorder encountered during pregnancy. This is the most common reason for significant thrombocytopenia in the first trimester.[29] Female-to-male prevalence is 3:1. About 70% of women diagnosed with this are less than 40 years of age.

Diagnosis

Common signs and symptoms include petechiae, ecchymoses, easy bruising, menorrhagia, epistaxis and gingival bleeding. There are no definitive symptoms, signs, or diagnostic tests for ITP. The diagnosis is one of the exclusion.

Immune thrombocytopenia purpura is suspected, if the first trimester platelet count is less than 100,000 mm^3 and declines during pregnancy. The differential diagnosis for thrombocytopenia in pregnancy is extensive.

- Gestational thrombocytopenia is the most common cause:
  - It accounts for 74% of pregnant women with thrombocytopenia
  - It is a diagnosis of exclusion
  - The typical woman has platelet counts between 100,000 and 150,000 mm^3
  - Women with platelet counts less than 70,000 mm^3 are less likely to have gestational thrombocytopenia
  - Usually it occurs in the late second or third trimester
  - The patient has no prior history suggestive of thrombocytopenia such as ecchymoses
- Preeclampsia can be associated with low-platelet count. Usually accompanying hypertension and proteinuria:
  - Infection, such as human immunodeficiency virus or malaria, can cause thrombocytopenia
- Some drugs are associated with thrombocytopenia:
  - Heparin, sulfonamides, penicillin, rifampin and quinine
- Thrombocytopenia can be caused by diseases, such as SLE, APS and thrombotic thrombocytopenic purpura[30]

Treatment is recommended in patients with platelet counts less than 30,000 mm^3 or with active bleeding. As a pregnant patient approaches term, the platelet count should be 50,000 mm^3 to ensure adequate hemostasis at delivery.[29]

Corticosteroids may be used. These are efficacious and inexpensive. 1–2 mg/kg/day is usually started. Once the platelet count reaches 75,000–100,000 mm^3, the dose is reduced to maintain the platelet count in this range. Side effects include hypertension and glucose intolerance:[30]

- High-dose intravenous immunoglobulin (IVIg)
- The typical dose is 1–2 per kg infused over 6–8 hours[30,31]
- Effective in two-thirds of patients
- Effective for a month
- More expensive than corticosteroids, but fewer side effects: these are usually mild and include headache, chills and nausea.

Splenectomy

- Considered when refractory to corticosteroids and IVIg
- Ideally, performed in the second trimester.[30]

Platelet Transfusion

- Recommended when a patient is actively bleeding or when the platelet count is less than 20,000 mm^3.

Complications

- Maternal hemorrhage from vaginal lacerations or cesarean section
- Can be minimized, if the platelet count is greater than 50,000 mm^3.

Neonatal thrombocytopenia: it occurs in 3–4% of newborns. Bleeding complications are uncommon in newborns with mildly depressed platelet counts. Intracranial hemorrhage, a very serious complication, occurs in less than 1% of infants. Maternal platelet count correlates poorly with neonatal platelet counts. The best method of obstetrical management to prevent intracranial hemorrhage is controversial. Ideally, the practitioner needs the fetal platelet count. Currently, we do not have a safe method of determining the fetal platelet count.

- Fetal scalp sampling in early labor has been advocated:
  - This technique is difficult in early labor because the presenting part is usually at a high station
  - Sampling can lead to a falsely low-platelet count as clumping of the platelets can be problematic
  - The fetus has already been subjected to the potential ill-effects of labor before the platelet count is determined
- Periumbilical blood sampling has been utilized to determine fetal platelet counts:
  - It does provide an accurate platelet count
  - It is expensive and requires personnel and equipment that are not available at most hospitals
  - It has largely been abandoned because the complication rate may be as high as high as 4.6% (fetal hemorrhage)
- Some authors advocate performing a cesarean section only for obstetrical indications since the incidence of intracranial hemorrhage is so low
- At the root of the controversy is that cesarean section has not been proven to reduce the incidence of intracranial hemorrhage
- A cesarean section does contribute to increased cost and maternal morbidity
- Intracranial hemorrhage may actually precede intrapartum events.[32]

SCLERODERMA

Scleroderma is an uncommon autoimmune disorder that usually affects women in the 4th decade of life. It may be divided into two forms:

1. Calcinosis, Raynaud phenomenon, esophageal hypomotility, sclerodactyly and telangiectasia (CREST) is the localized form
2. Systemic or generalized form involves skin, joints, gastrointestinal tract, lungs, heart and kidneys.

Evaluation

Systemic scleroderma can cause damage to multiple organs.

- Pulmonary: fibrosis
- Vital capacity should be assessed with pulmonary function tests as these patients are at risk for restrictive lung disease:
  - Cardiac: cardiomyopathy
    - Use echocardiogram to estimate the ejection fraction
    - Gastrointestinal: malabsorption and reflux
    - Weight and nutritional parameters can be determined
  - Kidneys: renal insufficiency
  - Renal function should be measured before conception
  - Hypertension.

Complications

- Gastrointestinal reflux: may be treated with histamine blockers or proton pump inhibitors.
- Renal crisis:
  - Antihypertensive therapy may be used to ameliorate
  - The most effective antihypertensive therapy is an angiotensin-converting-enzyme (ACE) inhibitor.

Because of a high associated maternal and fetal mortality, this may be one indication for ACE inhibitors in pregnancy.[33]

CONCLUSION

Immunological disorders in pregnancy present a challenging situtuation to the obstetrician, with the potential to affect both the mother and the fetus. An optimisation of the disease process before conception, early antenatal registration and monitoring throughout pregnancy, delivery and postpartum in conjunction with a multidisciplinary team of rheumatologists, intensivists and paediatriacian can ensure the best possible outcome for the mother and the baby.

REFERENCES

1. Miyakis S, Lockshin MD, Atsumi T, Branch DW, Brey RL, Cervera R, et al. International consensus statement on an update of the classification criteria for definite antiphospholipid syndrome (APS). J Thromb Haemost. 2006;4(2):295-306.
2. Giannakopoulos B, Passam F, Ioannou Y, Krilis SA. How we diagnose the antiphospholipid syndrome. Blood. 2009;113(5):985-94.
3. Branch DW, Silver RM, Blackwell JL, Reading JC, Scott JR. Outcome of treated pregnancies in women with antiphospholipid syndrome: an update of the Utah experience. Obstet Gynecol. 1992;80(4):614-20.
4. Lima F, Khamashta MA, Buchanan NM, Kerslake S, Hunt BJ, Hughes GR. A study of sixty pregnancies in patients with the antiphospholipid syndrome. Clin Exp Rheumatol. 1996;14(2):131-6.
5. Holers VM, Girardi G, Mo L, Guthridge JM, Molina H, Pierangeli SS, et al. Complement C3 activation is required for antiphospholipid antibody-induced fetal loss. J Exp Med. 2002;195(2):211-20.
6. Robertson L, Wu O, Langhorne P, Twaddle S, Clark P, Lowe GD, et al. Thrombophilia in pregnancy: a systematic review. Br J Haematol. 2006;132(2):171-96.
7. Di Simone N, De Carolis S, Lanzone A, Ronsisvalle E, Giannice R, Caruso A. In vitro effect of antiphospholipid antibody-containing sera on basal and gonadotrophin releasing hormone-dependent human chorionic gonadotrophin release by cultured trophoblast cells. Placenta. 1995;16(1):75-83.
8. Bates SM, Greer IA, Middeldorp S, Veenstra DL, Prabulos AM, Vandvik PO, et al. VTE, thrombophilia, antithrombotic therapy, and pregnancy: Antithrombotic therapy and prevention of thrombosis, 9th edition American College of Chest Physicians Evidence-Based Clinical Practice Guidelines. Chest. 2012;141(2 Suppl):e691S-736S.
9. The Royal College of Obstetricians and Gynaecologists (RCOG). (2015). Thrombosis and Embolism during Pregnancy and the Puerperium, Reducing the Risk (Green-top Guideline No. 37a). [online] Available from www.rcog.org.uk/womens-health/clinical-guidance/reducing-risk-of-thrombosis-greentop37a. [Accessed December, 2015].
10. The American College of Obstetricians and Gynecologists (ACOG). (2015). Practice Bulletin No. 132: Antiphospholipid syndrome. Obstet Gynecol. 2012;120:1514-21.
11. Harris EN, Spinnato JA. Should anticardiolipin tests be performed in otherwise healthy pregnant women? Am J Obstet Gynecol. 1991;165(5 Pt 1):1272-7.
12. Infante-Rivard C, David M, Gauthier R, Rivard GE. Lupus anticoagulants, anticardiolipin antibodies, and fetal loss. A case-control study. N Engl J Med. 1991;325(15):1063-6.
13. Mintz G, Niz J, Gutierrez G, Garcia-Alonso A, Karchmer S. Prospective study of pregnancy in systemic lupus erythematosus. Results of a multidisciplinary approach. J Rheumatol. 1986;13(4):732-9.
14. Ruiz-Irastorza G, Khamashta MA. Lupus and pregnancy: ten questions and some answers. Lupus. 2008;17(5):416-20.
15. Julkunen H, Kaaja R, Palosuo T, Grönhagen-Riska C, Teramo K. Pregnancy in lupus nephropathy. Acta Obstet Gynecol Scand. 1993;72(4):258-63.
16. Tandon A, Ibañez D, Gladman DD, Urowitz MB. The effect of pregnancy on lupus nephritis. Arthritis Rheum. 2004;50(12):3941-6.
17. Buyon JP, Cronstein BN, Morris M, Tanner M, Weissmann G. Serum complement values (C3 and C4) to differentiate between systemic lupus activity and pre-eclampsia. Am J Med. 1986;81(2):194-200.
18. Clark CA, Spitzer KA, Laskin CA. Decrease in pregnancy loss rates in patients with systemic lupus erythematosus over a 40-year period. J Rheumatol. 2005;32(9):1709-12.
19. Izmirly PM, Kim MY, Llanos C, Le PU, Guerra MM, Askanase AD, et al. Evaluation of the risk of anti-SSA/Ro-SSB/La antibody-associated cardiac manifestations of neonatal lupus in fetuses of mothers with systemic lupus erythematosus exposed to hydroxychloroquine. Ann Rheum Dis. 2010;69(10):1827-30.
20. Izmirly PM, Costedoat-Chalumeau N, Pisoni CN, Khamashta MA, Kim MY, Saxena A, et al. Maternal use of hydroxychloroquine is associated with

a reduced risk of recurrent anti-SSA/Ro-antibody-associated cardiac manifestations of neonatal lupus. Circulation. 2012;126(1):76-82.
21. Drugs and Lactation Database (LactMed) of the United States National Library of Medicine. (2015). [online] Available from toxnet.nlm.nih.gov/cgi-bin/sis/htmlgen?LACT. [Accessed December, 2015].
22. Lockshin MD, Sammaritano LR. Lupus pregnancy. Autoimmunity. 2003;36(1):33-40.
23. Hench PS. The ameliorating effect of pregnancy on chronic atrophic (infectious rheumatoid) arthritis, fibrosis and intermittent hydrarthrosis. Mayo Clin Proc. 1938;13:161.
24. Persellin RH. The effect of pregnancy on rheumatoid arthritis. Bull Rheum Dis. 1976;27(9):922-7.
25. Silman A, Kay A, Brennan P. Timing of pregnancy in relation to the onset of rheumatoid arthritis. Arthritis Rheum. 1992;35(2):152-5.
26. Kaplan D, Diamond H. Rheumatoid arthritis and pregnancy. Clin Obstet Gynecol. 1965;17:286-303.
27. Morris WI. Pregnancy in rheumatoid arthritis and systemic lupus erythematosus. Aust NZJ Obstet Gynaecol. 1969;9(3):136-44.
28. Guidelines for monitoring drug therapy in rheumatoid arthritis. American College of Rheumatology Ad Hoc Committee on Clinical Guidelines. Arthritis Rheum. 1996;39(5):723-31.
29. McCrae KR. Thrombocytopenia in pregnancy: differential diagnosis, pathogenesis, and management Blood Rev. 2003;17(1):7-14.
30. Kam PC, Thompson SA, Liew AC. Thrombocytopenia in the parturient. Anaesthesia. 2004;59(3):255-64.
31. Gill KK, Kelton JG. Management of idiopathic thrombocytopenic purpura in pregnancy. Semin Hematol. 200;37(3):275-89.
32. Silver RM. Management of idiopathic thrombocytopenic purpura in pregnancy. Clin Obstet Gynecol. 1998;41(2):436-48.
33. Steen VD. Scleroderma and pregnancy. Rheum Dis Clin North Am. 1997;23(1):133-47.

CHAPTER 57

Vascular Complications

Navneet Takkar

INTRODUCTION

The important vascular complications seen in pregnancy are vasculitis and cerebral vascular lesions in the form of aneurysms and arteriovenous malformations (AVMs).

VASCULITIS IN PREGNANCY

Within the past decade, vasculitis has become a major topic of interest. Ideally, pregnancy should be planned when the vasculitis is in remission. Every pregnant women with vasculitis in pregnancy needs to be monitored by a specialized multidisciplinary team consisting of obstetricians specialized in high risk pregnancies, internists and rheumatologists. Awareness and understanding regarding pregnancy in vasculitis is gradually increasing. At present, the overall risk of poor pregnancy outcome does not seem to be high with vasculitis as compared with systemic lupus erythematosus or antiphospholipid syndrome. When vasculitis is known before pregnancy and is in remission without or with appropriate maintenance therapy, outcomes for mother and newborn are usually good. When the disease is still active at pregnancy initiation, outcomes are more uncertain and decisions about treatment and/or pregnancy continuation can be difficult.[1-4] A single center experience from North India of pregnancy with Takayasu's arteritis (TA) reported hypertension as the most common presenting feature. Superimposed pre-eclampsia was seen in 62% of the pregnancies.[5] Vasculitis sequela, like hypertension, renal insufficiency or asthma, must also be taken into account and managed appropriately throughout pregnancy, delivery and thereafter. Vasculitis manifestations in newborns from mothers with vasculitis are very rare and usually transient.

Definition

The vasculitides are defined by the presence of inflammatory leukocytes in vessel walls with reactive damage to mural structures. Loss of vessel integrity may lead to bleeding. A compromise of the lumen leads to downstream tissue ischemia and necrosis. Vasculitis may occur as a primary process or may be secondary to another underlying disease. In general, affected vessels may vary in size, type and location in association with the specific vasculitis disorders.

Classification

The vasculitis syndromes have been categorized by the predominant sizes of the blood vessels and types of vessels must commonly affected among patients with the disorder.[6,7] The presence or absence of antineutrophil cytoplasmic antibodies (ANCA) has been added to the proposed classification. The notable changes suggested by the 2012 International Chapel Hill Consensus Conference (CHCC) on nomenclature of vasculitides were the use of term eosinophilic granulomatosis with polyangiitis (Churg-Strauss) (EGPA), in place of Churg-Strauss syndrome (CSS), and formal adoption of the term ANCA-associated vasculitis (AAV) for the three disorders: (1) microscopic polyangiitis (MPA), (2) granulomatosis with polyangiitis (GPA) (Wegener's); and (3) EGPA.[8]

Large Vessel Vasculitis

- Takayasu's arteritis: Takayasu's arteritis primarily affects the aorta and its branches. The inflammation may be localized to a portion of the thoracic aorta or abdominal aorta and branches or may involve the entire vessels.

Giant cell arteritis: giant cell or temporal arteritis (GCA) is a chronic vasculitis of large and medium sized vessels. The vessel inflammation prominently involves the cranial branches of arteries originating from the aortic arch.

Medium Vessel Vasculitis

- Polyarteritis nodosa (PAN): polyarteritis nodosa is a systemic necrotizing vasculitis that typically affects medium and small sized muscular arteries
- Kawasaki disease (KD): kawasaki disease is an arteritis of large, medium and small arteries, particularly the coronary arteries. The disease usually occurs in children and is often associated with a mucocutaneous lymph node syndrome. A small number of cases have been reported in adults
- Primary central nervous system vasculitis: primary or isolated central nervous system vasculitis (PCNSV) affects medium and small arteries over a diffuse area of central nervous system, without symptomatic involvement of extracranial vessels.

Small Vessel Vasculitis

- Eosinophilic granulomatosis with polyangiitis (Churg-Strauss): eosinophilic granulomatosis with polyangiitis, also called Churg-Strauss syndrome and allergic granulomatosis and angiitis, is a vasculitis of the medium and small sized muscular arteries and is often found with vascular and extravascular granulomatosis. The vasculitis classically involves the arteries of the lung and skin, but may be generalized
- Granulomatosis with polyangiitis (Wegener's): granulomatosis with polyangiitis, is a systemic vasculitis of medium and small arteries, as well as venules and arterioles. It typically produces granulomatous inflammation of the upper and lower respiratory tracts and necrotizing, power immune glomerulonephritis in the kidneys, GPA is usually associated with ANCA. MPA: microscopic polyangiitis or polyarteritis is a vasculitis that primarily affects capillaries, venules or arterioles. Involvement of medium and small arteries may be present. Henoch-Schönlein purpura (HSP); also termed as IgA vasculitis is a systemic vasculitis, is characterized by the complexes. Biopsy of lesions reveals inflammation of the small blood vessels (most prominent in postcapillary venules
- Cryoglobulinemic vasculitis: cryoglobulinemic vasculitis, previously termed as essential cryoglobulinemic vasculitis, is characterized by the presence of cryoglobulins, which are serum proteins that precipitate in cold and dissolve upon rewarming. In this disorder, which is most often due to hepatitis C infection, immune complexes are deposited in the walls of capillaries, venules, or arterioles and thereby causing small vessel inflammation
- Hypersensitivity vasculitis: the term hypersensitivity vasculitis has been used to include vasculitis of small blood vessels. These have included HSP, mixed cryoglobulinemia, allergic vasculitis and serum sickness. However, the term "hypersensitivity vasculitis" is most properly used to refer to vasculitis that occurs as a hypersensitivity reaction to a known or suspected substance, such as a vasculitic drug reaction
- Vasculitis secondary to connective tissue disorders: a subset of patients with systemic lupus erythematosus, rheumatoid arthritis, relapsing polychondritis, Behçet's disease (BD) and other connective tissue disorders may have or develop vasculitis. The vasculitic process in this setting most commonly involves small muscular arteries, arterioles and venules. A propensity for involvement of particular organs varies with the underlying autoimmune disorder
- Vasculitis secondary to viral infections: a number of viral infections may cause vasculitis of medium and/or small vessels. The commonly associated viral infections are hepatitis B and C, cytomegalovirus (CMV), human immunodeficiency virus (HIV), Ebstein-Barr virus and Parvovirus B19.

PREPREGNANCY COUNSELING OF PATIENTS WITH VASCULITIS

Procreation is an important issue in patients with vasculitides and use of cytotoxic therapies raises critical concerns regarding fertility and fetal toxicity when these drugs are administered to mothers during gestation. The immunological changes induced by pregnancy could improve maternal disease in primarily Th-1-mediated vasculitides, such as Takayasu is arteritis and BD and worsen ANCA-associated vasculitides that are mainly Th-2 mediated.[9]

Takayasu's Arteritis

Takayasu's arteritis typically occurs in women during their childbearing age and therefore it is more common to observe pregnancy in these patients. The risk of TA associated with pregnancy seems to be mainly due to arterial hypertension and/or pre-eclampsia and risk is greater in more severe and extensive cases. Spontaneous abortion is reported in 8–16% of cases. Severe aortic valve disease and aortic aneurysm are risk factors for maternal morbidity and mortality, therefore patients with these complications should be discouraged from pregnancy.

Behçet's Disease

Behçet's disease is a chronic, multisystemic disorder characterized by recurrent oral and genital ulcers, ocular, gastrointestinal and neurological manifestations. It affects young women in childbearing age and preconception counseling is important. Noel et al. home reported that disease course in BD seems to improve during pregnancy, mostly in patients treated with colchicine. Pregnancy in patients with BD appears not to be associated with increased rate of pregnancy related complications.[10]

Polyarteritis Nodosa

Few case reports on pregnancy with PAN are available and only two cases have been exported in World literature. Pregnancy outcome was poor when PAN was diagnosed during pregnancy versus a favorable outcome in patients who conceive during disease remission. There is a high risk of death in patients who are diagnosed with PAN during pregnancy and therapeutic abortions may be considered in early pregnancy.[11]

Churg–Strauss Syndrome

It is a disorder with systemic small vessel vasculitis, extravascular granulomas and hypereosinophilia seen in patients with asthma and allergic rhinitis. Patients with disease onset during pregnancy had a poor prognosis.[12] CSS relapse was reported in 50% of women who conceived while the disease was in remission. During relapse the prevalent manifestations were worsening of asthma, mononeuritis multiplex and skin rash.

Prematurity was a common feature and majority of the patients delivered normal but low-birth weight infants.

Wegener's Granulomatosis

The disease usually peaks after the age of 40 years and therefore, pregnancies in women with Wegener's granulomatosis (WG) are uncommonly seen. Tuin et al. have reported that pregnancies in women with WG and MPA (ANCA-associated vasculitides) have excellent outcome if the disease is in remission. Pregnancy in women with these vasculitides in remission does not show an increased risk of relapse.[3] Pagnoux et al. have reported pregnancy outcomes in patients with systemic necrotizing vasculitides and in patients with WG, risk of preterm birth and miscarriages is not uncommon.[13] Renal impairment and severe pneumonia have been observed in women with WG during pregnancy. Hence, appropriate counseling and multidisciplinary approach is needed in the preconception period.

PREGNANCY AND INDIVIDUAL VASCULITIS

Ideally, pregnancy should be planned in consultation with the rheumatologist or the referring physician in women with vasculitis. Patients need to be referred to tertiary care centers or dedicated clinics where a multidisciplinary approach is available to optimize their chances of successful pregnancy outcome. Patients with active disease may have several contraindications to pregnancy, like renal impairment, cardiac insufficiency, uncontrolled asthma in EGPA, and erratic blood pressure (BP) in TA or PAN. Treatment for vasculitis usually lasts more than 2 years and therefore pregnancy should be planned when vasculitis shows minimum activity and patient is on pregnancy-safe medication for 6 months. Among the medications regularly used to treat vasculitis, only corticosteroids, colchicine, intravenous immunoglobulin and azathioprine are considered safe at the timing of conception and throughout pregnancy.[14-16] If patients on these medications conceive and want to continue pregnancy, the therapy must be continued during pregnancy to limit the risk of flare. Pregnancy is not a known trigger for vasculitis onset. When vasculitis is known before pregnancy and is in remission or on maintenance treatment, outcomes for the mother and newborn are usually good. When the disease is still active at pregnancy initiation, outcomes are more uncertain. With the exception of BD for which case reports suggest improvement in up to 60% of women, pregnancy does not seem to improve vasculitis.[17]

TAKAYASU'S ARTERITIS AND PREGNANCY

Takayasu's arteritis is a chronic idiopathic vasculitis affecting aorta and its primary branches and was first recognized by a Japanese ophthalmologist, Dr Mikoto Takayasu in 1908. It commonly affects young women of Asian or oriental origin during childbearing years. Only a few Caucasian cases of TA and pregnancy have been published. The American College of Rheumatology (ACR) has devised classification criteria for TA and for diagnosis at least three of the six criteria must be present in a patient.[7]

1. Age of disease onset 40 years or younger
2. Claudication of extremities
3. Decreased pulsation of one or both brachial arteries
4. Difference of at least 10 mm Hg in systolic BP between the arms
5. Bruit over one or both subclavian arteries or abdominal aorta
6. Arteriographic narrowing or occlusion of entire aorta, its primary branches, or large arteries in the proximal upper or lower extremities, not due to arteriosclerosis, fibro-muscular dysplasia, or other causes.

Symptoms range from fever, fatigue, weight loss, abdominal pain, life-threatening hemoptysis, and heart failure from aortic regurgitation. Physical examination may lead to detection of reduced pulse rate, difference of BP between the two arms, bruit over neck, supraclavicular area and abdomen. Diagnosis is usually confirmed by computed tomography (CT), magnetic resonance imaging (MRI) or digital subtraction angiography (DSA).

Pregnancy with TA can be complicated by hypertension (up to 75% of patients, pre-eclampsia (up to 45%), preterm birth (15–20%), intrauterine growth restriction 10–25% and need for cesarean section (>35%).[4,5,18-22] Fetal losses up to 15–25% have been reported. A single center experience from North India based on a retrospective analysis of 9 years showed that hypertension was the most common presenting feature (27%) and superimposed pre-eclampsia complicated 62% of pregnancies.[5] An analysis of TA in pregnancy from Eastern India concluded that antenatal and intrapartum control of BP played a pivotal role in pregnancy outcome.[23] The risk of new vasculitis flare during pregnancy seems low for TA (<5%). Many of the potential maternal complications during pregnancy are due to damage from previous disease flares. With TA, severe complications are mainly due to hypertension because of renal artery stenosis and/or aortic value disease with cardiac insufficiency. Aortic dissection (spontaneous or on pre-existing aneurysm) or complications of pulmonary artery involvement and cardiac failure may occur. Anesthesia for patients with TA is an important aspect due to hypertension and risk of hemodynamic instability. Epidural, low dose spinal anesthesia rather than general anesthesia are often favored.[24] Management during pregnancy involves close watch for hypertension, worsening of cardiovascular hemodynamic status, worsening of cardiovascular hemodynamic status, cerebral ischemia and rupture of aneurysms. Hypertension is a serious complication and can lead to aneurysm rupture, aortic dissection and maternal heart failure. Antihypertensive agents that are safely used with proven success in pregnancy are labetalol, alpha-methyldopa and hydralazine. For monitoring of pregnancy, serial ultrasound for fetal growth assessment, umbilical artery Doppler studies and biophysical profile assessment from 24 weeks of gestation is recommended. Risk of vasculitis flare is <5% in TA and may be managed by lowest possible dose of corticosteroids and azathioprine should be considered in few cases that might not respond to steroids. The presence of aortic regurgitation should encourage the use of antibiotic prophylaxis against endocarditis at the time of delivery. Aspirin may be used during pregnancy to prevent pre-eclampsia, although the benefit remains unproven.[25]

To conclude, TA is not a major contraindication for pregnancy in either Asian or Caucasian patients, as long as the disease is clinically stable. The disease usually does not worsen because of pregnancy, although it conveys substantial morbidity and hence requires close monitoring and a multidisciplinary approach.

MEDIUM SIZED VESSEL VASCULITIS

Polyarteritis nodosa and KD are rare vasculitis and few cases (<15) of pregnancy after diagnosis of PAN have been reported.[1,2,4] Few severe cases (<5) of PAN diagnosed during pregnancy have been reported. The disease is associated with risk of hypertension, preterm birth (50–100%) and fetal loss (0–25%). Poor maternal outcome with PAN diagnosed *de novo* during pregnancy; some with maternal death have been reported.[26] KD is a disease of childhood, usually not relapsing. Exceptional cases (<5) of KD, have been reported *de novo* during pregnancy or postpartum. Very few data on patients with childhood KD with coronary aneurysms who later become pregnant.[27,28] Gordon et al. reported 10 women with history of KD in childhood carried a total of 21 pregnancies to term.[29] No cardiovascular complications during labor despite important cardiovascular abnormalities in 4 of the 10 subjects. Pregnancy was complicated by pre-eclampsia and postpartum course by hemorrhage in one subject. 2 of the 21 newborns subsequently developed KD. Hence, pre-pregnancy counseling, women's current cardiovascular status and an increased genetic risk of KD in offspring borne to these mothers needs attention.

SMALL SIZED VESSEL VASCULITIS

The International CHCC 2012 formally adapted to the term ANCA-associated vasculitis for three disorders: (1) GPA (Wegner's), (2) MPA, and (3) EGPA, also known as Churg-Strauss syndrome.

Wegner's Granulomatosis

Wegner's granulomatosis or GPA is an uncommon, small vessel, necrotizing vasculitis, which usually affects the upper respiratory tract, lungs and the kidney. The disease peaks after the age of 40 and thus, pregnancies are uncommonly observed. Pagnoux et al. have reported 20 pregnancies in 12 women with systemic necrotizing vasculitis and two life-threatening complications were noted in women with wegener's granulomatosis (WG).[13] One WG patient had vasculitis related renal damage and developed thrombotic microangiopathy associated renal impairment at 32 weeks and another patient had severe pneumonia at 37 weeks. Apart from this, about 40 pregnancies have been reported in WG patients with 41% of them ending in preterm delivery.[3,30-33] When WG was in remission, complications or vasculitis flares occurred in only 25% of the pregnancies. Conversely, outcomes were poorer when the pregnancies stared during active WG and some of them ending in miscarriage or therapeutic abortion or even maternal death. Kayatas et al. have reported subglottic stenosis as an important complication in pregnancy with WG and in these patients general anesthesia should not be preferred due to probability of difficult intubation.[34]

Treatment of disease relapse during pregnancy depends on the extent of disease and its manifestations. For features limited to upper airways, antibiotics, local treatment and low dose prednisone is recommended. Systemic manifestations require more aggressive treatment with high dose oral prednisone (1 mg/kg) or IV pulse methylprednisolone 0.5–1 g daily for three consecutive days. In case of insufficient response to corticosteroids, azathioprine should be started. In the presence of life-threatening manifestations during second or 3rd trimester of pregnancy cyclophosphamide may be given.

Microscopic Polyangiitis

Microscopic polyangiitis is a systemic, AAV and was initially recognized as a subset of PAN from which it may be difficult to distinguish. Unlike PAN, patients with MPA can develop severe renal disease and pulmonary hemorrhage. Only four case reports have been described in literature on pregnancy with MPA.

In 2011, Pagnoux et al. have reported two pregnancies in one patient with MPA, the first pregnancy ended up in miscarriage at 6 weeks and in the second pregnancy in the same patient had a good outcome with vaginal delivery at 39 weeks of gestation.[13] Two other case reports, on by Cetinkaya et al. described a patient at 16 weeks of gestation, treated with high dose methylprednisolone and cyclophosphamide but died due to pulmonary infection.[35] Milne et al. reported another case in whom MPA occurred at 24 weeks period of gestation with a good outcome.[36]

Churg-Strauss Syndrome

Churg-Strauss syndrome also known as eosinophilic granulomatosis with polyangiitis is a vasculitis of medium and small sized muscular arteries. The vasculitis classically involves arteries of the lung and skin, but it may be generalized. Extravascular granulomas and hypereosinophilia, occurring in patients with asthma and allergic rhinitis can be seen in these patients. The ACR has formulated 6 criteria for diagnosis of EGPA which are as follows:

1. Asthma (a history of wheeze or finding of diffuse high pitched wheezes on expiration)
2. Eosinophilia of >10% on differential white blood cell count
3. Mononeuropathy or polyneuropathy
4. Migratory or transient pulmonary opacities detected radiographically
5. Paranasal sinus abnormality
6. Biopsy containing a blood vessel showing accumulation of eosinophils in extravascular areas.

The presence of four or more of these criteria is usually diagnostic of EGPA. 21 pregnancies have been reported in literature, 19 of them concluding in a healthy offspring.[13,32,37-39] One twin pregnancy among them was complicated by transient maternal cardiac failure at 32 weeks. Maternal complications are mainly due to background asthma flare and cardiac damage.

Pre-eclampsia is seen in <5% while prematurity in about 10–40% and low birth weight in about 25% of pregnancies. Patients with disease onset during pregnancy had a very poor prognosis.[38,39] Treatment of CSS relapses during pregnancy consists of prednisone, where dose has to be adjusted according to severity of manifestations. Special care should be taken in monitoring bronchospasm during pregnancy and postpartum.

Behçet's Disease

Behçet's disease is a chronic, multisystemic inflammatory process characterized by recurrent oral and genital ulcers, ocular, gastrointestinal, neurological manifestations and thrombosis. The average age at disease onset is 20–30 years up to 60% of patients with BD report some improvement in pregnancy (but up to 30% can experience relapse, which can be severe).[40,41] Risk of preterm birth and intrauterine growth restriction are low (<5%). Complications which can occur especially around delivery are venous thrombosis (including cerebral, deep vein thrombosis, ovarian). Spectrum of disease and severity are wide, published data on pregnancy with poor outcomes are seen in patients with severe form of disease. Noel et al. have reported that BD seems to improve during pregnancy especially in patients treated with colchicine. The overall rate of complications during pregnancy was 15.8% which included miscarriage, low platelet count, elevated liver enzymes, hemolysis and immune thrombocytopenia.[42] Rare cases of minor and transient neonatal Behçet's, like disease (oral aphthous lesions) have been reported.[43] Treatment with colchicine, corticosteroids can be safely used in pregnancy without teratogenic risk. These medications taken before pregnancy, usually for remission maintenance, should not be stopped abruptly so as to limit the risk of disease flare. Enoxaparin may be used, where there is a risk of thrombosis. New drugs used in the treatment of BD are infliximab and tacrolimus. Their safety in pregnancy needs further evaluation, however, the few case reports in literature have not shown any teratogenic potential.[44-47]

SUMMARY

The incidence of vasculitis in women of childbearing age is low but prepregnancy diagnosis, planning of conception and multidisciplinary approach are associated with good outcomes. From the available data, most pregnancies in vasculitis have favorable outcomes for both the mother and the newborn. Pregnancy should be planned when the vasculitis is in remission and with no or little organ damage, off treatment or with drugs compatible with pregnancy. Pregnant patients must be monitored by physicians, rheumatologists including perinatologists (maternal-fetal medicine subspecialists) with experience in vasculitis and high-risk pregnancies.

CEREBRAL VASCULAR COMPLICATIONS

The other vascular complications apart from vasculitis in pregnancy are very rare and may be (1) aneurysmal subarachnoid hemorrhage, (2) cerebral AVM rupture. These two cerebral vascular conditions can present as subarachnoid hemorrhage or as hemorrhagic stroke both in pregnancy and puerperium. Pregnancy is a recognized risk factor for aneurysmal subarachnoid hemorrhage. Controversy exists regarding AVM and risk of hemorrhage in pregnancy. Bateman et al. found that pregnancy did not increase AVM bleed rates, but risk of intracranial hemorrhage was increased during the postpartum period.[48] A large retrospective study from Beijing Tiantan Hospital reported an annual AVM hemorrhage rate of 3.11% during pregnancy and puerperium. There was no increased risk of hemorrhage found in patients with cerebral AVM during pregnancy and puerperium and therefore this study did not advise against pregnancy in women with intracranial AVM.[49]

- Aneurysmal subarachnoid hemorrhage: pregnancy and in particular the puerperium are associated with an increased risk of intracerebral hemorrhage. The two most common causes of this bleed are eclampsia and ruptured vascular malformations. Telling the difference between eclampsia and cerebral hemorrhage due to aneurysmal rupture can prove to be difficult. The clinical features closely resemble and may be headache, seizures, systemic hypertension and altered consciousness. The confirmation of diagnosis is made with neuroimaging (CT scan, MRI and cerebral angiography). When CT and MR images are negative and clinical findings are very suggestive of subarachnoid hemorrhage, lumbar puncture should be performed
- Management: in pregnant women management is multidisciplinary (intensivist, neurosurgeon, neuro-radiologist, obstetrician, neonatologist). It is very important to obtain a prompt neurosurgical consultation and treatment of patient in a tertiary center with a team approach. For pregnancy management, it is better to perform cesarean section before neurosurgical treatment of aneurysm except in early pregnancy when the patient is treated like not pregnant. In these cases aneurysm is successfully clipped and the pregnancy is allowed to progress to term and vaginal delivery is preferred by most clinicians.[50] Cesarean section would be indicated in several circumstances, like when the clinical state of the mother is severe (coma, brainstem damage), if the aneurysm is diagnosed at term in labor, if the interval between the neurosurgical treatment of aneurysm and labor is less than 8 days.[50] Neurosurgical treatment can be surgical clipping of the aneurysm and endovascular coil treatment. Several studies in the last decade have established the efficacy and safety of endovascular coiling in treatment of cerebral aneurysms[51,52]
- Cerebral AVM rupture: women with an AVM face a 3.5% risk of hemorrhage during pregnancy. Pregnancy per se does not significantly increase the rate of first cerebral hemorrhage from an AVM. Therefore, pregnancy is not a risk factor for hemorrhage in women without a previous hemorrhage.[53] Another large retrospective study from Tiantan Hospital Beijing found no increased risk of hemorrhage in patients with cerebral AVM during pregnancy and the puerperium and therefore would not advise against pregnancy in women with AVM.[49] Predictors of hemorrhage in patients with untreated cerebral AVM's are age, AVM location and deep venous drainage. Although most studies show no increased risk of AVM rupture during pregnancy and puerperium but AVM rupture is seen more frequently in the late gestational age. This may be correlated with the more extensive changes of hemodynamic parameters, coagulative function and vessel wall in the 3rd trimester of pregnancy.

Spetzler and Martin proposed a simple and broadly applicable grading system to predict risk of morbidity and mortality attending the operative treatment of AVM's.[54] The lesion is graded on the basis of size, pattern of venous drainage and neurological eloquence of the adjacent brain. All AVMs fall into one of the six grades. Low grade AVMs (I, II, III), high grade AVMs (IV, V) and grade VI, lesions are essentially inoperable AVMs. Timely and accurate diagnosis of intracranial AVM is of utmost importance. At present DSA is the gold standard in diagnosing AVM and CT scan is the preferred method of diagnosing intracranial hemorrhage. Several studies have indicated that the effective radiation dose to fetus during DSA was very small and the radiation exposure can be minimized with lead shielding of the abdomen and pelvis.[55,56] The radiation dose to the fetus from CT and DSA under lead shielding might be small, especially during middle to late pregnancy but further studies are needed to confirm this.

At present, there is no class I or II evidence to guide the treatment of intracranial AVM in women during pregnancy. For patients with Spetzler-Martin grade V or VI, conservative management was preferred because of very high morbidity and mortality associated with operating these lesions.[49] For patients with grade I to IV AVM, urgent surgical evacuation of the intracranial hematoma and resection of AVM should be performed if signs of brainstem herniation occur. For patients of later pregnancy, surgical intervention can be performed after cesarean section.[49] The other treatment modalities are embolization and gamma knife radiotherapy.[57]

AVM rupture usually occurs in late gestational age and more attention should be provided to these patients during mid to late pregnancy. CT scan and DSA are needed for diagnostic evaluation of AVM. Treatment modalities for AVM are surgical, embolization and gamma knife radiotherapy which still need further evidence for standardization of treatment during pregnancy.

Aneurysms of the Aorta and its Branches

An aneurysm is the presence of a focal dilatation of a vessel wall, in direct communication with the lumen, due to congenital or acquired weakness in the vessel wall. Dissection is present when an intimal rear occurs in a major vessel, allowing formation of an aneurysm.

Pathophysiology

All of the following factors have been reported to play a role in the risk of aortic dissection and rupture of arterial aneurysms during pregnancy:

- Congenital disorders including Marfan syndrome, Ehlers-Danlos syndrome, aortic coarctation, and the mucopolysaccharidoses
- Takayasu's arteritis, a progressive granulomatous vaso-occlusive disorder of unknown etiology[58]
- Trauma or infection
- Increased wall pressure in the proximal aorta, especially in late pregnancy, which may occur due to cardiovascular changes associated with pregnancy:[59]
  - Increased cardiac output
  - Increased stroke volume
  - Increased blood volume
- Changes in progesterone concentrations may alter vessel wall integrity.

In the absence of Marfan syndrome or Ehlers-Danlos syndrome, arterial aneurysms are uncommon in people less than 40 years of age. The most common times for presentation of dissection or rupture during pregnancy are the 3rd trimester, labor, or the puerperium.

Evaluation

Common symptoms of aortic aneurysm rupture or dissection include:

- Chest or abdominal pain, often described as severe or "tearing"
- Nausea, vomiting, lightheadedness, and other vasovagal symptoms
- Pain or tingling in extremities.

The rupture of a splenic artery aneurysm will be associated with severe left upper quadrant pain.[60]

Physical findings with dissection or ruptured aneurysm may include:

- Tachycardia, hypotension or hypertension
- Anxiety
- Decreased pulses and BP differences between extremities.

Various imaging modalities are used to diagnose dissection and aneurysm rupture. As this condition threatens maternal and fetal well-being, timely imaging is indicated, and modalities that utilize ionizing radiation are not contraindicated.[59]

- Chest radiography may show mediastinal widening
- Echocardiography will demonstrate abnormalities of the thoracic aorta
- Abdominal ultrasound does not require radiation, but in late pregnancy the gravid uterus may impede imaging of the abdominal aorta and its branches
- Computed tomography of the chest (with shielding of the uterus) results in little fetal radiation exposure.

Treatment

Immediate management should be aimed at maternal stabilization, including aggressive treatment of hypertension if present; administration oxygen by face mask to optimize placental gas exchange; obtaining blood products for possible transfusion; and close maternal and fetal observation.

When aortic dissection is diagnosed before the 3rd trimester, surgical repair should be performed, but if the diagnosis is made in the 3rd trimester and the dissection is stable, expectant management is preferred. Repair should be undertaken after cesarean delivery, either at or near term, or if maternal condition worsens.[61] Splenectomy is the treatment of choice for a ruptured splenic artery aneurysm.

Complications

- Aortic rupture is frequently catastrophic and mortality is high; as many as 50% of aortic dissections in women younger than 40 occur during pregnancy.[62]
- Splenic artery aneurysms are associated with 75% maternal mortality and 95% fetal mortality; combined maternal and fetal survival is rare.[60]
- Renal artery aneurysms are rare. Rupture leads to retroperitoneal hemorrhage and is associated with a high mortality rate. This entity should be considered among the causes of retroperitoneal hemorrhage in pregnancy.[63]

ARTIFICIAL HEART VALVES

Another serious vascular complication is thrombosis of an artificial heart valve. The topic of artificial heart valves is emphasized here due to the high propensity to thromboembolism and the competing needs for maternal and fetal health. Pregnant women with mechanical prosthetic heart valves are at significant risk for thromboembolism (approximately 25%) and death (5%).[64]

In addition, pregnant women with bioprostheses who have atrial fibrillation and a large left atrium require anticoagulation.[65]

There is strong evidence that warfarin is most teratogenic during the 6th–12th week of gestation[66], whereas use of warfarin late in pregnancy predisposes to fetal intracranial hemorrhage. The risk for pregnancy complications in patients treated with sodium warfarin is higher when the mean daily dose exceeds 5 mg daily.[67]

Low molecular weight heparin should not be used for anticoagulation in patients with mechanical prosthetic heart valves, as reports of thrombosis and stroke in both pregnant and nonpregnant women have been published.[68]

In a systematic review of the literature of warfarin use (garget INR 2.5–3.0) throughout gestation, the risk of thrombosis was reasonably low (3.9%), but a 6.4% incidence of congenital fetal anomalies and a 1.8% risk of maternal death were reported.[64] Alternatively, adjusted-dose unfractionated heparin (UFH) [between weeks 6 and 12 of pregnancy, target a partial thromboplastin time (PTT) is not stated] followed by warfarin (target INR 2.5–3.0) thereafter with or without heparin and near term, was associated with a 9.2% incidence of thrombosis, a 3.4 incidence of congenital anomalies (0% if heparin was started before week 6), and a 4.2% incidence of maternal death.[64] While data do not exist from clinical trials to determine the optimal regimen to minimize both maternal and fetal risks, the following regimen could be considered:

- Adjusted dose UFH every 12 hours to prolong the 6-hour postinjection a PTT at 2.0–2.5 times baseline
- Conversion to warfarin for weeks 13–35 (target INR 2.5–3.0)
- Adjusted does unaccounted for gas (UFG) thereafter until warfarin is reinitiated following delivery[66]
- The addition of low-dose aspirin should be considered in high-risk women with prosthetic heart valves.[69]

REFERENCES

1. Pagnoux C, Mahendira D, Laskin CA. Fertility and pregnancy in vasculitis. Best Pract Res Clin Rheumatol. 2013;27(1):79-94.
2. Pagnoux C. Pregnancy and vasculitides. Presse Med. 2008;37(11):1657-65.
3. Tuin J, Sanders JS, de Joode AA, Stegeman CA. Pregnancy in women diagnosed with antineutrophil cytoplasmic antibody-associated vasculitis: outcome for the mother and the child. Arthritis Care and Res (Hoboken). 2012;64(4):539-45.
4. Gatto M, Iaccarino L, Canona M, Zen M, Nalotto L, Ramonda R, et al. Pregnancy and vasculitis: a systematic review of the literature. Autoimmun Rev. 2012;11(6-7):A447-59.
5. Suri V, Aggarwal N, Keepanasseril A, Chopra S, Viyayvergiya R, Jain S. Pregnancy and Takayasu arteritis: a single centre experience from North India. J Obstet Gynaecol Res. 2010;36(3):519-24.
6. Watts RA, Scott DG. Recent developments in the classification and assessment of vasculitis. Best Pract Res Clin Rehumatol. 2009;23(3):429-43.
7. Hunder GG, Arend WP, Bloch DA, Calabrese LH, Fauci AS, Fries JF, et al. The American College of Rheumatology 1990 criteria for the classification of vasculitis. Introduction. Arthritis Rheum. 1990;33(8):1065-7.
8. Jennette JC, Falk RJ, Bacon PA, Basu N, Cid MC, Ferrario F, et al. 2012 revised International Chapel Hill Consensus Conference Nomenclature of Vasculitides. Arthritis Rehum. 2013;65(1):1-11.
9. Doria A, Bajocchi G, Tonon M, Salvarani C. Pre-pregnancy counselling of patients with vasculitis. Rheumatology (Oxford). 2008;47 (Suppl 3):iii13-15.
10. Noel N, Wechsler B, Nizard J, Costedoat-Chalumeau N, Boutin du LT, Dommergues M, et al. Behcet's disease and pregnancy. Arthritis Rheum. 2013;65(9):2450-6.
11. Doria A, Laccarino L, Ghirardello A, Arienti S, Zampieri S, Rampudda ME, et al. Rare autoimmune rheumatic illnesses during pregnancy. Systemic sclerosis, polymyositis/dermatomyositis and vasculitis. Z Rheumatol. 2006;65(3):200-8.
12. Connolly JO, Lanham JG, Partridge MR. Fulminant pregnancy-related Churg-Strauss syndrome. Br J Rheumatol. 1994;33(8):776-7.
13. Pagnoux C, Le Guern V, Goffinet F, Diot E, Limal N, Pannier E, et al. Pregnancies in systemic necrotizing vasculitides: report of 12 women and their 20 pregnancies. Rheumatology (Oxford). 2011;50(5):953-61.
14. Ostensen M. Treatment with immunosuppressive and disease modifying drugs during pregnancy and lactation. Am J Reprod Immunol. 1992;28(3-4):148-52.
15. Ostensen M, Lockshin M, Doria A, Valensini G, Meroni P, Gordon C, et al. Update on safety during pregnancy of biological agents and some immunosuppressive anti-rheumatic drugs. Rheumatology (Oxford). 2008;47(Supple 3):iii28-31.
16. Elefant E, Cournot MP, Assari F, Vauzelle C. Immunosuppressants for autoimmune diseases and pregnancy. Presse Med. 2008;37(11):1620-6.
17. Marsal S, Falgá C, Simeon CP, Vilardell M, Bosch JA. Behcet's disease and pregnancy relationship study. Br J Rheumat. 1997;36(2):234-8.
18. Ishikawa K, Matsuura S. Occlusive thromboaortopathy (Takayasu's disease) and pregnancy. Clinical course and management of 33 pregnancies and deliveries. Am J Cardiol. 1982;50(6):1293-300.
19. Aso T, Abe S, Yaguchi T. Clinical gynecologic features of pregnancy in Takayasu arteritis. Heart Vessels Suppl. 1992;7:125-32.
20. Hidaka N, Yamanaka Y, Fujita Y, Fukushima K, Wake N. Clinical manifestations of pregnancy in patients with Takayasu arteritis: experience from a single tertiary center. Arch Gynecol Obstet. 2012;285(2):377-85.
21. Sharma BK, Jain S, Vasishta K. Outcome of pregnancy in Takayasu arteritis. Int J Cardiol. 2000;75(Suppl 1):S159-62.
22. Papantoniou N, Katsoulis I, Papageorgiou I, Antsaklis A. Takayasu arteritis in pregnancy: safe management options in antenatal care. Case report. Fetal Diagn Ther. 2007;22(6):449-51.
23. Mandal D, Mandal S, Dattaray C, Banerjee D, Ghosh P, Ghosh A, et al. Takayasu arteritis in pregnancy: an analysis from eastern India. Arch Gynecol Obstet. 2012;285(3):567-71.
24. Dutta B, Pandey R, Darlong V, Garg R. Low-dose spinal anaesthesia for a parturient with Takayasu's arteritis undergoing emergency caesarean section. Singapore Med J. 2010;51(6);e111-3.
25. Roberge S, Giguère Y, Villa P, Nicolaides K, Vainio M, Forest JC, et al. Early administration of low-dose aspirin for the prevention of severe and mild preeclampsia: a systematic review and meta-analysis. Am J Perinatol. 2012;29(7):551-6.
26. Clowse ME, Richeson RL, Pieper C, Merkel PA for the VCRC. Pregnancy in men and women with vasculitis. Arthritis and Rheumatism. 2011;63(Suppl 10):1537.
27. Tsuda E, Ishihara Y, Kawamata K, Tsukano S, Negi R, Echigo S, et al. Pregnancy and delivery in patients with coronary artery lesions caused by Kawasaki disease. Heart. 2005;91(11):1481-2.
28. Fason JT, Fry YW, Smith D. Kawasaki disease in a postpartum patient. J Natl Med Assoc. 2004;96(11):1499-502.

29. Gordon CT, Jimenez-Fernandez S, Daniels LB, Kahn AM, Tarsa M, Matsubara T, et al. Pregnancy in women with history of Kawasaki disease: management and outcomes. BJOG. 2014;121(11):1431-8.
30. Auzary C, Huong DT, Wechsler B, Vauthier-Brouzes D, Piette JC. Pregnancy in patients with Wegener's granulomatosis: report of five cases in three women. Ann Rheum Dis. 2000;59(10):800-4.
31. Dayoan ES, Dimen LL, Boylen CT. Successful treatment of Wegener's granulomatosis during pregnancy; a case report and review of medical literature. Chest. 1998;113(3):836-8.
32. Lima F, Buchanan N, Froes L, Kerslake S, Khamashta MA, Hughes GR. Pregnancy in granulomatous vasculitis. Ann Rheum Dis. 1995;54(7):604-6.
33. Bessias N, Moulakakis KG, Lioupis C, Bakogiannis K, Sfyroeras G, Kakaletri K, et al. Wegener's granulomatosis presenting during pregnancy with acute limb ischemia. J Vasc Surg. 2005;42(4):800-4.
34. Kayatas S, Asoglu MR, Selcuk S, Sargin MA. Pregnancy in a patient with Wegener's granulomatosis: a case report. Bull NYU Hosp Jt Dis. 2012;70(2):127-9.
35. Cetinkaya R, Odabas AR, Gursan N, Selcuk Y, Erdogan F, Keles M, et al. Microscopic polyangiitis in a pregnant woman. South Med J. 2002;95(12):1441-3.
36. Milne KL, Stanley KP, Temple RC, Barker TH, Ross CN. Microscopic polyangiitis: first report of a case with onset during pregnancy. Nephrol Dial Transplant. 2004;19(1):234-7.
37. Debby A, Tanay A, Zakut H. Allergic granulomatosis and angiitis (Churg-Strauss vasculitis) in pregnancy. Int Arch Allergy Immunol. 1993;102(3):307-8.
38. Connolly JO, Lanham JG, Partridge MR. Fulminant pregnancy-related Churg-Strauss syndrome. Br J Rheumatol. 1994;33(8):776-7.
39. Hiyama J, Shioto Y, Marukawa M, Horita N, Kanehisa Y, Ono T, et al. Churg-Strauss syndrome associated with pregnancy. Intern Med. 2000;39(11):985-90.
40. Marsal S, Falgá C, Simeon CP, Vilardell M, Bosch JA. Behcet's disease and pregnancy relationship study. Br J Rheumatol. 1997;36(2):234-8.
41. Kale A, Akyildiz L, Akdeniz N, Kale E. Pregnancy complicated by superior vena cava thrombosis and pulmonary embolism in a patient with Behcet disease and the use of heparin for treatment. Saudi Med J. 2006;27(1):95-7.
42. Noel N, Wechsler B, Nizard J, Costedoat-Chalumeau N, Bautin du LT, Dommergues M, et al. Behcet's disease and pregnancy. Arthritis Rheum. 2013;65(9):2450-6.
43. Fain O, Mathieu E, Lachassinne E, Buisson P, Bodemer C, Gaudelus J, et al. Neonatal Behcet's disease. Am J Med. 1995;98(3):310-1.
44. Takayama K, Ishikawa S, Enoki T, Kojima T, Takeuchi M. Successful treatment with infliximab for Behcet disease during pregnancy. Ocul Immunol Inflamm. 2013;21(4):321-3.
45. Mainini G, Di Donna MC, Esposito E, Ercolano S, Correa R, Stradella L, et al. Pregnancy management in Behcet's disease treated with uninterrupted infliximab. Report of a case with fetal growth restriction and mini-review of the literature. Clin Exp Obstet Gynecol. 2014;41(2):205-7.
46. Evereklioglu C. Current concepts in the etiology and treatment of Behcet disease. Surv Opthalmol. 2005;50(4):297-350.
47. Kainz A, Harabacz I, Cowlrick IS, Gadgil S, Hagiwara D. Analysis of 100 pregnancy outcomes in women treated systemically with tacrolimus. Transpl Int. 2000;13 (Suppl 1):S299-300.
48. Bateman BT, Schumacher HC, Bushnell CD, Pile-Spellman J, Simpson LL, Sacco RL, et al. Intracerebral hemorrhage in pregnancy: frequency, risk factors, and outcome. Neurology. 2006;67(3):424-9.
49. Liu XJ, Wang S, Zhao YL, Teo M, Guo P, Zhang D, et al. Risk of cerebral arteriovenous malformation rupture during pregnancy and puerperium. Neurology. 2014;82(20):1798-803.
50. Mosiewicz A, Jakiel G, Janusz W, Markiewicz P. Treatment of intracranial aneurysms in pregnancy. Ginokol Pol. 2001;72(2):86-92.
51. Meyers PM, Halbach VV, Malek AM, Phatouros CC, Dowd CF, Lawton MT, et al. Endovascular treatment of cerebral artery aneurysms during pregnancy: repot of three cases. AJNR Am J Neuroradiol. 2000;21(7);1306-11.
52. Shahabi S, Tecco L, Jani J, Pirotte B, Rodesch G, Baurain M, et al. Management of a ruptured basilar artery aneurysm during pregnancy. Acta Chir Belg. 2001;101(4):193-5.
53. Horton JC, Chambers WA, Lyons SL, Adams RD, Kjellberg RN. Pregnancy and the risk of hemorrhage from cerebral arteriovenous malformations. Neurosurgery. 1990;27(6):867-71.
54. Spetzler RF, Martin NA. A proposed grading system for arteriovenous malformations. J Neurosurg. 1986; 65(4):476-83.
55. Sanchez-Ramos L, Chami YG, Bass TA, DelValle GO, Adair CD. Myocardial infarction during pregnancy: management with transluminal coronary angioplasty and metallic intracoronary stents. Am J Obstet Gynecol. 1994;171(5):1392-3.
56. Mc Collough CH, Schueler BA, Atwell TD, Braun NN, Regner DM, Brown DL, et al. Radiation exposure and pregnancy: when should we be concerned? Radiographics. 2007; 27(4):909-17.
57. Deruty R, Pelissou-Guyotat I, Mottolese C, Bascoulergue Y, Amat D. The combined management of cerebral arteriovenous malformations. Experience with 100 cases and review of literature. Acta Neurochir (Wien). 1993;123(3-4):101-12.
58. Vanoli M, Daina E, Salvarani C, Sabbadini MG, Rossi C, Bacchiani G, et al. Takayasu's arteritis: A study of 104 Italian patients. Arthritis Rheum. 2005;53(1):100-7.
59. Robinson R. Aortic aneurysm in pregnancy: a case study. Dimens Crit Care Nurs. 2005;24(1):21-4.
60. Hillemanns P, Knitza R, Müller-H cker J. Rupture of splenic artery aneurysm in a pregnant patient with portal hypertension. Am J Obstet Gynecol. 1996;174(5):1665-6.
61. Zeebregts CJ, Schepens MA, Hameeteman TM, Morshuis WJ, de la Rivière AB. Acute aortic dissection complicating pregnancy. Ann Thorac Surg. 1997;64(5):1345-8.
62. Williams GM, Gott VL, Brawley RK, Schauble JF, Labs JD. Aortic disease associated with pregnancy. J Vasc Surg. 1988;8(4):470-5.
63. Yang JC, Hye RJ. Ruptured renal artery aneurysm during pregnancy. Ann Vasc Surg. 1996;10(4):370-2.
64. Chan WS, Anand D, Ginsberg JS. Anticoagulation of pregnant women with mechanical heart valves: a systematic review of the literature. Arch Intern Med. 2000;160(2):191-6.
65. Salazar E, Izaguirre R, Verdejao J, Mutchinick O. Failure of adjusted doses of subcutaneous heparin to prevent thromboembolic phenomena in pregnant patients with mechanical cardiac valve prostheses. J Am Coll Cardiol. 1996;27(7):1698-703.
66. Reimold SC, Rutherford JD. Valvular heart disease in pregnancy. N Engl J Med. 2003;349(1):52-9.
67. Cotrufo M, De Feo M, De Santo LS, Romano G, Della Corte A, Renzulli A, et al. Risk of warfarin during pregnancy with mechanical valve prostheses. Obstet Gynecol. 2002;99(1):35-40.
68. Rowan JA, McCowan LM, Raudkivi PJ, North RA. Enoxaparin treatment in women with mechanical heart valves during pregnancy. Am J Obstet Gynecol. 2001;185(3):633-7.
69. Bates SM, Greet IA, Hirsh J, Ginsberg JS. Use of antithrombotic agents during pregnancy: the Seventh ACCP Conference on Antithrombotic and Thrombolytic Therapy. Chest. 2004;126 (3 Suppl):627S-644S.

CHAPTER 58

Thromboembolic Disorders

Pratik Tambe, Pooja K Bandekar

INTRODUCTION

The risk of venous thrombosis and pulmonary embolism in otherwise healthy women is considered highest during pregnancy and puerperium.

The risk of pulmonary embolism has been estimated to be as much as 4- to 6-fold higher during pregnancy.[1,2] The incidence of all thromboembolic events averages about 1 per 1000 pregnancies and about an equal number are identified antepartum and in the puerperium. The frequency of venous thromboembolic disease during the puerperium has decreased remarkably as early ambulation has become more widely practiced. Pulmonary thromboembolism still remains a leading cause of maternal death in the United States.

PATHOPHYSIOLOGY

In 1856, Rudolf Virchow postulated the conditions that predispose to the development of venous thrombosis. The Virchow's Triad consists of:

- Stasis.
- Local trauma to the vessel wall.
- Hypercoagulability.

The risk for each increases during normal pregnancy. Compression of the pelvic veins and the inferior vena cava by the enlarging uterus renders the venous system of the lower extremities particularly vulnerable to stasis. This stasis is the most constant predisposing risk factor for venous thrombosis. Venous stasis and delivery may also contribute to endothelial cell injury. Also, marked increase in the synthesis of most clotting factors during pregnancy favor coagulation.

As seen in Box 1, there are a number of risk factors associated with an increased risk of developing thromboembolism during pregnancy. The risk approximately doubled

Box 1: Risk factors for development of thromboembolism[3]

Risk factor

Obstetrical

- Cesarean delivery
- Diabetes
- Hemorrhage and anemia
- Hyperemesis
- Immobility: prolonged bed rest
- Multifetal gestation

Some risk factors associated with an increased risk for thromboembolism

- Multiparity
- Pre-eclampsia
- Puerperal infection

General

- Age 35 years or older
- Cancer
- Connective-tissue disease
- Dehydration
- Immobility: long-distance travel
- Infection and inflammatory disease
- Myeloproliferative disease
- Nephrotic syndrome
- Obesity
- Oral contraceptive use
- Orthopedic surgery
- Paraplegia
- Prior thromboembolism
- Sickle cell disease
- Smoking
- Thrombophilia

in women with multifetal gestation, anemia, hyperemesis, hemorrhage and cesarean delivery. The risk is far greater in pregnancies complicated by postpartum infection. It is also significantly increased with maternal body mass index (BMI) >30 kg/m^2 or with multiparity.

The likelihood of developing thrombosis during pregnancy is especially increased in women with certain genetic risk factors. The American College of Chest Physicians (ACCP) now estimates that approximately half of pregnant women with thrombosis have an identifiable underlying genetic disorder. Importantly, 50–60% of patients with a hereditary basis for thrombosis probably do not experience a thrombotic event until one of the risk factors is present.[4]

THROMBOPHILIAS

Several important regulatory proteins act as inhibitors in the coagulation cascade. Inherited or acquired deficiencies of these inhibitory proteins are collectively referred to as thrombophilias (Table 1). These can lead to hypercoagulability and recurrent venous thromboembolism. Although these disorders are collectively present in about 15% of the European population, they are responsible for more than 50% of all thromboembolic events.[5]

The current recommendation of the American Academy of Pediatrics (AAP) and the American College of Obstetricians and Gynecologists (ACOG)[3] is that women with a personal or family history of venous thromboembolic disease be evaluated for hereditary and acquired thrombophilic disorders.

Antithrombin Deficiency (Fig. 1)

Antithrombin III, is one of the most important inhibitors of thrombin in clot formation. Antithrombin functions as a natural anticoagulant by binding to, and inactivating thrombin and the activated coagulation factors IXa, Xa, XIa and XIIa according to Franchini and coworkers.[6] Antithrombin deficiency may result from numerous mutations that are almost always autosomal dominant. Homozygous antithrombin III deficiency is lethal.[7]

Antithrombin III deficiency is rare. It affects about 1 in 5000 individuals and is the most thrombogenic of the heritable coagulopathies. The risk of thrombosis during pregnancy among antithrombin III deficient women without a personal or family history is 3–7% and it is 11–40% with such a history.[5] It is recommended that these women be treated during pregnancy with heparin regardless of whether a prior thrombosis has occurred.

Protein C Deficiency (Fig. 1)

When thrombin is bound to thrombomodulin on endothelial cells of small vessels, its procoagulant activities are neutralized. It also activates protein C, a natural anticoagulant, which in the presence of protein S controls thrombin generation in part by inactivating factors Va and VIIIa. Activated protein C also inhibits the synthesis of plasminogen activator inhibitor 1.

More than 160 protein C gene mutations have been described. The prevalence of protein C deficiency is 2–3 per 1000 and inheritance is autosomal dominant. These prevalence estimates are associated with a 6- to 12-fold increased risk for venous thromboembolism.[5]

Protein S Deficiency (Fig. 1)

This circulating anticoagulant is activated by protein C to decrease thrombin generation. Protein S may be caused by more than 130 different mutations with a prevalence of about

TABLE 1: Inherited thrombophilias[3]

Inherited thrombophilias and their association with venous thromboembolism (VTE) in pregnancy			
Thrombophilia	Percentage of VTE during pregnancy	Relative risk (95% CI) of VTE during pregnancy	Probability of VTE during pregnancy and postpartum in patients without personal or family history (%)
Factor V Leiden (homozygous)	<1	25.4 (8.8–66)	1.5
Factor V Leiden (heterozygous)	44	6.9 (3.3–15.2)	0.26
Prothrombin G20201A (homozygous)	<1	NA	2.8
Prothrombin G20201A (heterozygous)	17	9.5 (2.1–66.7)	0.37
Factor V Leiden and prothrombin G20201A (compound heterozygous)	<1	84 (19–369)	4.7
Hyperhomocysteinemia			
Antithrombin deficiency (heterozygous)	1–8	119 (N/A)	3–7.2
Protein S deficiency (heterozygous)	12.4	NA	<1–6.6
Protein C deficiency (heterozygous)	<14	13 (1.4–123)	0.8–1.7

2 per 1000. Protein S deficiency is measured by antigenically determined free, functional and total S levels. All three of these levels decline substantively during normal gestation, thus the diagnosis in pregnant women as well in those taking certain oral contraceptives is difficult. The detection of free protein S antigen levels of less than 55% in nonpregnant patients and less than 30% in pregnant women appears to most closely correlate with a mutated gene. Using such criteria, the prevalence of free protein S deficiency is low, 0.03–0.13% and its degree of thrombogenicity is modest.[5]

Activated Protein C Resistance (Factor V Leiden Mutation) (Fig. 1)

This is the most prevalent of the thrombophilic syndromes. This condition is characterized by resistance of plasma to the anticoagulant effects of activated protein C. A number of mutations have been described, but the most common is the factor V Leiden mutation, which is named after the city where it was first described. This mutation in the factor V protein retains its procoagulant activity and predisposes to thrombosis.

Heterozygous inheritance for factor V Leiden is the most common heritable thrombophilia. It is found in 3–15% of select European populations, 3% of African Americans and it is virtually absent in African blacks and Asians. The mutation is found in up to half of nonpregnant women with thromboembolic disease. Homozygous inheritance of two aberrant copies is rare and increases risk of thrombosis during pregnancy by almost 10-fold.[5]

Diagnosis is made in one of two ways. In the bio assay, resistance to activated protein C is measured. Activated protein C resistance can also be caused by antiphospholipid antibody syndrome. Resistance is normally increased after early pregnancy because of alterations in other coagulation proteins. Thus, during pregnancy, deoxyribonucleic acid (DNA) analysis for mutant factor V gene is used to confirm diagnosis. Hence, universal antenatal screening for the Leiden mutation and prophylaxis for carriers without a prior venous thromboembolism is not indicated and is not cost effective.

Prothrombin G20210A Mutation (Fig. 1)

This mutation in the prothrombin gene leads to excessive accumulation of prothrombin, which may then convert to thrombin. It is found in approximately 2% of white population and not at all found in the nonwhite population. Case control studies suggest that relative risk of thromboembolism is increased 3- to 15-fold during pregnancy. Homozygous patients and those who coinherit this mutation along with factor V Leiden mutation have an even greater risk of thromboembolism. The carriers of this mutation are candidates for life long anticoagulation after first thrombotic episode.

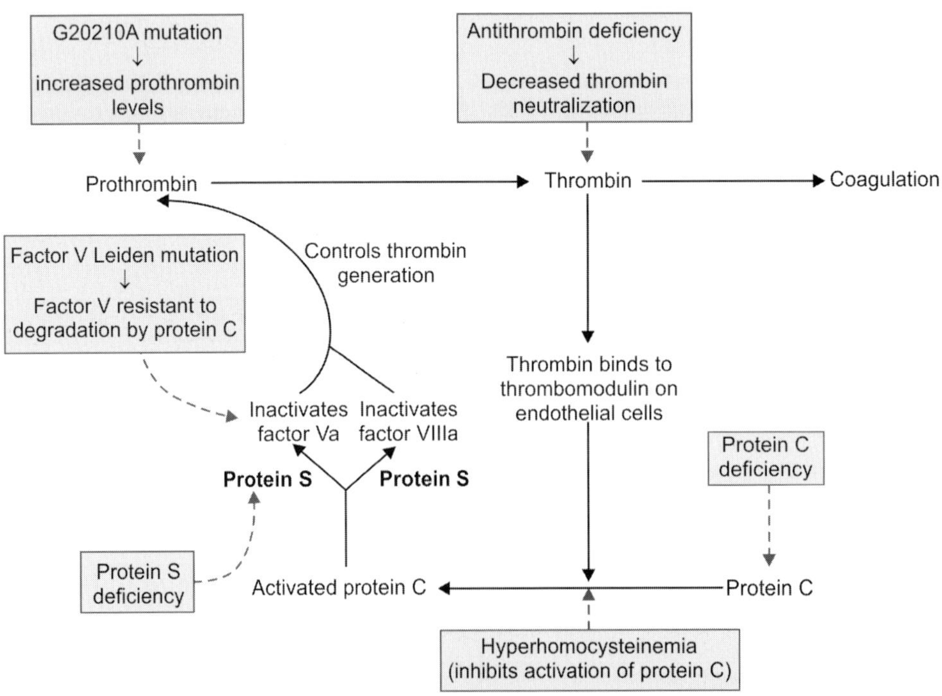

FIG. 1: Pathogenic cascade leading to thrombophilias.

Hyperhomocysteinemia (Fig. 1)

The most common cause of elevated homocysteine is the C667T thermolabile mutation of the enzyme 5, 10 methylene tetrahydrofolate reductase which has autosomal recessive inheritance. Kupferminc and coworkers found a homozygote prevalence of 8% in normally pregnant women.[8] Elevated levels of homocysteine may also result from deficiency of one of the several enzymes of methionine metabolism and from nutritional deficiencies of folic acid, vitamin B6 or vitamin B12. During normal pregnancy, mean homocysteine plasma concentrations are decreased. Thus, to make a diagnosis in pregnancy, Lockwood[5] recommends a fasting cut off level of > 12 μmol/L to define hyperhomocysteinemia.

The precise pathological mechanisms by which high level of homocysteine increases the risk of thromboembolism remains undefined. Possible pathways include decreased activation of protein C and interference of with ability of activated protein C to inactivate factor 5a. Although hyperhomocysteinemia is associated with an increased risk of venous thromboembolism in nonpregnant patients, it is unclear whether MTHFR C667T homozygotes have an increased risk during pregnancy. Physiologically lower homocysteine levels are seen during pregnancy. Also, most pregnant women take folic acid supplementation. Folic acid serves as a cofactor in the remethylation reaction of homocysteine to methionine. Hyperhomocysteinemia increases the lifetime risk of having a fetus with neural tube defect and premature atherosclerosis.

OTHER THROMBOPHILIA MUTATIONS

Protein Z Deficiency

This vitamin K dependant protein serves as a cofactor in activation of factor Xa. In nonpregnant patients, low levels of protein Z are associated with increased risk of thromboembolism.

Antiphospholipid Antibodies

These antibodies are detected in 2% of patients who have nontraumatic venous thrombosis. The antibodies are directed against cardiolipins or against phospholipid binding proteins, such as β-2 glycoprotein 1. They are commonly found in patients with systemic lupus erythematosus. Women with moderate to high levels of these antibodies may have antiphospholipid antibody syndrome which is defined by a number of clinical features, such as thromboembolism or obstetric complications:

- At least one otherwise unexplained fetal death at or beyond 10 weeks
- At least one preterm birth before 34 weeks
- At least three consecutive spontaneous abortions before 10 weeks.

In these patients, thromboembolism either venous or arterial involves lower extremities. The syndrome should also be considered in women with thromboses at unusual sites, such as portal, mesenteric, splenic, subclavian and cerebral veins.[4]

These antibodies are a predisposing factor for arterial thromboses. They may interfere with the normal function of phospholipids or phospholipid binding proteins involved in coagulation regulation, including prothrombin, protein C, Annexin 5 and tissue factor. These antibodies may promote thromboses through augmented platelet and/or complement.

Thrombophilia Prophylaxis

There are no randomized trials to guide prophylaxis to prevent recurrent adverse pregnancy outcome in women with any of the inherited thrombophilias. Empirical aspirin and/or low molecular weight heparin is recommended.[5]

Superficial Thrombophlebitis

Thrombosis limited strictly to the superficial veins of the saphenous system is treated with analgesia, elastic support and rest. If it does not subside soon or if deep venous involvement is suspected, appropriate diagnostic measures are performed. Heparin is given if deep venous involvement is confirmed. Superficial thrombophlebitis is typically seen in association with varicosities or indwelling intravenous catheter.

PULMONARY EMBOLISM

Although it causes about 10% of maternal deaths, pulmonary thromboembolism is relatively uncommon during pregnancy and the puerperium. The incidence averages about 1 in 7000 pregnancies. There is almost equal prevalence for antepartum and postpartum embolism; however, mortality is more for postpartum embolism. About 70% of women presenting with pulmonary embolism have associated clinical evidence of deep venous thrombosis. In women presenting with deep venous thrombosis, almost half will have silent pulmonary embolism.

Clinical Presentation

Common symptoms include:

- Dyspnea (82%)
- Chest pain (49%)
- Syncope (14%)
- Hemoptysis (7%)

Other predominant clinical findings include:
- Tachypnea
- Tachycardia
- Apprehension
- Accentuated pulmonic closure sound
- Rales and/or
- Friction rub.

Right axis deviation and T-wave inversion in the anterior leads may be evident on the electrocardiogram. On chest radiography, there may be loss of vascular markings in the region of lungs supplied by the obstructed artery. Although most women are hypoxemic, a normal arterial blood gas does not exclude pulmonary embolism. The alveolar–arterial oxygen tension difference is a more useful indicator of disease, as more than 86% of women with acute pulmonary embolism will have an alveolar–arterial difference of more than 20 mmHg.[9]

Even with massive pulmonary embolism, signs, symptoms and laboratory data to support the diagnosis may be deceptively nonspecific.

MASSIVE PULMONARY EMBOLISM

This is defined as embolism causing hemodynamic instability.[10] Acute mechanical obstruction of the pulmonary vasculature causes increased vascular resistance and pulmonary hypertension. Acute right ventricular dilatation follows. In otherwise healthy patients, significant pulmonary hypertension does not develop until 60–75% of pulmonary vascular tree is occluded. A circulatory collapse requires 75–80% obstruction. Most acutely symptomatic emboli are large and likely a saddle embolism. These are suspected when pulmonary artery pressure is substantively increased as estimated by echocardiography. If there is evidence of right ventricular dysfunction, the mortality rate approaches 25% compared to 1% without such dysfunction.[11] It is important in these cases to infuse crystalloids carefully and to support blood pressures with vasopressors. Oxygenation involves thrombolysis, filter placement or embolectomy.[10]

Diagnosis

It requires an initial high index of suspicion followed by objective testing. The current opinion of AAP and ACOG is that in contemporary practice, pulmonary embolism is commonly diagnosed with multidetector row spiral computed tomography (CT) pulmonary angiography.

Computed Tomographic Pulmonary Angiography

Multidetector spiral CT will replace pulmonary angiography as the gold standard for diagnosis of pulmonary embolism. Except in late pregnancy, fetal exposure is less than with ventilation/perfusion (V/Q) scanning. Also, better resolution allows detection of previously inaccessible smaller distal emboli that have uncertain clinical significance.

Ventilation Perfusion Scintigraphy: Lung Scan

It is less commonly used since past 5 years. It may be used if compression ultrasonography results are negative. The technique involves a small dose of radiotracers, such as intravenously administered -99m technetium macroaggregated albumin. There is negligible fetal radiation exposure. The scan may not provide a definite diagnosis because many other conditions may cause perfusion defects. Ventilation scans with inhaled xenon-133 or technetium-99m were added to perfusion scans to detect abnormal areas of ventilation in areas of normal perfusion, such as pneumonia or hypoventilation. However, a normal V/Q scan does not exclude pulmonary embolism.

Because of these uncertainties, the National Heart, Lung and Blood Institute commissioned the PIOPED, 1990: Prospective Investigations of Pulmonary Embolism Diagnosis to determine sensitivities and specificities of V/Q scan.

A low probability scan, combined with strong clinical impression that embolism is unlikely, makes the possibility of embolism, remote. Also normal and near normal scans make the diagnosis very unlikely. An intermediate scan is of no help in making diagnosis. Thus, V/Q scan combined with clinical assessment permits a noninvasive diagnosis or exclusion of pulmonary embolism for only a minority of patients. Two-thirds of nonpregnant women with a suspected pulmonary embolism have a nondiagnostic scan and require additional testing.

Magnetic Resonance Angiography

Although conventional magnetic resonance angiography has a high sensitivity for detection of central pulmonary emboli, the sensitivity for detection of subsegmental emboli is less precise.

Pulmonary Angiography

This requires catheterization of heart and is the most definitive study for pulmonary embolism. In addition to being invasive, it is also time consuming, uncomfortable and associated with dye-induced allergy and renal failure.

Management

Immediate treatment for pulmonary embolism is full anticoagulation, similar to that for deep venous thrombosis. A number of complementary procedures are indicated.

Vena Caval Filters

Placement of vena caval filters should be considered before surgery.[1] Routine filter placement has no added advantage to heparin given alone. In the very infrequent circumstances where heparin alone fails to prevent recurrent pulmonary embolism from the pelvis or legs or when embolism develops from these sites despite heparin treatment, a vena caval filter may be indicated. Filters can also be used with massive emboli in patients who are not candidates for thrombolysis. The device may be inserted through either the jugular vein or femoral vein. Retrievable filters may be used as a short-term protection against embolism. These may be removed till they become endothelialized, or they can be left in place permanently.

Thrombolysis

Compared with heparin, thrombolytic agents provide more rapid lysis of pulmonary clots and improvement of pulmonary hypertension.[10] There are very few studies of thrombolysis during pregnancy. Also, tissue plasminogen activator does not cross the placenta.

Embolectomy

Surgical embolectomy is uncommonly indicated with use of thrombolysis and filters.

DEEP VEIN THROMBOSIS

Clinical Presentation

Most cases of thrombosis during pregnancy are probably confined to the deep veins of lower extremities. Preliminary observations indicate that the iliac vein thrombosis may be frequent in those after cesarean delivery. The signs and symptoms vary greatly and depend in large measure on the degree of occlusion and the intensity of inflammatory response. Interestingly, most cases during pregnancy occur in the left leg (Fig. 2).

Classical thromboses involving the lower extremity are abrupt in onset and there is pain and edema of the leg and thigh. The lower extremity thrombus typically involves much of the deep venous system to the iliofemoral region. Conversely, there may be appreciable clot, yet little pain, heat or swelling. Importantly, calf pain either spontaneous or in response to squeezing or to stretching the Achilles tendon; Homan's sign, may be caused by a strained muscle or a contusion. About 25% of untreated cases have an associated pulmonary embolism. Anticoagulation reduces the risk to less than 5%.

Diagnosis

Because clinical diagnosis of deep venous thrombosis is difficult, other methods are imperative for confirmation.

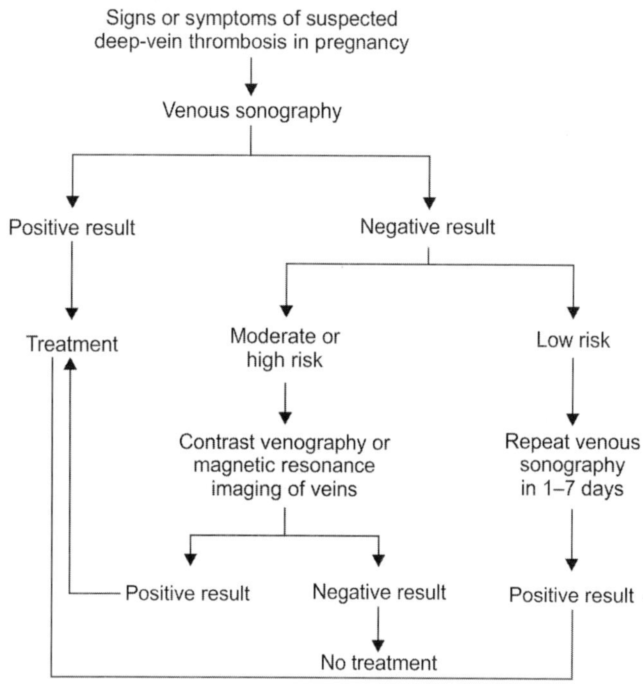

FIG. 2: The signs and symptoms of suspected deep vein thrombosis in pregnancy.

Venography

Invasive contrast venography remains the standard to exclude lower extremity deep venous thrombosis. It has a negative predictive value of 98%. Fetal radiation exposure without shielding is only about 300 mrad, but venography is associated with severe complications including thrombosis; it is time consuming and cumbersome. Hence, noninvasive methods are usually used to confirm the clinical diagnosis.

Impedance Plethysmography

This is an extremely accurate test to determine thromboses in the lower iliac, femoral and popliteal veins. It is based on the observation that alterations in venous return in the calf, produced by inflation and deflation of a pneumatic thigh cuff, result in changes in electric resistance detected at skin surface. These changes occur when popliteal or more proximal veins are obstructed.

Impedance plethysmography is only 50% sensitive for detection of clots in the small calf veins. Also, because of the decreased venous return of the lower extremities, it is associated with increased false positive results during pregnancy. Given these limitations and due to the wide availability of ultrasonography, it is seldom used today.

Compression Ultrasonography

This noninvasive technique is currently the most used first-line test to detect deep vein thrombosis.[12] The diagnosis is based on the noncompressibility and typical echo architecture of thrombosed veins. In symptomatic nonpregnant patients, examination of femoral, popliteal and calf trifurcation veins is more than 90% sensitive and more than 99% specific for proximal thrombosis. Moreover, it has a negative predictive value of 98%.

In pregnant patients, normal findings with venous ultrasonography results do not always exclude a pulmonary embolism. This is because the thrombosis may have already embolized or because it arose from deep pelvic veins inaccessible to ultrasound evaluation. In pregnant women thrombosis associated with pulmonary embolism frequently originates from iliac veins. Also, the natural history of calf deep venous thromboses during pregnancy is unknown. Thus, the safety of withholding anticoagulation with negative compression ultrasonography has not been evaluated in pregnant women who may have an isolated iliac vein thrombosis that is less accessible for imaging.[13]

Computed Tomography

Spiral CT scanning is widely available and very useful for detecting lower extremity deep venous thrombosis as well as those within the vena cava and iliac and pelvic venous systems. Although radiation and contrast agents are required, the benefits of CT outweigh any theoretical risks if shielding is used. Fetal radiation exposure is negligible unless pelvic veins are imaged.

Magnetic Resonance Imaging

This imaging technique allows excellent delineation of anatomical detail above the inguinal ligament. Thus, in many cases magnetic resonance (MR) imaging is immensely useful for diagnosis of ileofemoral and pelvic vein thrombosis. The venous system can also be reconstructed using MR venography.

D-dimer Screening Tests

These fibrin degradation products are generated when fibrinolysin degrades fibrin, as occurs in thromboembolism. Their measurement is frequently incorporated into diagnostic algorithms for venous thromboembolism in non-pregnant patients. Screening with d-dimer test in pregnancy is problematic for a number of reasons. Depending on assay sensitivity, d-dimer serum levels increase with gestational age, along with elevated plasma fibrinogen concentrations. D-dimer concentrations can also be elevated in certain complications of pregnancy, such as placental abruption, pre-eclampsia and sepsis. For these reasons, their use in pregnancy remains uncertain, but a negative d-dimer test should be considered reassuring.[1,10]

Management

Optimal management of venous thromboembolism during pregnancy has not undergone major clinical studies to provide evidence-based practices. There is, however, consensus for treatment with anticoagulants and limited activity. If thrombophilia testing is performed it is done before anticoagulation because heparin induces a decline in antithrombin levels and warfarin decreases protein C and S concentrations.[5]

Anticoagulation is initiated with either unfractionated or low molecular weight heparin. During pregnancy, heparin therapy is continued. For postpartum women, anticoagulation is begun simultaneously with warfarin. Over several days leg pain dissipates. After symptoms have abated, gradual ambulation should be started. Elastic stockings are fitted. Anticoagulation is continued. Recovery to this stage takes around 7–10 days.[14]

HEPARINIZATION

Treatment of thromboembolism during pregnancy is with either unfractionated or low molecular weight heparin (Table 2). Although either type is acceptable, most recommend low molecular weight heparin. In its recently revised guidelines, ACCP suggests preferential use of this heparin class during pregnancy, but scores this recommendation as grade 2c, the lowest quality level of evidence.[15]

UNFRACTIONATED HEPARIN

Treatment is with an intravenous heparin bolus followed by continuous infusion titrated to achieve full anticoagulation. The AAP and ACOG recommend an initial bolus of intravenous unfractionated heparin (UFH) at a dose of 80 units/kg. This is followed by continuous infusion of at least 30,000 IU for 24 hours, titrated to achieve an activated partial thromboplastin time (aPTT) of 1.5–2.5 times control values.

Intravenous anticoagulation should be maintained for at least 5–7 days, after which, treatment is converted to subcutaneous heparin. Injections are then given every 8 hours to maintain the aPTT to at least 1.5–2.5 times control throughout the dosing interval. For women with antiphospholipid syndrome, aPTT does not accurately assess heparin anticoagulation, and thus antifactor Xa levels are preferred.

The duration of full anticoagulation varies, and there are several acceptable schemes. The AAP and ACOG recommend therapeutic anticoagulation for at least 3 months after the acute event. The ACCP recommends anticoagulation throughout pregnancy and for 6 weeks postpartum but for a minimum total duration of 6 months. Lockwood recommends full anticoagulation be continued for at least 20 weeks followed by prophylactic doses if the woman is still pregnant.[9]

TABLE 2: Heparin infusion protocol[3]

Protocol for continuous heparin infusion for patients with venous thromboembolism		
Initial heparin dose:		
Units IV push (recommended 80 units/kg rounded to nearest 100, maximum 7500 units), then		
Units/hour by infusion (recommended 18 units/kg/hour rounded to nearest 50)		
Infusion rate adjustments; based on partial thromboplastin time (PTT):		
PTT (sec)*	**Intervention†**	**Baseline infusion rate change‡**
<45	80 units/kg bolus	by 4 units/kg/hour
45–54	40 units/kg bolus	by 2 units/kg/hour
55–84	None	None
85–100	None	by 2 units/kg/hour
>100	Stop infusion 60 minutes	by 3 units/kg/hour

Note:
*PTT goal 55–84.
†Rounded to nearest 100.
‡Rounded to nearest 50.

Prophylactic doses of subcutaneous UFH can range from 5000 to 10,000 units every 12 hours titrated to maintain an antifactor Xa level of 0.1–0.2 units, measured 6 hours after the last injection. If the venous thromboembolism occurs during the postpartum period, Lockwood recommends a minimum of 6 months of anticoagulation treatment.[9]

LOW-MOLECULAR-WEIGHT HEPARIN

This is a family of derivatives of UFH, and their molecular weights average 4,000–5,000 daltons compared with 12,000–16,000 daltons for conventional heparin. None of these heparins cross the placenta, and all exert their anticoagulant activity by activating antithrombin. The primary difference is in their relative inhibitory activity against factor Xa and thrombin. UFH has equivalent activity against factor Xa and thrombin, but low-molecular-weight heparin (LMWH) has greater activity against factor Xa than thrombin. They also have a more predictable anticoagulant response and fewer bleeding complications than UFH because of their better bioavailability, longer half-life, dose-independent clearance, and decreased interference with platelets.[10]

A number of studies have shown that venous thromboembolism is treated effectively with LMWH. Using serial venograms, Breddin et al.[15] observed that LMWHs were more effective than the unfractionated form in reducing thrombus size without increasing mortality rates or major bleeding complications.

Pharmacokinetics in Pregnancy

Several LMWHs are available for use in pregnancy and including enoxaparin, dalteparin, and tinzaparin. Enoxaparin pharmacokinetics show that owing to increased renal clearance, twice-daily dosing may be necessary to maintain anti-factor Xa activity. Optimal dosing was best achieved with periodic monitoring of peak activity, about 3.5 hours after a dose, and predose antifactor Xa activity.

Dalteparin pharmacokinetics show that women given once-daily dalteparin subcutaneously had mean antifactor Xa levels that were significantly lower across pregnancy compared with levels measured 6 weeks' postpartum.

The AAP and ACOG recommend that antifactor Xa levels be periodically re-evaluated during pregnancy in a woman fully anticoagulated with these agents. Monitoring anti-Xa levels during pregnancy is especially important in women who also have impaired renal or hepatic function, weigh less than 50 kg or greater than 100 kg, or have risk factors for bleeding. Dosing should be enough to achieve a peak anti-factor Xa level of 0.5–1.2 U/mL.

For women given thromboprophylaxis, most authorities do not recommend monitoring antifactor Xa levels.

Safety in Pregnancy

The ACOG concluded that these risks were rare, that their incidence was not higher than expected, and that no cause-and-effect relationship had been established. The committee further concluded that enoxaparin and dalteparin could be given safely during pregnancy. Caveats are that LMWHs should not be used in women with prosthetic heart valves because of reports of valvular thrombosis. They also should be avoided in women with renal failure.

Use of LMWHs may also increase the risk of spinal hematoma associated with regional analgesia. As a result, the AAP and ACOG advise that women receiving once-daily prophylactic low-dose LMWH not be offered regional analgesia until at least 10–12 hours after the last injection. In addition, LMWH should be withheld for at least 2 hours after the removal of an epidural catheter. The safety of regional analgesia in women receiving twice-daily therapeutic LMWH has not been studied sufficiently, and it is not known whether delaying regional techniques for 24 hours after the last injection is adequate. Protamine sulfate may help partially reverse the effects of LMWH.

Anticoagulation with Warfarin

Warfarin derivatives are generally contraindicated because they readily cross the placenta and cause fetal death and malformations from hemorrhages. Like unfractionated and LMWH, they are safe during breast feeding (AAP and ACOG).

Postpartum venous thrombosis is usually treated with intravenous heparin and oral warfarin initiated simultaneously. Patients are maintained on therapeutic doses of unfractionated or LMWH for 5 days and until the international normalized ratio (INR) is in a therapeutic range. The initial dose of warfarin is usually 5–10 mg for the first 2 days. Subsequent doses are titrated to achieve an INR of 2–3.

Duration of Therapy

The optimal duration of continued anticoagulation after delivery is uncertain, but anticoagulation with warfarin is continued for at least 4–6 weeks. Most recommendations have been extrapolated from studies in nonpregnant patients.

The current consensus of ACCP is that warfarin anticoagulation be given for at least 6 weeks postpartum, but to complete a minimum 6-month course following the initial episode.[15] Lockwood recommends a minimum of 6 weeks. Most authorities agree that deep-venous thrombosis that develops postpartum requires a minimum of 6 months of anticoagulation.[9]

Complications of Anticoagulation

Three significant complications associated with anticoagulation are (1) hemorrhage, (2) thrombocytopenia, and (3) osteoporosis. The latter two are unique to heparin, and their risk may be reduced with LMWHs. The most serious complication is hemorrhage, which is more likely if there has been recent surgery or lacerations. Troublesome bleeding also is more likely if the heparin dosage is excessive.

Heparin-induced Thrombocytopenia

There are two types of heparin-induced thrombocytopenia (HIT). The most common is a nonimmune, benign, reversible form that occurs within the first few days of therapy and resolves in about 5 days without cessation of therapy. The second is the more severe form of HIT, which results from an immune reaction involving IgG antibodies directed against complexes of platelet factor 4 and heparin.

When most severe, HIT paradoxically causes thrombosis, which is the most common presentation. The ACCP advises that the diagnosis of HIT be considered when the platelet count decreases by 50% between 5 and 14 days after the initiation of heparin therapy.[15] The incidence of HIT is approximately 3–5% in nonpregnant individuals. The ACOG recommends that platelet counts be measured on day 5 and then periodically for the first 2 weeks of heparin therapy.

If thrombocytopenia is severe, heparin therapy must be stopped and alternative anticoagulation initiated. LMWH may not be an entirely safe alternative because it has some cross reactivity with UFH. In these cases, many recommend danaparoid, a sulfated glycosaminoglycan heparinoid.

Heparin-induced Osteoporosis

Bone loss may develop with long-term heparin administration, usually 6 months or longer and is more prevalent in cigarette smokers. LMWHs can cause osteopenia although this is less likely than with UFH. Women treated with any heparin should be encouraged to take a daily supplement of 1500 mg of calcium LMWHs may cause less adverse effects.

Anticoagulation and Delivery

The effects of heparin on blood loss at delivery depend on a number of variables:
- Dose, route, and time of administration.
- Number and severity of incisions and lacerations.
- Intensity of postpartum myometrial contractions.
- Presence of other coagulation defects.

Heparin therapy generally is stopped during labor and delivery. If the uterus is well-contracted and there has been negligible trauma to the lower genital tract, it can be restarted after about 12 hours. Otherwise, a delay of 1 or 2 days may be prudent.

Protamine sulfate administered slowly intravenously generally reverses the effect of heparin promptly and effectively. It should not be given in excess of the amount needed to neutralize the heparin, because it also has an anticoagulant effect. Serious bleeding is likely when heparin in usual therapeutic doses is administered to a woman who has undergone cesarean delivery within the previous 24–48 hours.

Thromboprophylaxis

Either antepartum surveillance or heparin prophylaxis is recommended for women without a recurrent risk factor, including no known thrombophilia (Table 3). Women with a prior thrombosis in association with a thrombophilia or in the absence of a temporary risk factor generally should be given both antepartum and postpartum prophylaxis.

Cesarean Delivery and Antepartum Bed Rest

The use of thromboprophylaxis for women undergoing cesarean delivery or antepartum bed rest is not widely employed. The risk for deep-venous thrombosis and especially for fatal thromboembolism is increased many fold in women following cesarean compared with vaginal delivery. It is easily understandable that pulmonary embolism is a major cause of maternal mortality. Royal College of Obstetricians and Gynaecologists (RCOG) now recommends risk assessment for women undergoing uncomplicated cesarean delivery. The ACCP suggests risk assessment with thromboprophylaxis; mechanical, pharmacological, or both. They note this to be Grade 2C level of recommendation because of "low- or very-low quality evidence".

TABLE 3: Postpartum risk assessment[2,15]

Risk assessment to determine thromboprophylaxis following uncomplicated cesarean delivery	
Risk	**Intervention**
Low	• Early ambulation • In hospital, consider compression stockings
Medium or high	Early ambulation
Age older than 35 years	In hospital, consider compression or pneumatic stockings
BMI >30	Or
Multiparity (? 3)	In hospital, consider prophylactic LMWH or UFH
Varicosities	
Pre-eclampsia	
Postpartum hemorrhage	
Emergency delivery	
Hysterectomy	
Very high	Consider stockings as above and prophylactic heparin. For persistent risks, consider prophylactic heparin for 4–6 weeks
Multiple risk factors	

BMI, body mass index; LMWH, low-molecular-weight heparin; UFH, unfractionated heparin.

CONCLUSION

Pregnancy is a hypercoagulable state and thromboembolic disorders are a part and parcel of the complications encountered in the peripartum period. Current diagnostic modalities and treatment guidelines provide excellent and detailed information on how to treat venous thromboembolism and pulmonary embolism, even if the evidence behind may not be all that robust.

Low-molecular-weight heparins are easily available and inexpensive and the monitoring required to titrate the dose is not cumbersome and easily accessible. With a high index of suspicion and timely interventional with a multidisciplinary approach can go a long way towards curbing the morbidity and mortality once associated with these conditions.

REFERENCES

1. Christiansen LR, Collins KA. Pregnancy-associated deaths: a 15-year retrospective study and overall review of maternal pathophysiology. Am J Forensic Med Pathol. 2006;27(1):11-9.
2. Marik PE, Plante LA. Venous thromboembolic disease and pregnancy. N Engl J Med. 2008;359(19):2025-33.
3. James DK, Steer PJ, Weiner CP, Gonik B (Eds). High Risk Pregnancy: Management Options, 4th edition. Elsevier Health Sciences; 2010.
4. Committee on Practice Bulletins--Gynecology, American College of Obstetricians and Gynecologists. ACOG Practice Bulletin No. 84: Prevention of deep vein thrombosis and pulmonary embolism. Obstet Gynecol. 2007;110(2 Pt 1):429-40.
5. Lockwood CJ. Inherited thrombophilias in pregnant patients: detection and treatment paradigm. Obstet Gynecol. 2002;99(2):333-41.
6. Franchini M, Lippi G, Manzato F. Recent acquisitions in the pathophysiology, diagnosis and treatment of disseminated intravascular coagulation. Thromb J. 2006;4:4.
7. Katz DS, Hon M. Current DVT imaging. Tech Vasc Interv Radiol. 2004;7(2):55-62.
8. Kupferminc MJ. Thrombophilia and pregnancy. Reprod Biol Endocrinol. 2003;1:111.
9. Rosenberg VA, Lockwood CJ. Thromboembolism in pregnancy. Obstet Gynecol Clin North Am. 2007;34(3):481-500, xi.
10. Tapson VF. Acute pulmonary embolism. N Engl J Med. 2008;358(10):1037-52.
11. Kinane TB, Grabowski EF, Sharma A, Nimkin K, King ME, Cornell LD. Case records of the Massachusetts General Hospital. Case 7-2008. A 17-year-old girl with chest pain and hemoptysis. N Engl J Med. 2008;358(9):941-52.
12. Greer IA, Barry J, Mackon N, Allan PL. Diagnosis of deep venous thrombosis in pregnancy: a new role for diagnostic ultrasound. Br J Obstet Gynaecol. 1990;97(1):53-7.
13. Bates SM, Ginsberg JS. How we manage venous thromboembolism during pregnancy. Blood. 2002;100(10):3470-8.
14. Breddin HK, Kadziola Z, Scully M, Nakov R, Misselwitz F, Kakkar VV. Risk factors and coagulation parameters in relationship to phlebographic response and clinical outcome in the treatment of acute deep vein thrombosis. Thromb Haemost. 2003;89(2):272-7.
15. Bates SM, Greer IA, Pabinger I, Sofaer S, Hirsh J. American College of Chest Physicians. Venous thromboembolism, thrombophilia, antithrombotic therapy, and pregnancy: American College of Chest Physicians Evidence-Based Clinical Practice Guidelines (8th Edition) Chest. 2008;133(6 Suppl):844S-886S.

CHAPTER 59

Neurological Complications in Third Trimester of Pregnancy

Hema J Shobhane

INTRODUCTION

A wide range of neurological problems can complicate pregnancy and the puerperium. The frequent overlap of symptoms associated with common pregnancy complaints, the sometimes disabling and lethal consequences of the disease, the fetal effects of maternal treatment make the diagnosis and management of neurologic disease during pregnancy a challenging task. Central neurologic complications of pregnancy can present clinically in a variety of ways, ranging from transient focal symptoms to coma and death. The average age of pregnancy has increased from 24.6–27.2 in the past 30 years, increasing pregnancy-associated complications, such as eclampsia, gestational diabetes, and hypertension.[1,2] However, headache is a common complaint in pregnant women and distinguishing the benign headache from one that is a sign of serious disease is often not considered until serious neurological complications develop. As neurological diseases contribute to approximately 20% of maternal deaths,[3] many of these neurological diseases can lead to devastating complications if not recognized early. The pregnant woman is vulnerable in that many medications and diagnostic evaluations are avoided due to concerns of causing harm to the fetus. There are few randomized clinical trials to guide evidence based medicine in the field of neurological complications of pregnancy.

HEADACHE

Experiencing headaches during pregnancy is one of the most common discomforts and complaints. The most common categories are tension and migraine type. Headaches may occur at any time during pregnancy, but they tend to be most common during the first and third trimester. Headaches during the third trimester may also be caused by a condition called pre-eclampsia, which is high blood pressure during pregnancy, if headaches are accompanied by: blurry vision, sudden weight gain, pain in the upper right abdomen, and swelling in the hands and face and is not diagnosed promptly can end up in eclampsia and many of times death.

Management

Headache during pregnancy: "Headaches are a common complaint during pregnancy, and several treatments are contraindicated in pregnancy due to the side effects on fetus", thus many use a 'wait and see' treatment philosophy given that headache frequency is often reduced later in pregnancy. The drug combination of metoclopramide and diphenhydramine (MAD) is a safe, effective headache treatment for pregnant women, especially when acetaminophen fails to provide relief, according to new research presented today at the Annual Clinical Meeting of the American College of Obstetricians and Gynecologists. Metoclopramide is a prescription drug commonly used to treat heartburn due to gastroesophageal reflux. Diphenhydramine is an antihistamine found in several over-the-counter allergy medications and sleep aids.[4]

MIGRAINE

Migraine is three times more common in women (3:1 ratio) and female headache prevalence is highest during childbearing years.[5] However, studies have shown that the incidence of migraine headache is often reduced during the second 2 trimesters of pregnancy.[5,6] Migraine has not been shown to significantly affect fertility or pregnancy outcomes, but it is associated with a risk of developing pre-eclampsia or stroke.[5-7]

Management

Management of migraine during pregnancy should first focus on avoiding potential triggers. The mainstay of preventing and treating migraine pain during pregnancy involves nonpharmacological methods including maintaining a consistent sleep schedule, stress management, regular meals, and remaining hydrated.[8] Additionally, studies have shown that biofeedback therapy and moderate consistent exercise can reduce headache and its frequency.[8,9] Medical therapy is more limited in pregnancy but often include analgesics, such as acetaminophen, steroids, and if necessary, opiate medications.[7] Adequate treatment of nausea can be instrumental in helping the patient maintain nutrition and hydration as well as facilitate sleep. Antiemetic therapy may include treatment with metoclopramide (may cause akathisia, consider pretreatment with diphenhydramine, which may help abort migraine), ondansetron (does not particularly affect headache), and sedating agents, such as promethazine and chlorpromazine (suppository formulations can be helpful in severely nauseated patients).[7,8] Triptans, a mainstay of acute migraine treatment in non-pregnant patients, are probably safe in pregnancy but may slightly affect preterm labor rates.[10] Unfortunately, given the limited safety data available, triptan therapy cannot be recommended. In some refractory cases, dexamethasone or prednisone can be considered. Should prophylactic treatment become indicated, the beta-adrenergic receptor antagonists (e.g. propranolol) can be used.[11]

SEIZURE DISORDERS

Over 90% of women with epilepsy (WWE) have a normal pregnancy. This point should be emphasized to the patient who is likely to have many fears and anxieties regarding the risks. Nonetheless, there are a number of fetal and obstetrical complications associated with WWE. With close cooperation and communication among the obstetrician, neurologist, pediatrician, and patient, most women with idiopathic epilepsy who become pregnant will have an uneventful pregnancy with an excellent outcome.

Management

Comprehensive care of WWE during the reproductive years must include effective preconceptional counseling. The woman's antiepileptic drug (AED) regimen should be optimized and folate supplementation should be begun prior to pregnancy. A common but erroneous reason to change medications is that the woman presents to the neurologist after she has discovered she is pregnant. In many cases, she is already in or past the critical period of organogenesis. If a woman with epilepsy presents after conception and is taking a single AED that is effective, her medication should usually not be changed. The teratogenic risk is only increased by exposing the fetus to a second agent during a crossover period of AEDs, and seizures are more likely to occur with any abrupt medication changes. If a woman is receiving polytherapy and is seizure free, it may be possible to switch safely to monotherapy. However, changes in the total and free levels of the remaining drug will need to be monitored closely. Seizure control remains an important goal during pregnancy. Convulsive seizures in particular place the mother and fetus at risk. Nonconvulsive seizures may also be harmful, especially if they involve falling or other forms of trauma. Because each of the major AEDs is teratogenic, the medication that is most effective for the woman's epilepsy and seizure type should be prescribed. AED monotherapy is recommended and should be used at the lowest effective dose. If a large daily dose is needed, frequent smaller doses may be helpful to avoid high peak levels. Folate supplementation should begin prior to conception and is crucial during the first 30 days of gestation to protect against neural tube defects. The optimal dosage has not been established for WWE, and recommendations vary between 0.4 mg/day and 5 mg/day.[12]

Pregnancy can affect the pharmacokinetics of AEDs at any level from absorption, distribution, metabolism, to elimination. The effect varies depending on the type of AED. The most pronounced decline in serum concentrations is seen for AEDs that are eliminated by glucuronidation, in particular lamotrigine where the effect may be profound. Serum concentrations of AEDs that are cleared mainly through the kidneys, for example, levetiracetam, can also decline significantly. Some AEDs, such as carbamazepine seem to be affected only marginally by pregnancy. Data on pharmacokinetics during pregnancy are lacking completely for some of the newer generation AEDs: pregabalin, lacosamide, retigabine, and eslicarbazepine acetate. Consensus that monitoring could be important, in particular when women have been titrated to the lowest effective AED dose and serum concentration before pregnancy, and when that individual optimal concentration can be used as reference.[13]

CEREBROVASCULAR DISEASES

Cerebrovascular disease during pregnancy can be divided into two major categories: (1) thrombosis/ischemia (including arterial and venous infarction) and (2) hemorrhage (including intracerebral and subarachnoid hemorrhage). Normal physiologic changes associated with pregnancy, combined with pathophysiologic processes unique to pregnancy, predispose women to develop stroke during pregnancy and the puerperium.

Hemodynamic Changes

The drop in sustained virological response (SVR) is accompanied by a fall in the systolic and diastolic blood pressure. It reaches a nadir in the third or late second trimester, about 20–32 weeks, after which it rises until term to levels at or slightly above the normal nonpregnant blood pressure. There is increased venous capacitance and reduced blood flow (i.e. relative venous stasis), often accompanied by orthostatic intolerance. The volume increase tends to increase preload. However, preload is heavily dependent upon position, with reduced preload and orthostasis resulting from the higher venous capacitance and from compression on the inferior vena cava in the supine position.

Vascular and Connective Tissue Changes

Pregnancy causes remodeling of the heart and all blood vessels. The walls of systemic arteries show a reduction in collagen and elastin content and a loss of distensibility. The hemodynamic changes near term combined with these structural changes of blood vessels to result in a state in which more vulnerable vascular walls experience greater hemodynamic stress, possibly contributing to the risk of hemorrhage in late pregnancy.

Changes in the Coagulation System

Both hemodynamic and biochemical changes make pregnancy a state of hypercoagulability. Decreased venous compliance results in venous stasis and congestion. Compression of the inferior vena cava, aorta, and blood supply of the gravid uterus can cause vascular injury. Levels of procoagulant factors, coagulation inhibitors, and other mediators of clot formation and lysis are altered by pregnancy resulting in a state of increased hypercoagulability in late pregnancy.

Pre-eclampsia/Eclampsia

The criteria for diagnosis depend on the definition of the clinical syndrome. Modern consensus definitions all endorse pregnancy-induced hypertension beginning after the 20th week with proteinuria as pre-eclampsia, and generally accept the inclusion of women with pregnancy-induced hypertension without proteinuria but with other common manifestations, including (1) cerebral symptoms, (2) epigastric or right upper quadrant pain with nausea or vomiting, or (3) thrombocytopenia and abnormal liver enzymes.[14] It has been claimed that although pregnancy-induced hypertension is the cornerstone of clinical diagnosis, a significant proportion of women who develop hemolysis, elevated liver enzymes, and low platelet count (HELLP) syndrome or eclamptic seizures do not have hypertension. Endothelial dysfunction contributes to increased capillary permeability that underlies proteinuria, edema, and, most important among our concerns, brain edema at relatively modest elevations of blood pressure.

ISCHEMIC STROKE ASSOCIATED WITH PREGNANCY

The data estimate the incidence of all types of pregnancy-associated stroke, including ischemic and hemorrhagic strokes, subarachnoid hemorrhage, and cerebral venous sinus thrombosis, to be 25–34 per 1,00,000 deliveries. This analysis compares data from 1994 and 1995 to data from 2006 and 2007. Between these intervals, antenatal hospitalizations increased by 47% (from 0.15–0.22 per 1,000 deliveries), and postpartum hospitalizations by 83% (from 0.12–0.22 per 1,000 deliveries), with the increases largely explained by concurrent hypertensive disorders or heart disease.[14]

Mechanisms

When mechanisms of ischemic stroke are identified, the major ones are arterial or venous thrombosis or arterial embolism. Pre-eclampsia/eclampsia appears to be a major contributor to stroke risk. In studies in which pre-eclampsia/eclampsia is reported, it is present in 11–47% cases of stroke. Other well-established causes of stroke in young patients, such as arterial dissection and moyamoya syndrome, can present during pregnancy and should be consider. Other pregnancy-specific causes, such as peripartum cardiomyopathy, choriocarcinoma, and embolization of amniotic fluid or air, are very rare and should be considered based on the clinical presentations. Amniotic fluid embolism should be considered when evidence of diffuse or multifocal brain ischemia is present and accompanied by features of pulmonary embolism.

Evaluation

Stroke is suspected clinically based on the sudden onset of a neurologic deficit suggestive of a focal lesion and without an alternative cause. Properly timed neuroimaging will confirm the great majority of ischemic strokes. In general, with proper precautions, computed tomography (CT) and magnetic resonance imaging (MRI) should be used as with nonpregnant patients to identify areas of infarction and to investigate the cerebral vasculature. Cerebral vessel imaging with magnetic resonance (MR) angiography, CT angiography, or transfemoral catheter angiography is indicated to assess for cerebral arterial dissection, reversible cerebral vasoconstriction syndrome, moyamoya disease, or other arteriopathies. Cardiac ultrasound should be performed in patients with embolic infarctions, and should include agitated saline injection (bubble study) to investigate for a right-to-left shunt from a patent foramen ovale, the presence of which may suggest paradoxical embolism and warrant further testing for lower extremity or pelvic deep vein thrombus.[15] As with any patient with stroke, blood tests, such as lipid panel, hemoglobin A1C, erythrocyte sedimentation rate, C-reactive protein, and others should be routinely performed, with additional tests, such as hemoglobin electrophoresis for sickle cell disease or antiphospholipid antibody panel performed on a case by case basis. Genetic testing for thrombophilia (prothrombin G20210A mutation, factor V Leiden mutation, methylenetetrahydrofolate reductase mutation) can be performed during pregnancy, but testing for other hypercoagulable states (protein C, protein S, and antithrombin III deficiency) should be performed at least 6 weeks after delivery when physiologic changes due to pregnancy will have normalized.

Management

Intravenous (IV) recombinant tissue plasminogen activator (tPA) is a US Food and Drug Administration (FDA); approved thrombolytic drug that remains the only proven efficacious therapy for acute ischemic stroke.[16] Many large stroke centers offer intra-arterial thrombolysis as a salvage therapy in severe stroke cases. Intra-arterial thrombolysis typically involves mechanical clot retrieval using FDA-approved devices. Recent phase III clinical trials showing no benefit of intra-arterial over IV thrombolysis[17] will prompt a reassessment of the role of catheter-based therapies, but evidence exists that improved outcomes depend on early recanalization of occluded arteries, and FDA-approved devices will continue to find use as research proceeds on this issue.

Intravenous tPA has a very short serum half-life of less than 5 minutes. However, it binds to newly formed fibrin clots, where its lytic effect lasts for many hours. It is a large molecule that does not cross the placenta in animals, and so it should not be expected to place the fetus at risk of teratogenicity. The potential risks of real concern are maternal hemorrhage, placental hemorrhage and abruption, fetal loss, and preterm delivery. Obstetric consultation should be sought from the outset for careful monitoring and decision making. Care in facilities with experience both in advanced stroke care and high-risk obstetrics is optimal, and the cause and mechanism of the stroke should be carefully determined to the extent possible before therapy is prescribed. For example, women with stroke as a result of amniotic fluid embolism would not benefit from tPA. Additionally, given the known risk of cerebral hemorrhage from hypertensive encephalopathy in the setting of pre-eclampsia/eclampsia, patients who have strokes complicating pre-eclampsia or eclampsia should not receive tPA.

Pre-eclampsia/Eclampsia Hypertensive Encephalopathy, and Postpartum Cerebral Angiopathy

Pre-eclampsia/eclampsia contributes to cerebrovascular events in two major ways. First, as noted above, pre-eclampsia/eclampsia causes many pathophysiologic changes in blood vessels and the thrombotic system and in this way accounts for a large proportion of ischemic strokes in pregnancy. Second, one direct consequence of pre-eclampsia/eclampsia is the posterior reversible encephalopathy syndrome (PRES). PRES involves a neurotoxic state most often characterized by headaches, confusion, seizures, and visual changes. Additionally, there are characteristic imaging features associated with the syndrome which often include focal regions of symmetric edema in the posterior brain parenchyma.[18]

Pre-eclampsia/Eclampsia and Posterior Reversible Encephalopathy Syndrome

Pathophysiologic Mechanisms

The features of pre-eclampsia/eclampsia directly relevant to PRES and probably also to eclamptic seizures are: (1) an abnormal increase in vascular tone; and (2) dysfunction of endothelial cells. Patients with pre-eclampsia/eclampsia have heightened sensitivity to mediators of vasoconstriction, such as angiotensin II. This resultant increase in vascular tone is responsible for systemic hypertension and for the vasomotor instability that underlies vasospasm. Endothelial dysfunction is in part responsible for the instability of vascular tone, and it also results in increased vascular permeability that underlies the development of edema and proteinuria that characterize pre-eclampsia/eclampsia. The syndrome commonly called PRES results from the development of cerebral edema. Fluid crosses from the intravascular to the interstitial space as a result both of an increase in capillary filtration pressure caused by hypertension and of loss of integrity of the blood-brain barrier caused by endothelial dysfunction. Animal models of the blood-brain barrier's response to severe acute hypertension have shown both increased pinocytosis and flow across impaired endothelial gap junctions.[19]

Therapies and Outcomes

The goals of therapy are to control elevated blood pressure, control seizures, and minimize vasospasm and risk of secondary infarct and hemorrhage. The treatment of PRES in the pregnant patient mirrors that of eclampsia and, as noted above, these may not represent distinct syndromes in the pregnant patient. The patients' obstetrician may consider emergent delivery if feasible and appropriate. Magnesium sulfate is often utilized for seizure control. As with eclampsia, hypertension management is generally achieved with hydralazine or labetalol. Patients should be monitored closely and magnesium sulfate stopped if deep tendon reflexes are lost, if respirations are depressed, or if urine output falls below 100 mL in 4 hours. Calcium gluconate 1 g slow IV push can be given to reverse severe toxicity. In addition, patients with eclamptic syndromes should be treated urgently with IV antihypertensive agents and with additional antiepileptic agents if needed for seizure control. Most women with pre-eclampsia/eclampsia are volume contracted and will benefit from volume replacement and maintenance.

Cerebral Venous Sinus Thrombosis

Cerebral venous and sinus thrombosis (CVST) is a subtype of stroke which may result in ischemic and/or hemorrhagic complications and is more common in women than in men (~3:1 ratio). Mortality related to CVST is estimated at 9% and is primarily due to intracerebral hemorrhage.[20] The development of CVST has been related to a number of factors including hypercoagulable states, inflammatory disorders, and infection. Pregnancy, in and of itself, induces a degree of physiologic hypercoagulability in order to prepare for delivery and reduce the chance of maternal hemorrhage. Other genetic causes of hypercoagulability including antiphospholipid syndrome, prothrombin gene mutations, and factor V Leiden/MHTFR deficiency are associated with the development of CVST.[21] Hypertension, cesarian section, infection, obesity, hyperemesis, dehydration, and prolonged bed rest may also further increase the risk of developing a thrombosis. Women, although not pregnant women, may have exposure to oral contraceptive pills which have also been associated with an increased risk of developing CVST.[21,22]

Evaluation

Women with cerebral venous thrombosis may present with headaches, focal neurologic deficits, depressed level of consciousness, or seizures, and the pregnant state should greatly heighten the index of suspicion for this diagnosis. Examination of the patient suspected of having a venous thrombosis should include a complete neurological examination as well as a good fundoscopic examination to evaluate for papilledema. If papilledema is identified, then cerebral imaging to evaluate for a source of increased intracranial pressure must be performed. Cerebral venous sinus thrombosis can be detected on noncontrast CT as hyperdensity in the region of thrombosis or as parenchymal hypodensity from edema or infarction or hyperdensity from hemorrhage. Contrast CT may show a filling defect within the thrombosed sinus surrounded by the enhancing dura of the sinus wall (empty delta sign). Contrast CT venography may show the thrombosis as a filling defect in the region of the affected sinus. On MRI, venous sinus thrombosis can be seen directly as thrombus with signal characteristics appropriate to the time since onset.

Lumbar puncture may be indicated as a therapeutic measure in patients with elevated intracranial pressure (ICP) as long as imaging does not reveal a large intracranial mass lesion (including stroke or hemorrhage). Elevated D-dimer levels may help identify patients more likely to have CVST but levels below an identified threshold of 500 ng/mL do not rule out the diagnosis.

Treatment

Treatment of CVST in the first trimester with warfarin is not recommended (teratogenic) but the American Heart Association recommendations identify warfarin as safe in the second and third trimester, with the caveat that it must be discontinued late in the pregnancy in anticipation of delivery.[23] Low-dose aspirin is felt to be safe, particularly after the first trimester, as per the American College of Chest Physicians 2008 guidelines.[24] Additionally, both groups suggest that unfractionated heparin or low-molecular weight heparin can be utilized in pregnancy either as a bridge to warfarin therapy or as a stand-alone treatment. Following delivery, warfarin can be utilized for anticoagulation which is generally continued for a 3- to 6-month period with repeat imaging to establish the status of recanalization.

HEMORRHAGIC STROKE AND VASCULAR MALFORMATIONS

Hemorrhagic, like ischemic, stroke is uncommon during pregnancy and the puerperium and ranges from 5–35 per 100,000. Despite its rarity, because of the severe implications of cerebral hemorrhage, hemorrhagic stroke is also an important cause of pregnancy-related mortality. The major established causes of pregnancy-related cerebral hemorrhage are pre-eclampsia/eclampsia, followed by arteriovenous malformations (AVMs) and aneurysms.

The physiologic changes of pregnancy reviewed above include expansion of blood volume, increased stroke volume and cardiac output, rise of blood pressure from its nadir in the late second or early third trimester to near or slightly above normal as term approaches, and remodeling of vascular tissue with loss of collagen and elastin content and loss of distensibility. One might expect these changes to underlie an increased risk of hemorrhage near term. The strain and trauma of labor might be expected to add to the increased risk.

In case of a ruptured aneurysm if left unsecured surgically, rates of recurrent hemorrhage and maternal and fetal mortality are very high. This mortality may be greatly reduced by early surgery, open or endovascular, to secure ruptured aneurysms leads to better maternal and fetal outcomes, recommended that therapy for women after aneurysmal rupture proceed as it does for all patients as dictated by neurosurgical principles. Therefore, if aneurysmal subarachnoid hemorrhage occurs during pregnancy, the patient should proceed to surgery immediately, if feasible. Endovascular coiling may be an alternative with proper shielding to minimize fetal radiation exposure. If urgent obstetric issues (such as active labor, eclampsia, or fetal distress) prevent immediate surgery, then the woman should undergo urgent cesarean delivery followed by surgical control of the aneurysm. Because of the severe morbidity and high mortality rate of subarachnoid hemorrhage and the increased risk of rupture near term, it is recommended that unruptured aneurysms at significant risk of rupture be secured before pregnancy, whenever possible. With the high rate of screening by MR angiography for headaches and other common disorders, it is not uncommon to find small, asymptomatic, unruptured aneurysms. The best policy for management of such aneurysms is lacking; however, it is often considered prudent to deliver such women by cesarean delivery or by vaginal methods that interrupt the second stage of labor. Therapeutic decisions concerning AVMs discovered during pregnancy are lacking; however, based on the above considerations, expert recommendations are that (1) if a woman with known AVM anticipates pregnancy, the AVM should be treated before pregnancy; (2) if an AVM is discovered during pregnancy and has not bled during the pregnancy, conservative observation is usually recommended, with plans to proceed to definitive treatment after delivery; (3) if an AVM bleeds during pregnancy, consideration should be given to treatment during the pregnancy, taking into account the grade of the lesion and the expected timing of benefit in lowering risk (immediate for low-grade lesions amenable to complete surgical excision or embolization but delayed by up to 1–3 years for higher-grade lesions requiring radiosurgery and combination therapies).

NEUROPATHIES

Neuropathies in third trimester and in postpartum period are uncommon and has less incidence of 0.25% likely due to the shortened second stage of labor in postpartum period.[25] The most common injury is lateral femoral neuropathy, a purely sensory nerve from L2 and L4 innervating the anterolateral thigh, which can also occur during pregnancy itself, most frequently after 30 weeks of gestation. Palsies of the femoral, obturator, sciatic, common peroneal nerve, and lumbrosacral plexus also occur with decreasing frequency. Most injuries resolve by 6–8 weeks postpartum and can be confirmed with electromyography (EMG) if necessary.

Idiopathic Peripheral Facial Nerve Palsy or "Bell's Palsy"

Idiopathic peripheral facial nerve palsy or "Bell's palsy" is the most common cause of unilateral acute facial paralysis during pregnancy, and is most commonly presents during the third trimester or in the peripartum period.[26] The etiology of Bell's palsy does not appear to be significantly different in pregnant women although there is an association with pre-eclampsia. Treatment of Bell's palsy with corticosteroids appears to be effective, but is often avoided in the first trimester due to potential adverse effects on the fetus. Antiviral medications, such as valacyclovir and famciclovir are pregnancy category B and may be of benefit if started within 3 days of onset of the facial paralysis in conjunction with corticosteroid therapy.

Acute Inflammatory Demyelinating Polyneuropathy or Guillain-Barré Syndrome

Guillain-Barré syndrome (GBS) is a rare complication of pregnancy which, in a typical case, involves progressive motor weakness and areflexia. In some cases, antecedent infection with *Campylobacter jejuni* or cytomegalovirus (CMV) can be identified and is associated with a more severe disease course.[27] CMV infection is important to identify as this may confer significant risk to the fetus via intrauterine transmission. Treatment for acute inflammatory demyelinating polyneuropathy (AIDP) does not differ in the pregnant population and both plasmapheresis and intravenous immunoglobulin (IVIG) have been utilized. Additional considerations in the management of the AIDP patient include deep vein thrombosis (DVT) prophylaxis and nosocomial infections including pneumonia and urinary tract infections. AIDP does not appear to affect uterine contractile activity and delivery of the fetus in a patient with AIDP; should be based on obstetrical indications. Delivery should also be coordinated with anesthesiology as autonomic instability in some patients may complicate anesthetic care. Additionally, there are reports of succinylcholine administration precipitating hyperkalemia and use should be avoided.[27]

Myasthenia Gravis

Myasthenia gravis (MG) is a chronic autoimmune disorder affecting neuromuscular transmission which results in fatigable weakness of the skeletal muscles. The muscles of the face and orbit in addition to the extremities can be affected. Azathioprine can induce fetal leukopenia but is often maintained for severe disease. The management of pre-eclampsia in myasthenic patients presents a challenge as magnesium sulfate is contraindicated due to potential worsening of muscle weakness; and if seizures occur, phenobarbital or dilantin can be substituted. Close consultation with the obstetrical team and anesthesiology team should dictate the manner of delivery and anesthetics utilized. Vaginal delivery is not contraindicated but a myasthenic patient may not be able to tolerate full labor due to fatigue.[28] Following delivery, the infant must be closely evaluated for neonatal MG. However, as in MG and AID, immunosuppressive therapies (except corticosteroids), interferons, and biological agents (antibody therapies) are relatively contraindicated in pregnant and breast-feeding women in an attempt to reduce fetal toxicity.

DIAGNOSTIC CONSIDERATION IN THE PREGNANT WOMAN

Neuroimaging

Magnetic resonance imaging is often the preferred imaging study for a pregnant patient as there is no radiation involved. Paramagnetic contrast agents are to be avoided; however, as they cross the placenta with an unknown rate of clearance from the amniotic fluid. The effects of gadolinium-based agents on the fetus are not understood, but limited data in animal models reveal potential teratogenicity. MRI studies of the brain parenchyma can be very helpful in detecting both ischemic changes as well as hemorrhage. During an imaging study in involving radiation, care must be taken to shield the fetus from radiation exposure as much as possible. CT angiography and perfusion studies, which are increasingly utilized in a stroke evaluation, involve higher doses of radiation as well as the use of iodinated contrast and should be avoided unless deemed critical to the mother's evaluation. In the same vein, conventional cerebral angiography involves both radiation exposure and contrast administration but may, in some cases, be utilized as both a diagnostic and therapeutic intervention (e.g., aneurismal rupture, proximal cerebral embolism). Iodinated contrast is felt to be reasonably safe when utilized during pregnancy although there is a small concern related to induction of neonatal hypothyroidism.[29]

CONCLUSION

Any woman with an existing neurologic condition should consult her obstetrician and her neurologist before she becomes pregnant. During this consultation, the patient can be advised about the possible risks associated with her condition during pregnancy and about the possible teratogenic effects of her medications. If the woman is already pregnant and did not consult her physician in advance, she must alert her obstetrician and neurologist as soon as possible. Her physicians should review her current medications for their teratogenic potential, and drugs that pose a significant teratogenic risk should be discontinued if possible. It is important, however, that medications be discontinued only when doing so makes good clinical sense for the mother, not solely because they may be associated with congenital anomalies. For example, if antiseizure medications are stopped prematurely, seizure activity may increase during the pregnancy and eventually expose the fetus to several medications at doses higher than those originally used to control the condition.

REFERENCES

1. Silversides CK, Colman JM. Physiological changes in pregnancy. In: Oakley C, Warnes CA (Eds). Heart Disease in Pregnancy. Malden, MA: Blackwell Publishing; 2007. pp. 6-17.
2. Hull AD, Long DM, Longo LD, et al. Pregnancy-induced changes in ovine cerebral arteries. Am J Physiol. 1992;262:(1 Pt 2):R137-R43.
3. Sibai BM. Etiology and management of postpartum hypertension-preeclampsia. Am J Obstet Gynecol. 2012;206(6):470-5.
4. American Congress of Obstetricians and Gynecologists (ACOG). A 501(c)(6) organization, is its companion organization. [online] www.acog.org [Accessed December 2015].
5. Goadsby PJ, Goldberg J, Silberstein SD. Migraine in pregnancy. BMJ. 2008;336(7659):1502-4.
6. Sances G, Granella F, Nappi RE, Fignon A, Ghiotto N, Polatti F, et al. Course of migraine during pregnancy and postpartum: a prospective study. Cephalalgia. 2003;23(3):197-205.
7. Loder E. Migraine in pregnancy. Semin Neurol. 2007;27(5):425-33.
8. Marcus DA. Managing headache during pregnancy and lactation. Expert Rev Neurother. 2008;8(3):385-95.
9. Airola G, Allais G, Castagnoli Gabellari I, Rolando S, Mana O, Benedetto C. Non-pharmacological management of migraine during pregnancy. Neurol Sci. 2010;31(Suppl 1):S63-5.
10. Soldin OP, Dahlin J, O'Mara DM. Triptans in pregnancy. Ther Drug Monit. 2008;30(1):5-9.
11. Aubé M. Migraine in pregnancy. Neurology. 1999;53(4 Suppl 1):S26-8.
12. Pennell PB. Pregnancy in the woman with epilepsy: maternal and fetal outcomes. Semin Neurol. 2002;22(3):299-308.
13. Tomson T, Landmark CJ, Battino D. Antiepileptic drug treatment in pregnancy: changes in drug disposition and their clinical implications. Epilepsia. 2013;54(3):405-14.
14. Feske SK, Singhal AB. Cerebrovascular disorders complicating pregnancy. Continuum (Minneap Minn). 2014;20(1 Neurology of Pregnancy):80-99.
15. Colletti PM, Lee KH, Elkayam U. Cardiovascular imaging of the pregnant patient. AJR Am J Roentgenol. 2013;200(3):515-21.
16. Tissue plasminogen activator for acute ischemic stroke. The National Institute of Neurological Disorders and Stroke rt-PA Stroke Study Group. N Engl J Med. 1995;333(24):1581-7.
17. Hacke W, Kaste M, Bluhmki E, Brozman M, Dávalos A, Guidetti D, et al. Thrombolysis with alteplase 3 to 4.5 hours after acute ischemic stroke. N Engl J Med. 2008;359:(13):1317-29.
18. Hinchey J, Chaves C, Appignani B, Breen J, Pao L, Wang A, et al. A reversible posterior leukoencephalopathy syndrome. N Engl J Med. 1996;334(8):494-500.
19. van den Bergh WM, van der Schaaf I, van Gijn J. The spectrum of presentations of venous infarction caused by deep cerebral vein thrombosis. Neurology. 2005;65(2):192-6.

20. Cantú C, Barinagarrementeria F. Cerebral venous thrombosis associated with pregnancy and puerperium. Review of 67 cases. Stroke. 1993;24(12):1880-4.
21. Dentali F, Crowther M, Ageno W. Thrombophilic abnormalities, oral contraceptives, and risk of cerebral vein thrombosis: a meta-analysis. Blood. 2006;107(7):2766-73.
22. Canhão P, Ferro JM, Lindgren AG, Bousser MG, Stam J, Barinagarrementeria F, et al. Causes and predictors of death in cerebral venous thrombosis. Stroke. 2005;36(8):1720-5.
23. Hirsh J, Fuster V, Ansell J, et al. American Heart Association/American College of Cardiology Foundation. American Heart Association/American College of Cardiology Foundation guide to warfarin therapy. J Am Coll Cardiol. 2003;41(9):1633-52.
24. Bates SM, Greer IA, Pabinger I, et al. American College of Chest Physicians. Venous thromboembolism, thrombophilia, antithrombotic therapy, and pregnancy: American College of Chest Physicians Evidence-Based Clinical Practice Guidelines (8th Edition). Chest. 2008;133(6 Suppl):844S-886S.
25. Wong CA. Nerve injuries after neuraxial anaesthesia and their medicolegal implications. Best Pract Res Clin Obstet Gynaecol. 2010;24(3):367-81.
26. Shapiro JL, Yudin MH, Ray JG. Bell's palsy and tinnitus during pregnancy: predictors of pre-eclampsia? Three cases and a detailed review of the literature. Acta Otolaryngol. 1999;119(6):647-51.
27. Chan LY, Tsui MH, Leung TN. Guillain-Barré syndrome in pregnancy. Acta Obstet Gynecol Scand. 2004;83(4):319-25.
28. Kalidindi M, Ganpot S, Tahmesebi F, Govind A, Okolo S, Yoong W. Myasthenia gravis and pregnancy. J Obstet Gynaecol. 2007;27(1):30-2.
29. Kanal E, Barkovich AJ, Bell C, Borgstede JP, Bradley WG Jr, Froelich JW, et al. ACR guidance document for safe MR practices: 2007. AJR Am J Roentgenol. 2007;188(6):1447-74.

CHAPTER 60

Psychiatric Disorders

Sangeeta T Tajpuriya

INTRODUCTION

Pregnancy is generally thought to be a time of happiness and emotional wellbeing for a woman. However, for many women, pregnancy and motherhood increase their vulnerability to psychiatric conditions, such as depression, anxiety disorders, eating disorders, and psychoses. These conditions are often underdiagnosed because they are attributed to pregnancy-related changes in maternal temperament or physiology. In addition, such conditions are often undertreated because of concerns about potential harmful effects of medication. Reproductive events and process have profound psychological effects on the life of a woman, some of which can progress to overt psychopathological states. Motherhood confers a highly social and psychological impact on the life of a woman. Pregnant women undergoes marked hormonal, physical and psychological changes. Their attitudes toward pregnancy reflect deeply felt beliefs about all aspects of reproduction, including whether the pregnancy was planned and whether the baby is wanted.

According to psychoanalytical theorists, the child to be is a blank screen on which a mother projects her hopes and fears. In rare instances, these projections account for postpartum pathological states, such as mother's desire to harm her infant, whom she views as a hated part of herself.

Pregnancy and the puerperium are emotionally stressful periods for many women. Mood swings are commonly manifested by emotional liability, weepiness, irritability, and feeling blue or high. Prenatal assessment for psychological difficulties should include the following:

- Prior personal or family history of psychiatric illness.
- Psychiatric disorder.
- Psychological problems that accompanied maturational periods e.g., puberty.
- History of early maternal deprivation or mother's death.
- Difficulty about separating from parents.
- Conflicts about mothering.
- Marital or family difficulties, including separation.
- Past difficulty with pregnancy, delivery, or postpartum depression.
- Recent death of family member or close friend.
- Familial or congenital disorders.
- History of infertility.
- History of repeat abortion.
- History of pseudocyesis or hyperemesis.
- Prior fetal death, miscarriage, or congenital abnormality.
- History of sexual, physical, or emotional abuse, current or past.
- History of premenstrual syndrome.

Psychiatric disorders during pregnancy and in the puerperium have been described throughout the history, although there is disagreement as to whether these disorders are the same or different from those occurring at other times. Because untreated maternal mental illness is associated with deleterious effects on maternal-infant attachment and synchrony in child development, it is essential to diagnose and appropriately treat psychological disorders. Although some psychotropic medications appear to be safe when used in breastfeeding mothers, few randomized controlled trials have been performed. For this reason, it is important to involve a pediatrician in the infant's care when treating a breastfeeding mother with psychotropic medications.

PSYCHIATRIC ASPECTS OF PREGNANCY

The psychological reactions experienced following childbirth include the common, relatively mild, physiologic, and transient "maternity blues" (50–70% of women).

True depression occurs in 8–20%, and frank puerperal psychosis occurs in 0.14–0.26%.

Anxiety Disorders in Pregnancy

Anxiety during pregnancy and the puerperium is normal; its total absence is as pathologic as in its excess. When anxiety increases enough to be considered a disorder, there are two major classifications: (1) phobic disorders, and (2) anxiety state disorders. Phobic disorders include persistent and irrational fear of a specific object, activity, or situation that may lead to avoidance. In pregnancy, irrational fears are often related to the fetus (e.g., unsubstantiated worries about food that might harm the fetus). Treatment ranges from simple reassurance to behavior modification to medication.

Anxiety states are divided into three categories: (1) Panic disorders include recurrent attacks of anxiety with sudden onset of intense fear and apprehension. There may be physical symptoms, such as dyspnea, chest pains, palpitations, choking, and dizziness. Attacks may last minutes to hours with anxiety between attacks. They are thought to have biochemical basis, but there is often a precipitating event. Panic disorders may be part of the syndrome of depression. (2) Generalized anxiety disorders last a month or more with signs of motor tension, vigilance, scanning, autonomic hyperactivity, and apprehension. Other conditions causing anxiety must be ruled out. (3) Obsessive-compulsive disorder is characterized by repetitive behaviors that result from anxiety or preoccupation with particular irrational fears.

These disorders may interfere with function and compliance. Treatment of anxiety disorder is initiated with a psychiatric evaluation, reassurance, and behavioral modification. Cognitive behavioral therapy is an effective treatment for these syndromes, but requires patient commitment and compliance. Selective serotonin reuptake therapies, benzodiazepines are useful for an acute anxiety crisis, but should be avoided during pregnancy. They are highly addictive and there is some evidence that they are associated with fetal malformations.

Maternity Blues

The postpartum period may represent a time of increased vulnerability to depression for some women. Most of these women report symptoms consistent with "baby blues", "a transient mood disturbance characterized by mood liability, sadness, dysphoria, subjective confusion, and tearfulness. These feelings which may last several days, have been ascribed to rapid changes in women's hormonal levels, the stress of childbirth, and the awareness of the increased responsibility that motherhood brings.

There appear to be no obstetric, social, economic, or personality correlates for maternity blues. However, lower than expected tryptophan levels have been documented in association with the depressive symptoms in the immediate postpartum period, suggesting a role for neurotransmitters in the elaboration of puerperal mood changes.[1] Hyperactivity of the hypothalamic pituitary adrenal axis, *blunted* responsiveness of the hypothalamic-pituitary-thyroid axis, and altered central neurotransmitter function characterize postpartum depression as well as non-puerperal major depression.[2]

No professional treatment is required other than the education and support for the new mother. Some of the symptoms may be increased by exertion and sleep deprivation; hence, increased rest may be helpful. Family support and a sympathetic and understanding attitude of all family members are all which is required to tackle this troublesome and common mood change. If the symptoms persist longer than 2 weeks, evaluation is indicated for postpartum depression.

Postpartum Depression

Postpartum depression is characterized by insomnia, excessive anxiety, depressed mood, and change in weight. This affective disorder occurs after pregnancy of any duration, which is from spontaneous abortion to full-term deliveries. The onset is generally within 12 weeks, but can occur any time after delivery up to one year. No conclusive evidence indicates that postpartum blues will lead to postpartum depression. Several studies have indicated that an episode of postpartum depression does lead to an increased risk of lifetime episodes of major depression. However, changes in the hypothalamic-pituitary-adrenal axis, including corticotropin–releasing hormone, may occur in women with postpartum depression.[3]

The signs and symptoms of postpartum depression are not different from those in non-pregnant patients, but may be difficult to differentiate from normal involutional phenomenon (weight loss, sleeplessness). Behavioral psychiatrists have postulated that the increased stress associated with pregnancy complications (miscarriage. fetal death, neonatal death) leads to increased strain on the mother's compensatory defenses and thus depression develops.

Certain characteristics of antenatal patients put them under high risk for postpartum depression.[4,5]

Similarly to identify puerperal patients who are at high risk to develop postpartum depression is the Edinburgh Postnatal Depression Scale (EDPS)[6], shown below in Box 1. Women with a score of 12 or more are the high risk candidates for puerperal depression and need careful clinical evaluation to clinch the diagnosis.

Response categories are scored 0, 1, 2, and 3 according to increased severity of the symptom. Items in italics are reverse scored (3, 2, 1, 0). The total score is calculated by adding together the scores for each of the 10 items.

Risk of Recurrence

- 50–100% in subsequent pregnancies.
- 20–30% with previous history of other depressive episode.

Treatment

The treatment should be started earlier. Counseling and medications is the cornerstone of the treatment. Serotonin selective reuptake inhibitor (SSRI) medications are better tolerated and effective, while safe for breastfeeding too.

Less severe depression, as noted in several studies, have long-term effects on the infants of depressed mothers, in the form of cognitive changes, emotional reactions and behavioral changes.

The moderately depressed mother will often feel so much of guilt of not fulfilling her motherly role as expected, she would never admit the symptoms of depression.

Family plays a very important role. Husband along with all other family members is advised about the nature of the patient's illness, so that with their tender love and support she would be able to cope up the required motherly role with self-satisfaction and pride.

In women with a previous history of postpartum depression, it is advisable to start the SSRI medications 2–3 weeks prior to the delivery, so that an optimal drug level is maintained post delivery.

If there is no response to these general measures psychiatric consultation is advisable. Below shows the comparison between baby blues and postpartum depression.

Postpartum Psychosis

A woman is more likely to suffer from new-onset psychosis during the postpartum period than during any other time of her life. Interestingly, the antenatal period is not associated with increased risk of psychosis. Psychosis is a severe mental illness characterized by a false reality and can be associated with fear and impulsivity. Contributing factors include a family history of mental illness, past psychiatric disorders, marital and family problems, recent stressful life situations, and a lack of social supports, although none of these risk factors may be present. These individuals appear to be biologically vulnerable to mental disease. Risk of recurrence in subsequent pregnancies may be as high as 20–30%.

Box 1: Edinburgh postnatal depression scale

In the past 7 days:

- I have been able to laugh and see the funny side of things:
  - As much as I always could
  - Not quite so much now
  - Definitely not so much now
  - Not at all
- I have looked forward with enjoyment to things:
  - As much as I ever did
  - Rather less than I used to
  - Definitely less than I used to
  - Hardly at all
- I have blamed myself unnecessarily when things went wrong:
  - Yes, most of the time
  - Yes, some of the time
  - Not very often
  - No, never
- I have been anxious or worried for no good reason:
  - No, not at all
  - Hardly ever
  - Yes, sometimes
  - Yes, very often
- I have felt scared or panicky for no very good reason:
  - Yes, quite a lot
  - Yes, sometimes
  - No, not much
  - No, not at all
- Things have been getting on top of me:
  - Yes, most of the time I haven't been able to cope at all
  - Yes, sometimes I haven't been coping as well as usual
  - No, most of the time I have coped quite well
  - No, I have been coping as well as ever
- I have been so unhappy that I have had difficulty in sleeping:
  - Yes, most of the time
  - Yes, sometimes
  - Not very often
  - No, not at all
- I have felt sad or miserable:
  - Yes, most of the time
  - Yes, quite often
  - Not very often
  - No, not at all
- I have been so unhappy that I have been crying:
  - Yes, most of the time
  - Yes, quite often
  - Only occasionally
  - No, never
- The thought of harming myself has occurred to me:
  - Yes, quite often
  - Sometimes
  - Hardly ever
  - Never

Source: Cox JL, Holden JM, Sagovsky R. Detection of postnatal depression. Development of the 10-item Edinburgh Postnatal Depression Scale. Br J Psychiatry. 1987;150:782-6.

Schizophrenia is a psychiatric disorder of at least 6 months' duration, characterized in its acute phase by delusions, hallucinations, incoherent speech, catatonia, or flat affect. Schizophrenic women may have exacerbations during pregnancy and the puerperium and should be carefully monitored. Delusions in pregnancy often relate to bodily changes and fetal movements. The disease is considered to have an organic basis with biochemical abnormalities, and drug treatment is usually with neuroleptic antipsychotics, such as phenothiazines, butyrophenones, and thioxanthenes. A psychiatric referral is indicated. Suicidal risk should be assessed.

A medical and drug history should be obtained from the relatives or friends. Accuracy in diagnosis is essential (e.g., insulin shock in a diabetic may be confused with psychogenic seizures). If possible, a blood sample should be drawn for drug and toxicity screening. The patient is calmed and a relative or friend may remain with her unless she becomes violent. In such instances, security personnel should be alerted and the patient transferred to a psychiatric care facility as quickly as possible. Haloperidol may be given orally or parenterally to facilitate immediate management.

The incidence of postpartum psychosis is about 1–2 per 1,000 childbirths. About 50% affected mothers have family history of mood disorders. The most robust data indicate that it is essentially a mood disorder, usually a bipolar disorder but possibly a depressive disorder. The delivery process evokes a nonspecific stress that causes a major mood disorder, perhaps through a major hormonal mechanism. Symptoms usually manifest within 2–3 days to almost within 8 weeks of the delivery.

The onset of florid psychotic symptoms is usually followed by prodromal signs, such as insomnia, restlessness, agitation, fatigue, episodes of tearfulness and emotional liability. Once the psychosis develops, the patient is of danger either to herself or her infant. In one study, 5% of patients committed suicide and 4% infanticide.

Clinicians should take into consideration the possibility of psychotic disorder caused by general medical condition or substance induced. Hypothyroidism and Cushing's syndrome should be evaluated. Pain killers (pentazocine) and antihypertensive drugs can be considered for substance-induced psychotic disorder.

Treatment

Postpartum psychosis is a psychiatric emergency. Antipsychotic medications, lithium and antidepressant drugs are the treatment of choice. A suicidal patient is referred to psychiatric unit and is kept under supervision all the time. Psychotherapy is advised after the period of acute psychosis, and it is aimed at helping the patient to accept and adjust the new role of mother to be played with satisfaction. Most studies reported high rate of recovery from the acute illness.

Women with histories of psychiatric illness frequently come in for consultations regarding the use of psychotropic medications during pregnancy. Not infrequently, women present with the first onset of psychiatric illness while pregnant. Many pregnancies are unplanned and may occur unexpectedly while women are receiving treatment with medications for psychiatric disorders. Many women may consider stopping medication abruptly after learning they are pregnant, but for many women this may carry substantial risks.

Decisions regarding the initiation or maintenance of treatment during pregnancy must reflect an understanding of the risks associated with fetal exposure to a particular medication but must also take into consideration the risks associated with untreated psychiatric illness in the mother. Psychiatric illness in the mother is not a benign event and may cause significant morbidity for both the mother and her child; thus, discontinuing or withholding medication during pregnancy is not always the safest option.

RISKS OF MEDICATION EXPOSURE

All medications diffuse readily across the placenta, and no psychotropic drug has yet been approved by the Food and Drug Administration (FDA) for use during pregnancy. When prescribing medications during pregnancy, one must consider the following risks associated with prenatal exposure: risk of teratogenesis, risk of neonatal toxicity, and risk of long-term neurobehavioral sequelae.

Risk of Teratogenesis

During the earliest stages of pregnancy, formation of major organ systems takes place and is complete within the first 12 weeks after conception. Therefore, discussion around risks of exposures during pregnancy may be broken down by the timing of exposure or trimester, with particular vigilance around 1st trimester exposures.

A teratogen is defined as an agent that interferes the *in utero* development process and produces some type of organ malformation or dysfunction. For each organ or organ system, there exists a critical period during which development takes place and is susceptible to the effects of a teratogen. For example, neural tube folding and closure, forming the brain and spinal cord, occurs within the first 4 weeks of gestation. Most of the formation of the heart and great vessels takes place from 4–9 weeks after conception, although the entire 1st trimester is often considered pertinent.

Risk of Neonatal Symptoms

Neonatal toxicity or perinatal syndromes (sometimes referred to as neonatal "withdrawal") refer to a spectrum of physical and behavioral symptoms observed in the acute neonatal period that can be attributed to drug exposure at or near the time of delivery. Larger samples must be studied in order to establish a causal link between exposure to a particular medication and a perinatal syndrome.

Risk of Long-term Effects

Although the data suggest that some medications may be used safely during pregnancy if clinically warranted, but the long-term effects of prenatal exposure to psychotropic medications is incomplete. Because neuronal migration and differentiation occur throughout pregnancy and into the early years of life, the central nervous system (CNS) remains particularly vulnerable to toxic agents throughout pregnancy. While exposures to teratogens early in pregnancy may result in clear abnormalities, exposures that occur after neural tube closure (at 32 days of gestation) may produce more subtle changes in behavior and functioning.

CONCLUSION:

Although the overall prevalence of psychiatric disorders appears to be similar among currently pregnant, postpartum women and non-pregnant women, an important exception was the elevated risk of major depressive disorder during the postpartum period. Biological (e.g., hormonal) as well as psychological and social role changes associated with childbirth may increase the risk of major depressive disorder during postpartum. Furthermore, women with psychiatric illness who become pregnant may discontinue their psychiatric medication for fear of prenatal exposure to these agents, therefore increasing the risk of depressive relapse during pregnancy or the puerperium. We are not having any accurate national information on the mental health of pregnant women . Such information is needed for focused planning at the national and local level, and to inform the development of prevention and intervention programs for Mental disorders during pregnancy and the postpartum period.

REFERENCES

1. Handley SL, Dunn TL, WaldronG, Baker JM. Tryptophan, cortisol and puerperal mood. Br J Psychiatry. 1980;136:498-508.
2. Stowe ZN, Nemeroff CB. Women at risk for postpartum-onset major depression. Am J Obstet Gynecol. 1995;173(2):639-45.
3. Magiakou M-A, Matorakos G, Rabin D, et al. Hypothalamic corticotrophin-releasing hormone suppression during the postpartum period: implication for the increase in psychiatric manifestations at this time. J Clin Endocrinol. 1996;81:1912.
4. Posner NA, Unterman RR, Williams KN. Postpartum depression: the obstetrician's concerns. In: Inwood DG (Ed). Recent Advances in Postpartum Psychiatric Disorders. Washington, DC, American Psychiatric Press, Inc; 1985. p. 69.
5. Beck CT. The effects of postpartum depression on child development: a meta-analysis. Arch Psychiatric Nurs. 1998;12(1):12-20.
6. Cox JL, Holden JM, Sagovsky R. Detection of postnatal depression. Development of the 10-item Edinburgh Postnatal Depression Scale. Br J Psychiatry. 1987;150:782-6.

CHAPTER 61

Dermatological Complications

Mudita Gupta

INTRODUCTION

Pregnancy is a physiological state of multiple immunologic, metabolic, endocrine and vascular changes.[1] Virtually every organ undergoes some physiological or pathological changes to adjust the fetus in the mother's womb. Skin and cutaneous appendages are no exception.

Pregnancy is associated with a new endocrine organ: the placenta. Hormonal changes occurring during pregnancy are increased levels of estrogen, progesterone, β-human chorionic gonadotropin (hCG), prolactin, and a series of other hormones and mediators that affect various functions of the body.[2] Pituitary and thyroid gland enlarge leading to increased iodine uptake and increased output of adrenocorticotropic hormone (ACTH), prolactin and gonadotropins. Circulatory cortisol increases.

Also protein, carbohydrate, lipid metabolism is accelerated. Increase in cardiac output, blood volume and hemodilution occurs.

Maternal immunological alteration occurs to allow the fetus to survive. During pregnancy Th2 cytokines increase (IL-4, IL-5, IL-10, IL-13), while postpartum Th1 cytokines increase (TNF-α, IFN-γ, IL-2). Change in hormones can also lead to immunological alteration.[3] Increase in estrogen can suppress Th1 cytokine (IL-2). Increase in progesterone promotes Th2 cytokines. Increase in glucocorticoids causes decrease in Th1 cytokines and stimulate Th2 activity.

During pregnancy mother is not only bothered about her cosmetic appearance, but also about recurrence in subsequent pregnancy and the harm to the fetus. The dermatoses of pregnancy can be classified into 4 groups (Box 1) i.e., (1) physiological skin changes in pregnancy, (2) specific dermatoses of pregnancy, (3) diseases with uncertain association with pregnancy, and (4) dermatoses and cutaneous tumors affected by pregnancy.

PHYSIOLOGICAL CHANGES

There are certain cutaneous alterations that are so common that they are not considered as abnormal and accepted to be physiological.[4] Although these changes may be only cosmetic but they are of considerable anxiety to the patient. These changes do not harm the fetus. Broadly, they can be classified into five groups as shown below in Box 2.

Hyperpigmentation

Hyperpigmentation is seen in 90% pregnant females.[5] These changes are more common in dark skinned females. Hyperpigmentation of face, cheeks, nose, upper lip and chin forms the mask of pregnancy (Fig. 1). This is also known as melasma gravidarum or chloasma. Chloasma is seen in 75% of pregnant women.[5] Darkening of freckles, nevi and recent scars may occur uniformly.

Darkening of the skin adjacent to areola may result in formation of secondary areola (Fig. 2). Linea nigra is a dark line running from xiphoid process to pubic region seen during pregnancy[5] (Fig. 3).

It is pigmented linea alba. This is often accompanied by the displacement of the umbilicus to the right, known as the "ligamentum teres sign". This may persist postpartum till the muscles regain their tone. Hyperpigmentation usually affects the whole body, and areas normally more pigmented become darker, such as the areolae, genitalia, perineum, axillae and inner thighs. Group B pigmentary lines also known as voigt's

Box 1: Classification of skin diseases during pregnancy

- Physiological changes
- Pregnancy specific dermatosis
- Diseases of uncertain association with pregnancy
- Pregnancy aggravated dermatosis

Box 2: Physiological changes of pregnancy

- Pigmentary changes
    - Chloasma
    - Secondary areola
    - Linea nigra
    - Diffuse hyperpigmentation
    - Darkening of nevi, freckles and recent scars
    - Group B pigmentary lines
- Vascular changes
    - Spider nevi
    - Palmar erythema
    - Granuloma gravidarum
    - varicosities
    - Hemangioma and purpura
    - Vasomotor instability disorders
    - Physiological edema
- Structural changes
    - Striae
    - Skin tags
- Hair changes
    - Telogen effluvium
    - Hirsutism
    - Frontoparietal hair loss
- Nail changes
- Appendiceal changes
    - Increased eccrine gland activity
    - Decreased apocrine activity
    - Sebaceous gland activity increased/decreased

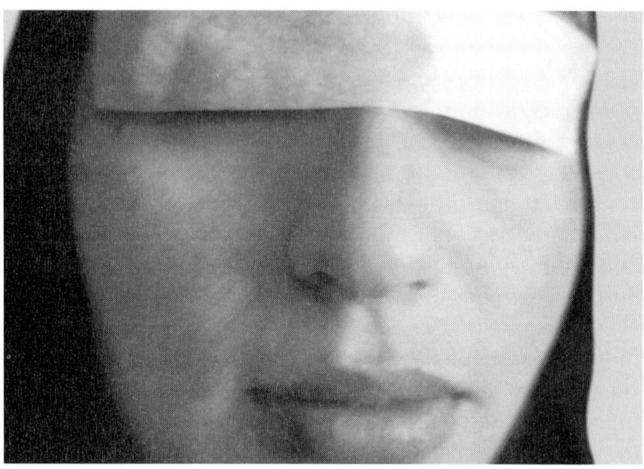

FIG. 1: Chloasma *(For color version, see Plate 6)*.

lines appear. Voigt lines are borders of abrupt transition between more deeply pigmented skin and that of lighter pigmentation.

Hyperpigmentation was previously thought to be due increase in melanocyte stimulating hormone (MSH) of pituitary origin, but the activity of this hormone does not

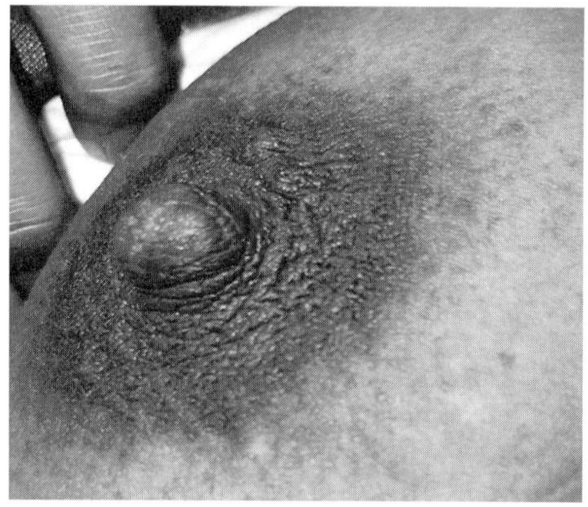

FIG. 2: Secondary areola *(For color version, see Plate 6)*.

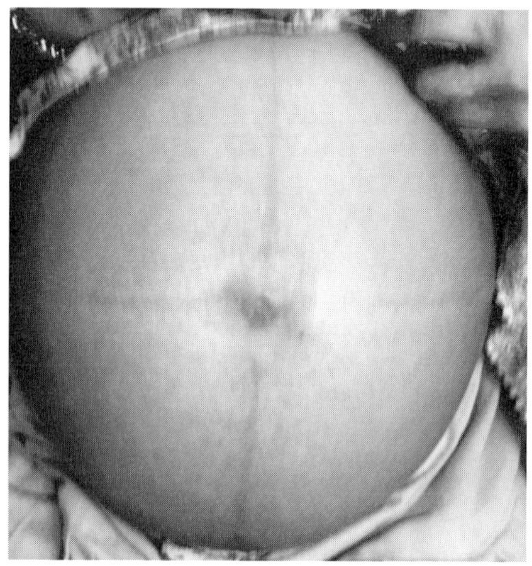

FIG. 3: Linea nigra *(For color version, see Plate 6)*.

coincide with hyperpigmentation appearance. Level of estrogen and progesterone have same pattern of rise and fall as hyperpigmentation.[6] Estrogen and progesterone level start increasing after 8th week and decrease after 30th week. Melanogenic enzymes (tyrosinase and tyrosinase-related proteins 1 and 2) are upregulated by bioactive sphingolipids secreted by placenta.[7] Increased number of melanocytes and sensitivity of receptors to estrogen and progesterone also increases.[7]

Hyperpigmentation gradually lightens but may persist in 30% cases. Chloasma recurs in subsequent pregnancies and with use of oral contraceptives (OCs). Use of broad spectrum sunscreens may have a protective effect. Treatment involves the use of bleaching agents, such as hydroquinone 2–4%

cream. Topical tretinoins can be added postpartum but are to be avoided during pregnancy to avoid possible teratogenicity. Ruby laser (694 nm) and the Q-switched alexandrite laser (755 nm) may be done postpartum.

Vascular Changes

Spider Nevi

Spider nevi also known as nevus araneus are bright red, blanchable, small arterioles with fine vessels radiating from the center (Fig. 4).

They appear during first trimester and gradually increase in size throughout pregnancy. These are usually seen on the skin drained by the superior vena cava, particularly around the eyes. Fair-skinned individuals (67%) are more predisposed while it is seen in only 11% of blacks.[8] Most spider nevi regress postpartum. A small percentage of persisting lesions can be ablated by electrocautery or laser.

Palmar Erythema

Palmar erythema is mottled erythema of the thenar and hypothenar eminences with sparing of the digits. It is seen in 66% of whites and 33% of blacks.[9]

Varicosities

Distension of the superficial venous vasculature of legs (i.e., varicose veins) (Fig. 5), vagina, vestibule (i.e., Jacquemier-Chadwick sign), and rectum (i.e., hemorrhoids) are common in pregnancy.

About 40% of pregnant women are affected. They develop secondary to hormonal factors and increased circulating maternal fluids.[10] Increased intra-abdominal pressure leading to compression of pelvic and abdominal vessels is also a major contributing factor. Elevation of the legs and trendelenburg position and compression stockings decrease the varicosity. Sustained sitting and standing should be avoided. Varicose veins often regress in the postpartum period; however, sclerotherapy may be necessary if varicosity persists.

Granuloma Gravidarum or Pyogenic Granuloma

Granuloma gravidarum (Fig. 6) is a benign, rapidly proliferating vascular lesion that commonly occurs at sites of previous trauma on the face, neck, and fingers. Pyogenic

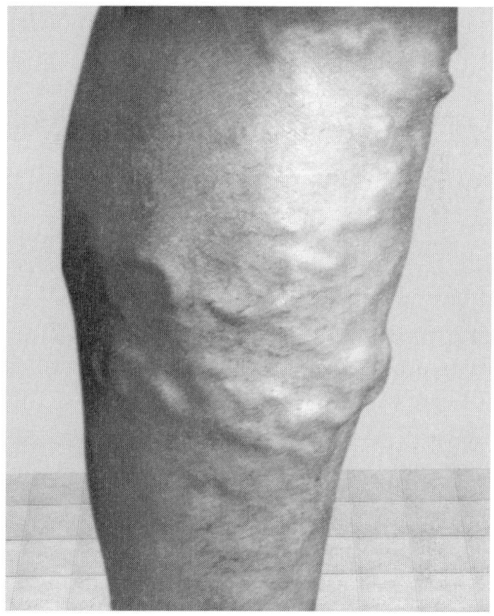

FIG. 5: Varicose veins *(For color version, see Plate 7)*.

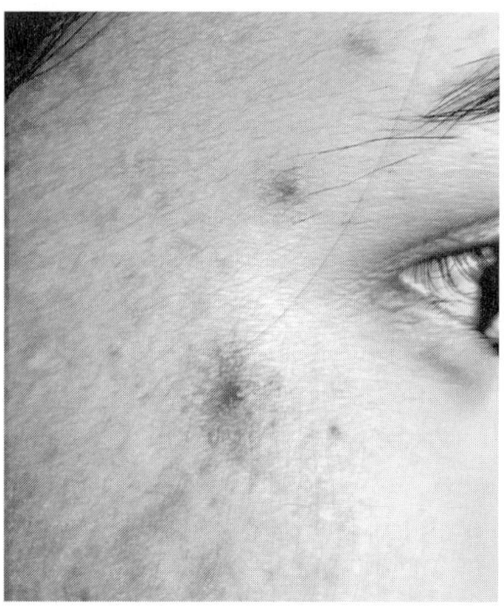

FIG. 4: Spider nevi *(For color version, see Plate 7)*.

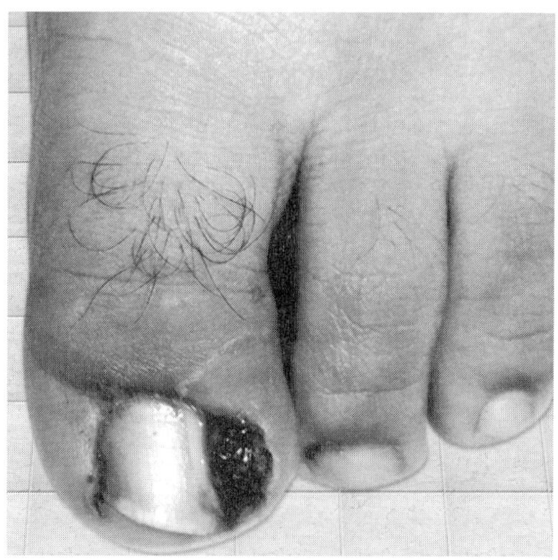

FIG. 6: Granuloma gravidarum *(For color version, see Plate 7)*.

granuloma is a misnomer. It is actually nodular granulation tissue. Surgical removal or electrocautery ablation can be done.

Vasomotor Instability Disorders

Cutis marmorata is intermittent reticulated cyanotic appearance that characteristically involves legs on exposure to cold. Facial flushing, pallor, hot and cold sensations can occur during pregnancy. Facial glow, dermatographism and itching on palms are other minor changes seen.

Hemangioma and Purpura

Hemangiomas occur spontaneously in 5% of pregnancies during the second or third trimesters generally on hands and neck (Fig. 7). Hemangiomas and purpura regress postpartum. Elevated hydrostatic pressure and increased capillary fragility may result in purpura of lower limbs.

Physiological Edema of Pregnancy

Increased capillary permeability and water and sodium retention contribute to nonpitting edema of the extremities and face. This is seen in 50% pregnant females particularly during the third trimester. Elevated hydrostatic pressure secondary to pressure of gravid uterus on inferior vena cava has additive effect.

Structural Changes

Striae Gravidarum

Striae gravidarum, or "stretch marks", occur commonly on the abdomen, thighs, buttocks and breast of pregnant women (Fig. 8). Striae are seen in 90% of fair-skinned individuals. These appear as atrophic, wrinkled, erythematous, purplish bands. Striae in primigravida are pink, shiny and in multigravida are white atrophic. The pathogenesis of striae formation is unclear. Physical factors and hormones (relaxin, estrogen, and corticosteroids) cause thinning of elastin fibers and fibrillin microfibrils in the dermis, and the fiber orientation shifts from perpendicular to parallel relative to the dermal-epidermal junction.[11] Risk factors for more severe striae include maternal family history, young maternal age, higher baseline and delivery body mass index (BMI), and increased abdominal and hip girth.[12] Currently, there is no effective treatment for striae. Contrary to popular belief, cocoa butter, massage, shea butter, and aloe vera preparations have no efficacy. Limited evidence suggests that two topical treatments may help prevent striae. One contains Centella asiatica extract plus α-tocopherol and collagen-elastin hydrolysates.[13] The other treatment contains tocopherol, essential fatty acids, panthenol, hyaluronic acid, elastin, and menthol. Tretinoins can be used in postpartum period.

Molluscum Fibrosum Gravidarum

Molluscum fibrosum gravidarum are benign, small, pedunculated, tan-to-brown, fleshy papules that are commonly seen on the neck (Fig. 9), axillae, inner aspects of the thighs, and inframammary folds. They frequently appear during the second half of pregnancy and may even regress postpartum. Their etiology is unclear. Treatment options include shave excision, electrocautery, cryosurgery, and scissors removal.

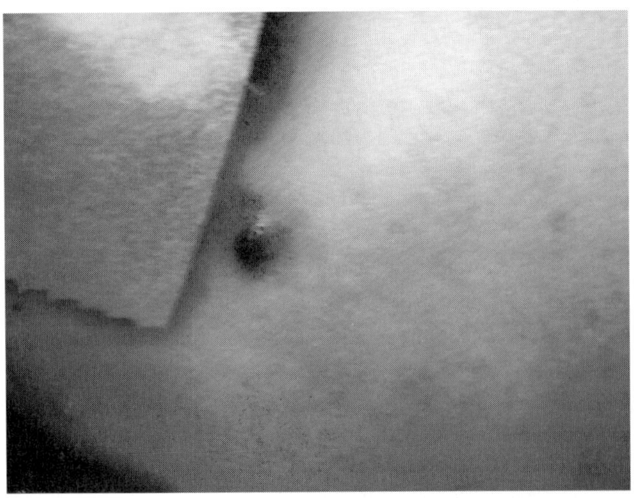

FIG. 7: Hemangioma *(For color version, see Plate 7).*

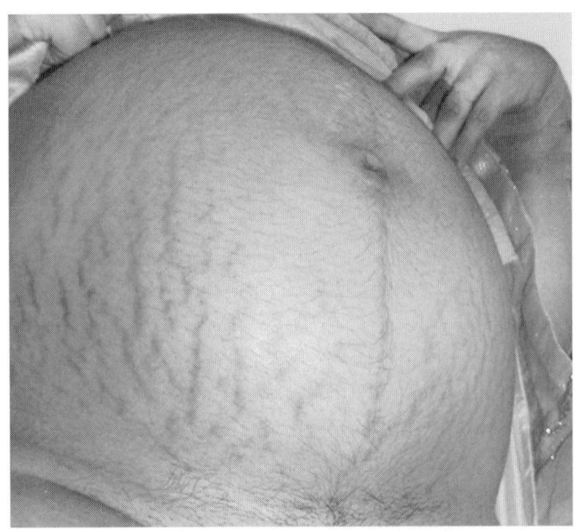

FIG. 8: Striae gravidarum *(For color version, see Plate 7).*

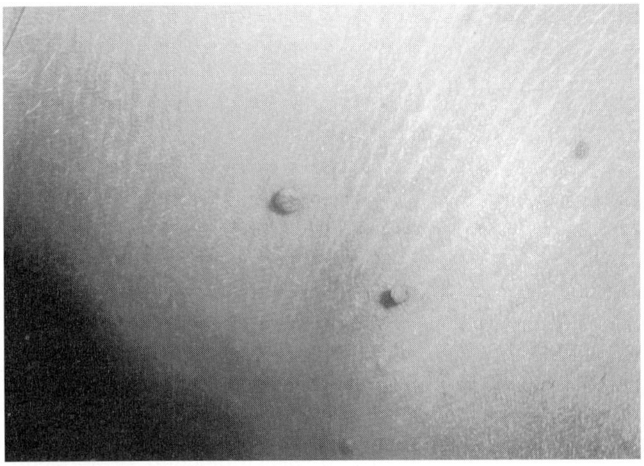

FIG. 9: Molluscum fibrosum gravidarum *(For color version, see Plate 7)*.

Appendageal Changes

Glandular Changes

The eccrine glands progressively enhance their activities, leading to hyperhidrosis, miliaria and dyshidrotic eczema. Symptoms may be treated with soaks of aluminum chloride hexahydrate (20%) in ethyl alcohol solution. Paradoxically, palmar sweating is decreased.

Apocrine glands have their activities reduced throughout pregnancy.

Sebaceous gland activity may decrease or increase.

Montgomery tubercles (Fig. 10) are small, papules appear on the areolae, occurring up to half of all pregnancies, and regress after childbirth (30–50%).

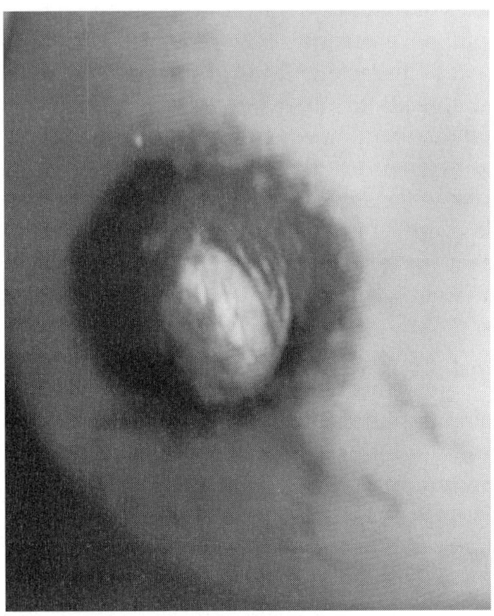

FIG. 10: Montgomery tubercles *(For color version, see Plate 8)*.

Hair Changes

Hypertrichosis mainly on face and arms is seen. Hypertrichosis results due to a reduced conversion of anagen into telogen hair. It usually disappears within six months after delivery and does not require specific therapy. Hirsutism is believed to result from increased ovarian and placental androgens acting on the pilosebaceous unit. Occasionally frontoparietal hair loss may occur.

Telogen effluvium (TE) is common and occurs between the first and fifth postpartum months. It is caused by the fast conversion of anagen into telogen hair. Most patients recover within 15 months of delivery.[14]

Nail Changes

Nails may become more fragile and brittle, with distal onycholysis and subungual onycholysis. Nail growth rate increases.

PREGNANCY SPECIFIC CUTANEOUS CHANGES

Pregnancy-specific dermatoses (PSD) are an ill-defined heterogeneous group of pruritic skin eruptions which are seen only in pregnancy. PSD has been variously termed and classified[15-17] in the past as shown in Box 3 and Table 1.

Pregnancy-specific dermatoses classified broadly into 4 types (Box 4). Atopic eruption of pregnancy (AEP) is the

Box 3: Historical review of pregnancy specific dermatoses

- Herpes gestationis (Milton 1874)
- Prurigo gestationis (Besnier 1904)
- Toxemic rash of pregnancy (Bourne 1962)
- Papular dermatitis of pregnancy (Spangler 1962)
- Prurigo of pregnancy (Nurse 1968)
- Early onset form
- Late onset form
- Pruritic folliculitis of pregnancy (1981)
- Linear IgM disease of pregnancy

TABLE 1: Historical classification of pregnancy specific dermatosis

Holmes and Black in 1983	Shornick in 1998	Ambros-Rudolph et al in 2006
PG	PG	PG
PEP	PEP	PEP
PP	PP	AEP (eczema, PP, PF)
PF	ICP	ICP

PG, pemphigoid gestationis; PEP, polymorphic eruption of pregnancy; PP, prurigo of pregnancy; PF, pruritic folliculitis of pregnancy; ICP, intrahepatic cholestasis of pregnancy; AEP, atopic eruption of pregnancy.

Box 4: Classification of specific dermatosis of pregnancy

- Pemphigoid gestationis
- Atopic eruption of pregnancy
- Pruritic urticarial papules and plaques of pregnancy
- Intrahepatic cholestasis of pregnancy

TABLE 2: Synonyms of pregnancy specific dermatoses

Names	Synonyms
Pemphigoid gestationis	• Herpes gestationis • Gestational pemphigoid
Pruritic urticarial papules and plaques of pregnancy	• Polymorphic eruption of pregnancy • Toxemic rash of pregnancy • Toxemic erythema of pregnancy • Late onset prurigo of pregnancy
Atopic eczema of pregnancy	• Prurigo of pregnancy • Prurigo gestationis • Early onset prurigo of pregnancy (Nurse) • Papular dermatitis of pregnancy (Spangler) • Pruritic folliculitis of pregnancy
Cholestasis of pregnancy	• Obstetric cholestasis • Intrahepatic cholestasis of pregnancy • Jaundice of pregnancy • Prurigo gravidarum

most common of these disorders. Different synonyms are used for PSD (Table 2). Diseases with uncertain association with pregnancy are an additional group.

PEMPHIGOID GESTATIONIS

Introduction

It is an intensely pruritic bullous eruption that may develop not only during pregnancy but also rarely associated with trophoblastic tumors, hydatidiform mole and choriocarcinoma. Initially, due to presence of bullous lesions it was known as herpes gestationis (HG). Due to its clinical and immunofluorescence similarities with bullous pemphigoid this condition was renamed pemphigoid gestationis (PG) in 1982 (Box 5).

Box 5: Key features of pemphigoid gestationis

- Intensely itchy vesiculo-bullous eruption
- Onset in late second trimester with aggravation during puerperium
- Increases in subsequent pregnancy
- Auto antibodies against BP Ag 2
- Direct immunofluorescence shows linear deposition of C3
- Fetal affection is seen

Epidemiology

It has an incidence rate between 1:50,000 and 1:60,000. It is associated with HLA-DR3 and HLA-DR4, and usually occurs during 12th–24th week of pregnancy.

Pathogenesis

Pemphigoid gestationis is an autoimmune disease associated with pregnancy. The major target antigen is the extracellular noncollagenous16A (NC16A) domain of the transmembrane hemidesmosomal glycoprotein, collagen XVII (BP180).[18] This antigen, is present on the amniochorionic stromal cells, trophoblast and basement membrane of skin.[19] When this antigen is presented to the maternal immune system by abnormally expressed MHC II class molecules an allogenic response is triggered. Immunoglobulin G (IgG) antibodies also known as HG factor are formed. IgG4 is the specific immunoglobulin that crosses the placenta.[20] Subsequent cross-reaction with maternal skin occurs. This leads to complement activation and chemo attraction of eosinophils. Degranulation of eosinophils and release of proteolytic enzymes dissolves the bond between epidermis and dermis leading to development of bulla.

Clinical Features

Pemphigoid gestationis usually presents in late second trimester of pregnancy. There is a phase of relative quiescence in late pregnancy with postpartum flares in 75% cases. Half the cases occur in first pregnancy. There is high risk of recurrence in subsequent pregnancies; the onset may be earlier and disease may be more severe. However, clinical presentation and course is variable. There be occasional skip pregnancies or milder disease in subsequent pregnancy.

Pemphigoid gestationis is extremely itchy condition with abrupt onset. Characteristically PG begins around umbilicus and then spreads to other parts of body including palms and soles. Face and mucous membrane are usually spared. Eruptions begin as urticated papules, plaques, target lesions and annular wheals with subsequent development of vesicles and bulla (Fig. 11) within days to weeks. Vesicles and bulla may appear on normal or urticated base and heal without scarring.

Differential Diagnosis

Pemphigoid gestationis has to be differentiated from other specific dermatosis of pregnancy, bullous drug rash and other autoimmune bullous disorders.

Risk to Fetus

Pemphigoid gestationis is associated with premature delivery and low birth weight. Risk of fetus is increased with early onset

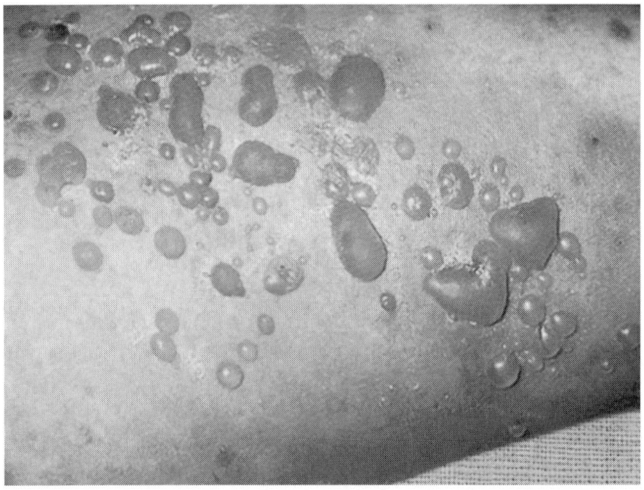

FIG. 11: Vesicles with urticated base in pemphigoid gestationis *(For color version, see Plate 8)*.

and severe disease. The fetal risks may not decrease with treatment and is due to low-grade placental insufficiency.[21] Neonatal PG may occur in 10% cases.[22] Regular fetal monitoring should be done and if growth restriction is found then decision of early delivery should be taken.[23]

Associated Diseases

Pemphigoid gestationis is associated with other autoimmune diseases in 14% cases.[24]

Pathology

Histopathology of early lesions shows epidermal and papillary edema with eosinophilic spongiosis. Bullous lesions are sub-epidermal and contain numerous eosinophils. Direct immunofluorescence shows C3 with or without IgG along basement membrane in a linear pattern in the perilesional skin. Indirect immunofluorescence (IIF) demonstrates HG factor. Auto antibodies bind to epidermal side of salt split skin. Immuno electron microscopy shows deposition of IgG at lamina lucida. Immunoblotting and enzyme-linked immunosorbent assay (ELISA) show BP180 to be the major antigen. IIF is not a marker of disease activity and severity while ELISA can be used for this purpose. ELISA was found to have a sensitivity of 93% and a specificity of 96%.[18]

Prognosis

Pemphigoid gestationis improves postpartum but may persist for few months or years. Flares may occur during menstruation or with use of OCs. OCs should be avoided till disease is active.

Treatment

The lesions may subside spontaneously weeks to months after delivery. Chronic PG is defined as disease persisting for longer than 6 months. Conversion to bullous pemphigoid is occasionally seen. Mild disease requires topical potent or very potent steroids. Bullous lesions need to be treated with systemic steroids 20–80 mg/day. Once flares are controlled maintenance with lower doses of steroids should be done. To prevent postpartum flares prophylactic systemic steroids should be given and dosage may be increased expecting a postpartum flare. Antihistamines can be given but are not of much benefit. Postpartum immunosuppressive treatment and plasmapheresis may be required in recalcitrant or chronic PG cases. Risk of therapy should be carefully weighed against the severity of disease.

PRURITIC URTICARIAL PAPULES AND PLAQUES OF PREGNANCY (POLYMORPHIC ERUPTIONS OF PREGNANCY)

Introduction

It is the second common pregnancy specific dermatoses. In 1979, Lawley et al clarified this disease presentation.

Epidemiology

Incidence is reported to be 1:160 pregnancies.[25]

Pathogenesis

The cause of polymorphic eruptions of pregnancy (PEP) is uncertain. PEP is a Th1 oriented disease (CD8+lymphocytes) in comparison to PG which is Th2 oriented (CD4+lymphocytes).[26] PEP is more commonly seen in multiple pregnancy and increased maternal weight gain.[27] Rapid late stretching of abdominal skin leads to connective tissue damage and provokes conversion of nonantigenic molecule to antigenic one.[28] Also increased progesterone in multiple gestation and peripheral chimerism favors skin with increased vascularity and damaged collagen. Increased activity of progesterone receptor has been found in skin lesions of PEP.[29] Finally, a small study demonstrated male fetal deoxyribonucleic acid (DNA) in skin lesions of PEP probably as a result from fetal cell migration to maternal skin secondary to peripheral blood chimerism, a phenomenon that is known to start early in gestation and increases as pregnancy progresses.[28]

Clinical Features

Pruritic urticarial papules begin in striae with periumbilical sparing (Fig. 12). Lesions appear on other parts of body but

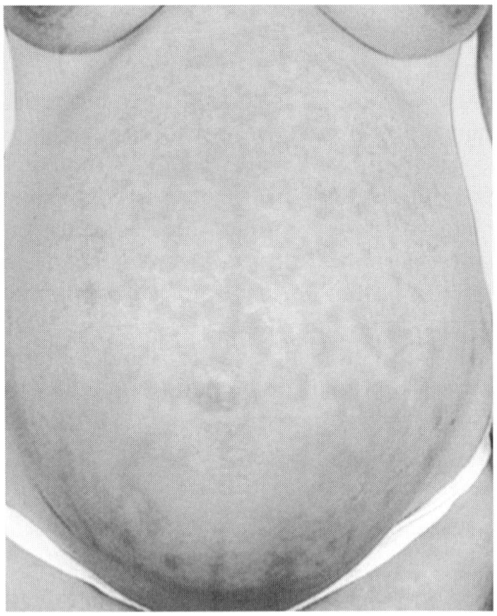

FIG. 12: Periumbilical sparing in pruritic urticarial papules and plaques of pregnancy *(For color version, see Plate 8)*.

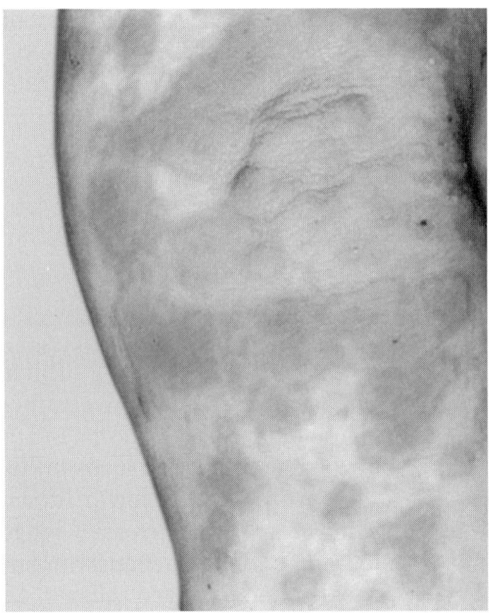

FIG. 13: Urticated papules and plaques in pruritic urticarial papules and plaques of pregnancy *(For color version, see Plate 8)*.

face, palms and soles are spared. Onset in late pregnancy or postpartum.[30] Lesions are often polymorphous (Fig. 13) consisting of urticarial (49%), vesicular (17%), targetoid (6%), polycyclic (6%).[24] Purpuric, eczematous, excoriated dyshidrotic and photo distributed lesions are also occasionally present. PEP may be generalized resembling toxic erythema. It does not recur in subsequent pregnancy. Even if it does the disease is less severe.

No biochemical abnormality is seen. Histopathology changes are nonspecific with epidermal and upper dermal edema. There is perivascular infiltration of lymphocytes, eosinophils and histiocytes. Eosinophil infiltration though is a prominent feature but it is less than in PG. No confirmatory diagnostic tests are available. Diagnosis is by exclusion. Immunofluorescence tests are negative.

Differential Diagnosis

Polymorphic eruption of pregnancy has to be differentiated from other specific pregnancy dermatosis.

Other diseases coinciding with pregnancy (nonspecific) are: scabies, eczema, drug rash, erythema multiforme, and urticarial.

Fetal risk: there is no substantial risk to the fetus.[31]

Treatment

Topical emollients, antipruritic topical medications (menthol and doxepin), and antihistamines are the mainstay of treatment for milder disease. Occasionally, topical or systemic steroids may be required. The condition resolves 2–3 weeks postpartum.

ATOPIC ERUPTION OF PREGNANCY

Vaughan-Jones et al. in a prospective study on pruritic skin diseases in pregnancy in 1999 reported a high prevalence of atopic eczema in pregnancy for first time.[32] AEP is a disease complex which includes eczema of pregnancy, prurigo of pregnancy and pruritic folliculitis.[33] Pruritic folliculitis of pregnancy (PF) was described by Zoberman and Farmer in 1981.[34]

Epidemiology

Atopic eruption of pregnancy is the most common pregnancy dermatosis; accounting for 36–49.7% of total cases.[17] Deterioration in pregnancy is seen in 50% cases, while improvement is seen in 25% cases. Personal history of atopy is seen in 27% cases and family history in 50% cases.[17] Prurigo of pregnancy has been reported to occur in approximately, 1 in 300 pregnancies.[1] Pruritic folliculitis is seen in the second and third trimester of pregnancy and affects an estimated one in 3,000 pregnancies.[35]

Pathogenesis

The Th2 shift associated with pregnancy may favor the exacerbation of atopic dermatitis (AD). Experimental studies indicate that estrogens may affect mast cell activation, while progesterone suppressed histamine release and potentiated IgE induction in animal studies.[17]

Clinical Features

The clinical features of gestational AD are identical to those seen in nonpregnant females.[36] Any part of body may be involved. Eczema may be of intrinsic or extrinsic type. Intrinsic AD is more commonly seen in pregnancy.[37] Intrinsic AD, as opposed to that with the extrinsic type, has no associated respiratory disease (bronchial asthma or allergic rhinitis), shows normal total serum IgE levels, no specific IgE and negative skin prick tests to aeroallergens or foods. The lesions in AEP may be eczematous/E type (75% cases) (Fig. 14) or papular type (P type) (Fig. 15).[17] Superadded *Staphylococcus* and herpetic infections are common. Prurigo of pregnancy is characterized by pruritic, often excoriated papules and nodules on the extensor surfaces of the legs and upper arms (Fig. 16). It can be seen in second and third trimester of pregnancy and is often associated with atopy.

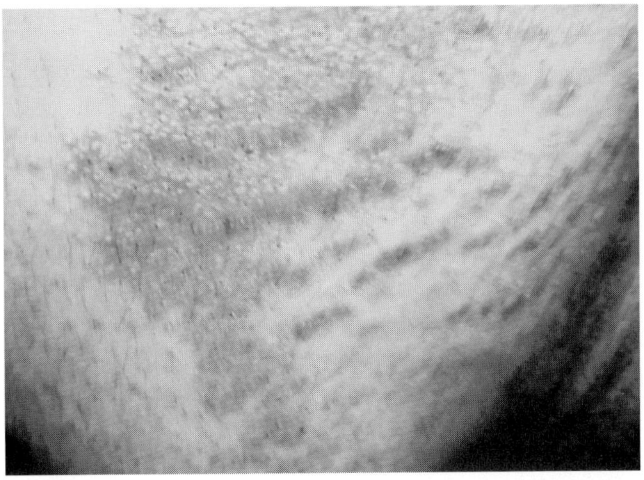

FIG. 14: Atopic eczema of pregnancy (E type) ***(For color version, see Plate 8).***

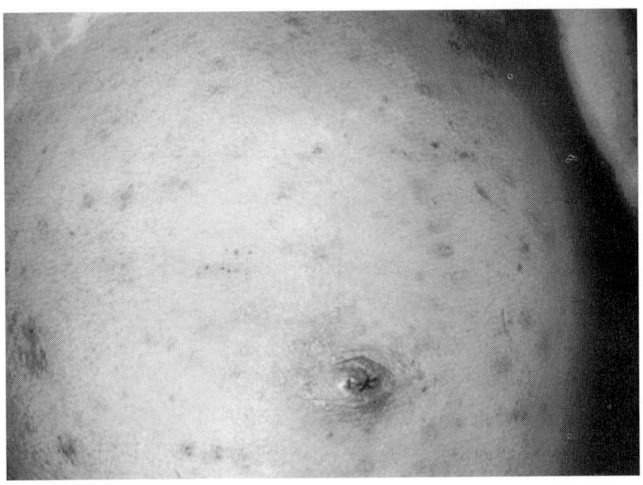

FIG. 15: Atopic eczema of pregnancy (P type) ***(For color version, see Plate 8).***

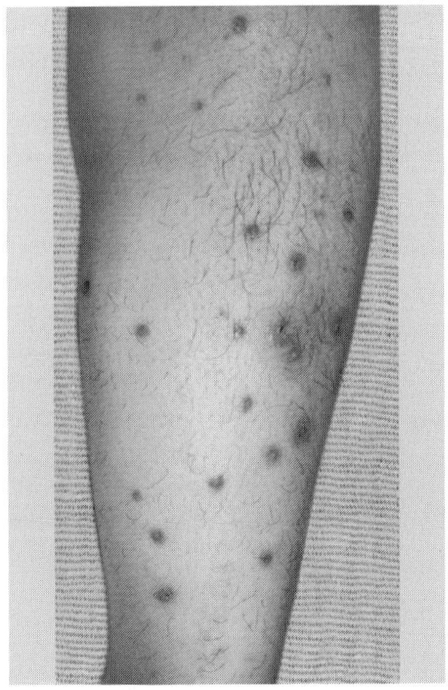

FIG. 16: Prurigo of pregnancy ***(For color version, see Plate 9).***

The name pruritic folliculitis is a misnomer as pruritus is not a major feature and it may be mistaken for acne or microbial folliculitis.[38] Acneiform eruption consisting of multiple, pruritic, follicular papules or pustules typically on the shoulders, upper back, arms, chest, and abdomen.[39] The diagnosis is made clinically after excluding other more common rashes.

Differential Diagnosis

Atopic eruption of pregnancy has to be differentiated from other specific dermatoses of pregnancy (Table 3) and dermatosis coinciding with pregnancy (e.g., scabies, allergic rash, drug rash, pityriasis rosea, etc.

Treatment

Dry skin care remains an integral part of eczema management. Emollients are to be applied immediately after bathing. Antipruritic additives, such as menthol and polidocanol can be used. First generation antihistamines or cetirizine and loratadine may be used. Mid or high potency topical steroids can be used for severe symptomatic AEP. For recalcitrant cases a short course of systemic steroids may be used in third trimester. For severe AEP narrow-band ultraviolet B (UVB) is effective.[20] If systemic agents are needed for severe or recalcitrant eczema, cyclosporine is the safest option and should be used for the shortest duration possible. Erythromycin and acyclovir can be used for superadded *Staphylococcus* infection and herpes simplex. PF lesions usually resolve spontaneously 1–2 months following delivery.

Fetal risk: there is no affection of the fetus.

TABLE 3: Differences between dermatoses of pregnancy

Character	Pemphigoid gestationis	Pruritic urticarial papules and plaques of pregnancy	Atopic eczema of pregnancy	Intrahepatic cholestasis of pregnancy	Impetigo herpetiformis
Incidence	1:50,000	1:160	AD 36–49.7% PP 1:300 PF 1:3000	1:1500	rare
Etiology	Autoimmune	Mechanical stretch Increased progesterone Fetal DNA chimerism	Immunological alteration in pregnancy	Genetic, environmental, alimentary, endocrinal, immunological	
Pruritus	Severe	Severe	Moderate	Severe	Mild
Time of onset	2first week/ postpartum 20% cases	34th week/ postpartum	Any trimester	30th week	third trimester
Site of onset	Umbilicus	Striae	AD: any site PP: extensors leg PF: upper back	Abdomen	Intertriginous areas
Classical morphology of lesion	Vesicles, bullae	Urticarial lesions	AD: E type (eczematous) P type (Papules) PP: papules PF follicular papules	No primary lesions. Secondarily, excoriations seen	Erythematous plaque studded with pustules at margins
Involvement of palms and soles		Spared	Involved	Present	Spared
Risk factors		Multiple pregnancies, increased maternal weight gain			
Classical lab finding	DIF shows linear C3 deposits	Diagnosis by exclusion		Increased serum bile acids	Subcorneal pustulosis and histopath consistent with psoriasis
Recurrence with subsequent pregnancy	Common and severer with early onset in next pregnancy	No recurrences		Seen in 40–50% cases	Common and severer with early onset in next pregnancy
Fetal risk	Increased prematurity, small for gestational age PG in newborn	No risk		Prematurity, meconium staining, fetal distress and death, vitamin K deficiency	Growth retardation and still births
Associated diseases	Other autoimmune diseases	None	Systemic atopy	Cholelithiasis, hepatitis C, pre-eclampsia, acute fatty liver of pregnancy, urinary tract infections, leaky gut and gestational diabetes Increased drug sensitivity	
Treatment of choice	Oral corticosteroids in a dose of 40–60 mg/kg	Antihistamines. Occasionally, topical steroids	Topical steroids and antihistamines	Ursodeoxycholic acid	Prednisolone 15–60 mg/day

AD, atopic dermatitis; PP, prurigo of pregnancy; PF, pruritic folliculitis of pregnancy; DNA, deoxyribonucleic acid; PG, pemphigoid gestationis; DIF, direct immunofluorescence test.

PRURITUS GRAVIDARUM (INTRAHEPATIC CHOLESTASIS OF PREGNANCY)

Pruritus gravidarum and intrahepatic cholestasis of pregnancy (ICP) are terms which have been used interchangeably. Both of them are not associated with primary skin lesions. While the former starts in first trimester ICP starts in third trimester.[39]

Introduction

Cholestasis of pregnancy was initially described by Svanborg and Thorling in 1954.[40] ICP is the most dangerous PSD as far as fetal prognosis is concerned.

Epidemiology: incidence of 1:1500.[41] Family history seen in 50% cases.

Pathogenesis

This disease has a multifactorial etiology. There is an interplay between genetic, immunological, environmental, alimentary and endocrine factors.[41] There is increased family history of ICP and cholelithiasis.[42] There is increased incidence in certain geographic areas suggesting that there may be some gene susceptibility.[42] Females heterozygous for progressive familial intrahepatic cholestasis mutations (Box 6), namely, ATP8B1, ABC11 (BSEP) and ABCB4 (encodes the multidrug resistance protein 3, a canalicular phosphatidylcholine translocase) have increased predisposition to develop ICP.[43] Mutations of ABC11 is thought to be especially responsible. Immunological factors implicated are variation in cytokines. Increased tumor necrosis factor-a and interferon-c, and decreased level of transforming growth factor-b2 and interleukin-4 is seen in ICP.[44] HLA-BW16 and HLA-DPB1*0402 are associated with ICP. These genetic changes are not significant when hormone levels are normal but lead to ICP when hormonal levels are high.

Endocrinal Changes

Estrogens interfere with bile acid secretion,[45] and progestins inhibit hepatic glucuronyl transferase.[46] Single nucleotide polymorphism of nuclear hormone pregnane X receptor (PXR) leads to increased risk of ICP and low fetal birth weight.

Box 6: Key features of intrahepatic cholestasis of pregnancy

- Pruritus without primary lesion
- Biochemical cholestasis with no definite etiology
- Spontaneous resolution after delivery
- Recurrence in 60–70% cases
- Fetal risk is there

PXR is involved in detoxification of bile acids.[47] ICP also shows decreased circulating levels of 1,25 dihydroxy vitamin D and increased endothelin-1 levels.[48]

Decreased selenium levels are also associated with this disease. ICP is more commonly seen in winters.[49]

Pruritus is secondary to an increase in the concentration of bile acids in serum and within the skin. There is a relative fall in the hepatic blood flow during pregnancy which leads to a decreased clearance of estrogens resulting in an increase in biliary cholesterol concentration and secretion. This also impairs the capacity of the liver to transport anions (bilirubin and bile salts). Lysophosphatidic acid (LPA) is activated by an enzyme autotaxin (ATX). LPA acts on different receptors that signal message that is interpreted as itch.[50]

Clinical Features

Intrahepatic cholestasis of pregnancy presents in second or third trimester with generalized pruritus with jaundice (20% cases)[51] or without jaundice. It is the second-most common cause of jaundice in pregnancy. Itching is more at night. No primary lesions are seen. Itching starts on abdomen later spreading to extremities and trunk. Palms and soles are also involved. Pruritus worsens with increased gestational period while jaundice remains the same. Pruritus may precede or lag behind the biochemical abnormalities. Increased risk of gall stones is associated. ICP is more common in multiple pregnancies. Recurrences are seen in subsequent pregnancies and with use of OCs. Pruritus improves within 48 hours of delivery.

Lab Diagnosis

For diagnosis serum bile levels should be >4.08 mcg per mL (11.0 μmol/L), conjugated fraction is particularly increased and can be used for monitoring disease activity.[20] Increased serum aminotransferases is seen. The serum cholic acid level increases, and an increase in the ratio of cholic acid to chenodeoxycholic acid is considered to be the most sensitive indicator for the early diagnosis of ICP.[20] A decreased glycine-to-taurine ratio is seen.[20]

Diagnostic criteria[51] for ICP are:

- Generalized pruritus with or without jaundice
- Absence of primary skin lesions
- Biochemical abnormalities consistent with cholestasis
- Resolution after delivery.

Recurrence with subsequent pregnancy occurs in 40–50% of patients.

Prognosis

Pruritus and biochemical abnormalities resolve spontaneously 2–3 weeks postpartum. Increased risk of meconium stained liquor, preterm labor (19–60%) and fetal arrhythmias/

distress (22–33%) and sudden intrauterine death (1–2%).[52] Decreased fetal elimination of toxic bile acids may cause vasoconstriction of placental chorionic veins and increased myometrial activity, thus increasing the risk of preterm labor. Also bile acids increase colonic motility thus increasing meconium passage. Meconium passage further can cause acute umbilical vein constriction.[53] Increased bile acid taurocholate in fetal circulation can cause fetal arrhythmias. Increased bile acid may cause bile acid pneumonia in the new born. Malabsorption of vitamin K may lead to intracranial hemorrhage.

Associated diseases-hepatitis C seropositivity, pre-eclampsia, acute fatty liver of pregnancy,[4] urinary tract infections,[54] increased permeability of gut (leaky gut)[55] and gestational diabetes.[54] There are increased chances of drug sensitivity especially to antibiotics.[55]

Treatment

Topical or systemic antihistamines and emollients are not very effective. Epomediol, silymarin, S-adenosyl-l-methionine, activated charcoal, phenobarbital and guar gum have also not found to be of much added benefit.[24] Suppression of feto-placental estrogen production and resolution of pruritic symptoms can be achieved by using 12 mg of dexamethasone daily for 6 days.[56] UVB phototherapy has been shown limited success.[16] Rest and low fat diet should be prescribed.

Cholestyramine binds bile acids and decreases their enterohepatic circulation. It may be used in mild to moderate ICP in a dosage of up to 18g/day. It needs to be administered for several days before pruritus improves. Cholestyramine are that it may be ineffective in severe ICP and there is no improvement in the biochemical abnormalities of ICP and fetal outcome.[57] Cholestyramine may deplete vitamin K and lead to coagulopathies.[58] Also there is relapse of pruritus after one week of treatment.[58] If cholestasis is prolonged, risk of intracranial hemorrhage in fetus and maternal prothrombin time has to be monitored.

Ursodeoxycholic acid (UDCA) is the most effective treatment of ICP given in a dose of 450–1200 mg/day. UDCA is a naturally occurring hydrophilic bile acid which enhances the excretion of hydrophobic bile acids and other hepatotoxic compounds and sulfated progesterone metabolites.[59] It also protects both cholangiocytes from cytotoxic bile acids and hepatocytes from apoptosis caused by bile acids.[39] It reduces the pruritus, improves liver function and decreases the frequency of premature labor.[58] UDCA is the only drug which helps to improve fetal prognosis.

A close obstetric surveillance is indicated in ICP. Weekly fetal cardiotocography (CTG) should be done at least from 34 weeks gestation onwards. Induction of labor should be done at 37–38 weeks.[60]

DISEASES WITH UNCERTAIN ASSOCIATION WITH PREGNANCY

Impetigo Herpetiformis

Introduction

Von Hebra in 1872 described impetigo herpetiformis (IH) as an acute pustular eruption arising usually in third trimester of pregnancy.[61] It is regarded as a variant of pustular psoriasis manifesting because of hormonal changes during pregnancy.[62] Thus, it is also known as generalized pustular psoriasis of pregnancy. It normally appears in a person with personal or family history of psoriasis.

Clinical Presentation and Course

Patient presents usually in third but rarely in late first trimester. Eruption usually originates in intertriginous areas (Fig. 17). It later spreads centrifugally and becomes generalized. The condition manifests as erythematous plaque studded with sterile subcorneal pustular at margins (Fig. 18).[63] Subungual involvement may lead to onycholysis. Mucosal lesions manifest as painful erosions. Face, hands and feet are usually spared. Constitutional symptoms like malaise, anorexia, nausea, vomiting, diarrhea, fever, muscle weakness, lymphadenopathy or chills may be present. Life-threatening maternal complication like septicemia, hyperparathyroidism with hypocalcemia[64] or hypoalbuminemia may occur.

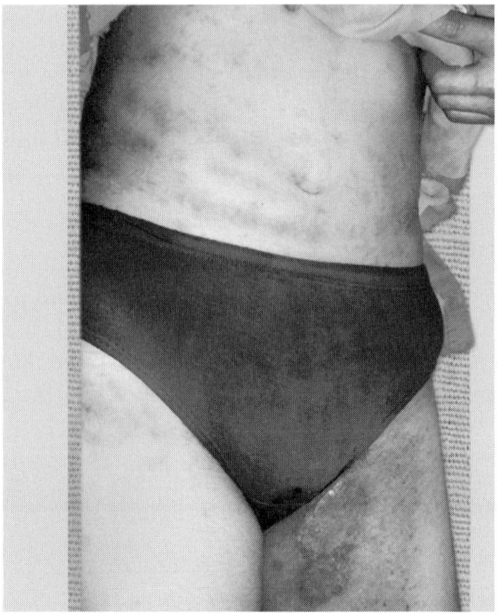

FIG. 17: Centrifugally spreading plaques in intertriginous areas in impetigo herpetiformis *(For color version, see Plate 9)*.

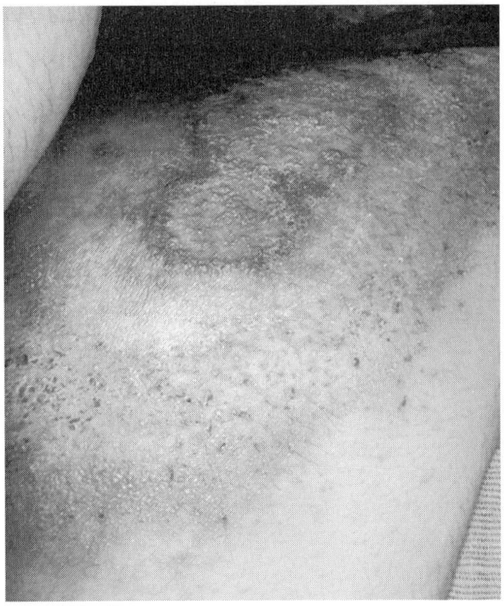

FIG. 18: Subcorneal pustulosis in impetigo herpetiformis *(For color version, see Plate 9)*.

Laboratory Investigations

Hematological investigations show leukocytosis with a neutrophilia, elevated erythrocyte sedimentation rate, hypo ferric anemia and hypoalbuminemia. Rarely there may be increased levels of blood urea nitrogen (BUN), increased levels of uric acid, hypocalcemia, and hyperphosphatemia as a manifestation of hypoparathyroidism.[65] Histopathologically, reveals features of pustular psoriasis.

Prognosis

Recurrences in subsequent pregnancies are common and more severe with onset in earlier gestation.

Fetal risk: growth retardation and still births may be seen.

Differential Diagnosis

Pustular drug eruption, pemphigoid gestationis, other immune bullous diseases, bullous impetigo, etc.

Treatment

Resolution after delivery is the norm. Systemic steroids (60–80 mg/day of prednisolone) are the mainstay of treatment.[66] Antibiotics are also required. Fluid and electrolyte balance should be monitored with rapid correction of imbalances. In severe cases, termination of pregnancy is advised.

Autoimmune Progesterone Dermatitis of Pregnancy

There is a single case report of autoimmune progesterone dermatitis of pregnancy presenting as nonpruritic acneiform eruptions on buttocks and extremities in two successive pregnancies.[67] There is hypersensitivity to endogenous progesterone. There was associated arthritis and skin reaction to progesterone was positive.

Linear IgM Dermatosis of Pregnancy

There is only a single case report of linear IgM dermatosis of pregnancy (LMDP).[58] LMDP is considered by some as a variant of PUPPP. It is characterized by intensely pruritic, red, follicular papules and pustules on the abdomen, forearms, thighs, and legs appearing after 36 weeks of pregnancy. Direct immunofluorescence test reveals linear IgM deposits at the basal membrane zone (BMZ). No pregnancy effects were observed in the patient. Histopathology showed perifollicular neutrophilic infiltration.

PREGNANCY AND ASSOCIATED DISEASE

Pregnancy is known to alter the course of pre-existing skin diseases in both positive and negative ways (Table 4 and Box 7).

Human immunodeficiency virus (HIV) does not get altered by pregnancy. But opportunistic infection, like pneumocystis carinii is fatal.

TABLE 4: Pregnancy modified skin diseases

Infections	• Candidiasis • Trichomoniasis • Condylomata acuminate • Pityrosporum folliculitis • Herpes simplex • Varicella zoster • Leprosy
Autoimmune	• Lupus erythematosus • Dermatomyositis • Pemphigus • Systemic sclerosis
Metabolic disease	• Porphyria cutanea tarda • Acrodermatitis enteropathica
Connective tissue disease	• Ehlers-Danlos syndrome • Pseudoxanthoma elasticum
Tumors	• Bowenoid papulosis, • Langerhans cell histiocytosis • Mycosis fungoides • Malignant melanoma • Neurofibromatosis
Miscellaneous	• Atopic dermatitis • Erythema multiforme • Erythrokeratoderma variabilis • Psoriasis • Acne vulgaris • Hidradenitis suppurativa • Fordyce disease

Box 7: Skin diseases improving with pregnancy
- Allergic contact dermatitis
- Fox–Fordyce disease
- Hidradenitis suppurativa
- Psoriasis (2/3 improves)
- Systemic sclerosis

During pregnancy there is decreased cell mediated immunity, neutrophil function, activity of natural killer cells and impairment of local antibody responses. All these immunological changes predispose the patient to certain diseases or others may improve or aggravate.

INFECTIONS DURING PREGNANCY

Candidal vaginitis is 10–20 times more common during pregnancy.[68] It presents as white curdy discharge (Fig. 19).

It is seen in 50% of infants born to infected patients. This can be treated with topical miconazole, nystatin or clotrimazole. Trichomoniasis can be seen in 60% pregnancies.[68] Fetus is not normally affected. This can be treated with metronidazole in symptomatic patents in second or third trimester. Incidence of Malassezia furfur infections also increases.

Infection with human papilloma virus can lead to exuberant warts. Viral DNA greatly increases. In anogenital area they present as cauliflower, like fleshy masses and are known as condylomata acuminate (Fig. 20).

These can be treated by chemical cautery with trichloroacetic acid electrodessication, cryosurgery or laser ablation. To decrease the risk of neonatal laryngeal warts elective cesarean has been suggested but not yet warranted.

Herpes simplex virus infections are not more common in pregnancy. When this infection manifests in pregnancy it has 50% chances of being transmitted to neonate on primary infections and 5% in recurrent one.[69] In neonatal infection may lead to neurologic squeal or death of the child.

Varicella in pregnancy may have increased risk of pneumonitis seen in 14% cases. Premature labor or maternal death may occur. Neonatal varicella syndrome may be seen if mother is infected in first trimester. Maternal herpes zoster does not affect pregnancy or its outcome.

Exacerbation occurs in one-third of leprosy disease activity. Type 1 reaction occurs in first trimester thereafter the incidence decreases and then again increases postpartum. Incidence of type 2 reactions increases in third trimester of pregnancy and persist till 9 months lactation.

Autoimmune Disorders

Systemic lupus erythematosus (SLE) in pregnancy leads to increased maternal risk of thrombosis and abortions due to antiphospholipid antibody. Neonatal lupus may develop in patients with anti-RO antibodies. Premature births may occur in 16–37% cases. During pregnancy there is suppression of Th1 and increase of Th2 cytokines. Though there are only minor flares of dermatologic, articular and hematologic manifestations of SLE. Renal flares may be life-threatening.[70] Antimalarial hydroxychloroquine (HCQ) given to control minor symptoms of SLE were once thought to cause fetal auditory and retinal toxicity. But long-term follow-up of these children has shown no adverse effect. Withdrawal of HCQ during pregnancy may aggravate disease activity. In severe SLE immunosuppressive treatment should be continued.

Progressive systemic sclerosis may improve during pregnancy. If there is renal involvement it may deteriorate during pregnancy.

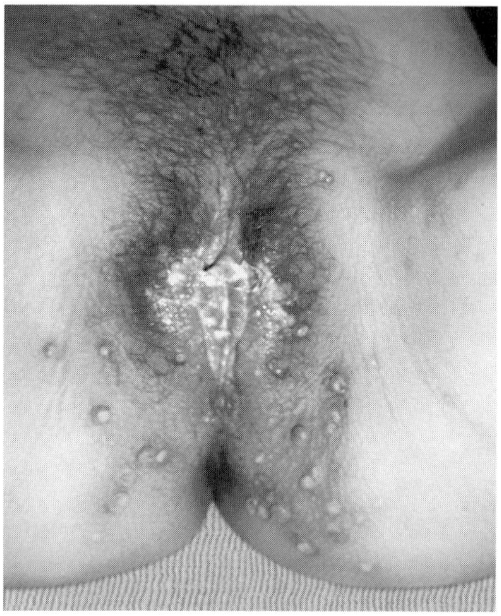

FIG. 19: Curdy discharge in candidiasis and pearly white umbilicated papules of molluscum *(For color version, see Plate 9).*

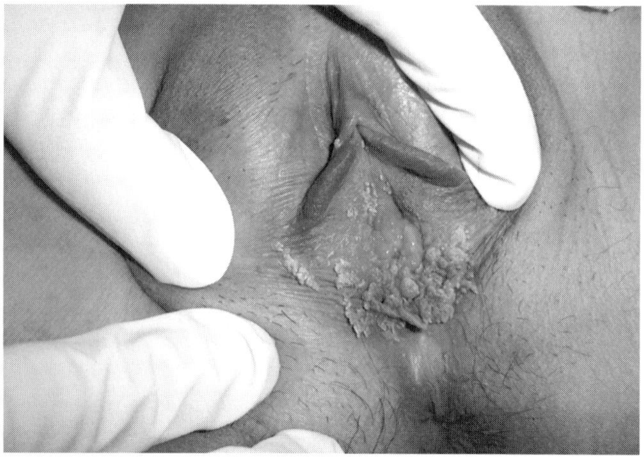

FIG. 20: Exuberant genital warts in pregnancy *(For color version, see Plate 9).*

Pemphigus

It may be precipitated or worsen during pregnancy. There is risk of transmission of IgG antibody in the fetus. The lesions appearing in newborn usually disappear in 2–3 weeks.[71] Fetal death may occur because of affection with disease, placental insufficiency or maternal infections.

Psoriasis Vulgaris

In 63% of pregnant women with psoriasis improve during pregnancy, while only 14% worsen.[72] This may be due to increased interleukin 10 in pregnancy, a cytokine which has a favorable effect on the course of the disease.

Metabolic Diseases

Porphyria Cutanea Tarda

Porphyria cutanea tarda (PCT) improves during pregnancy. Aggravating factors for PCT are estrogens, alcohol and iron. Early in pregnancy the skin fragility increases because of rise of estrogen level but later due to hemodilution and increased iron demand of the fetus the disease activity decreases.[1] Phlebotomy is the mainstay of treatment.

Acrodermatitis Enteropathica

Acrodermatitis enteropathica (AE) gets flared up during pregnancy because of the zinc deficiency resulting due to consumption of zinc by the fetus and also increased estrogen levels also.[68] There is diarrhea and skin rash which can be confused with impetigo herpetiformis. The disease flares during late first or early second trimester and progressively increases till term. Disease activity fades rapidly postpartum.

Ehlers-Danlos Syndrome

Ehler-Danlos Syndrome (EDS) type 1 (classic) and type IV (ecchymotic). These lead to joint hypermobility, skin fragility, easy bruising, skin hyperextensibility and rupture of arteries. These changes in pregnancy lead to increased risk of postpartum bleeding, poor wound healing, wound dehiscence, uterine lacerations, bladder and uterine prolapse, and abdominal hernias.[1] Pregnancy should be preferably avoided in this disease. Early termination should be considered if root of aorta is more than 4 cm dilated.

Pseudoxanthoma Elasticum

Pseudoxanthoma elasticum (PXE) is associated with elastic tissue degeneration of skin, eye, gastrointestinal tract and blood vessels. Effect of blood vessels particularly get aggravated leading to increased chances of hemorrhage, ventricular arrhythmias and congestive cardiac failure.[73]

Tumors

Malignant melanoma during pregnancy carries a worse prognosis.[74]

Neurofibroma may grow during pregnancy. Rupture of blood vessels may occur inside the tumor. Neurofibromas in renal artery may lead to hypertension. Pregnancy may exacerbate mycosis fungoides.

Acquired Immunodeficiency Disease

Pregnancy does not lead to aggravation of acquired immunodeficiency disease (AIDS). Opportunistic infections developing in pregnancy may be fatal.

APPROACH TO A PATIENT OF PRURITUS DURING PREGNANCY

Pruritus in pregnancy is a very common complaint. Itchy skin conditions not associated with pregnancy need to be excluded first (Flowchart 1). Severity of pruritus, trimester of onset, gestation of patient, parity, occurrence of symptoms in previous pregnancies, pruritus in nonpregnant state and in family are the questions which have to be dealt with. Patient has to be examined for the lesions if they are primary or secondary. The associated lesions, their evolution, morphology and distribution should be noted. Associated abnormality in liver function tests, albumin level or calcium levels may be seen. Histopathology may help in IH and direct immunofluorescence may be required in PG. For treatment of pruritus mild non-alkaline soaps should be used, too hot water for bathing should be avoided. Emollients should be used immediately after bathing. Emollients may contain 3% urea or polidocanol. Mild or moderate topical steroids, like desonide or mometasone can be used topically. When systemic steroids are required non-halogenated ones like cortisol, prednisone and prednisolone are used while betamethasone and dexamethasone are contraindicated. Prednisolone in a dose of 0.5–2 mg/kg can be for short duration (<4 weeks) with a lower maintenance dose of 10–15 mg/day. A longer course of steroids in addition to leading congenital abnormality like cleft palate may lead to adrenal insufficiency in the newborn. Antihistamines can control some pruritic conditions but are ineffective in others (as described earlier). Dimethindene, clemastine, pheniramine are preferable. Nonsedating ones like cetirizine and loratadine can be used in second and third trimester.

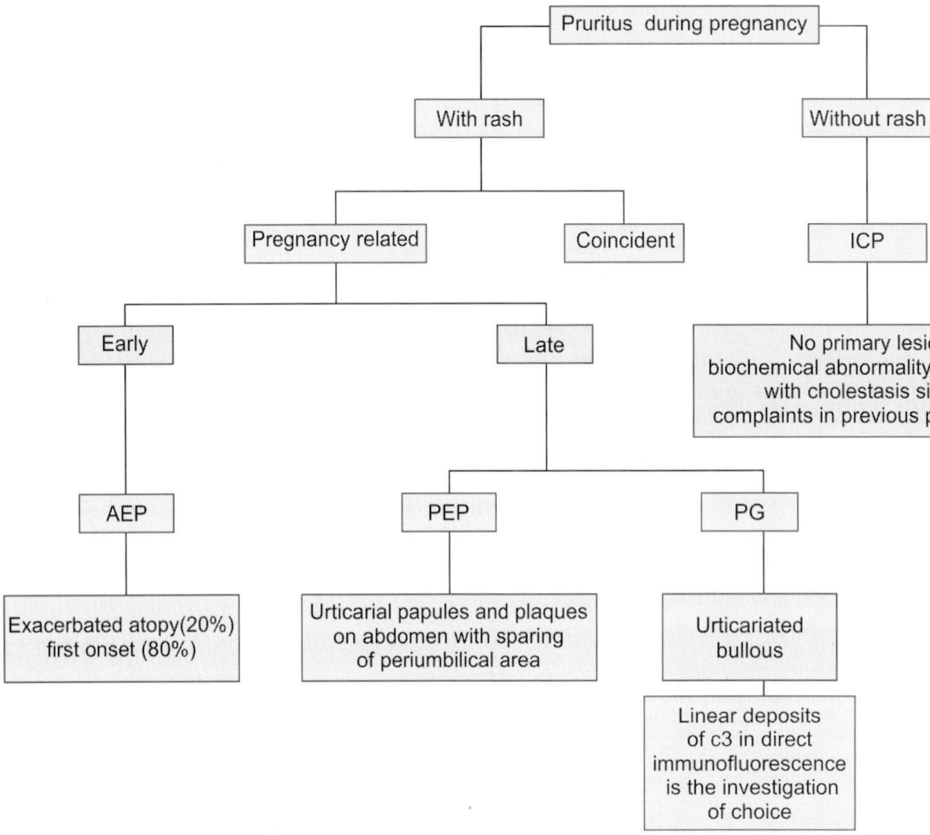

ICP, intrahepatic cholestasis of pregnancy; AEP, atopic eruption of pregnancy; PEP, polymorphic eruption of pregnancy; PG, pemphigoid gestationis.

FLOWCHART 1: Algorithm for diagnosing cause of pruritus in pregnancy.

REFERENCES

1. Kroumpouzos G, Cohen LM. Dermatoses of pregnancy. J Am Acad Dermatol. 2001;45(1):1-19.
2. Alves GF, Nogueira LSC, Varella TCN. Dermatology and pregnancy. An Bras Dermatol. 2005;80(2):179-86.
3. Warshauer E, Mercurio M. Update on dermatoses of pregnancy. Int J Dermatol. 2013;52(1):6-13.
4. Wade TR, Wade SL, Jones HE. Skin changes and diseases associated with pregnancy. Obstet Gynecol. 1978;52(2):233-42.
5. Wong RC. Physiologic skin changes in pregnancy. In: Harahap M, Wallach RC (Eds). Skin Changes and Diseases in Pregnancy. New York: Marcel Dekker, Inc; 1996. p. 37.
6. Wong RC, Ellis CN. Physiologic skin changes in pregnancy. J Am Acad Dermatol. 1984;10(6):929-40.
7. Mallick S, Singh SK, Sarkar C, Saha B, Bhadra R. Human placental lipid induces melanogenesis by increasing the expression of tyrosinase and its related proteins in vitro. Pigment Cell Res. 2005;18(1):25-33.
8. Muallem MM, Rubeiz NG. Physiological and biological changes in pregnancy. Clin Dermatol. 2006;24(2):80-3.
9. Winton GB, Lewis CW. Dermatoses of pregnancy. J Am Acad Dermatol. 1982;6(6):977-98.
10. Carvalho EV, Braga de Carvalho DS. Varices y embarazo. Rev Panam Flebol Linfol. 2001;40(1):25-30.
11. Geraghty LN, Pomeranz MK. Physiologic changes and dermatoses of pregnancy. Int J Dermatol. 2011;50(7):771-82.
12. Osman H, Rubeiz N, Tamim H, Nassar AH. Risk factors for the development of striae gravidarum. Am J Obstet Gynecol. 2007;196(1):1-5.
13. Ernst E. Herbal medicinal products during pregnancy: are they safe? BJOG. 2002;109(3):227-35.
14. Headington JT. Telogen effluvium. New concepts and review. Arch Dermatol. 1993;129(3):356-63.
15. Holmes RC, Black MM. The specific dermatoses of pregnancy. J Am Acad Dermatol. 1983;8:405-12.
16. Shornick JK. Dermatoses of pregnancy. Semin Cutan Med Surg. 1998;17(3):172-81.
17. Ambros-Rudolph CM, Müllegger RR, Vaughan-Jones SA, Kerl H, Black MM. The specific dermatoses of pregnancy revisited and reclassified: results of a retrospective two-center study on 505 pregnant patients. J Am Acad Dermatol. 2006;54(3):395-404.
18. Semkova K, Black M. Pemphigoid gestationis: current insights into pathogenesis and treatment. Eur J Obstet Gynecol Reprod Biol. 2009;145(2):138-44.
19. Huilaja L, Hurskainen T, Autio-Harmainen H, Hofmann SC, Sormunen R, Räsänen J, et al. Pemphigoid gestationis autoantigen, transmembrane collagen XVII, promotes the migration of cytotrophoblastic cells of placenta and is a structural component of fetal membranes. Matrix Biol. 2008;27(3):190-200.

20. Kroumpouzos G. Specific dermatoses of pregnancy: advances and controversies. Expert Rev. Dermatol. 2010;5:633-48.
21. Shornick JK, Black MM. Fetal risks in herpes gestationis. J Am Acad Dermatol. 1992;26(1):63-8.
22. Karna P, Broecker AH. Neonatal herpes gestationis. J Pediatr. 1991;119(2):299-301.
23. Semkova K, Black M. Pemphigoid gestationis: current insights into pathogenesis and treatment. Eur J Obstet Gynecol Reprod Biol. 2009; 145(2):138-44.
24. Kroumpouzos G, Cohen LM. Specific dermatoses of pregnancy: an evidence-based systematic review. Am J Obstet Gynecol. 2003;188(4):1083-92.
25. Vaughan Jones SA, Black MM. Pregnancy dermatoses. J Am Acad Dermatol. 1999;40(2 Pt 1):233-41.
26. Caproni M, Giomi B, Berti S, Bianchi B, Fabbri P. Relevance of cellular infiltrate and cytokines in polymorphic eruption of pregnancy (PEP). J Dermatol Sci. 2006;43(1):67-9.
27. Elling SV, McKenna P, Powell FC. Pruritic urticarial papules and plaques of pregnancy in twin and triplet pregnancies. J Eur Acad Dermatol Venereol. 2000;14(5):378-81.
28. Matz H, Orion E, Wolf R. Pruritic urticarial papules and plaques of pregnancy: polymorphic eruption of pregnancy (PUPPP). Clin Dermatol. 2006;24(2):105-8.
29. Im S, Lee ES, Kim W, Song J, Kim J, Lee M, et al. Expression of progesterone receptor in human keratinocytes. J Korean Med Sci. 2000;15(6):647-54.
30. Petropoulou H, Georgala S, Katsambas AD. Polymorphic eruption of pregnancy. Int J Dermatol. 2006;45(6):642-8.
31. Brzoza Z, Kasperska-Zajac A, Ole E, Rogala B. Pruritic urticarial papules and plaques of pregnancy. J Midwifery Womens Health. 2007;52(1):44-8.
32. Vaughan Jones SA, Hern S, Nelson-Piercy C, Seed PT, Black MM. A prospective study of 200 women with dermatoses of pregnancy correlating clinical findings with hormonal and immunopathological profiles. Br J Dermatol. 1999;141(1):71-81.
33. Roth MM. Atopic eruption of pregnancy: a new disease concept. J Eur Acad Dermatol. 2009;23:1466-7.
34. Zoberman E, Farmer ER. Pruritic folliculitis of pregnancy. Arch Dermatol. 1981;117(1):20-2.
35. Roger D, Vaillant L, Fignon A, Pierre F, Bacq Y, Brechot JF, et al. Specific pruritic diseases of pregnancy. A prospective study of 3192 pregnant women. Arch Dermatol. 1994;130(6):734-9.
36. Hanifin JM, Rajka G. Diagnostic features of atopic eczema. Acta Derm Venereol. 1980;92:44-7.
37. Cho S, Kim HJ, Oh SH, Park CO, Jung JY, Lee KH. The influence of pregnancy and menstruation on the deterioration of atopic dermatitis symptoms. Ann Dematol. 2010;22(2):180-5.
38. Kroumpouzos G, Cohen LM. Pruritic folliculitis of pregnancy. J Am Acad Dermatol. 2000;43(1 Pt 1):132-4.
39. Sachdeva S. The dermatoses of pregnancy. Indian J Dermatol. 2008;53(3):103-5.
40. Morrison JC, Parrish MR. Anemia associated with pregnancy. Glob Libr Women's Med. (ISSN: 1756-2228) 2011;DOI 10.3843/GLOWM.10164.
41. Lammert F, Marschall HU, Glantz A, Matern S. Intrahepatic cholestasis of pregnancy: molecular pathogenesis, diagnosis and management. J Hepatol. 2000;33(6):1012-21.
42. van der Woerd WL, van Mil SW, Stapelbroek JM, Klomp LW, van de Graaf SF, Houwen RH. Familial cholestasis: progressive familial intrahepatic cholestasis, benign recurrent intrahepatic cholestasis and intrahepatic cholestasis of pregnancy. Best Pract Res Clin Gastroenterol. 2010;24:541-53.
43. Oude Elferink RP, Paulusma CC. Function and pathophysiological importance of ABCB4 (MDR3 P-glycoprotein). Pflugers Arch. 2007;453(5):601-10.
44. Yayi H, Danqing W, Shuyun L, Jicheng L. Immunologic abnormality of intrahepatic cholestasis of pregnancy. Am J Reprod Immunol. 2010;63(4):267-73.
45. Stieger B, Fattinger K, Madon J, Kullak-Ublick GA, Meier PJ. Drug- and estrogen-induced cholestasis through inhibition of the hepatocellular bile salt export pump (Bsep) of rat liver. Gastroenterology. 2000;118(2):422-30.
46. Meng LJ, Reyes H, Axelson M, Palma J, Hernandez I, Ribalta J, et al. Progesterone metabolites and bile acids in serum of patients with intrahepatic cholestasis of pregnancy: effect of ursodeoxycholic acid therapy. Hepatology. 1997;26(6):1573-9.
47. Castaño G, Burgueño A, Fernández Gianotti T, Pirola CJ, Sookoian S. The influence of common gene variants of the xenobiotic receptor (PXR) in genetic susceptibility to intrahepatic cholestasis of pregnancy. Aliment Pharmacol Ther. 2010;31(5):583-92.
48. Beard MP, Millington GW. Recent developments in the specific dermatoses of pregnancy. Clin Exp Dermatol. 2012;37(1):1-4.
49. Reyes H, Báez ME, González MC, Hernández I, Palma J, Ribalta J, et al. Selenium, zinc and copper plasma levels in intrahepatic cholestasis of pregnancy, in normal pregnancies and in healthy individuals, in Chile. J Hepatol. 2000;32(4):542-9.
50. Oude Elferink RP, Kremer AE, Beuers U. Mediators of pruritus during cholestasis. Curr Opin Gastroenterol. 2011;27(3):289-93.
51. Shornick JK. Dermatoses of pregnancy. Semin Cutan Med Surg. 1998;17(3):172-81.
52. Joshi D, James A, Quaglia A, Westbrook RH, Heneghan MA. Liver disease in pregnancy. Lancet. 2010;375(9714):594-605.
53. Shaw D, Frohlich J, Wittmann BA, Willms M. A prospective study of 18 patients with cholestasis of pregnancy. Am J Obstet Gynecol. 1982;142(6 Pt 1):621-5.
54. Geenes V, Williamson C. Intrahepatic cholestasis of pregnancy. World J Gastroenterol. 2009;15(17):2049-66.
55. Reyes H, Zapata R, Hernández I, Gotteland M, Sandoval L, Jirón MI, et al. Is a leaky gut involved in the pathogenesis of intrahepatic cholestasis of pregnancy? Hepatology. 2006;43(4):715-22.
56. Diac M, Kenyon A, Nelson-Piercy C, Girling J, Cheng F, Tribe RM, et al. Dexamethasone in the treatment of obstetric cholestasis: a case series. J Obstet Gynaecol. 2006;26(2):110-4.
57. Laatikainen T. Effect of cholestyramine and phenobarbital on pruritus and serum bile acid levels in cholestasis of pregnancy. Am J Obstet Gynecol. 1978;132(5):501-6.
58. Kroumpouzos G. Intrahepatic cholestasis of pregnancy: what's new. J Eur Acad Dermatol Venereol. 2002;16(4),316-8.
59. Paumgartner G, Beuers U. Ursodeoxycholic acid in cholestatic liver disease: mechanisms of action and therapeutic use revisited. Hepatology. 2002;36(3):525-31.
60. Rioseco AJ, Ivankovic MB, Manzur A, Hamed F, Kato SR, Parer JT, et al. Intrahepatic cholestasis of pregnancy: a retrospective case-control study of perinatal outcome. Am J Obstet Gynecol. 1994;170(3):890-5.
61. Breier-Maly J, Ortel B, Breier F, Schmidt JB, Hönigsmann H. Generalized pustular psoriasis of pregnancy (impetigo herpetiformis). Dermatology. 1999;198(1):61-4.
62. Lotem M, Katzenelson V, Rotem A, Hod M, Sandbank M. Impetigo herpetiformis: a variant of pustular psoriasis or a separate entity? J Am Acad Dermatol. 1989;20(2 Pt 2):338-41.
63. Sasseville D, Wilkinson RD, Schnader JY. Dermatoses of pregnancy. Int J Dermatol. 1981;20(4):223-41.

64. Bajaj AK, Swarup V, Gupta OP, Gupta SC. Impetigo herpetiformis. Dermatologica. 1977;155(5):292-5.
65. Ott F, Krakowski A, Tur E, Lipitz R, Weisman Y, Brenner S. Impetigo herpetiformis with lowered serum level of vitamin D and its diminished intestinal absorption. Dermatologica. 1982;164(5):360-5.
66. Sauer GC, Geha BJ. Impetigo herpetiformis. Report of a case treated with corticosteroid-review of the literature. Arch Dermatol. 1961;83:119-26.
67. Bierman SM. Autoimmune progesterone dermatitis of pregnancy. Arch Dermatol. 1973;107(6):896-901.
68. Winton GB. Skin diseases aggravated by pregnancy. J Am Acad Dermatol. 1989;20(1):1-13.
69. McCormack WM. Genital infections of perinatal importance. Clin Obstet Gynecol. 1979;22(2):313-9.
70. Lockshin MD. Lupus pregnancy. Clin Rheum Dis. 1985;11(3):611-32.
71. Storer JS, Galen WK, Nesbitt LT, DeLeo VA. Neonatal pemphigus vulgaris. J Am Acad Dermatol. 1982;6(5):929-32.
72. Dunna SF, Finlay AY. Psoriasis: improvement during and worsening after pregnancy. Br J Dermatol. 1989;120(4):584.
73. Berde C, Willis DC, Sandberg EC. Pregnancy in women with pseudoxanthoma elasticum. Obstet Gynecol Surv. 1983;38(6):339-44.
74. Kjems E, Krag C. Melanoma and pregnancy. A review. Acta Oncol. 1993;32(4):371-8.

CHAPTER 62

Sexually Transmitted Diseases

Aswath Kumar, Anuradha Sood, Jay Mehta

INTRODUCTION

Women who are pregnant can become infected with pathogens causing sexually transmitted diseases (STDs) just as women who are not pregnant. STDs affecting pregnancy can be detrimental even to the baby as it may increase the risk of having a preterm birth as well as birth defects, some of which get diagnosed months following childbirth. This chapter aims to provide a broad overview on the clinical aspects to consider while approaching STDs in pregnancy and puerperium. Often, the state of pregnancy would allow the couple to resist sexual intercourse. However, having coitus during pregnancy may slightly increase the risk of abortions in the first trimester and may also have a role in increasing preterm labor.

Sexually transmitted diseases are a major public health problem in developed and developing countries. Both pregnant and nonpregnant females are at an equal risk of acquiring STDs. Pregnant females are in no way protected from STDs. The main STDs of concern in pregnancy include:

- Gonorrhea
- Chlamydia
- Trichomoniasis
- Bacterial vaginosis
- Syphilis
- Human papillomavirus (HPV)
- Hepatitis B virus (HBV)
- Herpes simplex virus (HSV) 1 and 2
- Human immunodeficiency virus (HIV).

IMPORTANCE

The primary role of a physician lies in not just diagnosing and treating the diseases, but also in the counseling and the testing to prevent the same. STDs can be more serious for the pregnant female and her baby. A pregnant woman with an STD can infect her baby before, during or after the baby's birth. She may have an abortion, early labor, or early rupture of the membranes leading to a premature birth. STDs affecting pregnancy can be detrimental to the baby as it may increase the risk of having a preterm birth as well as getting some birth defects, some of which get diagnosed months following childbirth. STD can make it easier for a person to get infected with HIV.[1]

If syphilis, chancroid and herpes are present in an individual the risk of acquiring HIV increases by 10-folds and by 4-folds if the patient has vaginal discharge due to gonorrhea, chlamydia, trichomoniasis and bacterial vaginosis.

Most of these problems can be prevented if the mother receives regular medical care during pregnancy. This includes tests for STDs starting early in pregnancy and repeated close to delivery, as needed.

BACTERIAL VAGINOSIS IN PREGNANCY

Causative Organism

Bacterial vaginosis is a STD caused by a close association of *Gardnerella vaginalis, Bacteroides* species and *Mobiluncus* species. The commensal lactobacilli are outgrown by these pathogenic microorganisms.

Signs and Symptoms

It is characterized by a foul smelling nonpurulent vaginal discharge with a raised pH or may have burning micturition or local vaginal and vulval discomfort.

The overall rate of affecting pregnancy is 12–22%.

Risk to Mother and Fetus

Bacterial vaginosis increases the risk of preterm labor by increasing incidence of preterm premature rupture of membranes (PPROM) and stimulating local prostaglandin release.

Diagnosis

It depends on three of the following four criteria which should be present for confirmation of bacterial vaginosis:

1. Presence of homogenous, white, noninflammatory discharge that smoothly coats the vaginal wall
2. Presence of clue cells which are vaginal epithelial cells that have a stippled appearance due to aggregates of coccobacilli. The lactobacilli present in normal vaginal secretions are either few or missing
3. Vaginal fluid pH of more than 4.5
4. A positive whiff test result, i.e. a fishy odor to the vaginal discharge after the addition of 10% potassium hydroxide solution.

Modified screening criteria for developing countries recommend that only two of the four conditions need be met for a diagnosis of bacterial vaginosis.[1]

Treatment

It includes metronidazole 500 mg orally twice per day for 7 days or clindamycin 450 mg orally twice per day for 7 days. Oral therapy and local therapy are both equally effective for pregnant women. Evidence is insufficient to assess whether the treatment of asymptomatic pregnant women with bacterial vaginosis who are at low risk for preterm delivery reduces adverse outcomes of pregnancy.[1]

CHLAMYDIAL INFECTION IN PREGNANCY

Causative Organism

Chlamydia trachomatis is an obligate intracellular gram negative bacterium with a unique biphasic life cycle. It has two morphological forms, elementary (extracellular form) and reticulate body. The elementary body is necessary for transmission. Upon uptake into a host cell, differentiation into the reticulate body occurs, which is the replicative form. After binary fission occurs, daughter reticulate bodies transform into elementary bodies, which are then released from the cell.

Mode of Transmission, and Signs and Symptoms

The usual mode of transmission to the fetus is vertical during the second stage of labor. The major routes of entry are the eye and the nasopharynx thus leading to neonatal conjunctivitis also called as ophthalmia neonatorum (inclusion blennorrhea) and pneumonia in the neonatal age group. Though approximately, 75% of women with *C trachomatis* infection are asymptomatic but they can still cause chorioamnionitis and postpartum endometritis which can be very severe in pregnant women. In pregnancy the disease manifests as urethritis, cervicitis, vaginal discharge, salpingitis and infertility.

Laboratory Diagnosis

Prenatal screening for chlamydia along with treatment of infected mothers is about 90% effective in preventing their infants from acquiring infection.[1]

Ocular, urethral, vaginal and cervical specimens should be collected by scraping the mucosa. Direct detection of chlamydia can be done by staining smears with Giemsa, Castaneda and Macchiavello stains and seeing for inclusion bodies.

Immunofluorescence staining is rapid and a more sensitive technique. Enzyme-linked immunosorbent assay (ELISA) for detection of antigens and antibodies, DNA probes, polymerase chain reaction (PCR) are the usual diagnostic methods performed.

Isolation of chlamydia in mice, yolk sac and tissue cultures can also be done but is labor intensive and requires specific facilities.

Though there is a doubt if chlamydia infection causes preterm labor, but infection has been surely found to lead to complications.[1] If a woman has symptoms of dysuria and frequency and urine culture results are negative, chlamydia is frequently the cause.

Centers for Disease Control and Prevention Recommendation for Chlamydial Screening

It includes:

- All pregnant women undergo screening early in pregnancy and pregnant women younger than 25 years and high-risk patients undergo screening again in the second trimester[1]
- Pregnant women who are found to have chlamydia during the first trimester should be retested 3–6 months later
- A nucleic acid amplification test (NAAT) performed on urine or an endocervical swab specimen: NAATs have the highest sensitivity for these specimens[1]
- Culture performed on endocervical swab.

Treatment

Azithromycin 1 g PO as a single dose is considered safe and effective for treating urogenital chlamydial infections in pregnancy and is now the first-line recommended therapy.[2] Tetracyclines and fluoroquinolones are contraindicated in pregnant women.

GONORRHEAL INFECTION IN PREGNANCY

Causative Organism

Neisseria gonorrhoeae is a Gram-negative cocci, 0.6–1.0 microns, present in pairs.

Mode of Transmission

A pregnant woman can transmit the infection to her infant at the time of delivery, causing life-threatening infections. Gonorrhea is transmitted vertically during the second stage of labor.

Signs and Symptoms

Signs and symptoms are usually asymptomatic in approximately 50% of patients. It gives rise to purulent urethral and vaginal discharge, increased frequency of micturition and dysuria. It can lead to ectopic pregnancy and infertility due to development of pelvic inflammatory disease (PID) in the mothers. The neonates can suffer due to premature birth, stillbirth, chorioamnionitis, postpartum sepsis and intrauterine growth retardation (IUGR). Neonates can also get conjunctivitis and meningitis.

Laboratory Diagnosis

Early detection and treatment lowers the likelihood of these complications and thus warrant screening in pregnancy. Swabs from endocervix, anal canal, vagina, urethra and oropharynx are to be collected. Smears are stained with Gram-stain and Gram-negative diplococci looked for under the light microscope. Culture can be done on Thayer Martin media. Serological tests like complement fixation tests and ELISA can also be done for detection of antigens and antibodies.

The American Congress of Obstetricians and Gynecologists (ACOG) recommends screening via endocervical culture in only high-risk pregnant women on their first antenatal visit. The Centers for Disease Control and Prevention (CDC) recommends screening all pregnant women "at risk for gonorrhea" and recommends rescreening in the second trimester among those at continued risk.[3]

Treatment

Due to widespread resistance to fluoroquinolones and the contraindication for using quinolones in pregnancy due to toxic effects, the current recommendations for treatment are cephalosporins. The treatment of choice for uncomplicated cervicitis is ceftriaxone, administered as a single intramuscular (IM) injection of 250 mg, plus azithromycin, 1 g as a single oral dose.[2,4-6]

SYPHILIS IN PREGNANCY

Early diagnosis and treatment are extremely important in preventing the potential effects of syphilis in pregnant women and their infants.

Causative Organism

Treponema pallidum is thin, motile spirochete which is 6–14 microns long and is twisted spirally round its long axis.

Mode of Transmission

Untreated primary or secondary syphilis in pregnant women leads to a fetal infection risk of almost 100% and a congenital infection in 40–50% of cases. Fetal complications include stillbirth and IUGR.

The stage of maternal disease during which the fetus is exposed to infection determines the morbidity risk; the earlier the stage of disease, the higher the risk of morbidity.

Signs and Symptoms

The clinical manifestations are divided into four stages:

1. Primary syphilis manifests as a hard, painless red ulcer typically forms on the vulva, cervix, or vagina
2. Secondary syphilis predominantly manifests as a nonpruritic rash that may involve the palms and soles along with fever, lymphadenopathy, and joint pain are less common manifestations of secondary syphilis
3. The latent stage causes no symptoms, and, although the disease may not be transmitted to sexual partners, it is still transmissible to the fetus
4. Tertiary syphilis characterized by slowly destructive disease affecting any organ. Gummata and aneurysms are formed, especially in heart and aorta.

Laboratory Diagnosis

Even when syphilis is considered unlikely, routine antenatal screening is warranted for all pregnant women for prevention and surveillance and it should be tested for at the first prenatal visit. If the patient is considered to be at high risk, tests should be repeated at 28 weeks' gestation and at delivery.[2] The testing for syphilis is extremely important as pregnant women do not usually have visible lesions.

Swabs from genital and rectal lesions can be subjected to dark ground microscopy to see for motile spirochetes.

Serological tests for diagnosis are divided into two main groups:

1. Nontreponemal tests (standard tests for syphilis) and
2. Treponemal tests.

The nontreponemal antibody tests are generally used for screening which include Venereal Disease Research

Laboratory (VDRL) tests, and are highly sensitive but nonspecific. Nontreponemal antibody test results are often false-positive in pregnant women; therefore, positive findings should be confirmed with specific anti-treponemal antibody tests.

Specific antitreponemal antibody tests such as the microhemagglutination assay—*T. pallidum* (MHA-TP) and the fluorescent treponemal antibody-absorption test (FTA-ABS). Antitreponemal antibody test findings are not indicators of current infection because results may remain positive for life. In primary syphilis, the diagnosis can be confirmed by identifying *T. pallidum* in dark-field examination of material taken from a lesion. Because most pregnant women do not have visible lesions, serologic screening is the primary means of establishing the diagnosis.

Treatment

Treatment in pregnant women consists of penicillin. Women who are found to be allergic to penicillin should be desensitized to it. A single dose of 2.4 million units of IM benzathine penicillin is for primary, secondary, and early latent syphilis. In late latent syphilis, treatment consists of 3 weekly doses of benzathine penicillin. Erythromycin does not prevent congenital syphilis.

GENITAL HERPES IN PREGNANCY

Causative Organism

Both HSV types 1 and 2 can cause genital herpes but mainly HSV 2 is responsible for genital and anal herpes.

Mode of Transmission

Neonatal infection occurs during their passage through infected birth canal and sometimes prenatally by transmission through placenta or ascending infection from cervix.

Signs and Symptoms

It manifests as painful vesicles on genitalia or anal region with regional lymphadenopathy. The fetal complications include neonatal herpes which can cause meningitis, encephalitis and pneumonia, especially, when the infection is acquired in the second trimester. This is because whenever the infection is acquired in the second trimester the mother is not able to provide for adequate immunoglobulin G (IgG) antibodies which can be protective for the fetus. If the infection occurs in the first and the second trimesters the chances for abortion are there but the chance for neonatal herpes is rare. Prenatal infections may lead to abortions or congenital defects. Overall, there is a risk of acquiring HSV infection in approximately 30–40% of neonates if the mother has primary herpes infection. Pregnant women who acquired HSV prior to pregnancy will already have IgG antibodies to HSV and will pass these antibodies to the fetus. Neonatal herpes is uncommon in this situation.

Laboratory Diagnosis

The diagnosis is confirmed by obtaining a swab from the base of an ulcer. Diagnosis can be done by examination of clinical specimen under the electron microscope and fluorescent microscope. HSV DNA detection by PCR is more sensitive than culture.[7] PCR can distinguish HSV-1 from HSV-2.

Treatment

Treatment of the patients includes local measures like adequate analgesia and topical applicants of anesthetic creams in order to reduce the pain. Suppressive acyclovir should be considered from 36 weeks until delivery in order to prevent clinical recurrences and, therefore, reduce the need for cesarean section. The standard dose for acyclovir in pregnancy is 400 mg tablets PO 3 times a day for 5 days. In the absence of lesions or prodromal symptoms at labor, vaginal delivery should be anticipated. All women having active infection at term or having had acquired herpes within 6 weeks should be offered elective cesarean section. The risk of neonatal herpes following vaginal delivery is small and one must balance this against the risk of cesarean section to the mother.[8-11]

HUMAN PAPILLOMAVIRUS INFECTION IN PREGNANCY

Causative Organism

Human *papillomavirus* belongs to the family papovaviridae and is a DNA virus with a size of 55 nm. There are over 70 types of HPVs. HPV type 11,16,18,31 are mainly responsible for cervical cancer.

Mode of Transmission

It could infect the neonate during the passage from the infected birth canal. *In utero* infection during second trimester could be due to ascending infection from an infected birth canal or through blood via the placenta.

Signs and Symptoms

It is responsible for cutaneous and genital warts, recurrent respiratory papillomatosis and cancer. Genital warts are caused by infection with HPV and are the most prevalent viral sexually transmitted infection (STI). Genital warts may increase in size and number during pregnancy. The diagnosis is usually made clinically upon visual inspection. Maternal infection is associated with juvenile laryngeal papillomatosis in the infant. This is a rare condition that can cause hoarseness and respiratory distress in children.

Treatment

Cesarean section is not indicated in mothers with genital warts as vertical transmission of HPV is rare.

Treatment is only really necessary in the unlikely event that the warts cause obstruction of the birth canal and impede vaginal delivery. Warts can be removed by surgery or cryotherapy. Cryotherapy with liquid nitrogen causes cytolysis at the dermo-epidermal junction and is safe for use in pregnancy. A freeze or thaw technique should be employed, whereby liquid nitrogen is applied for approximately 10 seconds until a halo of freeze develops a few millimeters around the wart. This is repeated three or more times for each lesion during the treatment session. Cryotherapy can be administered every 1–2 weeks. Lesions may regress after delivery without any treatment.

Podophyllin, podophyllotoxin and imiquimod are contraindicated in pregnancy.

HEPATITIS B IN PREGNANCY

As per CDC, approximately 350 million individuals worldwide are infected with HBV.

Causative Organism

Hepatitis B virus is a double-stranded DNA virus belonging to the Hepadnaviridae family. The average incubation period is 90 days from time of exposure to onset of symptoms, but may vary from 6 weeks to 6 months.

Mode of Transmission

It has three important modes of transmission: parenteral, perinatal and sexual. Sexual transmission accounts for most adult HBV infections. Hepatitis B infection in pregnancy poses a great threat to the neonate because if perinatally acquired an infant has approximately a 90% chance of becoming a chronic carrier. This leads to a 15–20% chance of dying from cirrhosis when he/she become an adult. In patients with acute hepatitis B, vertical transmission occurs in up to 10% of neonates when infection occurs in the first trimester and in 80–90% of neonates when acute infection occurs in the second trimester.[12]

Signs and Symptoms

In the pregnant females the picture is same as that of acute hepatitis in any other individual. Usually, the symptoms are mild during pregnancy but they may flare after delivery.

HBV infection does not appear to be cause birth defects, but there appears to be a higher incidence of low birth weight among infants born to mothers with acute infection during pregnancy.[12,13]

Management

As a routine all the patients are tested for hepatitis B surface antigen (HbsAg) at their first antenatal visit. More than 90% of women found to be HBsAg-positive on routine screening will be HBV carriers, routine follow-up testing later in pregnancy is not necessary for the purpose of screening. In special situations, such as when the mother is thought to have acute hepatitis, when there has been a history of exposure to hepatitis, or when, particularly, high-risk behavior such as parenteral drug abuse has occurred during the pregnancy, an additional HBsAg test can be ordered during the second trimester.[12] A positive HBsAg in the absence of IgM anti-HBc (hepatitis B core antigen) is indicative of chronic infection.

The most important goal in the management of hepatitis B in pregnancy is prevention of transmission to the neonate.[14] Infants of mothers with positive hepatitis B status should receive hepatitis B immunoglobulin and hepatitis B vaccine within 12-hour of birth. The dose of vaccine for neonates is 0.5 mL of given in the anterolateral part of the thigh at 0 month, 1 month and 6 months. Additionally, all neonates irrespective of hepatitis B status should be started with HBV vaccine schedule. Preterm infants with birth weight less than 4 lb, 6 oz (2,000 g) should receive modified dosing schedule.[15]

A dose of hepatitis B immune globulin (HBIG) 0.06 mL/kg IM into the contralateral arm along with the complete immunization as described above is needed in cases where the primary exposure has occurred causing acute hepatitis. For patients who are having chronic hepatitis, only active immunization is needed. Pregnant females with hepatitis b infection should be treated with several therapeutic agents like tenofovir or telbivudine under the guidance of a specialist. If started after 28 weeks of gestation it helps in reducing the viral load which may further reduce the perinatal transmission.

Cesarean section is not an indication in all patients who have stable and chronic disease. However, it is better to avoid artificial rupture of membranes (AROM) and usage of scalp electrode in patients with HBV infection. Breastfeeding is not a contraindication in patients with HBV.

HUMAN IMMUNODEFICIENCY VIRUS IN PREGNANCY

Causative Organism

Human immunodeficiency virus is a *Lentivirus* belonging to family *Retroviridae*. It is enveloped RNA virus about 90–12 nm in diameter and possesses two single-stranded RNA strands with reverse transcriptase enzyme.

Mode of Transmission

One of the mechanisms for transmission is sexual transmission apart from transmission by blood and blood products and breast milk. The risk of transmission is lower in vaginal intercourse (0.1% per episode) as compared to anal intercourse (1% per episode).This is primarily because virus laden lymphocytes from semen can directly enter through the mucosal tears which are more in anal intercourse. The chance of perinatal transmission is 13–40%.

The exact mechanism of mother-to-child transmission of HIV remains unknown. Transmission may occur during intrauterine life, delivery, or breast-feeding. The greatest risk factor for vertical transmission is thought to be advanced maternal disease, likely due to a high maternal HIV viral load.[16]

Signs and Symptoms

Though the virus as such does not cause an increase in maternal complications, there has been concern regarding the use of highly active antiretroviral therapy (HAART) increasing the medical complications of pregnancy like preterm labor, glucose intolerance and preeclampsia. However, the studies so far have not been able to conclusively demonstrate it.

Management

It is recommended that routine HIV screening for women aged 19–64 years and targeted screening for at-risk women outside of this age reference. All pregnant women should have their HIV serostatus evaluated when they first present for prenatal care. Women should have the right to refuse testing if they do not want it to be done.

Antenatal visits should be increased to a minimum of four in case a woman is found to be seropositive. Screening of Tuberculosis and other STDs are a must. Counseling for medical termination of pregnancy (MTP) and continuation of pregnancy in first 3 months and later on for safe delivery, birth planning and infant feeding options to be provided for all HIV infected females. According to the latest National AIDS Control guidelines (NACO) it is recommended to provide antiretroviral treatment (ARV) to all infected pregnant women regardless of CD4 results.[17] The preferred regimen includes triple drug therapy with tenofovir disoproxil fumarate, lamivudine and efavirenz.[18] Use of single dose nevirapine at onset of labor greatly reduces prepartum HIV transmission.

All neonates with a positive HIV status of mother should be started on nevirapine once daily for 6 weeks starting from birth.

Exclusive breastfeeding up to 6 months with complementary feeds after 6 months to 1 year is to be encouraged.

All infants HIV status should be confirmed by 18 months of age and cotrimoxazole prophylaxis should be started by 6 weeks of age.

REFERENCES

1. Rours GI, Duijts L, Moll HA, Arends LR, de Groot R, Jaddoe VW. Chlamydia trachomatis infection during pregnancy associated with preterm delivery: a population-based prospective cohort study. Eur J Epidemiol. 2011;26(6):493-502.
2. Centers for Disease Control and Prevention. Sexually transmitted disease guidelines. MMWR 2010. 2010;59:9.
3. Johnson RE, Newhall WJ, Papp JR, Knapp JS, Black CM, Gift TL, et al. Screening tests to detect Chlamydia trachomatis and Neisseria gonorrhoeae infections—2002. MMWR Recomm Rep. 2002;51:1-38.
4. Pitsouni E, Iavazzo C, Athanasiou S, Falagas ME. Single-dose azithromycin versus erythromycin or amoxicillin for Chlamydia trachomatis infection during pregnancy: a meta-analysis of randomised controlled trials. Int J Antimicrob Agents. 2007;30(3):213-21.
5. Workowski KA, Berman SM, Douglas JM Jr. Emerging antimicrobial resistance in Neisseria gonorrhoeae: urgent need to strengthen prevention strategies. Ann Intern Med. 2008;148(8):606-13.
6. Centers for Disease Control and Prevention (CDC). Update to CDC's Sexually transmitted diseases treatment guidelines, 2010: oral cephalosporins no longer a recommended treatment for gonococcal infections. MMWR Morb Mortal Wkly Rep. 2012;61(31):590-4.
7. Stokes JH, Beerman H, Ingraham N. Modern Clinical Syphilogy. In: Diagnosis, Treatment: Case Study, 3rd edition. Philadelphia: WB Saunders; 1945.
8. Wald A, Huang ML, Carrell D, Selke S, Corey L. Polymerase chain reaction for detection of herpes simplex virus (HSV) DNA on mucosal surfaces: comparison with HSV isolation in cell culture. J. Infect. Dis. 2003;188:1345-51.
9. Prober CG, Sullender WM, Yasukawa LL, Au DS, Yeager AS, Arvin AM. Low risk of herpes simplex virus infections in neonates exposed to the virus at the time of vaginal delivery to mothers with recurrent genital herpes. N. Engl. J. Med. 1987;316:240-4.
10. Brown ZA, Benedetti J, Ashley R, Burchett S, Selke S, Berry S, et al. Neonatal herpes simplex virus infection in relation to asymptomatic viral shedding at the time of labor. N Engl J Med. 1991;324(18):1247-52.
11. Sheffield JS, Hollier LM, Hill JB, Stuart GS, Wendel GD. Acyclovir prophylaxis to prevent herpes simplex virus recurrence at delivery: a systematic review. Obstet. Gynecol. 2003;102:1396-403.
12. American College of Obstetricians and Gynecologists. ACOG Practice Bulletin No. 86: Viral hepatitis in pregnancy. Obstet Gynecol. 2007;110(4):941-56.
13. Centers for Disease Control and Prevention, Workowski KA, Berman SM. Sexually transmitted diseases treatment guidelines, 2006. MMWR Recomm Rep.;55(RR-11):1-94. Erratum in. MMWR Recomm Rep. 2006;15;55(36):997.
14. Recommendations of the Immunization Practices Advisory Committee Prevention of Perinatal Transmission of Hepatitis B Virus: Prenatal

Screening of all Pregnant Women for Hepatitis B Surface Antigen MMWR. 1988;37(22):341-6,351.

15. Lam NC, Gotsch PB, Langan RC. Caring for pregnant women and newborns with hepatitis B or C. Am Fam Physician. 2010;82(10);1225-9.
16. Garcia PM, Kalish PA, Pitt J, Minkoff H, Quinn TC, Burchett SK, et al. Maternal levels of plasma human immunodeficiency virus type 1 RNA and the risk of perinatal transmission. Women and Infants Study group. N Engl J Med. 1999;341:385-93.
17. Tuomala RE, Shapiro DE, Mofenson LM, Bryson Y, Culnane M, Hughes MD, et al. Antiretroviral therapy during pregnancy and the risk of an adverse outcome. N Engl J Med. 2002;346(24):1863-70.
18. Ministry of Health and Family Welfare, Department of AIDS Control Basic Services Division, Government of India. (2013). Updated Guidelines for Prevention of Parent to Child Transmission (PPTCT) of HIV using Multi-drug Anti-retroviral Regimen in India. [online] available from naco.gov.in/upload/NACP%20-%20IV/18022014%20BSD/National_Guidelines_for_PPTCT.pdf. [Accessed December, 2015].

CHAPTER 63

Infectious Complications

Nishi Jaswal

INTRODUCTION

Pregnancy affects every physiological system of the body. Changes in immune system and hormonal imbalance make a pregnant woman more vulnerable to infections and serious complications. Some Infections are of particular concern as they are more severe in the pregnant state. It can be deleterious not only to the pregnant woman but also to the fetus, newborn or her partner. The management of infection in pregnancy aims mainly at improving the diagnosis and prognosis of congenital infections. Early diagnosis and treatment of infections not only prevents morbidity and mortality in the mother but also helps in neonatal treatment, prenatal diagnosis and interventions if needed. Some infections during pregnancy can even lead to miscarriage, preterm labor, birth defects or maternal death. To complicate matters, the drugs used to treat infections can cause serious side effects in the fetus or the neonate.

MATERNAL AND FETAL IMMUNOLOGY

The cell-mediated and humoral immunity in the fetus starts developing at the age of 9–15 weeks. The primary response is the development of immunoglobulin M (IgM) antibody and the delayed response is in the form immunoglobulin G (IgG) transferred across the placenta. At about 26 weeks the immunity of the child is as close to that of the mother. After birth, some infections are prevented by the breast milk. There are many changes to the genital tract that occur during pregnancy. There are hormonal, molecular, cellular and anatomic transformations that occur with conception and across gestation. The ability of the mother's body to tolerate a fetus that is not genetically identical to her has long been a topic of immunologic interest. While there are immunologic changes that occur at the maternal-fetal interface to allow the mother to tolerate her semiallogeneic fetus, there are also major components of the lower genital tract that play an important role in immunity and modification of these may not be beneficial to the mother. Almost all components of the innate immune system undergo some change during pregnancy.[1]

Any infection acquired in the third trimester of pregnancy or within 14 days of delivery due to any bacterial, viral, fungal infection or protozoal infestations has deleterious effects on both the mother and the child. Emerging infections also lead to complications in the mother and the neonate. The outcome depends upon the immunological status of the mother, timing of infection and the mode of acquiring the infection. The important causes of infections are listed in Table 1.

VIRAL INFECTIONS

The viral infections of concern during the third trimester of pregnancy and puerperium are those caused by rubella virus, *Cytomegalovirus* (CMV) and herpes simplex virus (HSV). The viruses known to cause congenital infections include Human parvovirus B19 (B19V), varicella-zoster virus (VZV), West Nile virus, measles virus, enteroviruses, adenovirus, and human immunodeficiency virus (HIV). Hepatitis B, C and E virus are also causes of the high mortality rate in pregnant women. Recently, lymphocytic choriomeningitis virus (LCMV) has been implicated as a teratogenic rodent-borne arenavirus.

Worldwide, congenital HIV infection is now a major cause of infant and childhood morbidity and mortality, responsible for an estimated 4 million deaths since the start of the HIV

TABLE 1: Important causes of infections

Viral Causes	Bacterial causes	Mycotic causes	Protozoal causes
• Varicella: Zoster • Coxsackievirus • Human parvovirus B19 (B19V) • Rubella • *Cytomegalovirus* (CVM) • HIV • Hepatitis B and C	• *Listeria* • Syphilis • *Borrelia* • Gonorrhea • Chlamydia • Group B streptococci • Tuberculosis • *Mycoplasma* • *Staphylococcus* • Coliforms	• Coccidioidomycosis • Blastomycosis • Cryptococcosis • Blastomycosis	• Toxoplasma • Malaria • Amebiasis

pandemic. With emerging influenza pandemic, attention has also now been directed to the effects of influenza on pregnant women. It is shown that influenza vaccination of high-risk pregnant patients also provides some protective immunity for newborns and reduces subsequent hospitalizations in the infants. Influenza has been shown to produce significant morbidity and mortality in pregnant women.

Varicella-Zoster Virus

Varicella-zoster virus is a double-stranded DNA virus that carries risks for both the mother and fetus during pregnancy. The incubation period is 10–21 days and it is contagious from 1 day prior to the onset of rash till the crusting of the lesions. Morbidity and mortality rates associated with this infection are much higher in adults than in children. Primary varicella infection during pregnancy is considered a medical emergency.[2]

Pneumonitis due to VZV infection is 25 times more common in adults than in children; in the third trimester, the risk for life-threatening ventilatory compromise is significant, with a mortality rate of 14%. Prior to the development of antiretrovirals, pneumonitis in pregnant women carried a mortality rate of 45%. Other risk factors for the development of pneumonitis include smoking and a large lesion burden (>100 lesions).

Clinical Picture

Congenital varicella syndrome (CVS) results in chorioretinitis, cataracts, limb atrophy, cerebral cortical atrophy, neurological disability. Spontaneous abortion has been reported in 3–8% of first trimester VZV infections, and CVS has been reported in 12%. Acquisition of infection by the mother in the perinatal period, specifically 5 days prior to delivery or 2 days afterward, poses a risk of severe neonatal varicella, which carries a mortality rate of 30%. Infection at this time prevents development of maternal antibodies that avert transplacental transfer of IgG antibodies, which confer passive immunity to the fetus.[3]

Diagnosis

The diagnosis is clinical. The laboratory tests available are Tzanck smear, tissue culture or direct fluorescent antibody tests performed on the scrapings obtained from the base of vesicle. Nucleic acid amplification techniques done on the amniotic fluid is a useful test for the diagnosis of congenital varicella infection.

Management

The exposed pregnant woman is given VariZIG within 96-hours of exposure to prevent the infection.[4] Women who are suffering with varicella infections the line of treatment is supportive. The patient should be kept in isolation and intravenous acyclovir therapy 10–20 mg/kg body weight 8 hourly is given.

Vaccination, a live attenuated vaccine Varivax are given in adolescents and adults with no active infection. The vaccine is contraindicated in pregnant women.

Influenza H1N1

Swine flu caused by the swine influenza virus is transmitted to humans via contact with infected pigs or environments contaminated with swine influenza viruses. It is caused by family Orthomyxoviridae which is a RNA virus causing influenza A and B infections. Influenza A is further classified on the basis of hemagglutinin (HA) and neuraminidase (NA) surface antigens.[3]

Signs and Symptoms

Manifestations of H1N1 influenza are similar to those of seasonal influenza. Patients present with symptoms of acute respiratory illness, including at least two of the following:
- Fever
- Cough
- Sore throat
- Body aches

- Headache
- Chills and fatigue
- Diarrhea and vomiting.

Diagnosis

The Centers for Disease Control and Prevention (CDC) criteria for suspected H1N1 influenza are as follows:

- Onset of acute febrile respiratory illness within 7 days of close contact with a person who has a confirmed case of H1N1 influenza A virus infection or
- Onset of acute febrile respiratory illness within 7 days of travel to a community where one or more H1N1 influenza A cases have been confirmed or
- Acute febrile respiratory illness in a person who resides in a community where at least one H1N1 influenza case has been confirmed.

Management

Treatment is largely supportive and consists of bed rest, increased fluid consumption, cough suppressants, and antipyretics and analgesics for fever and myalgias. Severe cases may require intravenous hydration and other supportive measures. Antiviral agents used are amantadine and rimantadine may also be considered for treatment or prophylaxis. The second class of drugs includes NA inhibitors in the early course of the disease. Antiviral drugs like oseltamivir orally and zanamivir by inhalation is used for the treatment as recommended by CDC (2009) to be started within 48 hours of the infection.[5]

Prevention

Vaccination is recommended for all women who are going to be pregnant in the influenza months. A trivalent cold attenuated vaccine for intranasal use is not recommended in pregnant women.[4]

Cytomegalovirus

Cytomegalovirus is a double-stranded DNA herpes virus and represents the most common congenital viral infection. The CMV seropositivity rate increases with age. Geographic location, socioeconomic class, and work exposure are other factors that influence the risk of infection. CMV infection requires intimate contact through saliva, urine or any other body fluids. Possible routes of transmission include sexual contact, organ transplantation, transplacental transmission and rarely by the breast milk or blood transfusion.

Fetal Effects

Primary or recurrent CMV infection can occur in pregnancy often leading to congenital CMV infection. Transplacental infection can result in intrauterine growth retardation, sensorineural hearing loss, intracranial calcifications, microcephaly, hydrocephalus, hepatosplenomegaly, delayed psychomotor development and optic atrophy.[6]

Vertical transmission of CMV can occur at any stage of pregnancy. The overall risk of infection is greatest in the third trimester. The risk of transmission to the fetus in primary infection is 30–40%. Most (90%) CMV infections cause no symptoms, but 10% result in signs and symptoms such as microcephaly, thrombocytopenia, hepatosplenomegaly, intrauterine growth retardation.

About 30% of infants with severe CMV infection die, more than half eventually develop neurological sequelae like microcephaly, mental retardation or sensorineural hearing loss. 7% of asymptomatic neonates develop sensorineural hearing loss or developmental delays during the first 2 years of life. 5% eventually develop microcephaly and neuromuscular defects. Only about 2% develop chorioretinitis. Congenital hearing loss is the most common sequel of recurrent CMV infection.

Diagnosis

Serological tests like identification of CMV specific IgG in paired and convalescent sera. CMV IgM is present in only 70–90% of infected pregnant women with acute infection.

Imaging studies like computed tomography (CT) and magnetic resonance imaging (MRI) are suggestive of fetal infection so along with nucleic acid amplification of the fetal amniotic fluid is the gold standard for the diagnosis of fetal infection in CMV infection.

Management

In the third trimester, passive immunization with CMV-specific hyperimmune globulin lowers the risk of congenital CMV infection when given to pregnant woman with primary disease.[4]

Management Scheme for Maternal Primary Cytomegalovirus Infections[7]

Cytomegalovirus IgM by immunoblot and IgG positive by enzyme-linked immunosorbent assay (ELISA) or avidity by ELISA:[7]

- If negative; no further evaluation
- In case positive; CMV specific IgG avidity index high
- *Cytomegalovirus* IgM negative means latent infection:
  - No further evaluation.
- In case positive, CMV specific IgG or seroconversion avidity index low:
  - *Cytomegalovirus* IgM positive means primary CMV infection
  - Invasive follow-up required

- In case positive, CMV specific IgG:
    - Immunoglobulin G avidity index high
    - *Cytomegalovirus* IgM positive means recurrent CMV infection
    - Noninvasive follow-up.

A positive test for CMV IgG indicates that a person was infected with CMV at sometime during their life but the IgG test cannot determine when a person was infected. However, if antibody tests of paired acute-phase and convalescent-phase serum samples show a four-fold rise in IgG antibody and CMV IgM antibody is present or CMV virus is cultured from a urine or throat specimen, an active CMV infection is present.

The presence of CMV IgM is not solely indicative of primary infection. CMV IgM is detectable when a person:
- Is newly infected,
- Has been infected in the past but recently re-exposed to CMV,
- Is undergoing reactivation of CMV infection that was acquired in the past
- Has a false-positive test result. The presence of CMV IgM should not be used by itself to diagnose primary CMV infection.

Recently, IgG avidity assays, which measure antibody maturity, have been shown to reliably, detect recent primary CMV infection. When a person is infected with CMV for the first time, the body produces low-avidity IgG. After 2–4 months, the body begins to produce high-avidity CMV IgG. Low CMV IgG avidity suggests a primary CMV infection occurred within the past 2–4 months. High CMV IgG avidity suggests that CMV infection occurred at some point in the past.[8]

Parvovirus B19

Parvovirus B19 causes erythema infectiosum or 5th disease. It is caused by small single-stranded DNA virus. Mode of infection is either respiratory route or hand to mouth contact. Although most adults with B19V infection are asymptomatic, the effects of this virus on the fetus are much greater and include fetal anemia, hydrops fetalis, myocarditis or intrauterine fetal death. B19V infection accounts for 15–20% of cases of nonimmune hydrops fetalis. 30–40% of pregnant women are seronegative for B19V and are susceptible to infection.

Fetal Effects

Various studies have estimated that 3–14% of intrauterine fetal deaths occur in the setting of B19V infection. second trimester infections have been studied most frequently because infection in this trimester carries a 1–3% risk of hydrops. But infection in any trimester may result in intrauterine fetal loss.[9] The critical period for the development of fetal hydrops is when maternal B19V infection is acquired between the 13th and 16th week of gestation, possibly because of the relative immaturity of the fetal immune response, as well as the shortened life span of the red blood cells at this gestational age.[10]

Herpes Simplex Virus

About 30–60% of women receiving obstetric care have serologic evidence of past HSV infection. Although both HSV-1 and HSV-2 may cause neonatal herpes, HSV-2 is responsible for 70% of cases. Neonatal herpetic infection is defined as infection within 28 days of birth. 90% of infections are perinatally transmitted in the birth canal. HSV infection acquired in this manner carries a 70% risk of dissemination and is associated with three distinct syndromes, each with its own typical outcome. The first and most common (45%) is localized skin, eye, or mouth disease. Approximately, 30% of cases manifest as central nervous system (CNS) disease, including meningitis or encephalitis, with evidence of HSV DNA in the cerebrospinal fluid (CSF). Finally, 25% of neonatal herpetic infections manifest as disseminated disease that involves multiple organs. Initial symptoms of this disease usually present during the first 4 weeks of life.[11]

Approximately, 10% of infections are congenital, usually a consequence of the mother acquiring primary HSV infection during pregnancy and the fetus acquiring the infection transplacentally or via an ascending infection from the cervix. Intrauterine infection is associated with intrauterine growth restriction, preterm labor, and miscarriage. The risk of neonatal herpes and death is highest in infants born to mothers who have not seroconverted by the time of delivery.

Mumps

Mumps is caused by RNA paramyxovirus. The virus primarily infects parotid gland but due to immunization in the childhood, 90% women in the third trimester and pregnancy are seropositive. The infection is via respiratory route. The average incubation period for mumps is 16–18 days, with a range of 12–25 days. Fever may persist for 3–4 days and parotitis, when present, usually lasts 7–10 days. Persons with mumps are usually considered most infectious from 1 to 2 days before until 5 days after onset of parotitis.

Laboratory Criteria for Diagnosis

- Isolation of mumps virus from clinical specimen or
- Detection of mumps nucleic acid [e.g., standard or real time-polymerase chain reaction (RT-PCR assays)], or
- Detection of mumps IgM antibody or
- Demonstration of specific mumps antibody response in absence of recent vaccination, either a 4-fold increase in IgG titer as measured by quantitative assays, or a

seroconversion from negative to positive using a standard serologic assay of paired acute and convalescent serum specimens.

Fetal Effects

- Severe complications of mumps are rare. Mumps can cause acquired sensorineural hearing loss in children and incidence is estimated at 1 in 20,000 cases. Mumps-associated encephalitis occurs in less than 2 per 100,000 cases and approximately 1% of encephalitis cases are fatal.[12]
- Some complications of mumps are known to occur more frequently among adults than among children. Adults have a higher risk for mumps meningoencephalitis than children.
- In addition, orchitis occurs in up to 30–40% of cases in postpubertal males. Although it is frequently bilateral, it rarely causes sterility.
- Mastitis has been reported in as many as 31% of female patients older than 15 years who have mumps. Other rare complications of mumps are oophoritis and pancreatitis. Aseptic meningitis occurs in 10% of cases and is associated with a good prognosis. Although mumps infection in the first trimester of pregnancy may result in fetal loss, there is no evidence that mumps during pregnancy causes congenital malformations.

Treatment

Treatment is symptomatic. Measles, mumps and rubella (MMR) vaccine is contraindicated in pregnancy but can be given to susceptible women postpartum. Breast-feeding is not contraindicated.

Rubella

Rubella is one of the more teratogenic viruses. Congenital rubella syndrome (CRS) is characterized by intrauterine growth restriction, intracranial calcifications, microcephaly, cataracts, cardiac defects (most commonly patent ductus arteriosus or pulmonary arterial hypoplasia), neurologic disease (with a broad range of presentations, from behavior disorders to meningoencephalitis), osteitis, and hepatosplenomegaly.

Neonates with rubella may have a "blueberry muffin" appearance caused by purpuric skin lesions that result from extramedullary hematopoiesis. Heart defects in these infants include ventricular septal defects, patent ductus arteriosus, pulmonary stenosis, and coarctation of the aorta. The presentation of rubella at birth varies greatly. Most of these complications develop in infants born to mothers who acquire rubella infection during the first 16 weeks of pregnancy. 90% of infants present with some finding of congenital rubella if infection occurs within the first 12 weeks, and 20% present with congenital disease if the infection occurs between weeks 12 and 16. Cataracts results when infection occurs between the third and eighth week of gestation, deafness between the third and 18th week, and heart abnormalities between the third and tenth week.

Enterovirus

Enterovirus infections are not believed to cross the placenta and cause fetal disease. However, some studies have linked coxsackievirus and echovirus to miscarriage, neurodevelopmental delay, myocarditis, and cortical necrosis. One study linked the presence of coxsackievirus in the third trimester with respiratory failure and global cognitive defects.

Measles Virus

Measles virus infection (rubeola) during pregnancy, as with VZV infection, tends to be severe, with pneumonitis predominating. Although it is not known to be teratogenic, rubeola has been associated with spontaneous abortion, premature labor, and low birth weight. Neonates born to mothers with active measles virus infection are at risk of developing neonatal measles, but no congenital syndrome has been described.[13]

Lymphocytic Choriomeningitis Virus

Lymphocytic choriomeningitis virus has been associated with sporadic cases of congenital infection worldwide. Affected infants demonstrate chorioretinitis, hydrocephalus, mental retardation, and/or visual impairment; in addition, intrauterine death is possible. Unlike congenital CMV and rubella infections, hearing deficits and hepatosplenomegaly are rarely seen in congenital LCMV.

Other Viruses

Other viruses postulated to cause congenital infections include echovirus, hepatitis B virus, hepatitis C virus, and adenovirus. In 2002, an article in morbidity and mortality weekly report discussed a single case of West Nile virus infection in a mother and associated chorioretinitis in her newborn. A causal link has not been determined. Since then, the CDC has maintained a registry of West Nile virus infections during pregnancy. Other congenital malformations have been described in this registry, but a direct cause-effect relationship has not yet been established. Infants born to mothers who develop symptomatic West Nile virus infection within 3 weeks prior to delivery may develop symptomatic West Nile virus disease shortly after birth.

BACTERIAL INFECTIONS

They can affect pregnant women from implantation of the fertilized ovum through the time of delivery and peripartum period. They may also affect the fetus and newborn. Many women with these infections are asymptomatic, necessitating both a high degree of clinical awareness and adequate screening.[14,15]

GROUP B STREPTOCOCCUS

Group B Streptococcus (*Streptococcus agalactiae*, GBS) is the most common cause of life-threatening infections in newborns and can also affect the mother. Features of GBS infection are as follows:[16]

GBS can be found as part of normal vaginal, rectal, and oral flora. Intrapartum transmission occurs via ascending spread or at the time of delivery. In pregnant women, GBS causes cystitis, amnionitis, endometritis, and stillbirth; occasionally, GBS bacteremia leads to endocarditis or meningitis. In postpartum women, GBS can cause urinary tract infections (UTIs) and pelvic abscesses. In newborns, early-onset GBS infection occurs before age 7 days (mean age at presentation is age 12 hours) and primarily manifests as nonfocal sepsis, pneumonia, or meningitis. Late-onset disease in neonates occurs at age 7–89 days, bacteremia and meningitis are the most common presentations.

Babies who survive the initial insult face possible hearing or vision loss, learning disabilities, and other neurologic sequelae.

Centers for Disease Control and Prevention Recommendations[17]

- At 35–37 weeks' gestation, all pregnant women should undergo screening with a vaginal and rectal swab for culture
- If the culture result is positive, the woman should be treated during labor
- If culture results are unknown at the time of delivery, a risk-based approach can be used, in which patients are deemed at high risk and receive treatment if they meet any of the following criteria:
  - Previously delivered infant with invasive GBS infection
  - Group B streptococcus bacteriuria during current pregnancy
  - Delivery before 37 weeks' gestation
  - Duration of ruptured membranes longer than 18 hours
  - Intrapartum temperature of more than 100.4°F (38°C).

High-risk women with negative screening culture results within 5 weeks of delivery do not require treatment.[18]

Treatment

- During labor and until delivery, IV penicillin G or ampicillin
- In penicillin-allergic patients at low risk for anaphylaxis, IV cefazolin; in those at high risk for anaphylaxis, IV clindamycin or erythromycin
- If susceptibility to clindamycin or erythromycin has not been established, IV vancomycin can be used
- The neonate must be carefully observed for signs and symptoms of disease.

URINARY TRACT INFECTIONS

Asymptomatic bacteriuria develops in 10–15% of pregnant women and can lead to complications such as pyelonephritis and premature labor, so all pregnant women should undergo screening with urine culture at least once during early pregnancy and should be treated if the results are positive. Significant bacteriuria is defined as more than 100,000 colony-forming units (CFU) of a single organism in a clean-catch specimen.[19]

Treatment

- Initial antibiotic therapy may be empirical
- Sulfonamides, amoxicillin, amoxicillin-clavulanate, cephalexin are acceptable
- Sulfonamides in the last few weeks of gestation may lead to kernicterus and hyperbilirubinemia in the newborn
- Trimethoprim is relatively contraindicated during the first trimester due to theoretical teratogenicity
- Nitrofurantoin may cause hemolysis in patients or fetuses with glucose-6-phosphate deficiency (G6PD)
- A 7-day regimen treats bacteriuria and acute cystitis; single-dose therapy is less effective
- Recurrent UTIs may warrant postcoital prophylaxis with single-dose cephalexin or nitrofurantoin macrocrystals
- Women treated for cystitis should be monitored with monthly urine cultures
- Apart from the need to avoid certain antibiotics, treatment of pyelonephritis in pregnant women mirrors that in nonpregnant patients
- Mild cases may be treated in an outpatient setting, but more severe cases may necessitate hospitalization and IV antibiotics plus IV hydration for nausea, vomiting, and dehydration
- Women who have had acute pyelonephritis should be monitored frequently with repeat urine cultures; if close follow-up care is not practical, continuous suppressive therapy can be considered.[20]

Listeriosis

Features of infection with *Listeria monocytogenes* are as follows:[21]

Approximately one-third of all reported cases of listeriosis occur during pregnancy, typically during the third trimester. Infection mainly follows ingestion of contaminated food, but rare cases following direct contact with infected animals and nosocomial transmission have been reported. The most common clinical presentation in pregnant patients with listeriosis is bacteremia, often asymptomatic; CNS *Listeria* infections are rare, unlike in other populations.[22] Symptomatic pregnant patients often have a febrile illness similar to influenza with fever, muscle aches, and, occasionally, nausea or diarrhea during the bacteremic phase of the disease. Although maternal symptoms may be mild, listeriosis can lead to amnionitis and result in either spontaneous septic abortion or premature labor with delivery of an infected baby, or even stillbirth. Fetal infection may manifest as septicemia, meningoencephalitis, or disseminated granulomatous lesions with microabscesses. Confirming a diagnosis of listeriosis requires a culture showing *L. monocytogenes* in blood or CSF. Serologic testing is not reliable for diagnosis, and stool cultures are not sensitive or specific. Treatment is with IV ampicillin or penicillin; patients with beta-lactam allergy should be desensitized.[23] Trimethoprim-sulfamethoxazole is the usual alternative for patients allergic to penicillin but can be problematic during the first or third trimesters.

Syphilis

Features of syphilis are as follows:

Untreated primary syphilis or secondary syphilis in pregnancy leads to a fetal infection rate of almost 100%. The disease can cause stillbirth; late abortion; or neonatal disease, death, or latent infection.[24] In primary syphilis, a hard, painless red ulcer typically forms on the vulva, cervix, or vagina. Secondary syphilis predominantly manifests as a nonpruritic rash that may involve the palms and soles; fever, lymphadenopathy, and joint pain are less common manifestations of secondary syphilis. The latent stage causes no symptoms and is still transmissible to the fetus. Tertiary syphilis can result in cardiovascular or gummatous disease. Neurosyphilis can occur at any stage, resulting in CNS or ophthalmic presentations. Serologic tests should be performed at the initial prenatal visit in all pregnant women; patients considered to be at high risk should have repeat testing at 28 weeks' gestation and at delivery. Nontreponemal antibody test results [e.g., rapid plasma reagin (RPR), Venereal Disease Research Laboratory (VDRL)] are often false-positive in pregnant women; therefore, positive findings should be confirmed with specific antitreponemal antibody tests such as the microhemagglutination assay-*Treponema pallidum* (MHA-TP) and the fluorescent treponemal antibody-absorption test (FTA-ABS). Once syphilis is diagnosed, consider other sexually transmitted diseases (STD), especially, HIV. Treatment is with a single dose of 2.4 million units of intramuscular (IM) benzathine penicillin for primary, secondary, and early latent syphilis, but some experts recommend a second dose of benzathine penicillin G 1 week after the initial dose, especially, in the third trimester or in patients with secondary syphilis. In late latent syphilis, treatment consists of 3 doses of benzathine penicillin, each one week apart; if results of subsequent quantitative VDRL or an equivalent test show a 4-fold increase, retreat the patient and perform a lumbar puncture to rule out neurosyphilis. Pregnant women who are allergic to penicillin must be desensitized and then treated with penicillin. Jarisch-Herxheimer reactions in pregnancy may involve uterine contractions, preterm labor, and premature delivery.

Chlamydia

Chlamydia trachomatis infection is the most common bacterial STD in the United States and continues to be a major cause of complications in pregnancy and disease transmission in newborns. Approximately, 75% of women with *C. trachomatis* infection are asymptomatic. *C. trachomatis* can cause endometritis, cervicitis, acute pelvic inflammatory disease (PID), and acute urethral syndrome in all women and chorioamnionitis, postpartum endometritis, and gestational bleeding in pregnant women. The usual mode of transmission to the fetus is vertical during the second stage of labor.[25] In neonates, *C. trachomatis* infection commonly causes conjunctivitis (ophthalmia neonatorum) and pneumonia. All pregnant women should undergo *Chlamydia* screening early in pregnancy; pregnant women younger than 25 years and high-risk patients should be screened again in the third trimester. Patients diagnosed with chlamydial infection in the first trimester should be retested 3–6 months later. According to the CDC, the following are the accepted screening methods. A nucleic acid amplification test (NAAT) performed on urine or an endocervical swab specimen. An unamplified nucleic acid hybridization test, an enzyme immunoassay, or direct fluorescent antibody test performed on an endocervical swab specimen.[26] Culture performed on an endocervical swab specimen.

Treatment

- Azithromycin (first-line recommended therapy)[27]
- Amoxicillin (alternative agent)
- Erythromycin (second-line agent because of compliance-limiting gastrointestinal adverse effects)
- Tetracyclines and fluoroquinolones are contraindicated in pregnant women
- Retest treated women 3 weeks after therapy to ensure therapeutic cure.

Gonorrhea

Gonococcal infections are second only to chlamydial infections in the number of cases of bacterial STDs. Gonococcal infections cause no symptoms in approximately 50% of patients. Pregnancy is a predisposing factor to the development of disseminated gonococcal infection, which classically presents as an arthritis-dermatitis syndrome. Newborns exposed to gonorrhea during vaginal delivery can develop an acute conjunctivitis (ophthalmia neonatorum), sepsis, arthritis, and/or meningitis. The screening via endocervical culture in high-risk pregnant women on their first antenatal visit is recommended. The CDC recommends screening all pregnant women "at risk for gonorrhea," with rescreening in the third trimester for those at continued risk. The recommended screening method remains endocervical culture; alternatives include the NAAT and the nucleic acid hybridization test. Culture, nucleic acid hybridization, and NAAT tests can all be used for diagnosis. The treatment of choice for uncomplicated cervicitis is single-dose IM ceftriaxone and oral azithromycin.[28]

Bacterial Vaginosis

Bacterial vaginosis is a clinical syndrome caused by excessive growth of bacteria that may normally be present in the vagina.[29] The etiology is polymicrobial in nature; with a pH of more than 4.5, *Gardnerella vaginalis* and anaerobes become the prominent-associated organisms. Women with bacterial vaginosis may be asymptomatic or may report an abnormal vaginal discharge with an unpleasant, fishlike odor, especially, after sexual intercourse. The discharge is generally white or gray, and women may experience burning during urination or itching around the vagina. Infection can lead to premature labor unresponsive to tocolytic therapy. Infection can be transmitted via the placenta to the fetus and can cause intrauterine fetal death.

A diagnosis of bacterial vaginosis can be confirmed via clinical or Gram stain criteria. When using the clinical criteria, three of the following four conditions should be present:[30]

1. A homogeneous, white, noninflammatory discharge that smoothly coats the vaginal wall. Clue cells (i.e., vaginal epithelial cells that have a stippled appearance due to aggregates of coccobacilli)
2. Vaginal fluid pH of more than 4.5
3. A positive whiff test result (i.e., a fishy odor to the vaginal discharge before or after the addition of 10% potassium hydroxide solution)
4. Oral metronidazole or clindamycin is recommended; clindamycin cream should be avoided during the second half of pregnancy.[31]

METHICILLIN-RESISTANT *STAPHYLOCOCCUS AUREUS*

It causes infection that is resistant to several common antibiotics. There are two types of infection. Hospital-associated methicillin-resistant *Staphylococcus aureus* (MRSA) happens to people in healthcare settings. Community-associated MRSA happens to people who have close skin-to-skin contact. 17% of pregnant women have vaginal-rectal colonization. The strains are resistant to penicillin and cephalosporin drugs. The infections involve skin and soft tissues. Invasive cellulitis is present in women with risk factors like diabetes mellitus, smoking, intravenous drug abuse and suffering with HIV infection.

Control of infection is key to stop MRSA in hospitals. To prevent community-associated MRSA:

- Practice good hygiene
- Keep cuts and scrapes clean and covered with a bandage until healed
- Avoid contact with other people's wounds or bandages
- Avoid sharing personal items, such as towels, washcloths, razors, or clothes
- Wash soiled sheets, towels, and clothes in hot water with bleach and dry in a hot dryer.

Treatments may include draining the infection and send for culture and sensitivity before the starting of antibiotics. Antibiotics such as clindamycin, vancomycin, fluoroquinolones can be used. Topical mupirocin nasal ointment applied twice daily for 5 days to decolonize the bacteria. Shower and shampoo with chlorhexidine 4% soap.[32]

TOXOPLASMOSIS

It is caused by infection with the protozoan *Toxoplasma gondii,* an obligate intracellular parasite has a life cycle in three forms:

1. Tachyzoite
2 Bradyzoite
3 Sporozoite.

The sexual cycle occurs only in cats, the definitive host. The asexual cycle occurs in other mammals (including humans). It consists of 2 forms:

Tachyzoites (the rapidly dividing form observed in the acute phase of infection) and bradyzoites (the slowly growing form observed in tissue cysts).The infection produces a wide range of clinical syndromes in humans, land and sea mammals.[33]

T. gondii infects a large proportion of the world's population but uncommonly causes clinically significant disease.[34] However, certain individuals are at high risk for severe or life-threatening toxoplasmosis. Individuals at risk for toxoplasmosis include fetuses, newborns, and immunologically impaired patients.

Congenital toxoplasmosis is usually a subclinical infection. Among immunodeficient individuals, toxoplasmosis most often occurs in those with defects of T-cell-mediated immunity, such as those with hematologic malignancies, bone marrow and solid organ transplants, or acquired immunodeficiency syndrome (AIDS). In most immunocompetent individuals, primary or chronic (latent) *T. gondii* infection is asymptomatic. A small percentage of these patients eventually develop retinochoroiditis, lymphadenitis, or, rarely, myocarditis and polymyositis.[35]

Diagnosis

It is rarely detected in the tissues or body fluids of the patient. The antibody IgG appears after 2 weeks peaks up to 1 month and persists up to lifetime. Other tests are IgM ELISA double sandwich test and Sabin Feldman dye test.[36]

Prenatally, it can be diagnosed by sonography and DNA amplification techniques.

Management

The drug of choice for toxoplasmosis is spiramycin. It reduces the risk of congenital infection. Pyrimethamine and sulfonamide is given in late pregnancy as a presumptive treatment.

Prevention

There is no vaccine. It can be prevented by eating properly cooked meat products and washing hands after handling cats. Primary prevention based on prenatal education could be an effective strategy to reduce congenital toxoplasmosis. Educate the public in toxoplasmosis-prevention methods, such as protecting children's play areas from cat litter. Mothers with toxoplasmosis must be completely informed of the disease's potential consequences to the fetus.

MALARIA

It is a life-threatening disease caused by infection with *Plasmodium* protozoa transmitted by an infective female *Anopheles* mosquito. *Plasmodium falciparum* infection carries a poor prognosis with a high mortality if untreated, but it has an excellent prognosis if diagnosed early and treated well in time.[37]

Guidelines for Laboratory Diagnosis of Malaria[38]

- Thick and thin films should be routinely used for malaria diagnosis; thick films should be stained with Giemsa or Field stain, thin films with Giemsa or Leishman stain
- Two observers should examine thick films, with each viewing a minimum of 200 high-power fields; if the films are positive, the species should be determined through examination of a thin film
- In cases of *P. falciparum* or *Plasmodium knowlesi* infection, the percentage of parasitized cells or the number of parasites per microliter should be estimated
- Rapid diagnostic tests for malarial antigen can be used on a supplementary basis when diagnosis is performed by inexperienced staff.

Signs and Symptoms

Patients with malaria typically become symptomatic a few weeks after infection, though the symptomatology and incubation period may vary, depending on host factors and the causative species.

- Clinical symptoms include the following:
    - Headache (noted in virtually all patients with malaria)
    - Cough
    - Fatigue
    - Malaise
    - Shaking chills
    - Arthralgia
    - Myalgia
    - Paroxysm of fever, shaking chills, and sweats (every 48 hours or 72 hours, depending on species).
- Less common symptoms include the following:
    - Anorexia and lethargy
    - Nausea and vomiting
    - Diarrhea
    - Jaundice.

Most patients with malaria have no specific physical findings, but splenomegaly may be present.

- Severe malaria manifests as the following:
    - Cerebral malaria (sometimes with coma)
    - Severe anemia
    - *Respiratory abnormalities:* Include metabolic acidosis, associated respiratory distress, and pulmonary edema; signs of malarial hyperpneic syndrome include alar flaring, chest retraction, use of accessory muscles for respiration, and abnormally deep breathing
    - Renal failure (typically reversible).

Diagnosis

The patient history should include inquiries into the following:[38]

- Recent or remote travel to an endemic area
- Immune status, age, and pregnancy status
- Allergies or other medical conditions
- Medications currently being taken.

The following blood investigations are requested:

- Blood culture
- Hemoglobin concentration

- Platelet count
- Liver function
- Renal function
- Electrolyte concentrations (especially sodium)
- Monitoring of parameters suggestive of hemolysis [haptoglobin, lactate dehydrogenase (LDH), reticulocyte count]
- In selected cases, rapid HIV testing
- White blood cell count: fewer than 5% of malaria patients have leukocytosis; thus, if leukocytosis is present, the differential diagnosis should be broadened
- If the patient is to be treated with primaquine, glucose-6-phosphate dehydrogenase (G6PD) level
- If the patient has cerebral malaria, glucose level to rule out hypoglycemia.

The following imaging studies may be considered:[39]

- Chest radiography, if respiratory symptoms are present
- Computed tomography of the head, if central nervous system symptoms are present.

Specific tests for malaria infection should be carried out, as follows:

- Microhematocrit centrifugation (sensitive but incapable of speciation)
- Fluorescent dyes or ultraviolet indicator tests (may not yield speciation information)
- Thin (qualitative) or thick (quantitative) blood smears (standard): note that 1 negative smear does not exclude malaria as a diagnosis; several more smears should be examined over a 36-hour period
- Alternatives to blood smear testing (used if blood smear expertise is insufficient): include rapid diagnostic tests, polymerase chain reaction (PCR) assay, nucleic acid sequence-based amplification, and quantitative buffy coat.

Histologically, various *Plasmodium* species causing malaria may be distinguished by the following:

- Presence of early forms in peripheral blood
- Multiply infected red blood cells
- Age of infected RBCs
- Schüffner dots
- Other morphologic features.

Management

Treatment is influenced by the species causing the infection, including the following:[40]

- *Plasmodium falciparum*
- *Plasmodium vivax*
- *Plasmodium ovale*
- *Plasmodium malariae*
- *Plasmodium knowlesi*

The patients with *P. falciparum* infection are often treated on an inpatient basis to allow observation for complications. Patients with non-*P. falciparum* malaria who are well can usually be treated on an outpatient basis.

General recommendations for pharmacologic treatment of malaria are as follows:[41]

- *P. falciparum* malaria: quinine-based therapy is with quinine sulfate or clindamycin or pyrimethamine-sulfadoxine; alternative therapies are artemether-lumefantrine, atovaquone-proguanil, or mefloquine
- *P. falciparum* malaria with known chloroquine susceptibility: Chloroquine
- *P. vivax, P. ovale* malaria: Chloroquine plus primaquine
- *P. malariae* malaria: Chloroquine
- *P. knowlesi* malaria: Same recommendations as for *P. falciparum* malaria.

Pregnant women (especially primigravidas) are up to 10 times more likely to contract malaria than nongravid women and have a greater tendency to develop severe malaria. Medications that can be used for the treatment of malaria in pregnancy include the following:

- Chloroquine
- Quinine
- Atovaquone-proguanil
- Clindamycin
- Mefloquine (avoid in first trimester)
- Sulfadoxine-pyrimethamine (avoid in first trimester)
- Artemether-lumefantrine
- Artesunate and other antimalarials.

AMEBIASIS

Amebiasis is caused by *Entamoeba histolytica* a protozoan that is found worldwide. The highest prevalence of amebiasis is in developing countries like India where barriers between human feces and food and water supplies are inadequate as in rural areas.[42]

Although most cases of amebiasis are asymptomatic, dysentery and invasive extraintestinal disease can occur. Liver abscess is the most common manifestation of invasive amebiasis, but other organs can also be involved like pleuropulmonary, cardiac, cerebral, renal, genitourinary, peritoneal and cutaneous sites.

E. histolytica is transmitted by ingestion of the cystic form (infective stage) of the protozoa. Viable in the environment for weeks to months, cysts can be found in fecally contaminated soil, fertilizer, or water or on the contaminated hands of food handlers. Fecal-oral transmission can also occur in the setting of anal sexual practices or direct rectal inoculation through colonic irrigation devices.

Excystation then occurs in the terminal ileum or colon, resulting in trophozoites (invasive form). The trophozoites can penetrate and invade the colonic mucosal barrier, leading to tissue destruction, secretory bloody diarrhea and colitis. In addition, the trophozoites can spread hematogenously via the portal circulation to the liver or even to more distant organs.

E. histolytica is capable of causing a spectrum of illnesses. Intestinal conditions resulting from *E. histolytica* infection include the following:[43]

- Asymptomatic infection
- Symptomatic noninvasive infection
- Acute proctocolitis (dysentery)
- Fulminant colitis with perforation
- Toxic megacolon
- Chronic nondysenteric colitis
- Ameboma
- Perianal ulceration.

Extraintestinal conditions resulting from *E. histolytica* infection include the following:

- Liver abscess
- Pleuropulmonary disease
- Peritonitis
- Pericarditis
- Brain abscess
- Genitourinary disease.

Laboratory diagnosis of amebiasis is made by demonstrating the organism or by employing immunologic techniques. In addition to standard blood tests, other laboratory studies employed for diagnosis include microscopy, culture, serologic testing, and PCR assay.[44]

Treatment of amebiasis includes pharmacologic therapy, surgical intervention and preventive measure. Most individuals with amebiasis may be treated on an outpatient basis, though severe clinical condition requires inpatient care.

FUNGAL INFECTIONS

Generally, pneumonia caused by due to coccidioidomycosis[45] caused by *Coccidioides immitis*, histoplasmosis caused by *Histoplasma capsulatum*, blastomycosis caused by *Blastomyces dermatitidis* and cryptococcus by *Cryptococcus neoformans*. It is difficult to diagnose pneumonias as the clinical picture is similar to community-acquired pneumonia. The vast majority of coccidioidal infections result from airborne transmission. Pulmonary infection can result from inhalation of a single spore in humans, but high inoculum exposures are more likely to result in symptomatic disease. Inhaled *C. immitis* or *Coccidioides posadasii* arthroconidia are deposited into the terminal bronchiole.

Treatment

Itraconazole is the drug of choice for disseminated fungal infections. Intravenous amphotericin B or ketoconazole can be given to pregnant females as it does not have teratogenic effects in fetus, especially, in the third trimester of pregnancy.[46]

URINARY TRACT INFECTIONS

Most common infection encountered in the third trimester of pregnancy is UTI. In the last trimester of pregnancy infection is mostly ascending due to pressure from the enlarged uterus. The UTI may be complicated or noncomplicated. Uncomplicated UTI can be treated with empirical antibiotic therapy without culture and drug sensitivity as mostly *Escherichia coli* is responsible in most of the cases. A urinalysis or test for leukocyte esterase should be performed;[47] if polymorphonuclear cells are absent then culture can be performed before the start of the treatment.

Clinical Symptoms

The cardinal symptoms are fever with chills and rigors and flank pain, though asymptomatic bacteriuria is common. Frequent and painful micturition with suprapubic heaviness may also be present.[48] Table 2 shows commensal flora and pathogens causing UTI.

Collection of Midstream Urine Sample

- Wash and be sure to rinse well before the sample is collected
- Use 4×4 inch soap sponges to wipe from front of the body backwards 4 times.
- Rinse well and discard the initial urine sample and collect the mid urine sample in the culture tube without soiling the mouth of the container.

Screening Tests for Urinary Tract Infections

Microscopic examination: Gram-stain revealing one bacterium per oil emersion field of uncentrifuged urine gives 94% sensitivity and 90% specificity.

Tests for bacterial products: common approach is Griess test which uses reagent impregnated dipsticks to detect urine nitrite and indirectly estimates the number of segmented neutrophils by detecting leucocyte esterase activity, as most of the UTIs are caused by nitrate reducing Enterobacteriaceae. False-positive results may result if the specimen has been delayed in transit or if the patient is on vegetable free diet.

TABLE 2: Commensal flora and pathogens implicated in urinary tract infections

Commensal flora	Pathogens causing urinary tract infections
Alpha hemolytic or beta hemolytic streptococci *Bacillus* spp., Coagulase-negative staphylococci (CONS), diphtheroids, *Lactobacillus* spp.	*Corynebacterium urealyticum*, *Enterococcus* spp, Enterobacteriaceae, *Pseudomonas* spp, *Staphylococcus aureus*, *Staphylococcus saprophyticus*

Detection by culture: rapid culture by urine dipslide. The advantages of screening methods is for the negative specimens.

INFECTIONS OF THE GENITAL TRACT

Table 3 shows the site of genital tract, their normal commensal flora, STD and non-STD causes.

DISEASES CAUSED BY SEXUALLY TRANSMITTED ORGANISMS

Cervicitis and Urethritis

Chlamydia trachomatis is the most common infection presents as mucopurulent discharge.

Genital Uler

- Herpes simplex virus type 1 and herpes simplex virus type 2 causing vesicular lesions with erythematous base on the vulva or cervix which are painful and ulcerative.
- Syphilis in which lesions are painless and have indurated margins and a clean base
- Chancroid (caused by *Haemophilus ducreyi*) in which the lesions are painful but do not have indurated margins
- Lymphogranuloma venereum (LGV) causes a pustule associated with bilateral necrotising inguinal adenopathy
- Granuloma inguinale (caused by *Calymmatobacterium granulomatis*) causes subcutaneous nodule that erodes the surface from which beefy red painless elevated granulomatous lesion develops.

INFECTIONS CAUSING DISCHARGE BY NONSEXUAL MEANS

- *Trichomonas vaginalis* a protozoan presents as vaginitis, vaginal discharge, generally, yellow green frothy collects in the posterior vaginal fornix and irritation
- *Candida* spp. cause thick curdy white discharge and vaginal mucosa turns erythematous
- Bacterial vaginosis caused by *G. vaginalis* and other anaerobic bacteria like *Bacteroides*, *Peptococcus*, *Mobiluncus* produces a malodorous discharge.

COLLECTION OF SPECIMEN

- The samples are most commonly taken from uterine cervix and urethra
- With the aid of the speculum clear the mucosa with the swab, the tip of the smaller swab preferably with Dacron tip is inserted a few millimeters in the os rotated firmly to obtain both exudate and the cervical cells
- Do not touch the lateral walls of the vaginal canal
- Urethral samples are obtained by taking the discharge if any or inserting urogenital swab in the urethra for a few seconds

TABLE 3: Infections of the genital tract

Site	Flora	Transmitted diseases	Non-STD causes
Urethra	Enterobacteriaceae, streptococci, *Enterococcus* spp, diphtheroids, coagulase-negative staphylococcus (CONS), anaerobes	*Chlamydia trachomatis, Neisseria gonorrhoeae*	
External genitalia	CONS, *Micrococcus* sp., yeast, *Acinetinobacter diphtheroids*	Herpes simplex type 1, human papillomavirus (HPV), *Treponema pallidum, Haemophilus ducreyi*, lymphogranuloma venereum (*Chlamydia trachomatis* serotypes L1 L2 L3), Granuloma inguinale	Herpes simplex type 1, *Candida* sp, *Streptococcus pyogenes*
Vagina	*Lactobacillus*, anaerobes, CONS, diphtheroids	HPV	*Candida* sp, bacterial vaginosis, *Staphylococcus aureus, Trichomonas vaginalis*
Endocervix	Minimally contaminated	Herpes simplex type 2, HPV, *Neisseria gonorrhoeae, Chlamydia trachomatis*	*Cytomegalovirus* (CVM), herpes simplex type 1
Endometrium fallopian tubes and ovaries	Sterile	*Neisseria gonorrhoeae, Chlamydia trachomatis*	Mixed aerobic and anaerobic ascending infections, *S. pyogenes, Listeria monocytogenes, Streptococcus agalactiae, Actinomyces israelii* [patients with intact intrauterine contraceptive devices (IUCDs)]
Systemic infections		HIV, hepatitis B, hepatitis C	

- Vaginal specimens are collected with a swab taking care not to contaminate the swab with the normal flora
- Endometrial swabs are best obtained by inserting a swab with a narrow bore catheter in the cervical canal
- For samples from fallopian tubes and ovaries laparoscopic approach is required
- Specimen from genital ulcer is obtained by cleaning and removing the debris and contaminating bacteria from the lesion. Scalpel blade is taken to abrade the base of the ulcer and to transfer the material to the slide
- For culture from the ulcer side the washing of the base or cotton swab is used
- In intact vesicles for herpes culture collect the vesicular fluid for Tzanck preparation
- Swabs are sent the laboratory in Amies' transport media.

DIAGNOSIS

Gram stain preparation of the discharge showing diplococcus gram-negative bacteria suggests the diagnosis of gonococcal urethritis.

Definitive diagnosis is by recovery of the bacteria on culture.

Wet preparation of unstained vaginal secretions can detect *Candida* spp. and motile *T. vaginalis*.

The pH estimation of the vaginal secretions (high pH) and high polyamine and fatty acid levels along with clue cells in small numbers suggests bacterial vaginosis.

Whiff Test

Amine production (fishy odor) on mixing 10% KOH with vaginal discharge rules out bacterial vaginosis.

Microscopic demonstration of clue cells and shift of Gram-positive bacilli to mixed flora indicates bacterial vaginosis.

Diagnosis of Genital Ulcer Disease

- Herpetic ulcers are diagnosed by viral culture or multinucleated giant cells with intranuclear inclusion bodies
- Donovan bodies by staining intranuclear bacteria in mononuclear cells
- *Haemophilus ducreyi* can be cultured but is labile so should be transported in the Amies' transport media
- Lymphogranuloma venereum is diagnosed serologically and can be also cultivated if the sample is taken from the suppurative lymph node
- Primary syphilis can be diagnosed by dark field microscopy of scrapings from ulcer base or serological tests like FTA-ABS may be done later in the illness
- Venereal warts are caused by human papillomavirus and the diagnosis is clinical.

BREAST COMPLICATIONS

Acute Mastitis

- Infection due to the cracking of the nipple which involves breast parenchymal tissue leading to cellulitis
- Infection through lactiferous glands leading to mammary adenitis.

Organisms Implicated

Mostly *Staphylococcus aureus*, the nursing mothers may get the infection from the nasopharynx of the baby.

Clinical Symptoms

Fever is generally high grade 102°F with chills with severe pain in the breast.

Signs

There is presence of swelling on the breast with its apex at the nipple.

Diagnosis

It is clinical.

Treatment

- Early administration of antibiotics, preferably, amoxicillin for at least 10 days
- Analgesics and sedatives
- Stop lactation
- Manual expression of milk.

TRAVEL PRECAUTIONS DURING PREGNANCY

It is safe to travel by air during pregnancy. The second trimester (weeks 14–27 of pregnancy) is the best time during pregnancy to travel. The reason being, most women experience morning sickness during the first trimester, which is likely to have subsided when they step in the second trimester. Moreover, energy level also increases during this trimester.

Preliminary Checks

- Before booking your tickets read up the airlines guidelines for pregnant women. Different carriers have different guidelines so it is better to check them up online before planning a trip
- It is also advisable to book in aisle seat for the travel to help to remain more comfortable

- Consider wearing maternity pants for the travel as it gives the baby some room to move
- It is essential to wear seat belts during take-off and landing. While buckling up your seat belt do remember to fasten the belt from under the abdomen
- Even while traveling, one should continue to do some activities that will help promote circulation
- During any form of travel, including air travel it is advisable to drink plenty of fluids
- Wear comfortable and sturdy foot wear during the journey as it will make it easier to maintain your balance in a moving train or aircraft.

REFERENCES

1. Stirrat G. The Immune System. In: Hytten F, Chamberlain G (Eds). Clinical Physiology in Obstetrics. London: Blackwell; 1991. pp. 101.
2. Plourd DM, Austin K. Correlation of a reported history of chickenpox with seropositive immunity in pregnant woman. J Repord Med. 2005;50(10):779-83.
3. American College of Obstetricians and Gynaecologists. Perinatal viral and parasitic infections (Practice bulletin No 171). Washington: ACOG; 1992.
4. American College of Obstetricians and Gynaecologists. Immunization during pregnancy (Committee Opinion No. 282). Washington: ACOG; 2003.
5. Centers for Disease Control and Prevention (CDC). Guideline for Prevention of Catheter-associated Urinary Tract Infections 2009. Atlanta: CDC; 2009.
6. Reef SE, Plotkin S, Cordero JF, Katz M, Cooper L, Schwartz B, et al. Preparing for elimination of congenital Rubella syndrome (CRS): summary of workshop on CRS elimination in the United States. Clin Infect Dis. 2000;31:85-95.
7. Spong CY, Cunningham F, Leveno K, Bloom S, Hauth J, Rouse D. Infectious diseases. In: Spong CY, Cunningham F, Leveno K, Bloom S, Hauth J, Rouse D (Eds). Williams Obstetrics, 23rd edition. New York: McGraw-Hill Education; 2009. pp. 1210.
8. Pereira LH, Embil JA, Haase DA, Manley KM. Cytomegalovirus infection among women attending a sexually transmitted disease clinic: association with clinical symptoms and other sexually transmitted diseases. Am J Epidemiol. 1990;131(4):683-92.
9. Young NS, Brown KE. Parvovirus B19. N Engl J Med. 2004;350:586-97.
10. Enders M, Weidner A, Zoellner I, Searle K, Enders G. Fetal morbidity and mortality after acute human parvovirus B19 infection in pregnancy: Prospective evaluation of 1018 cases. Prenat Diagn. 2004;24:513-8.
11. Wald A, Zeh J, Selke S, Warren T, Ashley R, Corey L. Genital shedding of herpes simplex among men. J infect Dis. 2002;186:S34-9.
12. American Academy of Pediatrics, American College of Obstetricians and Gynaecologists, and March of Dimes Birth Defects Foundation. Guidelines for Perinatal Care, 6th edition. Elk Grove Village, IL: American Academy of Pediatrics; 2007.
13. Ohji G, Satoh H, Satoh H, Mizutani K, Iwata K, Tanaka-Taya K. Congenital measles caused by transplacental infection. Pediatr Infect Dis J. 2009; 28(2):166-7.
14. Eschenbach DA, Wager GP. Puerperal infections. Clin Obstet Gynecol. 1980:23:1003-37.
15. Demmler GJ. Summary of a workshop on surveillance for congenital cytomegalovirus disease. Rev Infect Dis. 1991;13:315.
16. Lin Fyc, Philip JB 3rd, Azimi PH, et al. Level of maternal antibody required to protect neonates against early-onset disease caused by group B Streptococcus type La: a multicenter superspeciality study. J infect Dis. 2003;185:267.
17. Schrag S, Gorwitz R, Fultz-Butts K, Schuchat A. Prevention of perinatal group B streptococcal disease. Revised guidelines from the CDC. MMWR Recomm Rep. 2002;51:1-22.
18. American College of Obstetricians and Gynaecologists. ACOG Committee Opinion: number 279, December 2002. Prevention of early-onset group B streptococcal disease in newborn. Obstet Gynecol. 2002;100(6):1405-12.
19. Bradbury SM. Collection of urine specimen in general practice: to clean or not to clean? JR Coll Gen Pract. 1988;38:363-5.
20. U.S. Preventive Services Task Force. Screening for asymptomatic bacteriuria in adults: U.S. Preventive Services Task Force reaffirmation recommendation statement. Ann Intern Med. 2008;149(1):43-7.
21. Smaill F, Vazquez JC. Antibiotics for asymptomatic bacteriuria in pregnancy. Cochrane Database Syst Rev. 2007;CD000490.
22. Jackson KA, Iwamoto M, Swerdlow D. Pregnancy-associated listeriosis. Epidemiol Infect. 2010;138(10):1503-9.
23. Gellin BG, Broome CV, Bibb WF, Weaver RE, Gaventa S, Mascola L. The epidemiology of listeriosis in the United States--1986. Listeriosis Study Group. Am J Epidemiol. 1991;133(4):392-401.
24. Workowski KA, Berman S. Centers for Disease Control and Prevention. Sexually transmitted disease guidelines, 2010. MMWR Recomm Rep. 2010;59:1-110.
25. Geisler WM. Management of uncomplicated Chlamydia trachomatis infections in adolescents and adults: evidence reviewed for the 2006 Centers for Disease Control and Prevention sexually transmitted diseases treatment guidelines. Clin Infect Dis. 2007;44:S77-83.
26. Johnson RE, Newhall WJ, Papp JR, Knapp JS, Black CM, Gift TL, et al. Screening tests to detect *Chlamydia trachomatis* and *Neisseria gonorrhoeae* infections—2002. MMWR Recomm Rep. 2002;51:1-38.
27. Pitsouni E, Lavazzo C, Athanasiou S, Falagas ME. Single-dose azithromycin versus erythromycin or amoxicillin for *Chlamydia trachomatis* infection during pregnancy: a meta-analysis of randomised controlled trials. Int J Antimicrob Agents. 2007;30(3):213-21.
28. Workowski KA, Berman SM, Douglas JM Jr. Emerging antimicrobial resistance in *Neisseria gonorrhoeae*: urgent need to strengthen prevention strategies. Ann Intern Med. 2008;148(8):606-13.
29. U.S. Preventive Services Task Force. Screening for bacterial vaginosis in pregnancy to prevent preterm delivery: U.S. Preventive Services Task Force recommendation statement. Ann Intern Med. 2008;148(3):214-9.
30. Mittal V, Jain A, Pradeep Y. Development of modified diagnostic criteria for bacterial vaginosis at peripheral health centres in developing countries. J Infect Dev Ctries. 2012;6(5):373-7.
31. Marrazzo JM, Martin DH. Management of women with cervicitis. Clin Infect Dis. 2007;44(Suppl 3):S102-10.
32. Workowski KA, Berman SM. Sexually Transmitted Diseases Treatment guidelines, 2006. MMWR Recomm Rep. 2006;55:1-94.
33. Jones JL, Lopez A, Wilson M, Schulkin J, Gibbs R. Congenital toxoplasmosis: a review. Obstet Gynecol Surv. 2001;56(5):296-305.
34. Yamamoto JH, Vallochi AL, Silveira C, Filho JK, Nussenblatt RB, Cunha-Neto E, et al. Discrimination between patients with acquired toxoplasmosis and congenital toxoplasmosis on the basis of the immune response to parasite antigens. J Infect Dis. 2000;181(6):2018-22.
35. Freeman K, Tan HK, Prusa A, Petersen E, Buffolano W, Malm G, et al. Predictors of retinochoroiditis in children with congenital toxoplasmosis: European, prospective cohort study. Pediatrics. 2008;121(5):e1215-22.

36. Latkany P. Ocular disease due to *Toxoplasma gondii*. In: Weiss LM, Kim K (Eds). Toxoplasma gondii the Model Apicomplexan: Perspectives and Methods. London: Academic Press; 2007. pp. 101-31.
37. Dellicour S, Tatem AJ, Guerra CA, Snow RW, ter Kuile FO. Quantifying the number of pregnancies at risk of malaria in 2007: a demographic study. PLoS Med. 2010;7(1):e1000221.
38. McGregor IA, Wilson ME, Billewicz WZ. Malaria infection of the placenta in The Gambia, West Africa; its incidence and relationship to stillbirth, birthweight and placental weight. Trans R Soc Trop Med Hyg. 1983:77(2), 232-44.
39. Hänscheid T, Frita R, Längin M, Kremsner PG, Grobusch MP. Is flow cytometry better in counting malaria pigment-containing leukocytes compared to microscopy? Malar J. 2009;8:255.
40. Fotedar R, Stark D, Beebe N, Marriott D, Ellis J, Harkness J. Laboratory diagnostic techniques for Entamoeba species. Clin Microbiol Rev. 2007;20(3):511-32.
41. Tagbor H, Bruce J, Agbo M, Greenwood B, Chandramohan D. Intermittent screening and treatment versus intermittent preventive treatment of malaria in pregnancy: a randomised controlled non-inferiority trial. PLoS One. 2010;5(12):e14425.
42. van Hal SJ, Stark DJ, Fotedar R, Marriott D, Ellis JT, Harkness JL. Amoebiasis: current status in Australia. Med J Aust. 2007;186(8):412-6.
43. Aristizábal H, Acevedo J, Botero M. Fulminant amebic colitis. World J Surg. 1991;15(2):216-21.
44. Busse O. Ueber parasitare zelleninschlusse und ihre zuchtung. Zentralbl. Bakterial. 1894;16:175-80.
45. Buschke A. Ueber eine durch Coccidien Hervergerufene Krankheit des menschen. Deutsche Med. Wochenschr. 1895;21(3):14.
46. Lowell JR. Diagnosis of histoplasmosis. Ann Intern Med. 1983;98(2):260.
47. Wilson ML, Gaido L. Laboratory diagnosis of urinary tract infections in adult patients. Clin Infect Dis. 2004:38(8):1150-8.
48. Patterson TF, Andriole VT. Detection, significance, and therapy of bacteriuria in pregnancy. Update in the managed health care era. Infect Dis Clin North Am. 1997;11(3):593-608.

CHAPTER 64

Spine and Joint Disorders

Kiran Guleria, Esha Sharma

INTRODUCTION

The musculoskeletal system undergoes remarkable adaption during pregnancy. Hormonal changes cause relaxation of pelvic joints and modify the connective tissue response to mechanical stress during pregnancy.[1] Previously, it was thought that relaxin, which is a protein hormone secreted by corpus luteum, decidua and the placenta is responsible for these changes, but current literature does not support this as serum relaxin levels do not correlate with increasing peripheral joint laxity in pregnancy.[2]

As pregnancy advances, progressive lordosis occurs to accommodate the gravid uterus and thus shifting the center of gravity back over the lower extremities. The sacroiliac, sacrococcygeal and the pubic joints have an increased mobility which may contribute to the alteration in maternal posture leading to discomfort in the lower back.[3]

Women commonly present with musculoskeletal discomfort, which is temporarily disabling, but resolves spontaneously with completion of pregnancy. But there are certain chronic disorders which may affect the course of pregnancy.

DISORDERS OF SPINE

Scoliosis

Scoliosis is a three-dimensional deformity of spine, defined as a coronal spinal curvature of at least 10° with rotation of the vertebral bodies of unknown origin.[4]

It is more common in females; incidence being 2%.[5] Severity of the scoliosis is defined by "Cobb angle". More than 40° angle is considered severe which is associated with cardiac and pulmonary dysfunction.[6] Thoracic scoliosis causes a significant reduction in the number of alveoli predisposing these patients to impaired gas exchange and pulmonary hypertension.

Etiology

- Idiopathic (most common)
- Congenital
- Neuromuscular
- Degenerative

Idiopathic scoliosis is the most common and mostly occurs in the infantile, juvenile, and adolescent forms.

Diagnosis

Physical assessment

Height, weight and full musculoskeletal and neuromuscular assessment should be done to identify the etiology. Skin must be searched for hairy patch or dimples (spinal dysraphism) and *cafe-au-lait* spots (neurofibromatosis).

Adam's forward bend test: on bending forwards, curve of structural scoliosis is more apparent and imbalanced rib cage, with one-side being higher than the other, or other deformities can be noticed.

Curve assessment

Curve assessment includes curve location (thoracic, thoracolumbar, lumbar), convexity (right or left), flexibility of curves, extent of rib hump or lumbar bulge, shoulder level, pelvic obliquity, sagittal profile, sagittal balance, coronal balance.

The convexity of adolescent thoracic curves is mostly on right side (Fig. 1).

Diagnostic workup

Radiography remains the modality of choice (Fig. 2) but is generally avoided in pregnancy.

Magnitude of deformity is measured by Cobb angle i.e., angle of the two-end-vertebrae. Magnetic resonance imaging (MRI) is needed to detect intraspinal pathologies.

Effect on Pregnancy

- Previously, it was thought that there is an increased risk of progression of curve, but later studies suggested no effect on curve progression during pregnancy with regard to age of patient at the time of pregnancy or number of pregnancies. In the patients who have spine fusion, progression in the unfused portion of spine is negligible[7,8]
- Scoliosis can increase risk to pregnancy as the uterus expands, further impending the natural displacement of the diaphragm upwards and thus reducing vital capacity and residual volume of the lung. Women with scoliosis have difficulty in compensating for this displacement related to skeletal narrowing of the thoracic cavity. Loss of the normal adaptive mechanism leads to V/Q mismatch and increased work of breathing.[9]

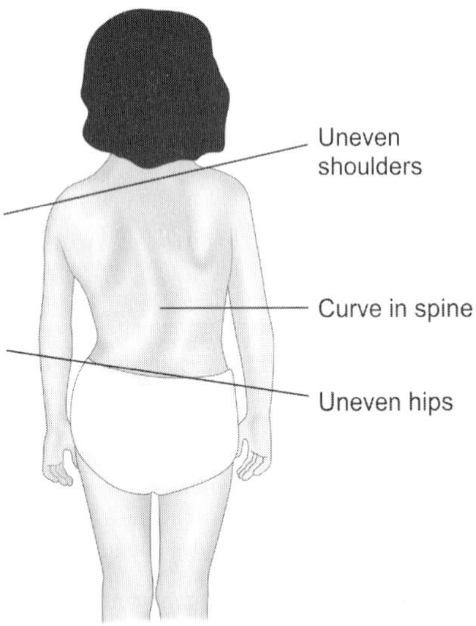

FIG.1: Signs of scoliosis.

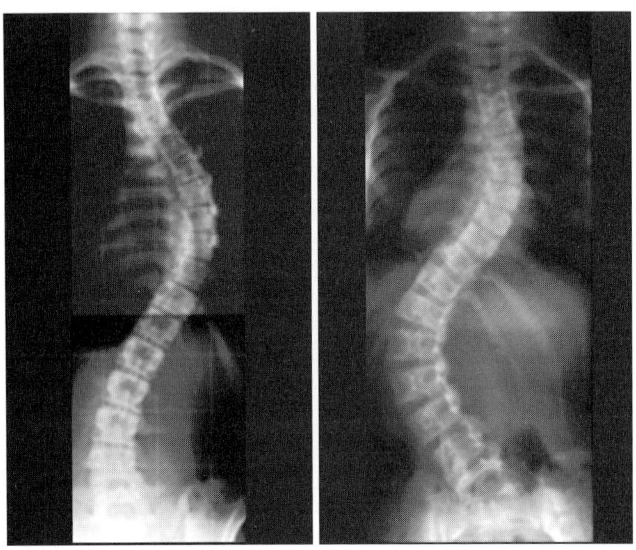

FIG. 2: X-ray showing thoracic and lumbar scoliosis.

Effect on Fetus

No major fetal complications are associated with maternal scoliosis.

Management

Labor and delivery: the incidence of cephalopelvic disproportion is increased in these patients and hence the instrumental and operative delivery rate is increased by 2.5 times the normal.[10]

Obstetric patients with thoracolumbar scoliosis or previous spinal surgery are a challenge. There is no accepted best practice to manage their care but there is a choice of available regional anesthetic technique, with different pros and cons that may be tailored to meet individual needs.

General anesthesia is preferred in scoliosis if there is maternal cardiopulmonary disease or difficulty in performing regional block.

Epidural, spinal and continuous spinal techniques can also be used for scoliotic women in labor and for operative delivery. The choice of technique will depend upon the clinical assessment and individual requirement. Continuous spinal anesthesia may overcome some of the problems of epidural or spinal technique; produce good analgesia and anesthesia in women with severe scoliosis, cardiorespiratory compromise or previous spinal surgery.[11]

In pregnancy there is increased intra-abdominal pressure and presence of engorged veins in the epidural space causing decrease in the subarachnoid space, leading to higher levels of block which can cause hypotension even in normal doses of the local anesthetic. This is more so in cases of severe scoliosis, which can be associated with decreased volumes of cerebrospinal fluid (CSF).[12]

In cases of severe kyphoscoliosis deformity, risk of cardiorespiratory complications should be prognosticated to the patient.

KYPHOSIS

Kyphosis is characterized by spine curvature that results in a bowing of the back, causing a slouching posture or hunchback (Fig. 3). The diagnostic criteria are wedging of more than 5 degree in the three consecutive vertebrae with typical end plate irregularities on the lateral radiograph.[13] Lung function is impaired only in severe deformities.[14]

Etiology

It can be developmental, degenerative or traumatic. Kyphosis may appear during development as a result of certain birth defects such as spina bifida.

Incidence

The reported incidence of kyphoscoliosis in pregnancy varies from 1:1,471 to 1:12,000.[15]

Effect on Pregnancy

In kyphoscoliosis there is a fixation of the thoracic cage, and a reduction in total lung capacity, i.e., reduction in vital capacity and in residual volume. Pregnancy further embarrasses this situation, as further reduction in the functional residual capacity with elevation of the diaphragm will not be neutralized by an increased inspiratory capacity. The net result will be a further reduction in the vital capacity which was already reduced before the pregnancy.[9] Kyphoscoliosis in pregnancy thus requires careful evaluation of the cardiorespiratory state.

Diagnosis

A spinal X-ray is essential to demonstrate the exact site of the vertebrae involved which in pregnancy can be performed with an abdominal shield.

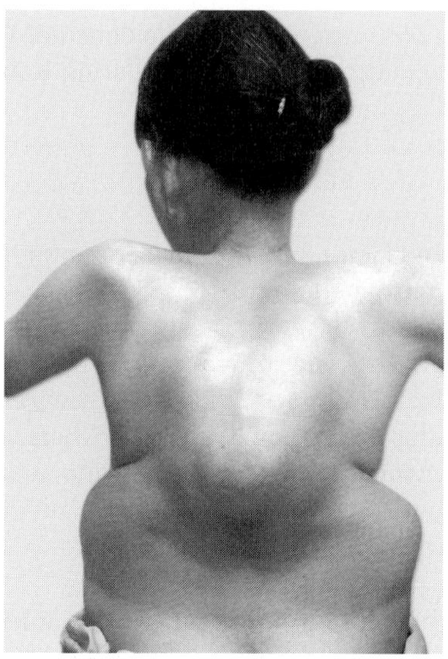

FIG. 3: Kyphosis.

Management

Hospitalization is essential as soon as pregnancy is diagnosed, in order to asses a baseline of the cardiorespiratory status.

Dyspnea at rest is a reflection of the energy cost of respiration or the ability of the patient to ventilate her lungs in the presence of restrictive lung disease in pregnancy. This is the most important criteria to be considered in deciding on termination.

The mode of termination will depend upon the clinical state of the patient, the adequacy of the pelvis and the ripeness of the cervix. If planned for vaginal delivery, careful monitoring of progress of labor is done. Continuous fetal monitoring is also considered during labor although kyphosis does not prove to be a threat to the fetus.

SPONDYLOLYSIS AND SPONDYLOLISTHESIS

Spondylolysis is a bony insufficiency at the pars interarticularis of the spine. and spondylolisthesis is the slipping forward of one vertebra on another.

Types of Spondylolisthesis

- Isthmic spondylolisthesis
- Degenerative spondylolisthesis
- Traumatic spondylolisthesis
- Pathologic spondylolisthesis
- Dysplastic spondylolisthesis

Degenerative spondylolisthesis is four times more common in women than in men, and six times more common at L4/L5 than at L3/L4. The reason for its location at L4/L5 level includes more sagittal orientation of L4/L5 facet joints in relation to the coronal placement of the L5/S1 joints.[16]
Grading of spondylolisthesis (Meyerding classification):

- Grade 1: 0–25% vertebral slippage
- Grade 2: 26–50% vertebral slippage
- Grade 3: 51–75% vertebral slippage
- Grade 4: 76–99% vertebral slippage
- Grade 5: >100% vertebral disk has slipped completely off.

Effect of Pregnancy

During pregnancy, the large flexion movement on the lower back is reported to be equivalent to the load imposed on the spine of a non-pregnant woman with her trunk flexed. This increase in loading of the lumbar spine may influence the development of degenerative spondylolisthesis.

Possibly the most important factor is the effect of pregnancy in reducing the tone of the abdominal muscle. Poor muscle tone may be a contributing factor in joint hypermobility.[17] Weak muscles may allow an increase in sheer forces on the L4/L5 joints, and lead to the rotatory deformity seen in degenerative spondylolisthesis

Pregnancy does not contribute to progression of spondylolisthesis, or for increased low-back symptoms in a woman with spondylolysis. Nor is spondylolysis, with or without olisthesis, a risk factor for pregnancy complications.

Symptoms

Predominantly backache, numbness and weakness of lower limb with or without bladder dysfunction because of compression of nerve roots.

Diagnosis

The primary role of imaging studies is to confirm the clinical diagnosis of degenerative spondylolisthesis, although advanced imaging studies are also essential for preoperative planning.

X-ray: radiographic features include the essential finding on a lateral view of forward displacement of L4 on L5 or rarely, L5 on S1 or L3 on L4 in the presence of an intact neural arch.

Magnetic resonance imaging: it may be warranted depending on the patient's presentation and the clinical findings.[18] Factors that speak about the need for further imaging include significant and progressing neurologic claudication or radiculopathies and the clinical suspicion that another condition, such as metastatic disease, may be the cause. An absolute indication is the presence of bladder or bowel complaints (Fig. 4).

Management

Symptomatic relief can be obtained by rest and immobilization.

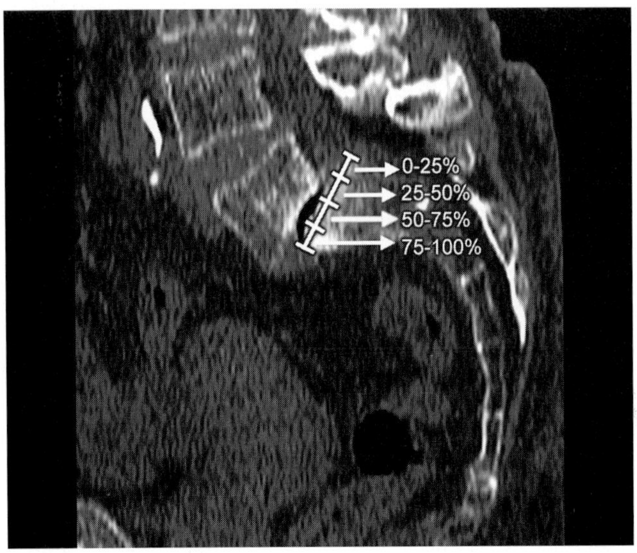

FIG. 4: Magnetic resonance imaging grading of spondylolisthesis.

In case of severe neurological symptoms, surgical intervention can be taken up.

ANKYLOSING SPONDYLITIS

Ankylosing spondylitis is an inflammatory condition with unknown etiology. It has a strong genetic predisposition and association with human leukocyte antigen (HLA)-B27. It most frequently affects axial skeleton; however, 30% can develop peripheral arthritis[19] and presents during the reproductive age.

Symptoms

Lumbar pain and morning stiffness are main symptoms. As the disease progresses, there is decrease in spinal mobility.
Diagnostic criteria:
- History of inflammatory back pain
- Limitation of motion of the lumbar spine in the sagittal and the frontal planes
- Limited chest expansion
- Evidence of sacroiliitis.

The presence of the first with any other criteria is sufficient for the diagnosis.[20]

Effect on Pregnancy

No remission occurs during pregnancy. Literature suggests mean age of patients with ankylosing spondylitis is 23 years with 21% presenting in pregnancy.[21] Disease activity remains unchanged in about 33%, improves in 31% and worsens in 33%. Women with history of peripheral arthritis and who give birth to a female show improvement. 60% of patients with active disease at conception present with postpartum flare within 6 months of delivery. Cesarean section is required in more than 50% cases. Higher incidence of the disease is found in the children of women suffering from ankylosing spondylitis.[20]

Diagnosis

- Rheumatoid factor and antinuclear antibodies (ANA) are negative in isolated case
- Positive for HLA-B27 and C-reactive protein
- X-ray: shows evidence of symmetric erosion and sclerosis of sacroiliac joint, loss of lordosis and squaring of vertebral bodies with calcification of the outer fibers of the annulus fibrosus giving the "bamboo spine" appearance (Fig. 5).

Treatment

Symptomatic treatment is required to ameliorate pain. Nonsteroidal anti-inflammatory drugs (NSAIDs) can be given with caution.

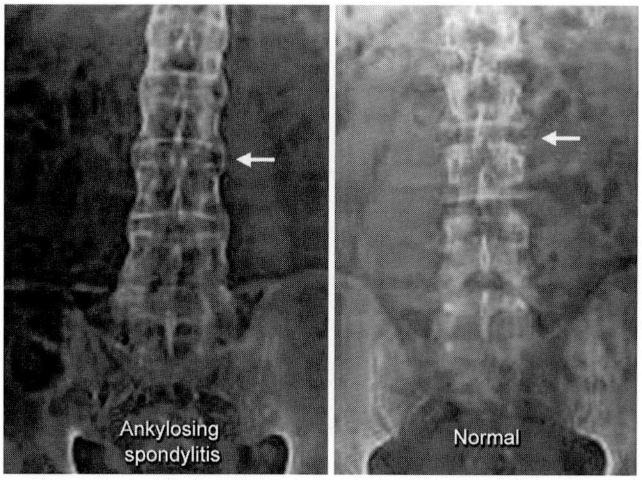

FIG. 5: There is a ligament (arrow head) on sides of the vertebrae which is not seen in normal person. In ankylosing spondylitis it becomes thick and calcified.

TUBERCULOSIS OF SPINE (POTT'S SPINE)

Spinal tuberculosis also known as Pott's disease, results from hematogenous spread of tuberculosis (TB) from other sites, usually pulmonary. The infection then spreads from two adjacent vertebrae into intervertebral disks and surrounding structures forming a paravertebral abscess.

Due to vertebral body and disk destruction, there is a cord compression which may lead to paraplegia and quadriplegia. It is a rare disease in developed world but still occurs in pregnancy in developing nations and most is commonly localized to the lower thoracic and upper lumbar vertebrae and intervertebral disks.[22] Due to delay in diagnosis, patient usually presents when paraplegia has already occurred.

Spinal tuberculosis is the most common form of skeletal involvement which accounts for 1–2% of all extra pulmonary cases.[23]

Signs and Symptoms

Localized backache (spinal or radicular) is the earliest and commonest symptoms which may worsen on weight bearing. As the disease progresses, pain increases, and paraspinal muscle spasm occurs which obliterates the normal spinal curves. In rare circumstances, patient may present with neurological signs, weakness, bowel and bladder involvement, paraplegia or quadriplegia.[24] Physical examination of the spine reveals localized tenderness and paravertebral swelling lump in a groin due to psoas abscess or kyphosis.

The most often involved areas in nonparalytic group is from T9–L2 vertebrae and T5-T9 thoracic vertebrae in paralytic group because the spinal canal is smallest at this level. Therefore, cord compression due to the products of inflammation would be maximum.[25]

Effect on Pregnancy

Low back pain (LBP) caused by spinal tuberculosis is often mistaken for a physiologic change associated with pregnancy which may delay diagnosis. Pregnancy minimally impacts disease progression but often obscures initial diagnosis leading to greater complications ranging from subclinical course in early pregnancy to the worsening of the disease in late pregnancy, leading to paraplegia or quadriplegia, pyelonephritis, decubitus ulcer, psoas abscess and meningitis. Autonomic dysreflexia can be a life-threatening complication secondary to hyperstimulation of the splanchnic nerves and loss of central control over sympathetic spinal reflexes when the lesion is above T6.[26]

Effect on Fetus

Premature or precipitate labor may occur in paraplegic patients.

Diagnosis

- Blood investigation: complete blood count with erythrocyte sedimentation rate (ESR) which may be markedly elevated
- Tuberculin test
- Imaging
- Plain radiographs:
  - X-ray chest: to look for any primary focus
  - X-ray spine: although not advocated in pregnancy but can be done with an abdominal shield. It shows earliest radiological features of narrowing of the joint space and indistinct paradiscal margin of vertebral bodies. Also seen are concave erosions around the anterior margins of the vertebral bodies producing a scalloped appearance called the aneurysmal phenomenon due to long standing abscesses and wedging of vertebral leading to kyphotic deformity
- Magnetic resonance imaging is the gold standard for evaluating disk space infection and osteomyelitis of the spine. The extension of disease into soft tissues and the spread of tuberculous debris under the anterior and posterior longitudinal ligaments are also demonstrated better. MRI is most-effective for demonstrating neural compression. Serial MRI can be used to assess the response to treatment and regression (Fig. 6)
- Histopathology and microbiology

In cases of doubtful clinic radiological findings, suspicion of drug-resistant strains and lack of proper response to drug therapy, a biopsy or aspiration can be done and sent for culture, antibiotic sensitivity and histopathology.

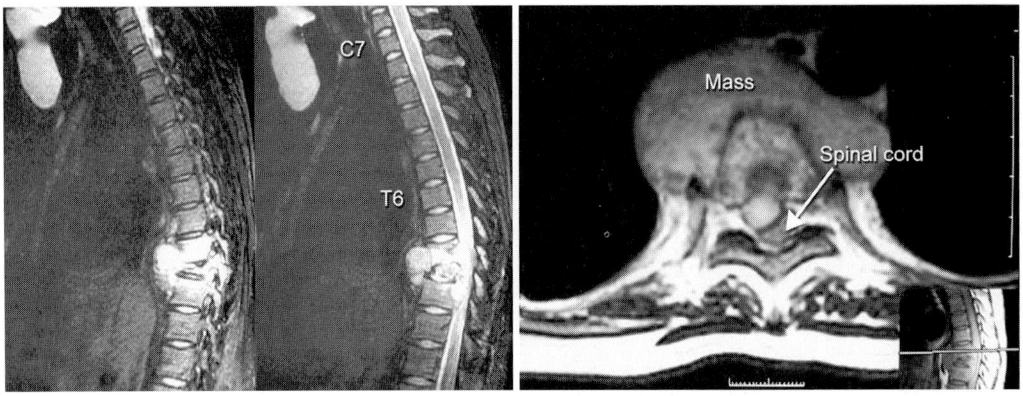

FIG. 6: Spinal magnetic resonance imaging showing collapse of T9 body with a soft tissue prevertebral and paravertebral mass (abscess) resulting in severe spinal cord compression.[26]

Treatment

Therapy should be started as soon as diagnosis of TB is confirmed. The World Health Organization (WHO) or Revised National Tuberculosis Control Programme (RNTCP) guidelines consider spinal tuberculosis with neurological deficit to be severe extra pulmonary (category 1) and should receive treatment for 6 months. In rare and exceptional cases of relapse or treatment failure, treatment should be given according to category 2, i.e., for 9 months.[27] Drug used are isoniazid 300 mg, rifampicin 450 mg, ethambutol 800 mg, pyrizinamide 1500 mg and pyridoxin 50 mg daily along with a short course of steroids (40 mg/kg/day) for 4 weeks and gradually tapered within 2 weeks.

In Pott's paraplegia, patient should not be allowed to remain in a paraplegic state indefinitely. Surgical intervention is considered in neurological deficit, spinal deformity with instability, severe or progressive kyphosis, retropulsed bone fragments in the canal, large abscess causing respiratory embarrassment, and no response to medical therapy of 3 to 4 months duration.[28]

Labor Management

Paraplegia is not a contraindication to vaginal delivery. The onset and detection of labor poses a problem in paraplegic woman. When the lesion is above the T-11 spinal level, premature labor tends to be more common due to painless labor.[29] Kyphosis due to disease process leads to diminished vertical diameter of the abdominal cavity. In kyphotic pelvis, only the voluntary forces of labor are affected and delay usually occurs in second stage of labor. The essential involuntary muscles are not much affected by the disease of the spine and the uterus may be excited to contraction by the most varied peripheral and the central influence.[30]

Caesarean section is done for obstetrics indication only. Cases have been reported where cesarean section was done without anesthesia and no analgesia used postoperatively.[31]

After surgical decompression, postoperatively the patient is advised absolute bedrest for 3 months, and continued antitubercular therapy and then gradually mobilized in a spinal brace.

PELVIC GIRDLE PAIN

Pelvic girdle pain (PGP) is defined as a pain experienced between the posterior iliac crest and the gluteal fold, particularly in the vicinity of the sacroiliac joints (SIJ). The pain may radiate in the posterior thigh and can also occur in conjunction with/or separately in the symphysis. The endurance capacity for standing, walking, and sitting is diminished. PGP generally occurs due to pregnancy, trauma or reactive arthritis. The diagnosis of PGP can be reached after exclusion of lumbar causes. LBP is usually defined by pain between the 12th rib and the gluteal fold.[32]

It is divided into five subgroups; pelvic girdle syndrome (pain in both SIJ and the symphysis), symphysiolysis, one-sided SIJ syndrome, double-sided SIJ syndrome and miscellaneous. A study showed a point prevalence of PGP as 20.1%. In the diagnostic subgroups, the point prevalence was: pelvic girdle syndrome 6%, symphysiolysis 2.3%, one-sided SIJ syndrome 5.5% and double-sided SIJ syndrome 6.3%.[33]

Etiology

- Hormonal: during pregnancy, the female body is exposed to certain factors that have an impact on the dynamic stability of the pelvis. Relaxin is a polypeptide hormone secreted from the decidua, corpus luteum and the chorion and targets the uterine cervix, the myometrium, the endometrium and the decidua. Other probable targets are pubic symphysis and SIJ. This results in the laxity of ligaments of the pelvic girdle as well as ligaments in the rest of the body. The effect of increased ligament laxity is a slightly larger range of movement (ROM) in the pelvic joints. If this is not compensated for by altered neuromotor control, pain may result. Although the relationship between hormone level and joint pain is not clear[34]

- Mechanical: during pregnancy, a woman develops postural changes that are necessary for her to maintain balance in the upright position. As pregnancy advances the abdominal muscles are stretched and tone is diminished, they lose their ability to contribute effectively to the maintenance of neutral posture. With these structural changes lumbar lordosis is increased. In the lumbar spine, joint laxity is most notable in the anterior and posterior longitudinal ligaments. This weakens the ability of static supports in the lumbar spine to withstand the shearing forces. As a result, there may be an increase in discogenic symptoms and/or pain coming from the facet joints[35]

  Sometimes "Parietal neuralgia of pregnancy" which is a radicular pain due to compression of nerves; lumbar and sacral plexi is often noted.[36]
- Vascular congestion: pain is a predominant symptom, due to increase in venous flow through the lumbar vein, the vertebral venous plexus, paraspinal veins and azygos veins that occurs at right. This may be owing to vena caval compression by the gravid uterus in a spine patient[35]
- Disk disease: relaxin weakens the annulus of the intervertebral disk.[35] The potential of disk herniation and nerve root compression with radicular pain should be considered
- Sacroiliac pain: during pregnancy, mechanisms stabilizing the SIJ is affected. This instability allows for increased motion, stressing the SIJ. Moreover, the additional weight and altered walking pattern associated with pregnancy can cause significant mechanical strain on the SIJ, which may result in SIJ inflammation, giving a deep ache in the posterior pelvis.[35]

Risk Factors

- Increasing parity
- Older maternal age
- Back pain during previous pregnancy
- History of trauma to the back or pelvis.

Diagnosis

It is strongly recommended that a pain history be taken with special attention paid to pain arising during prolonged standing, walking and/or sitting. To ensure that the pain is in the pelvic girdle area, it is important that the precise area of pain be indicated. The patient should either point out the exact location on his/her body or preferably, indicate the painful area on a pain location diagram.

The following tests are recommended for clinical examination of PGP:

- SIJ pain: posterior pelvic pain provocation test (P4/thigh thrust),[36] Patrick's Faber test,[37] palpation of the long dorsal SIJ ligament,[38] and Gaenslen's test[39,40]
- Symphysis: palpation of the symphysis and the modified Trendelenburg test of the pelvic girdle[41]
- Functional pelvic test: active straight leg raise test
- Radiographic evaluation is not warranted unless the exact mechanism could not be explained although no harm to the fetus has been demonstrated by exposure less than 5 rads. MRI is helpful in diagnosis of tumor, infection or herniated vertebral disk.

Treatment

Only symptomatic care is required in majority of complaints.

The institution of individualized physical therapy may be useful option to alleviate the intensity of pelvic pain:

- Exercise: exercise may play a role in altering the relationship between flexibility of the spine and LBP during pregnancy. A study by Stuge and colleagues showed a significant improvement in pain, functional status and health-related quality in a study group performing stretching and strengthening of the abdominal musculature, the lumbar multifidus, gluteus maximus, latissimus dorsi, erector spine, quadratus lumborum, hip adductors and abductors[42,43]
- Massage: massage might be helpful but there is no evidence to recommend massage as a stand-alone treatment for PGP.[44]
- Pelvic belt: a pelvic belt may be fitted to test for symptomatic relief, but should only be applied for short periods[45]
- Acupuncture: despite the moderate to low quality of some of the studies, there is evidence that acupuncture seems to alleviate LBP and pelvic pain during pregnancy[45]
- Sacroiliac joints therapeutic injection: different guiding techniques for intra-articular injections in the SIJ were used either under fluoroscopy or with CT or MRI guidance. All studies showed immediate pain relief with decreasing effects over time. Local injection appears promising in patients with inflammatory diseases[46]
- Drugs: prescribe medication, if necessary, for pain relief (preferably to be taken at regular intervals); first choice paracetamol, second NSAIDs.[47]

DISORDER OF JOINTS

Avascular Necrosis of Hip

Osteonecrosis (ON) is thought to result from the temporary or permanent loss of the blood supply to the bones. This disease is also known as avascular necrosis (AVN), aseptic necrosis, and ischemic bone necrosis.[48]

Avascular necrosis of femoral head, which is aseptic ischemia of cellular bone marrow, is fairly common in pregnancy. Since the femoral head is deficient in blood supply, it is particularly vulnerable for AVN.[49] The pathophysiology is thought to be due to venous stasis and increased intramedullary pressure.

It commonly involves the left femoral head because the growing fetus and uterus compress the left common iliac vein, which is directly posterior to the uterus on the left side.

As pregnancy-related ON seems rare, the causative role of pregnancy is not well-established. Several putative mechanisms have been evoked.[48]

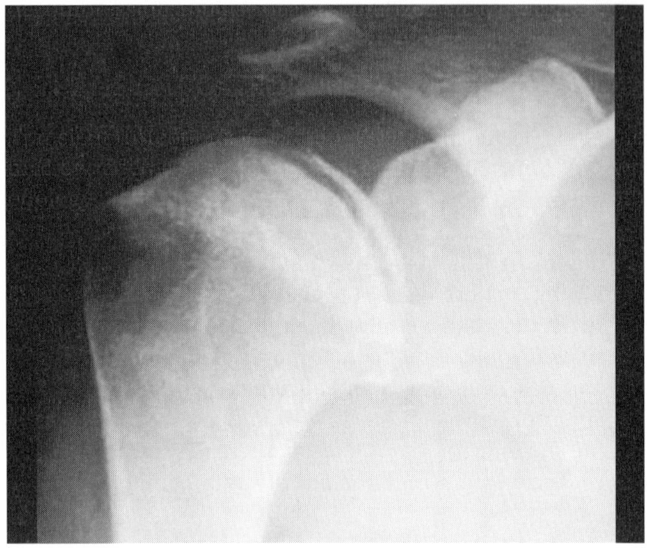

FIG. 7: Lateral radiographs of the pelvis demonstrating superolateral collapse of the right femoral head.[49]

Etiology

The relationship between AVN of the femoral head and pregnancy can result from:

- High level of adrenocortical activity
- Elevated maternal parathyroid hormone and its adverse effects on bone, and
- Mechanical stress, especially, due to excessive gain during the last trimester of pregnancy in women with a small body frame.[50] High levels of estrogen and progesterone may also be contributing factor. Another theory implicates fat embolism to the femoral head.

Symptoms

The pain begins in third trimester and is commonly localized to the groin area but it may also manifest in the ipsilateral buttock, knee, or greater trochanteric region.

Musculoskeletal examination is normal except for discomfort in extremes of hip motion. Painful symptoms are usually exacerbated with weight bearing but are relieved by rest.

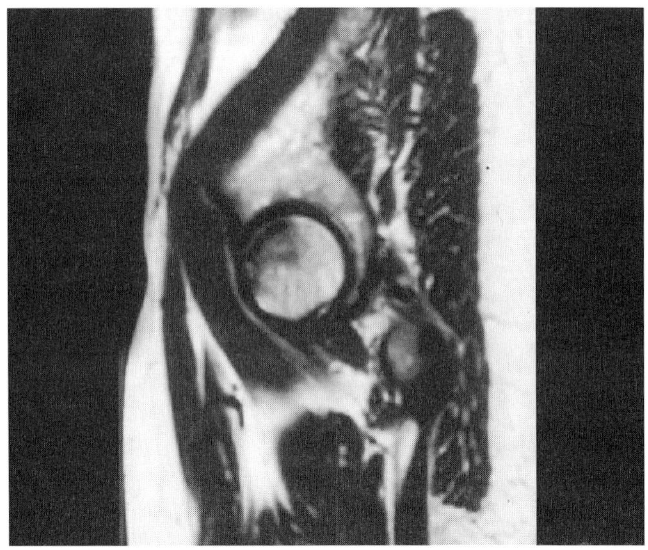

FIG. 8: Lateral spine echo T1-weighted MRI shows typical osteonecrosis of the femoral head.[51]

Diagnosis

X-ray shows subchondral lucency or subchondral collapse of dome of femoral head seen as "crescent sign" (Fig. 7).

Magnetic resonance imaging shows focal lesions in the anterolateral femoral head with decreased signal intensity on both T1 and T2 weighted images. Double density signal surrounding the lesion may also be seen (Fig. 8).

Treatment

Although the treatment of AVN of hip in pregnancy is controversial, conservative treatment consisting of reduction in weight bearing has been found to be effective.

Osteonecrosis of the femoral head, treated conservatively, usually progresses to collapse of the femoral head in 70–80% of patients with eventual development of osteoarthritis of the affected of the affected hip joint.[52]

Other options include osteotomy, use of non-vascularized structural graft, electrical stimulation, and core decompression and use of a vascularized structural graft.[53]

TRANSIENT OSTEOPOROSIS OF HIP

Transient osteoporosis of hip (TOH), also called "bone marrow edema syndrome", is a rare disorder of unknown etiology. It is a self-limiting skeletal disease that is both reversible and painful. The most common site affected is the hip joint, with the left hip more frequently involved than the right.[53]

Bilateral involvement occurs in only 25–30% of cases.[54,55] Involvement of other joints, such as lower-extremity joints, upper-extremity joints, and the spine, with migration to multiple sites is up to 40% of patients. Recurrence is seen in 25–50% of this population. The disorder primarily affects women in the third trimester of pregnancy.[56]

Etiology

Etiology includes neural, vascular, chemical, and hormonal mechanisms. Possible neural mechanisms include a variant of reflex sympathetic dystrophy, pathology of the peripheral nerves, compression of the obturator nerve, and irritation or compression of the pelvic nerves. Suggested vascular mechanisms include ischemia of the small vessels proximal to the nerve roots, obstruction of venous return, transient ischemia, and decreased fibrinolytic potential. Proposed chemical and hormonal mechanisms include factors associated with pregnancy and increased maternal demand for calcium, protein, and minerals.[56,57]

It may also be associated with liver cirrhosis, disorders related to increased bone turnover, or hypercalciuric osteoporosis. Genetic predisposition and osteogenesis imperfecta have also been associated with this disease. Viral, arthritic, and inflammatory factors have also been considered. But these factors are yet to been confirmed.[58]

Symptoms

Sudden onset of pain is usually located at the lateral aspect of the hip, the front of the thigh, buttocks, or the groin. The pain gradually increases over a period of weeks or months and may eventually become disabling. There is usually no history of trauma to the joint that would trigger pain. Alteration of gait may be observed as the patient tries to protect the joint and ease the pain.

Transient osteoporosis occurs in three phases:

- Stage 1 (first 1–2 months) features a rapid increase in pain and functional disability but normal radiographic findings
- Stage 2 (after 2–3 months) features maximal symptoms and signs, with osteopenia noted on radiographs
- Stage 3 (up to 6 months) involves gradual regression of the disease and radiographic changes, the latter taking longer.[59]

Diagnosis

Diagnosis is made by exclusion of other possible causes of hip pain. The most important differential diagnosis is AVN, in which the pain has an insidious onset and typically occurs at rest.[54]

Except for an elevated ESR, laboratory data are within the normal ranges, but this is a common finding during pregnancy as well.

X-ray: hip may not show radiolucency until the condition is advanced (usually 1–2 months after the pain starts). Remineralization usually occurs within 2 years. TOH may be confused with AVN or femoral neck stress fracture, but the joint space is preserved (Fig. 9).[60,54]

Magnetic resonance imaging (MRI) is the best tool currently available for detection of TOH. It typically shows bone marrow edema within 48 hours after the onset of symptoms and resolution within 6–8 months (Fig. 10). It shows decreased signal intensity of bone marrow on T1-weighted images, increased signal intensity of bone marrow on T2-weighted images, and surrounding soft-tissue edema and joint effusion on T2-weighted images. If the patient is pregnant, the image studies should be delayed until the last stages or after delivery.[61]

Bone densitometry shows 3–24% bone loss after 3–5 months from the onset of symptoms, with a return to normal bone density within 2 years.[62]

Treatment

Treatment is mainly conservative and symptomatic that includes reduction of weight bearing activities, analgesic medication, and physical therapy. Use of crutches, a cane, or other walking aids helps relieve the stress of weight bearing.

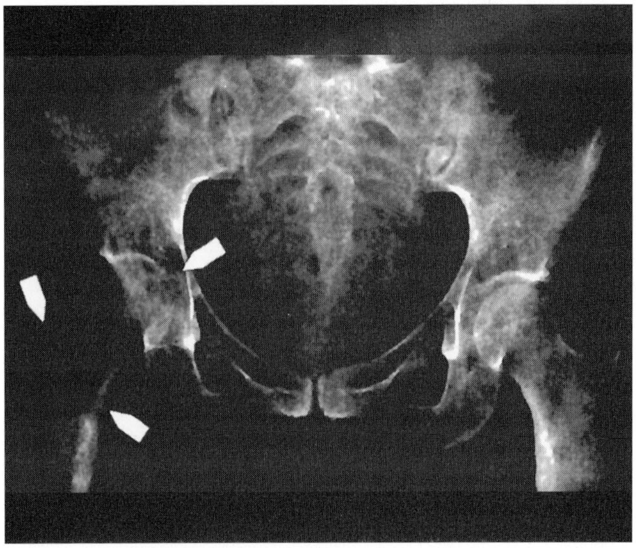

FIG. 9: Conventional radiograph of the pelvis and hips. The 3 arrows identify the osteopenia of the right proximal femur and acetabulum when compared with the corresponding areas of the left hip. No evidence of fracture or avascular necrosis.[60]

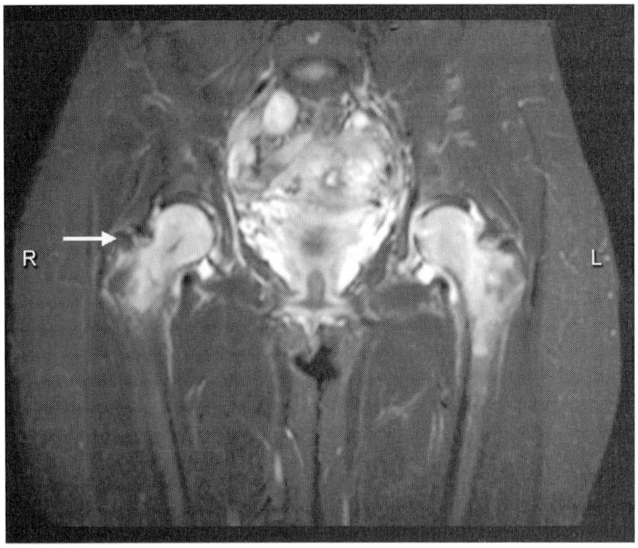

FIG. 10: Magnetic resonance imaging of pelvis showing marked bone marrow edema at femoral head and neck bilaterally (arrows), mild bilateral hip joint effusion, no definite abnormal signal at soft tissues bilaterally, and no definite osteolytic lesion.[62]

Nonsteroidal anti-inflammatory drugs can be administered to relieve pain. Physical therapy, including exercises to increase flexibility and ROM, is helpful. Pharmacological treatments such as bisphosphonates and calcitonin can also help. Surgical treatment such as core decompression is controversial as this is a benign process.

Elective cesarean section and cessation of breastfeeding may relieve the symptoms, but there are no controlled studies to support these suggestions.

Transient osteoporosis is self-limiting, with spontaneous resolution within 1-year in the majority of cases.

Prevention of damage to bones weakened by osteoporosis is important; the most severe possible complication is stress fracture of the hip.

RUPTURE OF PUBIC SYMPHYSIS

The symphysis pubis joint is a fibrocartilaginous structure which holds the two innominate bones of the pelvis together and keeps them steady during activity. Of the four ligaments enveloping the joint, the inferior or arcuate ligament is the strongest and contributes most to joint stability but, together, all four neutralize the shear and tensile stresses. In nonpregnant woman's symphysis pubis gap is 4–5 mm and it is normal for it to widen 2–3 mm, without discomfort, during the last trimester of pregnancy. This increases the diameters of the pelvic brim and cavity outlet to facilitate delivery of the fetus.[63]

Rupture of pubic symphysis is an uncommon event after vaginal delivery.

Incidence varies from 1 in 300 to 1 in 30,000 deliveries.[64] While a mild diastasis of the pubic symphysis (i.e., <10 mm), is considered to be physiological in pregnancy, greater separation can lead to tenderness of palpation and disability to ambulate. Where the gap increases to more than 10 mm this is known as diastasis of the symphysis pubis (DSP).

Separation of as much as 120 mm has been reported; the sacroiliac joint becomes affected with more than 40 mm of separation.[65]

Etiology

Multiparity, macrosomia accompanied by cephalopelvic disorder, McRoberts maneuver, forceps, maternal connective tissue disorders, prior pelvic trauma, and hyper-flexed legs may predispose to pubic symphysis diastasis.[66,67]

Symptoms

It shows immediate onset of suprapubic and/or sacroiliac pain within the first 24 hours of delivery often accompanied by an audible click.

Also there difficulty in walking, ascending or descending stairs, rising from a chair, impaired weight bearing activities, e.g., standing on one leg or lifting or parting the legs and turning in bed is seen complication.

Cases of bladder incarceration and bowel herniation have been reported in traumatic symphysis pubis diastasis.

Diagnosis

Tenderness over the symphysis pubis and SIJ is the commonest.

On palpation, anteroposterior or superoinferior displacement of the upper border of the pubic symphysis or pubic tubercle can be felt.

Imaging is the only way to confirm DSP. It may also prove a useful tool for monitoring progress of DSP and assisting in the exclusion of other differential diagnoses.

Plain radiographs (anteroposterior view in the "flamingo position" or single-leg standing position) are needed to assess vertical mobility (Fig. 11).

Computerized tomography (CT), MRI and ultrasound scans have all been used to assess the misalignment of the pelvic bones.

Management

Several reports have shown that a conservative therapy is a reasonable approach. Even in cases of large symphyseal ruptures measuring 5 cm tight pelvic binding and rest in lateral decubitus position is recommended.

Surgical treatment like internal fixation is recommended in case extensive anterior separation of the pubic symphysis

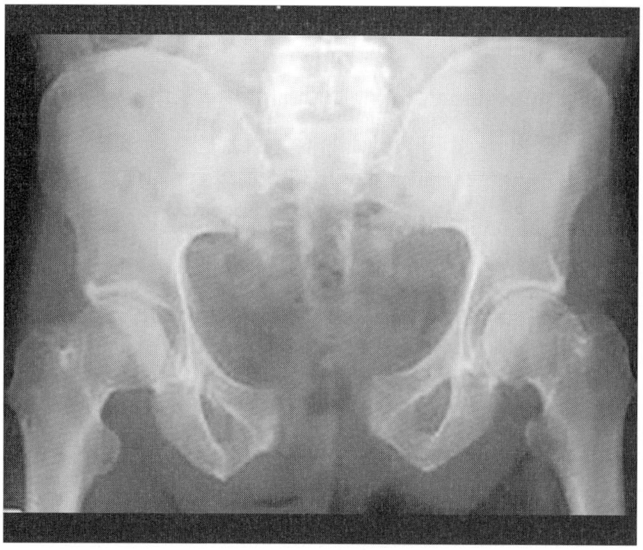

FIG. 11: Separation of the symphysis pubis.[68]

greater than 40 mm and vertical instability of the dorsal pelvic ring causing pelvic dislocation, recurrent or persistent diastasis.[68]

There is a significant risk of repeat symphyseal rupture with subsequent vaginal delivery thus it may be reasonable to offer cesarean to patient who sustained severe symphyseal disruption during previous vaginal delivery.

However, cases of successful and uneventful vaginal delivery following a rupture have been reported.[69]

POSTPARTUM OSTEITIS PUBIS

Osteitis pubis is a self-limited, apparently non-infective ON that begins at the public symphysis and extends into the public bones. It is rarely associated with pregnancy, either antepartum or postpartum. It is similar to pelvic arthropathy in its presentation, with accompanying public tenderness and pain that may prevent ambulation. It is differentiated from pelvic arthropathy and symphyseal disruption by radiographic rarefaction of the public bones, without symphyseal widening. It is differentiated from septic symphysitis by its lack of fever, leukocytosis, and radiographic bony sequestrum. Steroids and nonsteroidal anti-inflammatories have been recommended for treatment.[70] Treatment of symptomatic osteitis pubis with intravenous pamidronate has been reported.[71]

SEPTIC PUBIC SYMPHYSITIS AND SACROILIITIS

Osteomyelitis in or adjacent to the public symphysis has rarely been reported in association with pregnancy. Fever is not universal, though leukocyte count, erythrocyte sedimentation rate, and C-reactive protein levels are usually elevated. Surgical drainage and antibiotics should be curative.[72]

STRESS FRACTURES OF THE PUBIC BONE

Stress fracture of the body of the pubic bone has rarely been reported during pregnancy, unrelated to athletics or physical training. In the few cases reported, no underlying pathologic process has been found. The cause is thought to be due to ligament laxity, muscle imbalance, and increased load. Pain is usually insidious in onset. There is tenderness at the fracture. Radiography is diagnostic, but not usually until some healing has occurred. MRI has been suggested to diagnose pelvic stress fractures immediately.[73] Management is usually directed toward symptomatic relief.

PELVIC TRAUMA AND PREGNANCY

In a study of 34 women who had a displaced pelvic ring fracture, all of whom had at least one full-term pregnancy after healing, only two required elective cesarean section, and the need for the cesarean section was determined at the first presentation by pelvimetry. Of these 34 women, 17 had healed with displacement of fracture involving the birth canal. Of eigh,t who had previous traumatic pubic symphyseal disruption, two had recurrence of pain during pregnancy.

In a case of trauma very shortly after delivery, there is a report of a very wide traumatic diastasis of the pubic symphysis, which was "surprisingly easy" to reduce, with apparently no lasting injury sacroiliac ligaments. It was reasoned that the physiologic relaxation of the pelvis during pregnancy protected the ligaments from gross disruption during the injury. Successful surgical fixation of a severely displaced acetabular fracture has been reported in a patient 20 weeks pregnant, without affecting the pregnancy.[74]

TRANSIENT OSTEOPOROSIS OF THE HIP

Transient osteoporosis of the hip is a rare condition. It has been defined by multiple case reports over the last 41 years.[75] It is characterized by a gradually developing pain of the hip with weight bearing. Symptoms begin in the third (or late second) trimester. The pain is predominant in the anterior thigh and the groin. For unknown reasons, the left hip is affected more often than right, though both may be affected.[75] The pain is relieved by rest. There is no associated history of trauma or illness. Musculoskeletal examination is normal, except for discomfort at the extremes of hip motion and a slight decrease in total range of hip motion.[76] Other areas affected may include knee, ankle, foot, ribs, shoulders and spine.[75]

Management

The condition is self-limiting. Treatment is conservative, including protection from weight bearing, maintenance of joint motion, and analgesic medications.[76] In cases in which joint aspiration has been performed, the effusion is sterile, and the joint fluid is normal.[75]

Various treatments have been used, including limitation of weight bearing by wheelchairs, crutches, or canes. Corticosteroids, phenylbutazone, and calcitonin have been tried without beneficial effect.[76] After the delivery, symptoms completely resolve over 3–9 months.

REFERENCES

1. Borg-Stein J, Dugan SA, Gruber J. Musculoskeletal aspects of pregnancy. Am J Phys Med Rehabil. 2005;84(3):180-92.
2. Marnach ML, Ramin KD, Ramsey PS, Song SW, Stensland JJ, An KN. Characterization of the relationship between joint laxity and maternal hormones in pregnancy. Obstet Gynecol. 2003.101(2):331-5.
3. Mens JM, Pool-Goudzwaard A, Stam HJ. Mobility of the pelvic joints in pregnancy-related lumbopelvic pain: a systemic review. Obstet Gynecol Surv. 2009;64(3):200-8.
4. Cob J. Outline for study of scoliosis. AOS Instruct Course Lecture 5. 1948:261-75.
5. Rinsky LA, Gamble JG. Adolescent idiopathic scoliosis. West J Med. 1988;148(2):182-91.
6. Reisner LS, KuczKowski KM. Anesthetic considerations for complicated pregnancies. In: Creasy, Resnik, Iams (Eds). Meternal-fetal medicine. Philadelphia: Elsevier; 2003. pp 1243-60.
7. Betz RR, Bunnell WP, Lombrecht-Mulier E, MacEwen GD. Scoliosis and pregnancy. J Bone Joint Surg Am. 1987;69(1):90-6.
8. Josh E S, Joseph R D, Erika E, Leon K. Systematic review-Does pregnancy increase curve progression in women with scoliosis treated without surgery? Evidence-Based Spine-Care Journal. 2011;2(3):43-50.
9. Widlund G. The cardiopulmonal function during pregnancy. Acta Obstet Gynecol Scand. 1945;25(Suppl 1):7-125.
10. Cochran T, Irstam L, Nachemson A. Long-term anatomic and functional changes in patients with adolescent idiopathic scoliosis treated by Harrington rod fusion. Spine (Phila Pa 1976). 1983;8:576-84.
11. Smith PS, Wilson RC, Robinson AP, Lyons GR. Regional blockade for delivery in women with scoliosis or previous spinal surgery. Int J Obstet Anesth. 2003;12:17-22.
12. Kardash K, King BW, Datta S. Spinal anaesthesia for caesarean section after Harrington instrumentation. Can J Anaesth. 1993;40:667-9.
13. Braford DS. Juvenile kyphosis. Clin Orthop Relat Res. 1977;128:45-55.
14. Murray PM, Weinstein SL, Spartt KF. The natural history and long-term follow-up of Scheuermann kyphosis. J Bone Joint Surg Am. 1993:75(2):236-48.
15. Mendelson, CL. Pregnancy and kyphoscoliotic heart disease. Am J Obstet Gynecol. 1948;56:457-67.
16. Grobler LJ, Robertson PA, Novotny JE, Pope MH. Etiology of spondylolisthesis. Assessment of the role played by lumbar facet joint morphology. Spine (Phila Pa 1976). 1993;18:80-91.
17. Beimborn DS, Morrissey MC. A review of the literature related to trunk muscle performance. Spine (Phila Pa 1976). 1988;13:655-60.
18. Butt S, Saifuddin A. The imaging of lumbar spondylolisthesis. Clin Radiol. 2005;60:533-46.
19. Gran JT, Skomsvoll JF. The outcome of ankylosing spondylitis: a study of 100 patients. Br J Rheumatol. 1997;36:766-71.
20. Østensen M, Fuhrer L, Mathieu R, Seitz M, Villiger PM A prospective study of pregnant patients with rheumatoid arthritis and ankylosing spondylitis using validated clinical instruments. Ann Rheum Dis. 2004;63(10):1212-7.
21. Lui NL, Haroon N, Carty A, Shen H, Cook RJ, Shanmugarajah S, et al. Effect of pregnancy on ankylosing spondylitis: a case-control study. J Rheumatol. 2011;38(11):2442-4.
22. Govender S, Moodley SC, Grootboom MJ. Tuberculous paraplegia during pregnancy: A report of 4 cases. S Afr Med J. 1989;75(4):190-2.
23. Tuli SM. Textbook- Tuberculosis of the skeletal system (Bones, Joints, Spine and Bursal sheaths), 3rd edition. New Delhi: Jaypee Brothers; 2004.
24. Comaar AE. Observations on menstruation and pregnancy among female spinal cord injury patients. Paraplegia. 1966;3:263-66.
25. Goller H, Paeslack V. Our experiences about pregnancy and delivery of the paraplegic woman. Paraplegia. 1970;8:161-5.
26. Luewan S, Bunmaprasert T, Chiengthong K, Tongsong T. Spinal tuberculosis in pregnancy. Int J Gynaecol Obstet. 2008;102(3):298-300.
27. Wares F, Balasubramanian R, Mohan A, Sharma SK. Tuberculosis Control in India. Elsevier. 2005;2:96-7.
28. P Sarat Chandra The changing trends in management of spinal tuberculosis: Are we hitting a better road? Indian Journal of Neurosurgery. 2013;2(3):221-5.
29. Myers TH. Pott's Disease and Pregnancy. J Bone Joint Surg Am. 1891;S1-4:124-13.
30. Vaidya MK, Shah GV, Bharucha KE. Pregnancy and its outcome in quadriplegia due to Pott's spine. Int J Gynaecol Obstet. 1995;49(3):319-21.
31. Yusuf N, Ali Ma, Ahmad Q, Rahman L, Nigar T. Pregnancy in Pott 's disease: A Case Report and Review. Bangladesh J Obstet Gynaecol. 2010;25(1):37-40.
32. Vleeming A, Albert HB, Ostgaard HC, Sturesson B, and Stuge B. European guidelines for the diagnosis and treatment of pelvic girdle pain. Eur Spine J. 2008;17(6):794-819.
33. Albert HB, Godskesen M, Westergaard JG. Incidence of four syndromes of pregnancy-related pelvic joint pain. Spine(Phila Pa 1976). 2002;27:2831-4.
34. Albert H, Godskesen M, Westergaard JG, Chard T, Gunn L. Circulating levels of relaxin are normal in pregnant women with pelvic pain. Eur J Obstet Gynecol Reprod Biol. 1997;74:19-22.
35. James DK, Steer PJ, Gonik B, Cowrther C, Tobson S. High risk pregnancy. In: James DK, Weiner CP, Steer PJ, Gonik B, editors. 4th ed. St. Louis: Elsevier. 2010. pp. 917-28.
36. Östgaard HC, Zetherström G, Roos-Hanssoon E. The posterior pelvic pain provocation test in pregnant women. Eur Spine J. 1994;3:258-60.
37. Albert H, Godskesen M, Westergaard J. Evaluation of clinical tests used in classification procedures in pregnancy-related pelvic joint pain. Eur Spine J. 2000;9:161-6.
38. Vleeming A, de Vries HJ, Mens JM, Wingerden JP. Possible role of the long dorsal sacroiliac ligament in women with peripartum pelvic pain. Acta Obstet Gynecol Scand. 2002;81:430-6.
39. Gaenslen FJ. Sacro-iliac arthrodesis. J Am Med Assoc. 1927;89:2031-5.
40. Wurff P, Hagmeijer RHM, Meyne W. Clinical tests of the sacroiliac joint. A systematic methodological review. Part 1: Reliability. Man Ther. 2000;5: 30-36.
41. Wurff P, Hagmeijer RHM, Meyne W. Clinical tests of the sacroiliac joint. A systematic methodological review. Part 2: Validity. Man Ther. 2000;5:89-96.
42. Dumas GA, Reid JG, Wolfe LA, Griffin MP, McGrath MJ. Exercise, posture, and back pain during pregnancy. Part 2. Exercise and back pain. Clin Biomech. 1995.
43. Stuge B, Veierød MB, Laerum E, Vøllestad N. The efficacy of a treatment program focusing on specific stabilizing exercises for pelvic girdle pain

after pregnancy: a two-year follow-up of a randomized clinical trial. Spine (Phila Pa 1976). 2004;29:E197-203.
44. Field T, Hernandez-Reif M, Hart S, Theakston H, Schanberg S, Kuhn C. Pregnant women benefit from massage therapy. J Psychosom Obstet Gynecol. 1999;20:31-8.
45. Wedenberg K, Moen B, Norling A. A prospective randomized study comparing acupuncture with physiotherapy for low-back and pelvic pain in pregnancy. Acta Obstet Gynecol Scand. 2000;79:331-5.
46. Maugars Y, Mathis C, Berthelot JM, Charlier C, Prost A. Assessment of the efficacy of sacroiliac corticosteroid injections in spondylarthropathies: a double-blind study. Br J Rheumatol. 1996;35:767-70.
47. European guidelines for the management of low back pain. Eur Spine J. 2006;Suppl 2.
48. Assouline-Dayan Y, Chang C, Greenspan A, Shoenfeld Y, Gershwin ME. Pathogenesis and natural history of osteonecrosis. Semin Arthritis Rheum. 2002;32(2):94-124.
49. Kay NR, Park WM, Bark M. The relationship between pregnancy and femoral head necrosis. Br J Radiol. 1972;45(539):828-31.
50. McCollum DE, Matthews RS, O'NEIL MT. Aseptic necrosis of the femoral head: associated diseases and evaluation of treatment. South Med J. 1970;63(3):241-53.
51. Guerra JJ, Steinberg ME. Distinguishing transient osteoporosis from avascular necrosis of the hip. J Bone Joint Surg Am. 1995;77(4): 616-24.
52. Aldridge JM 3rd, Urbaniak JR. Avascular necrosis of the femoral head: role of vascularized bone grafts. Orthop Clin North Am. 2007;38:13-22.
53. Cohen L, Melamed E, Lipkin A, Robinson D. Transient osteoporosis of pregnancy complicated by a pathologic subcapital hip fracture. J Trauma. 2007;62(5):1281-3.
54. Gunaratne I, Singh P, Dega R. Transient migratory osteoporosis of the foot. Foot Ankle Surg. 2007;13:51-4.
55. Ma FY, Falkenberg M. Case reports: transient osteoporosis of the hip: an atypical case. Clin Orthop Relat Res. 2006;445:245-9.
56. Chowdhury FU, Robinson P, Grainger AJ, et al. Transient regional osteoporosis: a rare cause of foot and ankle pain. Foot Ankle Surg. 2006;12:79-83.
57. Lloyd JM, Lewis M, Jones A. Transient osteoporosis of the knee in pregnancy. J Knee Surg. 2006;19(2):121-3.
58. Noorda RJ, van der Aa JP, Wuisman PI, David EF, Lips PT, van der Valk P. Transient osteoporosis and osteogenesis imperfect. A case report. Clin Orthop Relat Res. 1997;337:249-55.
59. Karagkevrekis CB, Ainscow DA. Transient osteoporosis of the hip associated with osteogenesis imperfecta. J Bone Joint Surg Br. 1998;80(1):54-5.
60. Axt-Fliedner R, Schneider G, Seil R, Friedrich M, Mink D, Schmidt W. Transient bilateral osteoporosis of the hip in pregnancy. A case report and review of the literature. Gynecol Obstet Invest. 2001;51(2):138-40.
61. Wood ML, Larson CM, Dahners LE. Late presentation of a displaced subcapital fracture of the hip in transient osteoporosis of pregnancy. J Orthop Trauma. 2003;17(8):582-4.
62. Niimi R, Sudo A, Hasegawa M, Fukuda A, Uchida A.. Changes in bone mineral density in transient osteoporosis of the hip. J Bone Joint Surg Br. 2006;88(11):1438-40.
63. Philipp E, Setchell M. The bones, joints and ligaments of the female pelvis. In: Philipp E, Setchell M, (Eds). Scientific Foundations of Obstetrics and Gynaecology. Oxford: Butterworth Heinemann; 1991. pp. 80.
64. Owens K, Pearson A, Mason G. Symphysis pubis dysfunction--a cause of significant obstetric morbidity. Eur J Obstet Gynecol Reprod Biol. 2002;105(2):143-6.
65. MacLennan AH, MacLennan SC. Symptom-giving pelvic girdle relaxation of pregnancy, postnatal pelvic joint syndrome and development dysplasia of the hip. The Norwegian Association for Women with Pelvic Girdle Relaxation (Landforeningen for Kvinner Med Bekkenløsningsplager). Acta Obstet Gynecol Scand. 1997;76(8):760-4.
66. Snow RE, Neubert AG. Peripartum pubic symphysis separation: a case series and review of the literature. Obstet Gynecol Surv. 1997;52(7):438-43.
67. Coldron Y. Margie Poldon Memorial lecture: 'Mind the gap!' Symphysis pubis dysfunction revisited. Journal of the Association of Chartered Physiotherapists in Women's Health. 2005;96:3-15.
68. Rommens PM. Internal fixation in postpartum symphysis pubis rupture: report of three cases. J Orthop Trauma. 1997;11(4):273-6.
69. Culligan P, Hill S, Heit M. Rupture of the symphysis pubis during vaginal delivery followed by two subsequent uneventful pregnancies. Obstet Gynecol. 2002;100:1114-7.
70. Gonik B, Stringer CA. Postpartum osteitis pubis. South Med J. 1985;78(2):213-4.
71. Lovisetti G, Sala F, Battaini A, Lovisetti L, Guicciardi E. Osteomyelitis of the pubic symphysis, abscess and late disjunction after delivery. A case report. Chir Organi Mov. 2000;85(1):85-8.
72. Mikawa Y, Watanabe R, Yamano Y, Miyake S. Stress fracture of the body of pubis in a pregnant woman. Case report. Arch Orthop Trauma Surg. 1988;107(3):193-4.
73. Yosipovitch Z, Goldberg I, Ventura E, Neri A. Open reduction of acetabular fracture in pregnancy. A case report. Clin Orthop Relat Res. 1992;282:229-32.
74. Funk JL, Shoback DM, Genant HK. Transient osteoporosis of the hip pregnancy: natural history of changes in bone mineral density. Clin Endocrinol (Oxf). 1995;43:373-82.
75. Bruinsma BJ, LaBan MM. The ghost joint: transient osteoporosis of the hip. Arch Phys Med Rehabil. 1990;71(5):295-8.
76. Bramlett KW, Killian JT, Nasca Rj, Daniel WW. Transient osteoporosis. Clin Orthop Relat Res. 1987;222:19.

CHAPTER 65

Trauma and Surgical Complications

Bali R Sharma, Keshav Benipal

TRAUMA OR INJURY

INTRODUCTION

Trauma or injury is defined as cellular disruption caused by an exchange with environmental energy that is beyond the body's resistance. As a disease, trauma is a major public health problem and the most common cause of non-obstetric death in pregnancy. Most injuries are caused by motor vehicle crashes, domestic violence, but penetrating trauma and head injuries are also seen. Trauma complicates at least 6–7% of all pregnancies. The emergency physician should be well versed with the standard evaluation of blunt and penetrating trauma and the diagnostic technique employed in evaluating these patients. The immediate deaths represent patients who die of their injuries before reaching the hospital. The early deaths that occur within the first few hours after injury and late deaths occur within days or weeks.[1] The physiological changes in pregnancy can challenge even the most experienced emergency physician.

ANATOMIC AND PHYSIOLOGICAL CHANGES IN PREGNANCY

Understanding the normal anatomic and physiological changes in pregnancy is important for trauma management. The heart rate increases 10–15 beats/min above baseline, and the cardiac output increases by 30–50% before it plateaus at the end of the second trimester. Vena cava compression in the supine position may reduce cardiac output by 30–40% causing supine hypotension. In case of blood loss and hypovolemia, blood flow from the placental circulation is diverted to brain and heart, in supine position may reduce it further. Progesterone-related smooth muscle relaxation leads to a significant decrease in the total peripheral resistance, and thus the central venous pressure slowly drops from 9 mmHg to a third trimester value of about 4 mmHg. Blood pressure gradually decreases in the first trimester, reaching its nadir towards the end of the second trimester, with the systolic and diastolic pressures decreasing by 5–15 mmHg. During the third trimester, the blood pressure gradually climbs, returning to nearly prepregnancy readings at term. During pregnancy, blood volume increases by 50%, while red blood cell volume increases only about 30%, resulting in erythrocyte dilution so-called "physiological anemia" of pregnancy and an average hematocrit of 32–34%. The average estimated blood losses for a vaginal delivery and cesarean section are approximately 500 mL and 1,000 mL, respectively. In term patients, this amount of hemorrhage typically causes no change in hemodynamic parameters. With significant blood loss, the maternal systemic blood pressure is preserved at the expense of the uteroplacental and splanchnic circulation. Thus, the pregnant trauma patient's vital signs may lead to a false sense of security, because changes in pulse and blood pressure may not occur until hemorrhage of 1,500–2,000 mL. Fetal heart rate deceleration may be the first sign of significant hemorrhage.

Oxygen consumption increases by 15–20% during pregnancy, pregnant women tolerate anoxia poorly. It is important that oxygen must be administered to all pregnant women with major injuries. The gradual 4 cm elevation of the diaphragm and increasing thoracic anteroposterior diameter contribute to a 20–25% decrease in functional residual capacity. Placement of thoracotomy tubes must be revised accordingly.

The potential for aspiration is markedly increased because of decreased gastric tone, delayed gastric emptying, cephalad displacement of intra-abdominal organs, and an increase in baseline gastric acid production. The pregnant trauma patient is more susceptible to genitourinary injury. The uterus displaces the bladder anteriorly, superiorly, so that the bladder becomes an intra-abdominal organ and the renal pelvises and ureters become dilated. Abdominal tenderness, rebound, and guarding may be absent in the trauma patient with significant injury. Gradual growth and stretching of the peritoneal cavity seems to desensitize the pregnant patient to peritoneal irritation. Most coagulation factor levels rise throughout pregnancy, although laboratory values remain unchanged, except for fibrinogen levels which nearly double in value.

PREHOSPITAL CARE

The emergency medical service personnel should follow standard guidelines for trauma care. The American College of Surgeon defines four levels of institutional trauma care. Level I trauma center provides 24 hours specialists facilities and research, teaching, community outreach or injury prevention. Level II provides same but no teaching or research. Level III trauma center provides prompt assessment, resuscitation, and stabilization followed by surgical treatment or interhospital transfer as appropriate. Level IV center provides advanced life support prior to transfer in remote areas.[2] Management out of hospital should be performed in normal fashion, like spinal immobilization should be employed in most patients, especially those with blunt trauma. Placing the patient on a board with a 15° angle to the left is a pregnancy-specific intervention that should be employed in all patients beyond 20 weeks' gestation to relieve the compressive effect of the gravid uterus on the vena cava, which can reduce maternal cardiac output up to 30%. The use of towels or blankets placed under the backboard is quick, easy and effective. Two large-bore intravenous catheters should be placed and the patient should be given supplemental oxygen. Gestational age can be estimated by the size of the gravid uterus or by the history obtained from the patient or attendants. Fetal viability is likely, if the uterine fundal height is between the umbilicus and the xiphoid. Pregnancy is an indication for prehospital trauma triage designation.[3-4]

GENERAL MANAGEMENT

The pregnant trauma patient is best managed by a team approach. The emergency physician should involve the trauma surgeon and obstetrician early in the care of these patients. The sequence of evaluation includes the primary survey, resuscitation, secondary survey and definitive treatment. The patient must be handled as if a severe injury has occurred. The perinatologist may also be an integral member of the team. Because the most common cause of fetal death is maternal death, efforts to assess fetal well-being are secondary to resuscitation of the mother. The health of the fetus may be the most accurate indicator of maternal health. Fetal heart tones can be used as part of the vital signs, and fetal assessment should be performed early as a part of the maternal secondary survey. Cardiotocographic monitoring (CTM) be initiated in the emergency department as soon as possible.[5]

The primary survey is rapid assessment to detect life-threatening injuries following ABCD. The "golden hour" concept that timely prioritized interventions is necessary to prevent death. Glasgow coma scale score of eight or less requires placement of definitive airway. When assessing the airway, recall the increased risk of aspiration and consider early endotracheal intubation. This precaution also benefits the fetus because hypoxia is a significant factor in fetal distress. As always, assume that the patient has a full stomach and may have a cervical spine injury.[6-7] Although the pregnant patient may be tachypneic in the first and early second trimester, look for other causes of respiratory compromise in patients closer to term. A chest tube thoracotomy needs to be placed 1 or 2 intercostal spaces higher than usual to avoid diaphragmatic injury. Adequate oxygenation and pulse oximetry monitoring need to be emphasized because oxygen reserve is significantly reduced.[8]

Assessment of circulation and interpretation of vital signs should also be done in the context of pregnancy-related changes. Patients at greater than 20 weeks' gestation should be placed in the left-lateral decubitus position. The evaluation of perfusion includes central and peripheral pulse quality, skin color and temperature, capillary refill, and patient agitation or anxiety. Doppler fetal heart tones should be obtained as an adjunct to the vital signs. Hypovolemic shock may occur with minimal change in pulse or blood pressure, and fetal distress may be the first sign of maternal hemodynamic compromise. Early crystalloid fluid replacement using at least two large-bore peripheral intravenous cannulae. As in the nonpregnant population, head injury is a major cause of maternal morbidity and mortality in trauma. In evaluating the disability of a pregnant trauma patient, seizures should raise the additional concern for eclampsia. Traumatic injuries may mask the expected hypertension and proteinuria, and edema can be overlooked in the face of distracting injuries.

In the stable pregnant patient, a rapid but thorough secondary survey must include a thorough fetal assessment, including a pelvic examination. Estimated gestational age and viability can be ascertained quickly. At 24 weeks' gestation, the fetus is generally considered to be viable, and the height of uterus can be palpated. The fundal height in centimeters measured from the pubic symphysis correlates well with gestational age. The uterus should be palpated carefully, as tenderness and contractions should be observed. CTM monitoring, often requested from labor and delivery, should be readily available to patients in the emergency department. A sterile per speculum examination should be done. The source of vaginal fluid by ferning and blue discoloration of nitrazine paper may help in distinguishing alkaline amniotic fluid from urine.

Vaginal bleeding may herald placental abruption, uterine rupture, pelvic fracture with vaginal injury, or other injuries. The cervix should be visually inspected for evidence of dilation and effacement. A bimanual examination is an integral part of the secondary survey that is sometime overlooked.

The laboratory tests should include hemoglobin, hematocrit, typing and cross matching, and urine for protein, sugar. A serum bicarbonate level, blood gas analysis, or lactate level may be considered because maternal acidosis may be linked to fetal outcome.[9-10]

Placental abruption may be added to the list of possible causes of disseminated intravascular coagulation (DIC) in trauma. A fibrinogen level that is normal in nonpregnant patient may be an early indicator of DIC and placental abruption in a pregnant trauma patient.[11] A Kleihauer-Betke (KB) test may be considered in an Rh-negative patient with significant trauma. Routine use of KB is not indicated in the emergency department and may not be indicated at all for most patients.[12-14] Sher's clinical grading system for placental abruption. Grade I patients have a retroplacental clot of approximately 150 mL, and not more than 500 mL. Fetuses are not at risk and favorable perinatal outcome occurs. Grade II patients have features of abruption placentae and fetus is alive. Retroplacental clot volume is usually 150–500 mL and approximately 27% of them having clot larger than 500 mL. 92% of patients have abnormal fetal heart rate patterns and perinatal mortality high on vaginal delivery. In grade III, fetal demise is confirmed. It is subdivided based on presence (A) or absence (B) coagulopathy.[15]

Evidence of initial maternal acidosis seems to be a useful indicator and the factor most consistently identified, the injury severity score, may be helpful to the trauma surgeon, but unfortunately it is not available to the emergency physician.

DIAGNOSTIC AND RADIOGRAPHIC STUDIES

The evaluation of the pregnant trauma patient should focus on the identification of maternal injuries and the evaluation of fetal well-being. In general, diagnostic studies should be obtained in the pregnant trauma patient for the same indications as in nonpregnant patients. Some special management options; however, should be considered in pregnant patients to assure good outcomes. Initial plain radiographs of the cervical spine, chest, and pelvis should be obtained in traumatized pregnant patients as usual.[16-17]

Radiographic studies should not be withheld because of concerns about radiation exposure. The risk of radiation to the fetus depends on multiple variables, including gestational age, shielding of the uterus, techniques used. As a general rule, it is assumed that the earlier in gestation and the higher the dose, the greater is the risk from radiation. The most sensitive time for the fetus to be exposed to significant radiation is from 2 to 7 weeks, during organogenesis.[18,19] Unfortunately, at this period of highest risk, the pregnancy may be unsuspected by the patient. A radiation dose of less than 1 cGy (rad) is believed to carry very little risk. Exposures of 15 cGy, however, carry a15% chance of microcephaly, 6% chance of mental retardation, and 3% chance of childhood cancer. After 20 weeks' gestation, radiation is unlikely to cause any fetal anomalies, particularly, if cumulative exposure is less than 10 cGy. Computed tomography (CT) is widely used in the evaluation of traumatic injuries, particularly in head, chest, and abdominal or pelvic trauma. A typical abdominal CT will expose fetus to 5–10 cGy. As a general rule, abdominal CT should be avoided in early pregnancy.[20] Diagnostic peritoneal lavage (DPL) is still commonly used in trauma canters to identify intra-abdominal injury. DPL has proven to be a safe and accurate alternative to diagnostic imaging for identification of peritoneal injury using the usual criteria.[21] Supraumbilical approach is indicated when the gravid uterus is palpable above the pubis. The open-technique or the minilaparotomy should be employed. DPL emphasizes the increased sensitivity for identifying hollow-viscous injuries and early identification for immediate laparotomy in the case of massive hemoperitoneum.

The focused abdominal sonogram of trauma (FAST) has been shown to be sensitive in identifying peritoneal fluid. The first trimester pregnant patient with an equivocal FAST examination may be a candidate for DPL, avoiding exposure to large amounts of radiation. Later in pregnancy, DPL may help differentiate between massive peritoneal bleeding from an uteroplacental source. A fetal assessment can be obtained quickly, using some or all of the components of the biophysical profile. Amniotic fluid volume can be assessed, if there is concern for rupture of membranes. The remaining three components are gross fetal movement, tone and respiratory activity. Although abruption cannot be ruled out with ultrasonography alone, visualization of subchorionic hemorrhage or a retroplacental clot may allow early diagnosis.[17-19]

BLUNT TRAUMA

Most cases of blunt trauma are related to motor vehicle accidents, followed by falls and direct assaults. Motor vehicle accidents account for nearly 60% of blunt traumas[6,7,9,10] (Table 1). Maternal mortality is uncommon and often, as in nonpregnant patients, is a result of significant head trauma. Pregnant women are less than other motorists likely to wear seat-belts, usually because of concerns for fetal injury. The American College of Obstetricians and Gynecologists fully

TABLE 1: Incidence of various types of blunt trauma in pregnancy

Type of blunt trauma	Total number (%)
Motor vehicle accidents/pedestrians	1,098 (59.6)
Falls	411 (22.3)
Direct assaults	308 (16.7)
Other	24 (0.1)

endorses the use of a three-point safety, with the lap belt over the hips, not the uterine dome. If the mother survives, placental abruption is the most common cause of fetal mortality. Shearing forces lead to a separation of the rigid placenta from the elastic uterus. Relatively, minor trauma may result in placental separation and fetal demise.[6,7,11]

The incidence of placental abruptions may be as high as 2–4% of patients with minor trauma and 30% or higher in mothers who survive major trauma.[6,7] Clinical signs and symptoms of abruption, such as vaginal bleeding, abdominal pain and tenderness, and uterine tenderness may present, but they are often absent and cannot be relied upon.[13,14] Only 6 of 16 trauma patients with placental abruptions had vaginal bleeding. Back pain may be the only sign of a posterior placental abruption. The uterine rupture is one of the most serious complications of blunt trauma in pregnancy. It occurs most frequently in patients who have had a previous cesarean section or myomectomy. On physical examination may include uterine tenderness with irregular contours and palpable fetal parts. Rupture of the unscarred uterus tends to occur posteriorly and is commonly associated with bladder injury, occasionally presenting with blood or meconium inurine.[22] Uterine rupture is devastating to the fetus, with fetal mortality approaching 100% and maternal mortality of 10%. CTM has shown excellent sensitivity in detecting placental abruption with negative predictive value of 100% for adverse outcomes when a lack of clinical early warning symptoms was combined with reassuring monitoring. Many sources recommend CTM beyond 20 weeks' gestation. Patients at less than 24 weeks' gestation need not be monitored by obstetricians; however, because delivery by cesarean section for fetal distress is not an option. Emergency physicians should be able to recognize obvious signs of fetal distress.

PENETRATING TRAUMA

Penetrating trauma in pregnancy is usually the result of gunshot or knife wounds. Gunshot wounds, which are more common than knife wounds, have a higher mortality for both mother and fetus. As pregnancy advances into the second trimester, the gravid uterus moves out of the relatively protected position in the bony pelvis into the abdominal cavity, and a pregnancy-specific pattern of injury develops. Superiorly displaced visceral organs are less likely to be injured but they are at greater risk when penetrating trauma involves the upper abdomen. Maternal visceral injuries are less common during pregnancy, complicating only 19% of cases and carrying a maternal mortality of 3.9%.[21] The disparity probably results from the protective effect of the large, muscular uterus on visceral organs. Gunshot wounds cause transient shock waves and cavitations as they impart their kinetic energy to the high-density tissues of the body, thus causing more severe injury patterns than low-velocity knife wounds. Fetal mortality ranges from 40 to 70% in cases of penetrating trauma and generally results from either premature delivery or direct fetal injury by the missile.[23] Stab wounds have a lower mortality for both mother and fetus. The management options include immediate surgical exploration, laparoscopy, DPL, contrast-enhanced CT scanning, local wound exploration, and observation. If the entrance wound of the bullet is below the uterine fundus and the bullet remains in the body of the uterus, the incidence of visceral injury is less than 20%.[24] The evaluation of penetrating trauma in the pregnant patient needs to be a coordinated, multidisciplinary effort. As in blunt trauma, the biophysical status of the fetus should be ultrasonographically evaluated early in the resuscitation once maternal injuries have been stabilized. Amniocentesis may provide additional information on the viability and possible injury of the fetus; however, carry a significant risk to foetal.[25]

DOMESTIC VIOLENCE

The pregnant women are at increased risk (0.9–20.1%) for domestic violence. This may be a result of increased incidence, or greater health care use and better detection. Common sites of physical abuse in pregnancy include the face, head, breasts, and abdomen. Domestic abuse may be a risk factor for low birth weight and delay in prenatal care.[4,26] There were 17% prevalence of physical or sexual abuse during pregnancy. A high suspicion and a concise screening tool may afford the emergency physician the unique opportunity to identify, intervene, and prevent reoccurrence of domestic violence. If domestic violence is suspected, consultation with social services should not be delayed.

BURNS

Maternal outcome in cases of significant burns is determined by burn severity and complications, independent of the gravid state.[27] Fetal outcomes are directly related to maternal burn severity and the development of maternal complications. Burn severity depends on both the depth and the size of the burn. Burns are classified as partial thickness (both superficial and deep) and full thickness. Total body surface area (TBSA) can be quickly estimated with the rule of nines and the TBSA of the maternal burn is directly correlated with fetal outcome. Intravascular depletion and third-spacing of fluids may result in uteroplacental hypoperfusion, fetal hypoxia, and distress. Premature labor and death may be the final outcome. The Parkland formula, 4 mL/kg/% TBSA burned, estimates additional fluid requirements for the first 24 hours, with half of the fluid infused over the first 8 hours. A urinary catheter should be placed to ensure urine output of at least 0.5 mL/kg/hour early in the course of therapy. Carbon monoxide crosses the placenta freely, fetal hemoglobin has a higher affinity for carbon monoxide than maternal hemoglobin, and the clinical condition of the fetus can be difficult to assess.[28] The hyperbaric oxygen therapy should be considered early in pregnant patients despite the carboxyhemoglobin level.

When fetal death occurs, it is usually within a week of the initial injury. If premature labor is present, tocolytic therapy should be considered judiciously because tocolytics can effect the fluid distribution.[25] Initial wound care should be undertaken as in nonpregnant patients, with the application of sterile dressings and topical antibiotics. Early debridement of burn tissue should be undertaken. All patients with significant burn should receive broad-spectrum antibiotic therapy to prevent sepsis, although this issue is still controversial.[26] Tetanus toxoid and immunoglobulin can be administered safely in pregnancy when indicated.

Electrical Burns

Electrical burns have the potential for cardiac arrhythmias and compartment syndromes with concurrent rhabdomyolysis. A baseline ECG is recommended in all cases of electrical injuries. Long-term neurological or visual symptoms are not uncommon with high voltage electrical injuries.

Blast Injuries

Blast injuries in civilian populations occur as a result of fireworks, household explosions or industrial accident. Terrorist activities may take the form of letter bombs, suitcase bombs, vehicle bombs and suicide bombers. Military blast injuries may involve the personnel submerged in water. Water increases energy transmission and possibility of injury to the viscera of thorax and abdomen.

PERIMORTEM CESAREAN SECTION

The perimortem caesarean section should be performed, if resuscitation was unsuccessful over a period of 4 minutes and baby delivered in 5 minutes for maximum chances of fetal survival. The time for the onset of neurological injury in mother after cessation of cerebral flow has been estimated to be 6 minutes. A return of maternal pulse and blood pressure is noted in several cases after emptying the uterus, thus benefit maternal and resuscitation.[29]

SURGICAL PROBLEMS IN OBSTETRICS

INTRODUCTION

Pregnant women will present with processes that require surgical treatment. Correct identification of surgical emergencies, i.e. acute abdomen can be more difficult in pregnancy. Coordination of all the members of the surgical team including surgery, obstetrics and anesthesia is imperative to correctly diagnose and treat surgical events while minimizing maternal and fetal morbidity.

Surgery will be required in 0.1–2.2% of pregnant woman[30] or a total of 75,000 pregnant woman each year.[31] Pregnancy poses several challenges to surgeon. Physiologic changes in pregnancy may require modifications of standard surgical and diagnostic procedures. Diagnosis can be more difficult as pregnancy may disguise or obscure some conditions. Unique ethical issues may be encountered as treatment decisions must balance the well being of both the mother and the fetus.

PATHOPHYSIOLOGY

Pregnancy cause changes in maternal physiology that may hinder appropriate and timely diagnosis of surgical situations. Pregnancy associated symptoms can also imply other disease processes, i.e., headache, syncope, nausea, vomiting, abdominal discomfort and pain. Normal hemodynamic parameters are altered in pregnancy. The appendix moves progressively cephalic as pregnancy progresses and will at the level of iliac crest by 6 months gestation.

ETIOLOGY OF ACUTE ABDOMEN

Surgical exploration is usually required to rule out major causes of maternal and fetal morbidity, establish the diagnosis and proceed with treatment. The most common entities diagnosed in pregnancy:[32]

- Appendicitis (1 in 1,500 pregnancy)
- Ectopic pregnancy (1 in 100)
- Cholecystitis (1 in 1,600 pregnancy)
- Bowel obstruction (1 in 2,500 pregnancy)
- Most commonly secondary to adhesions (60–70%)
- Volvulus is less likely cause
- Inflammatory bowel disease (1 in 1,000 pregnancy)
- Ovarian torsion (rare)
- Spontaneous hepatic rupture (rare).

There are other processes in the differential for acute abdomen that may only require medical management, gastroenteritis, kidney stones, pylonephritis, pancreatitis, peptic ulcer disease, pneumonia.

Other diseases that potentially require surgery during pregnancy, i.e., solid complex adnexal masses, cervical intraepithelial neoplasia, malignant diseases of breast, ovary, cervix, melanoma and bone cancer. Cardiac disease that is surgically correctable and has failed medical management during pregnancy.

EVALUATION

The history should focus on thorough evaluation of the present and past medical illness and current obstetric history. The physical examination includes all maternal systems as well as evaluation of fetal well being. Pregnant woman should receive the same laboratory tests that would normally be used to evaluate a nonpregnant woman with an acute abdomen. Radiographic tests appropriate for the nonpregnant women should be used in pregnancy, if their omission would delay or adversely affect diagnosis. Ultrasound is usually the first imaging study and magnetic resonance imaging (MRI) may be the back-up imaging study of choice as it affords excellent anatomic details, no radiation exposure and diagnostic accuracy in pregnant women with abdominal pain. CT scan is the third choice, due to fetal radiation exposure, if necessary for assessment, then it should be performed. Use of minimum X-ray exposure, avoidance of redundant studies and shielding of fetus is advisable.

DIAGNOSIS

Acute abdomen differential diagnoses that require surgery:
- Acute appendicitis
- Cholecystitis
- Ovarian torsion
- Bowel obstruction.

Clinical Manifestation

Most common symptoms of acute abdomen in pregnancy are abdominal pain (82%), tachycardia (82%), fever (75%), nausea or vomiting (63%).

Acute Appendicitis[33]

Majority (80%) will still present with right lower quadrant colicky pain although it can be epigastric or periumbilical region, nausea or vomiting, fever, rebound tenderness or guarding, leukocytosis. In acute cholecystitis murphy sign may be present. Ultrasound is 95% sensitive for gallstones even in pregnancy.

Acute Cholecystitis

- Nausea and vomiting
- Acute abdominal pain, usually colicky
- Pain is located in the mid-epigastrium and right upper quadrant and may radiate to the back.
- Murphy sign may be present.
- Fever
- Tachycardia
- Tachypnea
- May have increased bilirubin, liver function tests, and serum alkaline phosphatase. But these can also be falsely elevated in pregnancy.
- Ultrasound is 95% sensitive for gallstones even in pregnancy.

Ovarian Tube Torsion

Acute onsets of pain usually lower abdominal, may have fever or leukocytosis, may have mass or enlarged ovary and may have loss of ovarian blood flow on Doppler ultra sound.

Bowel Obstruction[34]

Abdomen is usually distended with potentially high pitched bowel sounds. Symptoms include nausea, vomiting, and crampy abdominal pain that are poorly localized. Fever and leukocytosis are usually present. Do not confuse this with hyperemesis, especially in the second and third trimester.

DECISION FOR SURGERY

Once a surgical acute abdomen has been diagnosed, surgery is necessary to reduce maternal and fetal complications. In these situations, the patients and family should receive as much counseling as possible about the surgery, the potential course of action and the risk and benefits. Delay of an indicated surgical procedure to allow for fetal maturity or delivery should not occur, if the delay is likely to have an adverse maternal impact. Elective surgery should be postponed until after delivery.

Some procedures, due to complexity or the need for patient directions may require more extensive counseling among the patient, her family, the obstetrician, the anesthesiologist, and the surgeon to discuss risks and benefits of surgery during pregnancy.

For nonemergent problems, a thorough discussion with the patient must be undertaken to discuss the risks and benefits of immediate surgery compared to waiting for either fetal viability or delivery.

PREOPERATIVE MANAGEMENT

- Timing of surgery
- Determined more by the severity and acuity of the surgical illness than by gestational age
- Delay of an indicated surgical procedure to allow for fetal maturity or delivery should not occur, if the delay is likely to have an adverse maternal impact
- Elective surgery should be postponed until after delivery

- Surgery that is not emergent, but that should not be delayed until the postpartum period, is best performed in the second trimester when the risk of spontaneous abortion is the least
- The highest risk of pregnancy loss and/or premature delivery is in the third trimester.

DEEP VENOUS THROMBOEMBOLISM RISKS[35-37]

Pregnancy is considered to be a hypercoagulable state. Surgical procedure during pregnancy further increases the risks for thromboembolism, other risk factor includes age over 40, surgical procedure lasting longer than 30 min, major orthopedic or pelvic surgery, previous myocardial infarction or thromboembolic event, malignant disease. Prophylaxis with pneumatic compression stockings or heparin should be strongly considered. Low molecular weight heparin is the prophylactic agent of choice because of once daily dosing and lower risk of bleeding complications.

Informed consent about the risks of spontaneous abortion or premature labor should be obtained. Fetal heart rate monitoring is appropriate for viable pregnancy before, during, and after surgery. If the risk of premature delivery is significant, arrangement for neonatal intensive care services should be made.

ANESTHETIC CONSIDERATIONS

Prevention of aspiration: pregnancy causes a delay in gastric emptying as well as an increase in influx so the following steps should be implanted to prevent it:

- Preoperative administration of antacids
- Use of cricothyroid pressure during induction
- Rapid sequence induction
- Intraoperative nasogastric suction
- Intraoperative monitoring issue in pregnancy

Must maintain the best physiological condition for mother to ensure adequate perfusion to the fetus.

COMPLICATIONS

Preterm delivery is increased with intraperitoneal surgeries and disease processes. Delay in surgical intervention with appendicitis and bowel movements may increase the risk of preterm delivery, however, risk does not appear to differ between laparoscopic and open abdominal procedures. Appendicitis was also associated with decreased birth weight and increased risk of neonatal death. Prophylactic tocolysis immediately following completion of surgery.[32,38]

Neonatal death: a large registry linked surgery during pregnancy with increased neonatal deaths (within the first 7 days of life), but the causality is unclear.[39] Other studies with appendicitis and acute abdomen also demonstrate an increased rate of neonatal death.[38] While an association exists, it is unclear whether the increased rate of neonatal death is secondary to the surgery itself or the underlying condition that necessitated surgery.

Maternal mortality or morbidity: this usually results from sepsis related to delay in diagnosis. In appendicitis, maternal mortality is now rare and appendiceal perforation usually occurs secondary to marked delay in time to surgical intervention.[32] Delay in surgical intervention in women with acute abdomen results in increased admissions and lengths of hospital stay.[38] Bowel obstruction is marked by higher maternal mortality rate (6% in 66 cases) and 26% fetal mortality.[34]

Pregnant women should be encouraged to not delay seeking evaluation for potential surgical symptoms or problems just because they are pregnant. Surgical consent during pregnancy requires a definitive explanation and discussion of the risks to the pregnancy and fetus from both surgery and delay of surgery. When fetal viability is present, the patient and family should meet with neonatal intensive care unit personnel to discuss the implications of postpartum thyroid dysfunction at that gestational age.

CONCLUSION

Any female patient brought to trauma ward in reproductive age group pregnancy should be ruled out. Management of trauma is like in nonpregnant state, evaluation and stabilization of maternal injuries is the main goal. Extra care for fetus and judicious use of radiological investigations is required. Anti-D should be given to Rh-negative mother. Intravenous line, maintenance of airways, oxygen therapy and shifting to a proper hospital is done.

REFERENCES

1. Brunicardi F, Andersen D, Billiar T, Dunn D, Hunter J, Matthews J, et al. Schwartz's Principles of Surgery, 9th edition. USA: The McGraw-Hill Education Companies, Inc; 2009. p. 136.
2. Hemmila MR, Wahl WL. Management of the Injured Patient: Current Diagnosis and Treatment, 13th edition. Tata McGraw-Hill Education Pvt. Ltd; 2010. pp. 176-209.
3. Fort A, Harlin R. Pregnancy outcome after noncatastrophic maternal trauma during pregnancy. Obstet Gynecol. 1970;35(6):912-5.
4. Parker B, McFarlane J, Soeken K. Abuse during pregnancy: effects on maternal complications and birth weight in adults and teenage women. Obstet Gynecol. 1994;84(3):323-8.
5. Peckham CH, King RW. A study of intercurrent conditions observed during pregnancy. Am J Obstet Gynecol. 1963;87(5):609-24.
6. Rothenberger D, Quattlebaum FW, Perry JF Jr, Zabel J, Fischer RP. Blunt maternal trauma: a review of 103 cases. J Trauma. 1978;18(3):173-9.
7. Goodwin T, Breen M. Pregnancy outcome and fetomaternal hemorrhage after noncatastrophic trauma. Am J Obstet Gynecol. 1990;162(3):665-71.
8. Schneider R. Muscle relaxants. In: Walls R (Ed). Emergency Airway Management. Philadelphia: Lippincott Williams & Wilkins; 2000. pp. 121-8.

9. Hoff W, D'Amelio L, Tinkoff G, Lucke JF, Rhodes M, Diamond DL, et al. Maternal predictors of foetal demise in trauma during pregnancy. Surg Gynecol Obstet. 1991;172(3):175-80.
10. Scorpio R, Esposito T, Smith G, Gens DR. Blunt trauma during pregnancy: factors affecting foetal outcome. J Trauma. 1992;32(2):213-6.
11. Shah K, Simons R, Holbrook T, Fortlage D, Winchell RJ, Hoyt DB, et al. Trauma in pregnancy: maternal and foetal outcomes. J Trauma ICC. 1998;45(1):83-6.
12. Connolly A, Katz V, Bash K, McMahon MJ, Hansen WF. Trauma and pregnancy. Am J Perinatol. 1997;14(6):331-6.
13. Dahmus M, Sibai B. Blunt abdominal trauma: are there any predictive factors for abruption placentae or maternal-fetal distress? Am J Obstet Gynecol. 1993;169(4):1054-9.
14. Towery R, English P, Wisner D. Evaluation of pregnant women after blunt injury. J Trauma. 1993;35(5):731-5.
15. Bleeding during pregnancy. In: Arias F, Daftary SN, Bhide AG (Eds). Practical Guide to High Risk Pregnancy and Delivery, 3rd edition. Reed Elsevier India Pvt. Ltd; 2008. pp. 343-4.
16. Ali J, Yeo A, Gana T, McLellan BA. Predictors of fetal mortality in pregnant trauma patients. J Trauma. 1997;42(5):782-5.
17. Baerga-Varela Y, Zietlow S, Bannon M, Harmsen WS, Ilstrup DM. Trauma in pregnancy. Mayo Clin Proc. 2000;75:1243-8.
18. Kissinger D, Rozycki G, Morris J, Knudson MM, Copes WS, Bass SM, et al. Trauma in pregnancy. Predicting pregnancy outcome. Arch Surg. 1991;126:1079-86.
19. Morris J, Rosenbower T, Jurkovich G, Hoyt DB, Harviel JD, Knudson MM, et al. Infant survival after cesarean section for trauma. Ann Surg. 1996;223(5):481-91.
20. American College of Obstetricians and Gynecologists. Automobile passenger restraints for children and pregnant women. Washington (DC): ACOG Technical Bulletin 151; 1991.
21. `Neufeld J, Moore E, Mars J, Rosen P. Trauma in pregnancy. Emerg Med Clin North Am. 1987;5(3):623-40.
22. Lavery J, Staten-McCormick M. Management of moderate to severe trauma in pregnancy. Obstet Gynecol Clin North Am. 1995;22(1):69-90.
23. Buchsbaum H. Penetrating injury of the abdomen. In: Buchsbaum H (Ed). Trauma in Pregnancy. Philadelphia: WB Saunders; 1979. pp. 82-100.

24 Vaizey C, Jacobson M, Cross F. Trauma in pregnancy. Br J Surg. 1994;81: 1406-15.

25. Kuhlmann R, Cruikshank D. Maternal trauma during pregnancy. Clin Obstet Gynecol. 1994;37(2):274-93.
26. McFarlane J, Parker B, Soeken K, Bullock L. Assessing for abuse during pregnancy. Severity and frequency of injuries and associated entry into prenatal care. JAMA. 1992;267(23):3176-8.
27. Amy BW, McManus WF, Goodwin CW, Mason A, Pruitt BA. Thermal injury in the pregnant patient. Surg Gynecol Obstet. 1985;161:209-12.
28. Tibbles P, Edelsberg J. Hyperbaric-oxygen therapy. N Engl J Med. 1996;334(25):1642-8.
29. Katz VL, Dotters DJ, Droegemueller W. Perimortem caesarean delivery. Obstet Gynecol. 1986;68:571-6.
30. Beery PR, Ellision EC. Surgery in pregnant patient. In: Townsend C, Beauchamp RD, Evers BM, Mattox KL (Eds). Sabiston Textbook of Surgery. 17th edition. Philadelphia: Elsevier Saunders; 2004. pp. 2269-82.

31 Kuczkowski KM. Nonobstetric surgery during pregnancy: what are the risks of anaesthesia? Obstet Gynaecol Surv. 2003;59:52-6.

32. Sharp HT. The acute abdomen during pregnancy. Clinical Obstet Gynaecol. 2002;45:405-13.
33. Horowitz MD, Gomez GA, Santiesteban R, Burkett G. Acute appendicitis during pregnancy. Arch Surg. 1985;120:1362-7.
34. Perdue PW, Johanson HW, Stafford PW. Intestinal obstruction complicating pregnancy. Am J Surg. 1992;164:384-8.
35. Daskalakis G, Antsaklis A, Papageorgiou I, Michalas S. Thrombosis prophylaxis after treatment during pregnancy. Eur J Obstet Gynecol Reprod Biol. 1997;74:165-7.
36. Greer IA, Nelson-Piercy C. Low molecular heparins for thromboprophylaxis and treatment of venous thromboembolism in pregnancy: a systematic review of safety and efficacy. Blood. 2005;106:401-7.
37. Robertson L, Geer I. Thromboembolism in pregnancy. Curr Opin Obstet Gynaecol. 2005;17:113-6.
38. El-Amin AM, Yahia Al-Shehri M, Zaki ZM, Abu-Eshy S, Albar H, Sadik A. Acute abdomen in pregnancy. Int J Gynaecol Obstet. 1998;62:31-6.
39. Mazze RI, Kallen B. Reproductive outcome after anesthesia and operation during pregnancy: a registry study of 5405 cases. Am J Obstet Gynecol. 1989;161:1178-85.

CHAPTER 66

Gynecological Complications

Anita Pal

INTRODUCTION

One cannot easily separate gynecologic and the obstetric patient when she is one and the same. Pregnancy does not prevent or protect a woman from developing common gynecologic problems and complications. One has to be vigilant to these gynecological problems because untreated gynecologic problems can adversely affect obstetric care and exacerbate obstetric complications. Treatment of these problems is usually the same for the pregnant and the nonpregnant patient.

VULVAR ABNORMALITIES

A number of acute and chronic vulvar conditions are present during pregnancy.

Edema

Vulvar edema to some degree is present in pregnant women. Other causes are nephrotic syndrome and hypoproteinemia. During labor the vulva may become edematous in women with severe pre-eclampsia. Venous thrombosis and hematomas cause edema and pain. In postpartum women edema associated with a paravaginal, vulvar or perineal hematoma arising from lacerations or an episiotomy.

Inflammatory Lesions

Extensive perineal inflammation and scaring from hidradenitis suppurativa, lymph granuloma venereum or Crohn's disease may create difficulty with vaginal delivery, episiotomy and repair.

Careful inspection of the external genitalia before pregnancy, as well as at the initial prenatal visit, is crucial to the patient's health. Counseling about the signs and symptoms of external genital infections, as well as the risks of transmission with exposure of infectious organisms, should also be discussed.

Bartholin Abscess

Bartholin cysts are a common occurrence in the productive age female, and pregnancy can exacerbate their symptoms. Although asymptomatic cysts need not necessarily be treated, and abscess of the Bartholin gland usually requires immediate treatment.

A Bartholin gland abscess typically causes significant pain and inflammation. The diagnosis can often be made based solely on the patient's complaints. Patients will complain that they feel a large tender "bump" on their labia and have severe pain with standing, walking, or sitting. Although the symptoms are fairly classic, a thorough examination and evaluation must be performed.

Drainage via an incision on the mucosal side of the gland is appropriate when the area is fluctuant. Otherwise, sitz baths are recommended until the abscess is ready for drainage. Cultures obtained at the time of initial drainage are useful, as gonococcus is often the etiologic agent, and when suspected, antibiotics are appropriate. Once the abscess is incised, a Word catheter is placed for 4–6 weeks to allow adequate epithelialization of a drainage tract. Recurrent infection or development of recurrent symptomatic cysts warrants subsequent marsupialization (surgical exteriorization of the cyst for drainage).

Condyloma Accuminata

Condyloma acuminate has a classic "cauliflower-like" appearance and can protrude from the skin on stalks. The lesions appear fleshy and may cause some minor itching but are not painful. The clinician must clinically distinguish the very common condylomata acuminate (genital warts from the rare, wart-like growths of condyloma latum, which is caused by *Treponema pallidum)*. During pregnancy, genital warts may rapidly enlarge, and can obstruct the vaginal canal. *Human papillomavirus*, in rare cases, may be transmitted to the newborn, resulting in laryngeal papillomas. However, delivery by cesarean section is not indicated to prevent fetal intrapartum exposure.

Outpatient treatment of genital warts during pregnancy can be achieved by:

- Cryotherapy (liquid nitrogen application nitrous oxide cryoprobe)
- Carbon dioxide laser therapy
- Application of 50–80% trichloroacetic acid solution
- Imiquimod cream (Aldara R, which has been used with some success but should be used only when benefits outweigh risks, as it is a category C drug in pregnancy)
- Podophyllin is currently not advised for use in pregnancy because of anecdotal reports of birth defects, fetal death, stillbirth and maternal toxicity
- Removal of condyloma via electrocautery is an alternative that may require general anesthesia
- Both cryotherapy and carbon dioxide laser therapy appear to be highly effective in pregnancy, with no significant fetal, neonatal or maternal morbidity
- The recurrence rate of genital warts appears to be the lowest when treated in the third trimester
- Genital warts are not considered an indication for cesarean delivery unless they are so large as to constitute physical obstruction or significant risk for vagina or cervical lacerations.

VAGINAL ABNORMALITIES

Acquired vaginal abnormalities are uncommon. Even after major trauma, long-term sexual and reproductive function is usually normal.

Partial Atresia

"Incomplete atresia" may result from infection or trauma that leads to extensive scarring. During labor, this is overcome by pressure from the presenting part, occasionally incisions or even cesarean delivery is necessary.

Vaginal Plastic Operation

Patients with previous vaginal plastic operations should be delivered in hospital. Patients with repair of stress incontinence, vesicovaginal and rectovaginal fistula should have elective cesarean section.

ABNORMAL VAGINAL DISCHARGE

There is an increased vaginal transudate during pregnancy due to increased vascularity and hyperestrogenic state. Discharge is mucoid and nonirritating. Except for personal hygiene, no treatment is required.

TRICHOMONAS VAGINALIS

Infection is not increased in pregnancy. C/F are foul smelling frothy discharge with vaginal irritation. Diagnosis is by per speculum examination and wet smear for motile trichomonads. Culture can be performed. Metronidazole single dose 2 g is recommended by Centers for Disease Control and Prevention (CDC).[1]

Vulvovaginal Candidiasis

It is due to *Candida albicans* and is more common during pregnancy due to acid state of vagina during pregnancy. The patient complains of thick curdy white vaginal discharge with/without dysuria. The vulva may become extensively swollen and excoriated. Local antifungal vaginal tablets or pessaries containing imidazole antifungal (clotrimazole, miconazole, econazole or terconazole) are more effective than polyene (Nystatin)[2] Table 1. Same antifungal preparations can be used for local application as cream twice a day for 7–14 days.

Oral fluconazole is a class C drug and is not routinely recommended in pregnancy.

Bacterial Vaginosis

It is a condition in which the normal vaginal flora (lactobacilli) is replaced by anaerobes like *Gardnerella varginalis*, *Mycoplasma hominis*, and anaerobes including *Mobiluncus*, *Bacteroides* and *Peptostreptococcus* species. Woman may complain of whitish or greyish discharge with fishy odor. The Amsel criteria are the standard criteria used for clinical diagnosis which include a milky homogeneous discharge;

TABLE 1: Antifungal preparations and dosage for vaginal conditions

Antifungal preparations	Dosage
Clotrimazole vaginal cream	5 g intravaginally/per day for 7 days
Clotrimazole 100 mg vaginal tablet	One tablet per vaginum per day for 7 days
Miconazole 2% vaginal cream	5 g intravaginally/day for 7 days

Miconazole 100 mg vagina suppository One suppository intravaginal/day for 7 days

Nystatin 100,000 units' vaginal tablet One tablet intravaginally/day for 14 days.

vaginal pH is more than 4.5, release of a fishy odor on adding 10% KOH or the positive whiff test, and the presence of clue cells.[3] Three out of four criteria should be met to make a diagnosis that these women are associated with increased risk of preterm labor. Routine screening and treatment is not recommended in low risk women.[4] Symptomatic women should be treated by metronidazole tablets 250 mg 3 times a day for 7 days or clindamycin tablets 300 mg twice daily for 7 days.

CERVICAL ABNORMALITIES

Cicatricial cervical stenosis is uncommon. But it is rarely produced by cryotherapy, loop electrosurgical excision procedure (LEEP) and laser surgery.[5,6] Cervical stenosis undergoes complete effacement and no dilatation during labor. Pressure with fingertip, manual dilatation or cruciate incision, or cesarean section is required.

CERVICAL ECTOPY

Hormonal ectopy*:* during pregnancy as a result of hyper-estrogenism, there is marked hyperplasia of the endocervical mucosa. There is down growth of the columnar epithelium replacing the squamous epithelium producing pregnancy ectopy. It is circumoral in position and does not bleed on touch. It may cause copious non irritating mucoid discharge and regress in 6–8 weeks postpartum.

Cervical polyp: due to increased vascularity and pre-existent polyp, it constitutes extraplacental cause of antepartum hemorrhage (APH) in later months of pregnancy. Diagnosis is by per speculum examination and removed as in nonpregnant state and sent for histopathological examination.

CONGENITAL MALFORMATIONS OF THE UTERUS AND VAGINA

Severe degrees of congenital malformations of the uterus usually lead to infertility. It is the moderate degree of malformations which has got an adverse effect on pregnancy and labor. The diagnosis is made during (i) abdominal inspection—fundal notching, (ii) cesarean section, (iii) manual removal of placenta or evacuation operation, (iv) hysterosalpingography, (v) laparoscopy for infertility investigation. The adverse effects are: (i) malpresentations as breech, transverse lie, (ii) abnormal uterine action as uterine inertia or asymmetrical uterine contractions, (iii) prematurity, (iv) dysmaturity, (v) postpartum hemorrhage (PPH), (vi) retained placenta, (vii) increased incidence of operative interference, (viii) obstructed labor by the nonpregnant horn of a bicornuate uterus.

The common type of malformations are: (i) arcuate uterus, (ii) subseptate uterus, (iii) bicornuate uterus with equal or rudimentary horn.

Septate vagina hardly produces any difficulty during delivery but a transverse septum or partial atresia may be the cause of cesarean delivery.

ACQUIRED UTERINE ABNORMALITIES

A number of acquired uterine abnormalities may adversely affect pregnancy as well as fertility.

Anterior Sacculation of the Uterus

Severe anteflexion of the uterus caused by poor abdominal muscle tone or diastasis recti in the late third trimester may result in abnormal presentation and lack of engagement of the presenting part. This abnormality is seen almost exclusively in the grand multiparous but is also common in African-American females. Correction of the abnormal orientation of the fetus with abdominal pressure provided by a well-fitting girdle or other binding support may allow pushing in the second stage.

Antiflexion

In later months when the abdominal wall is lax, the uterus may fall forward. This may be so exaggerated that the fundus lies below the lower margin of the symphysis. Marked anti-flexion is usually associated with diastasis of recti and a pendulous abdomen. Abnormal uterine position prevents proper transmission of contractions which is prevented by repositioning and abdominal binder. The condition has nuisance value. The patient becomes uncomfortable due to extrastress on back and sacroiliac joints.

Retroflexion

Retrodisplacement of the uterus is common in early pregnancy, but the enlarging uterus nearly always assumes a more anteverted position by 12 weeks of pregnancy. Rarely, the retroflexed enlarging uterus may become incarcerated in the hollow of the sacrum, with resulting edema from venous obstruction, marked pain and notably, an inability to void because of urethral obstruction. The normally growing retroflexed uterus will occasionally remain incarcerated in the hollow of sacrum. It may cause anterior uterine sacculation due to dilatation of lower uterine segment to accommodate the growing fetus. Sonography and magnetic resonance imaging (MRI) are required to define anatomy.[7,8] Elongated vagina is palpated passing above the fetal head and balloon of the Foleys catheter is palpated above the umbilicus. The soft boggy pulsatile uterus is felt through the posterior fornix. In cesarean section the abdominal incision is given above umbilicus and uterus is delivered. First anatomy is to be restored to prevent the incision in vagina.

Patients with an incarcerated, retroflexed uterus should be placed in the knee-chest position, and the anterior lip of the cervix should be grasped and pulled with a ring forceps. Simultaneously, the posterior surface of the uterus is pushed ventrally by exerting pressure though the posterior fornix. This procedure typically requires anesthesia.

Torsion of Uterus

Uterine torsion is defined as rotation of the uterus on its long axis of more than 45 degree and blood supply is hampered and fetal death occurs.[9] Minor degree of rotation along the longitudinal axis is common during pregnancy. But major degree of rotation producing symptoms is rare. The cases are associated with presence of either fibroid uterus or ovarian tumor or bicornuate uterus or adhesions of previous pregnancy. The diagnosis is confused with abruption placentae in later months. The presenting features are of acute abdomen and shock. The uterus is tense and tender. The per-vaginum examination reveals spiraling of vagina. X-shaped vagina instead of usual H-shaped vagina.[10] Cesarean delivery by posterior hysterotomy may need to be performed.

UTERINE PROLAPSE

Uterine prolapse during pregnancy is uncommon with an estimated incidence rate of 1 per 10,000–15,000;[11] the main cause is failure of supportive ligaments of the uterus, such as Mackenrodt's or cardinal ligaments, leading to prolapse of uterus and vaginal vault. However physiological changes of pregnancy, in terms of cervical elongation, and hypertrophy can also contribute to uterine prolapse.[12,13]

The condition is usually first noted in the third trimester and disappears after labor and delivery.[14,15] On the contrary, pre-existing uterine prolapse usually resolves spontaneously during pregnancy but it persists or recurs after delivery.[14-17]

Effects on Prolapse of Pregnancy

Venous obstruction and stasis lead to acute edema and hypertrophy of the protruding cervix in addition to this the mechanical trauma causes ulceration and infection of the edematous cervix.[18] Vaginal discharge may be copious.

Effect of Prolapse on Pregnancy

Increase the risk of urinary tract infection, acute urinary retention, preterm labor, premature rupture of membranes and even maternal death. Preterm labor is one of the serious complications due to impaired blood flow induced by cervical trauma and vascular congestion. There is no evidence that chorioamnionitis could be a significant causative factor in prematurity.[19]

Management

Management options like gynecological hygiene and bed rest in slight Trendelenburg position are mandatory to allow prolapse replacement. These precautions protect the cervix from trauma and desiccation and reduce the incidence of preterm labor. Vaginal pessary support is more helpful in women with pre-existing prolapse rather than in those in whom the condition presents during mid to late pregnancy;[17] there may be early rupture of membrane and prolonged labor. During labor cervical dystocia is managed with Dührssen's incision in order to prevent stretching of the lower segment to a point of rupture.[20] If managed appropriately, the patients without obstetric complications considered to have favorable outcomes of achieving a spontaneous vaginal delivery rate of 84.8%.[21,22] Cervical lacerations are very common. Maternal mortality is rare and is due to obstructed labor with rupture uterus and sepsis. If prolapse persists in puerperium then it is managed with pessary.

PREMALIGNANT AND MALIGNANT LESIONS OF THE CERVIX

Carcinoma cervix is the most common genital tract malignancy encountered in pregnancy with an estimated incidence of 1 in 1,200 to 1 in 10,000.[23]

However, the epidemiology of both cervical cancer is changing. In most western countries with organized screening, the incidence of cervical cancer has dropped dramatically in the last 20 years. There has also been a significant stage shift to earlier stage disease.[24]

One to three percent of women diagnosed with cervical cancer are pregnant or postpartum at the time of diagnosis.[23,25] About one-half of these cases are diagnosed prenatally and the other half are diagnosed with in 12 months following delivery.[26]

Clinical Presentation

Presenting symptoms depends on clinical stage and lesion size.[27,28] Majority of the patients in stage 1 are diagnosed on routine examination. When symptomatic patients present with bleeding or discharge then pelvic examination and inspection of the cervix must be performed, if symptoms are more than 5-7 days. But it should be restricted in later months for the risk of placenta previa. Hardness of cervix is very characteristic as cervix is soft during pregnancy. Cervical biopsy is essential to confirm diagnosis. Clinical manifestations in patients with more advanced disease also include pelvic pain, sciatica type leg pain, flank pain, chronic anemia and shortness of breath.

Diagnosis of cervical cancer is often delayed in pregnant women since many symptoms are similar to those associated with normal pregnancy. Average duration of symptoms before diagnosis in pregnancy is 4.5 months.[29]

Diagnosis

Pregnancy presents a unique opportunity to screen women for cervical neoplasia, particularly in developing countries where routine screening is not available to the community at large. Visual inspection with or without acetic acid (VIA) should be offered to all pregnant women in low resource setting for screening. Other diagnostic modalities include cytology, colposcopy and colposcopic directed biopsy.

In women who have had regular Pap smears and the tests are normal then it should be repeated in pregnancy preferably in second trimester.[30] The reliability of the Pap smear is the same as in the nonpregnant provided the cytopathologist is aware of the pregnant state and is well versed with the normal changes of pregnancy. The columnar cells are exposed much more to the acidic pH of vagina and undergo metaplasia which may be mistaken for dysplasia. The hyperplastic changes in the endocervical glands may also mimic neoplastic changes.

The incidence of abnormal smear in pregnancy has been reported as 5–8% of which 1.2% have cancer.[31] Any abnormality reported on the Pap smear must be followed by colposcopy and directed biopsy.

Concordance between cytology and final diagnosis has been shown to be complete or within one degree of severity in 55.6% and 77.8% patients respectively,[32] whereas colposcopic biopsy is in complete concordance within one grade of severity in 95%.[33] Patients with preinvasive lesion can be followed with repeat Pap smear 6–8 week's interval. To deliver patients with cervical neoplasia require a careful and complete colposcopic evaluation 6 weeks postpartum.

- Endocervical curettage: endocervical curettage (ECC) is not recommended during pregnancy because columnar cells are sampled easily from the surface smear and this increase the risk of rupture membranes
- Conization: indications are very limited in pregnancy. It is performed only in cases where there is a suspicion of invasive cancer which cannot be ruled out on colposcopic biopsy, or in case of microinvasive carcinoma. It should ideally be performed in second trimester to reduce the risk of rupture of membranes or premature labor in third trimester.[34] Major risks are 5–15% preterm labor and infection. Cone biopsy can be done using a laser, large loop excision of transformation zone (LLETZ) or with knife.

Therapeutic conization for intraepithelial lesions is contraindicated in pregnancy. A shallow disc like cone is usually satisfactory for diagnosis with minimum of morbidity. Patients who have conization during pregnancy are at higher risk of residual disease. Therefore, close fellow-up is necessary to decrease morbidity. Flowchart 1 shows the protocol for evaluation of abnormal cytology.[35]

Lack of prenatal care, failure to obtain cervical cytology or to biopsy gross cervical abnormalities, false negative cytology, or failure to evaluate abnormal cytology or vaginal bleeding contributes to delay in diagnosis. So, cervical cancer is commonly diagnosed in postpartum rather than during pregnancy and although stage 1B is most common.

Management

- Premalignant lesions: a close follow-up throughout pregnancy must be maintained with cytology and colposcopy every 6–8 weeks, and biopsy is performed if suspicion of progression. When 62 women with high-grade squamous intraepithelial lesion (HSIL) were followed, the lesion regressed in 50% (complete regression in nearly half of the case) persisted in 40.3% and progressed to microinvasive carcinoma in 9.7%.[36] Of the 82 women followed during pregnancy with diagnosis of low-grade squamous intraepithelial lesions (LSIL), complete regression in 48.8%, persistence in 29.2% and progression to HSIL in 22%
- Microinvasion: in patients with a microinvasive squamous carcinoma with negative margins on cone biopsy conservative management should be done till delivery. The risk of occult metastasis depends on the depth of invasion and the presence or absence of lymphovascular space involvement[37,38]

  Postpartum hysterectomy with or without lymphadenectomy should be performed in postpartum period.
- Invasive carcinoma: when the diagnosis of invasive cervical cancer is established, the different members of the health-care team (obstetricians, gynecologist, oncologist, surgeon, radiation oncologists, neonatologists and pathologists) must discuss each case taking into account the multidisciplinary evaluation. Treatment modalities are based on essential questions: (i) is the prognosis of cervical cancer different during pregnancy, and (ii) under which conditions can the delivery be delayed to obtain sufficient fetal maturity. Accurate staging is important in view of pregnancy. In pregnant patients the standard staging evaluation is modified. Chest radiograph is done with abdominal shielding. Sonography for hydronephrosis and MRI for lymph node evaluation is done
- Invasive 1A2 1B 2A: in third trimester, the radical hysterectomy and pelvic ± para-aortic lymphadenectomy are performed after completion of a high classic cesarean section.[39] Although pelvic vessels are large, but dissection is enhanced by more easily defined tissue planes[39]

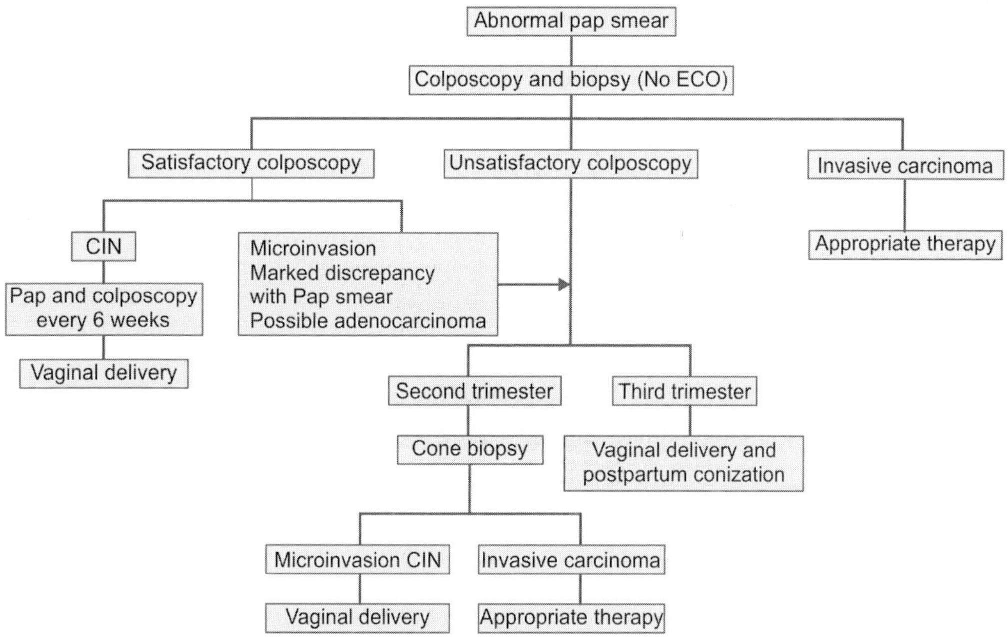

CIN, cervical intraepithelial neoplasia; ECC, endocervical curettage.

FLOWCHART 1: Protocol for evaluation of abnormal cytology.[35]

- Invasive locally advanced disease (stage 2B, stage 3 and stage 4A): management is challenging. Patients either in their second or third trimester should have a high classic cesarean delivery before starting standard chemotherapy or radiotherapy. If further fetal maturity is required then neoadjuvant chemotherapy is considered
- Invasive and distant metastasis: metastatic disease to extra pelvic sites carries poor prognosis. Personal patient's choices are the major factor in guiding the treatment in these situations. Neoadjuvant or adjuvant chemotherapy with cisplatin, etoposide and doxorubicin is recommended. However, each case should be individualized.[40,41]

CESAREAN VERSUS VAGINAL DELIVERY

Cesarean section is almost universally recommended in women with carcinoma cervix for the fear of hemorrhage and fear of dissemination of malignant cells as a result of cervical dilatation.[42] In a study which evaluated 56 women with cervical cancer with pregnancy or within 6 months of delivery, local and distant metastasis occur in 14% of those who delivered by cesarean section as compared to those who delivered vaginally.[43] There are reports of episiotomy implants of squamous cell carcinoma or adenocarcinoma after vaginal delivery.[44]

SURVIVAL

Although some authors have suggested that survival of patients with cervical cancer with pregnancy is compromised. Most reports indicate that the prognosis is not altered.[45]

FIBROID COMPLICATING PREGNANCY

Fibroids (leiomyomas) are benign smooth muscle cell tumors of the uterus. They are a common finding in the reproductive age group. The diagnosis of fibroids in pregnancy is neither simple nor straight forward. Only 42% of fibroids (>5 cm) and 12.5% of smaller fibroids (3–5 cm) can be diagnosed on the physical examination.46 The ability of ultrasound to detect fibroids in pregnancy is even more limited (1.4–2.7%) due to difficulty of differentiating fibroids from physiological thickening of the myometrium.[47,48]

The prevalence of uterine fibroids during pregnancy is underestimated. Incidence of fibroids in older women undergoing treatment for infertility is 12–25%.[49]

Effect of Pregnancy on Fibroids

Sixty to seventy eight percent of fibroids do not demonstrate any significant change in volume.[50,51] Increase in size is due to increase in vascularity, edema and hypertrophy and hyperplasia of fibromuscular tissue. Of the 22–32% of fibroids that increase in volume, the growth was almost exclusively in first trimester. Small and large fibroids (≥6 cm) have different growth patterns in the second trimester. Small fibroids grow whereas large remain unchanged or decrease in size in third trimester,[52] but all decrease in size in third trimester.

Majority of fibroids show no change in puerperium. Although, 7.8% will decrease in volume by up to 10%.

Changes in position and shape: fibroids become flattened.

Torsion of subserous pedunculated fibroids.

Infection and polypoidal changes are more common in puerperium.

Degenerative changes, especially red degeneration is more common. It predominantly occurs in large fibroids during the second half of pregnancy and puerperium. Cause is not known, but vascular is the most important cause. Pain is most common in large fibroids in second and third trimester.[53]

Causes of Pain

- Rapid fibroid growth results in the tissue out growing its blood supply leading to tissue anoxia or necrosis[54]
- Growing uterus results in a change in the architecture (kinking) of the blood supply to the fibroid leading to ischemia and necrosis even in the absence of growth[55]
- Release of prostaglandins.

On ultrasound, they show heterogeneous echogenic pattern or cystic change indicating red degeneration.

Naked eye appearance: tumor shows dark red areas in cut section and red beef appearance with cystic spaces. The color is due to hemolyzed red cells and presence of hemoglobin. The odor is fishy.

Microscopic: evidence of necrosis is present. Vessels are thrombosed but extravasation of blood is unlikely.

Clinical features: (i) Acute onset of pain, (ii) malaise or rise of temperature, (iii) dry or furred tongue, (iv) rapid pulse, (v) constipation, (vi) tenderness or rigidity over tumor, (vii) blood count shows leukocytosis.

Differential diagnosis: (i) Acute appendicitis, (ii) twisted ovarian cyst.

Diagnosis is on laparotomy.

Management in Pregnancy

Pain is managed conservatively by bed rest, hydration and analgesics. Prostaglandin synthetase inhibitors should be used with caution, especially if used more than 48 hours. In the third trimester where it is associated with premature closure of the fetus ductus arteriosus, pulmonary hypertension, necrotizing enterocolitis, intracranial hemorrhage, or oligohydramnios. Rarely for severe pain, narcotic analgesia is epidural analgesia or surgical management myomectomy done.

Myomectomy: in antenatal period can be done in first and second trimester. Pedunculated subserous fibroid can be removed.

Diagnosis of fibroid: with ultrasound mostly the fibroids are diagnosed in first trimester. Marked softening and change of shape make it difficult to differentiate from pregnant uterus. In uncomplicated tumors, it is confused with retroverted gravid uterus, ovarian tumors and nongravid half of pregnant uterus. Sonography confirms the diagnosis.

Treatment: Principle is to not to do anything to fibroid in pregnancy.

- During pregnancy: uncomplicated usual antenatal care and all cases are to be reassessed at 38 weeks to decide mode of delivery

  Place of cesarean section: (i) cervical or broad ligament fibroid, (ii) associated complicating factors like elderly prime gravida and malpresentations.
- During labor:
  - Fibroid above presenting part—usually results in uneventful delivery
  - Fibroid below the presenting part—vaginal delivery is difficult, so cesarean section is indicated. Myomectomy can be done if it is subserous pedunculated fibroid or fibroid is in the incision line. Otherwise if myomectomy is done, there is risk of bleeding and depends on expertise of the surgeon.

Effect of Fibroids on Pregnancy

May be none, but yes there are certain effects which are enlisted below:

Pressure symptoms:

- Bladder-retention of urine
- Rectum-constipation.

Preterm labor and preterm premature rupture of membranes (PPROM):

- Incidence of preterm labor is higher (16.1%) with fibroids than without fibroids (8.7%).[49] Multiple fibroids and fibroids contacting the placenta are independent risk factor[52,56,57]
- Fibroids do not appear to be risk factor for PPROM.

Placental abruption: risk of placental abruption is increased 3-fold. Submucous fibroids, retroplacental fibroids and fibroids volumes more than 200 cm^3 are independent risk factors.[58] Possible mechanism of placental abruption may be diminished blood flow to the fibroid and the adjacent tissues which results in partial ischemia and decidual necrosis in the placental tissues overlying the leiomyoma.

Placenta previa: 2-fold increased risk of placenta previa.[58]

Fetal growth restriction and fetal anomalies: women with fibroids are slightly increased risk of fatal growth restriction.[59] Rarely, large fibroids can compress and distort the intrauterine cavity, leading to fetal deformities including dolichocephalic, torticollis and limb reduction defects.[60,61,62]

Labor and delivery: large fibroids, multiple fibroids and fibroids in the lower segment are the risk factors for abnormal presentation, labor dystocia, and cesarean section.[63,64]

PPH: fibroids may distort the uterine architecture and interfere with myometrial contractions leading to uterine atony and PPH,[65] retained placenta is more common in all women with fibroids as compared with control subjects (1.4% vs 0.6%).[49]

Puerperium: subinvolution, sepsis, secondary PPH, lochiometra and pyometra.

DISEASE OF THE FALLOPIAN TUBE

Acute Salpingitis

Acute or chronic pelvic inflammatory disease (PID) is very rare in pregnancy.

Other conditions are far more common and should be considered before a diagnosis of PID is entertained. When PID does occur during pregnancy, it is associated with a high risk for septic abortion or fetal loss.

The diagnosis is difficult to make and easily confused with other entities, such as appendicitis, torsion of the adnexa, threatened abortion, and ectopic pregnancy. All of these conditions should be excluded before considering a diagnosis of PID. Laparoscopy would be performed if the suspicion for appendicitis, torsion, or ectopic pregnancy is high. In many cases, infection may have been present before conception. One theory holds that pathogenic organisms may be able to ascent from the cervix to the upper tract early in pregnancy, contrary to the thought that the conceptus acts as a barrier to the development of salpingitis. The presence of *gonococcus* or Chlamydia should be confirmed by cervical culture.

Pelvic inflammatory disease during pregnancy should be treated with gentamicin and clindamycin to avoid potential fetal effects of the other treatment regimens recommended by the CDC.

In subclinical disease, vaginal delivery puts the fetus at risk for contracting gonococcal or chlamydial ophthalmia or chlamydial pneumonia if the mother is not treated prior to delivery.

Torsion of the Fallopian Tube

Torsion of the fallopian tube has been described in pregnancy and should be included in the differential diagnosis of the abdominal pain during pregnancy.

The patient presents with pain, generally sudden in onset, located in the quadrant of the involved tube and perhaps radiating to the flank or thigh. Tenderness usually is present, but signs of peritoneal irritation are variable. Other symptoms include nausea, vomiting, and bladder or bowel irritability. Temperature, white blood cell count, and erythrocyte sedimentation rate usually are normal or slightly elevated.
Differential diagnosis includes:
- Torsion or degeneration of an ovarian cyst
- Torsion or degeneration of a uterine leiomyoma
- Ureteral or renal colic
- Acute appendicitis
- Placental abruption
- Inflammatory peritoneal processes
- Intraperitoneal bleeding.

Therapy is surgical. If the affected tube is beyond recovery, it is excised. Normal ovaries are not removed. If torsion is incomplete or recent, and if tissue distal to the torsion remains viable, detorsion of the tube with stabilization by suture may be considered.

OVARIAN TUMOR COMPLICATING PREGNANCY

The incidence of ovarian masses complicating pregnancy is one in one thousand to one in two thousand pregnancies. Any type of ovarian mass can be encountered but most common are dermoid, simple serous and pseudomucinous cyst adenoma. Because pregnant women are young, malignant tumors, including those with malignant potential are relatively uncommon. In California hospital discharge data, they found only 1% of 9,375 ovarian masses in pregnant women were frankly malignant and other 1% were of low malignant potential.[66]

Tumors Unique to Pregnancy

Luteomas: are unique to pregnancy and may be virilizing.[67] They are seen with high human chorionic gonadotropin (hCG) secretion—gestational trophoblastic disease, twins and other situations with increased placental mass.

Ovarian hyperstimulation syndrome: it is caused by ovulation induction. But it may develop spontaneously in pregnancy. This phenomenon is caused by mutation in the receptors.[68]

Complications: complications of tumor masses during pregnancy are torsion, hemorrhage, rupture or infection. Apart from these tumors may suffer incarceration with in the pelvis causing acute retention of urine. In third trimester, they may cause malpresentation or obstructed labor.

Diagnosis

The safety of diagnostic ultrasonography (USG) as well as its ability to delineate anatomic relationship and characterize the morphology of ovarian masses makes it ideal for diagnosis. The use of color flow Doppler to differentiate between benign and malignant is other option. But there is sufficient overlap in blood flow patterns and false positive rate is 50%.[69] MRI can be safely used in pregnancy.

Role of Tumor Markers

Cancer antigen 125 (CA125) is elevated in 80% of epithelial ovarian malignancies. CA125 values are highest during the first trimester, levels as high as 1250 U/mL have been reported.[70] It decreases during the late first trimester and remains below 35 IU/mL until delivery. They increase within hour of delivery and decrease rapidly.

In pregnant patients with marked elevation of α-fetoprotein (AFP) levels, germ cell cancers should be considered in the differential diagnosis. The yolk sac form of AFP contains an additional sugar and is the type produced by endodermal sinus tumor. With the exception of pre-eclampsia, lactic dehydrogenase (LDH) values change little with pregnancy and the puerperium. Beta-hCG and AFP have limited role in pregnancy. Tumor markers should be obtained before any surgical intervention.

Management

Cyst 5 cm or less should be observed and they may undergo spontaneous resolution.

In 5–10 cm cyst, management is controversial. If cyst contains septa, nodules, papillary excrescences or solid components then resection is recommended.[71] Improved resolution of the ultrasound machines, the use of transvaginal transducer and color Doppler can predict the malignancy with greater accuracy.

Elective surgical removal of persistent masses during second trimester or immediate surgery done in case of complications

Treatment of Ovarian Cancer

Most malignant tumors diagnosed in pregnancy are detected incidentally on clinical or ultrasound examination. Germ cell and low malignant potential tumors can be treated conservatively with unilateral oophorectomy or adnexectomy with appropriate staging. Invasive epithelial cancers have the worst prognosis .Optimum debulking surgery should be done followed by chemotherapy except for well differentiated stage 1A disease. Several authors have stated that once the existence of ovarian malignancy, especially epithelial origin, immediate laparotomy is indicated regardless of the stage of the disease,[72,73] problem arises in patients with stage 1B disease in the second trimester—whether surgery or chemotherapy should be given. Antineoplastic drugs are teratogenic or cause fetal growth retardation or fetal death when used in first trimester.[74] Several reports have documented the use of chemotherapeutic agents during second trimester and delivery of normal infant.[75,76] However, the potential risk of antineoplastic therapy must be weighed against the lethality of the maternal disease.

After 20 weeks, preservation of pregnancy is experimental though possible. Surgery should be limited to establish the diagnosis. Any debulking procedure is incomplete if preservation of pregnancy is aimed for. Incomplete surgery during pregnancy should be avoided. Paclitaxel-carboplatin chemotherapy until fetal maturity is the regimen of choice for preoperative chemotherapy. Vaginal delivery followed by final surgery in the postpartum period or planned laparotomy for cesarean delivery and debulking may be considered.

CONCLUSION

Women should understand that they can expect to experience most of the same gynecologic problems during pregnancy that they would when they are not pregnant. Women with PID and endomentriosis can be informed that they will likely experience an improvement or disappearance of their symptoms during pregnancy. Pregnant women should receive information about the continued risk for breast findings or Papanicolaou test.

REFERENCES

1 Centres for Disease Control and Prevention, MMWR Recommendations and Reports 2002;51(RR06):1-80. (2002). Sexually transmitted diseases treatment guidelines 2002. [online] Available from http://www.cdc.gov/mmwr/preview/mmwrhtml/rr5106a1.htm [Accessed December, 2015].
2 Young GL, Jewell D. Topical treatment for vaginal candidiasis (thrush) in pregnancy. Cochrane Database Syst Rev. 2001;(4):CD000225.
3 Amsel R, Tottem PA, Spiegel CA, Chen KC, Eschenbach D, Holmes KK. Nonspecific vaginitis. Diagnostic criteria and microbiological and epidemiological association. Am J Med. 1983;74 (1):14-22.
4 McDonald H, Bracklehurst P, Parsons J. Antibiotics for treating bacterial vaginosis in pregnancy. Cochrane Database Sys Rev. 2005;(1):CD000262.
5 Mathevet P, Chemali E, Roy M, Dargent D. Long-term outcome of a randomized study comparing three techniques of conization: cold knife, laser, and LEEP. Eurp J Obstet Gynecol Reprod Biol. 2003;106:214-8..
6 Alberchtsen S, Ramussen S, Thoresen S, Irgens LM, Iversen OE. Pregnancy outcome in women before and after cervical conisation: population based cohort study. BMJ. 2008;337:a1343.
7 Gottschalk EM, Siedentopf JP, Schoenborn I, Gartenschlaeger S, Dudenhausen JW, Henrich W. Prenatal sonographic and MRI findings in a pregnancy complicated by uterine sacculation: case report and review of the literature. Ultrasound Obstet Gynecol. 2008;32(4):528-6.
8 Lee SW, Kimmy MY, Yang JH, Moon MH, Cho JY. Sonographic findings of uterine sacculation during pregnancy. Ultrasound Obstet Gynecol. 2008;32(4):595.
9 Kaul RPM. A case of torsion of a gravid uterus caused by leiomyoma. Case Rep Obstet Gynecol. 2011;2011:206.
10 Nicholson WK, Coulson CC, McCoy MC, Semelka RC. Pelvic magnetic resonance imaging in the evaluation of uterine torsion. Obstet Gynecol. 1995;85(5 pt 2):888-90.

11 Keetel WC. Prolapse of uterus during pregnancy. Am J Obstet Gynecol. 1941;42:121-6.

12 Sawyer D, Frey K. Cervical prolapse during pregnancy. J Am Board Fam Pract. 2000;13:216-8.

13 Lavery JP, Boey CS. Uterine prolapse with pregnancy. Obstet Gynecol. 1973;42:681-3.

14 Horwitz ER, Yogev Y, Hod M, Kaplan B. Prolapse and elongation of the cervix during pregnancy. Int J Gynecol Obstet. 2002;77:147-8.

15 Gauriglia L, Carducci B, Botta A, Ferrzzani S, Caruso A. Uterine prolapse in pregnancy. Gynecol Obstet Invest. 2005;602:192-4.

16 Hill PS. Uterine prolapse complicating pregnancy. A case report. J Reprod Med. 1984;29:631-3.

17 Brown HL. Cervical prolapse complicating pregnancy. J Natl Med Assoc. 1997;89:346-8.

18 Piver MS, Spezia J. Uterine prolapse during pregnancy. J Obstet & Gynec. 1968;32(6):765-9.

19 Yogez Y, Harowitz ER, Ben- Haroush A, Kaplan B. Uterine cervical elongation and prolapse during pregnancy: an old unsolved problem. Clinical and Experimental Obstetrics and Gynaecology. 2003;30:183-5.

20 Findley P. Prolapse of the uterus complicating pregnancy. JAMA. 1911;57:2131.

21 Eddib A, Allaf MB, Lele A. Pregnancy in a woman with uterine procidentia: a case report. J reprod. Med. 2010;55:67-70.

22 Spezia J, Piver MS. Uterine prolapse during pregnancy. Obstet & Gynaec. 1968;32:765-9.

23 Nguyen C, Montz FJ, Bristaw RE. Management of stage 1 cervical cancer in pregnancy. Obstet Gynecol Surv. 2000;55(10):633-43.

24 Gershenson DM, McGuire WP, Gore M, Quinn MJ, Thomas G (Eds). Gynaecologic Cancer: Controversies in Management. New York, London, Edinburgha: Elsevier Churchill Livingstone; 2004.

25 Creasman WT. Cancer and Pregnancy. Ann NY Acad Sci. 2001;943:281.

26 Smith LH, Dalrymple JL, Leiserwoitz GS, Danielsen B, Gilbert WM. Obstetrical deliveries associated with maternal malignancy in California. 1992 through 1997. Am L Obstet Gynecol. 2001;184:1504-12.

27 Duggan B, MuderspachLI, Roman LD, Curtin JP, d'Ablaing G 3rd, Morrow CP. Cervical cancer in Pregnancy: reporting on planned delay in therapy. Obstet Gynecol. 1993;82:598-602.

28 Lee RB, NegliaW, Park RC. Cervical carcinoma in pregnancy. Obstet Gynecol. 1981;58:584-9.

29 Hannigan EV. Cervical cancer in pregnancy. Clin Obstet Gynecol. 1990;33:837-45.

30 NHSCSP. Publication 20: Colposcopy and Programme Management, 2nd edition. 2010.

31 Von Calstern K, Vergote I, Amant F. Cervical neoplasia during pregnancy: diagnosis, management and prognosis. Best Pract Res Clin Obstet Gynecol. 2005;19(4):611-30.

32 Baldauf JJ, Dreyfus M, Ritter J, Philippe E. Colposcopy and directed biopsy reliability during pregnancy: a cohort study. Eur J Obstet Gynecol Reprod Biol. 1995;62(1):31-6.

33 Economos K, Prez Verdiana N, Delke I, Collado ML, Tancer ML. Abnormal cytology in pregnancy: a 17-year experience. Obstet Gynecol. 1993;81(6):915-8.

34 Hannigan EV. Cervical cancer in pregnancy. Clin Obstet Gynecol. 1990;33:837.

35 Hacker NF, Berek JS, Lagasse LD, Charles EH, Savage EW, Moore JG. Carcinoma of the cervix associated with pregnancy. Obstet Gynecol. 1982;59:735-46.

36 Rebova H, Rob L, Kacirak J, Halaska M Jr, Strnad P, Schlegerova D. Squamous intraepithelial lesion-microinvasive carcinoma of the cervix during pregnancy. Eur J Gynecol Oncol. 2005;26(6): 611-14.

37 Copeland LJ, Silva EG, Gershenson DM, Morris M, Young DC, Wharton JT. Superficially invasive squamous cell carcinoma of the cervix. Gynecol Oncol. 1992;45:307-12.

38 Sorosky SJ, Squatrio R, Ndubisi BU, Anderson B, Podczaski ES, Mayr N, et al. Stage 1 squamous cell carcinoma in pregnancy: planned delay in therapy awaiting fetal maturity. Gynecol Oncol. 1995;59:207-10.

39 Sood AK, Sorosky JI, Krogman S, Anderson B, Benda J, Buller RE. Surgical management of cervical cancer complicating pregnancy: a case-control study. Gynecol Oncol. 1996;63(3):294-8..

40 Amont F, Von Calsterenk, Halaska M, Beijnen J, Lagae L, Hanssens M, et al: Gynecological cancers in pregnancy: guidelines of international consensus meeting. Int J Gynecol Cancer. 2009;19 Suppl 1:S1-12.

41 Balderstan KD, Tewari K, Gregory WT, Berman ML, Kucera PR. Neuroendocrine small cell cervix cancer in pregnancy: long term survivor following combined therapy. Gynecol Oncol. 1998;71:128-32.

42 Hunter MI, Tewari K, Monk BJ. Cervical neoplasia in pregnancy. Part 2: current treatment of invasive disease. Am J Obstet Gynecol. 2008;199(1):10-8.

43 Sood A, Sorosky JI, Mayr N, Anderson B, Buller RE, Niebyl J. Cervical cancer diagnosed shortly after pregnancy: prognostic variables and delivery route. Obstet Gynecol. 2000;95(6):832-8.

44 Cliby WA, Dodson WA, Podratz KC. Cervical cancer complicated by pregnancy: episiotomy site recurrences following vaginal delivery. Obstet Gynecol. 1994;84:179-82.

45 Greer BE, Easterling TR, McLennan DA, Benedetti TJ, Cain JM, Figge DC, et al. Fetal and maternal considerations in the management of stage 1-B cervical cancer during pregnancy. Gynecol Oncol. 1984;34:61-5.

46 Muram D, Gillieson M, Walters JH. Myomas of uterus in pregnancy: ultrasonographic follow-up. Am J Obstet Gynecol. 1980;138:16-9.

47 Rice JP, Kay HH, Mahony BS. The clinical significance of uterine leiomyomas in pregnancy. Am J Obstet Gynecol. 1989;160:1212-6.

48 Cooper NP, Okolo S. Fibroids in pregnancy--common but poorly understood. Obstet Gynecol Surv. 2005;60:132-8.

49 Klotsky PC, Tran ND, Caughey AB, Fujimoto VY. Fibroids and reproductive outcomes: a systemic literature review from conception to delivery. Am J Obstet Gynecol. 2008;198:357-66.

50 Aharoni A, ReiterA, Golan D, Paltiely Y, Sharf M. Patterns of growth of leiomyomas during pregnancy, a prospective longitudinal study. Br J Obstet Gynaecol. 1988;95:510-3.

51 Rosati P, Exacoustoc C, Mancuso S. Longitudinal evaluation of uterine myoma growth during pregnancy. A Sonographic study. J Ultrasound Med. 1992;11:511-5.

52 Lev-Toaff AS, Coleman BG, Arger PH, Mintz MC, Arenson RL, Toaff ME. Leiomyomas in pregnancy: sonographic study. Radioplogy. 1987;164:375-80.

53 Katz VL, Dotters DJ, Droeglmueller W. Complications of uterine leiomyomas in pregnancy. Obstet Gynecol. 1989;73:593-6.

54 De Carolis S, Fatigante G, Ferrazzoni S, Trivellini C, De Santis L, Mancuso S, et al. Uterine myomectomy in pregnant women. Fetal Diagn Ther. 2001;16:116-9.

55 Parker WH. Etiology, symptomology and diagnosis of uterine myomas. Fertil Steril. 2007;87:725-36.

56 Winer-Muran HT, Muram D, Gillieson MS. Uterine myomas in pregnancy. J Can Assoc Radiol. 1984;35:168-70.

57 Exacoustos C, Rosati P. Ultrasound diagnosis of uterine myomas and complications in pregnancy. Obstet Gynecol. 1993;82:97-101.

58 Vergani P, Ghidini A, et al. Large uterine leiomyomata and risk of cesarean delivery. Obstet Gynecol. 2000;95:764-9.
59 Corenado GD, Marshall LM, Schwartz SM. Complications in pregnancy, labor and delivery with uterine leiomyomas: a population based study. Obstet Gynecol. 2000;95:764-9.
60 Chuang J, Tsai HW, Hwang JL. Fetal compression syndrome caused by myoma in pregnancy: a case report, Acta Obstet Gynecol Scand. 2001;80:472-73.
61 Grahm JM Jr, Miller ME, Stephen MJ, Smith DW. Limb reduction anomalies and early in utero limb compression. J Pediatr. 1980;96:1052-56.
62 Remero R, Chervenac FA, DeVare G, Tortora M, Hobbins JC. Fetal head deformities and congenital torticollis with uterine tumor. Am J Obstet Gynecol. 1981;141:839-40.
63 Phelan JP. Myomas and pregnancy. Obstet Gynecol Clin North Am. 1995;22:801-5.
64 Vergoni P, Ghidini A, Storbelt N, Roncaglia N, Locatelli A, Lapinski RH, et al. Do uterine leiomyomas influence pregnancy outcome? AM J Perinatol. 1994;11:356-8.
65 Szamatowicz J, Laudanski T, Bulkzas B, Arerlund M. Fibromyomas and uterine contractions. Acta Obstet Gynecol Scand. 1997;76:973-6.
66 Leiserowitz GS, Xing G, Crens R, Brahmbhatt B, Dalrymple JL, Smith LH. Adnexal masses in pregnancy: how often they are malignant. Gynecol Oncol. 2006;101:315-21.
67 Wang YC, Su HY, Liu JY, Chang FW, Chen CH. Maternal and female fetus virilization caused by pregnancy leuteomas. Ferti Steril. 2005;84:509.
68 Vasseur C, Rodien P, Beau I, Desroches A, Gérard C, de Poncheville L, et al. A chorionic gonadotrophin-sensitive mutation in the follicle stimulating hormones as a cause of familial gestational spontaneous ovarian hyperstimulation syndrome. N Eng J Med. 2003;349:753-9.
69 Wheeler TC, Fleischer AC. Complex adnexal mass in pregnancy: predictive value of color Doppler sonography. J Ultrasound Med. 1997;16: 425-8.
70 Look KY. Epidemiology, etiology, and screening of ovarian cancer. In: Rubin SC, Sutton GP (Eds). Ovarian Cancer, 2nd edition. Philadelphia: Lippincott Williams & Williams; 2001. pp. 167-80.
71 Caspi B, Levi R, Appleman Z, Rabinerson D, Goldman G, Hagay Z. Conservative management of ovarian cystic teratoma during pregnancy and labor. Am J Obstet Gynecol. 2000;182:503;.
72 Jubb ED. Primary ovarian carcinoma in pregnancy. Am J Obstet Gynecol. 1963;85:345-54.
73 Chung A, Birnbaun SJ. Ovarian cancer associated with pregnancy. Obstet Gynecol. 1964;90:511-6.
74 Barber H. Fetal and neonatal effects of cytotoxic agents. Obstet Gynecol. 1981;58:415-47.
75 Weed JC, Roh RA, Mondenhall HW. Recurrent endodermal sinus tumor during pregnancy. Obstet Gynecol. 1979;54:653-6.
76 Malfetano JH, Goldcrand JW. Cis-platinum combination chemotherapy during pregnancy for advanced epithelial ovarian carcinoma. Obstet. 1990;75:545-7

CHAPTER 67

Malignant or Neoplastic Diseases

Niranjan N Chavan, Shubhrita Gupta

INTRODUCTION

Cancers that complicate pregnancy and lactation are generally defined as those that occur during gestation or within 1 year postpartum. It is the second most common cause of death during reproductive years. It complicates between 0.02% and 0.1% of all pregnancies.[1,2] Frequency and localization are comparable to those of nonpregnant women of the same age. The incidence is expected to rise with the increasing age of childbearing. The most common malignant tumors associated with pregnancy include cervical cancer, breast cancer, malignant melanoma, colorectal cancer, Hodgkin's disease and leukemia. The prognosis of cancer in pregnant women is same as in nonpregnant women, if the cancer stage and therapy are comparable. Treatment can be derived from the guidelines that apply for nonpregnant women. Close fetomaternal surveillance including serial Doppler measurement is necessary to recognize fetal impairment in advance. The delivery is scheduled accordingly to avoid life-threatening consequences to mother and child.

EPIDEMIOLOGY

Pregnancy-associated malignancies are all malignancies that are diagnosed during pregnancy or within 1 year postpartum. Estimations on the basis of age-adjusted incidences are shown in Table 1.

In total, the predicted number of malignancies complicating pregnancy amounts to 700 per year, given an average of 700,000 live births per year and an estimated rate of malignancies of 1 in 1,000 pregnancies.

TABLE 1: Estimated incidence of malignancies during pregnancy

Disease	Incidence
Cervical cancer	1/2,000–1.2/10,000
Breast cancer	1/3,000
Hodgkin's disease	1/1,000–6,000
Ovarian cancer	1/10,000–100,000
Malignant melanoma	2.6/1,000
Colorectal carcinoma	1/13,000
Leukemia	1/75,000–100,000

DRAWBACK: DELAYED DIAGNOSIS

Cancer in pregnancy is often diagnosed late and at an advanced stage. Nonspecific symptoms such as fatigue, development of anemia, constipation or lymph node swelling are easily attributed to the physiological changes occurring during pregnancy. In addition, specific symptoms such as vaginal bleeding or a palpable mass in the breast are frequently disregarded until invasive diagnostics are initiated.

If indications are there, all diagnostic noninvasive and invasive procedures, including inevitable biopsies, can also be carried out in pregnant women. Due to hormonal induced alterations, cytology and tissue examinations are more demanding in pregnant women and it is thus essential to inform the pathologist. Magnetic resonance imaging (MRI) can very often replace radiological diagnosis. However, if necessary, radiological diagnosis can be applied from the second trimester onwards. Postponement of diagnosis can worsen the prognosis in pregnant women.

ETHICAL AND MORAL CONSIDERATIONS

A desired pregnancy is a positive event. If cancer is diagnosed during the early stages of pregnancy, the prolongation of pregnancy depends on the stage and prognosis of the disease. Chemotherapy during the first trimester often causes intrauterine death of the fetus. During the second trimester, surgery and chemotherapy are the only available safe cancer therapies. It is essential to provide the pregnant woman with a multidisciplinary team of physicians, including gynecologists, medical oncologists and obstetricians as well as neonatologists. After having reached viability, it is necessary that the fetus and the mother to be monitored in a perinatological intensive care unit in the course of therapy. The goal would be to reach the maximum health for the fetus without endangering the prognosis for the mother and, on that basis, decide on the optimum delivery date.

THERAPEUTIC MODALITIES

Chemotherapy[3]

During the first trimester, it is suggested that pregnant women should not be exposed to chemotherapy due to the mutagenic and teratogenic potential resulting in up to 25% of miscarriage (Table 2).

Chemotherapy during the first trimester raises the percentage of miscarriages to 20% compared to an average of 3–4% in the general population. Safety for systemic chemotherapy is approved from the second trimester onwards. The therapy regimens in most cases are based on established therapy guidelines.

From the 5th week of gestation onwards, all chemotherapeutic agents can cross the placenta. Their teratogenic potential is highest between the 5th and 10th week of gestation and then decreases until organogenesis is completed in the 13th week of pregnancy. However, at this stage, the central nervous system and the genitals are not yet fully developed. From the second trimester onwards, growth restriction is the main risk of chemotherapy. In addition, myelosuppressive effects can occur in the mother as well as in the fetus.

Chemotherapy should be completed 2–3 weeks before delivery in order to avoid myelosuppression in the newborn or in the mother. The placenta is the metabolizing and excreting organ of the fetus and thus is significant for detoxification. The nadir of classical chemotherapy protocols usually is in between the 7th and the 10th day.[4]

Nevertheless, it is important to bear in mind that so far, no pharmacokinetic studies on pregnant women exist. The applied therapeutic regimens and dosages do neither consider the increased blood volume (50%) nor the higher drug clearance or the increased oxidase function of the liver that occur during pregnancy. For this purpose, prospective studies would be essential.

Follow-up after Intrauterine Chemotherapy[5,6]

In literature, only very few long-term follow-up data on children whose mothers received chemotherapy during pregnancy, exist. So far, the majority of the followed up children has not displayed any abnormalities. In a few cases secondary malignomas, growth retardation, intellectual impairment and reduced fertility have been reported.

Surgery

Depending on the localization of the tumor, surgery is possible at any stage during pregnancy. If the patient's prognosis is not impaired, the operation should only be carried out when the fetus has reached viability. If there is a risk for a preterm

TABLE 2: Teratogenicity of chemotherapeutic drugs during pregnancy

Substance group	Medication	Application during pregnancy
Alkylating agents	• Cyclophosphamide	• Rate of malformations can reach 14% during the first trimester
Antitumor antibiotics	• Doxorubicin (cardiotoxic) • Daunorubicin • Mitomycin • Bleomycin • Actinomycin D	• No increased risk for malformations from the second trimester onwards, successful single case reports during the first trimester, no cardiotoxicity for the fetus
Vinca alkaloids	• Vincristine • Vinblastine, neurotoxic	• No malformations—also in the first trimester
Antimetabolites	• 5-fluorouracil, methotrexate	• Contraindicated in pregnancy • High correlation with malformations
Platinum analogs	• Cisplatin, carboplatin	• Hearing test in the newborn; carboplatin not recommended due to thrombocytopenia
Taxanes	• Paclitaxel, docetaxel	• Case reports: first and second trimesters without any significant problems, available data is scarce

delivery before 34 weeks of gestation, lung maturation is stimulated with 12 mg intramuscular betamethasone, twice within a 24-hour interval. Usually, if the fetus has reached viability, the surgery in the small pelvis is combined with a cesarean section.

Radiotherapy[7-10]

Radiotherapy during pregnancy is contraindicated. Usually, a delay in therapy for several weeks does not aggravate the prognosis for the mother. Delivery can thus be awaited until tolerated by both the mother and fetus. If there is a vital indication such as the constriction of the mediastinum by extensive lymphomas, local radiotherapy has to be initiated during pregnancy. Tables 3 and 4 depict the radiation dose effect on fetal life and the adverse effects of radiation in relation to gestation stage respectively.

Endocrine Therapy, Monoclonal Antibodies

Endocrine therapy like tamoxifen or aromatase inhibitors should not be administered during pregnancy. Likewise, monoclonal antibodies such as bevacizumab or trastuzumab are contraindicated due to the risk of bleeding and cardiovascular complications.

Supportive Measures[11]

An effective antiemetic therapy is safe and particularly essential during pregnancy. Ondansetron, a serotonin (5-HT3) receptor antagonist, can be safely administered during the first trimester. In contrast, tropisetron is contraindicated as it causes malformations in animal experiments. If necessary, steroids can be administered. Therapy with granulocyte stimulating factor has no proven negative impact on pregnancy.

TABLE 3: Radiation dose effect on fetal life

Dose	Effect on fetus
<0.1 Gy (<10 rad)	No major effect
0.1–0.15 Gy (10–15 rad)	Increased risk
2.5 Gy (250 rad)	Malformation in most
>30 Gy (>300 rad)	Abortion

TABLE 4: Adverse effect of radiation in relation to gestation stage

Stage	Period	Adverse effect
Preimplantation/ immediate postimplantation	From conception to day 9–10	Lethal
Early organogenesis	Weeks 2–6	Teratogenesis and growth retardation
Late organogenesis/ early fetal period	Weeks 12–16	Mental retardation, growth retardation and microcephaly
Late fetal period	From weeks 20–25 till birth	Sterility, malignancies, genetic defects

Breastfeeding and Chemotherapy

Many chemotherapeutic agents, including doxorubicin with or without pegylated liposomal formulation, cisplatin, cyclophosphamide as well as methotrexate are excreted into breast milk.

Metastases of Maternal Tumors via the Placenta[12-15]

The placenta possesses very effective protective mechanisms against circulating tumor cells, which effectively reduce the risk of placental transmission of metastases in hematologic malignant diseases. The placenta itself is more often affected by metastases.

CERVICAL CANCER

Incidence

Pregnancy-associated cervical cancer (PACC) is the most common malignant tumor encountered throughout gestation, the estimated incidence ranging from 1.2 in 10,000 pregnancies.[16-18] Cervical cancer commonly occurs during the reproductive years. About 2–5% of these tumors are diagnosed during pregnancy.[19,20] The median age of women with cervical cancer diagnosed during pregnancy is in the early-thirties (about 10 years earlier than nonpregnant women) (Figures 1A to F).[21]

Diagnosis

The presenting symptoms of cervical cancer may vary depending mostly on the extent of the disease. Unspecific symptoms of cervical carcinoma are excessive discharge and vaginal bleeding. Pregnancy represents an ideal time for a routine physical and pelvic examination, and obtaining Papanicolaou (Pap) smear for cytology. Diagnosis can be safely performed by colposcopy and colposcopy-directed biopsy. However, endocervical curettage is not indicated during pregnancy.

Confirmed cervical intraepithelial neoplasia (CIN) II and III should be examined with colposcopy every 3 months. Conization and loop excision are usually associated with a higher risk of bleeding in up to 15% of patients and an abortion rate of up to 25%. The MRI is the preferred imaging method as there is no radiation. Apart from the first trimester, computed tomography can also be carried out during pregnancy.

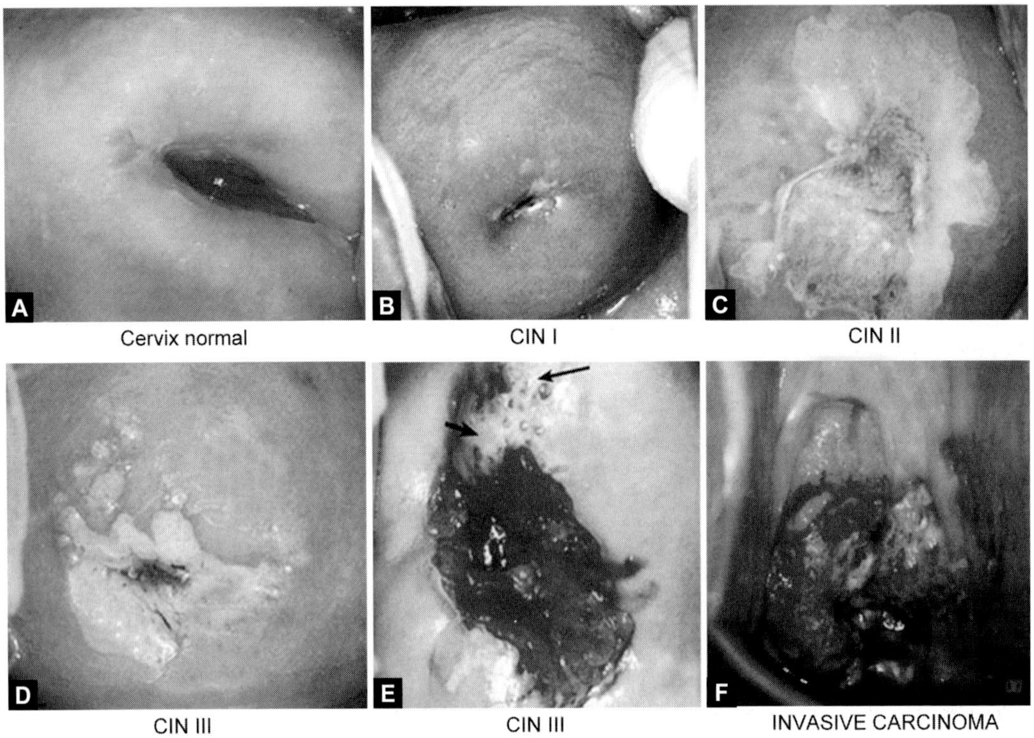

FIGS 1A TO F: Cervical cancer *(For color version, see Plate 10).*

Therapy

Surgery

Except for the early stages of malignancy, cervical cancer is always associated with the termination of pregnancy. However, a delay in the initiation of treatment is recommended during the early stages and with no impact on the course of disease.

If cervical cancer is diagnosed in stage II or higher, an immediate initiation of therapy is indicated. Scheduled therapy postponement requires regular clinical checkups of the local findings (palpation, inspection and colposcopy).

Early stages of the disease (I and IIA) are usually treated either by radical hysterectomy and pelvic lymph node dissection, or by radiation. Recent studies recommend the use of concurrent radiochemotherapy, followed by hysterectomy for bulky stage IB carcinoma. Patients with an advanced disease (stage IIB and higher) are usually treated by radiation.

Fertility-conserving surgery of cervical cancer stage IA1 by local tumor excision in young women with the desire for a child is not associated with a higher recurrence of disease or a worsened prognosis.

Radical trachelectomy is an alternative to radical hysterectomy performed during pregnancy and represent a pregnancy and fertility-maintaining alternative for cervical cancer at stages IA2 to IB1.

Chemotherapy, Radiochemotherapy and Radiotherapy

Platinum-based therapeutic schemes are effective in squamous cell carcinoma and adenocarcinoma. So far, curative treatment consists of combined radiochemotherapy including cisplatin as a radiosensitizer. This approach is compatible with the continuation of pregnancy.

So far, data on neoadjuvant chemotherapy prior to surgery are incoherent.

Cervical Cancer and Mode of Delivery

A strict surveillance during the course of pregnancy with an early induction of lung maturation if surgery is scheduled before week 34 of pregnancy is absolutely essential. A cesarean section, usually followed immediately by radical hysterectomy and pelvic and para-aortal lymph node dissection is the preferred surgical treatment in operable cervical cancer during pregnancy.

Few studies showed that vaginal delivery has a poorer prognosis than cesarean section. Malignant cell spreading in the episiotomy has been described and is associated with an unfavorable prognosis.

There is no difference in maternal survival between pregnant and nonpregnant women when matched by age, stage and the year of diagnosis.

OVARIAN CANCER

Incidence

The incidence of ovarian malignancies during pregnancy is estimated to be between 1 in 10,000 and 1 in 100,000. Around 40% of these tumors are germ cell tumors. Epithelial ovarian tumors are usually of low stage and low grade (Fig. 2).

Ovarian cancer in pregnant women is different from non-pregnant women in the following aspects:

- Mostly younger patients affected
- Confirmed diagnosis mostly at stage I or II
- More often ovarian borderline tumors
- No studies on long-term outcome.

Diagnosis

Ovarian cancer usually causes unspecific symptoms, which are easily attributed to the physiological changes occurring during pregnancy. Ultrasonography checkups are compulsory allowing an early detection of tumor especially during the first trimester.

Treatment

Expectant management is contraindicated at an advanced stage, considering the poor prognosis of ovarian cancer. If the fetus has reached viability at the time of diagnosis, the stimulation of lung maturity has got to be completed prior to surgery until the 34th week of gestation.

Surgery

The primary treatment is surgery, which only in the rare case of stage Ia1 permits the continuation of pregnancy. Prerequisite for this is the resection of the tumor in toto in negative intraoperative staging (peritoneal biopsy, biopsy of the contralateral ovary, omentum, Douglas aspiration cytology and negative pelvic and para-aortic lymph nodes).

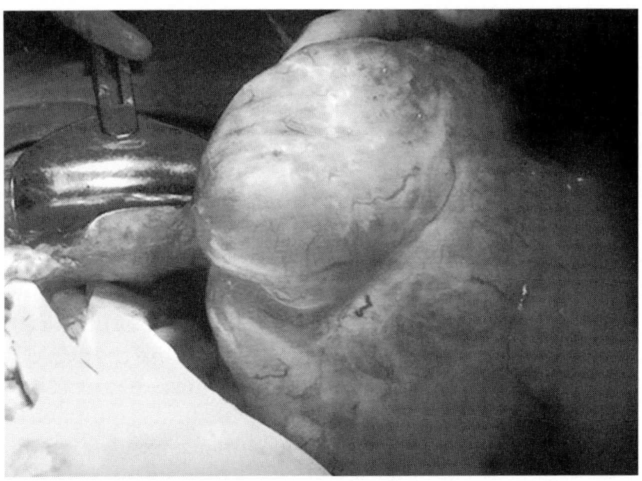

FIG. 2: Ovarian tumor ***(For color version, see Plate 10).***

Adjuvant Chemotherapy

Current data on neoadjuvant chemotherapy with carboplatin (paclitaxel) during pregnancy suggest that the use of taxane analogs is unfavorable. Thus, this therapy should only be used if the woman has the strong desire to continue pregnancy.

BREAST CANCER

Incidence

Pregnancy-associated breast cancer (PABC) is the second most common malignancy in pregnancy, complicating 1 in 3,000 pregnancies.[22] About 3% of all breast carcinomas are diagnosed during pregnancy. Median age is 33 years (23–47 years).

Symptoms

Most patients present with painless masses 90% of which are detected by self-examination.

Diagnosis

Diagnosis of breast cancer during gestation is often delayed for up to 11 months. This is due to the physiologically occurring hypervascularity and the hyperproliferative state of the breast during pregnancy.

Most carcinomas in pregnant and nonpregnant women are detected by self-examination. Diagnosis consists of ultrasonography and mammography as well as a biopsy (fine needle aspiration or excisional) to confirm diagnosis.[23] The maximum radiation dose for the fetus is 10 rad. Mammography with appropriate protection is equivalent to a radiation dose of 50 mrad. Magnetic resonance imaging represents a supplementary means of diagnosis.

Tumor Characteristics and Prognosis

Due to the delayed diagnosis, 70–80% of breast cancer in pregnant women is detected in advanced positive lymph node stages. The risk for peripheral metastases appears to be 2-fold. 70% of specimens are estrogen or progesterone receptor negative.

Therapy

Strategies of therapeutic management of PABC are mainly dependent on disease stage.

Early Breast Cancer (Stages I and II)

Modified radical mastectomy is the treatment of choice. Radiotherapy should be delayed until after delivery in order to avoid harmful effects on the fetus. Adjuvant chemotherapy if indicated should not be administered during the first trimester.[24-26]

Advanced Breast Cancer (Stages III and IV)

Radiation therapy should be avoided completely for the benefit of fetus. Chemotherapy is still indicated after the first trimester of pregnancy.

Endocrine therapy as well as monoclonal antibody therapy with trastuzumab are contraindicated during pregnancy.

Therapeutic Abortion

Therapeutic abortion was advocated due to concerns for hormonal stimulation of tumor growth. Oncologists consider therapeutic abortion during first and second trimesters only in aggressive primary breast cancer or in patient with advanced disease in which prompt treatment is recommended.

Metastatic spread to placenta is extremely rare and to fetus is never documented.

Pregnancy after Breast Cancer

The effect on pregnancy is related to stage of the disease. Patient with early stages I, II show no difference. Patients with stage III should consider deferring pregnancy for at least 5 years after treatment and women with stage IV disease should not conceive at all.[27]

MALIGNANT MELANOMA

Incidence

The incidence of malignant melanoma is estimated to be 2.8 per 1,000 pregnancies.[28] About 8% tumors arising during gestation and 30–35% women are of childbearing age.[29]

Diagnosis

During pregnancy, any abnormal skin alterations have to be examined by a dermatologist (Fig. 3). The local invasion depth can be visualized by ultrasonography and determines the margin of safety of the excision. Diagnosis is always made by tumor excision and pathological examination.[30]

Treatment and Outcome

Treatment is always surgical tumor excision.

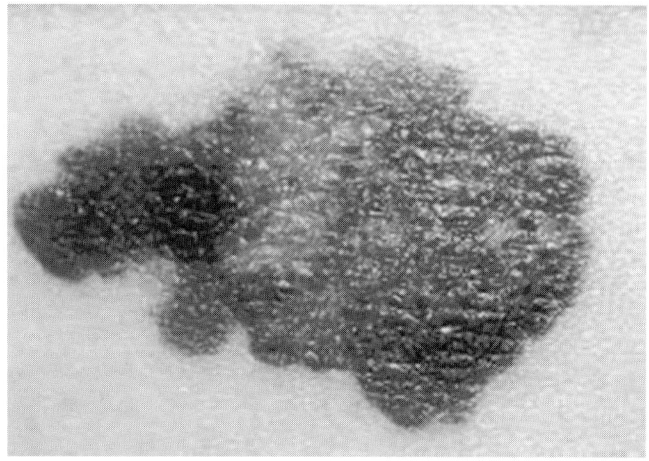

FIG. 3: Malignant melanoma *(For color version, see Plate 10)*.

In early primary lesion, adequate surgical excision has a good prognosis. These cases do not need therapeutic abortion. A sentinel lymph node biopsy during pregnancy is not contraindicated, as the fetal radiation dose is below 5 mGy. In high-risk melanomas with a poor prognosis, adjuvant therapy, which is limited during pregnancy, should be initiated within 6 weeks. Pregnancy itself does neither increase the risk nor worsen the prognosis of malignant melanoma.

COLORECTAL CANCER

Incidence

The incidence of colorectal cancer is estimated to be 1 in 13,000 pregnancies.[31]

Diagnosis

An average of 83% of colorectal cancers are rectal tumors and only 17% located in the colon (Fig. 4).

Symptoms are nonspecific like constipation, diarrhea, abdominal pain, bleeding, and mucus secretion. There is probably delay in diagnosis results in a poorer prognosis for the patient. Diagnosis is confirmed by endoscopy and additional imaging techniques.

Treatment

Within the first trimester, a curative resection of the locally circumscribed tumor can be carried out without endangering pregnancy. At more advanced stages of pregnancy or in case of a widespread tumor, pregnancy should be discontinued by a primary cesarean section. In order to assign the ideal date for delivery, the tumor stage and growth and thus the prognosis for the patient as well as the maturity of the fetus have to

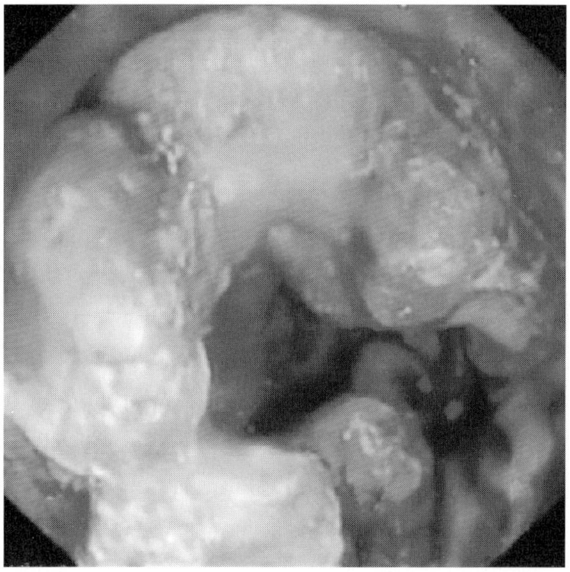

FIG. 4: Colorectal cancer *(For color version, see Plate 11)*.

be outweighed. In the case of colon cancer, simultaneous surgery should be considered. Chemotherapy with platinum analogs and 5-fluorouracil is indicated postoperatively if the diagnosis is a histologically confirmed stage IIB. Neoadjuvant radiochemotherapy for the treatment of a locally advanced rectal carcinoma is not compatible with pregnancy.

HEMATOPOIETIC TUMORS

Lymphomas

Hodgkin's disease: Incidence—1 in 1,000 to 1 in 6,000 pregnancies. Hodgkin's disease stage IA-IIA treated with radiotherapy.[32,33]

Non-Hodgkin's lymphoma (NHL) is very rare.[34]

Diagnosis and Staging

Limited staging workup is mandatory during pregnancy. Staging includes physical examination, blood test, chest X-ray, bone marrow biopsy and abdominal ultrasound. Tomographic and isotope scans are contraindicated.[35]

Treatment and Outcome

Pregnancy does not affect the course of lymphoma and survival while therapeutic abortion does not improve the course of the disease. Chemotherapy can be safely utilized as the primary treatment of Hodgkin's disease after completion of the first trimester. If the clinical presentation of the patient is acceptable, a delayed initiation of therapy without aggravating the prognosis of the patient is possible. If indicated, radiotherapy should be scheduled after delivery.

Leukemias

Acute Myelogenous Leukemia

Acute myelogenous leukemia (AML) is the most frequent type of leukemia diagnosed in pregnant women with an incidence of 3 in 100,000.[36-38] AML does not allow for a delay in treatment. At the time of diagnosis, the patient is at a great risk for bleeding due to impaired intravascular coagulation.

Induction therapy consists of a combination of cytarabine with an anthracycline. From the second trimester onwards, this combination is considered as sufficiently safe, but during the first trimester often leads to abortions or intrauterine fetal death. In addition, this combination therapy can cause growth retardation and, occasionally, myelosuppression in the child. If responsiveness to treatment is satisfying, premature termination of pregnancy before the initiation of consolidation therapy can be considered after having reached fetal viability.

Acute Lymphoblastic Leukemia

Treatment of acute lymphoblastic leukemia (ALL) requires the administration of methotrexate. Thus, the prolongation of the pregnancy has got to be discussed prior to therapy initiation.

Acute Promyelocytic Leukemia

Acute promyelocytic leukemia (APL) is usually associated with disseminated intravascular coagulopathy (DIC) at the time of diagnosis. Chemotherapy requires the administration of cytarabine, all-trans retinoic acid (ATRA) and an anthracycline. ATRA exposure is associated with a high rate of teratogenicity and is thus contraindicated in early pregnancy.

Chronic Myelogenous Leukemia

Interferon-alpha has no known teratogenic effect and is thus the treatment of choice for chronic myelogenous leukemia (CML) during pregnancy. Imatinib mesylate and hydroxyurea are not recommended during pregnancy due to their proven teratogenicity. Leukapheresis quickly reduces leukocytosis and can be a temporary alternative for chemotherapy.

Chronic Lymphocytic Leukemia

Usually, treatment of chronic lymphocytic leukemia (CLL) can be postponed until postpartum. Leukapheresis can temporarily reduce severe leukocytosis.

ENDOMETRIAL CANCER

It occurs very rarely during pregnancy.

THYROID CANCER

It is very rare during pregnancy; no hormonal association between maternal hormonal changes and thyroid cancer. Lobectomy with cervical lymph node dissection can be performed. Radioactive iodine should be avoided and chemotherapy is not effective.[39,40]

CONCLUSION

Malignant disease during pregnancy presents an extreme stress to both patient and physician, and its occurrence raises a conflict between optimal maternal therapy and fetal well-being. The most common malignancies (cervix, breast, lymphoma and melanoma) account for about 70–80% of pregnancy-associated tumor. Many other sites of primary tumors have been reported in the literature, mainly leukemia, ovary and thyroid carcinoma. Many reports and reviews have noted that pregnant patients tend to have a worse outcome when compared with nonpregnant women. Some have postulated that the altered hormonal environment of pregnancy may adversely influence the course of the disease. However, based on contemporary well-controlled studies, it seems that pregnancy *per se* should not be considered as a poor prognostic factor. However, since the gestational status might interfere with correct diagnosis and treatment, the result might be an inferior outcome.

REFERENCES

1. Kennedy S, Yudkin P, Greenall M. Cancer in pregnancy. Eur J Surg Oncol. 1993;19:405-7.
2. Murphey GP (Ed). CA-Cancer statistics. CA. 1999;49:20-1.
3. Zemlickis D, Lishner M, Degendorfer P, Panzarella T, Burke B, Sutcliffe SB, et al. Maternal and fetal outcome after breast cancer in pregnancy. Am J Obstet Gynecol. 1992;166:781-7.
4. Sorosky JI, Squatrito R, Ndubisi BU, Anderson B, Podczaski ES, Mayr N, et al. Stage I squamous cell cervical carcinoma in pregnancy; planned delay in therapy awaiting fetal maturity. Gynecol Oncol. 1995;59:207-10.
5. Reynoso EE, Shepherd FA, Messner HA, Farguharson HA, Garvey MB, Baker MA. Acute leukemia during pregnancy: the Toronto Leukemia Study Group experience with long-term follow-up of children exposed in utero to chemotherapeutic agents. J Clin Oncol. 1987;5(7):1098-106.
6. Aviles A, Neri N. Hematological malignancies and pregnancy: a final report of 84 children who received chemotherapy in utero. Clin Lymphoma. 2001;2:173-7.
7. Doll R, Wakeford R. Risk of childhood cancer from fetal irradiation. Br J Radiol. 1997;70:130-9.
8. Ogris E. Exposure to radioactive iodine in pregnancy: significance for mother and child. Acta Med Austriaca. 1997;24:150-3.
9. Langagergaard V, Horvath-Puho E, Norgaard M. Hodgkin's disease and birth outcome: a Danish nationwide cohort study. Br J Cancer. 2008;98(1):183-8.
10. Wyatt RM, Dale RG. The effect of delay in radiotherapy treatment on tumour control. Phys Med Biol. 2003;48:139-55.
11. Cardonick E, Lacobucci A. Use of chemotherapy during human pregnancy. Lancet Oncol. 2004;5:283-91.
12. Rothman LA, Cohen CJ, Astarloa J. Placental and fetal involvement by maternal malignancy: A report of rectal carcinoma and review of the literature. Am J Obstet Gynecol. 1973;116:1023-34.
13. Osada S, Horibe K, Oiwa K, Yoshida J, Iwamura H, Matsuoka H, et al. A case of infantile acute monocytic leukemia caused by vertical transmission of the mothers leukemic cells. Cancer. 1990;65:1146-9.
14. Sheikh SS, Khalifa MA, Marley EF, et al. Acute monocytic leukaemia (FAB M5) involving the placenta associated with delivery of a healthy infant: case report and discussion. Int J Gyn Path. 1996;15:363-6.
15. Green A. Oral contraceptives and skin neoplasia. Contraception. 1991;43(6):653-66.
16. Nevin J, Soeters R, Dehaeck K, Bloch B, van Wyk L. Cervical carcinoma associated with pregnancy. Obstet Gynecol Surv. 1995;50:228-39.
17. Hacker NF, Berek JS, Lagasse LD, Charles EH, Savage EW, Moore JG. Carcinoma of the cervix associated with pregnancy. Obstet Gynecol. 1982;59:735-46.
18. Norstorm A, Jansson I, Andersson H. Carcinoma of the uterine cervix in pregnancy. A study of the incidence and treatment in the western region of Sweden 1973 to 1992. Acta Obstet Gynecol Scand. 1997;76:583-9.
19. Duggan B, Muderspach LI, Roman LD, Curtin JP, d'Ablaing G, Morrow CP. Cervical cancer in pregnancy: reporting on planned delay in therapy. Obstet Gynecol. 1993;82:598-602.
20. Sivanesaratnam V, Jayalakshmi P, Loo C. Surgical management of early invasive cancer of the cervix associated with pregnancy. Gynecol Oncol. 1993;48:68-75.
21. Jones WB, Singleton HM, Russell A, Fremgen AM, Clive RE, Winchester DP, et al. Cervical carcinoma and pregnancy. A national patterns of care, study of the American College of Surgeons. Cancer. 1996;77:1479-88.
22. Advisory Committee on the Biological Effects of Ionizing radiation, National Research Council, National Academy of Sciences. The effect on populations of exposure to low levels of ionizing radiation. Washington, DC: National Academy Press; 1980.
23. Ishida T, Yokoe T, Kasumi F, Sakamoto G, Makita M, Tominaga T, et al. Clinicopathological characteristics and prognosis of breast cancer patients associated with pregnancy and lactation: analysis of case control study in Japan. Jpn J Cancer Res. 1992;83:1143-9.
24. Zemlickis D, Lishner M, Degendorfer P, et al. Maternal and Fetal outcome following breast cancer in pregnancy. In: Korean G, Lishner M, Farine D (Eds). Cancer in Pregnancy. Maternal and Fetal Risks. Cambridge: Cambridge University Press; 1996. pp. 95-106.
25. Byrd BF, Bayer DS, Robertson JC, et al. Treatment of breasts tumours associated with pregnancy and lactation. Ann Surg. 1962;155:940-7.
26. Berry DL, Theriault RL, Holmes FA, Parisi VM, Booser DJ, Singletary SE, et al. Management of breast cancer during pregnancy using a standardized protocol. J Clin Oncol. 1999;17:855-61.
27. Avertte HE, Mirhashemi R, Moffat FL. Pregnancy associated breast carcinoma: the ultimate medical challenge. Cancer. 1999;85:2301-4.
28. Smith RS, Randall P. Melanoma during pregnancy. Obstet Gynecol. 1969;34:825-9.
29. Garbe C. [Pregnancy, hormone preparations and malignant melanoma]. Hautarzt. 1993;44:347-52.

30. Antonelli NM, Dotters DJ, Katz VL, et al. Cancer in pregnancy: a review of the literature. Part I-II. Obstet Gynecol Surv. 1996;51:125-42.
31. Wood JB, Martin JN, Ingram FH, Odom CD, Scott-Conner CE, Rhodes RS. Pregnancy complicated by carcinoma of colon above the rectum. Am J Perinatal. 1992;9:102-10.
32. Riva HL, Anderson PS, O'Grady JW. Pregnancy and Hodgkin's disease: a report of eight cases. Am J Obstet Gynecol. 1953;66:866-70.
33. Stewart HL, Monto RW. Hodgkin's disease and pregnancy. Am J Obstet Gynecol. 1953:66:570-8.
34. Ward FT, Weiss RB. Lymphoma and pregnancy. Semin Oncol. 1989;16:397-409.
35. Lishner M, Zemlickis D, Degendorfer P, et al. Maternal and fetal outcome following Hodgkin's disease in pregnancy. In: Korean G, Lishner M, Farine D (Eds). Cancer in Pregnancy. Maternal and Fetal Risks. Cambridge: Cambridge University Press; 1996. pp. 107-15.
36. Yahia C, Hyman GA, Phillips LL. Acute leukemia and pregnancy. Obstet Gynecol Surv. 1958;13:1-21.
37. Catanzarite VA, Ferguson JE 2nd. Acute Leukemia and Pregnancy: a review of management and outcome, 1972-1982. Obstet Gynecol Surv. 1984;39:663-78.
38. Haas JF. Pregnancy in association with a newly diagnosed cancer: a population-based epidemiologic assessment. Int J Cancer. 1984;34:229-35.
39. Kobayashi K, Tanaka Y, Ishiguro S, et al. Rapidly growing thyroid carcinoma during pregnancy. J Surg Oncol. 1994;55:61-4.
40. Ringenberg QS, Doll DC. Endocrine tumours and miscellaneous cancers in pregnancy. Semin Oncol. 1989;16:445-55.

CHAPTER 68

Oro-dental Care

Nisha Thakur, Narotam K Ghezta, Pratibha Sharma

INTRODUCTION

Pregnancy is characterized by complex physiological changes which can adversely affect oral health.[1-4] The oral cavity may present both transient and irreversible changes as well as modification that are considered pathologic. Pregnant women are particularly susceptible to gingival and periodontal disease. Different oral lesions are reported to be common during pregnancy. Increased prevalence of dental alteration has also been documented including particularly caries and erosion. The biochemical and hormonal changes of pregnancy enhances the risk.[4] Routine dental care should not be deferred in pregnancy and necessary treatment for oral health problems should be given to a pregnant woman.[5] Pregnant women need more prenatal dental attention because they are more prone to develop certain pregnancy-associated lesions.[6] The physicians and dentist are cautious and often avoid treatment of oral health issues during pregnancy. This problem result from a lack of clinical guidelines for the prevention and management of common oral condition in pregnancy.[4] Health care professionals should make certain that need for dental care during pregnancy and early childhood is met.[5] This chapter reviews the commonly occurring oral problems during pregnancy and their management guidelines for prenatal counseling, dental procedures that can be carried out during pregnancy and preventive strategies that could be helpful in preventing the commonly occurring disease such as dental caries and periodontal diseases.

MANAGEMENT OF PHYSIOLOGIC CHANGES DURING PREGNANCY

Pregnancy leads to various changes in almost all the organ system. The common complaints include nausea, vomiting, food craving, heart burn, shortness of breath and fatigue. These changes may pose challenge in providing dental care for pregnant patient. Therefore, understanding physiologic changes of the body and effect of certain dental procedures, dental radiation, and medication used in dentistry on pregnant patients and fetus is essential for the management of the pregnant woman.[7]

Cardiovascular Changes

There is an increase in cardiac output by 30–50% during pregnancy. Heart rate increases by 20–30% and the stroke volume increases by 20–50%.[8,9] In 90% of the women these changes produces tachycardia and functional heart murmur which disappears shortly after delivery.[9] There is a decrease in blood pressure and cardiac output during the second and third trimesters when the patient is in supine position (lies flat on her back) in dental chair due to decrease in venous return to the heart. This results because of the compression of inferior vena cava by the gravid uterus. It can result in a 14% reduction in cardiac output.[8,9] There is decreased oxygen to the brain and uterus due to decrease in the venous return. In the supine position, women may complain of nausea or dizziness when hypotension is present.[5] The right hip of the pregnant women should be elevated by 10–12 cm.[7,9] Pregnant woman can be tilted in 5–15% tilt on her left side by placing a pillow or rolled towel under her right hip in order to elevate it and asking her to roll on her left side. This maneuver helps in lifting uterus off to the vena cava and also re-establishes aortocaval patency.[1,7-9] If hypotension is still not relieved, a full lateral position may be needed.[9]

Respiratory System Changes

There is an increase in the demand of oxygen during pregnancy. The changes seen are dyspnea, hyperventilation which is due to oxygen demand or decrease in the residual capacity of the lungs. Estrogen is increased leading to engorgement of nasal capillaries and rhinitis which can lead to nosebleed and predisposes the pregnant women to various upper respiratory infections.[7] Capillaries in the mucosa of the nasopharynx becomes engorged due to an increased estrogen production. This results in edema, nasal congestion, and predisposition to epistaxis.[1,3,7-9] There is a tendency to breathe with the mouth open as nasal breathing becomes more difficult, especially at night. Sometimes xerostomia or dryness of mouth develops in which patient looses the protection against dental decay provided by saliva. Pregnant women who are experiencing these problems especially those with a high caries index should undergo caries control to minimize the deleterious effect on the dentition.[1]

Hematologic System Changes

There is an increase in the maternal plasma volume and red blood cell changes resulting in overall increase in blood volume during pregnancy. There is a 25–52% increase in maternal blood volume and red blood cell mass increases by 20% over non-gravid values by late pregnancy.[8] There is an increase in red blood cells, white blood cells and erythrocyte sedimentation rate (ESR) whereas there is decrease in hemoglobin.[7] This disproportionate rise results in hemodilution or physiologic anemia of pregnancy that is maximum by the 30–32 weeks of gestation. There are two clinically significant reasons for blood volume changes. The first reason is to protect the mother from volume depletion resulting due to excessive peripartum hemorrhage and the second is to minimize the chance of thrombotic event occurrence.[8] In pregnancy, all coagulation factors except XI and XIII are increased.[7] Hypercoagulable state of pregnancy results from increase in thrombin-mediated fibrin generation, increased amount of clotting factors and increased hematocrit leading to deep vein thrombosis and pulmonary edema.[7,8] Compression of the inferior vena cava by the gravid uterus causes venous obstruction which leads to stasis. Endothelial cell wall damage results from venous stasis, which leads to thrombus formation. During pregnancy, an overall incidence of 0.09% has been reported. Pulmonary embolism (PE) has been reported in 15–25% of patients with untreated deep venous thrombosis (DVT), resulting in a 12–15% mortality rate.[8] Before carrying out any surgical procedure in the oral cavity, the practitioner should review hemoglobin level and red blood cell count of the pregnant women to prevent any further complications.[7]

Gastrointestinal System Changes

Gastrointestinal disorders in pregnancy are mainly due to the displacement of stomach by the enlarging uterus onto the spleen and liver which leads to high intragastric pressure. There is a decrease in the lower esophageal sphincter tone occurring because of the inhibition of production of peptide hormone motilin by the increased amount of progesterone. Stimulatory effect on the smooth muscle of the gastrointestinal tract is caused by motilin. These two mentioned disorders cause pyrosis (heartburn) in approximately 70% of all pregnant women as well as increased gastric emptying time. Gastric reflux and regurgitation is caused by the lowered esophageal sphincter tone, the elevated gastric pressure and the slowing of gastric emptying stage causes.[8] Nausea and vomiting during pregnancy is thought to be due to the hormonal effect of estrogen and progesterone.[9] Many pregnant patients experience morning sickness (hyperemesis gravidarum) in which they experience bouts of nausea and vomiting.[3] Pregnant patients should always be seated in a semisupine or comfortable position during a dental procedure. If the patient experiences nausea, the procedure should be stopped immediately and the chair should be repositioned upright.[9] In dental office, a dental surgeon should always be prepared by having the oropharyngeal suction readily available. If any object is lodged in the airway after vomiting, the dentist can use only chest compression during advanced stages of pregnancy to remove the foreign body blocking the airway (American Heart Association guidelines).[3] Morning appointments should be avoided for pregnant women with hyperemesis. Citrus drinks or fatty foods should be avoided by them as these may cause gastric upset or delay gastric emptying time. Salty liquids such as sport beverages should be given to the pregnant women to prevent dehydration due to recurrent vomiting.[9] Pregnant women suffering from nausea often leads to ptyalism or excessive secretion of saliva. Inability of the nauseated women to swallow normal amount of saliva rather than a true increase in production leads to excessive saliva in the mouth. Sometimes 2L of saliva per day is lost through drooling. Reducing the intake of complex carbohydrates may improve this condition.[1]

Renal and Genitourinary Changes and its Implication

In pregnancy, the length of the urethra increases by 4–7 mm. As the uterus enlarges, the bladder is drawn passively upwards and anterior. It becomes more an abdominal organ rather than a pelvic organ. There is an increased glomerular filtration rate (GFR). There are biochemical changes in the urine and blood, tendency to urinate more frequently and a greater risk of urinary tract infection. By the third trimester in 90% of the pregnancies there is hydroureter or ureteral dilation. Pyelonephritis may be caused by urinary stasis during pregnancy. If drugs with renal clearance are used in pregnancy, the doses of the drugs need to be increased. Just prior to starting the dental procedure, ask the patient to empty the bladder.[9]

Endocrine Changes and its Implications

Female sex hormones like estrogen, progesterone and human gonadotropin are secreted by placenta and are responsible for the various physiologic changes occurring during pregnancy. There is also an increase in thyroxine, steroids and insulin levels.[7,9] To overcome the antagonist action of estrogen and progesterone about 45% of pregnant women are unable to produce sufficient amounts of insulin which results in the development of gestational diabetes. Gestational diabetes develops in females who are obese and have a positive family history of type II diabetes mellitus. Increased levels of hormones estrogen and progesterone lead to insulin resistance as these hormones are insulin antagonists. Thus insulin levels are elevated in pregnant women to compensate for this resistance.[9] Hence practitioner should perform tests to check the blood sugar level before carrying out any dental procedures.[7]

Oral Changes during Pregnancy

The levels of hormones progesterone and estrogen increases during pregnancy. By the third trimester they can reach levels 30% higher than occurring during the menstrual cycle.[10] These increased hormones during pregnancy causes changes in mother's body and oral cavity is no exception[11] (Flowchart 1).

Common oral problems seen in pregnancy are:

Pregnancy Gingivitis

Elevated level of circulating estrogen causes increase in capillary permeability.[9,11] This results in exacerbation of pre-existing gingivitis or the production of a generalized gingivitis in patients with poor oral hygiene.[10] Gingivitis is the inflammation of the superficial gum tissue.[4] Plaque may get trapped underneath the swollen area because of this.[6] During pregnancy, gingivitis is aggravated due to increase in hormone (estrogen and progesterone) levels, alteration in oral flora and a decreased immune response, thus reducing the body's ability to repair and maintain healthy gingival tissue (Fig. 1). Frequent oral hygiene measures which include individual practices such as regular tooth brushing, flossing and use of mouthwashes and professional measures such as oral prophylaxis and oral irrigation can minimize

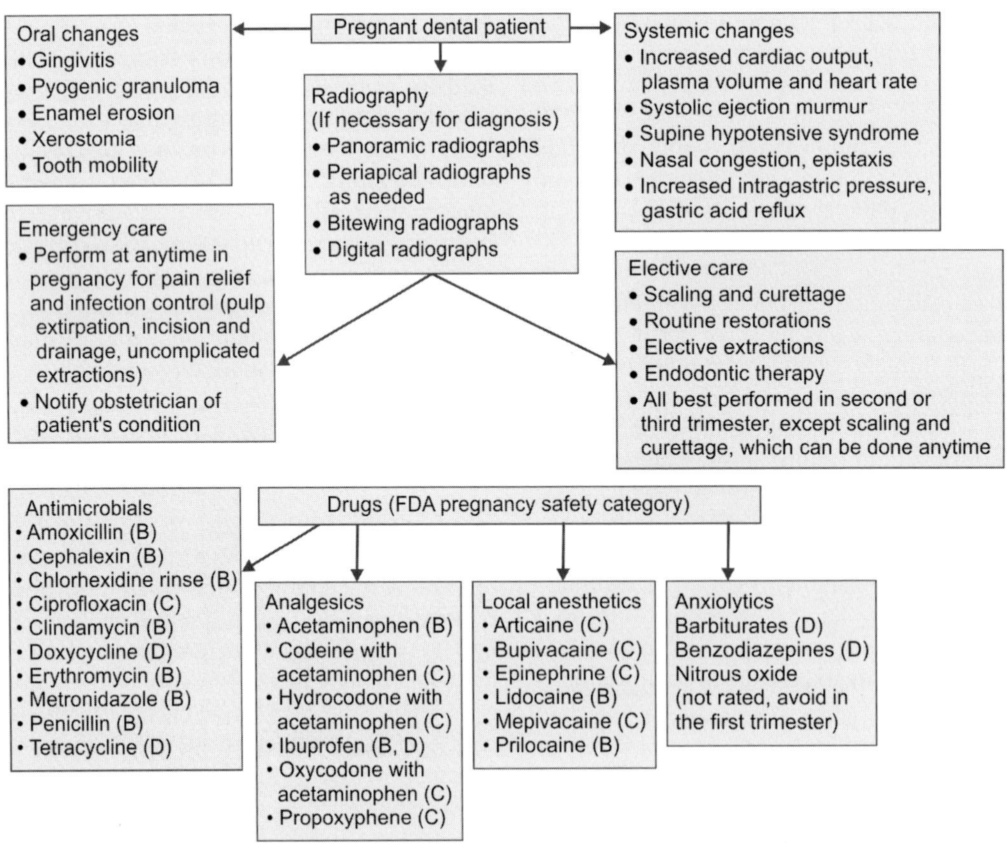

FLOWCHART 1: Summary of somatic changes with their diagnostic and treatment options in dental management of pregnant women.[1]

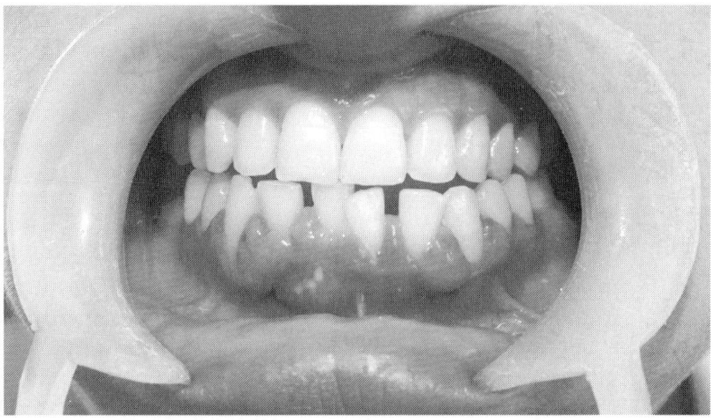

FIG. 1: Pregnancy gingivitis—gingivitis is aggravated due to increase in hormone *(For color version, see Plate 11)*.
Courtesy: Dr Amit Kumar, MDS-Periodontics.

the severity of gingivitis.[4] This condition is ephemeral and recedes after delivery. Good oral hygiene can help in the prevention of gingivitis during pregnancy.[7] At any time of pregnancy, coronal scaling, polishing and root planing may be performed but in the second and third trimesters of pregnancy only routine general dentistry should be done.[1] All tooth whitening (bleaching) procedure contains chemicals. There is a risk that if a pregnant woman has pregnancy gingivitis, the gingivitis will be worsened by the bleaching chemicals. As there is no body of evidence proving that bleaching procedures are safe during pregnancy, many authorities believe that such cosmetic procedures should be postponed until the postpartum period.[10]

Periodontal Disease

Periodontitis is a destructive inflammation of the periodontal apparatus affecting many women of childbearing age.[4] Pregnancy does not cause periodontal disease but it worsens an existing condition.[11] The process begins with inflammation followed by bacterial infiltration into the periodontal fibers. Chronic inflammatory response is stimulated by the toxins released by the infiltrated bacteria resulting in breakdown and destruction of the periodontium creating loss of attachment (pocket) which eventually gets infected. Finally the tooth becomes mobile. This can induce recurrent bacteremia, which indirectly triggers the hepatic phase response, resulting in production of cytokines, prostaglandins (i.e., PGE2), and interleukins (i.e., IL-6, IL-8), all of which can affect pregnancy.[4] Periodontitis if left untreated has been shown to contribute to preterm, low birth weight infants.[12] Significant reduction of preterm birth or low birth weight in children were seen in the pregnant women for whom dental treatment such as plaque control, scaling and daily rinsing using 0.12% chlorhexidine (category B antimicrobial mouthwash[1]) and maintenance therapy such as oral hygiene instructions were performed.[4]

Pregnancy Tumor (Pyogenic Granuloma)

In 1-5% of the pregnant women, pyogenic granuloma occurs. Pyogenic granuloma (Fig. 2) is caused by increased angiogenesis, which is caused by sex hormones, coupled with local factor like plaque. It mainly occurs on the labial aspect of the interdental papilla.[7,11] It can occur anytime in pregnancy but occurs most commonly during the first and second trimesters of pregnancy. However, it regresses after child birth.[11] No treatment is required unless some complications like bleeding from tumor or difficulty in mastication occurs. In such cases, tumor can be surgically removed. Oral prophylaxis coupled with good patient education and oral hygiene minimizes the frequency and severity of the lesion.[7]

Erosion

Some pregnant women are prone to develop morning sickness. Enamel demineralization is caused by the regurgitation of gastric acids. To compensate for the decreased stomach capacity, mothers are advised to eat frequent, smaller amount of carbohydrate-containing food. This leads to more frequent exposure to acid challenges. Some pregnant women have a craving for specific foods like sour foods. These foods contain high level of acid or sticky food with a high concentration of sucrose. Oral hygiene procedures and frequent water rinses will help prevent decalcification due to morning sickness or exposure to lots of acidic food. If vomiting continues, the dentist is able to provide daily topical application of fluoride gels that will reduce enamel decalcification. Flexible mouth guards can also be fabricated for the application of neutral sodium or stannous fluoride gels.[6] Application of fluoride varnish

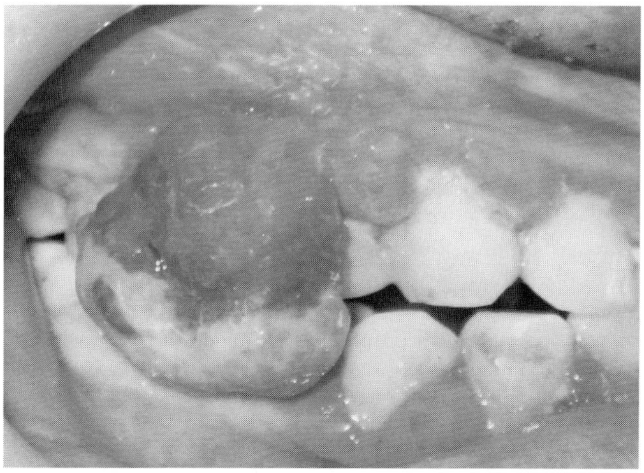

FIG. 2: Pregnancy tumor—it is caused by increased angiogenesis, which is caused by sex hormones, coupled with local factor like plaque *(For color version, see Plate 11)*.
Courtesy: Thakur M, et al. Pregnancy tumor. Kerala Dental Journal. 2012; 35(3):308-10.

may be better tolerated as topical fluoride gel may cause nausea.[1] Erosion of the enamel can also easily be controlled by advising the patient to rinse their mouth thoroughly after vomiting with a solution that contains sodium bicarbonate. Sodium bicarbonate neutralizes the acids and prevents the damage caused by the residue which remains on the teeth.[11]

Tooth Mobility

During a late pregnancy, tooth mobility may increase.[6,11] Changes in lamina dura, changes in the attachment apparatus or any underlying pathology which is unrelated to pregnancy causes increased tooth mobility.[1,11] Tooth mobility may be caused by vitamin C deficiency. Removal of the local irritants, therapeutic doses of vitamin C results in reversal of the tooth mobility.[1] Tooth mobility typically resolves postpartum.[6,11]

Dental Caries

An increased prevalence of dental alteration has been documented, particularly caries (99.38%).[4] Increased proliferation and desquamation of the oral mucosa and an increase in the subgingival crevicular fluid levels is caused by salivary estrogen. The desquamating cells provide suitable environment for bacterial growth which predisposes the pregnant women to dental caries.[11] The other reasons for pregnant women for a higher caries risk is an increased pH in the oral cavity due to frequent vomiting, craving towards sugary snacks and less attention towards oral health. Active dental caries should be treated as it can lead to local as well as systemic complications.[4] The most common restoration material used is dental amalgam. There is insufficient evidence to support or refute that mercury exposure from restorative material dental amalgam contributes to adverse pregnancy outcomes.[5,10,12] Mercury vapor released during the removal or placement of amalgam restoration may be inhaled and absorbed into the bloodstream and does cross the placental barrier. The use of rubber dam and high speed suction can reduce the risk of vapor inhalation.[5,12] In dental amalgam, elemental mercury is found which is different from methylmercury, a form of organic mercury. Major source of organic mercury is fish and seafood. The ingestion of methylmercury during pregnancy is a major public health concern, while evidence of the adverse effect of mercury released from dental amalgams during pregnancy is lacking.[5]

Tooth Pain

Many expectant mothers are worried about the adverse outcome of root canal treatment to their fetus. Severe tooth pain due to inflammation is a common reason for root canal therapy. Persistent pain during pregnancy is a stressful condition which can have lack of sleep, restlessness and distress from toothache may have negative outcomes to both mother and the fetus. Dental extraction these days is painless, produces least stress.[4]

Infection

Infection is another serious condition which can lead to significant danger for both the expectant mother and the fetus. If left untreated and is localized it can spread to surrounding spaces causing space infections and can end up spreading to the circulation causing septicemia.[4] Management of mild infection should be managed via incision/drainage under local anesthetic with subsequent antibiotic coverage. It is essential to aggressively treat the gravid patient to minimize the risk of infection spreading to the fascial spaces. Fascial space infection should be handled in a standard fashion: airway assessment (if any doubt, intubate), imaging (computed tomography scan) and to the operating room for adequate incision and drainage. Postoperatively, if the patient is unable to maintain oral intake, parenteral nutritional support must be instituted. Until the results of the culture/sensitivity are returned, empirical penicillin therapy is appropriate. More severe infections should be managed in the operating room under general anesthesia with intravenous antibiotics and incision and drainage.[8]

RADIOGRAPHS IN PREGNANCY

If protective measures such as high speed film, a lead apron and a thyroid collar are used, oral radiography is safe for pregnant patients. In case of X-ray radiation exposure less than 5–10 centigrays (cGy), no increase in congenital anomalies or intrauterine growth retardation has been reported.[1,3,13] Thus generally for a patient with a spreading odontogenic infection, a single orthopantomogram (OPG) will provide sufficient information at an acceptable radiation exposure. With advanced spreading odontogenic infection into the neck, generally this is best demonstrated by a computed tomography (CT) scan. A single CT scan has less than normal safe level of irradiation (e.g. 5–10 cGy) but is greater than for an OPG. Thus, CT scanning is best avoided in pregnant patient and only used if strongly clinically indicated, such as to define a pus collection in patients not responding to surgical management. Ultrasound has a place in defining moderate to large pus collection in the neck and it should be considered over and above a CT scan.[13]

LOCAL ANESTHESIA IN DENTISTRY

Lidocaine is one of the most common local anesthetic used during dental treatment. Lidocaine along with epinephrine when used in the correct dosage is safe during pregnancy.[7] Lidocaine and prilocaine are category B drugs. Epinephrine, mepivacaine, articaine and bupivacaine are in category C.

Epinephrine has been studied in amount of up to 0.1 mg added to local anesthetics used for epidural anesthesia (administered for pain relief during labor). No unusual side effects or complications have been reported in this context. Intravascular administration of a local anesthetic with epinephrine may cause insufficiency of uteroplacental blood flow. However for a healthy pregnant patient, if epinephrine is administered by proper aspiration technique and limited to the minimal dose required, the 1:100,000 epinephrine concentration used in dentistry is safe.[1]

ANTIBIOTIC USED IN DENTISTRY

Most antibiotics cross the placenta and have the potential to affect the fetus. Penicillin, a β-lactam structured cell wall inhibitor, has been used in clinical practice since the 1940s. In treating the gravid patient with an oral infection, penicillin remains the antibiotic of choice. The most commonly prescribed antibiotic in general use today is the cephalosporin. All the generations of cephalosporins have a Food and Drug Administration (FDA) classification B, which is presumed to be safe based on animal models.[8] Antibiotic ciprofloxacin a broad-spectrum fluoroquinolone is used to treat periodontal disease associated with *Actinobacillus actinomycetemcomitans* which is a category C drug. It causes arthropathy and adverse effects on cartilage development in immature animals. Its use in pregnancy has been restricted. There is not enough data to definitively determine its safety in humans. Metronidazole is a category B drug and recent studies have shown no definitive teratogenic effects. However, some authors caution against its use in the first trimester because of potential harm to the fetus. The obstetrician should be consulted before prescribing the drug and the risk-benefit ratio for the patient should be determined.[1] Erythromycin, clindamycin, azithromycin and clarithromycin are the macrolide family of antibiotics. The macrolides cross the placenta only minimally. In patients with allergies to penicillin or with resistant bacteria, erythromycin and clindamycin are used extensively for oral infection.[8] Hepatic toxicity is more likely to be induced in pregnant mother by the estolate form of erythromycin and is, therefore not recommended.[1,14] All the macrolides, except clarithromycin are FDA class B. Clarithromycin is a category C drug. Streptomycin, gentamycin, tobramycin, kanamycin, amikacin, netilmicin are the aminoglycosides. Widely used aminoglycoside during pregnancy is the gentamicin which is a category C drug. Gentamicin rapidly crosses the placenta. No congenital and no reports of neonatal ototoxicity or nephrotoxicity after *in utero* exposure have been reported with gentamicin.[8] Category D drugs are the barbiturates and benzodiazepines and they should be avoided during pregnancy. Cleft lip and palate are caused by the benzodiazepines. In the FDA classification system, nitrous oxide is not rated and its use during dental treatment is still controversial.[1] Skeletal and behavioral teratogenic effects have been demonstrated by prolonged high-dose exposures to nitrous oxide in rats. Occupational exposure to nitrous oxide has been implicated with spontaneous abortions and reduced fertility. The opioid analgesics should be used cautiously. Multiple congenital defects including heart defects and cleft lip/palate have been associated with codeine. Little is known about their potential fetal risks associated with other opioids like oxycodone and hydrocodone as they are administered infrequently during pregnancy. With opioid use neonatal respiratory depression as well as opioid withdrawal has been reported. Both aspirin and nonsteroidal anti-inflammatory drugs (NSAIDs) have a common mechanism of inhibiting prostaglandins synthesis. Prostaglandin E2 is involved in the induction of labor. NSAIDs may prolong labor by blocking the production of prostaglandins. Prostaglandin inhibitors also raise concerns about premature fetal ductus arteriosus constricture. This results in pulmonary hypertension in the fetus. Bleeding tendencies specifically intracranial hemorrhage have been associated with the newborns of the mothers who have ingested 5–10 g of aspirin 5 days before delivery. No bleeding tendencies were found if aspirin was taken no fewer than 6 days prior to delivery. In the third trimester of pregnancy, aspirin and NSAIDs should be avoided. Acetaminophen should be given as an alternative to aspirin and other NSAIDs. It causes less gastric irritation and does not cause bleeding tendencies. Hepatic toxicity is produced by acetaminophen so its dosage should be carefully monitored.[14] The maximum recommended daily dose of acetaminophen should be no more than 4 g/day for adults. Ibuprofen is a category B analgesic in the first and second trimesters, but it is a category D drug during the third trimester because it has been associated with lower levels of amniotic fluid, premature closure of ductus arteriosus and inhibition of labor when taken during this time. It should only be prescribed after consultation with an advice from the obstetrician.[1]

INTRAUTERINE DENTISTRY

It is a highly relevant subject. The use of preventive measures in the intrauterine stage can avoid several diseases like dental caries. The World Health Organization (WHO) has advised that from 4th month of pregnancy onwards women should avoid the consumption of sugar so that the fetus (future child) does not develop attraction for these types of food, thus becoming susceptible to caries.[3,15]

CONCLUSION

Prenatal oral health counseling for parents is an important factor because infant oral health begins at this stage. The main goal is to create awareness among the expectant mothers about the importance of prevention of dental disease by means of oral prophylaxis and restoring carious teeth. These procedures will decrease the microorganism in the oral cavity of the mother thereby reducing transmission to the child.[4] Mutans streptococci (MS) are found in all children with early childhood caries, and recent research demonstrates that transmission to mother to child is a common pathway to MS. Reducing maternal microflora by preventive measures lowers the level of dental caries in children. In pregnant women with high level of salivary MS, researchers encourage the use of chlorhexidine varnish and xylitol consumption after delivery.[16] Dental appointments should be short. Patient should be properly positioned to prevent supine hypotension. In early part of the third trimester it is safe to perform routine dental treatment, but from middle of the third trimester routine dental treatment should be avoided. In conclusion, it should be remembered that treatment is rendered to mother and fetus. Avoid the drugs which will put fetus at risk. Elective surgery in pregnant patients should be avoided by the oral and maxillofacial surgeons, if possible. Emergency cases involving trauma, infection and pathology should be treated by them whose treatment cannot be postponed. Active treatment is directed towards optimizing maternal health while minimizing fetal risk.

REFERENCES

1. Giglio JA, Lanni SM, Laskin DM, et al. Oral health for the pregnant patient. J Can Dent Assoc. 2009;75(1):43-8.
2. Ritter AV, Southerland JH. Pregnancy and oral health. J Esthet Restor Dent. 2007;19(6):373-4.
3. Antony VV, Khan R. Dentistry for the pregnant patient. J Dent Med Sci. 2014;13(1):83-90.
4. Kandan PM, Menaga V, Kumar RR. Oral health in pregnancy. J Pak Med Assoc. 2011;61(10):1009-14.
5. Kumar J, Samelson R. Oral Health Care During Pregnancy-Recommendations for Oral Health Professional. N Y State Dent J. 2009;75(6):29-33.
6. Ngeow WC, Chai WL. Understanding the dental need and care during pregnancy—a review. Med J Malaysia. 1999;54(1):146-50.
7. Kanotra S, Sholapurkar AA, Pai KM. Dental consideration in pregnancy: review. Rev Clin Pesq Odontol. 2010;6(2):161-5.
8. Turner M, Aziz SR. Management of the pregnant oral and maxillofacial surgery patient. J Oral Maxillofac Surg. 2002;60(12):1479-88.
9. Kurien S, Kattimani VS, Sriram RR, Sriram SK, Rao VK, Bhupathi A, et al. Management of pregnant patient in dentistry. J Int Oral Health. 2013;5(1):88-97.
10. Amerena VC. Oral care during pregnancy. Australian Dental Practice. 2010;102-4.
11. Hemalatha VT, Manigandan T, Sarumathi T, et al. Dental Consideration in Pregnancy—A Critical Review on the Oral Care. J Clin Diagn Res. 2013;7(5):948-53.
12. American Academy on Pediatric Dentistry Council on Clinical Affairs Committee on the Adolescent. Guidelines on oral health care for the pregnant adolescent. Pediatr Dent. 2008-2009;30(7):102-6.
13. Wong D, Cheng A, Kunchur R, Lam S, Sambrook PJ, Goss AN. Management of severe odontogenic infections in pregnancy. Aust Dent J. 2012;57(4):498-503.
14. Mendia J, Cuddy MA, Moore PA. Drug therapy for the pregnant dental patient. Compend Contin Educ Dent. 2012;33(8): 568-70, 572, 574-6 passim; quiz 579, 596.
15. Gonzaga HF, Buso L, Jorge MA, et al. Intrauterine dentistry: An integrated model of prevention. Braz Dent J. 2001;12(2):139-42.
16. Cengiz SB. The pregnant patient: considerations for dental management and drug use. Quintessence Int. 2007;38(3):e133-42.

CHAPTER 69

Obesity

Geeta Doppa, Ravikanth O Gowder

INTRODUCTION

Obesity is a challenge which every obstetrician is facing nowadays. Number of women who are overweight or obese getting pregnant is on a rise. Adverse effects of obesity on pregnancy begin prior to conception as obesity reduces fertility, also affects health of human oocyte quality and development of embryo in early gestation.[1,2] Obesity in pregnancy is also associated with increased chances of miscarriage.[3,4] It is associated with various health problems in mother and fetus throughout pregnancy and puerperium. Many women are not aware of these complications and they conceive when obese also, they do not know about the weight gain in pregnancy and after delivery also do not lose weight and conceive again with the same obesity. It is the duty of healthcare takers to give them the advice in this aspect of importance of weight reduction. Also the specialists who take care of these obese pregnant women must be aware of the complications of obesity to mother and fetus and also how to prevent and manage these complications.

INCIDENCE

In a recent survey it has been found that in the United States more than one-third of women are obese, more than half of pregnant women are overweight or obese and 8% of reproductive aged women are extremely obese.[5,6] This rising trend of obesity is seen in developed as well as in developing countries like India.[5] The prevalence of obesity has trebled in UK since 1980 and continues to rise. In UK 22% men, 24% women and 10% of children are obese.[7] The World Health Organization (WHO) describes obesity as: one of the most blatantly visible, yet most neglected, public health problems that threatens to overwhelm both more or less developed countries. A recent study showed that 1 in 5 women booking for antenatal care in 2002–2004 were obese.[8] Beginning of 21st century, morbid obesity population in India is estimated to be attributed to multiple factors like lack of physical activity and excessive consumption of diet rich in calories and added to this is genetic predispositions which lead to increased fat deposition and obesity.

Obesity is defined in terms of body mass index (BMI). It is calculated as weight in kilograms (kg) divided by height in meter square (m^2). Obesity during pregnancy is defined as BMI more than 30 kg/m^2 or more calculated using a prepregnancy weight but many times it is unknown so the weight at first antenatal visit is taken.[3] Table 1 shows categorization of maternal BMI by WHO.

COMPLICATIONS OF OBESITY IN PREGNANCY

Antenatal

Maternal

- Impaired glucose tolerance and gestational diabetes[3]
- Pre-eclampsia[3]
- Thromboembolism[3]

TABLE 1: Maternal body mass index categorized by World Health Organization[9]

S. no.	Types	Body mass index
1.	Underweight	<18.5 kg/m^2
2.	Normal	18.5–24.9 kg/m^2
3.	Overweight: Body mass index	25–29.99 kg/m^2
4.	Obese class 1	30–34.99 kg/m^2
5.	Obese class 2	35–39.99 kg/m^2
6.	Obese class 3	>40 kg/m^2

- Obstructive sleep apnea[10]
- Maternal death.[3]

Fetal[11,12]

- Prematurity
- Stillbirth
- Increased incidence of congenital anomalies
- Macrosomia
- Small for gestational age and intrauterine death.

Intrapartum

- Induction of labor, prolonged labor and failure to progress[13]
- Increased incidence of instrumental delivery, cesarean sections and postpartum hemorrhage[13-15]
- Shoulder dystocia[16]
- Difficulty in fetal heart rate monitoring[17]
- Difficulty in labor analgesia,[3] general anesthesia is also risky.

Anesthetic Risks[3]

- Difficulty in positioning for anesthesia, obscured landmarks, excessive adipose tissue and edema
- Difficult intubation, difficult to maintain adequate airway, sleep apnea occurring in these cases may further complicate anesthetic management and postoperative care
- Increased risk of need for intensive care unit (ICU) care postoperatively[14]
- Obese women have associated comorbidities like hypertension, diabetes, cardiac ailments, etc. which makes anesthesia more risky.

Postpartum

- Increased risk of thromboembolism[18]
- Postpartum hemorrhage[19]
- Delayed wound healing, increased chances of wound infection and endometritis
- Postnatal depression[20]
- Problem in initiation and maintenance of lactation[21]
- Increased requirement of neonatal intensive care
- Low APGAR scores at 5 minutes and fetal distress
- Maternal mortality.

Long-term Effects[22]

Maternal

- Impaired glucose tolerance
- Type-2 diabetes mellitus
- Cardiovascular disease
- Hypertension.

Fetal

- Reduced breast-feeding
- Increased overfeeding
- Increased risk of developing childhood obesity
- Increased risk of cardiometabolic complications in adult life.

MANAGEMENT OF OBESE PATIENTS DURING THIRD TRIMESTER AND PUERPERIUM

Ideally obese women should receive preconceptional counseling to reduce weight and advice on nutrition and exercise. Ray et al.[23] and Watkins et al.[24] in their study conclude that great emphasis needs to be placed on ensuring that reproductive aged women are of healthy weight preconceptionally. The obesity in pregnancy is associated with increased incidence of neural tube defects along with many other problems.

The adverse effects of obesity on pregnancy must be explained to them. Some studies have reported a higher rate of premature delivery for obese women than for women of normal weight. A large Swedish cohort study reported a greater risk of antepartum stillbirth among obese patients than among women who had a BMI of less than 20.

Obese pregnant women are at increased risk to give birth to infant with congenital anomalies. A dedicated anomaly scan in second trimester during 18–20 weeks is essential. About 15% of normally visible structures will be suboptimally seen in women with a BMI above the 90th percentile. The anatomic structures commonly less seen with increasing BMI include fetal heart, spine, kidneys, diaphragm and umbilical cord. Nuthalapathy and Rouse[25] reviewed 17 studies which were published between 1978 and 2003 are associated with maternal prepregnancy BMI with congenital anomalies. They reported a 2-fold increase in neural tube defects in the offspring of woman. Weiss[26] and colleagues have reported adverse outcomes and maternal morbidity in a prospective multicenter study of more than 16,000 women with class 1 and 2 obesity in the First and Second Trimester Evaluation of Risk (FASTER) Trial. The trial shows a marked increase in gestational hypertension and diabetes; also there was an increase in cesarean section risks: 33.8% for obese and 47.4% for morbidly obese compared with 20.7% in controls.

The number of obese reproductive aged women undergoing bariatric surgeries is increasing. The pregnancies after bariatric surgery are less likely to be complicated by gestational diabetes, pre-eclampsia and macrosomia than obese women who have not undergone such surgery.

Metabolic Syndrome

It is defined by the US National Cholesterol Education Program as presence of any three of the following conditions:[27]

- Excessive weight around the waist (waist measurement of more than 40 inches for men and more than 35 inches for women)
- High levels of triglyceride
- Low levels of high-density lipoprotein good cholesterol (below 40 mg/dL for men and below 50 mg/dL for women)
- High blood pressure (130/85 mm Hg or higher)
- High fasting blood glucose levels (110 mg/dL or higher).

Boney et al. suggested that obese mothers who do not fulfill criteria for gestational diabetes might still have metabolic factors that affect fetal growth and postnatal outcomes.

ANTENATAL CARE

Antenatal facilities must be well equipped to give adequate care to obese patients. Weighing machines which are calibrated up to 200 kg, large BP cuffs (15 × 33 cm for arm), appropriate chairs for sitting and suitable tables for examination must be there.

Gestational Weight Gain

Body mass index should be calculated depending on prepregnancy weight. Women must be offered services of dietitian and exercise physiologist. Weight gain must be assessed in every visit. BMI is not the perfect measure given it does not take into account age or ethnicity; however, it is widely considered a good measure of obesity in general population.

Fat deposition is greater in women with high BMI and thus energy costs are significantly lower. Kinoshita and Itoh[28] studied regional fat distribution changes during pregnancy using ultrasonography. They found that in third trimester increases were mainly in visceral fat. Inspite these stores they found that maternal catabolism is not good for fetal growth and development. Thus, pregnant women should not lose weight in pregnancy but limit the weight gain to 20 pounds. Chu and associates[29] reported in US in 2004–2005 that 40% of normal weight and 60% of overweight women gained excessive weight in pregnancy.

Pre-eclampsia Screening

There is an increased risk of pre-eclampsia in obese women, so appropriate screening must be done. The majority of studies show that maternal obesity is an important factor for gestational hypertension. The literature shows that overall obese pregnant women have 14–25% of pre-eclampsia. Recent studies show that a low level of sex hormone binding globulin, a marker of insulin resistance in obese women, is an early predictor of pre-eclampsia, allowing preventive treatment.

There is no doubt that obesity is a consistent risk factor for pre-eclampsia [Cedergren (2004);[30] Jensen (2003);[31] Sebire (2001);[32] Weiss (2004)[26] and all their colleagues]. O'Brien[33] and associates (2003) found that pre-eclampsia risk doubled with each 5–7 kg/m^2 increase in prepregnancy BMI. Ramsay[34] and coworkers (2002) confirmed that obese pregnant women had significantly elevated serum levels of interleukin-6 and C-reactive protein as well as impaired endothelial function. They also found that obese pregnant women had significantly higher levels of triglycerides, very low-density lipoprotein cholesterol, insulin, and leptin compared with normal weight pregnant women.

Low-dose aspirin 75 mg can be started from 12 weeks if they have additional risk factors like primi, maternal age more than 40 years, family history of pre-eclampsia, and multiple pregnancy.

Ultrasound Examination

Obesity will make assessment of anatomy, fetal size and fetal well-being more difficult.

Maternal obesity can make clinical assessment of fetal growth difficult, liquor and fetal weight estimation, diagnosis of intrauterine growth restriction (IUGR) is difficult. Ultrasound can provide more accurate assessment despite its limitations. The Atlanta Birth Defect Risk Factor Surveillance population-based control study found that for every incremental unit increase in BMI the risk of neural tube defect increased by 7%.[24] Hendricks et al.[35] showed that hyperinsulinemia was an independent risk factor for neural tube defects but, even for adjustment for hyperinsulinemia, obesity continued to be the modest risk factor. Other possible mechanisms in association between obesity and neural tube defects include increased triglycerides, uric acid, and endogenous estrogen levels in addition to insulin resistance. Werler et al.[36] in their study of neural tube defects and other congenital malformations and maternal prepregnant weight concluded that the risk of neural tube defects increases with increasing prepregnant weight, independent of the effects of folate intake.

Screening for Gestational Diabetes

Gestational diabetes is defined by the American Diabetes Association[37] as any degree of glucose intolerance with onset or first recognition during pregnancy. Ethnicity, prepregnancy weight, previous gestational diabetes mellitus, age, parity and family history of diabetes are factors related to development of gestational diabetes. Approximately 1–3% women compared to 17% of obese women develop gestational diabetes during pregnancy. Obese women with this problem have twice the risk of delivering children with chromosomal defects than those without. Overweight and obese women must be screened for gestational diabetes in early weeks and repeat at 28 weeks and later.

Anesthetic Assessment

Women who are obese must be referred for anesthetic assessment prior to delivery or at least during first stage of labor. These patients are at risk of anesthesia problems; both regional and general anesthesia.

Previous Cesarean Section Cases

Vaginal birth after cesarean is less likely to be successful in the obese gravid cases [Bujold (2005);[38] Goodall (2005);[39] Hibbard (2006);[40] Robinson (2005),[41] and all their colleagues]. Hence these women must be counseled regarding mode of delivery in antenatal period. The decision on mode of delivery is taken by considering the risk factors during labor. During the antenatal visits, identification of any complication must be done at earliest.

Postbariatric Surgery Cases

A number of surgical procedures are done to treat morbid obesity by either decreasing gastric volume or bypassing gastrointestinal absorption. Three procedures are commonly performed: (1) vertical gastroplasty, (2) gastric banding, and (3) Roux-en-Y gastric bypass. Older procedures no longer in use include jejunoileal bypass and upper gastrojejunostomy bypass.

Pregnant patients who have undergone bariatric surgery need to be supplemented with folate, vitamin B12, vitamin D, and calcium. Women with gastric banding should be monitored by surgeons whether adjustment of band required. These cases must be monitored for development of IUGR in fetus. Bariatric surgery itself is not an indication for cesarean section.

Intrauterine Death

Study of Sebire et al. showed that obese parous women had a significantly increased risk of late fetal death relative to women of normal weight (BMI 20–25 kg/m^2) after adjustment for obesity-related diseases in pregnancy. Also Cedergren found that morbidly obese women (BMI >40 kg/m^2) had an almost 3-fold increased risk of antepartum stillbirth. Nohr et al.[42] stated that the stillbirth may be due to rapid fetal growth due to fetal hyperglycemia, which may lead to fetal hypoxia and death if placenta cannot transfer sufficient oxygen for metabolic requirements.

INTRAPARTUM CARE

Vaginal delivery: women with BMI more than 40 kg/m^2 should have an intravenous (IV) line placed on admission to labor ward. More personnel must be available during delivery to tackle problems which may arise like shoulder dystocia, postpartum hemorrhage. Active management of labor must be done in all cases. Shoulder dystocia is defined as a delivery in which additional maneuvers are required to deliver the fetus after normal gentle downward traction has failed. It occurs after the anterior shoulder impacts against the maternal symphysis following the delivery of vertex. Risk factor associated with shoulder dystocia are fetal macrosomia, maternal diabetes mellitus, post-term pregnancy, prolonged second stage of labor, history of previous macrosomic infant, instrumental delivery, advanced maternal age, multiparity and maternal obesity. The shoulder dystocia results in maternal complications like postpartum hemorrhage, rectovaginal fistula, perineal tears, uterine rupture and symphyseal diathesis or separation. In fetus it leads to brachial plexus injury, fracture of clavicle or humerus, fetal hypoxia or fetal death, all these leading to increased neonatal ICU admissions.

Cesarean Section

Haeri and coworkers[43] have found increased rates of cesarean sections in obese adolescents. Lynch and associates (2008),[44] showed that obese women have increased rate of emergency cesareans.

Operating tables should be of adequate size. Arrangement of blood and blood products is to be made as obese women have increased rates of excessive blood loss. Surgery may take long operating time. Antimicrobial prophylaxis should be given using a higher dose before cesarean section. Maternal obesity is independent risk factor for cesarean section. Sheiner et al.[45] found that the association between obesity and cesarean section remained significant after controlling variables recognized to coexist with obesity. They also found that obese women were more likely to have labor induction, failure to progress during first stage of labor, meconium-stained amniotic fluid, malpresentations and so more cesarean sections than non-obese women. Usha et al. study shows that woman with BMI 30 kg/m^2 have a 1–2 fold higher risk of cesarean section. The cause for increased cesarean section may be large for gestational age infants leading to disproportion during labor; they also suggest that it may be possible that uterine contractility may be suboptimal in a subgroup of obese women, or there may be increased fat deposition in the soft tissues of the pelvis. They also state that higher rates of cesarean sections may be due to higher incidence of post term and difficulty with induction leading to other interventions. Similarly Sebire et al. showed that cesarean section rate for obese women was over 20% compared to near 10% for normal weight women.

Placement of pneumatic compression devices before cesarean delivery is recommended for all women who are not receiving thromboprophylaxis due to increased risk of thromboembolism.

Alexander and Liston (2006)[46] stated that for cesarean delivery forethought must be given to optimal placement and type of abdominal incision to allow access to the fetus and for effective wound closure with the least intervening tissue.

Correct decision regarding placement of surgical incision is essential that is placing incision above the panniculus adiposus. Wall and colleagues (2003)[47] reported a 4-fold wound complication rate when a vertical abdominal incision was compared with transverse incision (31% versus 8%). Studies have shown that suture closure of the subcutaneous layer after cesarean delivery in obese may lead to significant reduction in incidence of postoperative wound disruption.

Chelmow and associates (2004)[48] performed a meta-analysis of subcutaneous closure in 887 women undergoing cesarean delivery and whose wound thickness was greater than 2 cm. They reported that subcutaneous closure showed 6% decrease in wound disruption. National Institute for Health and Care Excellence (NICE) guideline 13 recommends to suture the subcutaneous tissue space in woman who have more than 2 cm subcutaneous fat to reduce risk of wound infection and separation.

POSTPARTUM

Postpartum Hemorrhage

Studies have shown that obese women have higher rates of postpartum hemorrhage. Usha et al. showed that obese women who had a vaginal delivery had a greater than 500 mL blood loss compared to those with a BMI of 20–30 kg/m^2. Sebire et al. noted a 44% increased risk of postpartum hemorrhage in gravidas with a BMI 30 kg/m^2. They suggested that it might be explained by excessive bleeding from the relatively larger area of implantation of the placenta usually associated with a large for gestational age fetus. Nuthalapathy and Rouse told the possibility of relatively larger volume of distribution related to obesity and resultant decreases in bioavailability of uterotonic agents may be another cause.

Thromboembolism Prophylaxis

Obese hospitalized and immobile patients are at risk of thromboembolism. Their risks have to be individualized and plan for thromboprophylaxis must be done. Pneumatic compression devices and unfractionated heparin or low-molecular weight (LMW) heparin may be used. Postpartum prophylaxis with heparin has also been recommended for patients thought to be at risk for venous thromboembolism. All women receiving LMW heparin antenatally should continue prophylactic doses till 6 weeks postpartum but risk assessment must be done. Women with BMI greater than 30 kg/m^2 should be encouraged to mobilize as early as possible following childbirth to reduce risk of thromboembolism. All women with BMI greater than 40 kg/m^2 should be advised post-thromboprophylaxis regardless of mode of delivery.

Breastfeeding

Maternal obesity reduces the rates of initiation and duration of breastfeeding. Ruowei and coworkers (2003)[49] reported that obese women were less likely to breastfeed. The causes may be difficulty with correct positioning of the baby, possibility of impaired prolactin response to suckling. Armstrong and colleagues (2002)[50] reported that breastfeeding decreases the risk of childhood obesity. So these women must be counseled regarding the benefits of breast-feeding during each antenatal visit.

Perinatal Morbidity

Fetal and neonatal complications are increased in obese women. Rasmussen and associates (2008)[51] found that 1.2-, 1.7-, and 3.1-fold increased risks of neural tube defects in overweight, obese and severely obese women compared with controls of normal weight. Watkins and associates (2003)[52] reported 3.5-fold increase in rates of neural tube defects. They also found a 2–3 fold increased incidence in omphalocele, heart defect and multiple anomalies in obese women.

Obesity in pregnancy is associated with chronic hypertension and diabetes. Chronic hypertension is a well-known cause of fetal growth restriction. Pregestational diabetes increases the rate of birth defects and gestational is complicated by large for gestational age and macrosomia. Bianco and coworkers (1998),[53] Cedergren (2004); Isaacs et al. (1994)[54] stated that even without diabetes the prevalence of macrosomic newborn is increased in obese women.

Postpartum Care

Obese women should receive advice from trained professionals regarding diet and exercise even during postnatal period. They should reduce their weights if planning next pregnancy; gestational diabetics should have their sugars tested at 6 weeks postpartum. They should regularly follow-up with physicians to screen for development of type 2 diabetes.

Linne et al.[55] followed up 28 women with gestational diabetes mellitus and a control group for 15 years and found that women with gestational diabetes mellitus who developed type 2 diabetes mellitus gained significantly more weight 15.1 kg following birth of their first child compared to women without gestational diabetes mellitus and women with gestational diabetes mellitus who did not develop type-2 diabetes mellitus. So even after delivery gestational diabetic patients should follow strategies for weight control and exercise regularly to prevent type-2 diabetes in future and associated morbidity and mortality.

During pregnancy, 2–10 kg of fat is stored in women's bodies; 14–20% of women are unable to lose this weight, on average gaining about 5 kg or more weight post pregnancy. But this excess is to be reduced as obesity leads to chronic morbidities like cardiovascular diseases and type-2 diabetes mellitus in future life.

CONCLUSION

Obesity in pregnancy is a major problem obstetricians are facing nowadays. Preconceptional counseling is important in obese women. Pregnancy and puerperium are associated with various risks like pre-eclampsia, gestational diabetes mellitus, increasing rates of cesarean section, more chance of postpartum hemorrhage, anesthetic problems, postoperative wound infections, venous thromboembolism, more chances of neural defects in fetus, breastfeeding problems, etc. So they should receive proper antenatal care; nutritionist and exercise physiotherapist also play an important role. Patients undergone bariatric surgery need nutritional supplementation and we have to watch for IUGR in fetus. Post-delivery, obese women should continue diet and exercise and reduce weight especially if they are planning another pregnancy. Modification of diet and physical activities are associated with significant reduction in body weight.

REFERENCES

1. Robker RL. Evidence that obesity alters the quality of oocytes and embryos. Pathophysiology. 2008;15(2):115-21.
2. Wu LL, Norman RJ, Robker RL. The impact of obesity on oocytes: evidence for lipotoxicity mechanisms. Reprod Fertil Devel. 2011;24(1):29-34.
3. National Institute of Health and Clinical Excellence. Weight management before, during and after pregnancy. 2010.
4. The American College of Obstetricians and Gynecologists. Obesity in Pregnancy: Committee Opinion Number 548. 2013.
5. Flegal KM, Carroll MD, Kit BK, Ogden CL. Prevalence of obesity and trends in the distribution of body mass index among US adults, 1999–2010. JAMA. 2012;307(5):491-7.
6. The American College of Obstetricians and Gynecologists. Obesity in Pregnancy: Committee Opinion Number 549. 2013.
7. Vlad I. Obesity costs UK economy 2bn pounds sterling a year. BMJ. 2003;327:1308.
8. Kanagalingam MG, Forouhi NG, Greer IA, Sattar N. Changes in booking body mass index over a decade: retrospective analysis from a Glasgow Maternity Hospital. Br J Obstet Gynaecol. 2005;112:1431-3.
9. World Health Organization. Global Database on Body Mass Index: BMI Classification 2006. [cited September 2013].
10. Maasilta P, Bachour A, Teramo K, Polo O, Laitinen LA. Sleep-related disordered breathing during pregnancy in obese women. Chest. 2001;120(5):1448-54.
11. Crane JM, Murphy P, Burrage L, Hutchens D. Maternal and perinatal outcomes of extreme obesity in pregnancy. J Obstet Gynaecol Can. 2013;35(7):606-11.
12. Salihu HM. Maternal obesity and stillbirth. Sem Perinat. 2011;35(6):340-4.
13. Yu CK, Teoh TG, Robinson S. Obesity in pregnancy. BJOG. 2006;113(10):1117-25.
14. Chu SY, Kim SY, Schmid CH, Dietz PM, Callaghan WM, Lau J, et al. Maternal obesity and risk of cesarean delivery: a meta-analysis. Obes Rev. 2007;8(5):385-94.
15. McIntyre HD, Gibbons KS, Flenady VJ, Callaway LK. Overweight and obesity in Australian mothers: epidemic or endemic? Med J Aust. 2012;196(3):184-8.
16. Gherman RB. Shoulder dystocia: an evidence-based evaluation of the obstetric nightmare. Clin Obstet Gynecol. 2002;45(2):345-62.
17. Fraser R. CK. Problems of obesity in obstetric care. Curr Obstet Gynaecol. 2003;13(4):239-43.
18. Thromboembolism in pregnancy. Practice Bulletin No. 123. American College of Obstetricians and Gynecologists. Obstet Gynecol. 2011;118:718-29.
19. Usha KT, Hemmadi S, Bethal J, Evans J. Outcome of pregnancy in a women with increased body mass index. Br J Obstet Gynecol. 2005;112:768-72.
20. Institute of Medicine (US) and National Research Council (US) Committee to Re-examine IOM Pregnancy Weight Guidelines. Weight Gain During Pregnancy: Re-examining the Guidelines. Washington DC: National Academy of Sciences; 2009.
21. Amir LH, Donath S. A systematic review of maternal obesity and breastfeeding intention, initiation and duration. BMC Pregnancy Childbirth. 2007;7:9.
22. Kriplani G. Current Progress Obstet Gynecol, Polyscystic ovarian syndrome. Infertility and Obesity. 2012:1;403-4.
23. Ray JG, Wyatt PR, Vermeulen MJ, Meier C, Cole DE. General maternal weight and the ongoing risks of neural tube defects after folic acid flour fortification. Obstet Gynecol. 2005;105:261-5.
24. Watkins ML, Rasmussen SA, Honein MA, Botto LD, Moore CA. Maternal obesity and risk of birth defects. Pediatrics. 2003;111:1152-8.
25. Nuthalapathy FS, Rouse DJ. The impact of obesity on obstetrical practise and outcome. Clin Obstet Gynaecol. 2004;47:898-913.
26. Weiss JL, Malone FD, Emig D, Ball RH, Nyberg DA, Comstock CH, et al. Obesity, obstetric complications and cesarean delivery rate—a population based screening study. Am J Obstet Gynecol. 2004;190:1091-7.
27. National Cholesterol Education Program. Third Report of the Expert Panel on Detection, Evaluation, and Treatment of High Blood Cholesterol in Adults (Adult Treatment Panel iii. Bethesda, MD: National Heart, Lung, and Blood Institute; National Institutes of Health; 2001.
28. Kinoshita T, Itoh M. Longitudinal variance of fat mass deposition during pregnancy evaluated by ultrasonography: the ratio of visceral fat to subcutaneous fat in the abdomen. Gynecol Obstet Invest. 2006;61:115-8.
29. Chu SY, Callaghan WM, Bish CL, D'Angelo D. Gestational weight gain by body mass index among US women delivering live births, 2004-2005: fueling future obesity. Am J Obstet Gynecol. 2009;200:271.e1-7.
30. Cedergren MI. Maternal morbid obesity and the risk of adverse pregnancy outcome. Obstet Gynecol. 2004;103:219-24.
31. Jensen DM, Damm P, Sorensen B, Mølsted-Pedersen L, Westergaard JG, Ovesen P, et al. Pregnancy outcome and prepregnancy body mass index in 2459 glucose-tolerant Danish women. Am J Obstet Gynecol. 2003;189:239-44.
32. Sebire NJ, Jolly M, Harris JP, Wadsworth J, Joffe M, Beard RW, et al. Maternal obesity and pregnancy outcome: A study of 287,213 pregnancies in London. Int J Obes Relat Metab Disord. 2001;25:1175-82.

33. O'Brien TE, Ray JG, Chan WS. Maternal body mass index and the risk of preeclampsia: A systematic overview. Epidemiology. 2003;14:368-74.
34. Ramsay JE, Ferrell WR, Crawford L, Wallace AM, Greer IA, Sattar N. Maternal obesity is associated with dysregulation of metabolic, vascular, and inflammatory pathways. J Clin Endocrinol Metab. 2002;87:4231-7.
35. Hendricks KA, Numo OM, Sourez L, Larsen R. Effects of hyperinsulinemia and obesity on risk of neural tube defects among Mexican Americans. Epidemiology. 2001;12:630-5.
36. Werler MM, Louik C, Shappiro S, Mitchell AA. Prepregnant weight in relation to risk of neural defects. JAMA. 1996;275(14):1089-92.
37. American Diabetic Association. Gestational diabetes mellitus. Diabetes Care. 2003;26:S103-5.
38. Bujold E, Hammoud A, Schild C, Krapp M, Baumann P. The role of maternal body mass index in outcomes of vaginal births after cesarean. Am J Obstet Gynecol. 2005;193(4):1517-21.
39. Goodall PT, Ahn JT, Chapa JB, Hibbard JU. Obesity as a risk factor for failed trial of labor in patients with previous cesarean delivery. Am J Obstet Gynecol. 2005;192:1423-6.
40. Hibbard JU, Gilbert S, Landon MB, Hauth JC, Leveno KJ, Spong CY, et al. Trial of labor or repeat cesarean delivery in women with morbid obesity and previous cesarean delivery. Obstet Gynecol. 2006;108(1):125-33.
41. Robinson HE, O'Connell CM, Joseph KS, McLeod NL. Maternal outcomes in pregnancies complicated by obesity. Obstet Gynecol. 2005;106(6):1357-64.
42. Nohr EA, Bech BH, Davies MJ, Frydenberg M, Henriksen TB, Olsen J. Pregnancy obesity and fetal death: a study within the Danish National Birth Cohort. Obstet Gynecol. 2005;106:250-9.
43. Haeri S, Guichard I, Baker AM, Saddlemire S, Boggess KA. The effect of teenage maternal obesity on perinatal outcomes. Obstet Gynecol. 2009;113:300-4.
44. Lynch CM, Sexton DJ, Hession M, Morrison JJ. Obesity and mode of delivery in primigravid and multigravid women. Am J Perinatol. 2008;25(3):163-7.
45. Sheiner E, Levy A, Menes TS, Silverberg D, Kartz M, Mazor M. Maternal obesity as an independent risk factor for caesarean delivery. Paediatr Perinat Epidemiol. 2004;18:196-201.
46. Alexander CI, Liston WA. Operating on the obese woman—A review. BJOG. 2006;113(10):1167-72.
47. Wall PD, Deucy EE, Glantz JC, Pressman EK. Vertical skin incisions and wound complications in the obese parturient. Obstet Gynecol. 2003;102:952-6.
48. Chelmow D, Rodriquez EJ, Sabatini MM. Suture closure of subcutaneous fat and wound disruption after cesarean delivery: A meta-analysis. Obstet Gynecol. 2004;103:974-80.
49. Li R, Jewell S, Grummer-Strawn L. Maternal obesity and breast-feeding practices. Am J Clin Nutr. 2003;77:931-6.
50. Armstrong J, Reilly JJ; Child Health Information Team. Breastfeeding and lowering the risk of childhood obesity. Lancet. 2002;359:2003-4.
51. Rasmussen SA, Chu SY, Kim SY, Schmid CH, Lau J. Maternal obesity and risk of neural tube defects; a metaanalysis. Am J Obstet Gynecol. 2008;198(6):611-9.
52. Watkins ML, Rasmussen SA, Honein MA, Botto LD, Moore CA. Maternal obesity and risk for birth defects. Pediatrics. 2003;111:1152-8.
53. Bianco AT, Smilen SW, Davis Y, Lopez S, Lapinski R, Lockwood CJ. Pregnancy outcome and weight gain recommendations for the morbidly obese woman. Obstet Gynecol. 1998;91:97-102.
54. Isaacs JD, Magann EF, Martin RW, Chauhan SP, Morrison JC. Obstetric challenges of massive obesity complicating pregnancy. J Perinatol. 1994;14:10-4.
55. Linne Y. Effects of obesity on women's reproduction and complications during pregnancy. Obes Rev. 2004;5:137-43.

CHAPTER 70

Human Immunodeficiency Virus

Rashmi Bagga, Parul Arora

INTRODUCTION

Human immunodeficiency virus (HIV) infection is associated with significant morbidity and mortality. Antiretroviral therapy (ART) with a combination of three or more antiretroviral (ARV) drugs is the current standard of care in HIV-infected individuals and this helps to improve the length as well as the quality of life. Besides concerns for an HIV-infected woman's health, if she gets pregnant, the issue of perinatal transmission and methods to reduce it assumes significant importance. The risk of perinatal transmission ranges from 15 to 20% in nonbreastfeeding populations in Europe and from 25 to 40% in breastfeeding African, populations.[1] Perinatal transmission can be reduced to less than 2% with suitable measures such as ART, delivery by elective cesarean section (CS), and giving replacement feeds to the baby. Some of these interventions may not be feasible for resource-poor countries, like India and Sub-Saharan Africa and are modified to be implemented in such countries.[2] But, even with best possible measures taken to prevent perinatal transmission, no intervention guarantees a zero transmission rate of HIV infection to the baby.

MAGNITUDE OF THE PROBLEM

Global

The reported global estimate of 35.3 million people living with HIV in 2012, showed an increase from previous years (30 million in 2001) as more people are receiving lifesaving ART. There were 2.3 million new HIV infections in 2012, showing a 33% decline from 3.4 million in 2001. The number of acquired immunodeficiency syndrome (AIDS) deaths is also declining with 1.6 (1.4–1.9) million AIDS deaths in 2012, down from 2.3 (2.1–2.6) million in 2005.[3]

National

In India, there were 22.5 lakhs people living with human immunodeficiency virus (PLHIV) in 2007, which reduced to 20.9 lakhs in 2011. The HIV prevalence among adults in India has declined over the last decade (0.4% in 2000 to 0.27% in 2011); women constitute 39% of PLHIV while children about 7%.[4] Based on HIV prevalence rates in the adult population estimated from the National Sentinel Surveillance rounds, India's states and union territories are divided into three groups:

1. High prevalence of HIV infection more than 1% among antenatal (AN) women (Maharashtra, Tamil Nadu, Karnataka, Andhra Pradesh, Manipur, and Nagaland),
2. Moderate prevalence less than 1% among AN women and more than 5% among high-risk groups (Gujarat, Goa, and Pondicherry)
3. Low prevalence or less than 1% among AN women and less than 5% among high risk groups.[5] The National AIDS Control Organization (NACO) launched a Prevention of Parent-to-Child Transmission (PPTCT) program for screening AN women and treating those who are HIV infected. National AIDS Control Organization had previously advocated prophylaxis with single dose nevirapine (sd-NVP) to the mother and baby which reduces perinatal transmission to about 10%.[4] Wider access to ART has resulted in around 30% reduction in mortality rates due to HIV-related causes. A total of 13,443

HIV-infected pregnant women and 11,639 HIV-infected children were detected at the integrated counseling and testing centers (ICTC) in India, in 2012–13.[4]

ETIOLOGY AND PATHOGENESIS

Human immunodeficiency viruses 1 and 2 are deoxyribonucleic acid (DNA) retroviruses which cause the immunodeficiency syndrome. Human immunodeficiency virus-1 causes most infections worldwide, including in India, whereas HIV-2 virus is endemic in West Africa. Retroviruses make DNA copies of its own genome within the host cells by transcription from ribonucleic acid (RNA) with the help of reverse transcriptase enzyme. Transmission routes are chiefly sexual (homo- or heterosexual), from blood or body fluids, and perinatal. The HIV virus attacks cells bearing the CD4 antigen, which are chiefly T-lymphocytes, some monocyte-macrophages, and microglial brain cells. After attaching to the CD4 receptors, the virus enters into the cells where it uses its reverse transcriptase enzyme to transcribe its genomic DNA. Viral DNA gets incorporated into cellular DNA and after cell death, many virions are released into the bloodstream which attack more T-cells. The cell life is shortened by this infection and the number of T-lymphocytes falls gradually, insidiously, and profoundly, leading to immunosuppression. Viremia can be detected and quantified by using viral RNA assay. The initial infection resembles an acute viral syndrome and lasts for a few days only. This is followed by a latency period (5–10 years) during which the HIV-infected individual is asymptomatic and ultimately, with profound immunosuppression, the clinical symptoms and signs of AIDS manifest. Antibodies can be detected 6 months after initial infection by enzyme-linked immunosorbent assay (ELISA).

HUMAN IMMUNODEFICIENCY VIRUS SCREENING DURING PREGNANCY

National AIDS Control Organization, India, recommends a routine voluntary screening for HIV infection with an "opt-out" approach in all pregnant women after counseling.[4] If a woman declines testing, she is counseled again during subsequent visits about the benefits of screening. Post-test counseling is offered to women who test positive. The "ANC centric" (antenatal care) approach is being replaced by the "family centric" approach by ensuring involvement of the spouse and other family members.

EFFECT OF PREGNANCY ON HUMAN IMMUNODEFICIENCY VIRUS DISEASE PROGRESSION

There has been concern that pregnancy itself, either because of associated hormonal changes or because of suppression of cellular immunity, leads to an acceleration in the disease progression. However, studies in developed countries, like United States and in Europe, have not shown any effect of pregnancy on disease progression.[6,7] Although CD4 count falls during pregnancy, it returns to prepregnancy level in the postpartum period and there is no increased risk of accelerated immunosuppression during pregnancy. An observational study of 140 HIV-seropositive asymptomatic women of childbearing age in Haiti (1984–92), in which 44 women were pregnant or became pregnant during the study period, showed that there was a trend toward earlier manifestation of HIV-related symptoms among the pregnant cohort, but no significant difference was observed in the rate of progression to AIDS or death between the pregnant and nonpregnant women.[8] A study among 71 tribal women with AIDS in Manipur, India (1992–96) showed that pregnancy had a detrimental effect on maternal and obstetric outcome and accelerated disease progression in women with AIDS.[9]

EFFECT OF HUMAN IMMUNODEFICIENCY VIRUS DISEASE ON PREGNANCY

Human immunodeficiency virus infection, especially when more advanced, may adversely affect pregnancy outcome. There is evidence of a possible increased risk of spontaneous abortion, fetal growth restriction, low birth weight, and preterm birth but no increase in congenital malformations.[10] More adverse outcomes were seen among women with advanced disease.[10] There is increased susceptibility to certain infections or alteration in their natural course or increased perinatal transmission. These include vulvovaginal candidiasis, bacterial vaginosis, genital herpes, syphilis, human papillomavirus infection, cytomegalovirus infection, toxoplasmosis, and hepatitis B and C.[11] Women with either HIV or malaria infection have a significantly increased risk of adverse outcomes of pregnancy and childbirth. Dual infection has additional detrimental effects on maternal and infant survival in an area where HIV and malaria coexist.[12]

TIMING OF VERTICAL TRANSMISSION

Mother-to-child transmission (MTCT) can occur during pregnancy, labor and delivery, and during breastfeeding. According to the Pediatric Virology Committee of the AIDS Clinical Trials Group in the United States, a child with a positive polymerase chain reaction (PCR) within 48 hours of birth has been affected *in-utero* and a positive PCR within 7–90 days of birth indicates an intrapartum infection.[13] Majority (65–75%) of the transmissions occur during the intrapartum period, the postulated mechanisms being maternofetal microtransfusions during uterine contractions and exposure of the baby's mucocutaneous surfaces to maternal blood and cervicovaginal secretions during delivery. Some proportion (25–35%) occur during antenatal period as HIV has been shown to cross the placental barrier early in pregnancy and most of these occur in the late third trimester (after 36 weeks).[14] Breastfeeding is associated with a twofold increase in transmission and it results in excess transmission rates of 12–16%, and the risk is maximum during the first 6 months of life.[10]

FACTORS INFLUENCING VERTICAL TRANSMISSION OF HUMAN IMMUNODEFICIENCY VIRUS

Human Immunodeficiency Virus-related Factors

The risk is reduced when the maternal plasma HIV-RNA level is low or undetectable and CD4 level is high. Reduced transmission is seen with HIV subtype 2 and T-cell tropic virus phenotype (more risk with macrophage tropic).

Maternal Factors

The risk is increased in the presence of AIDS-related symptoms, sexually transmitted infections (STIs), substance abuse, smoking, and unprotected sexual intercourse (by increasing STIs). A trial with vitamin A supplementation did not lower the overall MTCT but reduced the preterm births, and among the preterm babies, reduced HIV transmission.[15] A randomized trial in Tanzania showed that multivitamin supplementation during pregnancy, but not vitamin A, was associated with significant increase in CD4, CD8, and CD3 counts. The clinical relevance of multivitamin supplementation for reducing vertical transmission of HIV and disease progression was not known but this appeared to be a low cost measure of decreasing adverse pregnancy outcomes and increasing T-cell counts in HIV-infected women. The beneficial effects of multivitamins on birth outcomes may have been mediated through improved maternal immune status.[16]

Obstetric Factors

The risk is increased in prolonged labor, ruptured membranes (2% per hour of ruptured membranes), episiotomy, operative vaginal delivery, invasive fetal monitoring like scalp blood sampling, vaginal delivery, placental abruption, and chorioamnionitis.[17] Elective CS performed prior to ruptured membranes or labor onset (~38 weeks) reduces the vertical transmission in all HIV-infected women except in women with HIV-RNA levels less than 1,000 copies/mL at 36 weeks as in this situation, the rate of vertical transmission is already very low (<2%) and elective CS does not reduce it further. More advanced is the HIV disease status, more is the benefit obtained by elective CS for reducing perinatal transmission. But women with advanced disease themselves have more morbidity when delivered by CS.

Fetal and Neonatal Factors

The risk of perinatal transmission is higher in preterm babies as compared to term babies. It is also increased with breastfeeding especially mixed feeding, maternal breast infection or cracked nipples, and oral candidiasis in the infant. The risk is reduced by use of ART in the mother and neonate.

PREPREGNANCY COUNSELING

Before planning a pregnancy, the HIV disease status should be evaluated clinically, by CD4 count and HIV-RNA levels. If required, ART may be initiated as per guidelines in order to optimize the disease status. Sexually transmitted infections must be screened for and treated. Good general health and nutrition should be ensured, lifestyle modifications like avoidance of substance abuse encouraged. Hepatitis B immunization should be done.

TESTS FOR HUMAN IMMUNODEFICIENCY VIRUS

Human immunodeficiency virus infection is diagnosed by means of detecting antibodies to the virus in the blood of infected woman. These are commonly tested by rapid screening tests and confirmed by three different ELISA-based assays. Rapid screening tests are user-friendly and provide results within 30 minutes with a sensitivity of 99% and a false positive rate of less than 2%. These are available free of cost at the ICTC centers. Women screened by whole blood finger test at peripheral areas or in emergency require confirmatory testing at ICTC. National AIDS Control Organization recommends the use of rapid HIV kits in the ICTC. A client who has a negative result in one test is declared to be HIV-negative. When the same blood sample is tested three times using kits with different antigens/principles and the result of all three tests is positive, the client is declared to be HIV-positive. For indeterminate results (any two rapid tests positive but third negative), testing is repeated on a second sample taken after 14–28 days. In case the serological results continue to be indeterminate, then the sample is to be subjected to a Western blot/PCR if facilities are available or referred to the National Reference Laboratory for further testing. Sample for CD4 count is obtained at ART center where treatment is initiated and screening for tuberculosis (TB) and other infections is done. Both pretest and post counseling is provided at the ICTC and the spouse and children are screened for infection.

MANAGEMENT DURING PREGNANCY

These women are to be linked to the ART center and be managed by a team of an obstetrician, a physician conversant with HIV infection, a pediatrician, and a health counselor who coordinates her care. Counseling on choices of continuation or medical termination of pregnancy are undertaken within the first 3 months of pregnancy only. Management strategies during pregnancy are summarized below.

Assessment of Human Immunodeficiency Virus Disease Status and Antiretroviral Therapy

A physician classifies the pregnant women into asymptomatic HIV-positive [World Health Organization (WHO) clinical stage 1 and 2] or having advanced disease (WHO clinical stage 3 and 4). The need for initiating ART for the woman's own health was previously decided based upon HIV disease status. Women with WHO clinical stage 3 and 4 were started on triple drug ART irrespective of CD4 count. Women with WHO clinical stage 1 and 2 and CD4 less than or equal to 350 cells/mm^3 were also started on triple drug ART. Women who did not meet the criteria for ART were offered ARV prophylaxis to reduce perinatal transmission. National AIDS Control Organization, India had earlier recommended sd-NVP tablet 200 mg as ARV prophylaxis to the mother in labor and sd-NVP syrup to the newborn.

The 2010 WHO guidelines had recommended lifelong ART for women eligible for treatment (CD4 ≤350 cells/mm^3 or WHO clinical stage 3 or 4 disease) and ARV prophylaxis for prevention of MTCT for women with HIV not eligible for treatment. For those not eligible for treatment, two ARV prophylaxis regimens were recommended:[18]

Option A: zidovudine (AZT) for the mother during pregnancy, and sd-NVP plus AZT plus lamivudine (3TC) for the mother at delivery; AZT and 3TC continued for a week postpartum (tail); and

Option B: triple ARV drugs for the mother during pregnancy and breastfeeding.

Antiretroviral prophylaxis was recommended to start at 14 weeks of gestation, and both options included 4–6 weeks of NVP or AZT for the infant, regardless of breastfeeding. Countries were advised to choose a national approach for their ARV option based on operational considerations. Option A is no longer recommended due to its problems which include different treatment and prophylaxis regimens, need for CD4 level to decide treatment, and need for a postpartum ARV "tail" in mothers. In 2011, Malawi implemented a new approach of lifelong ART for all pregnant and breastfeeding women with HIV regardless of CD4 count or clinical stage, commonly referred to as Option B+ which was adopted by WHO in 2013.[19]

Recent Changes

The WHO guidelines for ART issued in 2013, focus on early initiation of ART using fixed dose combinations. In men and in nonpregnant women, ART is now recommended at CD4 less than or equal to 500 cells/mm^3, replacing the earlier threshold of less than or equal to 350 cells/mm^3. The WHO is moving away from the previous terms "Options A, B, and B+". The new WHO guidelines (2013) have two options:[20]

1. Providing lifelong ART (triple drugs) to all the pregnant and breastfeeding women living with HIV regardless of CD4 count or clinical stage, or
2. Providing ART (triple drugs) for pregnant and breastfeeding women with HIV during the MTCT risk period and continue lifelong for those eligible for treatment.

The first policy of providing lifelong ART to all the pregnant and breastfeeding women living with HIV regardless of CD4 count or clinical stage has been adopted by NACO, India in 2013 and has replaced the earlier sd-NVP prophylaxis.[4] The ART should preferably be initiated at an ART center and not delayed for want of CD4 report. The ART regimen recommended by NACO as the first line therapy is a fixed dose combination of two nucleoside reverse transcriptase inhibitor (NRTI) plus one non-nucleoside reverse transcriptase inhibitor (NNRTI). These are tenofovir 300 mg + lamivudine 300 mg in one tablet once daily and efavirenz 600 mg in another tablet once daily (TDF + 3TC + EFV). Antiretroviral therapy should be started as soon as possible even if the woman presents late in pregnancy and should be continued throughout pregnancy, delivery, breastfeeding, and lifelong thereafter.

The neonate is given syrup NVP once daily for 6 weeks (2 mg/kg if weight is <2,000 g; 10 mg if weight is 2,000–2,500 g; 15 mg for weight >2,500 g). The first dose is given within 6–12 hours after birth. The duration of NVP to infant is minimum of 6 weeks but more if ART to mother was started in late pregnancy, during or after delivery and has not been on adequate period of ART as to be effective to achieve optimal viral suppression (which is at least 24 weeks), then the duration of NVP in the infant should be increased to 12 weeks (Flowchart 1). This recommendation of extended NVP duration applies to infants of breastfeeding women only and not those on exclusive replacement feeding.

The benefits of lifelong ART for all pregnant and breastfeeding women with HIV are plenty especially in countries with high HIV rates, limited access to CD4 testing, limited partner testing, long duration of breastfeeding and high rates of fertility. This assures maximum coverage for those needing treatment for their own health, avoids stopping and starting drugs with repeat pregnancies, provides early protection against MTCT in future pregnancies, and reduces the risk of HIV transmission to HIV-serodiscordant partners.

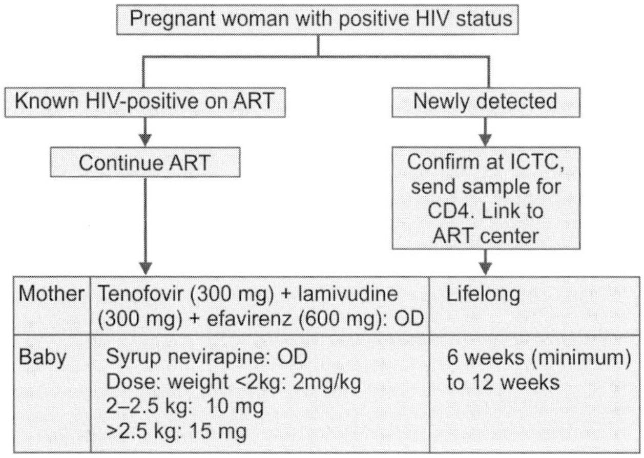

ART, antiretroviral therapy; NACO, National AIDS Control Organisation; HIV, human immunodeficiency virus; ICTC, integrated counseling and testing center; OD, once daily.

FLOWCHART 1: Antiretroviral therapy in pregnant women and neonates according to National AIDS Control Organization 2013 guidelines.

A fixed dose regimen has benefits like ease of implementation, more acceptability, increased coverage, maximum vertical transmission benefit, and maternal health benefit.

Drug Concerns

Efavirenz (NNRTI) was earlier thought to be teratogenic due to data from animal studies showing increased neural tube defects and hence, avoided in pregnancy. However, a systematic review studying the effect of EFV among 1,502 live births to women receiving EFV in the first trimester found no increase in overall birth defects.[21] If pregnancy is recognized before or after 28 days of gestation in women who are receiving an EFV-based regimen, there is no indication for abortion/termination of pregnancy due to EFV exposure in the first trimester of pregnancy. Because pregnancy is recognized at 4–6 weeks of gestation, and neural tube develops before 5–6 weeks of gestation, the women already on an EFV-based regimen should be allowed to continue the same. In a woman not on ART, an EFV-based regimen may be initiated after 8 weeks of gestation.[22]

Similarly, there were initial concerns about TDF usage include renal toxicity, adverse birth outcomes, and effects on bone density. A systematic review assessed the toxicity of fetal exposure to TDF and concluded that prevalence of all birth defects with TDF exposure in the first trimester was 2.4% which was similar to the background risk.[23] Limited studies showed no difference in fetal growth between women who were exposed to TDF and those who were not.

Zidovudine and 3TC have not been shown to be teratogenic in animals in concentrations similar to those used in humans. Zidovudine, 3TC, and NVP cross the placenta and provide prophylaxis to the fetus, unlike protease inhibitors (PIs) which do not cross the placenta.[2] Nucleoside reverse transcriptase inhibitors bind to mitochondrial DNA polymerase γ and cause mitochondrial dysfunction, which may be manifested as myopathy, cardiomyopathy, neuropathy, lactic acidosis, or fatty liver. Lamivudine is associated with mitochondrial dysfunction which may result in a clinical picture mimicking acute fatty liver of pregnancy or hemolysis, elevated liver enzymes, and low platelets (HELLP) syndrome. Nevirapine is associated with cutaneous rash and hepatotoxicity. Data from humans do not suggest an increase in the incidence of tumors in children with prenatal exposure to ARV drugs.[23]

Human immunodeficiency virus infected pregnant women who have had previous exposure to sd-NVP (or EFV) for PPTCT prophylaxis in prior pregnancies, an NNRTI-based ART regimen, such as TDF + 3TC + EFV, may not be fully effective due to persistence of archived mutation to NNRTIs (resistance to NVP and cross-resistance to EFV). Hence, these women will require a PI-based ART regimen viz.: TDF + 3TC + LPV/r (lopinavir/ritonavir). The dose will be TDF + 3TC (1 tablet daily) + LPV (200 mg)/r (50 mg) (2 tablets BD). This is called a "boosted PI" based regimen. The sd-NVP exposed cohort of mothers and babies who now require ART need to be given the boosted PI regimen as they are possibly resistant to the EFV or NVP-based ART regimens.

Phasing Out of Nevirapine

There are concerns about a higher risk of adverse events with NVP compared with EFV, and about the use of NVP in women with HIV with CD4 counts more than 250, with data showing an increased relative risk for severe hepatic and skin reactions in pregnant women using NVP at higher CD4 cell counts.[24-26] A review suggests that the frequency of adverse events with NVP is elevated but no higher than that observed in the general adult population.[27] The need for lead-in dosing for initial use of NVP and the fact that it is not available as a fixed dose combination with TDF + 3TC are important drawbacks. Sd-NVP increases drug resistance and cross-resistance with other NNRTIs. Nevirapine should be used with caution in pregnant women and only after considering the risk and benefits, and available alternatives.

Antenatal Evaluation

National AIDS Control Organization recommends at least four antenatal visits during pregnancy: registration and 1st check-up within 12 weeks, second between 14 and 26 weeks, third between 28 and 32 weeks, and fourth between 36 and 40 weeks.[4] At the initial visit, the obstetric and medical history are noted. A physical examination including an obstetric examination is performed. In addition, a pelvic examination is done to collect a Pap smear to screen for cervical dysplasia and to look for any STIs or vaginal infections which should be appropriately treated.

Investigations

These include blood group, hemogram, Venereal Disease Research Laboratory (VDRL), hepatitis B surface antigen, anti hepatitis C virus (HCV), urine routine analysis and culture, kidney and liver functions, toxoplasma serology, cytomegalovirus serology, and CD4 count. Complete blood counts and liver functions are repeated every 3–4 months. Screening for gestational diabetes is done at 24–28 weeks. Ultrasound to screen for congenital fetal malformations is desirable. It is likely that invasive procedures like amniocentesis or chorionic villus sampling for prenatal diagnosis carry a risk of HIV transmission, especially among untreated women and should be avoided.[28] Urine routine analysis is done at all antenatal visits and hemoglobin to be rechecked at 28–32 weeks. Routine iron, folic acid and calcium supplementation is advised as in antenatal women. A multivitamin supplement may be given especially among those with a poor nutritional status.

Clinical and Laboratory Monitoring

Women on ART in pregnancy should be monitored clinically by the WHO staging for disease progression or treatment failure. Weight loss (an indicator for deteriorating clinical stage) is difficult to assess in pregnancy. Antiretroviral therapy related side effects like nausea, and vomiting, usually overlap with those of pregnancy. Renal function test and CD4 count is done at baseline and thereafter 6 monthly. Liver function tests are repeated once after 2 weeks and 6 monthly thereafter or as and when clinically indicated. Lipid profile and blood sugars are retested at 6 months and 1 year if started on LPV/r based regime.

Prevention of Opportunistic Infections

If CD4 count is less than 250/mm^3, once daily tablet of double strength trimethoprim-sulfamethoxazole is given for prophylaxis of *Pneumocystis carinii* pneumonia (PCP), toxoplasmosis, diarrhea as well as other bacterial infections.[4] Folate supplements are to be ensured with cotrimoxazole prophylaxis.

Coinfections

Human Immunodeficiency Virus and Tuberculosis Coinfection

The risk of active TB is approximately 10 times higher in HIV-infected pregnant women compared to HIV-uninfected women and causes increased risk of maternal and neonatal morbidity and mortality. The WHO recommends TB prevention measures at HIV care settings like airborne infection control and isoniazid preventive therapy. All HIV-positive women should be evaluated for TB and started on treatment whenever indicated. In HIV-TB coinfection, treatment for TB should be started first and followed by ART as soon as feasible (usually 2 weeks later).[4] Rifampicin can cause drug interactions with ART; EFV is the preferred NNRTI in those receiving treatment for TB.

Hepatitis B and Hepatitis C Coinfection

Hepatitis B Virus

All women who screen negative for HBV infection should receive the hepatitis B virus (HBV) vaccine.[22] These women are negative for hepatitis B surface antigen, hepatitis B core antibody, and hepatitis B surface antibody. In women coinfected with HIV and HBV, the preferred ART regimen includes TDF + 3TC + EFV, if treatment is required for HBV infection. Women with low CD4 count should be monitored for immune-mediated flare in HBV disease following initiation of ART and may have elevated liver enzymes. If no treatment is required for HBV, routine monitoring for ART is recommended. Interferon-α and pegylated interferon are not recommended during pregnancy. Women with chronic HBV infection should also be screened for hepatitis A virus (HAV) by HAV immunoglobulin G antibodies.

Hepatitis C Virus

Hepatitis C virus-HIV coinfection is common in injecting drug abusers. Pregnant women with HIV-HCV coinfection do not require any changes in ART and require routine clinical and laboratory monitoring. Women with chronic HCV infection should be screened for HAV. Use of ribavirin, interferon-α and pegylated interferon is not recommended during pregnancy.

Immunizations

Pneumococcal and influenza vaccine are recommended before the flu season. Hepatitis B vaccine is to be given in anti-HBc-negative patients. Hepatitis A vaccine is given in women with chronic hepatitis C. Vaccination should ideally be administered after HIV-RNA has been suppressed to undetectable levels with ART, in order to prevent the increase in the risk of transmission that theoretically accompanies the transient increase in HIV-RNA after immunization.

MODE OF DELIVERY

Elective CS at 38 weeks lowers the MTCT (odds ratio 0.43) both in women receiving AZT monotherapy or no ARV but possibly not in women on highly active antiretroviral therapy with low or undetectable HIV-RNA level (<1,000 copies/mL).[24] However, the morbidity and mortality with CS is 5–7 times that of vaginal delivery, a fact to be remembered while discussing its benefits and risks with the patient. Its benefit in reducing MTCT is more in women with high viral loads.

Cesarean Section

NACO, India does not recommend elective CS to reduce MTCT; rather, CS is recommended only for obstetric indications.[4] For any planned (elective) CS, ART should be given prior to the CS. Women on lifelong ART should continue their standard ART regimen. In case of an emergency, CS in pregnant women who are not on ART, ensure that the women receive ART prior to the procedure and continues thereafter. During a CS, use round-tip blunt needles and use forceps to receive and hold the needle. The amniotic membrane is left intact until the head is delivered through the surgical incision and the cord is clamped as early as possible. A word of caution about using methylergonovine: EFV increases the levels of injection methylergonovine by slowing drug metabolism. Their combination may cause vasospasm and ischemia.

Vaginal Delivery

Care should be taken to minimize the duration of membrane rupture, avoid invasive monitoring (scalp electrodes, scalp blood sampling), minimize number of vaginal examinations, and avoid a routine episiotomy or operative delivery. If indicated, low cavity outlet forceps is preferable to ventouse, as it is generally associated with lower rates of fetal trauma than the ventouse. Artificial rupture of the membranes should be avoided, and labor may be augmented after spontaneous rupture of membranes to reduce the duration of ruptured membranes. In case an HIV-positive woman who is not on ART is encountered in labor, ART should be initiated as soon as possible and continued lifelong. Broad-spectrum antibiotics should be given intrapartum to prevent maternal infection. The infant should be wiped clean to remove maternal secretions and blood before suction or any invasive procedure is performed. Universal precautions should be followed in all deliveries.

ADVICE REGARDING INFANT FEEDING PRACTICES

Breastfeeding is known to increase MTCT. There is accumulative risk of HIV transmission with increasing duration of breastfeeding, 0.7% per month in the first 5 months, 0.6% during 6–11 months, and 0.3% between 12 and 17 months.[29] Breastfeeding is not recommended for HIV-infected women in the United States, including those receiving ART.[22] In developing (low and middle income) countries where infant mortality is more due to malnutrition and infection as compared to AIDS itself, WHO recommends that a choice of exclusive breastfeeding with gradual weaning (over 1 month) at 12 months of age can be offered. Complementary foods are added after 6 months and breastfeeding is stopped at 12 months or when nutritionally adequate diet is accessible. The option of exclusive replacement feed can be allowed only if it fulfills the AFASS criteria, provided, it is acceptable, feasible, affordable, sustainable, and safe (AFASS).[18] Mixed feeding in the first 6 months should not be allowed, as mixed-fed children are probably more likely to acquire HIV than exclusively breastfed children due to infection-related injuries in gastrointestinal mucosa.[2] The WHO recommends that each country should decide about feeding practices (replacement feeding or breastfeeding). In the first 12 months of life, exclusive breastfeeding is associated with the least risk of HIV transmission to infant in the presence of ARV drugs.[30] This also gives maximum benefit in preventing infant mortality from diarrhea, pneumonia, and malnutrition. If early infant diagnosis (EID) is positive, then stop breastfeeding at maximum 24 months and if EID is negative, stop breastfeeding at 12 months (maximum time).

National AIDS Control Organization, India (2013), recommends exclusive breastfeeding for 6 months and continuation of breastfeeds with introduction of complementary feeds thereafter till 12 months. In situations where breast-feeding cannot be done (maternal death, severe maternal illness) or individual mother's choice (at her own risk), then exclusive replacement feeding may be considered if AFASS criteria are met.[4] Mixed feeding is not allowed during the first 6 months as it may cause mucosal abrasions in the gut of the neonate which will facilitate entry of the HIV virus present in the breast milk into the mucosa, and increase the risk of HIV acquisition by the neonate.

POSTPARTUM FOLLOW-UP AND CONTRACEPTION

Assess wound healing and uterine involution. Discuss issues like contraception and need for lifelong follow-up with a physician. Consistent condom (both male and female) use must be stressed and hormonal contraception can be given in addition (combined oral pills or progestin only contraceptives). Though hormonal contraceptives can lead to increased virus shedding in the genital tract and increased cervical ectopy, but given their effectiveness and overall safety, they remain an appropriate option for these women. Estradiol levels from oral contraceptives are reduced by NVP, ritonavir and nelfinavir which may reduce the contraceptive efficacy.[7,17] Interactions between medroxyprogesterone acetate and ARV drugs are under study, but this agent is a reasonable choice. Intra-uterine contraceptive devices may be offered to HIV-infected women who have a low risk of

STIs and do not have severe immune suppression. These should be used with caution due to increased risk of pelvic inflammatory disease and increased duration and amount of bleeding. Spermicides, like nonoxynol-9, though HIV-cidal, negate this beneficial effect by local inflammation and mucosal injury by prolonged use and may increase HIV transmission.[10]

CARE OF THE HUMAN IMMUNODEFICIENCY VIRUS-EXPOSED INFANT

Human immunodeficiency virus DNA PCR test using dried blood spot (DBS) and whole blood specimen is being used for the EID of HIV infection in newborn with a sensitivity of 93% by 14 days of life. Cord blood sample is not to be taken due to chances of contamination with maternal blood. The neonate is tested at 6 weeks and 6 months of age by DNA-PCR. Human immunodeficiency virus can be excluded if these two tests are negative. The third test is, repeated at again 12 months if the 6 month test was negative. The third EID testing should be undertaken after 6 weeks of stopping breastfeeds which may not happen exactly at 12 months, but anytime after 6 months and before 13 months. Confirmation of HıV status is done using three rapid antibody HIV-ELISA tests at 18 months at the ICTC. All exposed infants are given cotrimoxazole prophylactic treatment prophylaxis beginning at 6 weeks till HIV infection is excluded at 18 months.[4] Immunization is as per the schedule starting with bacillus Calmette-Guérin (BCG), HBV, and oral polio vaccine at birth. If DBS is positive at 6 weeks, whole blood sample is tested. If positive, pediatric ART is initiated for babies less than 2 years irrespective of CD4 count.

CONCLUSION

The introduction of ART for the treatment of HIV has improved the expectancy and the quality of life of PLHIV. Instition of ART in pregnancy and its life long continuation has become the current standard of care for HIV infected women in developing women as advocated recently by the WHO. NACO, India recommends this lifelong treatment (with Tenofovir 300 mg , Lamivudine 300 mg and Efavirenz 600 mg) alongwith exclusive breastfeeding of infants; CS as a mode of delivery is reserved only for obstetric indications. Infant born to HIV infected mother is given syrup Nevirapine for a minimum 6 weeks. Adequate antenatal care, compliance with ART, monitored delivery, suitable contraception and regular follow-up care are essential for HIV infected women for an optimatal perinatal outcome.

REFERENCES

1. Working Group on Mother- to-Child Transmission of HIV. Rates of mother-to-child transmission of HIV-1in Africa, America and Europe: results from 13 perinatal studies. J Acquir Immune Defic Syndr Hum Retrovirol. 1995;8:506-10.
2. Antiretroviral drugs for treating pregnant women and preventing HIV infection in infants. Guidelines on care, treatment and support for women living with HIV/AIDS and their children in resource-constrained settings. Geneva: World Health Organization Expert Consultation; 2004.
3. UNAIDS. Global report: the UNAIDS report on global AIDS epidemic 2010. [online] Available from: www.unaids.org/globalreport/Global_report.htm. [Accessed December, 2015].
4. NACO. Updated Guidelines for the Prevention of Mother to Child Transmission (PPTCT) of HIV using Multi Drug Anti-retroviral Regimen in India, 2013. [online] Available from: www.naco.gov.in/upload/National_guidelines_for_PPTCT.pdf. [Accessed December, 2015].
5. Manual for Management of HIV/AIDS in Children. NACO, IAP, WHO, UNICEF; 2004.
6. Burns DN, Landesman S, Minkoff H, Wright DJ, Waters D, Mitchell RM, et al. The influence of pregnancy on human immunodeficiency virus type 1 infection: Antepartum and postpartum changes in human immunodeficiency virus type 1 viral load. Am J Obstet Gynecol. 1998;178:355-9.
7. Saada M1, Le Chenadec J, Berrebi A, Bongain A, Delfraissy JF, Mayaux MJ, et al. Pregnancy and progression to AIDS: results of the French prospective cohorts. AIDS. 2000;14:2355-60.
8. Deschamps MM1, Pape JW, Desvarieux M, Williams-Russo P, Madhavan S, Ho JL, et al. A prospective study of HIV-seropositive asymptomatic women of childbearing age in a developing country. J Acquir Immune Defic Syndr. 1993;6:446-51.
9. Kumar RM, Uduman SA, Khurrana AK. Impact of pregnancy on maternal AIDS. J Reprod Med. 1997;42:429-34.
10. Anderson JR. (2001). HIV and reproduction. A guide to the clinical care of women with HIV. [online] Available from: http://www.hab.hrsa.gov/. [Accessed December, 2015].
11. Ticconi C, Mapfumo M, Dorrucci M, Naha N, Tarira E, Pietropolli A, et al. Effect of maternal HIV and malaria infection on pregnancy and perinatal outcome in Zimbabwe. J Acquir Immune Defic Syndr. 2003;34:289-94.
12. Rouzioux C, Costagliola D, Burgard M, Blanche S, Mayaux MJ, Griscelli C, et al. Estimated timing of mother-to-child human immunodeficiency virus type 1 transmission by use of a Markov model: the HIV Infection in Newborns French Collaborative Study Group. Am J Epidemiol. 1995;142:1330-7.
13. Lewis SH, Reynolds-Kohler C, Fox HE, Nelson JA. HIV-1 in trophoblastic and villous Hofbauer cells, and haematological precursors in eight-week fetuses. Lancet. 1990;335:565-8.
14. Kapoor A, Kapoor A, Vani SN. Prevention of mother to child transmission of HIV. Indian J Paediatr. 2004;71:247-51.
15. Fawzi WW, Msamanga GI, Spiegelman D, Urassa EJ, McGrath N, Mwakagile D, et al. Randomised trial of effects of vitamin supplements on pregnancy outcomes and T cell counts in HIV-1-infected women in Tanzania. Lancet. 1998;351:1477-82.
16. International Perinatal HIV Group. Duration of rupture of membranes and vertical transmission of HIV-1: a meta-analysis from 15 prospective cohort studies. AIDS. 2001;15:357-68.
17. Report of the NIH panel to define principles of therapy of HIV infection and guidelines for the use of antiretroviral agents in HIV-infected adults and adolescents. MMWR Morb Mortal Wkly Rep. 1998;47:1-82.
18. Antiretroviral drugs for treating pregnant women and preventing HIV infection in infants: towards universal access: recommendations for a public health approach. 2010 revision. Geneva: WHO; 2010. Available from: http://whqlibdoc.who.int/publications/2010/9789241599818_eng.pdf. [Accessed December, 2015].

19. Integrated HIV program report July–September 2012. Lilongwe, Ministry of Public Health, Government of Malawi. Available from: http://www.hivunitmohmw.org/uploads/Main/Quarterly_HIV_Programme_Report_2012_Q3.pdf. [Accessed December, 2015].
20. WHO. Consolidated guidelines on the use of antiretroviral drugs for treating and preventing HIV infection: recommendations for a public health approach. Geneva: WHO; 2013. Available from: http://www.who.int/hiv/pub/mtct/en/arvdrugswomenguidelinesfinal.pdf. [Accessed December, 2015].
21. Ford N, Calmy A, Mofenson L. Safety of efavirenz in the first trimester of pregnancy: an updated systematic review and meta analysis. AIDS. 2011;25:2301-4.
22. Recommendations for Use of Antiretroviral Drugs in pregnant HIV-1 women for maternal Health and Interventions to reduce perinatal HIV transmission in the United States. Washington DC: United States Department of Health and Human Services Panel on Treatment of HIV infected Pregnant women and prevention of perinatal transmission; 2014. Available from: http://aidsinfo.nih.gov/guidelines. [Accessed December, 2015].
23. World Health Organization. (2013). Web annexes. [online] Available from: www.who.int/hiv/pub/guidelines/arv2013/annexes. [Accessed December, 2015].
24. Watts DH. Management of human immunodeficiency virus infection in pregnancy. N Engl J Med. 2002;346:1879-91.
25. Phanuphak N, Apornpong T, Teeratakulpisarn S, Chaithongwongwatthana S, Taweepolcharoen C, Mangclaviraj S, et al. Nevirapine-associated toxicity in HIV-infected Thai men and women, including pregnant women. HIV Med. 2007;8:357-66.
26. Jamisse L, Balkus J, Hitti J, Gloyd S, Manuel R, Osman N, et al. Antiretroviral-associated toxicity among HIV-1-seropositive pregnant women in Mozambique receiving nevirapine-based regimens. J Acquir Immune Defic Syndr. 2007;44:371-6.
27. Aaron E, Kempf MC, Criniti S, et al. Adverse events in a cohort of HIV infected pregnant and non-pregnant women treated with nevirapine versus non-nevirapine antiretroviral medication. PLoS One. 2010;5:e12617.
28. Mandelbrot L, Mayaux MJ, Bongain A, Berrebi A, Moudoub-Jeanpetit Y, Bénifla JL, et al. Obstetric factors and mother-to-infant transmission of human immunodeficiency virus type 1: the French perinatal cohorts. Am J Obstet Gynecol. 1996;175:661-7.
29. Miotti PG, Taha TE, Kumwenda NI, Broadhead R, Mtimavalye LA, Van der Hoeven L, et al. HIV transmission through breastfeeding: a study in Malawi. JAMA. 1999;282:744-79.
30. Gibb DM, Kizito H, Russell EC, Chidziva E, Zalwango E, Nalumenya R, et al. Pregnancy and infant outcomes among HIV-infected women taking long-term ART with and without tenofovir in the DART trial. PLoS Med. 2012;9:e1001217.

Section 8

Miscellaneous

CHAPTER 71

Critical Care

Sharda Patra, Indira Prasad

INTRODUCTION

Traditionally, critical care is defined as an intensive treatment of seriously ill patients with life-threatening illness or trauma that has potential to develop complications leading to significant morbidity and even mortality if not reversed in time. A critically ill obstetric patient is one who because of abnormal pregnancy, delivery, and puerperium or because of effects of a pre-existing systemic disease, anesthesia or surgery develops life-threatening complications for which intensive monitoring, therapy and/or life support system is required. Critical care of an obstetric patient is an area which is less discussed, however, of late there has been a growing need to address this issue in order to implement the most up-to-date standards to identify and treat with appropriate interventions and thus prevent maternal or perinatal mortalities or long-term organ dysfunctions.

WHAT IS CRITICAL CARE IN OBSTETRICS?

Care of critically ill patients is a unique challenge in obstetrics requiring thorough knowledge of maternal and fetal physiology. Pregnancy affects every organ system. Altered maternal physiology, presence of a fetus, and diseases specific to pregnancy pose various challenges in management of critically ill obstetric patients.

On one hand, medical conditions might present risk to the pregnancy and on the other, pregnancy itself may modify state of the medical disease. Drug therapy may be affected by altered pharmacokinetics or have impact on the developing fetus. Obstetric patients are generally young, healthy, and recover rapidly. However, the potential for catastrophic complications is really immense.

Majority of women during their pregnancy, labor, and postnatal period require care that can be met through routine obstetric care. However, a small but quite a significant number of women require critical care in some situations (Table 1).

Depending on methods and protocols at various institutions, approximately 1% of obstetrical patients need

TABLE 1: Types of obstetric patients in different intensive care units

MHDU	ICU
• Severe pre-eclampsia requiring IV antihypertensives • Eclampsia, HELLP syndrome • Severe renal impairment • Major hemorrhage due to abruption/placenta previa • Major PPH >1,500 mL, uterine balloon *in situ*, B-Lynch suture for atonic uterus • Hypovolemic shock • Sepsis syndrome and ARDS • Amniotic fluid embolism • Peripartum cardiomyopathy and cardiogenic shock • Severe anemia with CHF	• Pulmonary embolism • Bronchial asthma and status asthmaticus • Diabetic ketoacidosis • Thyroid storm • Epilepsy and status epilepticus

MHDU, medical high dependency unit; ICU, intensive care unit; PPH, postpartum hemorrhage; HELLP, hemolysis, elevated liver enzymes levels, low platelets; ARDS, acute respiratory distress syndrome; CHF, congestive heart failure.

some type of intensive care and management.[1] Women with complications specific to pregnancy have the greatest need for obstetrical intensive care. Hemorrhage and hypertension are the most common causes of intensive care unit (ICU) admission in obstetric patients. Approximately, 20–30% of obstetric ICU patients have nonobstetric causes for admission, such as sepsis, and about 75% of obstetric ICU patients admitted to the ICU are postpartum. Hence, operative intervention is required in only 10–15% cases. Reported maternal mortality in critically ill obstetric patients admitted to an ICU is approximately 8.4%.[2] There is, therefore, an urgent need to train more practitioners in obstetric critical care.

LEVELS OF CARE FOR OBSTETRIC PATIENTS

Care of critically ill obstetric patients is subdivided into three levels based on organ support and level of monitoring irrespective of underlying disease. The different levels of critical care in obstetrics was first defined in *Comprehensive Critical Care* and subsequently updated in 2009.[3] It may be at times difficult to distinguish between various levels of care as different hospitals have different service protocols under various levels. However, such a division is quite useful and helps in a more scientific allocation of resources. Patients who require admission to a medical high dependency unit (MHDU) are likely to require level 1 or 2 care, although some patients who require level 2 care may need transfer to an ICU. The Intensive Care Society (ICS) has further expanded this guidance to clarify exactly what may be expected in different levels of care (Table 2).[4]

TYPES OF OBSTETRICAL CRITICAL CARE UNITS

Obstetrical critical care includes maternal high dependency care unit, obstetrical ICU, and medical/surgical ICU[5] (Fig. 1).

Maternal High Dependency Unit

This is the type of care basically provided in specialized areas within the vicinity of labor room with availability of experienced personnel, which includes specially trained maternofetal medicine specialists and nurses with experience in critical care obstetrics, anesthesiologists with readily available pulmonologists, cardiologists, and other medical and surgical specialists. Pregnant women with high risk factors should be admitted in the MHDU.

Advantage of MHDU is that it provides a continuous care of the pregnant woman with high risk factors during her antenatal, intrapartum, and postnatal period by the same dedicated team and the delivery of the baby takes place in a more familiar and better-equipped environment with minimal disruption of mother-to-baby bonding. The risk of hospital acquired infection in a hazardous ICU environment is lowered in these critically ill pregnant mothers with her altered cell-mediated immunity and high levels of circulating corticosteroids. Patients are more satisfied as MHDU is less noisy and have more liberal family visitation policies. The women can breastfeed the child and last but not the least, high dependency unit (HDU) care is cheaper as compared to ICU care. It provides high level of individual, medical, and psychological care, delivered by staffs who understand the physiology and pathology unique to obstetric patients.

Obstetrical Intensive Care Unit (Obstetric Intensive Care Unit)

These are full-care ICUs as described above, but are operated by obstetrical and anesthesia personnel with experience in critical care in labor and delivery suites.

Medical/Surgical Intensive Care Unit (General Intensive Care Unit)

In most healthcare setups, women who require ventilatory support, invasive monitoring, or pharmacological support of circulation are transferred to a specialized medical/surgical ICU under the care of medical/surgical and anesthesia personnel.

MANAGEMENT OF OBSTETRIC PATIENT IN A CRITICAL CARE UNIT

Obstetric conditions that are likely to require HDU care have been illustrated in Table 1. Obstetric patients admitted in the MHDU should be initially assessed with a present and past medical and obstetric history, systemic examination with an individual organ-based approach with special consideration of the gestational age of the fetus. The management depends on the underlying condition complicating pregnancy.

INITIAL ASSESSMENT AND RESUSCITATION OF CRITICALLY ILL OBSTETRIC PATIENT

Management of an obstetric patient includes management both during antenatal period and in the postpartum period and that of an undelivered patient poses greatest challenge both to the obstetricians and the anesthesiologists. As for all critically ill patients, initial management begins with obstetric history and examination for finding out whether patient is in antepartum or postpartum period; and if antepartum then whether the baby is viable or not. A complete medical history and examination for evaluation

TABLE 2: Different levels of care in obstetric patients

Level of care	Conditions in obstetrics
• Level 0: routine care ○ Midwifery staff, interns, medical officers ○ Place: ward/labor suite	• Low risk pregnant woman • Women with normal labor
• Level 1: conditions where additional monitoring or intervention is required or patient transferred from ICU needing additional monitoring, clinical input, or advice obstetricians ○ Place: MHDU	• Women requiring labor induction/augmentation • Laboring women with epidural analgesia • Management of women with APH/PPH • Mild pre-eclampsia on oral antihypertensives • Women with medical condition such as congenital heart disease, diabetics on insulin infusion
• Level 2 : single organ support ○ Obstetricians and midwifery staff trained in the care of the critically ill women, anesthesiologists, pulmonologists, cardiologists, and other medical and surgical specialists ○ Place: MHDU	• Respiratory support • 50% or more oxygen via face mask to maintain oxygen saturation • Continuous positive airway pressure • Bi-level positive airway pressure • Extended postoperative care • Basic cardiovascular support (BCVS) • Intravenous antihypertensives, to control blood pressure in pre-eclampsia • Monitoring through CVP line to guide therapy • Advanced cardiovascular support • Simultaneous use of at least two intravenous, anti-arrhythmic/antihypertensive/vasoactive drugs, need to measure and treat cardiac output • Neurological support • Magnesium sulfate therapy to control convulsions in eclampsia • Intracranial pressure monitoring • Hepatic support • Management of acute fulminant hepatic failure, e.g., from acute viral hepatitis, HELLP syndrome or acute fatty liver
• Level 3: advanced respiratory support alone, or support of two or more organ systems above ○ Team of intensivists, obstetricians, and midwifery staff trained in the care of the critically ill women, anesthesiologists pulmonologists, cardiologists, and other medical and surgical specialists ○ Place: ICU	• Advanced respiratory support • Invasive mechanical ventilation • Support of two or more organ systems • Renal support and basic respiratory support • Basic respiratory support/BCVS and an additional organ supported

ICU, intensive care unit; MHDU, medical high dependency unit; APH, antepartum hemorrhage; PPH, postpartum hemorrhage; HELLP, hemolysis, elevated liver enzymes levels, low platelets; CVP, central venous pressure.

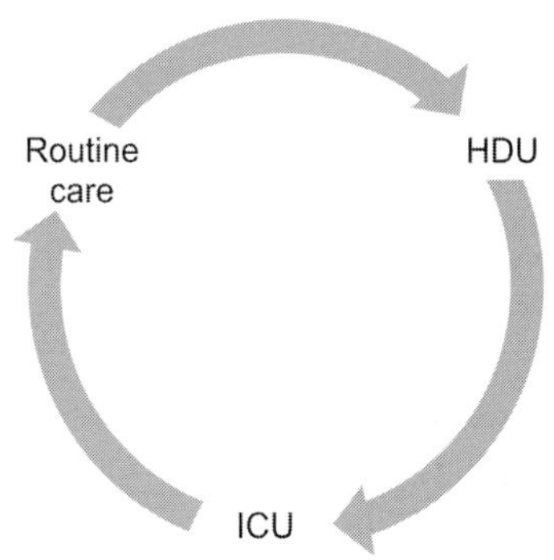

HDU, high dependency unit; ICU, intensive care unit.

FIG. 1: Types of obstetrical care.

of cardiovascular, renal, pulmonary, hepatic, and cerebral functions should be done. An initial baseline and specific investigations should be sent followed by a strict maternal observation to monitor organ functions—cardiovascular, renal, pulmonary, hepatic, and cerebral functions. Then, one must begin planning the treatment of the primary condition (e.g., severe pre-eclampsia, hemorrhage, sepsis) with supportive management and monitoring; adequate fluid therapy: crystalloid/colloid, blood component therapy with strict central venous pressure (CVP) monitoring, an hourly urine output, and chest condition. If the woman is antenatal, then check the fetal condition with cardiotocography and maintain uteroplacental oxygen delivery followed by plan for delivery as the case may be with an informed consent.

MONITORING REQUIRED IN A CRITICAL CARE UNIT

Monitoring in a critical care unit is extremely important as it ensures rapid detection of changes in the clinical status and allows for accurate assessment of progress and response to therapy. Advent of noninvasive techniques and alarms has enabled strict monitoring feasible.

Characteristics of a critically ill patient are variable and are related to complications of pregnancy or a pre-existing/co-existing disease causing specific organ dysfunction or hemodynamic instability and so warrant individualized monitoring and treatment.

Modified early warning obstetric charts called Worcestershire obstetric warning (WOW) charts allow smart recording of observations and is a precise monitoring tool. It should be used in all obstetric inpatient settings. Any abnormal observation in a WOW chart must trigger urgent action, i.e., specialist medical review and assessment.[6]

The parameters for monitoring basically includes hemodynamic monitoring (blood pressure, CVP, pulmonary artery wedge pressure, cardiac output, electrocardiography), respiratory monitoring [arterial blood gas analysis, oxygen saturation by SpO_2, mixed venous O_2 saturation (SvO_2), lung function, respiratory compliance, and capnography], and monitoring of organ and tissue oxygenation (serum lactate levels and blood pH, SvO_2 ,urine output, temperature, neurological).[7] Any deviations in the above parameters in some cases/further progress of the disease leading to deterioration of the patient calls for a level 3 or an ICU care (Box 1).

Box 1: Suggested criteria for transfer to intensive care unit from medical high dependency unit[8]

- Respiratory distress: if the respiratory rate is <5 and >35 breaths per minute
- Abnormal ABG (PaO_2 <6.6 kPa and/or $PaCO_2$ >8.0 kPa, SaO_2 <90% on supplemental oxygen
- Severe acidosis (pH <7.1)/alkalosis (pH >7.7)
- Tachycardia/bradycardia: pulse rate <40 and >140 beats per minute
- Hypotension: systemic arterial pressure (systolic blood pressure) <80 mmHg
- Deranged kidney function: urine output <400 mL in 24 h unresponsive to simple measures
- Patient is unconscious/unarousable
- Severe dyselectrolytemia: serum sodium <110 and >160 mmol/L, serum potassium <2.0 and >7.0 mmol/L

ICU, intensive care unit; MHDU, medical highdependency unit; ABG, arterial blood gas; PaO2, partial pressure of arterial oxygen; PaCO2, partial pressure of arterial carbon dioxide.

MANAGEMENT OF CRITICALLY ILL OBSTETRIC PATIENT IN ICU

Generally, if two organ systems are failing with a need for ventilator support ICU admission becomes mandatory. There are no specific studies regarding various medications used for sedation in this group of patients and depending upon normal ICU practices usual sedatives could be used. It is advisable not to use propofol for sedation in these patients as its risks would outweigh benefits and can lead to propofol infusion syndrome.[9] The treating team should at all times involve the obstetricians as the intensive care team may be ignorant in monitoring the fetal well-being. The viability of the fetus, advantages and disadvantages in continuation of the pregnancy, and the mode of delivery, if required are some of the important issues that need to be discussed at the outset. All medications used in an ICU are categorized from A to D (in order of increasing fetal risk) and X (contraindicated); such a list should be readily available for the ICU team. A multidisciplinary management plan should always be available in anticipation of a catastrophe for all critically ill pregnant patients. The management of a critically ill pregnant woman in ICU involves two categories of patients: obstetric patient not in labor and obstetric patient in labor.

MANAGEMENT OF A CRITICALLY ILL OBSTETRIC PATIENT NOT IN LABOR

The management of critically ill obstetric patient not in labor, basically, should take into account fetal considerations like assessment of gestational age, need for fetal surveillance, and need for termination of pregnancy.

The assessment of gestational age is crucial to determine whether the fetus is of gestational age sufficient to ensure a good chance of survival after birth. Wherever possible, antenatal care records should be obtained to establish the most accurate dating criteria. In the event that gestational age remains uncertain, prompt ultrasound evaluation should establish the best possible estimate with documentation of the potential range of uncertainty. If preterm delivery may be necessary, a course of antenatal corticosteroids should be given to promote fetal lung maturity in fetuses between 24 and 34 weeks of gestation, and are not contraindicated in an ICU setting even in the setting of sepsis.

Fetal surveillance often is used when a pregnant patient is admitted to the ICU. Because fetal heart rate monitoring reflects uteroplacental perfusion and maternal acid-base status, changes in baseline variability or the new onset of decelerations may serve as an early warning system for derangements in maternal end-organ status. Changes in fetal monitoring should prompt reassessment of maternal mean arterial pressure, hypoxia, acidemia, or compression of the inferior vena cava (IVC) by the gravid uterus. Correction of these factors may result in improvement of the tracing and every attempt should be made at intra-uterine fetal resuscitation.

In an antepartum patient, obstetrician must monitor the fetal heart and decide regarding termination of pregnancy after weighing the risks and benefits and assessing the fetal maturity. If a patient is found to be in heart failure, evaluation and diagnosis is imperative about the cause of failure; whether it is secondary to heart disease or pre-eclamptic pulmonary edema or fluid overload or adult respiratory distress syndrome. Diuretic (e.g., furosemide) should be administered in case of crepitations found in the chest, after checking the vitals (systolic blood pressure >100 mmHg) and according to its response, further management is decided. If with diuretic, chest clears and patient symptomatically improves, it is usually suggestive of pulmonary edema and warrants urgent termination of pregnancy. Thus, next step involves pelvic assessment and Bishop's scoring for finding out whether conditions are favorable for a vaginal delivery. If patient is stabilized and she comes out of failure (i.e., the chest gets cleared of crepitations) and the internal examination findings suggest that the vaginal delivery is feasible in next 6–12 hours, the labor induction or augmentation must be carried out. In a critical care unit, obstetrician monitors the progress of labor and level of uterine contractions in a patient laboring and decides whether vaginal delivery will be possible and takes a decision for cesarean delivery timely. However, if the patient does not come out of failure (i.e., the chest still has crepitations) or if the Bishop's score is poor; immediate cesarean delivery should be carried out.

MANAGEMENT OF A CRITICALLY ILL OBSTETRIC PATIENT IN LABOR

If a laboring patient requires critical care services, it is important to determine the optimal setting for her care. If the fetus is previable (<28 weeks) or the duration of ICU services is anticipated to be lengthy, the labor room is not the best option. However, if the patient is in active labor, the labor room may be the best choice if adequate maternal support can be provided there itself. Advantages of vaginal delivery in the ICU include the availability of critical care interventions and staff while disadvantages include lack of space and facilities to conduct a vaginal delivery accommodating pediatric personnel and equipment. The unfamiliarity of critical care personnel with obstetric interventions and management also acts as a disadvantage. Factors that will affect this decision include the degree of patient instability, interventions required, availability of staffing and expertise, anticipated duration of ICU stay and probability of delivery.

Delivery in the ICU is associated with an increased likelihood of operative vaginal delivery. In part, this is because patients with translaryngeal intubation cannot close the glottis to push; therefore, an assisted second stage of labor may be required. In addition, ICU patients often have underlying cardiac or neurologic processes where an assisted second stage of labor is recommended.

Cesarean delivery in the ICU is complex and has significant disadvantages compared with procedures performed in a traditional operating room. These disadvantages include inadequate space for anesthetic, surgical, and neonatal resuscitation equipment and attendant personnel unfamiliar with the operation. In addition, ICUs have the highest rates of healthcare associated infections in a hospital, so the risk of nosocomial infection with drug resistant organisms is increased.[10] Cesarean delivery in the ICU should be restricted to cases in which transport to the operating room or delivery room cannot be achieved safely or expeditiously, or to a perimortem cesarean delivery.

In the care of the postpartum ICU patient, obstetric input may include evaluation of vaginal or intra-abdominal bleeding, evaluation of obstetric sources of infection, duration of specific therapies such as magnesium therapy in eclampsia and feasibility of breastfeeding, especially compatibility of various medications with breastfeeding. There may also be issues related to surgical interventions, including re-exploration of the abdomen, or reclosure of abdominal or vaginal incisions. Under some circumstances, the obstetrician and the neonatologist will also need to advocate for bringing together the critically ill mother and her baby.

TRANSFER FROM CRITICAL CARE AREA (MEDICAL HIGH DEPENDENCY UNIT/ INTENSIVE CARE UNIT) TO WARD

When the disease process or physiological disturbance that led to MHDU/ICU admission has been reversed, the patient may be discharged from critical care area and transferred to ward (Box 2).

CRITICAL CARE IN SPECIAL SITUATIONS

Management of Sudden Cardiac Arrest in an Obstetric Patient

Cardiac arrest in pregnant patient is a rare and an unexpected event. It may arise due to a pathogenic process within a

Box 2: Suggested discharge criteria from critical care area to general ward[11]

- Patient is conscious and alert
- Stable and normal respiratory status
- Stable and normal hemodynamic parameters with no evidence of hemorrhage
- Intensive/invasive monitoring is no longer required
- Four hourly recording of vital signs is considered appropriate

patient or may result due to iatrogenic factors or trauma. Successful resuscitation of a pregnant woman and survival of the fetus require prompt and excellent cardiopulmonary resuscitation (CPR) with some modifications in techniques. Appropriate decision making for emergency cesarean delivery can increase the infant's survival in the following situations:

- Short interval between the mother's arrest and the infant's delivery
- No sustained pre-arrest hypoxia in the mother
- Minimal or no signs of fetal distress before the mother's cardiac arrest
- Aggressive and effective resuscitative efforts for the mother
- Delivery to be performed in a medical center with a neonatal intensive care unit.

CARDIOPULMONARY RESUSCITATION IN AN OBSTETRIC PATIENT

Cardiopulmonary resuscitation refers to the application of both basic life support (BLS) and advanced life support (ALS) algorithms. Both BLS and ALS follow a streamlined format designed to intervene on life-threatening disorders that could potentially be reversed. A simple and easy to recall starting point is to approach each unstable or cardiopulmonary arrest victim in an "ABCDE" method which becomes the basis for resuscitative evaluation, critical decision-making, and intervention. In 2010, there has been a change in this paradigm. The new first step is doing chest compressions instead of first establishing the airway and then doing mouth to mouth. The new guidelines apply to adults, children, and infants but exclude newborns. The old way was ABC—for airway, breathing, and compressions. The new way is CAB—for compressions, airway, and breathing.[12]

ABCDE paradigm is to be followed while resuscitating any unstable or unresponsive patient.[13] This helps in identification of reversible life threats and its appropriate management which includes the following:

Airway assessment in a crisis includes a quick check whether patient is phonating. Stridor, snoring, or gurgling sounds suggest that patient's airway is compromised. A patient in cardiac arrest may have no spontaneous respiration and may need BLS maneuvers and bag mask ventilation. Chin lift and jaw thrust maneuvers help in removing airway obstruction caused by loose pharyngeal musculature. After this, mouth is opened and a bag mask device attached to a high flow oxygen source is applied to the patient's face and two breaths are delivered to see if the patient's chest rises. No chest rise means persistent airway obstruction which needs to be relieved by maneuvers like Heimlich or laryngoscopy and foreign body removal.

Breathing assessment includes assessment of presence, speed, and depth of spontaneous respiration. Regular respiratory rates for the pregnant patients increase up to 20 breaths per minute. Patients without spontaneous respiration need oxygenation and ventilator support. Both lung fields must be auscultated to check whether breath sounds are equal. If they are not so, it may indicate tension pneumothorax and will require needle decompression (with wide bore 12–14 gauze needle, in the second intercostal space in midclavicular line).

Circulation assessment includes determination of pulse rate and rhythm along with blood pressure estimation. In cardiac arrest, patients tend to lose peripheral pulses and if radial pulses are palpable, patient has a minimum blood pressure of 70 mmHg. An absence of pulsations mandates chest compressions.

Chest compressions should occur with patient lying on a flat surface and uterus displaced to the right by an assistant or a 15 degree left tilt position by using a backboard or tilt table. Compressions must be 1.5–2 inch deep and about 100 per minute.

Drugs, fluids are to be given after establishing a large bore (18-gauge needle) intravenous access. External defibrillation is to be used if compressions are ineffective. There is no contraindication to external defibrillation during pregnancy and direct current (DC) shocks up to 400 J have been used without adverse fetal effects. Current basic cardiac life support (BCLS) guidelines recommend monophasic defibrillation at 200, 300, and 360 J for the initial three shocks and all subsequent shocks with 360 J and biphasic defibrillation at 100, 200, and 200 J for first three shocks and subsequent shocks with 200 J.

ADVANCED LIFE SUPPORT

Emergent laryngoscopy and intubation, use of medications, use of noninvasive positive pressure devices, and mechanical ventilation are included in advanced life support.

Pregnancy is associated with changes in maternal anatomy and physiology. Some of these factors that limit the effectiveness of standard CPR regimens are:

- Altered airway anatomy: the more anterior and cephalad larynx, friable tissues, enlarged breasts, edema, obesity—all lead to increased incidence of failed intubation
- Increased oxygen consumption: basal metabolic rate (BMR) and oxygen consumption is increased by 20%
- Altered respiratory mechanics: displacement of diaphragm by 4–7 cm cephalad due to pressure of the gravid uterus leads to decrease in functional residual capacity and chest compliance. Most critical respiratory concern is the decrease in functional residual capacity (by about 10–15%) near term

- Decreased buffering capacity: changes in BMR, oxygen demand, and carbon dioxide production induce hyperventilation and a state of compensated respiratory alkalosis which produces low bicarbonate levels and thus decreased buffering capacity
- Circulatory changes: maternal blood volume increases during pregnancy and serves to protect maternal cardiovascular physiology in the face of hypovolemia. However, the uterine circulation is passive and dependent on normal blood volume and flow, as it is in parallel circuit with the maternal circulation
- Aortocaval compression: by the 20th week of gestation, the gravid uterus can compress the IVC and aorta, obstructing venous return and arterial blood flow. The gravid uterus also impacts maternal circulation by its size and weight. It can compress the IVC and the distal aorta during later pregnancy and cause decrease in cardiac output. A critical maneuver in case of maternal shock or cardiac arrest is to either manually displacing the uterus to the patient's left or to roll the patient into the left lateral decubitus position. These maneuvers will serve to decompress the great vessels and augment cardiac return. Rescuers can relieve this compression by positioning the woman on her side or by pulling the gravid uterus to the right side during CPR.

CONDITION OF THE FETUS DURING MATERNAL CARDIAC ARREST

The oxyhemoglobin dissociation curve of fetal hemoglobin is shifted to the left when compared to maternal hemoglobin, yielding a greater oxygen saturation of fetal hemoglobin at any given partial pressure of oxygen to protect the fetus during maternal arrest. But if asphyxia persists, such physiologic adjustments become inadequate and neurologic damage or death of the fetus will occur. It is best to remember that best chance for fetal survival is with a resuscitated mother; however, experience with perimortem section indicates that fetal survival and neurologic outcome are best if delivery is conducted within 5 minutes of maternal arrest.[14]

PERIMORTEM CESAREAN DELIVERY

These days, perimortem cesarean delivery (PMCD) is rarely performed. In literature, about 300 cases have been reported of PMCD.[15] During 1980s, several authors reported unexpected recoveries after PMCD which led to consideration of the possibility that PMCD actually improve, rather than worsen chance of survival during a collapse.

Uteroplacental blood flow requires up to 30% of a woman's cardiac output during pregnancy, some of which may be retrieved for other visceral organ perfusion after delivery. There is a 30% decrease in stroke volume and cardiac output in a pregnant woman who lies supine, largely because there is a vena-caval compression. In addition, there is a 20% reduction in functional residual capacity at term and there is high metabolic rate leading to decreased oxygen reserves and faster onset of anoxia following apnea. Delivery of the near term fetus provides 30–80% improvement in cardiac output and in conjunction with other resuscitative measures, may provide sufficient circulatory improvement to adequately support central nervous system during arrest. This has led a school of thought that PMCD can prove to be an appropriate resuscitative intervention for maternofetal survival.

Anticipation of potential cardiopulmonary arrest in a pregnant patient adds an additional burden of ensuring fetal well-being and survival. Apart from usual understood principles of CPR, few already discussed modifications must be applied carefully during resuscitation of pregnant patients. The CPR guidelines for antepartum and postpartum women are shown in flowcharts 1 and 2.[16] A multidisciplinary management plan should always be available in anticipation of a catastrophe for all critically ill pregnant patients.[3]

Most women experience a normal pregnancy. However, there is a small percentage of women who experience life-threatening complications that may result from the pregnancy itself or may be part of a pre-existing medical or surgical condition. Such critically ill pregnant women provide unique challenge to obstetricians. It is absolutely essential for all obstetricians and other members of the healthcare team to have a working knowledge of unique considerations of an obstetric patient requiring critical care.

CONCLUSION

A critically ill obstetric patient is one who because of abnormal pregnancy, delivery and puerperium or because of effects of a pre-existing systemic disease, anesthesia or surgery develops life-threatening complications for which intensive monitoring, therapy and/or life support system is required. On one hand, medical conditions might present risk to the pregnancy and on the other, pregnancy itself may modify state of the medical disease. Approximately 1% of obstetrical patients need critical care and reported maternal mortality in critically ill obstetric patients admitted to an ICU is approximately 8.4%. Care of critically ill obstetric patients is subdivided into three levels based on organ support and level of monitoring irrespective of underlying disease. It includes Maternal High-Dependency Care Unit, Obstetrical Intensive Care Unit and Medical/surgical Intensive Care Unit. Monitoring in a critical care unit is extremely important as it ensures rapid detection of changes in the clinical status and allows for accurate assessment of progress and response to therapy. Advent of non-invasive techniques and alarms

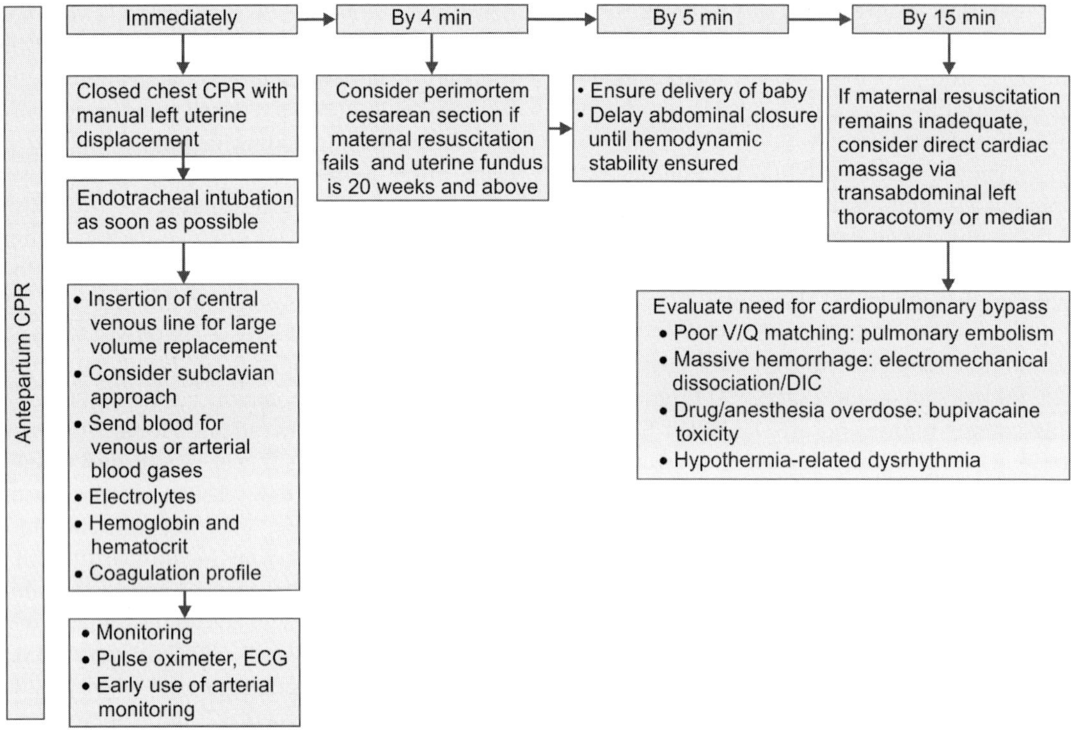

ECG, electrocardiogram; DIC, disseminated intravascular coagulation.

FLOWCHART 1: Algorithmic representation of antepartum cardiopulmonary resuscitation.

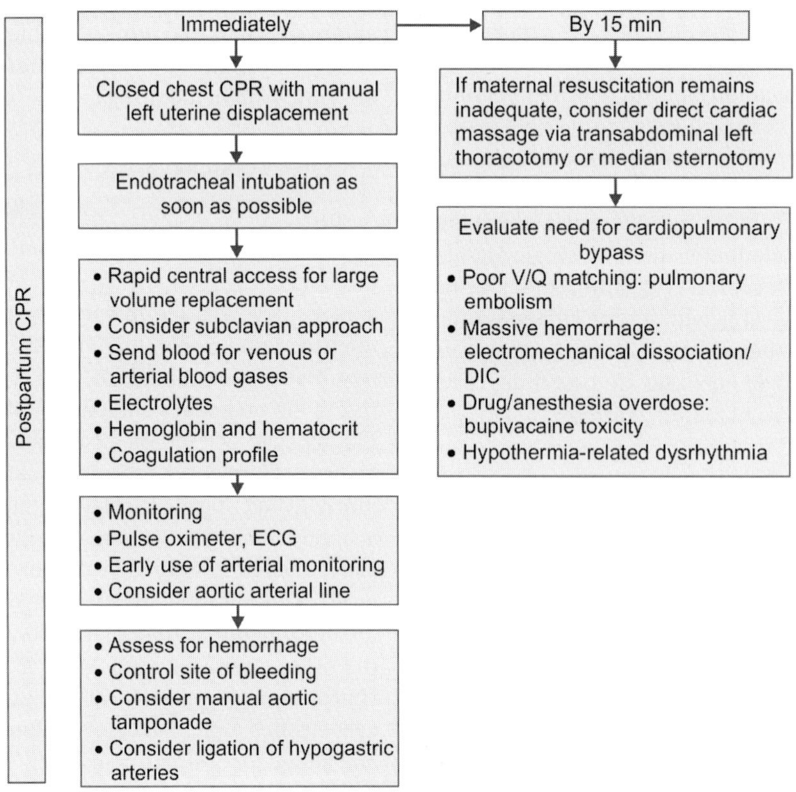

ECG, electrocardiogram; DIC, disseminated intravascular coagulation.

FLOWCHART 2: Algorithmic representation of postpartum cardiopulmonary resuscitation.

has enabled strict monitoring feasible. Generally, if two organ systems are failing with a need for ventilator support ICU admission becomes mandatory. The management also depends on whether patient is in labor or not in labor, the fetal gestational age and need for termination of pregnancy. Cardiac arrest in pregnant patient is a rare and an unexpected event. It may arise due to a pathogenic process within a patient or may result due to iatrogenic factors or trauma. Successful resuscitation of a pregnant woman and survival of the fetus require prompt and excellent CPR with some modifications in techniques.

REFERENCES

1. Kuklina EV, Meikle SF, Jamieson DJ, Whiteman MK, Barfield WD, Hillis SD, et al. Severe obstetric morbidity in the United States: 1998-2005. Obstet Gynecol. 2009;113:293-9.
2. Ananth CV, Smulian JC. Epidemiology of critical illness in pregnancy. In: Belfort M, Saade G, Foley M, Phelan J, Dildy G (Eds). Critical Care Obstetrics, 5th ed. Blackwell Publishers; 2010.
3. Comprehensive Critical Care—a review of adult critical care services. London: DH; 2000. Available from: www.dh.gov.uk/en/Publicationsandstatistics/Publications/PublicationsPolicyAndGuidance/DH_4006585. [Accessed December, 2015].
4. Levels of Critical Care for Adult Patients. Standards and Guidelines. London: ICS; 2009. [Online] Available from: www.ics.ac.uk/intensive_care_professional/standards_and_guidelines/levels_of_critical_care_for_adult_patients. [Accessed December, 2015].
5. Critical care and trauma. In: Cunningham FG, Leveno KJ, Bloom SL, Hauth JC, Rouse DJ, Spong CY (Eds). Williams Obstetrics, 23rd ed. McGraw Hill Publishers; 2010. pp. 926-7.
6. L Moorcroft RM/SoM & H Cooper RN. Severely Ill Women Using the Physiological Observation Track & Trigger System, POTTS (Modified Early Obstetric Warning Score). Version 4.0. June 2013.
7 Joseph V, Fromm RE. Critical care of a pregnant patient. Handbook of Practical Critical Care Medicine, 1st ed. Springer; 2003. p. 315.
8 Guidelines for the transport of the critically ill adult. London: ICS; 2002. [Online] Available from: www.ics.ac.uk/intensive_care_professional/standards_and_guidelines/transport_of_the_critically_ill_2002. [Accessed December, 2015].
9 Kam PC, Cardone D. Propofol infusion syndrome. Anaesthesia. 2007;62;690-701.
10 Vincent JL, Rello J, Marshall J, Silva E, Anzueto A, Martin CD, et al. International study of the prevalence and outcomes of infection in intensive care units. EPIC II Group of Investigators. JAMA. 2009;302:2323-9.
11 The maternity high dependency unit. In: Vaughan D, Robinson N, Lucas N, Arulkumaran S (Eds). Handbook of Obstetric High Dependency Care, 1st edition. John Wiley & Sons Ltd, McGraw Hill Publishers; 2010. pp. 13-25.
12 Peripartum cardiomyopathy: National Heart, Lung, and Blood Institute and Office of Rare Diseases (National Institutes of Health) workshop recommendations and review. JAMA. 2000;283(9):1183-8.
13 Caro D, Topp S. Cardiopulmonary resuscitation during pregnancy. In: Benrubi GI (Ed). Handbook of Obstetric and Gynecologic Emergencies, 4th ed. Lippincott Williams & Wilkins; 2012. pp. 78-80.
14 Royal College of Anaesthetists. Providing equity of critical and maternity care for the critically ill pregnant or recently pregnant woman. Guidelines. 2011.
15 Lyon DS. Perimortem cesarean delivery. In: Benrubi GI (Ed). Handbook of Obstetric and Gynecologic Emergencies, 4th ed. Lippincott Williams & Wilkins; 2012. pp. 90-6.
16 Gombar KK, Gombar S. Resuscitation and care of critically ill obstetric patients. In: Gupta S (Ed). Obstetric Anaesthesia, 1st ed. Arya Publications; 2008. p. 667.

CHAPTER 72

Anaphylaxis

Rashmi Bagga, Aashima Arora

INTRODUCTION

Anaphylaxis is defined as a serious allergic reaction that is rapid in onset and might be fatal. The prevalence of anaphylaxis in community settings is estimated to be 0.05–2%.[1] However, its true incidence during pregnancy is unknown because of paucity of data in literature on anaphylaxis in pregnancy. In one review, the prevalence of anaphylaxis occurring during pregnancy is reported as approximately 3 cases per 100,000 deliveries.[2] Although uncommon, it might be increasing in parallel with the increased incidence of anaphylaxis in the general population. Anaphylaxis during pregnancy can be catastrophic both for the mother and the fetus. It places the mother and especially the baby at high risk of permanent central nervous system (CNS) damage. Similar to infancy and old age, pregnancy also increases the risk of severity and fatality of anaphylaxis.

ETIOLOGY AND PATHOGENESIS

The most common mechanism underlying anaphylaxis in humans involves an immunologic mechanism in which immunoglobulin E (IgE) is synthesized in response to an allergen and becomes fixed to mast cell IgE receptors. On re-exposure to the same allergen, cell activation occurs leading to sudden release of histamine, tryptase, leukotrienes, prostaglandins, platelet-activating factor, and other mediators. The tissue effects of these mediators result in bronchospasm, laryngeal edema, myocardial ischemia, peripheral vasoconstriction, and anaerobic metabolism. Majority of the deaths occur due to circulatory collapse and respiratory arrest. Immunoglobulin E independent immunologic mechanisms are rare in human anaphylaxis. In addition, nonimmune disturbances of mast cells and basophils may also lead to anaphylaxis. The etiology of anaphylaxis in all the three trimesters of pregnancy is similar to that in general population, with food allergens being the most common triggers. The other commonly implicated allergens are medications, venoms, and biological agents, such as natural rubber latex. The medicines usually involved in triggering anaphylaxis in pregnancy are nonsteroidal anti-inflammatory drug (NSAIDs), intravenous iron, and injectable vitamins (mainly B1, B6 and B12). During labor and delivery, the most common etiology of anaphylaxis is antibiotics. The rampant uses of prophylactic injection of penicillin or cephalosporin to prevent maternal infection after cesarean delivery or to prevent neonatal group B streptococcal infection are most commonly implicated. Two large reviews of anaphylaxis in pregnancy and postpartum women, one multicentric and the other from Texas, have found the triggering allergen to be a β-lactam antibiotic in around 35 and 60% women, respectively.[3,4] The other common etiologies found in these two reviews were antigens such as oxytocic agents, antiemetics, antihypertensives, and antirheumatic medications. Less common causes may be bee sting, radiocontrast medium, or local anesthetic agent. Rapid changes in the level of progesterone may be the underlying cause of an increased incidence of anaphylaxis, both in late pregnancy and in immediate postpartum period.[5-7]

DIAGNOSIS

The diagnosis of anaphylaxis is primarily clinical and valid even if the results of laboratory tests are normal. Clinical diagnosis is based on detailed history and recognition of characteristic symptoms which must be sudden in onset and rapid in progression. The symptoms occur characteristically within minutes to a few hours after exposure to a known or likely antigen and typically involve more than one organ system. Symptoms may vary between individuals and even from one anaphylactic episode to another in the same individual. Skin symptoms and signs are reported in 80–90% of patients and hence, anaphylaxis may not be identified in their absence. Respiratory tract involvement is seen in up to 70% of cases while gastrointestinal and cardiovascular symptoms each are reported in 45% of cases. Characteristic symptoms in pregnancy include intense vulvar itching, low back pain, preterm labor, and evidence of fetal distress. The episode of anaphylaxis may vary in severity from being a transient and unrecognized episode, to respiratory or cardiac arrest, and death within minutes. The World Allergy Organization developed anaphylaxis guidelines in 2011 to facilitate its prompt recognition and management.[8-10] According to these guidelines, the clinical criteria for diagnosis of anaphylaxis during pregnancy is highly likely when the following criteria are fulfilled. The first criterion is applicable in women with no prior history of anaphylaxis. The second criterion is for women who develop symptoms after exposure to a likely allergen while the third criterion is for women who develop symptoms after exposure to known allergen.

- Acute onset of an illness (minutes to several hours) with involvement of the skin, mucosal tissue, or both (generalized urticaria, itching or flushing, swollen lips-tongue-uvula) and at least one of the following:
    - Respiratory compromise (dyspnea, wheeze or bronchospasm, stridor, reduced peak expiratory flow, hypoxemia)
    - Reduced blood pressure or associated symptoms of end-organ dysfunction (hypotonia or collapse, syncope, incontinence)
- Two or more of the following that occur rapidly after exposure to a likely allergen for that patient (minutes to several hours):
    - Involvement of the skin-mucosal tissue (e.g., generalized urticaria, itch-flush, swollen lips-tongue-uvula)
    - Respiratory compromise (e.g., dyspnea, wheeze-bronchospasm, stridor, hypoxemia)
    - Reduced blood pressure or associated symptoms (e.g., hypotonia and collapse, syncope, incontinence)
    - Persistent gastrointestinal symptoms (e.g., crampy abdominal pain, vomiting)
- Reduced blood pressure after exposure to known allergen for that person (minutes to several hours) defined as systolic blood pressure of less than 90 mmHg or more than 30% decrease from that person's baseline value.

Serum total tryptase measurement is a useful test for confirming the diagnosis of anaphylaxis in general population, there is no specific literature on the utility of this laboratory test in pregnant women.[11] These serum tryptase levels may be useful for confirmation of the diagnosis in some pregnant women like those with medication induced anaphylaxis. Serial measurements are more sensitive than single blood levels. Also, the samples should optimally be obtained 15 minutes to 3 hours after the onset of symptoms.

DIFFERENTIAL DIAGNOSIS

The differential diagnoses of anaphylaxis in the first three trimesters of pregnancy are similar to that in general population. The more common conditions, like acute asthma, acute generalized urticaria, or syncopal attack, pose significant diagnostic dilemmas. Other forms of shock like hypovolemic, septic, or cardiogenic and rare conditions, like hereditary angioedema, also need to be considered in patients who present with anaphylaxis like clinical picture. It is important to differentiate the above mentioned conditions from anaphylaxis based upon the history or clinical setting for these conditions. However, during labor and delivery, there are certain differentials which may closely mimic an anaphylactic reaction. Pulmonary embolism and cardiac conditions are the most common differential diagnosis in these patients. Pregnant women with heart disease may manifest for the first time during labor because the physiological cardiovascular changes during pregnancy, labor, and delivery can lead to decompensation in these women with coexisting heart disease. Also, specific obstetric conditions, like pre-eclampsia/eclampsia-associated symptoms, abruptio placenta, or uterine rupture may also have a clinical presentation overlapping with anaphylaxis. These conditions need to be diagnosed timely because they require urgent management which is different from that of anaphylaxis. Rarer differentials may be myocardial infarction and amniotic fluid embolism. They may be difficult to diagnose, especially because these conditions are also associated with increased total tryptase levels, as found in anaphylaxis. Amniotic fluid embolism has a case fatality rate of more than 20% and the diagnosis is mainly clinical with patient presenting with one or more of profound hypotension, cardiovascular collapse, arrhythmias, cyanosis, dyspnea, respiratory distress, hemorrhage, disseminated intravascular coagulation, and altered mental status, in the absence of other medical explanations for this clinical course.

MANAGEMENT

The management of anaphylaxis in pregnancy is same as that in nonpregnant population. A written emergency anaphylaxis protocol must be displayed at all medical and surgical settings and must be rehearsed by the medical staff. Removal of exposure to the antigen must be expedited, if possible for example stopping an intravenous drug being administered. Senior help should be immediately sought for, and should preferably include an anesthesiologist, obstetrician, and neonatologist in hospital setting. Simultaneously, maternal airway, breathing, circulation, and mental status must be assessed. Adrenaline (epinephrine) is the treatment of choice for anaphylaxis and must be administered intramuscularly using a first aid dose of 0.3 mg. Epinephrine for intramuscular injection contains 1 mg/mL and may also be labeled as 1: 1,000. For adults, the recommended dose of epinephrine (1 mg/mL) is 0.3–0.5 mg per single dose, injected intramuscularly into the mid-outer thigh (vastus lateralis muscle). Intramuscular injection is recommended over subcutaneous because it provides a more rapid increase in the plasma and tissue concentrations. This may be repeated after 5–15 minutes, if required. It decreases mediator release from mast cells, prevents and reverses obstruction in the upper and lower respiratory tracts, and prevents or reverses cardiovascular collapse.[12] High flow humidified oxygen should be administered through a close fitting face mask or oropharyngeal airway. Two large 16 G intravenous lines should be secured and saline should be infused rapidly. The patient should be placed in left lateral position to prevent the gravid uterus from compressing the inferior vena cava and obstructing venous return to the heart. Personalized written instructions about avoidance of confirmed or relevant trigger(s) and safe alternatives should be provided for patients who have had an episode of anaphylaxis. Regarding the role of glucocorticoids and antihistamines, two Cochrane reviews were unable to make any recommendations for their use in the treatment of anaphylaxis.[13,14] The onset of action of glucocorticoids takes several hours and they do not relieve the initial symptoms and signs of anaphylaxis. The rationale for giving them is to prevent the delayed or biphasic reactions that occur in some cases of anaphylaxis. For relieving itching and urticaria, H1-antihistamines may be useful, but they do not relieve bronchospasm, gastrointestinal symptoms, hypotension, or shock. Diphenhydramine (50 mg intravenously) or oral cetirizine/loratidine may be given during pregnancy. Bronchodilators (e.g., nebulized albuterol) may help in severe bronchospasm but these do not relieve upper airway edema, and should not be substituted for epinephrine in the treatment of anaphylaxis. During pregnancy, besides maternal monitoring, continuous electronic fetal heart monitoring (EFM) of viable fetuses is to be done. Emergency cesarean may be required for a persistent nonreassuring EFM trace. In a review describing anaphylaxis in the setting of obstetric anesthesia, fetal outcomes were normal in cases in which epinephrine was administered promptly and at appropriate doses, and cesarean delivery was performed within 10–15 minutes after the onset of anaphylaxis.[2] However, before resorting to an emergency cesarean, the fetal benefits must be balanced against the anesthetic and surgical risks to the pregnant woman experiencing anaphylaxis.[15]

CONCLUSION

Anaphylaxis in pregnancy may be life threatening both for the mother and the fetus. Its true incidence in pregnant population is not known but is expected to be rising. The condition is primarily clinical and usually presents within of minutes of exposure to a known or a likely antigen. WHO has issued anaphylaxis guidelines in 2011 to aid prompt diagnosis and management. The differential diagnosis in the antenatal period are similar to the non pregnant population; however, during labour and delivery, pulmonary embolism and cardiac conditions closely mimic anaphylactic reaction. Conditions specific to obstetrics, like pre-eclampsia/eclampsia, abruptio, uterine rupture or amniotic fluid embolism must be differentiated from anaphylaxis timely in view of different management. The primary treatment of anaphylaxis in pregnancy is same as non-pregnant which include prompt removal of exposure to antigen, intramuscular adrenaline and supportive care.

REFERENCES

1. Lieberman P, Camargo CA, Bohlke K, Jick H, Miller RL, Sheikh A, et al. Epidemiology of anaphylaxis: findings of the American College of Allergy, Asthma and Immunology Epidemiology of Anaphylaxis Working Group. Ann Allergy Asthma Immunol. 2006;97(5):596-602.
2. Hepner DL, Castells M, Mouton-Faivre C, Dewachter P. Anaphylaxis in the clinical setting of obstetric anesthesia: a literature review. Anesth Analg. 2013;117(6):1357-67.
3. Chaudhuri K, Gonzales J, Jesurun CA, Ambat MT, Mandal-Chaudhuri S. Anaphylactic shock in pregnancy: a case study and review of the literature. Int J Obstet Anesth. 2008;17(4):350-7.
4. Mulla ZD, Ebrahim MS, Gonzalez JL. Anaphylaxis in the obstetric patient: analysis of a statewide hospital discharge database. Ann Allergy Asthma Immunol. 2010;104(1):55-9.
5. Villalta D, Martelli P. A case of breastfeeding anaphylaxis. Eur Ann Allergy Clin Immunol. 2007;39(1):26-7.
6. McKinney KK, Scranton SE. A case report of breastfeeding anaphylaxis: successful prophylaxis with oral antihistamines. Allergy. 2011;66(3):435-6.
7. Shank JJ, Olney SC, Lin FL, McNamara MF. Recurrent postpartum anaphylaxis with breast-feeding. Obstet Gynecol. 2009;114(2 Pt 2):415-6.
8. Simons FE, Ardusso LR, Bilo MB, El-Gamal YM, Ledford DK, Ring J, et al. 2012 Update: World Allergy Organization Guidelines for the assessment and management of anaphylaxis. Curr Opin Allergy Clin Immunol. 2012;12(4):389-99.
9. Sampson HA, Munoz-Furlong A, Campbell RL, Adkinson NF, Bock SA, Branum A, et al. Second symposium on the definition and management

of anaphylaxis: summary report--Second National Institute of Allergy and Infectious Disease/Food Allergy and Anaphylaxis Network symposium. J Allergy Clin Immunol. 2006;117(2):391-7.

10. Braveman FR. Pregnancy-associated diseases. In: Hines RL, Marschall KE (Eds). Stoelting's Anesthesia and Coexisting Diseases, 5th edition. Philadelphia, PA, USA: Churchill Livingstone; 2008. pp. 557-80.
11. Schwartz LB. Diagnostic value of tryptase in anaphylaxis and mastocytosis. Immunol Allergy Clin North Am. 2006;26(3):451-63.
12. Vadas P, Perelman B. Effect of epinephrine on platelet-activating factor-stimulated human vascular smooth muscle cells. J Allergy Clin Immunol. 2012;129(5):1329-33.
13. Choo KJ, Simons FE, Sheikh A. Glucocorticoids for the treatment of anaphylaxis. Cochrane Database Syst Rev. 2012;4:CD007596.
14. Sheikh A, Ten Broek V, Brown SG, Simons FE. H1-antihistamines for the treatment of anaphylaxis: Cochrane systematic review. Allergy. 2007;62(8):830-7.
15. Simons FE, Schatz M. Anaphylaxis during pregnancy. J Allergy Clin Immunol. 2012;130(3):597-606.

CHAPTER 73

Blood Component Therapy

Jai B Sharma, Manisha Yadav

INTRODUCTION

Blood transfusion (BT) is a lifesaving procedure. Obstetric hemorrhage is a major cause of maternal morbidity worldwide and is more common in the developing countries. It significantly reduces mortality and morbidity if used where indicated. But transfusion of blood and its various components also has many risks associated with it which includes immunological and nonimmunological complications.

PURPOSE OF BLOOD TRANSFUSION

Principles of blood transfusion are mentioned below.
It is primarily used for three main reasons:
1. For replacement of vascular volume
2. For replacement of clotting factors
3. For maintenance of oxygen carrying capacity of blood.

PRINCIPLES OF BLOOD TRANSFUSION

- At the first antenatal check-up, all females should have their blood group determined and at 28 weeks of gestation, the antibody status should be checked
- Do not use blood samples more than 7 days old for crossmatching red blood cells (RBCs). Prefer a fresh blood sample
- There are two main indications for BT in obstetric patients: anemia and hemorrhage
  - Indications of transfusion in anemic patients include:
    - In healthy antenatal women, there is no need of BT
    - If hemoglobin (Hb) levels drop to 7 g/dL, the possibility of transfusion should be taken based on individuals' medical history, age, and clinical condition of the patient
    - If Hb levels falls less than 5 g/dL, BT is definitely indicated
  - In patients with hemorrhage or blood loss, transfusion depends upon the blood volume lost by the patient. Refer to table 1 for management.

Volume occupied by both cells and plasma in the vascular system constitutes total blood volume. In an adult, about 7% of body weight or 70 mL/kg is total blood volume.
Blood is a fluid connective tissue composed of:
- Plasma:
  - Proteins
  - Coagulation factors
  - Metabolic substances

TABLE 1: Management of patient with blood loss

Blood volume lost		Treatment
(%)	(mL)	
≥40	≥2,000	Rapid volume replacement,* RBC transfusion
30–40	1,500–2,000	Rapid volume replacement,* ± RBC transfusion
15–30	800–1,500	± Rapid volume replacement, ± RBC transfusion
≤15	≤750	No transfusion indicated except in rare cases

Note: Transfusion of 1 unit of whole blood or RBCs increases hematocrit by 3% or Hb by 1 g/dL in a non-bleeding adult.
*With crystalloids or synthetic colloids.
RBC, red blood cell.

- Cells:
  - Red blood cells
  - White blood cells
  - Platelets.

BLOOD PRODUCTS

These are classified as blood components prepared in the BT center [red cells, platelets, fresh frozen plasma (FFP) and cryoprecipitate] or plasma derivatives manufactured from pooled plasma donations in plasma fractionation centers (such as albumin, coagulation factors, and immunoglobulins). Plasma derivatives are covered by the Medicines Act and, like any other drug, must be prescribed by a licensed practitioner.

Blood Components

Whole blood is now rarely used for transfusion. Blood component therapy makes clinical sense as most patients require a specific element of blood, such as red cells or platelets, and the dose can then be optimized. Each component is stored under ideal conditions (e.g., red cells must be refrigerated, platelets must not) and the use of precious blood donations becomes more efficient. Flowchart 1 shows various blood components.

Whole Blood

- A bag of whole blood contains: 450 mL donor blood and 63 mL anticoagulant
- Hemoglobin is approximately 12 g/dL and hematocrit is 35–45%. There are no functional platelets and no labile coagulation factors (V and VIII)
- Unit of issue: one donation, also referred to as a unit or pack
- Infection risk: not sterilized.

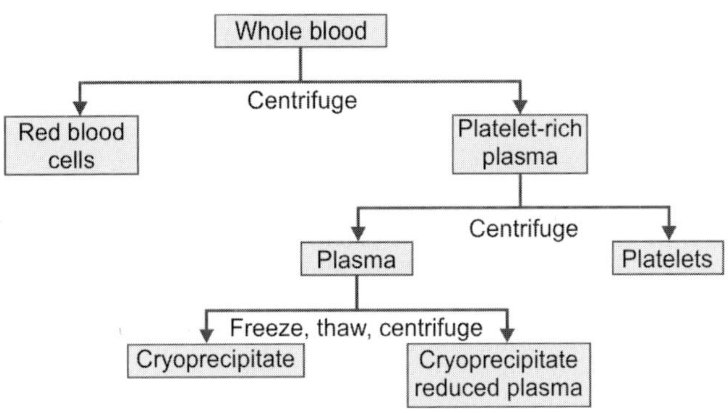

FLOWCHART 1: Blood components.

Indications

- Improve oxygen delivery over a short time where there is no facility for blood component
- Maintain blood volume after massive hemorrhage
- Exchange transfusion.

Storage

- Between 2 and 6°C.

Contraindications

Risk of volume overload in patients with:
- Chronic anemia
- Incipient cardiac failure.

Administration

- Must be ABO and RhD compatible with recipient
- Never add medication to a unit of blood.

COMPONENT PREPARATION

Red Cell Components

Red Cell Concentrate

- 150–200 mL red cells from which most of plasma has been removed
- Hemoglobin level approximately 20 g/100 dL
- Hematocrit 55–75%
- 50–70 mL plasma
- One unit of red cell concentrates (pRBCs) should raise the Hb level by 1 g/dL and hematocrit by 3%.[1]

Indications:
- Thalassemia
- Hemoglobin less than 7 g/dL
- Aplastic anemia
- Congestive heart failure/chronic renal failure
- Blood loss more than 15% of blood volume.

Red Cell Suspension

- 150–200 mL red cells with 110 mL normal saline, adenine, glucose, and mannitol
- Hemoglobin 15 g/dL
- Hematocrit 50–70%
- 10–20 mL or less plasma.

Advantages:
- Lower packed cell volume, reduce viscosity, and easier to infuse
- Better preservation, longer shelf life than whole blood or packed cells:
  - Irradiated pRBCs are irradiated by using cesium 137 source
  - A dose of 2,500 cGy delivered to each unit

- After irradiation, storage time decreased to maximum of 28 days
- Purpose is to inactivate donors' immunocompetent lymphocytes and prevention of transfusion associated graft versus host disease.[2]

Platelet Concentrates

Single donor unit in a volume of 50–60 mL of plasma contains:
- At least 55 × 10^9 platelets
- Less than 1.2 × 10^9 red cells
- Less than 0.12 × 10^9 leukocyte.

Unit of issue

Supplied as either:
- Single donor unit (50,000–100,000)
- Pooled unit (10,000–20,000)
- Random donor platelet (4,000–5,000)
- Single donor platelets are also referred to as jumbo platelets or apheresis platelets
- 1 unit = 100 mL.

Advantage

- Less infectious risk
- Full and effective transfusion dose
- Less risk of human leukocyte antigen (HLA) allo-immunization.

Donor selection

- Hemoglobin more than 12.5 gm/dL
- Platelets counts more than 1.8 lacs
- Should be human immunodeficiency virus, hepatitis B surface antigen, hepatitis C virus, Venereal Disease Research Laboratory Test, and malaria negative.[3]

Storage

- At 20–24°C (with agitation) for up to 5 days (longer storage increases the risk of bacterial proliferation and septicemia in recipient).

Indications[3]

It is indicated for the treatment of bleeding due to:
- Thrombocytopenia
- Platelet function defects
- Prevention of bleeding in bone marrow failure.

Not generally indicated for prophylaxis of bleeding in surgical patients unless preoperative significant platelet deficiency.

Indications for transfusion

- Platelet count less than 20,000/μL
- Active bleeding and platelet count less than 50,000/μL
- Platelet count less than 50,000/μL and surgery without active bleeding
- Surgery with active bleeding and platelet count 50,000–100,000.

Platelets express ABO antigens and will get best increment with ABO compatible platelets.

They do not express Rh antigens and can be given regardless of Rh type. However, platelets contain a small amount of RBCs, so Rh-negative woman of childbearing age should receive Rh-negative platelets.

Leukodepleted Blood Products

Remove leukocytes prior to transfusion to reduce the incidence and severity of nonhemolytic febrile transfusion reaction and sensitization to blood products (HLA alloimmunization).

Technique of leukocyte reduction

- Centrifugation
- Removal of buffy coat
- Spin cool filter method (microaggregate).

Filters reduce leukocyte more than 99.9% with less than 10% depletion of RBCs. Prestorage leukocyte reduction is preferred to poststorage reduction.

Plasma (Pale Yellow Fluid)

One unit of plasma (180–300 mL) is defined as amount of plasma obtained from centrifugation of 1 unit of whole blood. It contains nearly normal levels of all factors except factor VIII.

Storage

- Indefinitely at –18°C.

Indication

- Invasive procedure or surgery with international normalized ratio (INR) more than 1.5
- Massive hemorrhage with INR more than 1.5
- Inherited coagulopathies, in which specific factor not available
- Emergency reversal of anticoagulant therapy
- Volume replacement as in trauma and burns.

Fresh Frozen Plasma

Plasma is separated from whole blood within 6 hour of collection and rapidly frozen to –25°C. It contains normal plasma levels of stable clotting factors, albumin, and immunoglobulin.

Storage

- At –25°C for up to 1 year.

Dosage

- Initial dose is 15 mL/kg.

Indications

Replacement of multiple coagulation factor deficiencies, e.g.:
- Liver disease
- Warfarin anticoagulant overdose
- Dilution-induced coagulopathy
- Disseminated intravascular coagulation
- Thrombotic thrombocytopenic purpura.

Administration must normally be ABO compatible to avoid risk of hemolysis in recipients.

Before use, thawed in water at 30–37°C and once thawed, stored at 2–6°C. Labile factors rapidly degrade, so should be used within 6 hour of thawing.

Cryoprecipitate[4]

Cold insoluble plasma proteins, precipitate in FFP when it is thawed at 1–6°C, then centrifuged, collected, and refrozen. Main constituents:
- Fibrinogen: 150–300 mg/pack
- Factor VIII: 80–100 IU/pack
- von Willebrand disease (vWF/vWD)
- Factor XIII and fibronectin (made from FFP within 12 months of collection).

Storage

- At –25°C or colder for up to 1 year and must be transfused within 4 hour.

Indications

- Disseminated intravascular coagulation with active bleeding or before invasive procedure and activated partial thromboplastin time (APTT) more than 1.5 normal
- Hypofibrinogenemia (<100 mg/dL) or dysfibrinogenemia with active bleeding or before scheduled invasive procedure
- von Willebrand disease unresponsive to desmopressin (1-deamino- 8-D-arginine vasopressin) with active bleeding or before scheduled invasive procedure
- Factor XIII deficiency.

Factor VIII Concentrate

Partially purified factor VIII prepared from large pools of donor plasma. One freeze dried vial contains 250 IU. It is stored at 2–6°C.

Indications:
- Treatment of hemophilia A
- Treatment of vWD

Alternatives:
- Cryoprecipitate
- Fresh frozen plasma.

Recombinant Activated Factor VII (NovoSeven)

Recombinant activated factor VII (rFVIIa) used to stop active bleeding in hemophilia patients with antibodies to factor VIII. Single dose of rFVIIa at 90–120 µg/kg intravenous over 3-5 minutes, induce immediate hemostasis.

Mechanism of action: Binds tissue factor and activates factor X directly.

Advantages of Component Therapy

- Specific portions of the blood that patients require can be administered, thereby allowing several patients to benefit from one donation
- Administration of unnecessary or unwanted components is avoided
- Chances of transfusion associated illness are less.

COMPATIBILITY TESTING

Compatibility testing is done in three steps:
1. ABO-Rh typing
2. Crossmatching
3. Antibody screening.

ABO-Rh Typing

Determination of the patient's correct blood type is exceedingly important and is done by testing RBCs for A and B antigens and the serum for A and B antibodies. Rh typing is also carried out.

Crossmatching

Crossmatching is essentially a trial transfusion in which donor cells are mixed with recipient serum to detect potential for serious transfusion reactions. It takes about 45-60 minutes for crossmatching and is carried out in three phases:
1. First phase is carried out at room temperature and is a check against errors in ABO typing and those naturally occurring antibodies in the mononuclear phagocytes and Lewis systems
2. Second phase involves incubation of the first phase reactions at 37°C in albumin which aids in detection of incomplete antibodies. This step primarily detects antibodies in Rh system
3. Third phase involves addition of antiglobulin sera to incubated test tubes. This antiglobulin phase detects most incomplete antibodies in the blood group systems including Rh, Kell, Kidd, and Duffy blood group systems.

While all the three phases are important, the first two stages are of prime importance in preventing serious hemolytic transfusion reactions.

Antibody Screening

This is also carried out in three phases and is similar to the length of crossmatching. The screen for unexpected antibodies is also carried out on donor serum. This screen is performed primarily to prevent reactions between transfused donor units.

TRANSFUSION REACTIONS

Acute Complications

- Mild reactions:
  - Allergic/urticarial reactions
- Moderately severe reactions:
  - Severe urticarial reactions
  - Febrile nonhemolytic reactions
- Possible bacterial contamination life-threatening reactions:
  - Acute intravascular hemolysis
  - Bacterial contamination and septic shock
  - Fluid overload
  - Anaphylactic reactions
  - Transfusion-associated lung injury.

Hemolytic Transfusion Reactions

The incidence of hemolytic transfusion reactions varies from 1:4,000–1:6,000. Fatal hemolytic transfusion reactions occur in about 1:100,000. Signs and symptoms include fever, chills, chest and flank pain, flushing, nausea, dyspnea, hemoglobinuria, and bleeding diathesis is how a patient with hemolytic transfusion reaction would present.

Treatment

- Stop the BT
- Maintain urine output at 75–100 mL/h by generously administrating intravenous fluids and possibly mannitol 2.5–50 g given over 5–15 minutes period. If this is ineffective in maintaining urine output, then administer furosemide 20–40 mg intravenous
- Alkalinize the urine since bicarbonate is preferentially exercised in the urine. Only 40–70 mEq/70 kg of sodium bicarbonate is required to raise the urine pH to 8
- Assay urine and plasma hemoglobin concentrations
- Determine platelet count, partial thromboplastin time, and serum fibrinogen level
- Return unused blood to the blood bank for recrossmatch
- Send patient's blood sample to blood bank for antibody screen and direct antiglobulin test
- Prevent hypotension to ensure adequate renal flow.

Delayed Hemolytic Transfusion Reactions

In many cases of hemolytic transfusion reaction, the transfused donor cells may survive well initially, but after a variable delay of 2–21 days will be hemolyzed. This type of reaction occurs usually in patients sensitized to red cell antigens by previous BTs or pregnancy. These patients manifest as decreased hematocrit, sometimes jaundice or hemoglobinuria. They can also sometimes cause impairment in renal function but rarely cause demise.

Unlike immediate transfusion reactions, antibodies most commonly involved in delayed hemolytic reactions is Rh and Kidd systems rather than the ABO systems.

Nonhemolytic Transfusion Reactions

These reactions are febrile or allergic in nature. The symptoms consist of chills, fever, headache, myalgia, nausea, and nonproductive cough occurring shortly after BT. Allergic transfusion reactions are mild and caused by foreign protein in transfused blood. The most common symptom is urticarial associated with itching. Three percent of all transfusions cause allergic reactions. Antihistaminics are used to relieve symptoms.

Transfusion-associated Acute Lung Injury

It is acute respiratory distress syndrome within 2–6 hours after transfusion in which:

- Chocking, noncardiogenic pulmonary edema occurs manifested as hypoxia
- Seen one in every 2,000–5,000 BTs
- Pathogenesis is antibody-mediated against HLA or granulocyte specific antibody. Treatment is supportive with the mechanical ventilation and intravenous fluid for hypotension
- Diuretic worsens the situation.

Delayed Complications

Transfusion-transmitted Infections

Transfusion-transmitted infections (TTIs) are infections transmitted by blood from donor to recipient. The incidence has decreased dramatically due to advanced technology and strict laws. The common TTIs are:

- Human immunodeficiency virus 1 and 2
- Human T-lymphotropic viruses I and II
- Viral hepatitis B and C
- Syphilis
- Chaga's disease
- Malaria cytomegalovirus
- Human parvovirus B19 and hepatitis A
- Delayed hemolytic reactions

- Post-transfusion purpura
- Graft-host disease
- Iron overload.

ALTERNATIVES OF BLOOD TRANSFUSION

Wherever possible, BT should be avoided and other alternatives are considered like the following:

- Treat anemia in all antenatal women
- Start with oral iron therapy if Hb level is less than 10.5 g/dL
- If oral iron is not well tolerated by the patient start on parenteral iron therapy. Advantage of the same includes a prompt response but the disadvantage is that it is more invasive and leads to increase in the treatment cost for the patient
- Recombinant human erythropoietin is indicated in anemia due to end-stage renal disease but is still under clinical trials
- All procedures to minimize blood loss should be undertaken, especially during delivery, third stage of labor, and during surgery. Active management of third stage of labor should be done. Decrease operative blood loss during surgery by prompt ligation of all bleeding points, diathermy, and use of local hemostatic agents
- All high risk patients should have their deliveries conducted in institutions with facilities for BT.

REFERENCES

1. Carson JL, Grossman BJ, Kleinman S, Tinmouth AT, Marques MB, Fung MK, et al. Red blood cell transfusion: a clinical practice guideline from the AABB*. Ann Intern Med. 2012;157(1):49-58.
2. World Health Organization (WHO). Blood Manual - 2006.
3. Sharma S, Sharma P, Tyler LN. Transfusion of blood and blood products: indications and complications. Am Fam Physician. 2011;83(6):719-24.
4. CHCSJ Health Bureau, Macau. Blood transfusion guidelines. 2005.

CHAPTER 74

Sexual Activity: Pre- and Postdelivery

Rohini Rao, Rajesh K Verma, Divya Yadav

INTRODUCTION

Pregnancy is the most wonderful experience which a women encounters in her lifespan. When a woman decides to carry a baby in her womb she puts aside all her priorities and interests for her health and physical appearance to have a healthy baby.

Pregnancy is a period in a woman's life which is punctuated by the emotional, psychological, and physical changes, which in turn, affect her sexual life.[1]

Sexuality during pregnancy and the postpartum was considered a taboo and many misconceptions, misinformation, and myths are also associated with it.[2]

Even in the present century, the topic for the sexuality during pregnancy and postpartum period is very deemed and untouched topic. Till the starting of the present era most of the health workers presumed that a pregnant woman is not comfortable having a discussion on sexuality during that period.

The information regarding sexuality during pregnancy and postpartum is lacking in the masses and not up to the mark even in this era of high level of education. This topic is hardly discussed during prenatal counseling or rather it is avoided to be discussed by the healthcare provider.[3]

PHYSIOLOGICAL CHANGES IN REPRODUCTIVE ORGANS IN PREGNANCY AND POSTPARTUM

From the inception of the pregnancy to the end of the postpartum, there are constant and continuous changes in her body which are influenced by many hormones.

Progesterone

The changes in the pregnant female's body by the hormones, especially due to progesterone, can cause physical and mental changes in the first trimester of pregnancy. These changes actually alter the female sexuality. The changes which occur are increased sensitivity and excitability of breasts, vagina, and vulva due to the tissue congestion, which in turn, sometimes can cause dyspareunia. There could be discharge which can be copious and even to the extent that some females have involuntary urine leakage that can cause negative effect on quality of sexuality.[4-7]

The vasodilatation effect of the progesterone causes lowering of the blood pressure and also fatigue, which in combination with discomfort, causes further reduction of sexual excitability. And last but not the least the central effect of progesterone causes dysphoria.[8,9]

Estrogen

As such pregnancy is considered a hyperestrogenic state. This elevated level of estrogens causes a risk of chronic vaginal mycotic infection, which in turn, leads to dyspareunia. There is a fall of estrogen level during first 6–8 weeks after the childbirth. This fall causes decrease in the sexual excitability decreases in orgasms and also there is thinning of vaginal wall which causes dyspareunia.[4,10]

Oxytocin

There are oxytocin receptors in the uterus and during intercourse in the latter half of the pregnancy it results in postorgasmic contractions. These contractions do not promote cervical ripening or preterm labour, they usually settle in 15 minutes.[11]

Prolactin

Breastfeeding is associated with decrease in coital activity and sexual desire. The negative effect which is caused by the breastfeeding is due to raised levels of prolactin, which in turn, suppresses the production of gonadotrophins and thus results in hypoestrogenic state. During breastfeeding, there can be milk ejaculation during orgasm. All these factors when combined leads to decrease in sexual excitability.

SEXUAL BEHAVIOR AND ACTIVITIES DURING PREGNANCY AND POSTPARTUM

Sexual desire fluctuates and varies a lot during pregnancy. It is admitted by most of the women that their libido changes to some degree throughout the pregnancy.[12]

The research done so far has indicated that there is no contraindication to coitus in a healthy pregnant woman.[13] Even the Holy Bible is not against the sexual intercourse during postpartum and pregnancy.

The sexual intercourse should be prohibited in complicated pregnancies such as in patients having placenta previa, premature dilatation of cervix, premature rupture of membranes, multiple gestational pregnancy, presence of some infection, and in engaged head. In these conditions, the effect of sexual activity on pregnancy must be discussed with the healthcare provider.[14]

The important components for the couples to have good sexual intimacy are that the intercourse should be painless and satisfactory, which in turn, is influenced by the emotional, physical, and gestational demands.[15]

Usually, the female sexual interest is not changed during first trimester. There is only a slight decrease in sexuality.[10,16]

The second trimester is emotionally most stable period of pregnancy. In this period, the pregnancy is clearly established and as the pregnancy advances the fear of fetal loss is decreased. Due to cessation of nausea and the pregnant pelvic-vascular changes, there is an increase in orgasmic quality and erotism level as well. Thus the sexual functions are best in second trimester.

In the third trimester, there are significant changes in the female body. These changes are responsible for the fall of libido and decrease in the sexual activity during this trimester. In this period, there is increase in abdominal volume and the fetal weight which causes lack of balance and discomfort in the change of posture, which leads to use of muscles which are seldom used before pregnancy and leading to lumbar pain. The other factors are anxiety, fatigue, and apprehension about the process of labor making the sexual relationship unattractive for pregnant woman. Another important factor which contributes is the partner's loss of sexual interest as he is more concerned for the health of woman and the baby. He has nonerotic effect because of the woman's appearance towards the end of pregnancy.

However, about 37% of females indicate that they have increase in the sexual interest throughout the pregnancy.[17]

In pregnancy, the partner also explores the non coital means of intimacy, such as cuddling, fondling, caressing, massaging, oral sex, masturbation, and many other gestures, to show the love and tenderness, to maintain the relationship, and to relieve the sexual tension in pregnancy.[18]

In postpartum, the noncoital activity invariably commence early, approximately 3 weeks after parturition. After the childbirth, the first orgasm is usually perceived by 7 weeks postpartum in most of the women. Most of the couples start their sexual life in the 6–8 weeks of puerperium. Maximum numbers of females (about 95%) have regular sexual intercourse till the end of 3 months after the parturition. There is a significant decrease in sexual activity in first year of the childbirth. Most of the couples use one or other method of contraception.[10,19]

SEXUAL PROBLEMS AND DYSFUNCTIONS

Epidemiology

Sexual problems and dysfunctions can have a huge impact on the couple's quality of life. The decrease in the sexual functions might have negative effect on self-esteem and the partner's interpersonal relationship. All these factors lead to emotional distress.[20]

About 30–50% of the couples are insecure about the safety and fear of insulting the fetus by sexual activity. The male partners are also afraid of hurting their female partners and the female partner is afraid and is motivated by the endeavor of insufficient satisfaction of her partner.[21,22]

Only 12–14% of couples do not have any sexual dysfunction or any problem after the childbirth. About half of the females have pain on their first sexual contact and with the passage of time the dyspareunia gradually decreases. Initially, after 3 months, about 41% have dyspareunia and it comes down to about 22% after the initial 6 months with a drastic fall to 19% after the first year of delivery. Nearly 57% of the females give a priority and are concerned about their male partner's satisfaction.[4,5,10,23,24]

The Female Sexual Function Index Questionnaire (FSFI) is the only index which can evaluate the prevalence of sexual dysfunction and sexual function in the teenagers and adults in all the three gestational trimesters. The FSFI is safe and valid index to measure the female sexual function. It also gives a reflection of female's sexual response and response to the pain as it is a multidimensional research instrument.[25] Using FSFI as tool in a meta-analysis of 59 studies, von Sydow made following observations:

- There is slight decrease in sexuality in first trimester
- A variable pattern of sexuality is observed in second trimester
- Significant decrease in sexuality is seen in third trimester.[4]

Etiology of Sexual Problems and Dysfunction

The problem of sexuality and dysfunction during the course of pregnancy is from time immemorial, and the human female is the only species on the earth to boast of sexuality during pregnancy.[26]

Broadly, the sexual problems and dysfunction or the decrease in the sexual activity, enjoyment, or the interest in these activities during the due course of pregnancy and postpartum period are mainly related to social and interpersonal relationship factors, psychological and physiological factors, and hormonal and biochemical factors.

Social and Interpersonal Relationship Factors

- Low satisfaction with the partner or vice versa
- Change in the attitude of the partner for women and child safety
- Feeling of inefficiency to give best at job.

Psychological and Physiological Factors

- Fear of damage or harm to the fetus
- Low physical attraction of the females
- Depressive mood
- Prepregnancy sexual behavior.

Hormonal and Biochemical Factors

- Exhaustion, fatigue
- Dyspareunia
- Back pain
- Alteration in mood.

The multifunctional aspects of the woman which includes taking care of the baby, house, husband, and last but not the least, her job are also the reasons for the poor sexual performance.

A positive attitude during pregnancy and postpartum has definitely a positive impact on sexual problems and dysfunction during that period. In the entire period of pregnancy and the postpartum, the woman is having a constant fear and feeling in her mind about the change in her identity as becoming a mother, physical changes in her body, health of the baby, harm to the unborn baby, and last but not the least, the fear about her partner's sexual interests and his reactions. All these factors affect her behavior towards sexuality.[1,27]

Factors, like lack of knowledge, fear, and sometime anger, are the facilitators to build the negative attitude towards sexuality in pregnancy and perpeurium.[28]

The other factors, such as cultural, social, and economical factors, are also likely to have changes in sexual behavior.[1]

SEXUAL PROBLEMS AND DYSFUNCTION: PREVENTION AND TREATMENT

The sexual problems and dysfunctions should be discussed beforehand by the healthcare providers either in the prenatal period counseling or in the pregnancy by the healthcare providers. Prenatal counseling is effective for helping couples to explore their physical communication and their understanding of what sexual intimacy means to them during this period. There are some of the issues that may be addressed in prenatal counseling to help couples become more aware of each other's needs, desires, and the problems they may encounter during pregnancy for maintaining their sexuality, thus be able to reach a solution that works best for both of them. They should also discuss the alternative coital positions or the alternatives of vaginal intercourse.

The main factors which cause problems are:

- Dyspareunia
- Breastfeeding directly or indirectly
- Fatigue.

Dyspareunia depends on the extent of injuries to the birth canal. About 11% of women who have no birth injury still have dyspareunia and about 15% who have only minor lacerations or first degree perineal tear that require no sutures have dyspareunia. Roughly about 21% of the women who need suturing of these defects and 40% of women who underwent episiotomy have dyspareunia.[19,24,29,30]

The patients who undergo cesarean section have less prevalence of dyspareunia.

Breastfeeding is also associated with low-sexual desire; the negative influence is caused by increased level of prolactin.

So, for the preventive measure, the episiotomy should be given to only those patients in whom it is strongly indicated to prevent the dyspareunia. The lubricants should be used.

CONCLUSION

Pregnancy is a period of various changes at different levels which includes emotional, psychological and physical changes. Pregnancy and perpeurium is hormonally mediated life event, associated with changes in sexual desire in most women. Various studies indicate that there is no contraindication to coitus in a healthy pregnant female until unless the associated complications of pregnancy are taken care of and discussed with the health care provider. Heath care providers should counsel the couple regarding sexual activity in pregnancy and perpeurium so the apprehension and anxiety of the couple is alleviated. The lines of communication should be open and should not ruin this time of joy.

REFERENCES

1. Gokyildiz S, Kizilkaya NK. The effects of pregnancy on sexual life. J Sex Marital Ther. 2005;31(3):201-15.
2. Read J. Sexual problems associated with infertility, pregnancy, and ageing. BMJ. 2004;329(7465):559-61.
3. Lewis JA, Black JJ. Sexuality in women of child-bearing age. J Perinat Educ. 2006;15(2):29-35.
4. Von Sydow K. Sexuality during pregnancy and after childbirth: a metacontent analysis of 59 studies. J Psychosom Res.1999;47(1):27-49.
5. Byrd JE, Hyde JS, Delamater JD, Plant EA. Sexuality during pregnancy and the year postpartum. J Fam Pract. 1998;47(4):305-8.
6. Scottner O, Zahumensky J, Kremar M, Brtnicka H, Kolarik D, Driak D, et al. Urinary incontinence in a group of primiparous women in the Czech Republic. Gynecol Obstet Invest. 2006;62(1):33-7.
7. Leeners B, Sauer I, Rath W. [Nausea and vomiting in early pregnancy/ hyperemesis gravidarum. Current status of psychosomatic factors]. Z Geburtshilfe Neonatol. 2000;204(4):128-34.
8. Conneely OM, Lydon JP. Progesterone receptors in reproduction: functional impact of the A and B isoforms. Steroids. 2000;65(10-11):571-7.
9. Conneely OM, Lydon JP, De Mayo F, O'Malley BW. Reproductive functions of the progesterone receptor. J Soc Gynecol Investig. 2000;7(1 Suppl):S25-32.
10. Zahumensky J, Zverina J, Sottner O, Zmrhalova B, Driak D, Brtnicka H, et al. Comparison of labor course and women's sexuality in planned and unplanned pregnancy. J Psychosom Obstet Gynecol. 2008;29(3):157-63.
11. Leeners B, Brandenburg U, Rath W. [Sexualitat in der Schwangerschaft: risiko oder Schutzfaktor?] Gynecol Obstet Invest. 2000;60:536-43.
12. Pillitteri A. Maternal and Child Health: Care of the Childbearing and Childrearing Family, 5th ed. Philadelphia: Lippincott Williams & Wilkins; 2007.
13. Wong DL, Perry SE, Hockenberry MJ, Lowdermilk DL, Wilson D. Maternal and Child Nursing Care. 3rd ed. Singapore: Elsevier; 2009.
14. Orshan SA. Maternity, Newborn, and Women's Health Nursing: Comprehensive Care Across the Lifespan. Philadelphia: Lippincott Williams & Wilkins; 2008.
15. Eryelmaz G, Ege E, Zincir H. Factors affecting sexual life during pregnancy in eastern Turkey. Gynecol Obstet Invest. 2004;57(2):103-8.
16. Regan PC, lyle JL, Otto AL. Pregnancy and changes in female sexual desire. Soe Behav Pers. 2003;31:603-11.
17. Khamis MA, Mustafa MF, Mohamed SN, Toson MM. Influence of gestational period on sexual behaviour. J Egypt Public Health Assoc. 2007:82(1-2):65-90.
18. Allen L, Fountain L. Sexuality in women of childbearing age. J Perinatal Education. 2007;15(2):29-35.
19. Von Svdow K, Ullmever M, Hann N. Sexual activity during pregnancy and after childbirth: results from the Sexual preferences Questionnaire. J Psychosom Obstet Gynaecol. 2001;22(1):29-40.
20. Laumann EO, Paik A, Rosen RC. Sexual dysfunction in the United States: prevalence and predictors. JAMA. 1999;281(6):537-44.
21. Alder EM. Sexual behaviour in pregnancy, after childbirth and during breast-feeding. Baillieres Clin Obstet Gynaecol. 1989;3(4):805-21.
22. Oruç S, Esen A, Laçin S, Adigüzel H, Uyar Y, Koyuncu F. Sexual behaviour during pregnancy. Aust N Z J Obstet Gynaecol. 1999;39(1):48-50.
23. Barret G, Victor C. Postnatal sexual health. BMJ. 1994;309(6968):1584-5.
24. Hyde JS, De Lamater JD, Plant DE. Sexuality during pregnancy and the year postpartum. J Sex Res. 1996;33:143-51.
25. Edwards WM, Coleman E. Defining sexual health: a descriptive overview. Arch Sex Behav. 2004;33(3):189-95.
26. Still H. Sexuality during and after pregnancy. Can Fam Physician. 1986;32:2177-9.
27. Taylor CM, Pernoll ML. Current Obstetric and Gynecologic Diagnosis and Treatment. 7th ed New York: NP: Appleton & Lange; 2009.
28. Brown CS, Bradford JB, Ling FW. Sex and sexuality in pregnancy. Glob Libr Women's Med. 2008. doi 10.3843/GLOWM.10111.
29. Glazener CM. Sexual function after childbirth: women's experiences, persistent morbidity and lack of professional recognition. Br J Obstet Gynaecol. 1997;104(3):330-5.
30. Barret G, Victor CR. Postnatal sexual health. Br J Gen Pract. 1996;46(402):47-8.

CHAPTER 75

Physiotherapy and Yoga in Pregnancy

Geetika G Gupta, Alok Sharma, Padam Sharma

INTRODUCTION

Physiotherapy or physical therapy is the management of disease, injury, or deformity by physical methods, such as massage, heat treatment, or exercise, rather than by drugs or surgery (Oxford Dictionary). Physiotherapy practice has expanded over time worldwide. The aim of this chapter is to highlight its importance in obstetrics and hence encourage use of physical therapy in obstetric patients. A number of physiological, biomechanical, and anatomical changes are seen in pregnancy which affects all systems of the body. The changes vary with the time of gestation and the knowledge is important to educate the patient on what she can expect and then how she can cope with the changes.

PHYSIOLOGICAL CHANGES DURING PREGNANCY

- Cardiac output increases by 40–50%, which is mainly due to increase in blood volume by 50% and increase in heart rate by about 20 beats per minute
- There is a decrease in blood pressure due to smooth muscle relaxation of blood vessels caused by progesterone and relaxin
- Delayed gastric emptying
- Increased tidal volume.

BIOMECHANICAL CHANGES IN PREGNANCY

Changes occur in muscle balance, control, and posture during pregnancy. These changes are not pathological but may lead to acute or chronic back pain syndromes if bad postures are used. The laxity of the ligaments and connective tissues caused by hormonal changes, mainly relaxin, and increase in weight of breasts, abdomen, fetus, and fluid retention are responsible for these changes.[1]

The postural changes in pregnancy are:

- Increased lordosis of cervical and lumbar spine
- Hyperextension of the knees
- Protraction of shoulder girdle.[2]

There occurs waddling gait in late pregnancy due to lengthening of the abdominals and increased pressures on the pelvic floor due to increased fetal weight, and of course the postural changes. There is loosening of the joint and ligament capsule due to the effect of relaxin.

Musculoskeletal Dysfunction

Certain musculoskeletal discomforts are common in pregnancy which may be treated by physiotherapy. Common problems are back pain, calf cramps, carpal tunnel syndrome, and varicosities. Postural changes, fluid retention, direct pressure on nerves, referred pain venous stasis, and congestion are the changes responsible for the above ailments.

Physical Therapy Modalities

Various physiotherapy modalities are available for management in nonpregnant patients. To enumerate them, they include massage, traction which may be manual or mechanical, diathermy, joint and soft-tissue mobilization, moist heat, the McKenzie approach for back care, transcutaneous electrical nerve stimulation, ultrasound, and whirlpool. However, many of these modalities are either contraindicated in pregnancy, or are to be used with caution.

- Massage and moist heat can be used in pregnancy, except in cases of thrombophlebitis[3,4]
- Traction is to be used with care because of increased joint mobility. The McKenzie approach for back care increases lumbar lordosis and is difficult to perform in the last trimester, and hence is not to be used during pregnancy.[5] Others, like diathermy, transcutaneous electrical nerve stimulation, and whirlpool, are contraindicated in pregnancy as their safety is not proven.

Exercises and Posture in Pregnancy

Before a health professional prescribes any exercise to the pregnant patient, her overall examination in reference to obstetric and medical risks must be made. Pregnant woman can be allowed moderate intensity exercises which could be similar to prepregnant state.

The exercises should be avoided in supine position and in prolonged standing positions due to decreased venous return and hence decreased cardiac output.

CONTRAINDICATIONS TO AEROBIC EXERCISE DURING PREGNANCY

American College of Obstetricians and Gynecologists recommendations.[6]

Absolute Contraindications

- Hemodynamically significant heart disease
- Restrictive lung disease
- Incompetent cervix/cerclage
- Multiple gestation at risk for premature labor
- Persistent second or third-trimester bleeding
- Placenta previa after 26 weeks of gestation
- Premature labor during the current pregnancy
- Ruptured membranes
- Pre-eclampsia/pregnancy induced hypertension.

Relative Contraindications

- Severe anemia
- Unevaluated maternal cardiac arrhythmia
- Chronic bronchitis
- Poorly controlled type 1 diabetes
- Extreme morbid obesity
- Extreme underweight (body mass index <12)
- History of extremely sedentary lifestyle
- Intra-uterine growth restriction in current pregnancy
- Poorly controlled hypertension
- Orthopedic limitations
- Poorly controlled seizure disorder
- Poorly controlled hyperthyroidism
- Heavy smoker.

Warning Signs to Terminate Exercise while Pregnant[6]

- Vaginal bleeding
- Dyspnea prior to exertion
- Dizziness
- Headache
- Chest pain
- Muscle weakness
- Calf pain or swelling (need to rule out thrombophlebitis)
- Preterm labor
- Decreased fetal movement
- Amniotic fluid leakage.

EXERCISES IN THIRD TRIMESTER OF PREGNANCY

- Swimming: it is the best exercise during pregnancy. Around 25–45 minutes swim is adequate. It puts no stress on the joints as it is a no impact activity
- Seated cable row: the patient takes a resistance band, and fixes it to any pole acting as an anchor. Then she sits on a chair around 2 feet away from it and holds one end of the band in each hand. Keeping the bands in the hands the shoulder blades are squeezed together and then hands pulled towards the chest
- Leg curls and extensions: the patient sits on the chair and extends the legs straight in front. Then the knees are bent and heels taken backwards to touch the seat on the underside
- Bicep curls: the patient takes a weight in her hand and moves the weight held hand towards the shoulder involving the biceps. She slowly lowers them back
- Lateral shoulder: raise one weight each is held in both hands. The arms are abducted up to shoulder level and slowly lowered down
- Pelvic floor exercises: these help not only to strengthen the pelvic floor muscles which aid during labor, but also prevent postnatal discomforts like incontinence of urine and pain. These and can relieve symptoms of hemorrhoids and vulvar varicosities by relieving increased venous return. The exercises also are preventive for uterine prolapse. These help in maintaining the tone of vagina for sexual activity.

The patient can do the pelvic floor exercises in standing, sitting, kneeling, or even in lying down position. The patient has to do the Kegel exercises, i.e., contraction of the pelvic floor muscles. The muscles should be squeezed initially for 2–3 breaths or for 5 seconds. These exercises can be done in five sets throughout the day.[7,8]

COMFORT POSITIONS DURING PREGNANCY

Standing

Because of lumbar lordosis and increased body weight, the patient is advised to avoid standing in the same position for a long time. A stool must be used to rest one foot on if prolonged standing is required. She must change feet every 5–15 minutes (Fig. 1).

Sitting

The patient must sit up with back straight and shoulders back. The buttocks must touch the back of the chair. A lumbar support can also be used (Figs 2 and 3).

Lying Down Position

The patient should lie in lateral position with knees slightly bent. She can keep pillows under her head, in between knees, and under the abdomen (Fig. 4).

Defecation Position

The knees should be higher than the hips, so a footstool can be used. The patient must lean forwards and rest the elbows on the knees. The back must be straight and the lower abdomen is pushed forwards (Fig. 5).

PHYSIOTHERAPY AFTER CHILDBIRTH

The body needs extra care in puerperium because of risk of injury due to hormonal changes. It includes maintaining good posture, good bladder and bowel habits, and some exercises to help body recover after pregnancy and childbirth.

Pelvic Floor Exercises

- Can be started within 24 hours even in the presence of episiotomy or abdominal incision
- Should start with few and in lying down position and then can be performed in sitting and standing position as tolerated.

Abdominal Exercises

These are important and can be done 10–15 times, once or twice daily as can be tolerated.

Strengthening of Abdominal Muscles

The patient sits upright, and relaxes the lower stomach into the hands (Fig. 6). The pelvic floor muscles and the abdominal muscles are drawn in synchronized with inspiration, held in position for 5 seconds and released. If the patient finds it difficult it can be done in lateral lying down position. If well tolerated, the amount, number, and duration can be increased.

Pelvic Rocking

It is done in lying down position. The knee and hip joints are flexed and keeping the bottom on the floor, the coccyx is lifted slightly and kept in position for 5 seconds (Fig. 7).

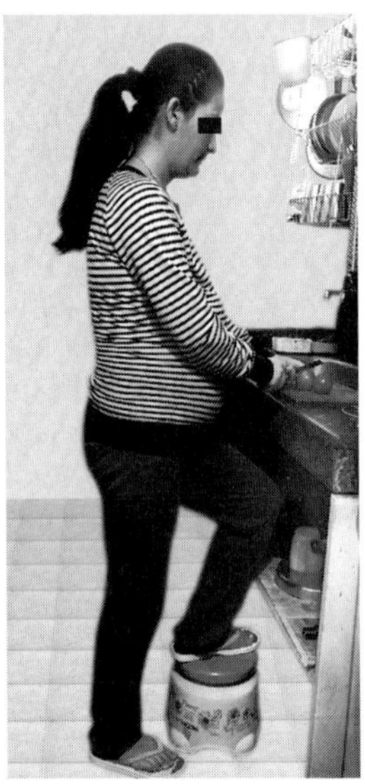

FIG. 1: Standing with stool.

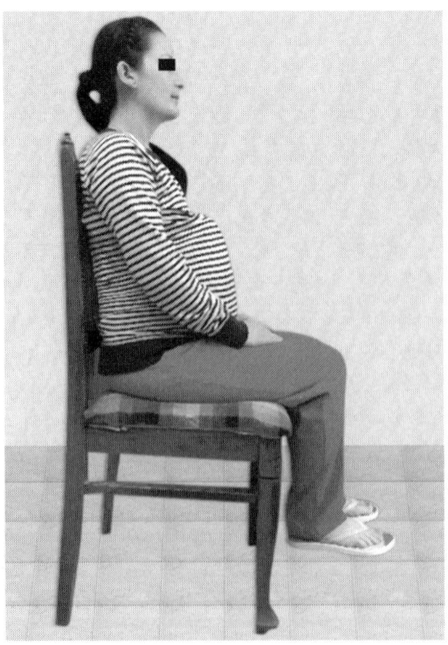

FIG. 2: Sitting.

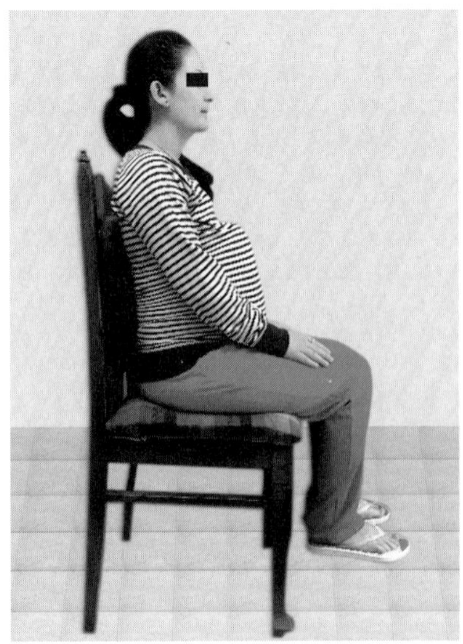

FIG. 3: Sitting with lumbar support.

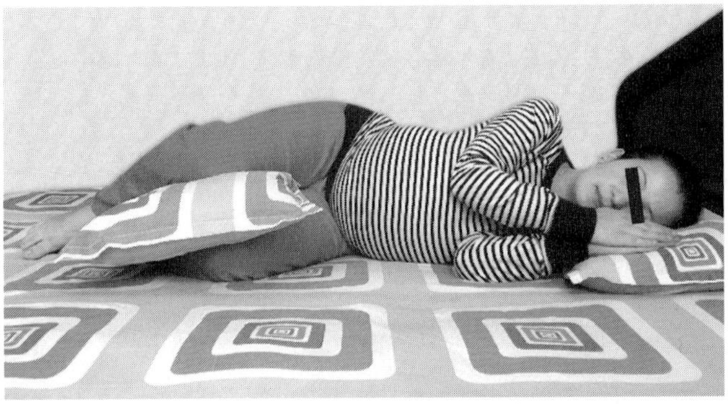

FIG. 4: Lying down position.

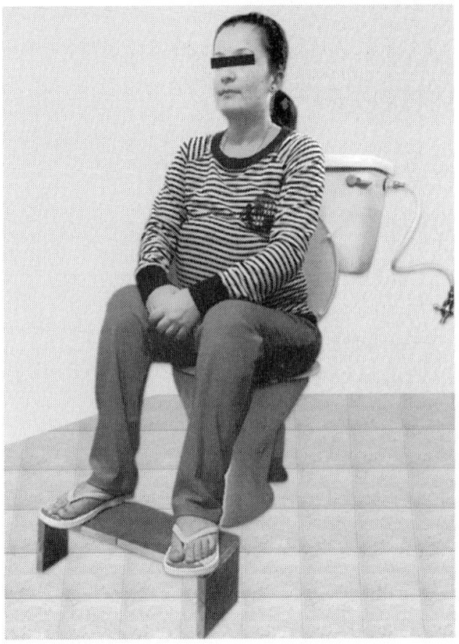

FIG. 5: Defecation position.

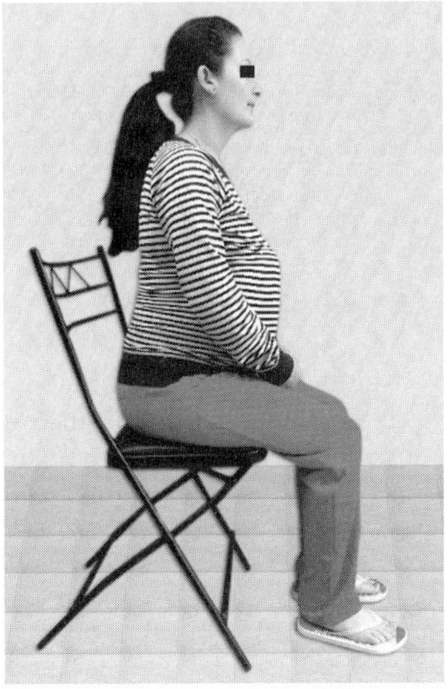

FIG. 6: Strengthening of abdominal muscles.

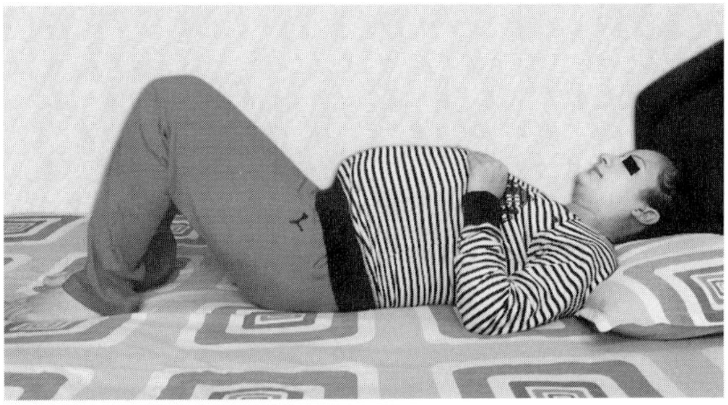

FIG. 7: Pelvic rocking.

Knee Rolling

The patient lies supine and rolls both knees gently to each side, keeping shoulders flat. This exercise strengthens the abdominal muscles and stretches the back (Fig. 8).

Butterfly

The patient sits tall on the chair and opens arms. The shoulder blades are squeezed together. This helps to open chest and strengthen upper back (Fig. 9).

After 6 weeks, the patient can start with swimming, walking for 30 minutes along with the above exercises. Jumping, jogging, and aerobics must be avoided for the first 3–6 months.

Back Care

The back is liable for injury in the puerperium because of the hormonal changes and more than usual lifting and bending involved in baby care.

Precautions

- Keep work surfaces at height of waist (Fig. 10)
- For low-level works, it is advisable to kneel down (Fig. 11)
- Tightening of abdominal and pelvic floor muscles during lifting must be done.

YOGA IN PREGNANCY

Yoga is derived from *Sanskrit* word "YUJ" meaning "to unite". Yoga is the control of mind which brings ease, peacefulness, and awareness of body and life. Hence it not only helps to maintain health, but also is useful for the development of the fetus.

Yogic Exercises during Pregnancy

Benefits

- Safe and effective
- Nausea and vomiting decreases

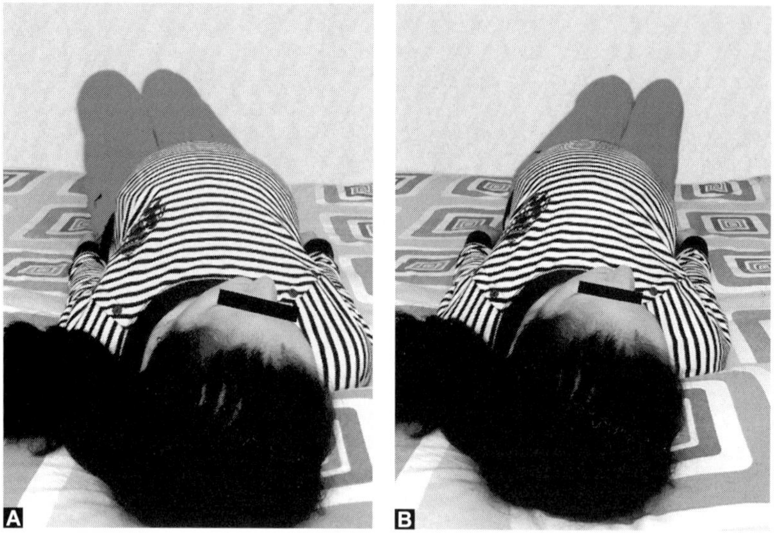

FIG. 8: Knee rolling: turn towards A, left; B, right.

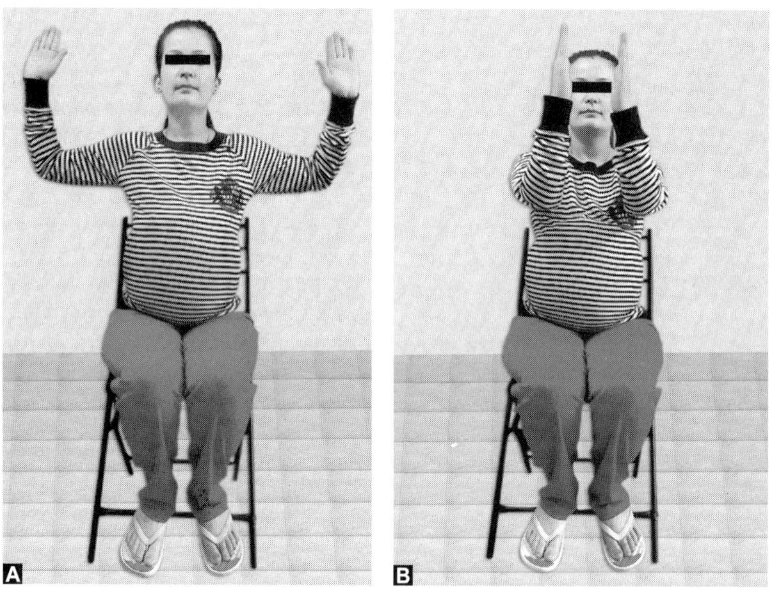

FIG. 9: Butterfly. A, open chest; B, strengthen upper back.

- Help to reduce morning sickness and mood swings in combination with *Pranayamas* (yogic breathing)
- Heart pumps effectively
- Tones up the elasticity and strengthen the spine
- The diaphragm is made elastic and strong, and can stretch to accommodate the uterus easily
- Healthy blood, oxygenation, and other fluids are circulated properly to the placenta and fetus
- Pranayama stabilize the nervous system
- Pain in joints and backache decreases
- Influences position of the baby. Strengthens and massages the abdomen, which helps in stimulating the appetite and bowel action, hence decreasing constipation
- Raises the level of energy and also helps in maintenance of the metabolism
- Anemia decreases
- Obesity is controlled
- Maintain the hormone balance
- Minor complaints, like varicose vein, piles etc., can be reduced

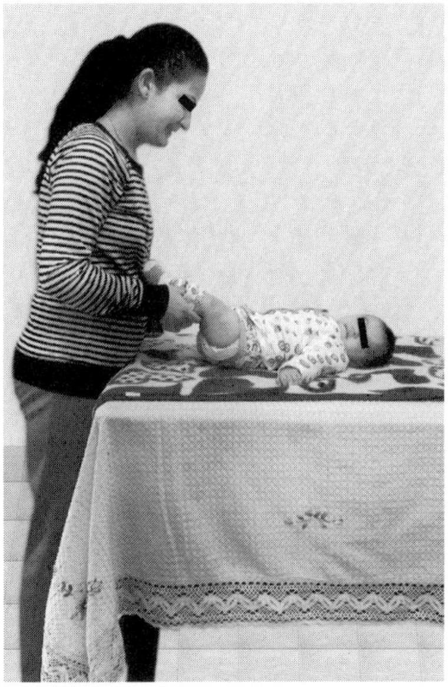

FIG. 10: Work surfaces at height of waist.

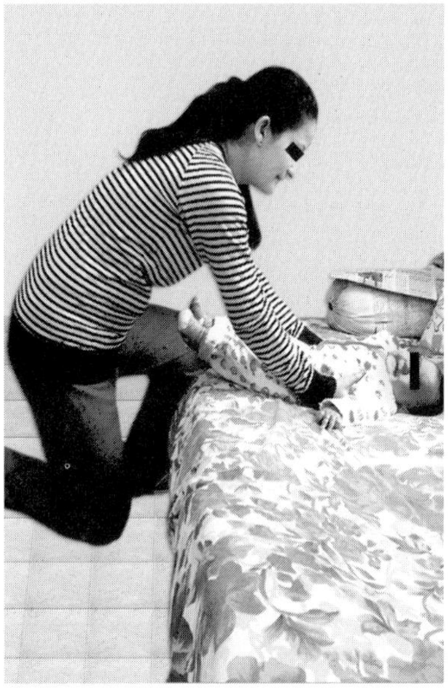

FIG. 11: Kneel down while you are working at low surface.

- The incidence of intrauterine growth retardation, pregnancy induced hypertension and complications due to gestational diabetes can be prevented or reduced
- Relieves swelling (fluid retention: edema and cramping which can be quite common in the later months)
- As the resilience's power is more, immunity increases and hence infections are reduced
- Focus on relieving tension around the cervix, birth canal, and pelvis, thereby preparing the body to make the process of labor easier
- Increase in the muscle tone decrease the prolapse of uterus
- Postpartum blues and psychosis decreased
- Cope with the stressful months of pregnancy and after delivery
- Cesarian deliveries are decreased
- Malpositions, malpresentations, and instrumental delivery decreased.

Yoga for Third Trimester of Pregnancy

Shoulder Rotation

The patient places the right fingertips on the right shoulder and rotates the shoulder joint as if making circles with the elbow. It is repeated with left side. The next step is to use both sides simultaneously. This yoga helps in improving circulation and breathing. It relieves neck tension. In puerperium, it helps in maintain lactation (Fig. 12).

Ankle Crank

The patient places the right foot over the left knee while in seated position. The right toes are held with left hand and the same foot's ankle with right hand. She rotates this ankle in all direction. It is repeated on the other side. This helps in improving circulation in the feet and is helpful in cramping and edema of feet (Fig. 13).

Ardha Baddha Konasana (Half Butterfly)

While in sitting position, the patient places the right foot on left thigh. The right knee is slowly moved up towards the chest while inhaling. The knee is pushed down while exhaling to touch the floor. It is repeated on the other side. It helps in loosening of hip and knee joints which aid in delivery (Fig. 14).

Baddha Konasana (Full Butterfly)

The patient sits with both legs outstretched. She is asked to bend both knees bringing both feet together. The feet are held with both hands. Both knees are bounced up and down. This asana relieves the tension of legs and improves circulation of pelvis (Fig. 15).

Marjari Asana (Cat Stretch Pose)

The patient bends on the knees and hands. She raises her head and depresses the spine making it concave while inhaling. Then she lowers the head and stretches the spine upwards while inhaling. This helps in improving the flexibility of neck, shoulders and spine (Fig. 16).

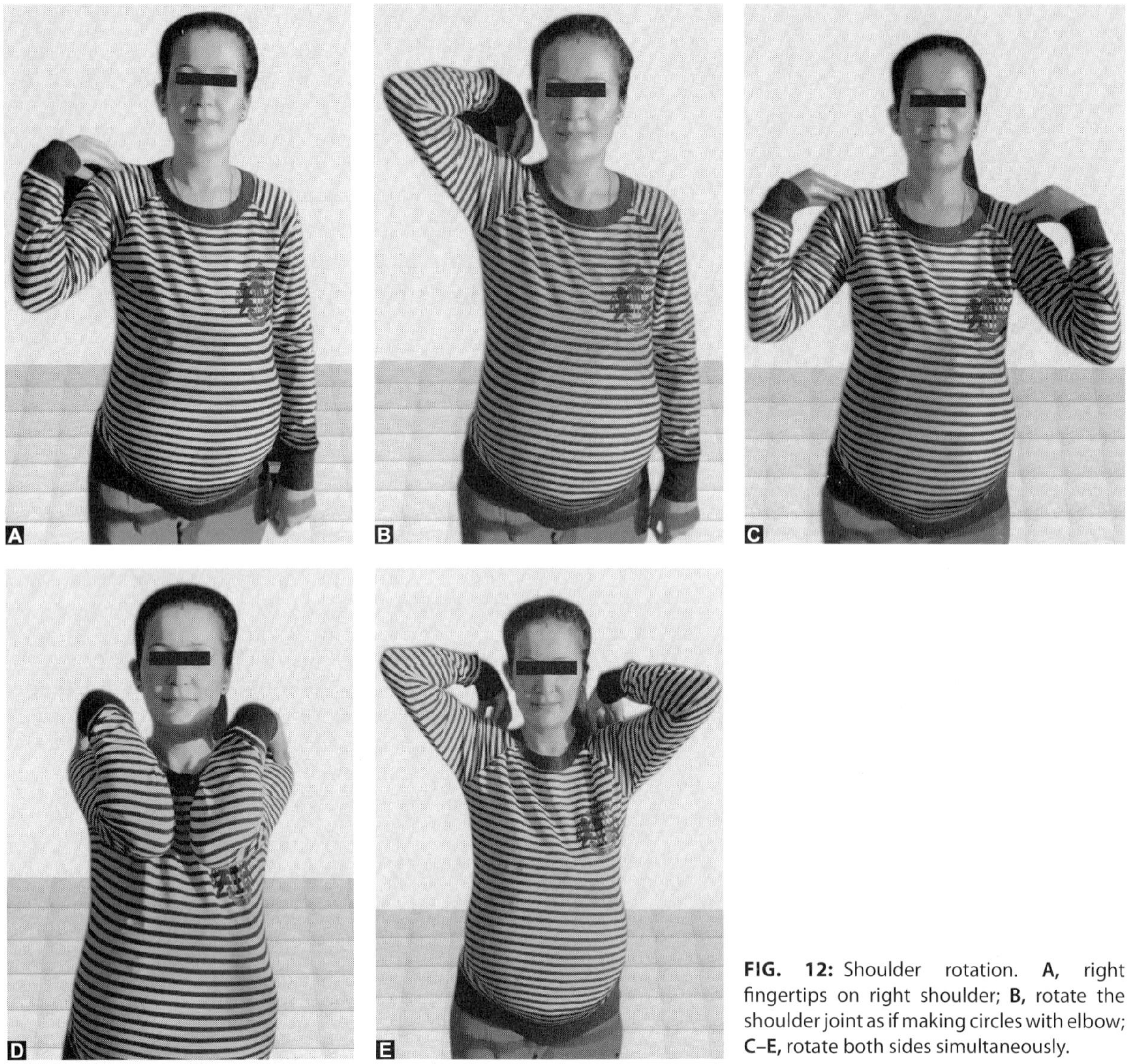

FIG. 12: Shoulder rotation. **A,** right fingertips on right shoulder; **B,** rotate the shoulder joint as if making circles with elbow; **C–E,** rotate both sides simultaneously.

Supta Udarakarshan Asana (Sleeping Abdominal Stretch Pose)

The patient lies laterally on one side. The right and left hands are placed on the head and thighs, respectively. The left knee is slightly bent. It is repeated on the other side. This helps to relieve constipation.

How Yoga Can Help in Postnatal Care

- Restoring the uterus, abdomen, and the pelvic floor
- Postnatal complications can be avoided
- Relieving body pain and breast discomfort
- Improve the milk production
- The major change that takes place is involution
- Stretch marks after delivery is reduced by maintaining the elasticity of the skin
- Yoga makes young mothers pretty, attractive, youthful, and more vibrant
- We have segregated these yoga exercises into trimester-wise sequences. However, it is recommended that you follow these under expert guidance.

Postnatal Asana

For normal delivery only practiced after 6 months under the guidance.

Baddhakonasana (Full Butterfly)

- Sit with legs outstretched
- Bend the knees and bring the soles of the feet together, keeping the heels as close to the body as possible

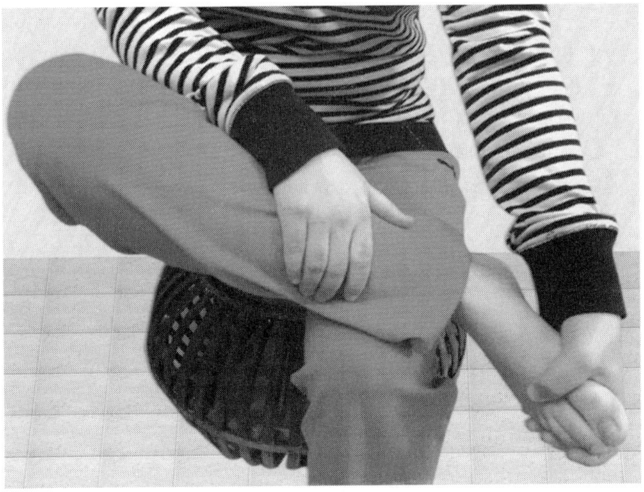

FIG. 13: Ankle crank.

- Fully relax the inner thighs
- Clasp the feel with the feet with both hands
- Gently bounce the knees up and down, using the elbows as levers to press the legs down
- Do not use any force
- Repeat up to 20–30 times
- Straighten the legs and relax
- By doing this tension from inner thigh muscles is relieved
- Removes tiredness from legs and improves blood supply to the uterine muscles and pelvic region (Fig. 17).

Marjari Asan (Cat Stretch Pose)

- Sit with buttocks on the heels (*Vajrasana*)
- Raise the buttocks and stand on the knees
- Lean forward and place the hands flat on the floor. This is the starting position

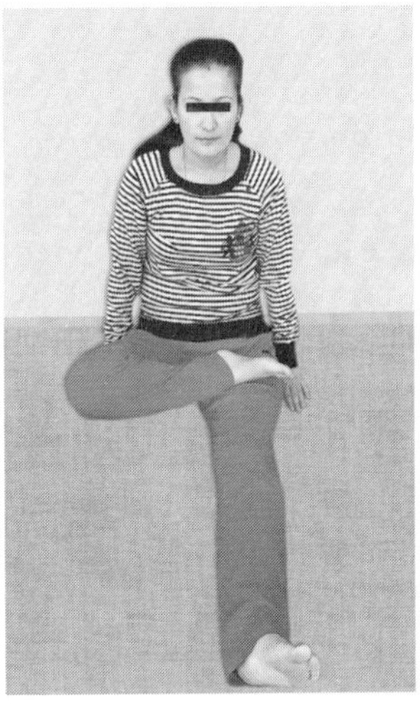

FIG. 14: *Ardha baddha konasana* (half butterfly).

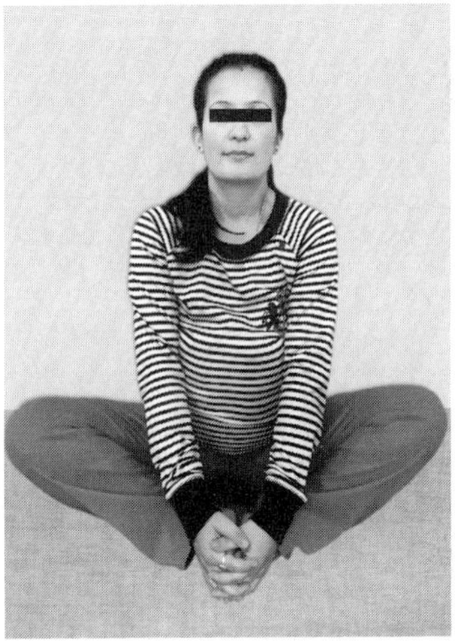

FIG. 15: *Baddha konasana* (full butterfly).

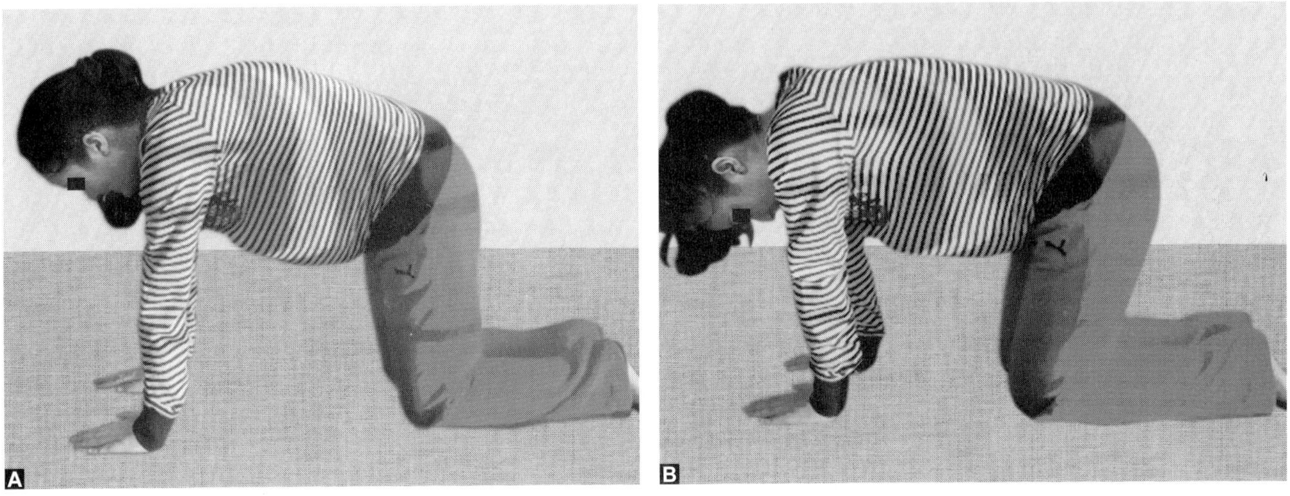

FIG. 16: *Marjari asana* (cat stretch pose).

- Inhale while raising the head and depressing the spine so that the back becomes concave
- Exhale while lowering the head and stretching the spine upward
- This asana improves flexibility of the neck, shoulders and spine
- Tones female reproductive system
- Can be safely practiced during first 6 months of pregnancy (Fig. 18).

Vakrasana

- Patient is asked to sit erect, keep the legs straight, and hands by the side of her body

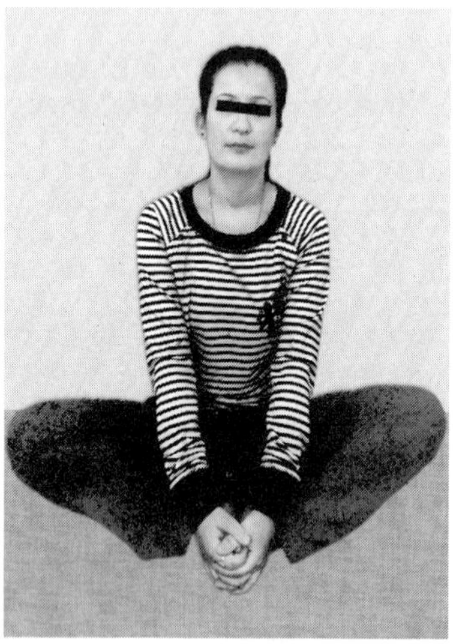

FIG. 17: *Baddha konasana* (full butterfly).

- Bend her left leg, keep the left foot near right knee, place left hand at the center of the back, place right across left bent legs; by pressing right hand and left leg twist and look back maintain for some time come back slowly
- Similarly, do other side starting with leg bending
- It gives flexibility to the spine (Fig. 19).

Eka Pada Uttanasana

- Lie on your spine
- Raise one leg up to 45° from the ground by partial inhale, other leg straight on the ground
- Fully inhale and raise the leg up to 90° and place the hands by the side of the body
- Maintaining the posture
- Repeat on the other side
- This asana tones up the pelvic organs and is good in varicose veins, constipation, and menstrual disorders (Fig. 20).

Dwi Pada Uttanasana

Patient is asked to lie on her spine. She is asked to raise both legs together up to 45° from the ground by partial inhale. Fully inhale and raise the legs up to 90° and place the hands by the side of the body. Maintaining the posture, this tones up the pelvic organs and is good in varicose veins, constipation, and menstrual disorders (Fig. 21).

Note: All these exercises given must be undertaken with the help of yoga therapist under the supervision and guidance of the doctor/consultant.

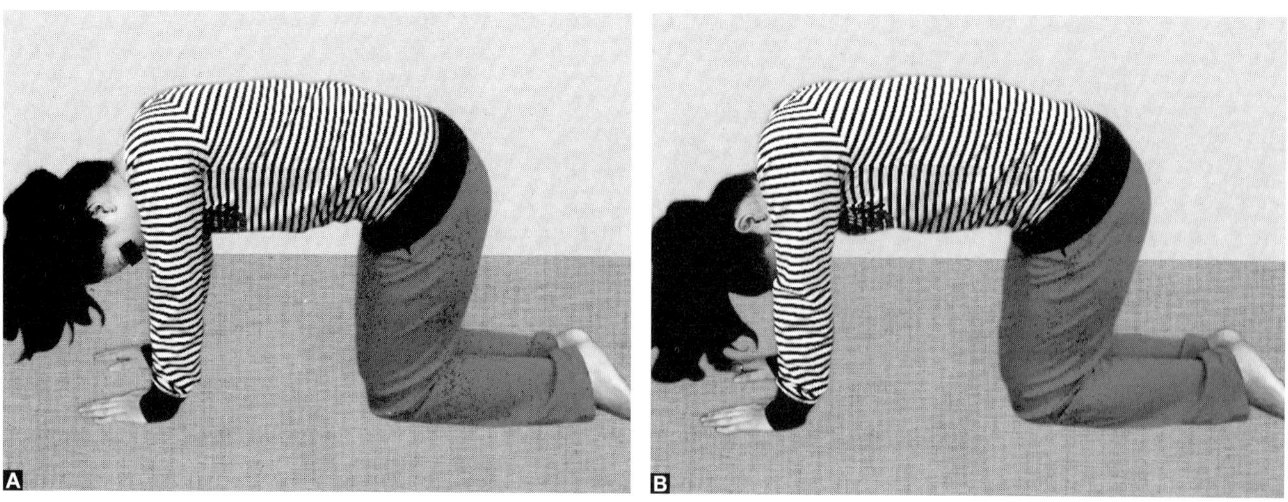

FIG. 18: *Marjari asana* (cat stretch pose).

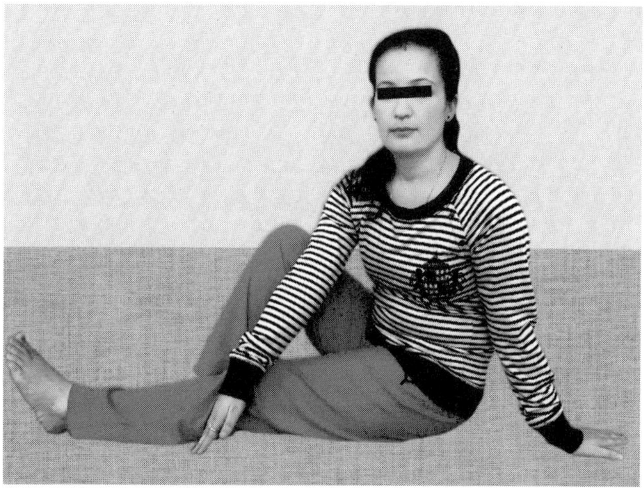

FIG. 19: *Vakrasana.*

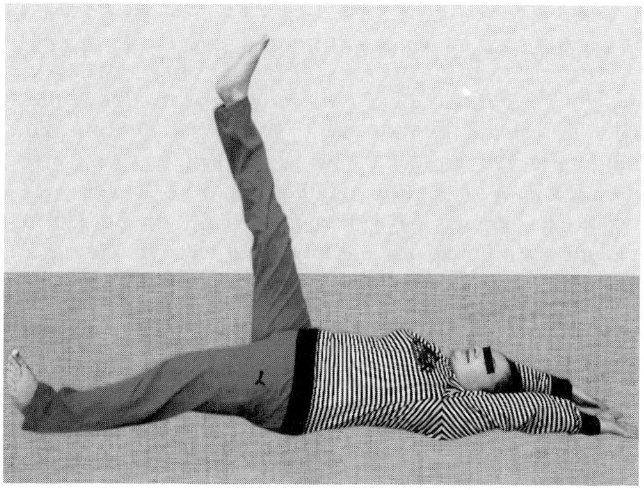

FIG. 20: *Eka pada uttanasana.*

CONCLUSION

Disorders of fetal growth brings the two ends of spectrum, from being less than normal to more than normal. Adequate fetal monitoring, clinically and sonographically can screen the conditions easily and measures to remedy the causes can be taken. Many cases can be managed well through screening, diagnosis of cause, interventions towards maternal causes and nutrition and timing of delivery.

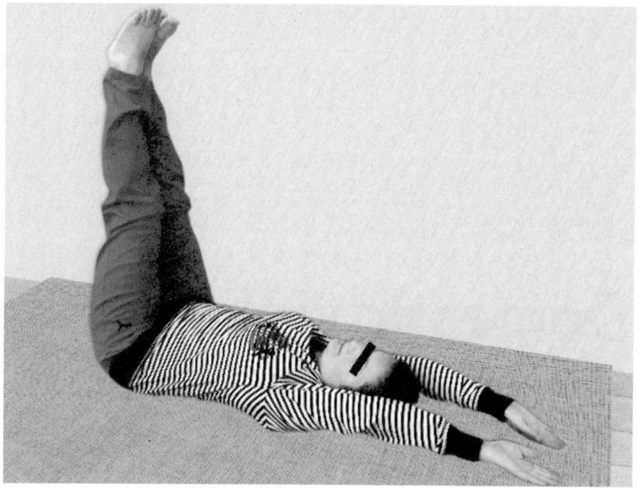

FIG. 21: *Dwi pada uttanasana.*

But even with these, complications due to fetal growth disorders may outpace the diagnosis and management interventions, thus this remains a challenge for the obstetrician even with good diagnostic facilities.

REFERENCES

1. Shrock P. (2008). Exercise and Physical Activity During Pregnancy. [online] Available from: www.glowm.com/section_view/heading/Exercise%20and%20Physical%20Activity%20During%20Pregnancy/item/98. [Accessed December, 2015].
2. Little J. Postural adjustments during pregnancy and implications for the childbearing woman. Bulletin of the Section on Obstetrics and Gynecology. Am Physical Ther Assoc. 1984;8(3):16-9.
3. Kessler RM, Hertling D. Management of Common Musculoskeletal Disorders: Physical Therapy, Principles and Methods. Philadelphia, PA, USA: Harper & Row; 1983. pp. 346-8.
4. Griffin JE, Karselis TC. Physical agents for physical therapists. Springfield: Charles C Thomas; 1978. pp. 232-3.
5. Pernoll ML, Metcalf J, Kovach PA, Wachtel R, Dunham MJ. Ventilation during rest and exercise in pregnancy and postpartum. Respir Physiol. 1975;25(3):295-310.
6. ACOG Committee Obstetric Practice. ACOG Committee opinion. Number 267. January 2002: exercise during pregnancy and the postpartum period. Obstet Gynecol. 2002;99(1):171-3.
7. Erkkola R. The influence of physical training during pregnancy on physical work capacity and circulatory parameters. Scand J Clin Lab Invest. 1976;36:747-54.
8. Maly BJ. Rehabilitation principles in the care of gynecologic and obstetric patients. Arch Phys Med Rehabil. 1980;61(2):78-81.

CHAPTER 76

Domestic Violence

Kawita Bapat, Pratik Tambe

INTRODUCTION

Domestic violence (DV) is a condition that transcends class, culture, and socioeconomic conditions. It is especially of relevance in today's times when women are increasingly becoming targets of mental, emotional, economic, physical and sexual violence. Domestic abuse, also known as spousal abuse, occurs when one person in an intimate relationship or marriage tries to dominate and control the other person. Domestic abuse that includes physical violence is called DV.

EPIDEMIOLOGY AND PATHOPHYSIOLOGY

Domestic violence and abuse are used to gain and maintain total control over the partner. An abuser uses fear, guilt, shame, and intimidation to wear his partner down and keep her under his thumb. Domestic violence and abuse can happen to anyone, yet the problem is often overlooked, excused, or denied. This is especially true when the abuse is psychological, rather than physical. Domestic violence and abuse does not discriminate. It occurs within all age ranges, ethnic backgrounds and economic levels. Domestic abuse often escalates from threats and verbal abuse to violence. While physical injury may be the most obvious danger, the emotional and psychological consequences of domestic abuse are also severe. Around the world, the events that trigger violence in abusive relationships are remarkably consistent. They include disobeying or arguing with the man, questioning him about money or girlfriends, not having food ready on time, not caring adequately for the children or the home, refusing to have sex, and the man suspecting the woman of infidelity.

INTIMATE PARTNER VIOLENCE

Violence against intimate partners occurs in all countries, all cultures, and at every level of society without exception, although some populations (e.g., low-income groups) are at greater risk of violence by an intimate partner than others. As well as acts of physical aggression such as hitting or kicking, violence by intimate partners includes forced intercourse and other forms of sexual coercion, psychological abuse such as intimidation and humiliation, and controlling behavior such as isolating a person from family and friends or restricting access to information and assistance.

Pregnancy when coupled with DV is a form of intimate partner violence (IPV) where health risks may be amplified. Abuse during pregnancy, whether physical, verbal or emotional, produces many adverse physical and psychological effects for both the mother and fetus.

Most victims of physical aggression are subjected to multiple acts of violence over extended periods of time. They also tend to suffer from more than one type of abuse, e.g., a study of 613 abused women in Japan found that less than 10% were victims of physical violence alone, while 57% had suffered physical, psychological, and sexual abuse. A study in Mexico found that over half of the women who had been physically assaulted had also been sexually abused by their partners.[1] McCauley J et al. conducted a survey on 1,952 women in four community-based practices to determine the prevalence of DV among female patients and to identify clinical characteristics that are associated with DV between February and July 1993. Out of 1952 respondents (5.5%), 108 had experienced DV in the year before presentation. 418 (21.4%) had experienced DV sometime in their adult lives,

429 (22.0%) before age 18 years, and 639 (32.7%) as either an adult or child.

Compared with women who had not recently experienced DV, currently abused patients were more likely to be younger than 35 years of age [prevalence ratio (PR), = 4.1; 95% confidence interval (CI) = 2.8–6.0]; were more likely to be single, separated, or divorced (PR = 2.5; CI = 1.7–3.6); were more likely to be receiving medical assistance or to have no insurance (PR = 4.3; CI = 2.8–6.6); had more physical symptoms (mean = 7.3 ± 0.38 compared with 4.6 ± 0.08; p <0.001); had higher scores on instruments for depression, anxiety, somatization, and interpersonal sensitivity (low self-esteem) (p <0.001); were more likely to have a partner abusing drugs or alcohol (PR = 6.3; CI = 4.4–9.2); were more likely to be abusing drugs (PR = 4.4; CI = 1.9–10.4) or alcohol (PR = 3.1; CI = 1.5–6.5); and were more likely to have attempted suicide (PR = 4.3; CI = 2.8–6.5).

They visited the emergency department more frequently (PR = 1.7; CI = 1.2–2.5) but did not have more hospitalizations for psychiatric disorders. In a logistic regression model into which nine risk factors were entered, the likelihood of current abuse increased with the number of risk factors, from 1.2% when 0–1 risk factors were present to 70.4% when 6–7 risk factors were present.

They concluded that in a large, diverse, community-based population of primary-care patients, 1 of every 20 women had experienced DV in the previous year; 1 of every 5 had experienced violence in their adult life; and 1 of every 3 had experienced violence as either a child or an adult. Current DV is associated with single or separated status, socioeconomic status, substance abuse, specific psychological symptoms, specific physical symptoms, and the total number of physical symptoms.[2]

DOMESTIC VIOLENCE DURING PREGNANCY

Domestic violence during pregnancy is categorized as abusive behavior towards a pregnant woman, where the pattern of abuse can often change in terms of severity and frequency of violence. Abuse may be a long-standing problem in a relationship that continues after a woman becomes pregnant or it may commence in pregnancy.

Domestic abuse can be triggered by pregnancy for a number of reasons. Pregnancy itself can be used as a form of coercion and the phenomenon of preventing one's reproductive choice is referred to as reproductive coercion. Studies on birth-control sabotage performed by males against female partners have indicated a strong correlation between DV and birth-control sabotage.

Pregnancy can also lead to a hiatus of DV when the abuser does not want to harm the unborn child. The risk of DV for pregnant women is greatest immediately after childbirth.

Domestic violence can increase a woman's chances of becoming pregnant and the number of children she has, both because the woman may be coerced into sex and because she may be prevented from using birth control. A correlation has been shown between large families and DV. Whereas previously it was thought that having many children and the resultant stress of large families increased likelihood DV, it has been shown that the violence commonly predates the births.

Pregnant women were also victimized by abusive behavior and by lack of emotional support. Such behavior was faced more frequently by women who experienced DV. Usually, the men who perpetrate violence tend to hold conventional gender role attitudes, expecting women to take sole responsibility for household chores. Also, the inability to perform routine household tasks due to physical exhaustion and reduced mobility due to pregnancy frequently resulted in violence.

Similarly, exerting pressure for male child was noticed more frequently among women who faced DV. This type of behavior is a form of psychological DV women experience. These abusive behaviors are also a risk factor for DV during pregnancy. These behaviors had a positive association with all the three forms of DV. Pregnancy does not protect women from violence. This is reflected by the alarming prevalence rates of physical abuse found in the pregnancy, ante- and postpartum periods. Women whose mother or mother in law had experienced physical spousal abuse have increased odds of experiencing abuse during pregnancy and all women of reproductive age are at risk for IPV.

Bachhus et al. conducted a cross-sectional survey in an Inner-London Teaching Hospital. Two hundred women aged 16 years and over, were interviewed between July 2001 and April 2002. The Abuse Assessment Screen was used to assess for experiences of DV. Depression was assessed using the Edinburgh Postnatal Depression Scale (EPDS). The analysis of predictors of obstetric complications grouped together those known to be associated with DV.

They found that 23.5% of women had lifetime experience of DV, 3% during the current pregnancy. Women with a history of DV were significantly more likely to be single, separated or in noncohabiting relationship and to have smoked in the year prior to and/or during pregnancy. Higher EPDS scores were significantly associated with DV, single, separated or noncohabiting status and obstetric complications. Both a history of DV and increased EPDS scores were significantly associated with obstetric complications after controlling for other known risk factors. They concluded that DV is as an important risk marker for the development of obstetric complications and depressive symptomatology. This finding itself justifies training and education of maternity health professionals to raise awareness.[3]

INJURIES UNIQUE TO THE PREGNANT PATIENT

Preterm Labor and Preterm Premature Rupture of Membranes

The prevalence of preterm labor (PTL) in prenatal populations has been estimated to be from 6.9% to 10.0%. It has been suggested that violence during pregnancy may be associated with an increase in antenatal complications. The hypothesis is that physical violence and verbal abuse in pregnancy lead to increased risk of PTL.

Shumway J et al. studied a cohort of 636 women attending the Adult Obstetrical Clinic for their first prenatal visit, between December 1989 and September 1990. These were 567 participants in the study. They were interviewed 3-times during the course of their prenatal care, and 401 participants successfully completed their third prenatal interviews. Violence data were obtained during the third interview. Obstetrical and neonatal outcome data were obtained by abstracting the maternal and neonatal medical records. When stratified by levels of violence, women who experienced moderate or severe violence had incidences of PTL of 15.4% and 17.2%, respectively. Chi-square test for homogeneity revealed a significant difference among these groups. They concluded that serious acts of verbal abuse and physical violence occurred with significant frequency. PTL was strongly correlated with increasing acts of violence with 4.1-times greater risk of PTL in women who experienced severe violence as compared to those who experienced no maternal abuse.[4]

Placental Abruption

Leone JM et al. examined prenatal and hospital obstetrical charts for 2,873 women who gave birth between January 2000 and March 2002 in a north-eastern city. They examined associations among sociodemographic characteristics, health-related variables, IPV and pregnancy trauma and placental abruption using univariate and multivariate logistic regression. Of the 2,873 women in the analyses, 105 (3.7%) reported IPV during prenatal care. After controlling for sociodemographic variables; tobacco, alcohol and drug use; preeclampsia; and gestational diabetes during pregnancy, women who reported IPV also had higher odds of pregnancy trauma and placental abruption [adjusted odds ratio (OR) = 32.08; 95% CI = 14.33–71.80; p <0.01, and OR = 5.17; 95% CI = 1.37–19.51; p <0.05, respectively]. They concluded that IPV is a significant and independent risk factor for pregnancy trauma and placental abruption after controlling for factors typically associated with these outcomes. This study has implications for partner violence screening and intervention policies among pregnant women and highlights the importance of making distinctions about the type of IPV that women experience.[5]

Placental abruption can occur even after minor abdominal trauma. It is the second most common cause of fetal mortality in this patient population; the incidence ranges between 1% and 60%. In minor trauma, the rate of placental abruption is between 1% and 5% with significant mechanisms associated with rates of 20–60%.

Placental abruption results from the placenta shearing away from the uterus with bleeding into this space and clot formation. The elasticity of the uterus, matched against the relative stiffness of the placenta, creates a vulnerable interface. A placental abruption can result in the patient experiencing abdominal pain, cramping, and vaginal bleeding. The clinician may detect uterine tenderness on physical examination. Unfortunately, the absence of these features does not exclude the diagnosis of placental abruption reliably.

Several diagnostic modalities may be used in the evaluation of placental abruption. Ultrasound may detect a placental abruption, has the benefit of the absence of ionizing radiation, and provides additional information about fetal well-being. Its sensitivity for placental abruption, however, is poor (~50%) so a negative ultrasound does not rule out a placental abruption.

Use of the Kleihauer-Betke (KB) test as an indicator of the fetomaternal hemorrhage likely to accompany abruption is not of great clinical utility because of its low specificity and currently is not recommended for this application by the American Congress of Obstetricians and Gynecologists.

Continuous fetal monitoring is the preferred test and should be initiated as early in the evaluation as possible. In the absence of symptoms consistent with placental abruption, an observation period of 4–6 hours is adequate. Because of the potential for delayed manifestation (24–48 hours) of significant placental abruption, the Eastern Association for the Surgery of Trauma recommends continuation of fetal monitoring in the presence of uterine contractions, a nonreassuring fetal heart rate pattern, vaginal bleeding, significant uterine tenderness or irritability, or serious maternal injury. This recommendation applies to even minor trauma, because these patients are particularly prone to delayed recognition of placental abruption.

Uterine Rupture

Uterine rupture is a rare consequence of maternal trauma, one that carries a grave outcome for the fetus. This diagnosis is present in less than 1% of blunt trauma and is found typically in patients who have had a previous cesarean section. Associated fetal mortality is nearly universal, with an associated 10% maternal mortality rate.

Presenting features may include uterine tenderness and variable shape, hemodynamic instability and the ability to palpate fetal parts on abdominal examination. In patients without a previous cesarean section, the uterus is more likely to rupture posteriorly, making detection of these physical examination findings more difficult.

Oxford CM et al. from Harvard note that in the United States (US), trauma is the leading nonobstetric cause of maternal death. The principal causes of trauma in pregnancy include motor vehicle accidents, falls, assaults, homicides, DV and penetrating wounds. The managing team evaluating and coordinating the care of the pregnant trauma patient should be multidisciplinary so that it is able to understand the physiologic changes in pregnancy.

Blunt trauma to the abdomen increases the risk of placental abruption. Evaluation of the pregnant trauma patient requires a primary and secondary survey with emphasis on airway, breathing, circulation, and disability. The use of imaging studies, invasive hemodynamics, critical care medications and surgery, if necessary, should be individualized and guided by a coordinating team effort to improve maternal and fetal conditions.[6]

Pelvic Fracture

As expected from proximity alone, injuries to the bony pelvis are complicated to manage in pregnancy. Leggon RE et al. described maternal and fetal mortality rates of 9% and 35%, respectively, in a retrospective review of 101 pelvic and acetabular fractures sustained during pregnancy. The major causes of fetal deaths were direct injury to the uterus, placenta, or fetus (52%) and maternal hemorrhage (36%).

Fatal insults to the fetus were identified in all three trimesters, with no significant difference in the distribution of fetal mortality by gestational age. In subanalysis of this population according to injury severity, a fetal mortality rate of 10% was discovered in patients who had injuries of minor severity. These results are significantly higher than the generally accepted fetal mortality rates of 1% in this subset of pregnant trauma patients.

Pelvic and acetabular fractures in pregnancy continue to be associated with a high fetal mortality rate. Mechanism of injury and injury severity appear to influence mortality rates, whereas the fracture classification, the fracture type, the trimester of pregnancy, and the era of literature reviewed did not.

Pelvic fractures are associated with the highest risk of placental abruption and maternal and fetal death. Women who had pelvic fractures and who were discharged without delivering, carried an increased risk of fetal, neonatal, and infant death, mostly attributed to abruption and low-birth weight.[7]

PSYCHOLOGICAL CONSEQUENCES

It was observed that partner violence against women is common during pregnancy and might have an adverse effect on the mental health of women after delivery. The association of postnatal depression with psychological, physical and sexual violence against women by their intimate partners during pregnancy was investigated. After controlling for age, education, race and gravidity, women who had experienced IPV were at an increased risk for adverse pregnancy outcomes. Women who had been a victim of sexual abuse as an adult were 50% more likely to have had a premature baby [risk ratio (RR) = 1.5; 95% CI = 1.1–1.8] and more than twice as likely to have had 3rd trimester bleeding (RR = 2.1; 95% CI = 1.5–3.1). Those who were stalked were 20% more likely to have had preeclampsia (RR = 1.2; 95% CI = 1.0–1.5), 40% more likely to have had a premature delivery (RR = 1.4; 95% CI = 1.2–1.7), and 90% more likely to have had 3rd trimester bleeding (RR = 1.9; 95% CI = 1.4–2.7). About 5% of the women experienced violence during their pregnancy.[8]

Physical violence in pregnancy was positively associated with perinatal mortality and neonatal mortality, but not with early pregnancy loss. The differences remained largely unchanged after adjustment for age, parity, education level, wealth status, marital status and place of residence: adjusted OR = 2.32; 95% CI = 1.34–4.01 for perinatal mortality; OR = 1.86; 95% CI = 1.05–3.30 for neonatal mortality; and OR = 1.16; 95% CI = 0.60–2.24 for early pregnancy loss.[9]

INTERVENTIONS FOR REDUCING DOMESTIC VIOLENCE

Violence during pregnancy is related to adverse pregnancy outcomes. Major efforts are needed to tackle violence during pregnancy. This can be achieved through measures that are directed towards the right target groups. Measures could include empowerment; upgrading the socioeconomic status of women; and education of cultural and traditional aspects with regard to human rights. Organizations which offer help to women should be more recognized and supported, so that victims know where to go for help.

Finally, an important obstacle is the silence surrounding the subject, in order to take measures to abate violence it is necessary to break this silence. DV is a multidisciplinary problem requiring coordination with the legal system (e.g., police, prosecutors and court system), the social system (e.g., legal aid, social services and shelters), the community at large (e.g., neighbors, families, friends, schools and churches), and the health profession (e.g., physicians, nurses, counselors, and social workers).

Routine screening of women for DV at initial office visits and annual examinations has been encouraged. Lack of knowledge and training in DV may contribute to the inability of providers to recognize and correctly interpret behaviors associated with DV. Deficiencies in the education of health-care provider (HCPs) listed by Holtz and Safran include the inability to identify, assess, document and manage the care of clients experiencing DV.[10]

Chambliss, Curtis-Bay, and Jones found limitations in the education of obstetrics/gynecology residents related to DV including:

- Lack of faculty interest
- Underestimated prevalence
- Failure to recognize common presentations.[11]

Primary Prevention

The goal of primary intervention is to prevent a detrimental health event from occurring. HCPs may become involved in primary intervention through political action, through the promotion of linkages with referral resources, and through the education of communities and professional colleagues. Education of communities and professionals about DV is a primary intervention. Health professionals may become involved in community forums, in their offices, in schools, or in the education of other health professionals.

Secondary Prevention

Secondary intervention is aimed at early identification and intervention of the health problem. Assessment for violence should be routine in annual and new client visits for prenatal or other health-related care. Asking specific questions about violence implies knowledge of the problem and a willingness to help. Women in violent relationships also should be assessed for the risk of homicide.

Tertiary Prevention

Tertiary intervention involves long-term planning related to a health problem that exists. For a woman in a violent relationship, the choice of leaving is hers. Leaving often places the woman at greater risk for homicide. Often the woman will remain because of financial, educational, family, or religious constraints. Tertiary intervention by the HCP involves accepting the women's decision for action or for lack of action; remaining supportive to the family; continuing to listen and to pursue alternative problem-solving methods.[12]

CONCLUSION

Domestic violence, a public health menace, is the largest cause of injury to women in the US. Between 2 million and 4 million women in the US alone are battered annually by their partners. DV often begins or escalates during pregnancy. It is the result of power, control and coercive behavior of one individual over another in a relationship. The abuse often involves repetitive battering and injuries, psychological abuse, sexual assault, progressive social isolation and intimidation. Approximately 90% of the victims of DV are females from all socioeconomic, educational, and ethnic backgrounds. Routine screening of women for DV at initial office visits and annual examinations has been encouraged and should be the norm.

The fetus is at risk because adverse pregnancy outcomes, such as miscarriage, stillbirths, and premature delivery, have been reported following battering episodes. Pregnant women are more likely to have multiple sites of injury than nonpregnant women and are more likely to suffer abdominal trauma. Two of the most common causes of blunt abdominal trauma to the pregnant woman are falls and assaults. Placental or direct fetal injury can occur with minor maternal injuries resulting in death of the fetus. PTL, preterm premature rupture of membranes (PPROM), placental abruption, uterine rupture and pelvic fractures resulting in fetal and maternal morbidity and mortality encompass the entire gamut of clinical scenarios which may present as a result of DV.

REFERENCES

1. World Health Organization. (2002). World Report on Violence and Health: Summary. [online] Available from www.who.int/violence_injury_prevention/violence/world_report/en/summary_en.pdf. [Accessed December, 2015].
2. McCauley J, Kern DE, Kolodner K, Dill L, Schroeder AF, DeChant HK, et al. The "battering syndrome": prevalence and clinical characteristics of domestic violence in primary care internal medicine practices. Ann Internal Med. 1995;123(10):737-46.
3. Bachhus L, Mezey G, Bewley S. Domestic violence: prevalence in pregnant women and associations with physical and psychological health. Eur J Obstet Gynecol Reprod Biol. 2004;113(1):6-11.
4. Shumway J, O'Campo P, Gielen A, Witter FR, Khouzami AN, Blakemore KJ. Preterm labor, placental abruption, and premature rupture of membranes in relation to maternal violence or verbal abuse. J Matern Fetal Med. 1999;8(3):76-80.
5. Leone JM, Lane SD, Koumans EH, DeMott K, Wojtowycz MA, Jensen J, et al. Effects of intimate partner violence on pregnancy trauma and placental abruption. J Womens Health (Larchmt). 2010;19(8):1501-9.
6. Oxford CM, Ludmir J. Trauma in pregnancy. Clin Obstet Gynecol. 2009;52(4):611-29.
7. Leggon RE, Wood GC, Indeck MC. Pelvic fractures in pregnancy: factors influencing maternal and fetal outcomes. J Trauma. 2002;53(4):796-804.
8. Garabedian MJ, Lain KY, Hansen WF, Garcia LS, Williams CM, Crofford LJ. Violence against women and postpartum depression. J Womens Health (Larchmt). 2011;20(3):447-53.
9. Pool MS, Otupiri E, Owusu-Dabo E, de Jonge A, Agyemang C. Physical violence during pregnancy and pregnancy outcomes in Ghana. BMC Pregnancy Childbirth. 2014;14:71.
10. Centers for Disease Control (CDC). Education and adult domestic violence in U.S. and Canadian medical schools, 1987-88. MMWR Morb Mortal Wkly Rep. 1989;38(2):17-9.
11. Chambliss LR, Curtis Bay R, Jones RF. Domestic violence: an educational imperative? Am J Obstet Gynecol. 1995;172(3):1035-8.
12. McClure BM. Domestic violence: the role of the healthcare professional. Michigan Fam Rev Spring 1996;2(1):63-75.

CHAPTER 77

Infection Prevention in Obstetrics

Anuradha Sood, Madhvi Kaistha, Aradhna Sharma, Rajneet Kaur

INTRODUCTION

Nosocomial infections (healthcare-associated infections, hospital-acquired infections) are infections which are a result of treatment in a hospital or a healthcare service unit, but secondary to the patient's original condition. They usually appear 48 hours or more after hospital admission. Although hospital infection control is important in every unit of a healthcare facility, it is of the utmost importance for the obstetric patients. Poor hospital-infection control in labor and delivery care units can result in puerperal sepsis and other infections of childbirth. Apart from the mothers, the neonates are at a risk since their new immune systems are not adequately developed to fight infections.

IMPORTANCE

India accounts for nearly a fifth of all maternal deaths worldwide with a maternal mortality ratio of 220 per 100,000 live births.[1] Antenatal cases are at a risk only if membranes have ruptured, which may lead to ascending type of infection. Many wound and genital tract infections can be introduced during childbirth.

Infections both to mothers and neonates can occur.

Infections in Mothers

In postnatal patients, puerperal sepsis and postpartum endometritis are the most serious and life threatening. Puerperal sepsis constitutes the second most common cause after hemorrhage for maternal deaths in India. It can progress very rapidly and is usually caused by group A *Streptococcus* (GAS). Other organisms include *Staphylococcus aureus*, group B, C, and G *Streptococcus, Escherichia coli, Enterobacter species*, and *Chlamydia trachomatis.*

Infections in Infants

Neonatal sepsis can occur, which can be broadly divided into two main categories, early- and late-onset septicemia. The preterm and low-birth babies are at an additional risk because of their immature immune system.

Early-onset Neonatal Sepsis

It most often appears within 72 hours of birth. The baby gets the infection from the mother before or during delivery.[2] The following increases an infant's risk of early-onset sepsis (EOS):
- Preterm delivery
- Rupture of membranes more than 24 hours before birth
- Infection of the placenta tissues and amniotic fluid
- Microorganisms associated with EOS include Group B *Streptococcus, E. coli,* coagulase negative *Staphylococcus* (CONS), *Haemophilus influenza, Listeria monocytogenes*[3]
- The neonates can also get infection from the mother through vertical transmission, e.g., cytomegalovirus, hepatitis B virus (HBV), human immunodeficiency virus (HIV), TORCH [Toxoplasmosis, Other (syphilis, varicella-zoster, parvovirus B19), Rubella, Cytomegalovirus and Herpes infections] group of infections etc.

Late-onset Neonatal Sepsis

Babies with late-onset neonatal sepsis get infected 72 hours after delivery. The following increase an infant's risk of sepsis after delivery:

- Staying in the hospital for an extended period of time
- The organisms are acquired from the environment
- The microbiological profile includes CONS, *Staphylococcus aureus, E. coli, Klebsiella speceis, Pseudomonas speceis, Enterobacter speceis, Candida speceis,* Group B *Streptococcus* and *Acinetobacter.*[3]

PREVENTIVE MEASURES FOR INFECTION CONTROL

There is a set of preventive measures which has to be taken by all healthcare workers at all times to minimize transmission of infections in health setup. These are called as "Universal work precautions" or "Standard precautions". One must assume that every person is infectious and can transmit the infections to others. These apply to blood and all body fluids, except sweat.

Standard Precautions

The standard precautions include the following:

- Handwashing
- Proper disinfection and sterilization
- Safe injection practices and safe handling of sharps
- Proper disposal of biomedical waste
- Use of personal protective equipment
- Isolation of the patient if she has air borne/contagious illness
- Management of spillages of blood and body fluids
- Management of needle-stick injuries
- Immunization against HBV
- Rationalization of admissions and reduction of trafficking in sensitive areas like major and minor operation theaters, labor rooms, and nurseries. Avoid overcrowding in these areas
- Minimize invasive procedures
- Rational use of antibiotics.

Handwashing

It is the single most effective measure to reduce healthcare infections. The rationale for handwashing/handrub is to reduce the transient microflora. It is of three main types:

1. Social handwashing
2. Hygienic handwashing
3. Surgical handwashing.

Social handwashing: here we use soap and water for a time period of 10 seconds. This type of handwashing is done before handling food, eating, before feeding patient, and after going to toilet. This handwashing is sufficient in most cases of obstetric care.

Hygienic handwashing: in this we use antiseptics/alcohol rub. The chemicals which can be used are:

- 2–4% chlorhexidine
- 5.0–7.5% povidone iodine
- 60–70% alcoholic rub.

These are used for a period of 30 seconds. This should especially be followed in handling of infectious patients, nurseries and in times of outbreak.

Surgical handwashing: we use the same agents except here which are used in hygienic handwashing. It includes wrist, and forearms for a minimum of 2–3 minutes. If alcohol rubs are to be used then 2 rubs of 5 mL each rubbed to dryness. This is undertaken before one does any kind of major or minor surgery.

Note: In case of visibly soiled hands always do handwashing first and then use alcoholic handrubs.

Steps of Handwashing

There are six basic steps in handwashing which are demonstrated in the Figures 1A to F. It includes:

- Step 1: wet hands with water and apply soap and make lots of lather. Rub right palm over left palm and vice versa
- Step 2: rub back of hands by palm of right hand over back of left hand and palm of left hand over back of right hand
- Step 3: rub between fingers on each hand, i.e., interdigital spaces
- Step 4: rub fingertips of each hand against the palm of the other hand
- Step 5: rub around each of your thumbs and wrists
- Step 6: finally scrub the nails of each hand.

The World Health Organization (WHO) has defined the key moments for all healthcare workers for performing hand hygiene. According to this, hand hygiene always has to be performed in the following circumstances:

- Before touching a patient
- Before clean/aseptic procedures
- After body fluid exposure/risk
- After touching a patient
- After contact with patient surroundings.

Personal Protective Equipment

Also called as barrier protection, it refers to variety of barriers used to protect oneself from contact with infectious agents. It includes:

- Gloves
- Gowns
- Masks
- Goggles

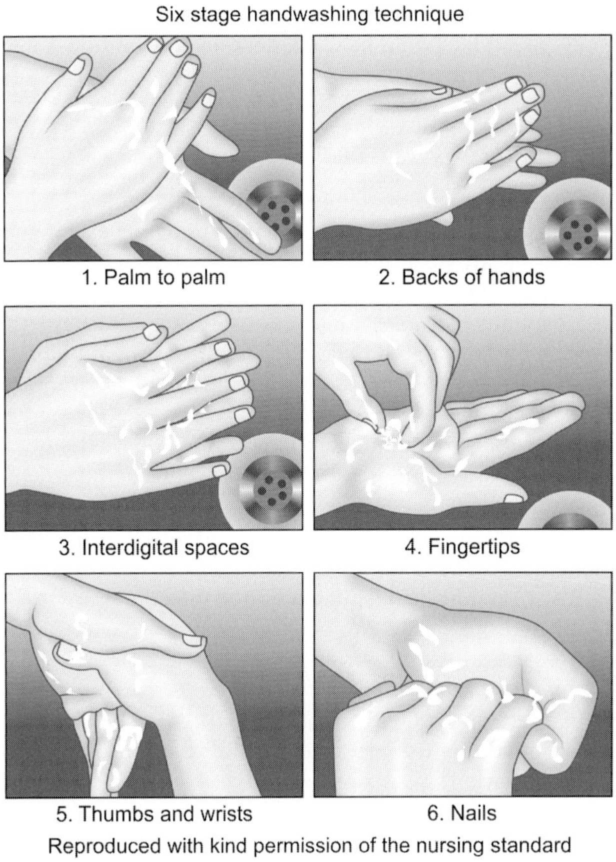

FIGS 1A TO F: Steps of handwashing (six-stage handwashing technique): **A,** Palm to palm; **B,** Backs of hands; **C,** Interdigital spaces; **D,** Fingertips; **E,** Thumbs and wrists and **F,** Nails.

Source: Reproduced with kind permission of the Nursing Standard.

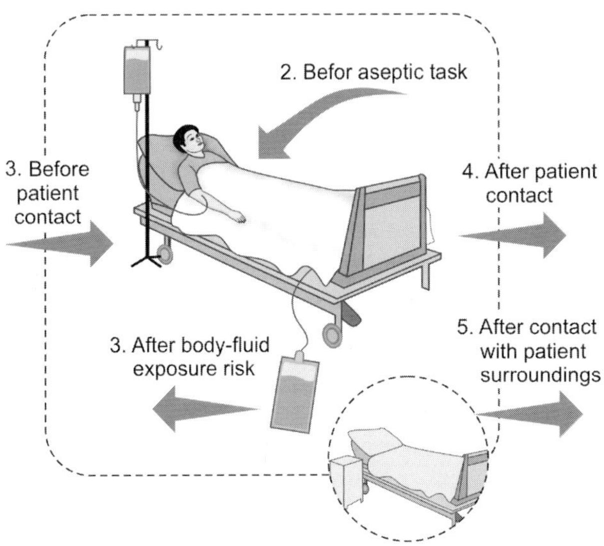

FIG. 2: Five moments of hand hygiene.

- Face shields
- Shoe covers.

Indications and precautions while using PPE: this should include the following:[4]

- Select PPE based on the anticipated level of exposure
- Personal protective equipment is to be worn only during patient care. Remove PPE once you leave the room of patient care
- Always perform hand hygiene after using PPE
- Wear gloves for contact with mucus membranes and nonintact skin of all patients
- Discard gloves, whenever they are contaminated or perforated
- Gloves are put on last while donning PPE
- Gowns are usually the first to be put on amongst all PPE
- Masks should be chosen so that they cover the nose and mouth properly to prevent infection from splashes and aerosols
- Face shields provide better protection than masks
- N-95 respirators are to be used for respiratory infections transmitted by aerosols, e.g., tuberculosis, severe acute respiratory syndrome, smallpox, avian influenza, etc.

Sequence of donning of PPE: while wearing PPE the following order should be followed:

- Gown first
- Mask or respirator
- Goggles or face shield
- Gloves last.

Sequence for removing PPE: the PPE has to be removed in the following order:

- Gloves
- Face shield or goggles
- Gown
- Mask or respirator.

Gloves are to be used in the following situations:

- Whenever an invasive procedure is to be undertaken
- Whenever contact with sterile sites and nonintact mucous membranes/skin is there
- Whenever there is risk of exposure to blood, excretions, secretions, and body fluids.

Note: Always wear sterile gloves if sterile areas have to be touched and any aseptic procedure has to be done.

Careful handling of sharps: to reduce the infections of HIV, HBV, hepatitis C virus (HCV), etc. one should take the following measures:

- Avoid recapping of used needles. Use a one-hand technique in which the needle is used to pick up the cap, and then the cap is pushed against a hard surface to ensure a tight fit onto the device
- Avoid breaking or bending of needles

- Destroy all needles by a needle destroying machine
- Collect all contaminated sharps in puncture-proof containers
- Pass all sharps in a tray and not directly to doctor or any other healthcare provider
- Containers for sharp collection should be easily accessible and sharps should be disposed off soon after use. All the sides and the bottom of the container should be leakproof. They should be filled only up to two-third level.

Proper Disinfection and Sterilization

Labor rooms and nurseries require that all items used for mother and child be clean and sterilized to prevent any kind of infections in both. For this the following things are of prime importance:

- Hospital Infection Control Committee should formulate a disinfectant policy for the use of type of disinfectant and the dilution of disinfectant to be used. This policy should be strictly adhered to especially in labor rooms, operation theaters, and nurseries
- All surgical instruments to be used should be properly sterilized. Steam sterilization or autoclave is the preferred method for sterilization. For heat-sensitive instruments ethylene oxide or high-level disinfection is preferred
- Do not allow blood/soil to dry on any instruments. If so, soak the instruments in detergent for prior cleaning
- During sterilization mechanical/chemical/biological indicators to be used for sterilization monitoring and to know the microbiological status of processed items
- Once sterilized, store the sterilized items in proper surgical trays in safe-storage places
- Towels and sheets used for babies must be sterilized by autoclaving and stored properly in a closed clean cupboard
- Umbilical stump of the neonates should be cut taking all aseptic measures and then cleaned with 70% ethanol
- If suction apparatus is to be used then use new sterilized, or disposable tube for each neonate
- Infant incubators should be wiped regularly with either 70% alcohol or freshly-prepared bleach solution [125 ppm (parts per million) available chlorine] and then aired thoroughly before use
- For disinfection of vaginal speculum, use 2% glutaraldehyde or 70% alcohol for 10 minutes before use in any other patient
- Glutaraldehyde 2% should be available for the disinfection of reusable items like oxygen tubes, etc.
- Items like endotracheal tubes, airways and face-shields which enter or come near the patients' respiratory tract should be disinfected after every use
- Ventilators, if used, should be cleaned as per needs. If it is visibly contaminated with blood or secretions, it should be cleaned before disinfection. Two methods of disinfection should be used: nebulization with hydrogen peroxide and the use of formaldehyde vapour.[5]

Biomedical Waste Management

Hospital waste can be defined as all waste generated from medical facilities. Its management is an integral part for good running of any institute as it is directly related to safety of healthcare workers, the patients, and their attendants.

Hospital waste can be hazardous, toxic, and even lethal because of their high potential for diseases transmission. In India, the rules are framed by the Ministry of Environment and Forests, Government of India, known as "Biomedical Waste (Management and Handling) Rules, 1998". The newer biomedical waste rules (2011) which replace the existing 1998 rules.

Health hazards associated with poor management of biomedical waste include:

- Risk of acquiring hospital-acquired infection (HAI)
- Injury from sharps can occur to healthcare workers and waste handlers
- Apart from the staff of hospital, there is risk of spreading of infection to general public
- Occupational risk associated with hazardous chemicals, drugs, etc.
- Repackaging and resale of used disposable items and unused/date expired drugs can also be very harmful.

Categories of waste and their disposal: previously in India, medical waste had been divided into 10 categories which now have been reduced to 8 categories. The first 7 categories are the same. Category 8 (liquid waste), 9 (incineration ash) have been deleted, and category 10 (chemical waste) has been renamed as category 8. Categories of waste are shown in Table 1.

Segregation of waste and color coding of bags: infectious and noninfectious wastes have to be segregated prior to disposal so that there is no mixing of the waste as they have to be disposed in different manners. One thing that has to be conveyed to all healthcare workers is that the generator of waste is responsible for the segregation of waste.

Different color bags are used for the segregation of waste. The color coding of the bags has been modified in newer rules and is shown in Table 2. There is no overlapping with regards to different categories, e.g., categories 3 and 6 previously could be collected in yellow or red bags and category 7 may be collected in red or blue bags.

Also remember that:

- For chemical treatment use at least 1% hypochlorite solution or any other equivalent chemical reagent
- There will be no chemical pretreatment before incineration
- Chlorinated plastics shall not be incinerated

TABLE 1: Categories of waste according to biomedical waste rules 2011

Category	Types of waste
1	Human anatomical waste (human tissues, organs, body parts)
2	Animal waste (animal tissues, organs, body parts, carcasses, waste generated by veterinary hospitals and colleges, animal houses)
3	Microbiology and biotechnology waste (cultures, stocks or specimen of live microorganisms or attenuated vaccines, human and animal cell cultures from research and industrial laboratories, wastes from production of biologicals, toxins, and devices used for transfer of cultures)
4	Waste sharps (needles, syringes, scalpels, blades, glass, etc. that may cause puncture and cuts: this includes both used and unused sharps)
5	Discarded medicine and cytotoxic drugs (wastes comprising of outdated, contaminated, and discarded medicines)
6	Soiled waste (items contaminated with body fluids including cotton, dressings, soiled plaster casts, lines, bedding, and other materials contaminated with blood)
7	Solid waste (waste generated from disposable items other than the waste sharps, such as tubing, catheters, intravenous sets, etc.)
8	Chemical waste (chemicals used in production of biologicals, chemicals used in disinfecting, as insecticides, etc.)

TABLE 2: Newer rules for color coding and disposal of waste

Color of bag	Container	Waste category (new)	Treatment
Yellow	Non-chlorinated plastic bag	1, 2, 5, 6	Incineration
Red	Plastic bag Puncture-proof container	3, 7 4	Autoclaving, microwaving or chemical treatment
Blue	Nonchlorinated plastic bag	8 (chemical waste)	Chemical treatment
Black	Nonchlorinated plastic bag	Household waste	Disposal in municipal sites

- Deep burial to be done only in rural/urban areas with less than 5 lakhs population
- Incineration generates highly toxic gases [dioxins and furans if polyvinyl chloride (PVC) plastics are there].

Management of Needle-stick Injuries

In 2002 WHO report it was observed that 2 million health providers (out of total 35 million) experience percutaneous exposure to infectious diseases each year exposing them to dangerous infections like HBV, HCV, HIV/acquired immunodeficiency syndrome (AIDS), etc.

- All needle-stick injuries to be reported to higher authorities
- Stop whatever procedure one is doing and remove gloves
- First aid includes washing wounds under tap water immediately and the wound allowed to bleed. Then dry and cover it with a sterile waterproof dressing
- Determine whether HIV, HBV, HCV exposure has occurred: it is known that the seroconversion rate due to needle-stick injuries for HIV is about 0.3%.[6] Determine the HIV, HBV, HCV status of the healthcare worker affected and that of the patient. If HIV exposure is likely postexposure prophylaxis (PEP) should be administered, preferably within an hour and not later than 72 hours before the virus has time to make too many copies in the body. PEP has to be taken for a period of 28 days. HIV-antibody test is to performed for at least 6 months thereafter, i.e. to be repeated at 6 weeks, 3months and 6 months[7]
- If there have been splashes to the nose or mouth they should be flushed with plenty of water
- Eye splashes, if there have to be irrigated immediately with clean water, saline, or a sterile irrigant.

MANAGEMENT OF SPILLS IN LABOR ROOM OR OBSTETRIC-CARE WARDS[8]

- Wear PPE (gloves, masks, gowns) for cleaning spills. Shoe covers to be used only for the large spills
- Table 3 shows type of spills and their management
- Finally mop with a gauze/cotton.

TABLE 3: Management of spills in labor room or obstetric-care wards

Category of spill	Management	Contact time
Small spills (≤10mL)	Sodium hypochlorite (5.00–6.15%) 1: 100 dilution	15–20 minutes
Large spills (≥10 mL)	Sodium hypochlorite (5.00–6.15%) 1: 10 dilution	15–20 minutes

USE OF PROPHYLACTIC ANTIBIOTICS

Indications include:
- Intrauterine procedures in which contamination by vaginal flora is there
- Cesarean section
- In immunocompromised antenatal cases
- In cases where inadequate infection-ontrol strategies are three.

Disadvantages include increased chances of antibiotic resistance and increased cost for treatment.

ISOLATION OF THE PATIENT

Isolation of both mother and the neonates born to them are required in certain circumstances which include:
- Puerperal sepsis
- Breast abscesses
- *Staphylococcus aureus*
- Any respiratory illness/communicable disease of the mother.

INFECTION CONTROL MEASURES TO PREVENT TETANUS

Tetanus (caused by *Clostridium tetani*) is transmitted in healthcare settings by use of contaminated instruments, improper handwashing techniques and use of unsterile hospital supplies in any invasive procedure during deliveries or medical termination of pregnancy. Table 4 shows methods to prevent tetanus.

HOUSEKEEPING SERVICES

Proper biomedical waste management has to be done according to the hospital-waste management guidelines. Pest-control strategies to be implemented.

All policies should be adhered to ensure proper cleaning of furniture, mattresses, beddings, linen, etc.; continued medical education and trainings to be imparted, especially for new staff; any problem related to sanitation to be related promptly.

All surfaces should be kept free of dirt and it is advised that in labor rooms and in operation theaters wet mopping should be done instead of brooming. Daily cleaning of shelves and ledges should be done by all concerned.

TABLE 4: Infection-control measures to prevent tetanus

In mothers	• Immunization of all antenatal cases with two doses of tetanus toxoid (TT), 0.5 mL intramuscularly (IM) at least 2 weeks apart • If there is unhygienic delivery/medical termination of pregnancy (MTP), give: ○ If lady is immunized, booster dose of TT, 0.5 mL IM ○ If lady is unimmunized, give antitetanus serum 1,500 U IM followed by booster injection of TT 0.5 mL IM after 4 weeks
In neonates	• Use of all aseptic techniques to cut the cord • Immunization of mothers during pregnancy as passively transferred maternal antibodies protect the child

REFERENCES

1. WHO, UNICEF, UNFPA, The World Bank, The United Nations Population Division. (2014). Trends in Maternal Mortality: 1990 to 2013. [online] Available from apps.who.int/iris/bitstream/10665/112697/1/WHO_RHR_14.13_eng.pdf. [Accessed December, 2015].
2. Ballot DE, Nana T, Sriruttan C, Cooper PA. Bacterial bloodstream infections in a developing country. ISRN Pediatr. 2012;2012:508512.
3. Hornik CP, Fort P, Clark RH, Watt K, Benjamin DK, Smith PB, et al. Early and late onset sepsis in very-low-birth-weight infants from a large group of neonatal intensive care units. Early Hum Dev. 2012;88(Suppl 2);S69-74.
4. World Health Organization. (WHO). (2002). Prevention of hospital-acquired infections. [online] Available from www.who.int/csr/resources/publications/whocdscsreph200212.pdf. [Accessed December, 2015].
5. Aylife GA, Fraise AP, Geddes AM, Mitchell K, Arnold M (Eds). Aylife's Control of Hospital Infections: A Practical Handbook, 4th edition. London, UK: Oxford University Press; 2000. p. 115-18.
6. Tokars JI, Marcus R, Culver DH, Schable CA, McKibben PS, Bandea CI, et al. Surveillance of HIV infection and zidovudine use among health care workers after occupational exposure to HIV-infected blood. The CDC Cooperative Needlestick Surveillance Group. Ann Intern Med. 1993;118(12):913-9.
7. Panlilio AL, Cardo DM, Grohskopf LA, Heneine W, Ross CS; U.S. Public Health Service. Updated U.S. Public Health Service guidelines for the management of occupational exposures to HIV and recommendations for postexposure prophylaxis. MMWR Recomm Rep. 2005;54(RR-9):1-17.
8. Mathur P (Ed). Cleaning, disinfection and sterilization. In: Hospital Acquired Infections: Prevention and Control, 1st edition. New Delhi, India: Wolters Kluwer Health; 2010. pp. 153-4.

CHAPTER 78

Demography and Vital Statistics

Anjali Mahajan, Alka Kuthe

INTRODUCTION

The word demography has a Greek origin-demos (people) and graphein (to draw, describe).[1] Therefore, by definition demography means the scientific study of human population. The term demography is based on observation of certain human phenomenon which includes:

- Alteration in population size that is growth or decline in population over the time
- Population composition in terms of age and sex
- Population distribution patterns.

It deals with five demographic processes namely fertility, marriage, migration, mortality, and social mobility and the interaction of all these with prevailing social and economic conditions.

The main sources of demographic statistics in India are: population census, National Sample surveys, registration of vital events and adhoc demographic studies. The Indian Census is the most authentic source of information on sociocultural and socioeconomic data of Indian population. This includes demographic details, fertility, mortality, economic activity, literacy and education, housing and household amenities, urbanization, disability, etc. The first regular census in India was carried out in 1881. Since it is a decennial event, therefore Census conducted in 2011 is the 15th National Census of the country. For obtaining information of the population at the grass root level that is wards, towns and villages the census is the only source of credible data. It is a source of valuable information for Central and the State Governments, so that they can formulate and implement policies accordingly. It is widely used by agencies working at national and international levels for research purposes by research scholars, business organizations, individuals, etc.

DEMOGRAPHIC CYCLE

All the nations in the world pass through a demographic cycle which typically consists of five stages. This fact has been proven historically since 1650. Table 1 below shows the stages and characteristics of demographic cycle.

India was in the high-stationary phase till 1920 and has now entered the late-expanding phase.

Low-stationary phase refers to zero population growth. This phase is also termed as replacement level of fertility. It is believed that to ensure environmental sustainability in the future, keeping in view the ever growing population of the world, all the nations should strive to attain this phase. China is believed to reach this phase by 2030 owing to stringent government policies of population control.

There are twenty countries in the world which exhibit negative or zero natural population growth as has been established by latest data available from the Population Reference Bureau.[2] Ukraine is the leading country in the list of top 20 countries with highest decrease in birth rate. The birth rate in Ukraine is decreasing at the rate of 0.8% per year. Out of the top 20 countries, 19 countries are European and Japan is the only country in the list which is non-European and exhibits 0% natural birth increase. Seeing the present trend of population decline, it is expected that Japan would lose 21% of its population by 2050.

DEMOGRAPHIC TRANSITION

Demographic transition or demographic revolution is the process when countries show a gradual drift from high-fertility and high-mortality situation to low fertility and low mortality situation. WHO defines it as "the process by which, over a number of years, continuous changes in one or more of

TABLE 1: Demographic cycle with its stages and characteristics

Stages	Name	Characteristics
First	High stationary	Very high birth and death rates, therefore growth cancels and population remains stationary
Second	Early expansion	Birth rate remains unchanged, death rate begins to decline
Third	Late expanding	Birth rate starts declining, death rate further declines, and therefore very slow expansion in population as births are still in excess of deaths
Fourth	Low stationary	Low birth and death rates, population remains stationary
Fifth	Declining	Birth rate further declines, which is more than death rate resulting in decline in population

the fertility, mortality and migration rates in the population produce alterations in the characteristics and structure of the population".

The Earth is inhabited by humans and the total number of humans living on this planet constitutes the world population. United States Census Bureau (USCB) estimated that the total world population was 7.158 billion[2] as on March 26, 2014. This agency estimated that the world population exceeded 7 billion on March 12, 2012. Another international agency—United Nations Population Fund reported that the world population achieved this milestone on October 31, 2011.[3]

The ever growing world population has registered an increase from 2.5 billion in 1950 to 7 billion people in 2011, i.e., 4.5 billion people have been added to Mother Earth in about 60 years. This is an alarming increase which can have adverse implications for development of the world. These points to an emerging serious situation where in sustainability, employment, food shortage, housing and shelter would be far from reach of each and every new individual added to the total world henceforth.

The Governing Council of the United Nations Development Program in 1989, recommended that 11 July should be observed by the international community as World Population Day so as to highlight the importance of issues related to growing population and draw attention of all to search for early redressal of these issues. Henceforth, this day is celebrated world over to create awareness amongst the masses which otherwise would have adverse impact on human survival on Mother Earth.

About 16 million adolescent girls under the age 18 years get pregnant each year, thereby resulting in sixteen million births. World-over, about 3.2 million teenager girls undergo unsafe abortions owing to some factors like lack of medical facilities, poor availability and utilization of health services. An alarming fact is that the vast majority of the pregnant adolescents in the developing world are married. Pregnancy in these adolescent girls is not as a result of informed choice. It is a consequence of illiteracy or inadequate education, female discrimination, child marriage, and sexual oppression. In developing countries including India, the leading causes of death among adolescent girls are the complications arising due to pregnancy and childbirth. Therefore, the theme for 2013 World Population Day was focussed upon dangers of adolescent pregnancy. The objective of 2013 World Population Day was to draw the attention towards the issue of adolescent pregnancy so that each and every pregnancy is wanted and every childbirth is safe, thereby ensuring well-being of each mother-child duo.

DEMOGRAPHIC TRENDS IN INDIA

India's population has been steadily increasing since 1921. The year 1921 is called the "big divide" because the absolute number of people added to the population during each decade has been on the increase since 1921. India's population is currently increasing at the rate of 16 million each year. This will make India the most populous country in the world surpassing China.

DEMOGRAPHIC INDICATORS

Demographic indicators can be divided into two parts:

1. Population statistics: these include indicators that measure the population size, sex ratio, density, and dependency ratio
2. Vital statistic: these include indicators such as birth rate, death rate, natural growth rate, life expectancy at birth, mortality and fertility rates. Ever since India attained independence from the British Empire 60 years ago, the country's population has more than tripled from a mere figure of 350 million. India crossed the one billion mark in the year 2000; 1 year after the world's population crossed the six billion threshold.

At present India with 1,270,272,105 (1.27 billion) people is the second most populous country in the world, while China is on the top with over 1,360,044,605 (1.36 billion) people. India represents almost 17.31% of the world's population which means that every sixth person in this world lives in India.

Although, at present China is the world's most populous country, yet India is all set to take this position by 2030. India has a population growth rate of 1.58%, therefore prediction is that India would have more than 1.53 billion people by the end of 2030. More than 50% of India's current population is below the age of 25 and over 65% below the age of 35. About 72.2% of the population is rural and the rest is urban i.e., 27.8%.[4] Illiteracy rates are highest in India in the world. Every year, India adds more people than any other nation in the world. The individual population of some of its states is equal to the total population of many countries. For example, Population of Uttar Pradesh almost equals to the population of Brazil. The population of the second most populous state Maharashtra in India is equal to that of Mexico's population. Bihar is the third most populous state in India and its population is more than Germany's.[4] As per Census 2011, India's population is 1210 million, of which the urban population is 377 million. The increase in migration rates of people from villages to urban agglomerations has resulted in rise of the level of urbanization from 27.8% in 2001 to 31.2% in 2011 (Fig. 1).[4] 15.4% of the total urban population of India is concentrated in the four major metropolitan cities in India, namely, Mumbai, Kolkata, Chennai, and Delhi.

SEX RATIO

Sex ratio is defined as the number of females per 1,000 males in a particular area. Child sex ratio is defined as the number of girl children aged 0–6 years per 1000 boy children aged 0–6 years in a defined geographical area. The sex ratio for the entire world is 101 males for 100 females. However, in India there is a disparity between male and female populations, thereby leading to gender imbalance (Table 2). Much attention these days is being given to improve the sex ratio in the entire world. In India, the sex ratio is generally adverse to women; meaning that the number. of women per 1,000 men is less than 1,000. To add to the woes, this sex ratio has been showing some decline over the decades. Census 2011 reports that the total female sex ratio in India is 940 per 1,000 males and the female-child sex ratio is 944 girl children per every 1,000 boy children of the same age group. Owing to rise in public awareness and stringent laws adopted by the Indian Government, the overall female sex ratio has increased by 0.75 % in the Census 2011 as compared to the previous Census conducted in 2001.[4]

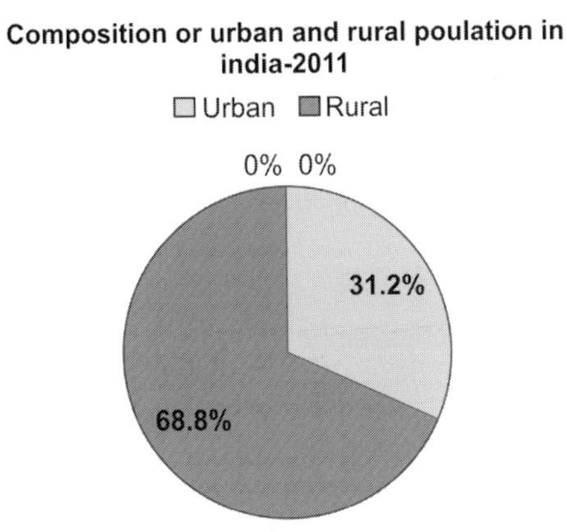

FIG. 1: Composition of urban and rural population of India.
Source: Census of India, 2011.

DEPENDENCY RATIO

It is defined as the proportion of persons above 60 years of age and children below 15 years of age who are considered to be dependent on the economically productive age group (15–59 years).

Total dependency ratio (Table 3) or societal dependency ratio is defined as the ratio of the combined age groups 0–14 years plus 60 years and above to the 15–59 years age group. Dependency ratio can be divided in 2 parts:

1. Young dependency ratio (0–14 years) (Table 4)
2. Old dependency ratio (60 years and more) (Table 5).

Dependency ratio gives the proportion of persons needs to be supported by the economically active age group. Reduction in dependency ratio indicates a phase of population transition where a higher percentage of persons in the working age group may translate into higher per capita income for the economy. This is also called the phase where a country may benefit from "demographic dividend".

AGE PYRAMID (POPULATION PYRAMID, AGE PICTURE DIAGRAM)

The age and sex distribution of a population can be most effectively represented graphically with the help of population

TABLE 2: Child sex ratio in India: A comparison

Census	Total	Rural	Urban
1991	945	948	935
2001	927	933	906
2011	914	919	902

TABLE 3: Dependency ratio in India

1991	2001	2011
794	752	652

TABLE 4: Young dependency ratio in India

1991	2001	2011
672	621	510

TABLE 5: Old dependency ratio in India

1991	2001	2011
122	131	142

Source: Census 2011

pyramids. A population pyramid consists of two bar graphs in which the population is plotted on the X-axis and age is plotted on the Y-axis. This takes the shape of a pyramid when the population it is representing, shows an increasing trend. The distribution of various age groups in a population of a particular country or region of the world can be easily gauged through this graphical illustration.

Uses of Age Pyramid

- A great deal of information regarding age and sex distribution of the population of a particular country or a region of the world can be easily obtained by mere look at a population pyramid. This information can be further utilized to assess the effectiveness of programs and policies devised and implemented by various agencies which are aimed at progress and development of the population in a region or a country
- The age range of people of each sex living in any particular area can also be deduced
- They are powerful means to gauge the dependency ratio in a particular region.

Types of Population Pyramids

On the basis of fertility and mortality rates of a country, four general types of population pyramids can be identified. These age pyramids show great deal of variation from one country to another owing to varying fertility and mortality rates. These population pyramids exhibit various shapes and therefore, in some countries they are referred to by a description of their shape. The pyramid is undoubtedly, the classic shape which geometrically consists of three triangular outer surfaces which meet at a single point at the top. The alterations in the shape of pyramid are described below:

Stable Pyramid

When the pattern of fertility and mortality in particular country or a region of the world remains unaltered, the resultant pyramid obtained is stable pyramid.

Stationary pyramid

It is very similar to a constrictive pyramid. This population pyramid is typically representative of countries which exhibit low fertility and low mortality rates. It is also referred to as a "clock-model" pyramid.

Expansive Pyramid

Gary Fuller (1995) described this particular form of pyramid as youth bulge. This population pyramid is of great width at the base thereby indicating high birth and death rates in a particular region.

Constrictive Pyramid (Onion-shaped, Urn-shaped)

The population which exhibits a low birth rate, a low death rate, the population in general has a long life expectancy and is generally older on average typically shows a constrictive pyramid (Fig. 2). This pyramid is becoming more common worldwide owing to the improvement in the delivery of health services to the masses. Developed countries with a high level of socioeconomic indicators, such as a high level of education, easy access to health facilities, good healthcare

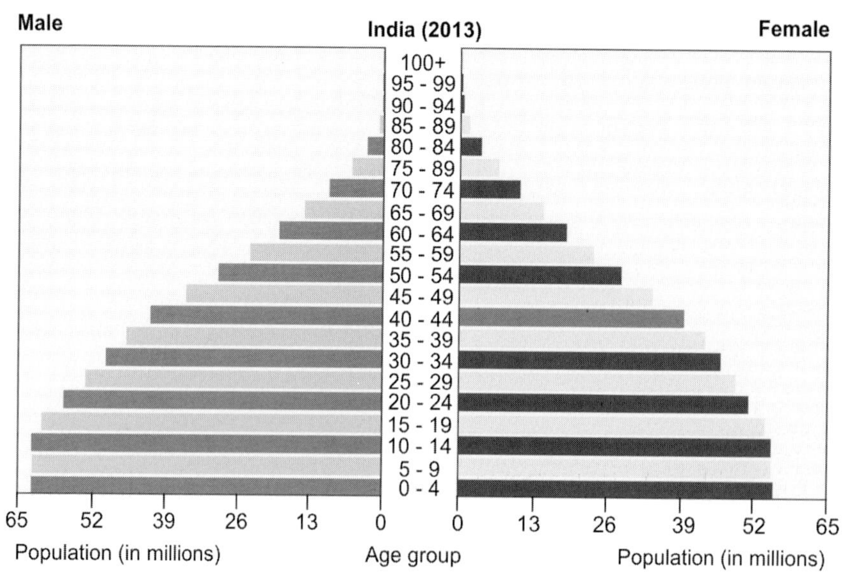

FIG. 2: Constrictive population pyramid.

provision to masses and favorable environmental factors are the ideal representatives of such a type of pyramid. In other words, it is indicative of excellent performance of the health services of a country.

VITAL STATISTICS

Vital statistics refers to the demographic data concerning all the events which happen and are related to individual's life events like birth and death, together with changes in civil status like marriages, separations and divorces, fetal deaths, maternal deaths, perinatal deaths, fertility rate, etc. The National Vital Statistics System of the United States is the oldest and most successful example of intergovernmental data sharing in public health. The National Centre for Health Statistics (NCHS) collects and disseminates official statistics through contractual agreements with vital registration systems operating in various jurisdictions legally responsible for the registration of events mentioned above. The division of vital statistics of NCHS which is a division of the centers for disease control and prevention (CDC) has been assigned the task of annual collection of vital statistics.

Obstetrics is largely preventive medicine, the aim being to ensure that throughout pregnancy and puerperium, the mother will have sound health and that every pregnancy would result in a healthy mother and a healthy child. The age old concept that obstetrics is mainly a technical skill concerned with antenatal, intranatal and postnatal care is now replaced by the broad concept of community obstetrics which takes in to account not only obstetric issues but also concepts of primary health care (PHC). The maternal and neonatal outcomes in forms of different indices indirectly reflect the quality of health and life in human society. Thus, indices that reflect poor obstetrical and perinatal outcomes would lead to the assumption that medical care for the entire population is lacking.

Definitions recommended by the NCHC and the CDC which are important from obstetric point of view are as follows:

- Birth: the complete expulsion or extraction from the mother of a fetus after 20-weeks gestation. In the absence of accurate dating criteria, fetuses weighing less than 500 grams are usually not considered as births but are termed as abortuses for the purpose of vital statistics
- Live Birth: the term used to record a birth whenever the new born at or sometimes after birth breathes spontaneously or shows any other sign such as a heartbeat or definite spontaneous movement of voluntary muscles Heartbeats are distinguished from transient cardiac contractions and respirations are differentiated from fleeting respiratory efforts or gasps
- Birth weight: the weight of neonate determined immediately after delivery or as soon thereafter as feasible. It should be expressed to the nearest gram
- Birth rate: the number of live births per 1,000 population
- Perinatal period: the period after birth of an infant born after 20 weeks and ending at 28-completed days after birth. When perinatal rates are based on birth weight, rather than gestational age, it is recommended that the perinatal period be defined as commencing at 500 grams
- Stillbirth or fetal death: the absence of signs of life at or after birth
- Early neonatal death: death of a live-born neonate during the first 7 days after birth
- Late neonatal death: death after 7 days but before 29 days
- Stillbirth rate or fetal death rate: the number of stillborn neonates per 1,000 neonates born, including livebirth and stillbirths
- Neonatal mortality rate: the number of neonatal deaths per 1,000 live births. It is calculated as:

  Neonatal mortality rate =

$$\frac{\text{Number of neonatal death (<28 days of age)}}{\text{Number of live births}} \times 1{,}000$$

- Perinatal mortality rate: the number of stillbirths plus neonatal deaths per 1,000 total births. Thus,

  Perinatal mortality rate (PMR) =

$$\frac{\text{Number of fetal deaths [>28-weeks gestation} + \text{early neonatal deaths (<7-days age)}}{\text{Number of live births} + \text{stillbirths}} \times 1{,}000$$

WHO definition:

For international comparison, WHO Expert Committee on the Prevention of Perinatal morbidity and mortality (1970) recommended a more precise formulation: 'Late fetal and early neonatal deaths weighing over 1,000 grams at birth expressed as a ratio per 1,000 live births weighing over 1,000 grams at birth. It is calculated as:

Perinatal mortality rate =

$$\frac{\text{Late fetal and early neonatal deaths weighing over 1000 g at birth} \times 1000}{\text{Total livebirths weighing over 1,000 grams at birth}}$$

- Infant death: all deaths of liveborn infants from birth through 12 months of age
- Infant mortality rate: the number of infant deaths per 1,000 live births. It is calculated as,

  Infant mortality rate (IMR) =

$$\frac{\text{Number of infant deaths during time period}}{\text{Number of livebirths during time period}} \times 1{,}000$$

- Low birthweight: a newborn whose weight is less than 2500 grams
- Very low birthweight: a newborn whose weight is 1500 grams

- Extremely low birthweight: a newborn whose weight is less than 1,000 grams.
- Term neonate: a neonate born any time after 37 completed weeks of gestation and up until 42 completed weeks of gestation (260–294 days)
- Pre-term neonate: a neonate born before 37 completed weeks (the 259th day)
- Postterm neonate: a neonate born any time after completion of the 42nd week, beginning with day 295
- Abortus: a fetus or embryo removed or expelled from the uterus during the first-half of gestation—20 weeks or less or in the absence of accurate dating criteria, born weighing less than 500 grams
- Nonmaternal death: death of mother that results from accidental or incidental causes not related to pregnancy, e.g., death from an automobile accident, burn, or concurrent malignancy
- Maternal mortality rate: it is a very sensitive indicator which points towards health status of women in reproductive age group. It also tells us about the provision of obstetric services in any area. Maternal death is defined as any death occurring to a woman, while pregnant or within 42 days of termination of pregnancy, irrespective of the duration, and site of pregnancy, from any cause related to or aggravated by pregnancy, but not from accidental or incidental causes.[6] Each product of such a birth is considered live born

Maternal mortality rate (MMR) =

$$\frac{\text{Number of deaths due to maternal causes during time period}}{\text{Number of live births during the same time period}} \times 1{,}000$$

It is very difficult to accurately measure MMR especially in those communities where comprehensive registration of deaths and of causes of death does not exist. Reproductive-age mortality studies (RAMOS) are considered the best way to estimate levels of maternal mortality (maternal mortality ratio). They use triangulation of different sources of data on deaths of women of reproductive age coupled with record review and/or verbal autopsy to identify maternal deaths. Elsewhere, census, surveys, or models have to be relied upon to estimate levels of maternal mortality. The high level of disparity in the number of maternal deaths in different areas of the world reflects gross inequitable access to health services world over by the masses and highlights the rich-poor divide as far as reach to the health services are concerned. Developing countries account for almost all maternal deaths (99%) occurring in the world. More than half of these deaths occur in sub-Saharan Africa and almost one-third occur in South Asia.

- Maternal mortality ratio: the number of maternal deaths that result from the reproductive process per 1,000 live births. Maternal mortality rate or maternal death rates are more commonly used terms but they are less accurate. The term ratio is more accurate because it includes in the numerator the number of deaths regardless of pregnancy outcome, e.g., live births, stillbirths, ectopic pregnancies, whereas the denominator includes the number of live births

  The maternal mortality ratio in developing countries is 240 per 100,000 births versus 16 per 100,000 in developed countries.
- Teenage Pregnancy: the risk of maternal mortality is highest for adolescent girls under 15 years of age. Complications in pregnancy and childbirth are the leading causes of death among adolescent girls in most developing countries.[7,8] Like abortion, teenage pregnancy is a complex situation influenced by strong rigid opinions and religious ideology that may lead to blocked access to family planning services for teenagers. The issue is also related to prevalence of sex education in schools. Despite the success of family-planning program, a number of states in the western hemisphere, usually driven by sociopolitical concern, have linked funding to "abstinence-only" counseling and to exclusion of family-planning counseling that include abortion topics. Even worse, some states have diverted funds from planning services and put them into program for abstinence-only counseling despite the fact: They do not work. They are actually counterproductive
- Pregnancy-associated death: the death of a woman from any cause while pregnant or within one calendar year of termination of pregnancy, regardless of the duration and size of pregnancy
- Pregnancy-related death: a pregnancy-associated death results from:
  - Complication of pregnancy itself
  - The chain of events initiated by pregnancy that led to death
  - Aggravation of an unrelated condition by the physiological or pharmacological effects of pregnancy that subsequently caused death.

Vital Statistics: Measures of Obstetrical Care[9]

The various indices mentioned above under vital statistics definitions are used as a yardstick of obstetrical and perinatal outcomes to assess quality of care.

Infant Deaths

Infant mortality rate is universally regarded not only as a most important indicator of the health status of a community but also the standard of living of people in general.

Causes of Infant Mortality

The three leading causes of infant death are congenital malformations, low birth weight, and sudden infant death syndrome. Infants born at lower gestational age birth weights are predisposed to higher mortality rates. In India, the principle causes of infant mortality are low birth weight; respiratory infections; diarrheal diseases; congenital malformation; and cord malnutrition; birth injury; and unclassified (about 18%).

PERINATAL MORTALITY

Fetal deaths after 20 weeks are an important public health issue. Although much importance is given to reduction in infant mortality rate, a focus on fetal mortality may provide further opportunities for prevention.

Causes of Perinatal Mortality[10]

About two-thirds of all perinatal deaths occur among infants with less than 2500 grams birth weight. The causes include one or more complications in the mother during pregnancy or labor, in the placenta or in the fetus or neonate.

Important causes: intrauterine and birth asphyxia, low birth weight, birth trauma and intrauterine or neonatal infections are important causes of perinatal deaths. The various causes leading to perinatal mortality can be categorized as mentioned below.

Antenatal Causes

- Maternal diseases: hypertension, cardiovascular diseases, diabetes, tuberculosis, anemia
- Pelvic diseases: uterine myomas, endometriosis, ovarian tumors
- Anatomical defects: uterine anomalies, incompetent cervix
- Endocrine imbalance
- Blood incompatibilities
- Malnutrition
- Pregnancy-induced hypertension
- Antepartum hemorrhage
- Congenital defects
- Advanced maternal age.

Intranatal Causes

- Asphyxia
- Birth injuries
- Prolonged labor
- Obstetric complications.

Postnatal Causes

- Prematurity
- Respiratory distress syndrome
- Respiratory and alimentary infections
- Congenital anomalies.

Unknown Causes

In some cases exact cause can not be ascertained.

Thus the etiology of perinatal and infant mortality is multifactorial. Therefore nothing less than a multipronged approach as stated below will reduce the mortalities.

Preventive and Social Measures

They include the following:[10]
- Improvement in prenatal nutrition
- Prevention of infection
- Optimum breastfeeding practices
- Growth monitoring
- Family planning
- Sanitation
- Provision of PHC
- Socioeconomic development
- Female literacy: it is a driving force for better health. Women who are educated do not have early pregnancies, can space their pregnancies appropriately, can take care of their children and have better access to information related to personal hygiene and make better use of healthcare services. It is well studied and documented that those women with higher literacy rates are associated with low fertility and low maternal mortality as well as low infant morbidity and mortality.

Rising Cesarean Delivery Rate

In the United States, the researchers found that there is significant increase in cesarean delivery rates in the year 2002 (26.1%) with the increase of 31.1% in 2006 (Martin and colleagues, 2009). This rise is found in both primary and the repeat cesarean rate. Infact, more than 90% of women with prior cesarean deliveries now undergo repeat cesarean. The multiple factors responsible for such rise in rate are:
- Increase in the diagnosis of dystocia, a major indication for primary cesarean
- The sharp decline in the vaginal birth after cesarean (VBAC) is likely related to the risk of uterine rupture associated with VBAC
- A new and controversial factor is cesarean delivery on maternal request (CDMR). This is defined as a cesarean delivery at term for a singleton pregnancy on maternal request in the absence of any medical or obstetrical

indication (Reddy and Spong, 2006). To address the issue, the National Institute of Child Health and Human Development (NICHD) convened a State-of-the-Science Conference in 2006 to provide an in-depth evaluation of evidence , raise public awareness, identify research goals and guide practitioners in assessing risks and benefits. In summary, it was concluded that there was insufficient evidence to evaluate fully the benefits and risks of CDMR versus planned vaginal delivery. Cesarean delivery on maternal request is not recommended for women desiring several children, since the risks of placenta previa and accreta increase with each cesarean delivery. Moreover, it was concluded that CDMR should not be performed before 39 completed weeks gestation or before verification of fetal lung maturity. Fertility means actual bearing of children. Various indices are used to measure fertility patterns of women in any particular area. These indices show varied values in different regions of the world. There is a gross difference of fertility patterns between developed and developing nations of the world.

Severe Maternal Morbidity

The concept of "near miss" maternal mortality has led to the statistical data systems that measure indicators of severe maternal morbidities. The investigators reported that for every maternal death, approximately 50 women experience severe morbidities in the form of need for transfusion, eclampsia, hysterectomy, cardiac or respiratory or renal event, septicemia, anesthetic complications, hemorrhagic shock, stroke, pulmonary embolism, etc. As with maternal deaths, these morbidities can be investigated to discover and correct systemic errors and to improve substandard care.

MATERNAL MORTALITY

India is among those countries which have very high maternal mortality rate. Most maternal deaths are preventable. The low status of women in the society coupled with their low literacy levels prevents the women from taking antenatal care even though services are easily available. In spite of the continued efforts by the government and the sanctioning of various welfare schemes to promote institutional delivery, there are deliveries which take place at home without the services of the trained midwife. The situation is tragic as these deaths are not caused by the disease but they occur during or following a natural physiological event of birth. It is one of the leading causes of death of a woman in the reproductive age group in developing countries.[10] Most maternal deaths and pregnancy complications can be prevented, if a pregnant woman has access to good quality of antenatal, natal, and postnatal care and if certain age-old harmful birthing practices are avoided. Misconceptions, misbeliefs, and superstitions deeply rooted in the community need to be tackled. For that, mass health education and awareness program needs implementation in full force.

The International Classification of Diseases (ICD) has recommended that maternal deaths may be disaggregated into two groups:[10]

1. Direct obstetric death: the death of the mother that results from obstetrical complications of pregnancy, labor, or the puerperium and from interventions, omissions, incorrect treatment or a chain of events resulting from these factors, e.g., maternal death resulting from exsanguination after uterine rupture
2. Indirect obstetric death: a maternal death that is not directly due to an obstetric cause but results from previously existing disease or a disease developing during pregnancy , labor or puerperium that was aggravated by maternal physiological adaptation to pregnancy, e.g., a maternal death from complications of mitral valve stenosis.

The MMR, the direct obstetric rate, and the indirect obstetric rate are fine measures of the quality of maternal services.

Causes[10]

Worldwide, about 80% of maternal deaths are due to direct causes i.e., obstetric complications of pregnancy, labor, and puerperium. The single most common cause accounting for a quarter of all maternal deaths is obstetric hemorrhage generally occurring postpartum which can lead to death very rapidly if prompt life saving measures are not instituted. Puerperal infection, eclampsia, unsafe abortion, prolonged or obstructed labor, ectopic pregnancies, embolism, and deaths related to interventions. About 20% of the maternal deaths are due to indirect causes such as anemia; hepatitis; cardiovascular diseases; diseases of the endocrine and metabolic system; and infections such as tuberculosis, malaria, and human immunodeficiency virus infection (HIV).

Preventive and Social Measures[10]

High maternal mortality reflects not only inadequacy of healthcare services for mothers but also a low standard living and socioeconomic status of the community. In the world as a whole the problem of maternal mortality is principally one of applying existing obstetric knowledge through antenatal, intranatal, and postnatal services rather than developing new skills. Efforts should be made to lower MMR by adopting following measures:

- Early registration of pregnancy
- At least three antenatal checkups
- Dietary supplementation including correction of anemia
- Prevention of infection and hemorrhage in puerperium
- Prevention of complications (eclampsia, malpresentation, rupture uterus)

- Treatment of medical conditions (hypertension, diabetes, tuberculosis)
- Antimalaria and tetanus prophylaxis
- Clean delivery practices
- Encouraging institutional deliveries especially with bad obstetric history and risk factors
- Training of local dais and female health workers
- Promotion of family planning to control the number of children to not more than two and spacing of births
- Identification of every maternal death and searching for its cause.

MILLENNIUM DEVELOPMENT GOALS FOR MATERNAL AND CHILD HEALTH[10]

Representatives from 189 countries met, at the Millennium Summit in New York in september, 2000 to adopt the United Nations (UN) Millennium Declaration. The goals in the area of development and poverty eradication are now widely referred to as "Millennium Development Goals" (MDGs). The MDGs place health at the heart of development and represent commitments by governments throughout the world. They are an integral part of the road map towards the implementation of the UN Millennium declaration. Governments had set a date of 2015, by which they would meet the MDGs, i.e., eradicate extreme poverty and hunger; achieve universal primary education; promote gender equality; improve maternal health; combat HIV or AIDS; malaria and other communicable diseases; ensure environmental sustainability, and develop a global partnership for development.

NATIONAL RURAL HEALTH MISSION[10]

Recognizing the importance of health in the process of social and economic development and to improve the quality of life of it is citizens, the Government of India launched "National Rural Health Mission"(NRHM) on 5th April 2005 initially for a period of 7 years (2005-2012). The main aim of mission is to provide accessible, affordable, accountable, effective, and reliable PHC and bridging the gap in rural healthcare through creation of Accredited Social Health Activist (ASHA). All district-level vertical-health and family-welfare programs will merge into one common "District Health Mission" and at state level into "State Health Mission". For improved outreach services at district level there will be provision of a mobile medical unit.

At national level, NRHM aims at reduction in, maternal mortality ratio, and total fertility rate in addition to other indicators of general health. It also aims at increased utilization of first referral units. At community level, it aims at fixed day or month program to provide immunization; antenatal or postnatal checkups and services related to mother; child healthcare and nutrition; and good hospital care through availability of doctors, drugs and quality services at PHC or community health centers (CHC) level and improved access to universal immunization through improved mobilization services under the program; improved facilities for institutional delivery through provision of referral, transport escort, improved hospital care subsidized under the "Janani Suraksha Yojna" for the below poverty line families improved outreach services through mobile medical unit at district level.

REPRODUCTIVE AND CHILD HEALTH PROGRAM[10]

Reproductive and child health (RCH) approach has been defined as "people have the ability to reproduce and regulate their fertility, women are able to go through pregnancy and child birth safely, the outcome of pregnancies is successful in terms of maternal and infant survival and well-being and couples are able to have sexual relations free of fear of pregnancy and of contracting disease".

The concept supports the integrated approach to the program aimed at improving the health status of young women and young children through various programs like family welfare program, universal immunization program, oral rehydration therapy, child survival and safe motherhood program, acute respiratory infection control, etc.

REPRODUCTIVE AND CHILD HEALTH PHASE I

This program incorporated the components relating child survival and safe motherhood and included two additional components one relating to sexually transmitting disease (STD) and other relating to reproductive tract infection (RTI). The RCH program is based on a differential approach. Inputs in all districts have not been kept uniform. While the care components are the same in all districts, the weaker districts get more support and sophisticated facilities are proposed for relatively advanced districts. On the basis of crude birth rate and female literacy rate, all the districts have been divided into three categories, i.e., category, category 2, and category 3. All the districts were covered in a phased manner over a period of 3 years. The program was formally launched on 15th October 1997. The RCH phase I launched various interventions related to safe motherhood, child survival, safe abortions, essential obstetric care, facility of referral transport, and RTI or STD clinic in all districts and selected states. Maternal healthcare was a part of Family Welfare Program from its inception. Interventions were introduced as vertical schemes, namely the National Nutritional Anemia Control Program, tetanus toxoid (TT) immunization of pregnant ladies (part of immunization program) and dais training program, etc. Family planning remained a separate intervention. In 1992, the Child Survival and Safe

Motherhood (CSSM) program integrated all the schemes for better compliance. The program had following components:

- Early registration of pregnancy
- To provide minimum three antenatal checkups
- Universal coverage of all pregnant women with TT immunization
- Advice on food, nutrition and rest
- Detection of high-risk pregnancies and prompt referral
- Clean deliveries by trained personnel
- Birth spacing
- Promotion of institutional deliveries.

The RCH program has integrated these services and the major interventions are essential obstetric care, 24-hour delivery services at PHCs or CHCs, emergency obstetric care, medical termination of pregnancy, prevention of RTI and STD, and district survey.

REPRODUCTIVE AND CHILD HEALTH PHASE II

The program started from first April 2005 to reduce the maternal and child morbidity and mortality with emphasis on rural health.

Under RCH-II more flexibility has been given to states for planning their own interventions to achieve the goals through their project implementation plan (PIP). Major interventions are included in the PIP of the state for which Government of India provide funds. The implementation of manual vacuum aspiration services at the level of the PHC is one of the important strategies under safe abortion services. The Government of India has given some broad guidelines and strategies to reduce maternal and infant mortality rate. The initiatives which have been covered under the program are:

- Essential obstetric care
  - Institutional delivery
  - Skilled attendance at delivery
  - The policy decision for auxiliary nurse midwife (ANMs) or lady health visitors (LHVs) or staff nurses (SN) to use drugs and to carry out certain emergency interventions in specific emergency situations to reduce maternal mortality
- Emergency obstetric care:
  - Operationalizing first referral units
  - Operationalizing PHCs and CHCs for round-the-clock delivery services
- Strengthening referral system.

JANANI SURAKSHA YOJNA10

The National Maternity Benefit scheme has been modified into a new scheme called Janani Suraksha Yojna (JSY). It was launched on 12th April 2005. The objectives of the scheme are reducing maternal mortality and infant mortality through encouraging delivery at health institutions and focusing at institutional care among women belonging to the category of below poverty line.

Salient Features

The salient features JSY of are as follows:

- It is 100% centrally-sponsored scheme
- Under National Rural Health Mission, it integrates the benefit of cash assistance with institutional care during antenatal, delivery and immediate postpartum care .Both rural and urban women belonging to below poverty line families and in the age group of 19 years and above and up to first two live births will get benefit from this scheme. However, with a view to give special focus in ten low performing states, the benefit will be extended to the third child if the mother of her own accord chooses to undergo sterilization in the health facility where she delivered immediately after delivery. The accredited social health activist (ASHA) would work as a link health worker between the poor pregnant women and public sector health institution in the ten low performing states. ASHA would be responsible for escorting the pregnant women to healthcenter and for making available institutional antenatal as well as postnatal care.

All below-poverty line (BPL) pregnant women would be eligible to get cash benefit of Rs 500 per live birth on registration, which is disbursed at the time of delivery irrespective of the place of delivery. They would get an additional amount of Rs 200, if the delivery takes place in health institution and if they belong to rural areas and Rs.100, if they in ten low performing states. Even the ASHA workers get the package of assistance for the services they render depending upon the area of their work (rural/urban). In case, the pregnant woman develops complications and she requires cesarean section, assistance up to Rs 1500 per case is provided for having services of private experts where government specialist is not available in government health institution. Since the infrastructural facilities in the public sector are not adequate, benefits under this scheme would also be available to eligible pregnant women delivering in the private hospitals or nursing homes or clinics duly accredited and recognized by the state or union territories or governments.

This scheme is implemented through the State and Union Territory Governments or State Committees on voluntary action.

FERTILITY-RELATED STATISTICS

Indices used for Measuring Fertility

Crude birth rate (CBR) =

$$\frac{\text{Number of live births during time period}}{\text{Total population at mid-point of time period}} \times 1{,}000$$

The denominator in CBR is the total population. A known fact is that the whole population does not contribute in adding new individuals to the total population, i.e., is not involved in giving births because this involves the male population as well. The denominator should therefore include only female population in the reproductive age group, i.e., 15–49 years. This shortcoming is overcome by using general fertility rate (GFR) where the denominator includes midyear population of females in the reproductive age group.

General fertility rate =

$$\frac{\text{Number of live births during time period}}{\text{Total population of females age 15–49 years at mid-point of time period}} \times 1{,}000$$

The main drawbacks of this index are that comparison between two different populations would not be possible as the number of females in the age group of 15–49 years may vary between any two populations. Secondly, it does not allow identification of females with the highest reproductive potential, i.e., those who are at potential risk of conception. This leads to inability to identify these target groups who are in dire need of usage of any kind of family-planning methods. Hence, it may be deterrent to provision of family-planning activities. This is handled by using age-specific fertility Rate.

Age-specific Fertility Rate

$$\frac{\text{Number of live births to women in a specific age group in a specific area during time period}}{\text{Total population of females in the same age group at mid-point of time period}} \times 1{,}000$$

This rate is useful in identification of those women who should be the actual candidates for the utilization of family-planning services.

Total Fertility Rate

This measure provides us with an accurate measure of fertility. The total fertility rate (TFR) is a more direct measure of the level of fertility than the crude birth rate, since it refers to births per woman. A rate of two children per woman is considered the replacement rate for a population, resulting in relative stability in terms of total numbers. This measure tells us that how many children 1,000 women would bear on an average in their life span, if they were to start their reproductive life at a common point of life and were to pass through their entire reproductive span, subject to the current age-specific fertility rates (ASFRs). It is calculated by summing up the ASFRs for the different age groups and multiplying such sum by the class interval on which the age groups have been formed. The midterm objective of National Population Policy was to bring the TFR to replacement level, i.e., 2 by 2010 and long-term objective is to attain stable population by 2045.[5] The TFR gives the approximate magnitude of the completed family size.

Gross Reproductive Rate

This measure tells us the average number of female births per new-born female, growing up and passing her entire reproductive age if subjected to current fertility rates. However, there is a shortcoming with this rate as it assumes that all females would live up to completion of childbearing age. The major shortcoming of this measure is that it is based on a hypothetical assumption that all women would survive through their entire reproductive life span.

Net Reproductive Rate

It is a sensitive demographic indicator of population growth. This measure tells us the average no. of female live births per new born female, growing up and passing her entire reproductive age, subject to application of current fertility and mortality rates. This rate is similar to the gross reproduction rate but it also takes into account that some females will die before completing their childbearing years. If net reproductive rate (NRR) is one, it means that each generation of mothers is having exactly enough daughters thereby replacing themselves in the population i.e., the number of females at any given time does not either increase or decrease. This leads to the maintenance of female population at any given time. If the NRR is less than one, the reproductive performance of the population is below replacement level.

Population Growth Rate

This rate measures the difference between crude birth rate and crude death rate. This difference is also expressed in the form of population gap. If CBR is more than crude death rate (CDR), it would lead to increase in total population.

FAMILY PLANNING[10]

The family planning program is not merely related with sterilization operations but it is now termed as family welfare program which is a very comprehensive term and is basically related with quality of life. It aims at achieving higher end that is to improve quality of life of people.

Small family norm: small difference in family size will make big difference in the birth rate, which will have tremendous impact on the population growth.

Eligible couples: the "eligible couple" refers to a currently married couple wherein the wife is in the reproductive age which is generally assumed between the ages of 15 years and 45 years.The eligible couple register is a basic document for organizing family-planning work.

Target couples: the term now is more widely used than past with a view to develop acceptance of the idea of family planning from the earliest possible stage that is right from the stage of newly married couple.

Couple protection rate (CPR): it is an indicator of the prevalence of contraceptive practice in the community. It is defined as percent of eligible couples effectively protected against childbirth by one or the other approved methods of family planning, i.e., condom, oral contraceptive pills, intrauterine device, or sterilization. Sterilization accounts for over 60% of effectively protected couples. Demographers are of the view that the demographic goal of NPR = 1 can be achieved only when if the CPR exceeds 60%. Thus, attaining a 60% CPR will be equivalent to cutting of almost all third or higher order births. In short, CPR is a dominant factor in the reduction of net reproduction rate.

CONCLUSION

Thus to conclude, the vital statistics plays a major role in maintaining the broader concept of family welfare. It gives momentum to building of policies that would move the nation and the whole world towards universal health insurance.

REFERENCES

1. Kishore JA. Dictionary of public Health. Edition. New Delhi: Century Publications; 2002. p. 135.
2. Population Reference Bureau http://www.prb.org/pdf13/2013-population-data-sheet_eng.pdf (Accessed March 2014).
3. "World Population Clock Worldometers". Worldometers.info. http://www.worldometers.info/world-population/ Retrieved [Accessed april, 2014].
4. Census India 2011 Report. Available from http: //www.censusindia.net. [Accessed March 2014).
5. Gupta VM, Sen P. National Population Policy 2000: An insight (Editorial). Indian Journal of Public Health. 2000:44(1):1-4.
6. WHO (2005). Regional Health Forum. Vol 9, No1, 2005.
7. Conde-Agudelo A, Belizan JM, Lammers C. Maternal-perinatal morbidity and mortality associated with adolescent pregnancy in Latin America: Cross-sectional study. American Journal of Obstetrics and Gynecology. 2004;192:342-9.
8. Patton GC, Coffey C, Sawyer SM, Viner RM, Haller DM, Bose K, et al. Global patterns of mortality in young people: a systematic analysis of population health data. Lancet. 2009;374:881-92.
9. International Institute for Population Sciences (IIPS) and Macro International. 2008 National Family Health Survey (NFHS-3), India, 2005-06.
10. Park K. Demography and Vital Statistics, Text Book of Preventive and Social Medicine. 20th edition. Jabalpur/s Banarsidas Bhanot; 2009.

CHAPTER 79

Legal and Ethical Issues

Sangeet K Dhillon, Alka Kuthe

INTRODUCTION

Litigation in obstetrics is far more common than in any other superspeciality or subspecialty of medicine. Obstetricians are at increased risk for claims of medical negligence. According to an American Congress of Obstetricians and Gynecologists (ACOG) survey, an obstetrician and gynecologist can expect an average of 2.5 liability claims over the course of his or her career or around 80% of obstetricians and gynecologist can anticipate being sued one or more times in their career. Around 25.6% of surveyed obstetricians decreased their high risk obstetric patients while 7.2% quit practicing obstetrics altogether, 28.5% of those who continue to deliver patients reported increasing number of cesarean section with 26.4% not performing vaginal birth after cesarean (VBAC).[1]

Obstetricians deal with two lives simultaneously; mother and her developing fetus. They have to predict the physiology and well-being of fetus based on the electronic gadgets such as cardiotocography (CTG), Doppler and ultrasound applied to mother. Thus, there is an obvious inherent potential for error or inability to diagnose certain fetomaternal disorders. Secondly, obstetrics patients are usually young and healthy. Hence, relatives find it difficult to accept mishap. Thirdly, the follow-up of an obstetric case lasts up to 46 weeks (40 weeks of gestation plus 6 weeks of postpartum phase). Any pathological condition can occur within such a prolonged condition resulting in poor outcome. In addition to this, pregnancy and child birth are considered as physiological processes. Therefore, the patient and the relatives are not ready to accept any adverse or unfavorable outcome while in other branches of medicine, the patient is already suffering with some pathological condition which often have a known poor course and that makes relatives and patient mentally prepared for mishap if it occurs.

With the application of Consumer Protection Act 1986 to medical fraternity one hears that litigations have increased and the litigants go to the courts at the slightest of mistakes of the doctor. Hence, as the litigations have increased the ethical and legal issues which come in different courts are also different and mind boggling at times and which were never thought of in earlier times. Third trimester of pregnancy and labor, especially is the crucial period of the pregnant state of woman which gives ultimate result in terms of healthy mother and healthy baby. Therefore, it is prudent to know the medico-legal aspects of third trimester and labor so that an obstetrician can offer standard care to the pregnant ladies without fear of litigations. In the present chapter, we will be discussing the medicolegal issues which can arise in the treatment in third trimester of pregnancy and labor.

AREAS OF SUES[2]

Some common areas of obstetric sues are mentioned below but any deviation from the standard approach may lead to medicolegal problems.

The areas of common obstetric sue are:

- Errors of omission in antenatal clinical/ultrasonographic screening and diagnosis
- Preterm labor
- Maternal injuries during delivery—vaginal delivery/instrumental vaginal delivery/lower (uterine) segment cesarean section (LSCS)

- Postpartum hemorrhage
- Perinatal death
- Birth asphyxia/neurologically impaired infant
- Swab retained after procedure

The above areas of obstetric sue can be very well prevented by focusing our attention on following medico-legal aspects in third trimester in pregnancy and labor:

Consent

Consent can be defined as "an agreement, compliance or permission given voluntarily without any compulsion. Section 13 of the Indian Contract Act defines consent as "two or more persons are said to consent when they agree upon the same thing in the same sense".[3] It is a legal basis that allows a surgeon to perform any surgery or invasive procedure. In the present scenario, it is the word prior informed consent which has been propagated of late. A proper consent is very important part of any procedure conducted on the patient as not taking consent and doing a procedure amounts to battery by the doctor.

Informed Consent

In this type of consent, the doctor explains to the patient relevant details regarding the nature of her disease, the diagnostic procedures involved, the course and alternatives to the treatment proposed, risk involved and the prognosis. The relative chance of success or failure is explained so that patient can take an intelligent decision. At times, it may happen that patient is in dire need of treatment but as per the law of "full disclosure" revealing the risks involved may frighten her resulting in her refusal to treatment.[3] A situation like this calls for the common sense and discretion of doctor. At this juncture, "therapeutic privilege" can play the role of exception to the rule of full disclosure. It is mandatory for the doctor to explain all the pertinent facts to the patient and the relatives in the language they can understand to help them in decision making. Informed consent has now become a must in all operative, anesthetic procedures, complicated therapeutic procedures, and any procedure that carries some risk.[3]

Consent for a Cesarean Section

It has to be taken before starting the procedure. At times, when cesarean section is being done, a complication is noticed like rupture of uterus and it becomes a risk for the life a patient. If the consent has been taken only for the cesarean section, now it becomes a dicey situation for the doctor as to the procedure to be adopted for the next step. The next step should be a procedure towards saving the life of a woman hence any step taken in emergency situation where there is no time to think about consent, is accepted by a court of law. However, such emergency treatment or surgery should be restricted only to the procedures absolutely necessary and lifesaving. Anything else that could be performed later or electively should be deferred, e.g., when an abdomen is opened for a cesarean section and the doctor comes to know that there is an ovarian cyst then she has to think whether it is an emergency situation or not. If such a cyst is not posing any immediate danger towards the health of the patient, it can be operated upon at a later stage when the lady recovers from the cesarean section and after taking the consent the cyst can be removed.

Where the situation is such that a person would need a blood transfusion, a written permission should be obtained from the person without which the procedure should not be done. If the written consent has been taken earlier for some other procedure and there is need for blood transfusion a separate consent specifically has to taken for the same said procedure.

Antenatal Checkup and Detection of High-risk Cases[4]

Proper antenatal checkup and detail history is the corner stone of achieving a satisfactory obstetric outcome. High risk cases should be screened through routine checkup including investigations like hemoglobin (Hb), blood group, Rh, hepatitis B surface antigen (HbsAg), veneral disease research laboratory (VDRL), human immunodeficiency virus (HIV), blood sugar level, routine urine examination and selective and discriminate use of modern gadget for prenatal, intranatal fetal surveillance. Otherwise, the obstetrician may face complications and thereby, litigations. Screening of high-risk cases, appropriate investigations, counseling and if needed timely referral to higher center, are the key words for managing such pregnancies. Inability in early diagnosis of such cases may end in to serious fetal and maternal complications and hence litigations. It is observed that hospitals not equipped with proper facility to handle high-risk cases or physicians who do not have proper qualification, experience and good communication or counseling skill, face more litigations.

Imaging in Obstetrics

Information about ultrasonography (USG) is so common that it is rare for an obstetric patient not to have at least one scan during the antenatal period. If not done earlier, third trimester USG can also prevent many mishaps. In high-risk cases, it has proved as a boon. Missed diagnosis of fetal anomalies accounts for over a quarter of obstetric suits.[1] Antepartum fetal surveillance, fetal heart monitoring, amniotic fluid index (AFI) study, bio-physical profile study, color Doppler study, etc., are essential in high-risk pregnancy cases. Proper use of such testing with indication and proper interpretation has been established as an accepted standard of care. Deviation from such norms may lead to errors in decision making with poor outcome. Explanation about the prognosis of mother and baby along with counseling on options of route of delivery may decrease litigations.

Wrongful Birth

A wrongful birth is an alleged claim against a clinician for the birth as opposed to a specific birth injury which is usually brought by patients after the birth of an infant with serious or disfiguring disabilities such as central nervous system defects, e.g., hydrocephalus, meningomyelocele, encephalocele or various chromosomal abnormalities, e.g., trisomy 21, Tay-Sachs disease, or cystic fibrosis. The patients usually allege that the genetic or hereditary basis for a potentially serious condition was not recognized by the clinician or that appropriate diagnostic technique was not offered early enough in pregnancy for prevention or termination. In these proceedings, parents of the deformed or abnormal child must prove that if they had been informed of the potential for a defective fetus prior to pregnancy or of an existence of an abnormal fetus during pregnancy, they would have ought to either avoid pregnancy altogether or to terminate the affected pregnancy. Allegations of this nature emphasize the importance of obtaining complete family or genetic history and informing and advising pregnant women of the available methods of genetic testing. At-risk families are nowadays are often referred to prenatal centers for genetic testing and evaluation by peri-natal geneticists. Routine referral to a genetic counselor for evaluation is not yet considered the standard of care.[5]

Wrongful Life

Wrongful life is an action claiming that negligent prenatal testing on the part of the health care provider resulted in the birth of a "damaged" child. Wrongful life differs from wrongful birth in that the claim is brought in the name of physically or mentally disabled child and not of the parents. Such claims usually involve devastated infants with serious genetic disorders or those born with major injuries as a result of early in utero exposure to drug or undiagnosed maternal disease. The legality behind this claim is that the duty of the clinician owed to the unborn child is similar to that owned to the parents.

Wrongful Death

Wrongful death is a cause of action arising when an otherwise normal pregnancy, which has reached viability, is terminated because of a missed diagnosis, e.g., a missed diagnosis of renal agenesis resulting in pregnancy termination.

Late Trimester Bleeding

Placenta previa and abruptio placenta are the major causes of late trimester bleeding. The role of USG or Doppler can never be overemphasized, though at times the diagnosis can be difficult or can be missed.

The communication made with the patient and/or her relatives about the potential seriousness of the condition needs to be documented. Their participation in the care of such patient needs to be discussed. The advice given to the patient in the form of complete bed rest, avoidance of strenuous work, abstinence and care by responsible attendant all the times should be noted down.[4] Any communication with the patient should be noted down in the language the patient can understand along with her and attending relatives' signatures in whose presence the counseling was done.

Premature Birth

Failure to diagnose and manage preterm labor may give grounds for law suits because of high incidence of complications in preterm infants. It is difficult to assign the cause of the preterm labor but for that matter newer tests such as fetal fibronectin can help to identify a population at high risk for preterm labor and delivery.[1] Use of corticosteroids to enhance lung maturity and role of tocolytic agents in such cases may decrease the complications with the preterm birth.

Multiple Pregnancy

Multiple gestations itself carry enormous risk both for the mother and the fetuses.[4] Any deficiency in services may create problem from medicolegal point of view.

Medical Disorder in Pregnancy

A physician reference for medical disorder to evaluate a pregnant woman is usually done by an obstetrician but many times they differ with the physician's management protocol because of the drug selection, and dose schedule which can be different in pregnancy and the fear of possible toxic effects on fetus and the surrounding environment. It would be preferable that both the specialties should manage the patient as a team.

Protocol for Induction and Augmentation

Protocols for induction and augmentation should be followed and their steps documented. The proper doses of appropriate drug should be used for induction or augmentation of labor at term.

Labor Monitoring

Proper monitoring of progress of labor and fetal well-being by clinical methods and in complicated cases with the help of modern gadgets like CTG would definitely add safety in obstetric practice from medicolegal point of view. Proper monitoring of labor with the help of standard partogram is essential for timely intervention and also to select right mode of delivery.

Assisted and Difficult Vaginal Delivery

Delayed or wrong decision and faulty technique may result into complicated or difficult vaginal delivery posing legal problems for the obstetrician. It should be practiced only after taking the informed consent in a good hospital set up. A genital fistula developed following a difficult or instrumental delivery may be the reason for the law suit.[4] Cesarean section is better option in selected cases instead of difficult or instrumental vaginal delivery.

Analgesia and Anesthesia

Complications may occur due to anesthesia during operative intervention. Obstetric analgesia can call forth legal problems.[4] An experienced, qualified anesthetist is the prerequisite for any operation.

Cesarean Section

In case of cesarean, obstetricians face litigations in either way, such as why cesarean section was performed or why there was delay in performing that. Threatened scar rupture, cord prolapse, placenta previa, placental abruption, or hand prolapse need prompt operative intervention, failure of which causes delay in LSCS and result in a poor outcome that can result into legal action.

Delay in the decision in indicated cases may lead to obstructed labor and the birth of asphyxiated newborn who may suffer from cerebral palsy or even result in to a fresh still-birth.[4] In many cases, relatives insist on a vaginal delivery for their patient or ask to wait for husband or in-laws to come. But the obstetrician must use his own judgment and explain the possible hazards in delaying the operation to patient and her relatives. It is important to note down refusal for the operation in the case paper as a safeguard. On the other hand, obstetricians should avoid unnecessary LSCS as sometimes it may also be challenged in the court of law if some mishap occurs and relatives file a case.

Forgotten foreign bodies in the form of instruments or swab left in the abdomen is a serious offence indicating shear negligence on the part of operating team, difficult to defend. The doctrine of "Res Ipsa Loquitur" which means, "the thing speaks for itself" is applied in such cases of obvious negligence.

Patients with Rare Blood Group

In rural areas and at remote places, availability of blood is always a tricky issue. Though obstetric emergencies are severe and many a times unpredictable, keeping blood ready for all patients is just not practicable. But in situations where blood loss is anticipated, the obstetrician should take reasonable care. It may mean taking informed consent, keeping blood ready, keeping alternative fluids ready, making enquiry about availability with a blood bank. If the patient's blood group belongs to a category of rare blood group and she is high risk patient, arranging blood will also go a long way in ensuring a reasonable care. Documenting each and every thing will protect the doctor from the claims against deficiency in services.

Mismatched Transfusion

If after transfusion, there follows a morbidity or mortality, the protocol for investigating transfusion reaction should be meticulously followed.[4] All samples from the patient, the blood bag and the transfusion set, etc., will become source of information.

Vaginal Birth After Cesarean

There is a need of documented discussion of the risks and benefits of VBAC with signature of patient at the end. If the patient or relative insists for vaginal delivery then their wish is put down on paper, signature is taken after an explanation of possible risk to both mother and baby. If they refuse to give written consent then they may be referred with findings and reason for referral.[1]

Whenever a patient is being allowed a trial of labor with a scarred uterus, the operation theatre should be alerted, equipment for emergency cesarean should be checked, blood should be kept ready, if the patient is anemic and her blood group is Rh negative. Informed high-risk consent should be taken.

Intrauterine Death

It is again very delicate issue and an emotional shock to the patient and the entire family. It can be prevented by proper clinical checkup and the necessary investigations including USG. The diagnosis of intrauterine device (IUD) must be done promptly and an effort should be done to deliver the baby as early as possible to prevent the future complications though in most of the cases the patient goes in spontaneous labor. Along with gross and microscopic examination of placenta, a fetal autopsy by an experienced pathologist is strongly indicated especially in cases where the cause of death is "unexplained". The issue of intrauterine death is dealt in detail in separate chapter in this book.

Brain Damage

In developed countries, brain damage is one of the most common factors leading to compensation claims. Delayed delivery either by LSCS or by forceps were the reasons for two-thirds of claims in UK in which it was alleged that intracranial injury and subsequent hemorrhage were the causative factors.[4] The failure on the part of an obstetrician to recognize and promptly react to highly significant evidences of fetal compromise was held responsible for the insult. The occurrence of fetal brain injury is generally attributed to intrapartum events. However, there are a few evidences that neurological damage unrelated to intrapartum events can occur during fetal life. Perinatal morbidity and mortality is a very important cause for medical litigations

Obstetric Hysterectomy

The decision of obstetric hysterectomy is solely the discretion of operating surgeon.[6] If massive hemorrhage is not controlled by any of the medical or surgical methods of hemostasis, it will land up in obstetric hysterectomy. The consent of the relatives or accompanying persons though desirable and important from medicolegal point of view, may not be possible in such dire emergency. To decide and execute the decision of obstetric hysterectomy to save the life of the woman is the priority and that is what demanded by court of the law, if the patient files the case. The written opinion of colleague to support the decision of emergency obstetric hysterectomy as lifesaving measure would also help when the indication is challenged in the court of law.

Maternal Death

Maternal death is a sensitive issue and is a matter of concern for everybody who are involved in patient's care. It has to be reported and a postmortem is insisted upon.

OTHER RELATED MEDICO-LEGAL ISSUES

Rape during Pregnancy[7]

As the lady is progressing towards third trimester, the hemodynamic are all altered and she is in a state where her body is adjusting to the altered hormonal and hemodynamic level. In such a condition, if a person commits rape on a woman knowing her to be pregnant shall be punished with rigorous imprisonment for a term which shall not be less than 10 years but which may extend to imprisonment for the remainder of that persons natural life and shall also be liable to fine.

If a pregnant woman is brought to the hospital with history of rape, police should be informed immediately and a medicolegal examination to be performed and lady has to be kept under observation along with all the necessary things to be sent for examinations to the forensic science laboratory. The examination should be elaborate and methodically written as the latest amendment states that a man is said to commit rape if he (a) penetrates his penis, to any extent in to the vagina, mouth, urethra or anus of a woman or makes her to do so with him or any other person; or (b) inserts to any extent any object or a part of the body, not being the penis, in to the vagina, urethra, or anus of a woman or makes her to do so with him or any other person; or (c) manipulates any part of the body of a woman so as to cause penetration in to the vagina, urethra, anus or any part of body of such body of such woman or makes her to do so with him or any other person; or (d) applies his mouth to the vagina, anus, urethra of a woman or makes her to do so with him or any person under the circumstances falling under seven descriptions. Hence, the entire definition should be kept in mind and a thorough examination of the body parts is to be done along with blood to be taken for analysis for any intoxicant administered during the act.

Before starting the examination, consent should be taken from the woman and if she is minor her parents' consent should be taken.

Surrogate Motherhood and the Issues

Surrogacy is a term when one woman lends her womb for bearing some other couples child. India has become the hub for surrogacy and couples from all over the world come to India for the same. The issues in surrogacy are more of an ethical nature than legal. Ethics include code of conduct, rules and obligations towards patients, society and nation.[1] Surrogacy raises various ethical problems, the main one is a commercial contract of renting of uterus for financial gain. Surrogacy can also disturb family harmony or integrity as it may affect maternal bonding and paternal caring. The surrogate mother may refuse to handover the child after birth due to greed for more money or genetic couple may not accept the child if handicapped or born with some disorder in case of financial bond. A well-detailed explained consent mentioning possible situations and their outcome may prevent such difficulties.

There are no laws for the artificial reproductive techniques framed in India, however an Artificial Reproductive Technique Bill 2008 is being followed for the cases done in India. The draft of the latest bill is ready for the parliament and is awaited for certain changes required in the 2008 bill.

Earlier, the clinics doing the artificial reproductive techniques were not required to be registered with the department of health and research but presently the scenario is changing and in the proposed bill it will be made compulsory for the clinics to be registered with the department of health and research. Presently, the ministry of external affairs has released a letter that the couples coming for the procedure will have to get a letter from the government of their country that the surrogacy is legal in their country and the child will be allowed inside their country and considered their citizen.[8]

In another letter issued, it was the couples coming in the country are allowed a stay of minimum 3 months and then have to return to their country and can apply again for their visit.

In the proposed bill, it is that the surrogate mother has to take care of herself and during delivery has to cooperate with the couple and after the baby is fit to be given to the couple should hand over the baby to them. Further, if nobody comes to take the child within the stipulated time should put the child for adoption in an adoption home. It is also proposed that a lady who will become a surrogate mother should not be more than 35 years. She should be having a living child of her own and can become a surrogate mother for a maximum of 3-times and the couple who is adopting the child should have been married since the last 2 years.

Measures for Prevention of Lawsuits[1]

Efforts should be made to prevent the litigations instead of fighting them in the court of law. Some important preventive measures are:

- Proper selection of patient as per the knowledge, expertise and skill
- Good communication and counseling skill
- Proper informed consent
- Good documentation and record keeping, preservation of medical records for an appropriate length of time, in case of pediatric patient till the child becomes major and a limitation period of 3 years for them to file a case (21 years)
- Fully equipped hospital with availability of qualified, appropriately trained & experienced specialist
- Provide standard medical care as per the guidelines and recommendations of standard textbooks/federations/organizations
- Timely referral to higher center, if required
- Evidence based practice
- Regular checking of expiry dates of medications in labor room, operation theatre, indoor wards, etc. In case of mishap, preserve the empty ampoules, vials, saline sets, urine catheter, etc., to avoid the allegations if any, in case of enquiry
- Management of high risk obstetric case by a multi-speciality approach preferably at fully equipped critical care center. Care should be taken to avoid any contradiction in the notes written by different specialists involved in the management which may complicate the issue if a case is filed in the court of law
- Regular updating of medical and legal knowledge by attending CMEs/workshops/conferences by referring standard books
- Awareness of potential litigation areas in obstetric practice
- Self and professional auditing: there is a balance between the input of services and the output of result in terms of patient satisfaction. In professional audit, the objective evaluation of the balance sheet of the cost-effectiveness and the patient benefit is done for the sake of rendering quality service and for competitive survival with dedication to the profession with a clear cut sense of objectivity. There is long-term advantage and benefit of auditing
- Medical indemnity insurance is a must
- Risk management strategies: it is a prospective process which identifies factors prompting legal action and aims at improving medical system to prevent future losses. It involves the participation of health care providers of all types, attorneys, various technicians, health insurance providers, hospital administrators and many others. One can opt for several possible resolutions once a potential risk is identified. The development of education programs, a review of the performance of clinicians, the purchase of new equipment or changes in existing protocols and practice as per guidelines or evidence based practice are some of the resolutions
- Documentation: like in other branches of medicine, the importance of documentation in obstetrics can not be stressed enough. It is the most important evidence in litigations. It also helps in the treatment of the patient. It is the evidence which justifies the diagnosis, warrants the treatment and follows the end result of all the patients treated in the hospital. Documents are the legal jackets offering strong defence in the court of law.

Role of Counseling

Counseling plays an important role in every branch of medicine but its role in obstetrics and gynecological situations is very crucial. It is a two-way process and helps to strengthen relationship between doctor and patient. Therefore, in addition to the knowledge of subject, an obstetrician should have communication skill to share this knowledge with the patients and help them in decision making to achieve the best possible outcome and best patient satisfaction. Timely communication about progress with frank discussion about the labor or the disease process, clinical situation and measures taken for prompt management can help to prevent law suits.

CONCLUSION

Legal problems in third trimester and labor, and obstetrics as a whole are more common than any other branch in medicine. Child birth is perceived as a much more awaited, a cheerful moment for everybody and normalcy is taken for granted. Any deviation from this may put the doctors to litigation. Hence, an obstetrician must be aware of the potential areas of litigation so that it would be easier for him to tackle the situation successfully.

To conclude, proper care, proper documentation, proper counseling, and empathetic approach towards patients may go a long way in averting any medicolegal problem in obstetrics.

REFERENCES

1. Mittal Prabhu. Medicolegal Aspects in Obstetrics and Gynecology Practice. Textbook on Medicolegal Issues, 1st Edition. In: Tiwari Satish, Baldwa Mahesh, Tiwari Mukul, Kuthe Alka (Eds). Jaypee Brothers Medical Publishers (P) Ltd, New Delhi; 2012, pp. 86-191,194.
2. The Gazette of India Extraordinary. The Criminal law Act, 2013. No 13 of 2013.
3. Kuthe Alka. Consent in Textbook on Medicolegal Issues. In: Tiwari Satish, Baldwa Mahesh, Tiwari Mukul, Kuthe Alka (Eds). 1st edition. New Delhi: Jaypee Brothers Medical Publishers (P) Ltd; 2012. pp. 53-6.
4. Mukherjee AK. Potential areas of litigation in Obstetrics. Medico-legal Aspects in Obstetrics and Gynecology. In: G Ganguly Mukherjee, Soonawala RP, Tank DK. A FOGSI Publication, 1st edition. New Delhi: Jaypee Brothers, Medical Publishers (P) LTD; 1997. pp. 114-9.
5. Satish Tiwari. Legal aspects in Medical Practice. Indian Paediatrics. 2000;37:961-6.
6. Abhyankar Shantanu. Medico-legal aspects of Obstetric bleeding. In: Textbook on Medicolegal Issues: (Editors) Tiwari Satish, Baldwa Mahesh, Tiwari Mukul, Kuthe Alka: 1st Edition: New Delhi, Jaypee Brothers Medical Publishers (P) Ltd, 2012: pp. 201-3.
7. The Assisted Reproductive Technologies (Regulation) bill. Ministry of health and Family Welfare, Government of India, ICMR, New Delhi.2010.
8. Reddy Narayan KS. The Essentials of Forensic Medicine and Toxicology. 25th edition.

Index

Page numbers followed by '*f*', '*t*', and '*fc*' indicate figure, table, and flowchart, respectively.

D

E

F

G

H